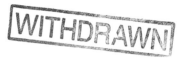

INTEGRATING COMPLEMENTARY MEDICINE INTO VETERINARY PRACTICE

INTEGRATING COMPLEMENTARY MEDICINE INTO VETERINARY PRACTICE

Edited by: **ROBERT S. GOLDSTEIN**, VMD
Paula Jo Broadfoot, DVM; **Richard E. Palmquist**, DVM; **Karen Johnston**, DVM;
Barbara Fougere, BVSc; **Jiu Jia Wen,** DVM; with **Margo Roman**, DVM

⊛WILEY-BLACKWELL

A John Wiley & Sons, Inc., Publication

Robert S. Goldstein is Director of Veterinary Services for Animal Nutritional Technologies, Healing Center for Animals, Northern Skies Veterinary Center and Director of Product Development for Earth Animal, all in Westport, Connecticut.

Paula Jo Broadfoot, DVM, graduated from Kansas State University School of Veterinary Medicine and has been studying and practicing therapeutic nutrition for the past 18 years.

Richard E. Palmquist, DVM, is currently the head of medicine at Centinela Animal Hospital in Inglewood, California. He is also currently a research chair for the American Holistic Veterinary Medical Association and a consultant in alternative medicine for the Veterinary Information Network (VIN).

Karen Johnston, DVM, works at Hampton Veterinary Hospital in the fields of small animal and exotic pet medicine, surgery, and acupuncture. She is also the co-owner of Natural Solutions, herbal supplements for veterinary use.

Jiu Jia Wen, DVM, is the owner of Hampton Veterinary Hospital in Speonk, New York. His hospital provides complete veterinary care for birds, reptiles, and small mammals using a combination of both Western style medicine and traditional Chinese modalities including herbal medicine and acupuncture.

Barbara Fougere, BSc BVMS (Hons), GDBus MOD&T CVA (IVAS), CVHM, CVCP, ACNEM, is the president of the Australian Veterinary Acupuncture Association and President for the International Veterinary Botanical Medicine Association.

Margo Roman, DVM, founded her own animal clinic in 1983. It originated as a mobile clinic and now is a full service holistic veterinary practice. In 2002 she opened the first holistic health center for animals offering chiropractic, cranial sacral, physical therapy, massage, reiki, and polarity in the lower level and in the main clinic homeopathy, acupuncture, herbs, surgery, and conventional medicine in an integrative method.

Edition first published 2008
© 2008 Wiley-Blackwell

Blackwell Publishing was acquired by John Wiley & Sons in February 2007. Blackwell's publishing program has been merged with Wiley's global Scientific, Technical, and Medical business to form Wiley-Blackwell.

Editorial Office
2121 State Avenue, Ames, Iowa 50014-8300, USA

For details of our global editorial offices, for customer services, and for information about how to apply for permission to reuse the copyright material in this book, please see our website at www.wiley.com/wiley-blackwell.

Library of Congress Cataloguing-in-Publication Data
Integrating complementary medicine into veterinary practice / by Robert S. Goldstein . . . [et al.]. – 1st ed.
    p.   ;   cm.
  Includes bibliographical references and index.
  ISBN-13: 978-0-8138-2020-0 (alk. paper)
  ISBN-10: 0-8138-2020-0 (alk. paper)
 1. Alternative veterinary medicine. I. Goldstein, Robert S., 1942–
  [DNLM: 1. Complementary Therapies–veterinary. 2. Animal Diseases–therapy. 3. Veterinary Medicine.   SF 745.5 I61 2007]

  SF745.5I58 2007
  636.089'55–dc22

                                                                    2007017470

A catalogue record for this book is available from the U.S. Library of Congress.

Set in 9.5/12 Sabon by SNP Best-set Typesetter Ltd., Hong Kong

Printed in Singapore by Markono Print Media Pte Ltd

Disclaimer
The contents of this work are intended to further general scientific research, understanding, and discussion only and are not intended and should not be relied upon as recommending or promoting a specific method, diagnosis, or treatment by practitioners for any particular patient. The publisher and the author make no representations or warranties with respect to the accuracy or completeness of the contents of this work and specifically disclaim all warranties, including without limitation any implied warranties of fitness for a particular purpose. In view of ongoing research, equipment modifications, changes in governmental regulations, and the constant flow of information relating to the use of medicines, equipment, and devices, the reader is urged to review and evaluate the information provided in the package insert or instructions for each medicine, equipment, or device for, among other things, any changes in the instructions or indication of usage and for added warnings and precautions. Readers should consult with a specialist where appropriate. The fact that an organization or Website is referred to in this work as a citation and/or a potential source of further information does not mean that the author or the publisher endorses the information the organization or Website may provide or recommendations it may make. Further, readers should be aware that Internet Websites listed in this work may have changed or disappeared between when this work was written and when it is read. No warranty may be created or extended by any promotional statements for this work. Neither the publisher nor the author shall be liable for any damages arising herefrom.

1 2008

Dedication

This book is dedicated to our fellow colleagues and all veterinary professionals who have the insight, motivation, and inspiration to reach out and find innovative therapies that improve the health and well being of animals everywhere. A special acknowledgement goes to our patients, past and present, and their human companions for their courage, fortitude, and ability to persist through these challenging times of transformation. They are our greatest teachers and rewards in this work. We also dedicate this work to the new patients who will benefit from the open mindedness of their veterinarians who begin to include nutritional, biological, and herbal therapies in their treatment regimes. God bless us all!

Table of Contents

Foreword

By Carvel G. Tiekert

About 30 years ago I became interested in the concepts of alternative and complementary veterinary medicine and in the course of things searched out names of veterinarians who had similar interests. One of those is the editor of this new book in veterinary medicine. At that time Dr. Bob Goldstein was a practitioner with his brother Marty in New York State. During a visit with Bob, he said to me, "We need somebody who can pull us all together and get the idea of complementary veterinary medicine going."

As a result, I sent letters around and in 1982 the American Veterinary Holistic Medical Association was formed at the Western States Veterinary Conference (now the Western Veterinary Conference). Over the course of time this organization's name changed to the American Holistic Veterinary Medical Association. At the time of that initial meeting we wrestled with the terms to describe what we wanted to do in the profession, and the word (w)holistic was chosen because then it seemed to be the most commonly used word. We didn't want "alternative" for obvious reasons, and "complementary" seemed too far away at the time.

Now things have changed, and veterinary medicine is looking to integrate these complementary and alternative veterinary protocols into mainstream veterinary medicine. We have sessions relating to alternative and complementary therapies at all the major meetings, and almost all state associations have had sessions at one time or another. Even the words have changed. Since many presentations frequently mention conventional medicine techniques along with the alternative techniques, the word "integrative" is one that is appropriately used.

This book is designed to answer the changing needs brought on by these developments. Its concept is to be in the line of *Conn's Current Therapy* for human medicine and Kirk's *Current Veterinary Therapy* for veterinary medicine, taking diseases and syndromes and examining diagnostic treatment techniques for each of them. We have a number of books currently available within the profession that present great discussions about particular modalities. This book allows us to integrate those conventional modalities of the profession with a number of the complementary and alternative modalities to provide better care for our patients. It is my hope that this book, like *Current Veterinary Therapy*, will be updated and expanded as new information and understandings in veterinary medicine become available.

Carvel G. Tiekert, DVM; Founder, American Holistic
Veterinary Medical Association

Foreword

By Martin Deangelis

Dr. Robert Goldstein and his contributing authors have written a book that bridges the gap between allopathic and complementary veterinary medicine, which many professionals consider opposing methods of treating disease. Allopathic and complementary medicine are methodologies that support each other in the quest to restore our patients to health and well being.

I am a board-certified surgeon and I have 42 years of experience as a veterinarian. I have worked closely with Dr. Goldstein and several other complementary practitioners for many years and I have come to greatly appreciate the benefits of these associations.

Over the years I have operated on animals that have been diagnosed with "inoperable" or "incurable" cancer. Many of these patients had tumor removal or debulking procedures followed by complementary medical treatment. A significant percentage of these individuals survived longer than expected, went into remission, or sometimes had no detectable cancer years after surgery. This experience has enabled me to recommend surgery in conjunction with complementary medicine for patients that in the past, without such support, I would have considered to be untreatable.

It is my experience that the importance of therapeutic nutrition and biological support in the management of serious and complicated disease is often unappreciated or given no credit. It is important for us to acknowledge that all drugs possess some degree of toxicity and potential for creating adverse side effects. When conventional drug therapy is chosen, side effects can be minimized and efficacy increased by integrating complementary medicine.

As an example, nutritional and biological therapies, when given in combination with chemotherapy, often-times protect the patient from toxic side effects. Also, the elements of treating degenerative joint disease include weight and exercise control and the use of therapeutic levels of antioxidants to neutralize free radicals and their inflammatory effect. Nutritional supplementation can aid cartilage protection and repair and help relieve pain and joint stiffness.

Integrating Complementary Medicine into Veterinary Practice is written by experienced practitioners and presents in modern and concise language a fully referenced book on the theory of alternative methods as well as individual disease treatment protocols. This book gives clinicians a guide so they can quickly access a knowledge base of alternative therapies and decide on a case-by-case basis whether to use conventional medical or alternative therapies alone or a combination of both.

Integrating Complementary Veterinary Medicine into Veterinary Practice is important because an increasing number of clients request complementary medicine for their pets' medical treatment as well as pre- and post-operative regimes. This book provides, in a clear and organized fashion, the indications and applications of complementary medicine for the general practitioner as well as the specialist.

Martin Deangelis, DVM; Diplomate, ACVS

Preface

The veterinary profession has made major diagnostic and therapeutic advances in the treatment of infectious and degenerative diseases. The incidence of chronic disease and cancer, however, has increased at alarming rates and is diagnosed at younger ages, even in puppies and kittens. Perhaps it is this rising incidence of degenerative diseases that has spawned an insatiable search by professionals, scientists, and animal guardians for alternative therapies. Such therapies are gentle in their action, more effective in their abilities to prevent disease, and hold the promise of true healing—a goal that modern medicine to date has only been able to control but not cure.

At this same time, there is a widening gap within the veterinary profession between the "conventional" and "holistic" practitioners. This gap is deep and has been fueled by misunderstandings in terms, evidence-based rules, and the sense that a clinician has to be either one type of practitioner or another, as well as an overall incorrect perception that one form of practice is right and therefore the other must be false or bogus.

Integrative veterinary medicine (IVM), as outlined in this book, defines one profession that uses a combination of alternative and conventional practice methods for the benefit of the patient. IVM seeks to remind veterinarians of their "oath" to use knowledge and skill for the protection of patients, to relieve suffering, to help advance medical knowledge and individual competency, and above all to do no harm.

Within the tenets of this oath and our intent to do right for our patients, we often run into the brick wall of evidence-based rules that prohibit the expanded use of alternative therapies because there is little statistical proof that they work. While the authors of this book do not challenge this "evidence-based filter," our 100-plus years of combined experience has shown us that these therapies are right for our patients and their companions.

At some point in our evolution as practitioners, we made a paradigm shift to expand our approach and care for our patients within the broad framework of our veterinary oath. Each author has had a personal journey that has led to the exploration of alternative therapies. At that point in time, there was no book nor reference nor scientific study that led to and opened the door. In our cases, "a light bulb went on" that brightened our way to explore alternative therapies with the ultimate goal of benefiting our patients and their companions. The intent of this "shift in perception" was not to abandon school and practice lessons, but rather to include therapies that we resonated with, that made sense, were requested by our clients, helped our patients, and improved our skills as medical healers.

We became proficient in these methods, but our profession as a whole did not embrace a unified vision, and many who were thought to be in opposing camps were choosing sides. The concept of one profession with multiple treatment choices was not materializing, and frustrated clients were forced to seek alternative solutions in areas such as the data-bloated Internet—fraught with misinformation—or from well intended but unqualified people. Our vision was to write a book for the professional that addressed these issues.

Integrating Complementary Medicine into Veterinary Practice was written in the convenient style of *Current Veterinary Therapy* or *Blackwell's Five-Minute Veterinary Consult*, offering clinicians fully referenced treatment protocols that address the clinical, emotional, and decisional situations that practitioners face daily. When this integrative veterinary concept was presented to Wiley-Blackwell, the publisher, they felt it was important to secure independent veterinary opinions as to the perceived need for a book of this type. This practitioner survey was overwhelmingly positive, indicating that the need for this book truly exists.

Chances are, if you are reading this preface, you too are wondering if there are other tools out there for your own personal toolbox of healing. Perhaps you hope for or envision a day when you can heal more patients with greater clarity in regard to this newly emerging field of practice. If so, we welcome you to our family and to the pages of this book. Holistic doctors believe that through natural methods much health can be rekindled and engaged, and through conventional medicine many miracles can occur.

We truly believe that integrative medicine is the movement of the future. It holds the experiential efforts of pioneering healers long gone and the promise of technologies we haven't yet dreamed of discovering, let alone implementing. It uses science to chart a path but never forgets its own ability to watch, listen, and know what it sees. Medicine is and always will be an art, and technology serves that art; however, it is the artist that applies the technology in ways that lead to success. We as authors of this book have worked diligently in our spare time to create this text, and we know that your experiences and comments will make the future editions even better. That is the reason that we came together to produce this text. It is our hope that this book brings you greater fulfillment and a new sense of joy in your work as veterinarians.

May your journey never end!

Respectfully,
Robert S. Goldstein, VMD, (editor); and
Rick Palmquist, DVM (writing for Paula J. Broadfoot, DVM; Karen Johnston, DVM; Barbara Fougere, BVSc; Jiu Jia Wen, DVM; and Margo Roman, DVM)

Acknowledgments

I would like to thank my wife Susan for her total support for the writing of this book. Thanks to Susan and Andes Best for the creation of the book's logo, which represents the guiding principle of integrative medicine. I thank Dan, who introduced Wiley-Blackwell to the data and concept that serve as the basis for this book. Thanks to Fred Best for his technical and editorial efforts and to Melissa, John, Betsy, Helmut, and Patricia for their ongoing support. I give my thanks to my family Abbey, Merritt, Jeff, Dan, Sam, Cooper, and Graham, and an extra special thanks to my brother Marty for his pioneering work in alternative veterinary medicine.

I give my thanks to PJ and Rick, who spent innumerable hours writing the homotoxicology sections of this book and also found the necessary time to assist me in the editing process, and to Jay and Karen for staying on course and especially for substantiating CHM clinical references under tremendous deadline pressure. A very special thanks goes to Barbara Fougere, who miraculously delivered the chapters on Western herbal medicine in an incredibly short amount of time, and to Margo Roman for her efforts and support of Barbara and the book. I thank Ray Kersey, Justin Jeffryes, Erica Judisch, Erin Magnani, and Antonia Seymour from Wiley-Blackwell—especially Erica and Justin, who smoothed the road to a larger and more comprehensive book. And finally a special thanks to Tracy Petersen whose editing and query expertise has transformed the raw manuscript into a professionally organized, readable textbook.

Robert S. Goldstein, VMD

I would like to thank, first and foremost, my husband Jeff, who kept the ship afloat while I was working to research this text. I thank my children Brannon, Barrett, Burke, and Brea, who are a constant affirmation of just how important is our quest for a gentler, more biological approach to medicine; my clinic staff Susan, Sonia, Ila, Sally, and Emily, who kept me grounded and managed the day-to-day work so that I could devote more time to writing; my parents, especially my mother, Benita, for allowing me to study and for instilling a thirst for knowledge and an abiding belief in my own abilities; Lauri Parent, for being a marvel of information and data gathering over the last decade; Carvel Tiekert, whose constant devotion to the furthering of integrative medicine—and in particular, homotoxicology—has made many of our advances possible; my co-authors—particularly Rick Palmquist—who remained steadfast in purpose and encouraged me to stay on task when I was weary of the work; and Bob Goldstein, without whom we would not have created this work. A particular tribute is owed to Susan Youngblood, my "girl Friday," who has been with me for 25 years of this long journey and adventure into complementary healing.

PJ Broadfoot, DVM

My eternal gratitude extends to my parents Mary and Allen, for showing me how to know truth; my wife MJ and my children Jessica, Jake, and Jared, for allowing me the time and support to write; to my staff for their endless support; my clients and patients, for teaching me how to apply the wonderful things I learned in veterinary school; Martin Goldstein, for showing me another way to practice; my co-authors—especially PJ Broadfoot and Robert Goldstein—who I am sure will remain lifelong friends in healing; and the American Holistic Veterinary Medical Association, for providing a safe place for the development of CAVM. Finally, I extend my gratitude to Dr. Alta Smit of Heel for her tireless support of biological therapy.

Rick Palmquist, DVM

It has been a great honor to be trusted with the lives of my patients and I am grateful for the faith their people have shown in me. I promise to continue to seek knowledge so that I may always provide them with my best care. I would like to thank my family for their support throughout my schooling, and my husband Jiu for introducing me to herbs and acupuncture. I also want to thank Jason,

Joshua, and Jacob for being the best sons a mother could have.

Karen Johnston, DVM

I want to thank my wife Karen for all her support.

Jiu Wen, DVM

I would like to acknowledge Drs. Susan Wynn, Bob Goldstein, and Margo Roman for their support in this project; my teachers—particularly Kerry Bone—and my

four-legged patients who have shown me the gentle power of plant-based medicine.

Barbara Fougere, BVSc

I thank all the animals that have given enlightenment to the doctors and their caretakers and my horse Champ who empowered me to seek integrative veterinary medicine for his care and for inspiring the DrDoMore project.

Margo Roman, DVM

Introduction: How to Use This Book

This book is a working manual for veterinarians who are interested in the integration of alternative methods into conventional veterinary practice.

Section 1 of the book covers the history, theory, evidence, and clinical references for therapeutic nutrition, Chinese herbal medicine/acupuncture, homotoxicology, and Western herbal medicine. In each modality there is an extensive reference section that substantiates the use of each of the methodologies in both human and veterinary medicine.

Sections 2 and 3 of the book contain disease protocols using combination therapies of therapeutic nutrition, Chinese herbal medicine/acupuncture, and homotoxicology. Section 2 covers chronic degenerative diseases and Section 3 covers infectious diseases. The disease protocols are all similarly formatted as follows: definition and cause, medical therapy and nutritional recommendations, anticipated prognosis, integrative veterinary medicine, therapeutic nutrition (general considerations and appropriate nutrients), Chinese herbal medicine/acupuncture (general considerations and appropriate Chinese herbs), homotoxicology (general considerations and appropriate antihomotoxic agents), the authors' suggested protocols (therapeutic nutrients, Chinese herbs, and homotoxicology), product sources, and references.

Section 4 is dedicated completely to Western herbal medicine. It lists similar diseases as found in Section 2 and 3 and specific Western herbal protocols for those diseases, followed by substantiating references.

Section 5 covers neoplastic processes and is similar in organization to Sections 2 and 3. The first chapter in this section is a discussion of the integrative veterinary therapies of therapeutic nutrition, Chinese herbal medicine, and introductory homotoxicology. There is a discussion on diet, elaborating upon the restrictions that are required when Chinese herbal protocols are used. The next chapter spells out cancer treatment protocols by cancer type, listing the recommended therapeutic nutrients, Chinese herbal formulas, and homotoxicology remedies. The following chapter provides more in-depth discussions on the autosanguis and advanced homotoxicology approach to cancer and a complete listing of references and scientific studies that support the recommendations.

Section 6 is a discussion of vaccinations, their impact upon the cause and prevention of diseases, and alternatives, as well as treatment protocols that are designed to prevent complications and future problems. This is followed by scientific references.

Section 7 is a glossary of the most common terms related to therapeutic nutrition and nutraceuticals, Chinese herbal medicine and acupuncture, homotoxicology, and Western herbal medicine.

Section 8 is a comprehensive set of resources. It includes organizations and advanced studies for alternative methods and an extensive listing of companies that manufacture the foods, nutraceuticals, homeopathics, Western herbs, and Chinese herbs that are presented in the disease protocols in Sections 2, 3, and 5.

The Appendix contains a list of acupuncture points mentioned in this text.

INTEGRATING COMPLEMENTARY MEDICINE INTO VETERINARY PRACTICE

SECTION 1

Introduction to Integrative Veterinary Medicine: The Integration of Old and Ancient Medical Practice Techniques into Conventional Veterinary Practice

Chapter One

Introduction to Integrative Veterinary Medicine

INTEGRATING ANCIENT MEDICAL PRACTICE TECHNIQUES INTO CONVENTIONAL VETERINARY PRACTICE

Integrative veterinary medicine (IVM) combines natural and alternative approaches with conventional veterinary practice methods for the benefit of the patient. IVM uses modalities such as therapeutic nutrition, Chinese herbal medicine, and homeopathy, along with a proper diagnosis, relying upon internal medicine, ultrasound, radiology, blood evaluation, and other recognized diagnostic techniques. The purpose of this book on integrative veterinary medicine is to define and blend conventional (allopathic) veterinary and alternative (holistic) practice methods along with traditional definitions of healing.

This book discusses the arts and practices of therapeutic nutrition, Chinese and Western herbal medicine, and homotoxicology (a combination form of homeopathy). Guidelines for practicing veterinarians to incorporate these treatment modalities into routine daily practice are outlined in modern terms. The book defines and clarifies terms and concepts of therapeutic nutrition and non-Western forms of medicine in more understandable language. As an example, fever, redness, inflammation, and thready pulse are commonly accepted terms that are often discussed in a clinical veterinary practice. Terms such as "Chi," "Yin and Yang," and "tongue or pulse diagnosis" often bring misunderstanding and confusion to conventionally trained clinicians.

The modern interpretation of alternative and ancient therapies allows them to be integrated into veterinary practice without years of intensive training or learning of new methodologies, terms, and procedures. The treatment protocols presented in this book have been used in a clinical setting and are specifically matched to the clinical condition. The goal is to improve therapeutic results when these treatment modalities are used alone or in combination with prescribed medications for the benefit of the patient. Also presented, when indicated, is a comparison of results when treating diseases with conventional medicine alone, with alternative medicines alone, and with a combination of conventional and alternative methods.

DESCRIPTION OF VETERINARY PRACTICES TODAY

The basis of conventional veterinary practice— diagnosis and pathology orientation and symptom-oriented drug therapies

Our veterinary education builds from the scientific basis of biochemistry and physiology, through disease definitions and histology, and finally into the clinical application of diagnosis and medical treatments. The more specialized our veterinary training, the further our focus shifts from underlying causes and prevention to diagnosis and appropriate medical therapies. Additionally, most pharmaceutical research is focused upon the treatment of existing disease and less upon prevention and wellness.

As busy veterinary practitioners, we often become overwhelmed with the case load of infectious and chronic degenerative diseases. Many times we barely have enough time to do more than treat and stop the bleeding, itching, chewing, vomiting, diarrhea, limping, eating, drinking, urinating, and so on. In many practices, this required focus upon medicating symptoms often leaves little time to discuss prevention, wellness, supplements, and natural remedies, all of which may help the pet's present situation.

Although this may be an exaggeration of day-to-day practice, as veterinarians, we often guide our clients on daily home care, diet, supplements, training, grooming, and so on. However, the fact remains that wellness and prevention methods often do not get the time that they deserve. The unfortunate result is that clients, when faced with recurring conditions and desiring options for alternatives to chronic medications, often seek answers to their questions from the Internet or from other potentially unreliable sources.

Holistic, alternative, and complementary veterinary practice

Many terms such as "holistic," "alternative," and "complementary" are often used interchangeably, leading to confusion and a breakdown in communication between animal companions, veterinarians, and animal health care personnel. Current terminology refers to such practices as complementary alternative veterinary medicine (CAVM), which includes a diverse group of therapies typically not taught in medical schools. (Some alternative modalities, such as acupuncture, therapeutic nutrition, and Chinese herbal medicine, are now being taught in a few veterinary schools and an increasing number of medical schools.) Because of these misunderstandings, veterinarians are often reluctant to speak highly of any alternative therapies until there is sound evidence-based proof that these treatment modalities are clinically beneficial.

Unfortunately, this lack of scientifically validated evidence has helped to fuel and widen the gap between conventional and holistic veterinarians, leading to more client confusion and perceived divergent types of veterinary practices available for the public to select, i.e., conventionally trained or holistically trained practitioners. Many clients are beginning to say they prefer medical professionals trained in both types of healing, i.e., integrative veterinarians.

Alternative veterinary therapies may augment, or in some instances replace, conventional medical therapy, depending upon the condition and the clinical status of the patient. In this book on integrative veterinary medicine, we present protocols for chronic and infectious diseases using therapeutic nutrition, Chinese and Western herbal medicine, and homotoxicology. These therapies are presented on an integrative basis for veterinarians to choose at their level of comfort and experience.

Clinical (academic) veterinary nutrition

Veterinary schools recognize and offer nutrition as part of their teaching curriculum. Although the importance of proper nutrition in the cause and treatment of diseases is recognized, graduate veterinarians have not totally embraced the concept of nutrition for the treatment of disease. Of the approximately 60,000 veterinarians in the United States, there are about 60 diplomates of the American College of Veterinary Nutrition (ACVN), and only about one-third of veterinary schools have a diplomate on faculty staff.

The trained or board-certified veterinary nutritionist assesses nutrition in a clinical setting by first assessing the animal's condition, i.e., physical, diagnostics (blood and so forth), current diet, body weight, and hydration. This is done to gain knowledge about the animal's nutritional requirements and adequacy of the current diet; it does not focus on the potential therapeutic value of food or supplements in the treatment of disease.

Please note that the disease protocols presented in Sections 2 and 3 (Chapters 6 through 18) of this book list nutrients based upon their therapeutic value in the treatment of that disease.

Integrative veterinary medicine

IVM incorporates a fair measure of the lost "art of medicine," in which the practitioner uses his or her senses in a more critical way to assess the totality of the patient being treated, by tapping into an expanded list of therapies based upon the following criteria:

- The clinical and physical condition of the animal
- The medical diagnosis
- An evaluation of the proper medical or surgical treatments available, including their effectiveness and prognosis
- A similar evaluation of alternative therapies, such as therapeutic nutrition, as well as herbal and homeopathic remedies that are appropriate for the condition
- An evaluation of the client's needs and wants

This expanded treatment option program is discussed with the client, who then, with all the facts in hand, makes the appropriate decision for the animal's health and well being.

INTEGRATIVE MEDICINE AND THE EVIDENCE-BASED MODEL

Evidence-based medicine in practice

According to the Evidence-Based Veterinary Medical Association (EBVMA 2006), evidence-based veterinary medicine (EBVM) is "the incorporation of evidence-based medicine principles (EBM) into veterinary practice." Evidence-based medicine relies upon the principle that "the practice of medicine should be based on valid, clinically relevant research data" with a footnote that states "to be accurate, this definition should include the phrase, 'whenever possible,' as medical ethics precludes conducting research that includes inhumane circumstances."

The EBVMA Web site goes on to say that this "is in preference to the traditional method of medical training—still in sway—that is weighted more toward authoritative 'experts,' espousing their best judgments, which are based on their experiences and their understandings of pathophysiology. Once fully integrated, EBM will place human medicine on a scientifically sound foundation so that decisions concerning diagnosis, prognosis, treatment, and risk can be made on the basis of more predictable outcomes."

As practicing veterinarians, we rely upon authoritative experts for our clinical, decision-making process. We also depend upon data from the pharmaceutical industry, veterinary journals, professional reference books, lectures, veterinary teaching schools and specialty groups, conventions, and the wealth of data that is available on the Internet. Another influence for veterinarians is our clients' wishes for their animals. We are often faced with decisions that alter the course of our recommendations because the client does not wish to pursue our medical or surgical recommendations. Veterinarians are often asked what alternative therapies are available for the animals. Currently in veterinary practice, unlike in human medicine, the decision makers are the clients, and they are free to make the choices that they feel will be best for their animals and their families.

Integrative veterinary medicine

The American Veterinary Medical Association (AVMA) guidelines for complementary and alternative veterinary medicine (CAVM) assist veterinarians in making choices related to CAVM techniques. The AVMA guidelines clearly state, "All veterinary medicine, including CAVM, should be held to the same standards. Claims for safety and effectiveness ultimately should be proven by the scientific method. Circumstances commonly require that veterinarians extrapolate information when formulating a course of therapy. Veterinarians should exercise caution in such circumstances. Practices and philosophies that are ineffective or unsafe should be discarded."

Therefore, veterinarians, confronted with the standards of EBVM and the AVMA guidelines for CAVM, face a dilemma when considering IVM therapies. To begin with, most current clinical research focuses upon the efficacy of a specific medical therapy for a disease condition, and little data has been published or peer reviewed on alternative veterinary therapies. To complicate matters further, although much data exists on alternative veterinary therapies, little has been published. There exists a much larger clinical pool of data in human medicine; however, many scientists and veterinarians correctly caution that human data is often not relevant for animals.

The practicing veterinarian is left to do the following:

1. Make the medical diagnosis.
2. Discuss the medical or surgical recommendation with the client.
3. Search out alternative methods when conventional therapy has no clear curative answers or when the client decides against conventional therapies.
4. Heed the precautions of the AVMA.

This book on integrative veterinary medicine helps practitioners who are interested in integrating alternative methods into their practices by compiling available, credible clinical research and authoritative data into a single resource.

Evidence-based history

The battle between evidentiary medicine and holistic medicine goes back hundreds of years. Factually, conventional doctors created the term "evidentiary" in their attack on homoeopaths. Homeopaths were concerned with results for individuals only and not on populations. Evidentiary doctors were worried about "broad-population" health issues, and at the time this term was coined, they were concerned with competition. As the medical and veterinary professions have progressed and become more sophisticated, so too has this evidentiary issue matured, such that today, it is a central issue in the growth and expansion of all healing professions.

The veterinary profession is broad in many opportunities for practicing and research veterinarians, from clinical small animal practice, food animal medicine, treatment of race and show horses, across the spectrum to zoo and laboratory animal medicine. These areas of specialties have a common thread as the basis for their teaching—there is evidence and research supporting their science and practice, but many things are not known and remain to be properly researched. Some alternative therapies, such as acupuncture and Chinese herbal medicine, are mainstream and being taught at veterinary schools, even though much evidentiary proof is scant or not available in the United States.

In homotoxicology and Traditional Chinese Medicine (TCM), for example, a large portion of the literature is not translated into English, which makes its pursuit even more challenging. Similarly, there is evidence and research on pharmaceutical agents, but that doesn't assure their safety or efficacy. Traditional Chinese Medicine has been practiced for more than 4,000 years, and it is firmly entrenched in a methodology that is fundamentally different from the evidenced-based theories and practices upon which conventional (Western) treatments are based. TCM relies upon a deep, astute observation of body systems and responses to manipulation with herbs and other interventions. As a result, these ancient therapies are quite often difficult to integrate or evaluate, because their foundation uses a different point of reference.

When integrating these conventional and alternative methods of healing, we must realize that both the known and unknown are important. As individual doctors we need to be professionally responsible and use techniques that are predictable in assisting our patients in their recovery. When these are known we should recommend them.

When they are not known, it becomes the professional's responsibility to apply his or her knowledge of fundamental theories and concepts to the case at hand to improve the patient's condition.

For example, when some NSAIDs cause illness from side effects, it makes sense to look for alternatives. Glucosamine, chondroitin, and similar natural products lead to improvement and have no major side effects. Once these alternatives are known to be safe and helpful, it makes sense to choose them before resorting to more dangerous agents. In this way alternative agents become therapeutic norms, based on evidentiary results. We currently know that glycosaminoglycans assist in control of arthritis, and they have become more mainstream therapeutic agents. Similarly, milk thistle and its components, as well as SAMe, have moved forward by this same logic.

Evidence—The evolution of scientific truth

Humans have long sought information in pursuit of improved survival (Hellemans, Bunch 1988). Resulting fields of knowledge grow and are organized, and when they are beneficial, become specialized areas of expertise. In this way, civilization grows and prospers on the accuracy of its knowledge base. Professionals are respected for their command of knowledge and their ability to apply it in such a way that it helps the survival of others. The field of medicine is simply one such field, and judging from the longevity statistics over the last few generations, medicine is assisting our population to live longer and more productive lives.

As with all professions, veterinarians continually strive to gain better perspectives and theories of health and disease, and as we gather better information, we constantly review our practices, abandoning the less successful ones and adding those techniques with better outcomes. This is an endless process for any sincere profession. A profession that succeeds in this is respected and loved, and the veterinary profession is currently enjoying rapid growth and high respect. Individual veterinarians who perform these functions effectively are found to have superior incomes and better quality of life.

Science is the orderly asking of questions and recording of data, which is then organized into specialized areas of knowledge. This scientific data can be verified and is repeatable. The word "science" literally means "to know," and the process involves looking at a specific area, deriving what is known, making hypotheses about that area, and then testing those hypotheses using the scientific method. The data achieved from that process are organized and evaluated until a theory, an idea that explains phenomena in a more correct way, can be put forth. This theoretical idea gives rise to models, and these are tested until they are proven or refuted. Achieving scientific

knowledge is a process. It is never static, but rather dynamic, and movements within the fields of knowledge arise and build agreement for their theories and models. Political and economic pressures and factors can enter into the field and block this process with a resulting decline in understanding and scientific discovery.

Technology takes the data that is discovered by scientific method and organizes it into workable means of improving life. The more a discovery improves life, the more valued it becomes. Technology is simply applied knowledge. Philosophy values these discoveries and technologies and examines how they are beneficial or damaging. A truly enlightened civilization will realize that the more ethically its citizens behave, the greater the value of its discoveries and technologies. For this reason, there must always be a conscious ethical arm of any profession, and discussion of ethics (those actions that bring maximal survival to self, groups, and other life forms) must prevail in any living and active profession.

Evidenced-based medicine is a simple concept. It states that a doctor and profession should strive to use technology and techniques that have been proven to be helpful. This keeps a profession on its healing course and preserves the ethical compass of its practitioners, which further ensures the survival of the profession and its clients. It would be ridiculous to fight evidenced-based medicine as a theory, but there can be much disagreement as to what is considered evidence acceptable to the profession. Just as we see in science, a profession must examine the evidence and measure the outcomes of its activity. In doing so we must realize that we will invariably encounter disagreements stemming from a wide variety of sources, not the least of which are economic, religious, and political. The idea of evidenced-based medicine is a good one and one that should be actively pursued, but the concept can become a trap as well, especially when methodologies and meaning of evidence are not properly understood, or when economic or political pressures are brought to bear on a body of knowledge with a purpose other than discovery of the truth.

The word "evidence" comes from "evident," which originates from Latin and literally means "to see out." Evidence is what we see, perceive, or can measure on instruments. A hidden thing is not evident until one removes the barrier to perception, at which time it become obvious. The hidden thing is always there and acting as itself, even though science or scientists do not recognize it, name it, or understand it. Consider, if you will, the concept of the zero net energy field, the variable in physics equations that is known to exist but at present is an unquantifiable entity. On Earth, the sun appears to rise in the east and set in the west; however, until more recently there were many opinions and theories about where the sun spent its time at night. In medicine, the scientific method has spent a considerable time understanding the events of the cell, but only recently did medicine begin to appreciate the massive contribution to the organism made by the space between cells and the connective tissue.

First proposed a century ago, this area of research has been hidden as the field of medicine that looked almost exclusively at cellular structural mechanics and the biochemical activity. Cellular study has been a most worthy study, with a host of lifesaving pharmaceuticals and techniques resulting. As we begin to delve into cellular energetics, field mechanics, and the actions of the connective tissue, we find a gold mine of information with which we may assist patients in recovery from disease, as well as create better states of health for our population.

The science of therapeutic nutrition

Therapeutic nutrition, of all the modalities discussed and explained in this book, is the most studied under the guidelines set by evidence-based standards. One simply has to go to a popular Web site, such as the Linus Pauling Institute at Oregon State University (http://lpi.oregonstate.edu/) or the Mayo Clinic (http://www.mayo.edu/), to find a wealth of credible information on the topic. Linus Pauling, the famous researcher most well known for his work with vitamin C, is referenced throughout chapter 2 of this book. Simply by going to the Linus Pauling Institute Web site and reviewing the micronutrient section one can find an extensive listing of references and clinical trials on vitamins, minerals, phytonutrients, antioxidants, foods, and so on.

In this age of the Internet and the overwhelming amount of credible and not-so-credible information, it is nearly impossible for the layperson, and somewhat difficult for the professional, to decipher truth from fiction. However, if one goes to credible sites such as the Pauling Institute, page after page of non-biased scientific research backs up the claims that various nutrients have been proven beneficial in medical conditions ranging from simple skin disease to cancer.

The one important difference in credible sites is the almost paranoid desire to get away from false and misleading claims and to state the true facts. For example, there is language such as: "while a specific clinical trial has definitively shown that a certain nutrient has been proven beneficial for a specific disease, there is equal and oftentimes more data that states that the specific clinical trial was not only flawed but that other clinical trials failed to prove what the original trial claimed."

Using The Pauling Institute and the medical benefits of vitamin C in treating cancer as an example, one can find the following published data on the Pauling Institute Web site (http://lpi.oregonstate.edu/):

"Studies in the 1970s and 1980s conducted by Linus Pauling and colleagues suggested that very large doses of vitamin C (10 grams/day intravenously for 10 days followed by at least 10 grams/day orally indefinitely) were helpful in increasing the survival time and improving the quality of life of terminal cancer patients (Cameron, Pauling 1976). However, two randomized placebo-controlled studies conducted at the Mayo Clinic found no differences in outcome between terminal cancer patients receiving 10 grams of vitamin C/day orally or placebo (Creagan 1979, Moertel 1985). There were significant methodological differences between the Mayo Clinic and Pauling's studies, and recently, two researchers from the NIH suggested that the route of administration (intravenous versus oral) may have been the key to the discrepant results. Intravenous (IV) administration can result in much higher blood levels of vitamin C than oral administration, and levels that are toxic to certain types of cancer cells in culture can be achieved with intravenous but not oral administration of vitamin C (Padayatty 2004). Thus, it appears reasonable to re-evaluate the use of high-dose vitamin C as cancer therapy."

This example shows the evidentiary process in action. Some clinical trials support the use of vitamin C as a treatment and some do not. The important point regarding this book on integrative veterinary medicine and the current status of the veterinary/client relationship relates to the statement mentioned above in the section on the evolution of scientific truth. What do we as veterinarians recommend for our client whose dog has cancer and who is morally or ethically against chemotherapy and is asking for alternative advice? Three choices:

1. Refer the client to a holistic veterinarian who is experienced in treating cancer but who uses modalities that have no evidence-based proof.
2. Suggest that the client search the Internet or other sources for alternative therapies to treat the animal that has cancer.
3. Suggest alternative therapies that have been used clinically, that may or may not have evidence-based proof, that do no harm, and that offer the client the veterinary-supervised alternative therapy to help in the animal's day-to-day battle against the disease.

Throughout this book's sections on therapeutic nutrition, we will present clinical proof, when available, and outline specific protocols that are designed to assist veterinarians in making therapeutic nutritional treatment decisions for the benefit of their patients and clients.

The science of Chinese herbal medicine

Traditional Chinese Medicine has historically been passed down from one person to the next. In fact, formulas from one region might be markedly different from formulas in another region. The doctors would use whichever herbs were available to them. Now we have classes and even entire schools dedicated to herbal medicine and acupuncture. This is an exciting development. Although some formulas may be proven to be ineffective, most have demonstrated efficacy in the laboratory and in practice.

Recent research has begun to assign Western indications to herbs. Not surprisingly, the Western and Eastern indications tend to match. In traditional Chinese medicine, ginseng (ren shen) is used for "wasting and thirsting disorder," which is a syndrome of polydipsia and weight loss, such as might be seen with diabetes mellitus. In experimental settings we find that ginseng improves clinical signs and lowers blood glucose levels (Chavez 2001). It is also known to benefit Heart Qi in TCM. It is indicated for calming the spirit and for palpitations with anxiety due to Qi and Blood deficiency (Bensky 2004). Modern research has demonstrated that it has inotropic effects similar to cardiac glycosides in dogs, cats, and rabbits (CA 1992). It is clear that although the terminology differs between the two modalities, both are describing the same effect upon the body.

The final stumbling block for acceptance by "modern" practitioners is the often-mentioned lack of scientific studies concerning herbs. Throughout this book, references are cited to demonstrate the use of herbs for each specific condition. The references cited are based upon in vitro laboratory experiments or studies in animals or humans. When the authors have been unable to find studies of acceptable quality, the herbs are listed in a separate paragraph with a statement that these herbs help increase efficacy of the formula.

Because traditional Chinese herbal medicine originated in Asia, many of the studies of herbs and acupuncture were first conducted and published in Asian countries. It is only in recent times that researchers and universities in the United States and other countries have begun to publish on these topics. As a result, more reference material is currently available in foreign language texts. This is changing rapidly, and in future writings, we expect to cite more clinical studies that are published in English and in the United States.

In addition, professional journals have been reluctant to publish articles about herbs, preferring a more progressive image. Just recently, veterinarians who use herbs have been given columns in professional journals. *Veterinary Forum*, the *Journal of the American Veterinary Medical Association*, and *Veterinary Practice News* have all published articles concerning herbal medicine and acupuncture.

There are now entire practitioner-oriented publications that carry studies about herbal medicine, homeopathic medicine, and acupuncture. For example, *Alternative Therapies in Health and Medicine* is a peer-reviewed journal that has been available at the National Library of Medicine since 1996. Books devoted to acupuncture and herbal medicine are being published in record numbers. Universities and government agencies are beginning to conduct research on the use and abuse of herbs. With this increase in research comes a greater understanding of the efficacy and safety of herbal therapy.

The science of homotoxicology

This text contains many studies regarding homotoxicology. Academic studies are desired in a scientific field, and homotoxicology has its share of them. The reader is referred to the evidence-based section (Chapter 4, introduction to homotoxicology) for more detail. Knowledge can be obtained in many ways. The simplest method is to ask the question and look at the material available. When we ask, "Does homotoxicology assist survival?" the answer is not clear to many people. This necessitates the application of scientific method and ethical discussion to the field, because it will be rapidly recognized that this question is simply too broad for inquiry. We must narrow the field and look at simpler systems to gain better understanding.

Analysis literally means "to break apart." Just as we gained understanding of the body by dissection, a healing profession gains professional data from breaking fields down and examining their parts. For a professional considering integrative practice, that process involves constantly evaluating information and choosing those factors that seem plausible to assist patients and then incorporating them into clinical practice. As evidence arises, it is then examined and decisions can be made. The entire profession is currently involved in this very activity.

Homotoxicology attempts to unite and integrate the fields of conventional Western medicine and homeopathy. Its discoveries are validated by normal physiological and biochemical sciences, but the validity of homotoxicology is linked to the question of the validity of homeopathy. A major problem in examining homeopathy for validity has been the lack of any theory that adequately explains the results observed. Many trained in Western medicine feel that they must understand these materials before using them. Although understanding is nice, it is not necessary for successfully using an area of technology. A person can use a computer to assist a veterinarian in running his practice without knowing how the computer works. Homeopaths frequently comment that it is not necessary to know the details of how something works if it can be established that it does work. There is much merit to this comment.

Penicillin kills many bacteria and was successful for years before we understood how it interfered with bacterial growth. As we learned more, science discovered enzymes and enzyme inhibition, and our knowledge base grew. Penicillin continued to kill bacteria in the same way as before, and doctors used it frequently because it accomplished the treatment goals, even though there were no random clinical trials done. Some areas of complementary alternative veterinary medicine and complementary alternative medicine (CAM) are more difficult to examine directly (Lewith, Jonas, Walach 2005). The anatomy of the spirit is a controversial concept, yet nearly half of our population believes that we are spiritual beings and resorts to prayer as part of the routine activity of living. Prayer is the most common form of CAM in human medicine.

Numerous studies have demonstrated benefits from prayer, and some of these are even blinded. This suggests that there is some phenomena, be it simply the power of positive thinking or something far greater, in action in this area. Fortunately for us, prayer rarely interferes with effective medical procedures; it is not required that we answer the exact mechanics involved in this area, because people do not routinely die from prayer; and involving prayer in a practice should not cause much harm to those involved! If a CAM procedure is not harmful in and of itself, then it may be criticized as an unnecessary expense, or it may cause the patient to seek out ineffective therapy over effective therapy, thus delaying needed treatment. For this last reason alone, it is wise for those seeking out CAVM to have an interest in the evidence for each aspect proposed for use in an animal hospital.

Homeopathy is a field that has suffered for lack of a concrete explanation of its method of action. Until recently no one really knew how a homeopathic remedy created its effect. Skeptics frequently state that homeopathy works as some sort of placebo, but one study demonstrated greater results than placebo alone, a fact that makes interested parties continue to investigate the field (Reilly, et al. 1986). Thanks to major attention from European universities, we are beginning to see that at least low-potency homeopathic agents create some of their beneficial effects by very conventional, scientific means (stimulation of cellular receptors and enzyme induction in accordance with the Arndt-Shultz and Michalis-Menton principles).

Perhaps we would be better served to discuss this new field as nanopharmacology, the study of the effects of low doses of substances on physiological systems. Such a change in semantics would likely end most of the misunderstandings between conventional medicine and homotoxicology. The new field that arises from these discoveries is rightly called "regulation medicine," and it seeks to handle disease by assisting the body in its efforts to properly regulate itself.

In the past, however, this information was not known, and even now it is not widely disseminated. Therefore, and quite understandably, conventional medicine, with its attention concentrated on cellular mechanics, tended to reject homeopathic thinking and its terminology of "vital force." Because classical homeopathy tended to be disagreeable to conventional practices of the late 1700s and dangerous medications (mercury and blood letting) due to their destructive and harmful natures, and because

classical homeopathy depended upon only one remedy being given at a time, there was natural disharmony between allopathic medicine and homeopathy.

The 2 fields separated early on, and the financial power lines followed allopathic research and development and the fundamental biological principles of enzyme suppression by large doses of biochemical agents. Pharmaceutical companies endowed modern medicine with billions of dollars to develop current medical practices based upon allopathic agents. Homeopaths, though, because of their ability to achieve results on seemingly difficult individual cases, weathered the storm and survived a period of extreme suppression. As research is conducted, more and more evidence exists to support the practice of homeopathy. Many clients seek out homeopathic doctors as their first choice because they feel they recover faster, better, and more naturally using this form of medicine.

Researching homeopathy is difficult, because no two identical patients exist. The allopathic method of diagnosis is not valid in homeopathy, because remedies are selected based upon symptoms and not classical Western pathological or etiological diagnosis. This makes it most challenging to design double-blind, controlled studies involving classical homeopathy.

In 1991, Kleijnen, et al. reviewed the literature and performed a meta-analysis of studies involving homeopathy. They examined 105 clinical trials involving homeopathic medicines and found positive results in 81 of the studies. Strong responses were identified in the treatment of respiratory disease (13/19 studies showed positive response) and trauma and pain management (18/20 studies indicated positive responses). A fairly large body of knowledge is building that shows some effects attributable to homeopathic agents in both humans and animals (Bellavite and Signorini 2002). Such studies are far from a final answer but indicate why clients seek out homeopathic doctors for their healthcare needs.

Something is working in these patients, and bearing in mind the safety records of homeopathic remedies, using homeopathics in the field of pain management becomes a very tempting impulse. Clients and professionals are well informed about the risks of NSAIDs and actively pursue alternatives (Barnard, Lavoie, Lajeunesse 2006; Lascelles, McFarland, Swann 2005). The most common way that conventional veterinarians enter the field of CAVM is in searching for safer, more effective ways to manage their patients' pain. This is another example of how truth spreads through good results, even in the absence of concrete understanding of a modality's method of action. This is good medicine, using a field with some clinical evidence and improved safety before using a method that is known to be potentially damaging and dangerous. Although classical homeopathy might not easily integrate with conventional allopathic medical practice, such studies should serve to indicate that homeopaths deserve respect as healers and medical professionals. They should also serve to interest medical practitioners in finding out more about these modalities, and statistics show more veterinarians are trained in homeopathy than at any time in modern history.

The field of homotoxicology has evolved because of the obvious improvement in patients receiving homeopathy after treatment failures in conventional medicine, and out of respect for the infinite value of scientific diagnostic processes. The founder of homotoxicology, Dr. Hans-Heinrich Reckeweg, sought to integrate the field of homoeopathy with Western scientific medicine. Through direct clinical observation and trial and error, he developed a series of formulas from mineral, plant, and animal components that assisted his patients in their recoveries. Homotoxicology contains a very active clinical research structure. Dr. Reckeweg was German, and so much of his writing and clinical research was not available in the United States. Recently, though, English material has become more available, and the work that is ongoing in Baden-Baden, Germany, continues to demonstrate the effectiveness and usefulness of homotoxicology remedies.

The presence of clinical research and the results of these studies, along with strong personal success stories of patients who have benefited through application of six-phase theory and antihomotoxic drugs, have led many human healthcare providers and veterinarians, as well as a large number of patients, to move toward use of homotoxicology remedies. In Dr. Reckeweg, once again we see the pattern of a single person who observed irregularities, created a theory explaining these irregularities, and then hypothesized a solution based on the theory. His clinical success led to the creation of a company to market his materials, and this company is the largest of its type worldwide. Currently more and more data are emerging to show that homotoxicology can integrate nicely into conventional veterinary practices and that these practices gain new tools to examine disease pathogenesis as well as therapy. The authors see this fact daily and hope that readers may benefit to the same degree from use of these gentle biological therapies.

It is only natural that veterinarians are becoming increasingly interested in this category of biological therapies. Only a few years ago, all seminars in homotoxicology were sponsored by the parent company, Heel, but homotoxicology is now taught at meetings sponsored by the American Veterinary Medical Association, the American Holistic Veterinary Medical Association, and a rapidly expanding number of local meetings, such as the North American Veterinary Medical Conference and the Annual Conference of the American Holistic Veterinary Medical Association.

Positive clinical results fuel this interest, but there are evidence-based reasons for selecting homotoxicology as

well. Many of these are discussed in the Chapter 4 later in this text.

REFERENCES

Barnard, L., Lavoie, D., Lajeunesse, N. 2006. Increase in non-fatal digestive perforations and haemorrhages following introduction of selective NSAIDs: a public health concern. *Drug Saf.* 29(7):613–20.

Bellavite, P., and Signorini, A. 2002. The Emerging Science of Homeopathy: Complexity, Biodynamics and Nanopharmacology. Berkeley: North Atlantic Books:37–83.

Bensky, D., Clavey, S., and Stoger, E. 2004. Materia Medica 3rd ed. Eastland Press:711.

CA, A. *Cancer Journal for Clinicians* 1992;116: 34223d.

Cameron, E., and Pauling, L. 1976. Supplemental ascorbate in the supportive treatment of cancer: Prolongation of survival times in terminal human cancer. Proc Natl Acad Sci U S A.;73(10):3685–3689.

Chavez, M. 2001. Treatment of Diabetes Mellitus with Ginseng. *Journal of Herbal Pharmacotherapy*, vol 1 (2):99–113.

Creagan, E.T., Moertel, C.G., O'Fallon, J.R., et al. 1979. Failure of high-dose vitamin C (ascorbic acid) therapy to benefit patients with advanced cancer. *N Engl J Med.*;301(13):687–690.

Evidence Based Veterinary Medicine Association (EBVMA), http://www.ebvma.org, P.O. Box 5444, Mississippi State, MS 39762, taken from site December 2006.

Food and Nutrition Board, Institute of Medicine. 2000. Vitamin C. Dietary Reference Intakes for Vitamin C, Vitamin E, Selenium, and Carotenoids. Washington D.C.: National Academy Press:95–185.

Food and Nutrition Board, Institute of Medicine. 1998. Folic Acid. Dietary Reference Intakes: Thiamin, Riboflavin, Niacin, Vitamin B-6, Vitamin B-12, Pantothenic Acid, Biotin, and Choline. Washington, D.C.: National Academy Press: 193–305.

Freudenheim, J.L., Graham, S., Marshall, J.R., et al. 1991. Folate intake and carcinogenesis of the colon and rectum. *Int J Epidemiol*;20:368–74.

Lascelles, B.D., McFarland, J.M., and Swann, H. 2005. Guidelines for safe and effective use of NSAIDs in dogs. *Vet Ther.* Fall;6(3):237–51.

Lewith, G., Jonas, W.B., and Walach, H. 2005. Clinical Research in Complementary Therapies: Principles, Problems, and Solutions. London: Churchill Livingstone.

Moertel, C.G., Fleming, T.R., Creagan, E.T., Rubin, J., O'Connell, M.J., and Ames, M.M. 1985. High-dose vitamin C versus placebo in the treatment of patients with advanced cancer who have had no prior chemotherapy. A randomized double-blind comparison. *N Engl J Med.*;312(3):137–141.

Padayatty, S.J., Sun, H., Wang, Y., et al. 2004. Vitamin C pharmacokinetics: implications for oral and intravenous use. *Ann Intern Med.*;140(7):533–537.

Reckeweg, H. 2000. Biotherapeutic Index: Ordinatio Antihomotoxica et Materia Medica, 5th ed. Baden-Baden, Germany: *Biologische Heilmittel Heel* GMBH;279, 333.

Chapter Two

A Modern Approach to Therapeutic Nutraceuticals

INTRODUCTION

Therapeutic nutrition is broadly defined as the use of nutrients, such as vitamins, minerals, amino acids, essential fatty acids, co-factors, enzymes, antioxidants, and phytonutrients, to support the body's immune and healing systems, thereby altering the course and outcome of a disease process. This is a different application of nutrition than that defined above as clinical or academic nutrition as practiced in veterinary schools. Many of the nutrients, antioxidants, vitamins, and phytonutrients referred to in this section of the book have therapeutic value for patients. Therapeutic nutrition can be used as a preventive, i.e., helping to reduce inflammation and correcting deficiencies and imbalances before they lead to a disease process. Or enzymes, antioxidants, phytonutrients, co-factors, vitamins, minerals, and so on can be used as therapeutic agents.

The word "nutraceutical" is a combination of terms describing nutrition or the use of nutrients and "ceuticals" (from "pharmaceutical"), simply meaning nutrients that have a therapeutic effect on the body. The American Holistic Veterinary Medical Association (AHVMA) and other holistically oriented groups and practitioners further define and refine nutrition according to such properties as having a "hot" or "cold" or "damp" effect on the body, which is similar to theories of Chinese herbal medicine. Modern therapeutic nutrition and nutraceutical therapies focus not on food types, nor calories nor minimum daily requirements, but rather on the metabolic and physiological effects of foods on the body's healing and immune systems.

Therapeutic nutrition action focuses upon the intracellular and intercellular spaces. Unlike drugs, nutritional products are not designed to, nor do they function to, address symptoms or diseases; rather, they are designed to "feed" and "fuel" the cells of the body, using or calling upon the cells' inherent ability to heal and achieve homeostasis.

The goals of therapeutic nutrition fall within 3 broad categories of body essential action, which directly help to improve cellular function and enhance healing:

- The supply of appropriate, bioavailable nutrients
- The reduction of inflammation
- The enhancement of elimination

Supplying appropriate, bioavailable nutrients (provides metabolic building blocks)

The pet food industry was greatly influenced by the guidelines created by the late Dr. Mark Morris, which attempted to help regulate and standardize commercially prepared pet foods. This method is based upon the chemical content and analysis of food (the actual levels of fats, proteins, carbohydrates, and moisture).

This regulatory methodology is accomplished via the guaranteed analysis of the food, which is required to be listed on all pet foods sold in the United States. To qualify as a pet food, the following 4 categories must be listed on the label: crude protein, crude fat, crude fiber, and moisture. A typical guaranteed analysis that is required to qualify as a canned pet food may look like this: crude protein, 10%; crude fat, 6.5%; crude fiber, 2.4%; moisture, 68%.

We veterinarians are familiar with the old shoes adage described by Dr. Morris, where he put together and chemically analyzed a mixture containing coal, shoes, and crankcase oil. (The full description is presented later in this chapter.) When chemically analyzed, this mixture met the minimum requirements of a pet food. Dr. Morris's goal was to dramatize that what is important in pet food is not only the chemical composition, but the bioavailability of the raw ingredients used.

The use of therapeutic nutrition as presented in this book adds the concept of the "biological" value of food, a premise touted by "anti-aging" scientists and doctors, which is covered in detail later in this chapter. For this current discussion of the supply of appropriate nutrients, therapeutic nutritional programs must ensure that beyond the chemical analysis (protein, fat, fiber, moisture, and carbohydrates), the biological value of food, i.e., the vitamin content and the presence of biologically active antioxidants, phytonutrients, enzymes, co-factors and so on, is considered when nutritionally addressing a disease condition.

Reducing inflammation

The cause and method used to reduce inflammation are similar from one organ system to another. It has been clinically proven that free radicals (reactive oxygen molecules with unpaired electrons) bond to tissues and initiate an oxidative process that evokes an inflammatory response.

This load of free radicals can be reduced and neutralized with sufficient dietary levels of antioxidant vitamins, minerals, phytonutrients, and co-factors. Free radicals are formed as a result of the normal metabolic process. Excessive free radicals form upon exposure to foreign substances, such as chemical preservatives, pesticides, herbicides, and environmental chemicals. These foreign substances contribute to the depletion of the body's antioxidant reserves, such as vitamins E and C, which normally function to control the free radical levels. The resulting inflammatory response, if left unchecked, can lead to degradation of tissue and impaired organ system function.

The question often asked, however, is "Why don't vitamin- and antioxidant-enhanced pet foods neutralize this building free radical load?" The simple answer relates to the heat of cooking and processing. Studies demonstrate that many of the important vitamins and antioxidants, which are required to neutralize free radicals, are inactivated by heat. The nutrient inactivation of various antioxidants was reported in several studies (BASF 1983, 1986). In one study it was shown that more than 75% of the available vitamin C, a potent antioxidant, was inactivated by heat (BASF 1998).

The inflammation referred to above that responds to therapeutic nutrition is cellular inflammation. It has been demonstrated that free radical reactions initiate and create a local cellular inflammation, which, if unchecked, quickly spreads to groups and sheets of cells, tissues, and organs. Detection of this inflammatory response, if addressed and neutralized early, helps prevent this cellular inflammation, organ degenerating, and eventual organ and tissue disease (Cerutti 1994, Charlton 1999, Davies 1991, Gilchrist 1997, Halliwell 1989, 1993, 1994).

Enhancing elimination

The final piece underlying the effectiveness of therapeutic nutrition, and one of the keys to healing, is the elimination of metabolic wastes and toxins from the body. When an organ or system is diseased, ridding the body of the metabolic wastes (toxins), as well as strengthening and supporting related organs and tissues, is beneficial to the overall healing process.

The enhancement of elimination is not confined to nutrition alone, as other modalities such as homotoxicology are built upon the concept of the body's ability to eliminate toxins. (See the homotoxicology section of this book on toxins, homotoxins, and detoxification.) The following is the basic underlying theory by which homotoxicology is built (Reckeweg 2000.):

"According to homotoxicology, all of those processes, syndromes, and manifestations, which we designate as diseases, are the expression, thereof that the body is combating poisons and that it wants to neutralize and excrete these poisons. The body either wins or loses the fight thereby. Those processes, which we designate as diseases, are always biological, that is natural teleological processes, which serve poison defense and detoxification."

FREE RADICALS, ANTIOXIDANTS, AND PHYTONUTRIENTS

Free radicals

Free radicals are reactive molecules that contain unbound or unpaired electrons that are initiated by metabolism or exposure to foreign materials, such as toxins and metabolic wastes. Formed on exposure to oxygen, these then reactive free radicals can initiate a local cellular inflammation that expands by a chain reaction to adjacent cells and tissues, and finally throughout the entire organ. There are 2 types of free radicals, endogenous and exogenous. Endogenous free radicals result from the body's normal day-to-day functioning, such as metabolism byproducts or the breakdown of bacteria and viruses by the white blood cell system. Exogenous free radicals are more well known and result from events such as exposure to environmental chemicals and toxins. One of the more studied is the effect of smog and secondhand smoke as a cause of free radical production and disease in people (Opara 1997).

The primary danger of these free radical complexes is that they can induce inflammation that can interfere with the DNA and the vital elements of the cell, causing improper functioning and even cellular death. In anti-aging human medicine, there is a popular theory that associates the process of aging directly with free radical production (Harman 1955, 1992, 1994; Masoro 1993).

Free radical formation is a normal, day-to-day occurrence. Free radicals are also normal byproducts of metabolism and serve physiological and biochemical purposes. However, research points to the fact that excessive formation of free radicals (the free radical load) for any number of reasons as explained below can lead to this oxidative state, which results in cell destruction, inflammation, organ degeneration, and the developments of degenerative diseases, such as heart disease, liver disease, kidney disease, arthritis, and cancer (Cochrane 1992; Davies 1991, 1995; Halliwell 1989, 1993; Harman 1994; Poli 1993; Sies 1985, 1991; Spatz 1992).

Antioxidants

Antioxidants (free radical scavengers) are compounds that slow or prevent oxidation, neutralize reactive free radicals, and help prevent the initiation of the inflammatory process. This inflammatory response is believed to be responsible for premature aging, organ degeneration, and cell death.

The body's antioxidant system is one of the primary defenses against free radical production and associated cellular damage. Antioxidants are naturally occurring in fresh fruits and vegetables. Many antioxidants are not produced by the body and therefore are a requirement in the diet. The more common and well-known antioxidants are the vitamins A, E, beta carotene, and C and minerals such as selenium.

The mechanism of action of antioxidants is the prevention of peroxidation. By stabilizing the free radicals, antioxidants indirectly reduce the initiating oxidation, the resulting inflammatory response, the spread of inflammation, and cellular and tissue death.

The antioxidant reserve (the levels of activated antioxidants that are found in the body) depends upon many factors, including the level of antioxidants found in the diet. Although this appears to be a simple case of just eating more antioxidants, building the reserve, and capping the free radical buildup, there are numerous factors that interfere with this neutralization process, such as: growing food on depleted soil; the heat of cooking and processing, which destroys most naturally occurring antioxidants (BASF 1983); and stress, disease, infection, overvaccination, chemical and toxin exposure, emotional issues, and so on (Opara 1997).

This balance between free radical load and depletion of antioxidants has broader implications. The Iams Company, at their symposium in 2000, presented proof that antioxidants such as vitamin E also play a direct role in immune system functioning, health maintenance, and disease prevention (Hayek 2000).

The importance of achieving the balance between antioxidant reserves and free radical load is one of the cornerstones of therapeutic nutrition. The addition of unprocessed, uncooked, unchemicalized, bioavailable antioxidants as part of a therapeutic nutritional program is essential for preventing the initiation and progression of degenerative diseases (Lindley 1998, Nicoli 1999).

Phytonutrients (phytochemicals)

Phytonutrients are chemical compounds that are produced by and help in the performance of the metabolic functions of the plant. New and growing research has proven that these nutrients, although not classified as essential nor required like foods and vitamins, act as antioxidants and prevent oxidative damage. They exert a positive and often dramatic effect on wellness, health, prevention and treatment of disease, and longevity (Broadhurst 2001, Duke 1992, Gaziano 1995, Shils 1994).

Phytonutrients, as they relate to health and nutrition, are activated plant compounds that, when eaten, are therapeutic and have beneficial effects on the physiology and metabolism of animals (Duke 1992, Hyson 2002). Described below are some of the more well-known and researched phytonutrients; however, literally thousands of phytonutrients have been discovered and are being researched for their health benefits.

Although phytonutrient compounds are not essential for life, they are beneficial for optimum health and are often classified with vitamins, minerals, and antioxidants. Recently, advanced scientific techniques and methodologies have allowed researchers to identify categories of phytonutrients and classify and define them according to their health benefits.

Categories of phytonutrients, such as amines, bioflavonoids, carotenoids, lignans, organosulfurs, phenols, phytosterols, sterols, sterolins, and terpines are being clinically proven to positively affect health and well being, reduce inflammation, and slow degenerative disease. They are also being shown to have a critical role in cancer prevention (Ames 1993, Block 1992, Carlton 2000, Duthie 1996).

Carotenoids

Carotenoids make up a category of phytonutrients that impart the yellow, red, or orange pigment color to fruits and vegetables. The most common and well known are alpha, beta, and gamma carotene, as well as lutein, lycopene, and xanthophylls. New and emerging research has identified hundreds of carotenoids, which are being studied in all categories of degenerative diseases and cancer (Agarwal 2000, International Agency for Research on Cancer 1998, Naguib 2003).

The earlier research on carotenes, and particularly beta carotene, was centered upon dogs' ability and cats' inability to convert beta carotene to vitamin A, thereby preventing deficiencies. More recent research, however, has focused in the area of degenerative disease and cancer prevention. Besides their potent antioxidant (anti-inflammatory) properties, research has uncovered their immune-enhancing function and their ability to help regulate cellular communications and division (Gaziano

1995, Ito 1999, Nishino 2000, Slattery 2000, Zeegers 2001).

Research shows that long-term dietary deficiency of carotenoids is associated with chronic degenerative diseases due to carotenoids' antioxidant properties. Although much of this research is focused on people, veterinarians should be aware that the majority of dog and cat foods fed over the past 35 to 50 years was highly processed and cooked (canned and extruded dry foods) at extremely high temperatures, which has been demonstrated to have a negative effect on the health benefits of antioxidants and phytonutrients (Nicoli 1999, Price 1998, Shahidi 1997, Lindley 1998).

Besides the adverse affects of high temperatures upon vital nutrients, dog and cat foods most often are devoid of phytonutrients. Coupling this with the statements that the addition of vitamins, minerals, and table scraps (such as vegetables) should be avoided stimulates inquiry concerning a link between the rising level of chronic diseases and cancer in dogs and cats and the feeding of antioxidant- and phytonutrient-deficient foods (Delgado-Vargas 2000, Goldstein 1999, Heaton 2002, Seddon 1994).

Flavonoids

Flavonoids are a large family of plant-derived chemicals that are mainly responsible for the colors and pigments of most fruits and vegetables. They were discovered in the 1930s by Albert Szent-Gyorgyi, who originally classified them as vitamin P. The more commonly know flavonoids are flavones, isoflavones, anthocyanins, anthocyanidins, and flavonols. Commonly named flavonols are rutin, heseridin, and quercetin. Some of the main health benefits of flavonoids are their function as potent antioxidants and their ability to help reduce inflammation.

Research has proven that flavonoids increase the body's level of the antioxidant glutathione, helping to control, reduce, and eliminate inflammation, pre-disease. Several studies indicate that flavonoids can help regulate the immune response and have a controlling effect over reactivity of immune-mediated cells, such as T and B lymphocytes, mast cells, and neutrophils (Middleton 1986, 1992; Myhrstad 2002; Panthong 1994; Roger 1998).

There is currently much investigation of flavonoids in disease prevention and treatment. Clinical evidence suggests that flavonoids' ability to reduce inflammation plays an important role in heart disease in humans (Blake 2003, Geleijnse 2002, Hertog 1997, Rimm 1996, Sesso 2003). Currently, the effects of flavonoids in prevention and treatment are not conclusive. Although some studies do show potential benefits, others have proven nonconclusive (Knekt 2002, Ross 2002).

Of primary importance for the health benefits of flavonoids is their susceptibility and inactivation secondary to processing, farming, and the high heat of cooking. Adding flavonoids to dog or cat foods does not necessarily guarantee the health benefits. This is an important point substantiating the addition of fresh foods, such as fruits and/or vegetables, to the daily feeding of dogs and cats (Gil 1999, Ioku 2001).

Lignans

Lignans are naturally occurring chemicals found in both plants and animals and are broadly considered to be phytoestrogens. They are found in abundance in flax seed, fruits, vegetables, and beans. Phytoestrogens are plant-derived chemicals that mimic the activity of animal estrogens. Research into lignans (and also soy isoflavonoids) is occurring in the field of human mammary cancer prevention. The research interest in phytoestrogens is based upon the fact that plant-derived compounds can compete with the body's hormonal estrogen, actually lessen phytoestrogens' effect, and help prevent hormonally aggravated mammary cancers (Brooks 2005; Kleinsmith 2003; Wang 2002; Serraino 1992; Sung 1998; Thompson 1996, 1998).

Other studies show lignans may also have additional cancer prevention benefits (Sung 1998). Lignans are also being studied in relationship to heart disease prevention. Lignan-rich foods such as fruits, vegetables, nuts, and seeds are being studied for their beneficial, cardioprotective effects (Adlercreutz 1997, Arjmandi 1998, de Kleijn 2002, Jenkins 1999, Prasad 1997, Vanharanta 2003).

Sterols and phytosterols

Sterols are plant-based lipid compounds that are chemically similar to cholesterol and are found in many seeds. The most commonly known and well-studied sterol is betasitosterol. Sterols are similar to and able to chemically compete with cholesterol, and much research is being conducted in humans in the area of cholesterol lowering and heart disease prevention. One study compared the cholesterol levels of Seventh-Day Adventists (vegetarians) with the non-vegetarian public and found a significant low ratio between phytosterols and cholesterol and a lower risk for heart disease (Nair 1984). This study also indicated a higher risk of colon cancer related to the ratio of phytosterols to cholesterol, as compared to the actual level of blood cholesterol, emphasizing the importance of these phytosterols in the diet. It is thought that the phytosterols somehow interfere with both the reduction of inflammation and the altering of the cell membrane in tumor growth.

Pegel (1997) feels that sterols are essential for a properly functioning immune system. Pegel believes that in cancer patients, sterols can directly reduce the adverse immune-suppressing effects of both chemo- and radiation therapies. In studies on cats with FIV, sterols are believed to have an immune-modulating effect and help to maintain proper lymphocyte levels (Bouic 1997). Treated cats showed a 20% mortality rate, as compared to the non-treated cat mortality rate of 75%. It was further reported that there were no deaths in surviving cats after 3 years with sterol treatment. Although the sterols have no direct antiviral properties, the balancing and modulation of the immune system are enough to control the spread and effects of the virus.

Other properties of plant-derived sterols are their anti-inflammatory and antipyretic properties, which appear to be similar to corticosteroids and aspirin (Gupta 1980). Sterols have been found to enhance T lymphocyte production and moderate B cell activity, thereby helping to balance the immune response and indirectly reducing the risk of an autoimmune reaction (Bouic 1996).

Awad (1999) proved that in the laboratory, the use of sterols reduced the number of breast cancer cells as compared to the controls. In another study Awad (1999) further proved that the sterols also enhanced intracellular communications in such a way that they inhibited cell growth, which can prevent the formation of cancer.

Antioxidants and phytonutrients: Their effect on aging and degeneration and their critical role in preventing degeneration and neoplasia

The theory that free radicals cause aging is quite popular and accepted, especially in human medicine. This theory, introduced in the 1950s, stated that highly reactive free radicals are directly linked to the aging process (Harman 1955). This theory states that free radicals are produced as a result of the metabolism, endogenously and exogenously, by exposure to foreign substances such as cigarette smoke. Left to accumulate into a free radical load, these reactive particles will initiate and damage cells, tissues, and organs. This theory is now being supported and proven by numerous clinical studies both in people and animals, which confirms the direct effect on the aging process and the formation of chronic degenerative diseases (Harman 1992). This theory also remains so popular because it integrates well with genetic and DNA research in which the free radicals, also called reactive oxygen species (ROS), alter the DNA and can cause mutations that in turn lead to diseases such as cancer (Opara 1997, Harman 1992, Masoro 1993).

Antioxidants, phytonutrients, free radicals, and their relationship to aging have spawned a tremendous amount of clinical research in both the medical and veterinary fields. The major dog food and cat food companies are funding research to prove that antioxidants and phytonutrients in their food have a beneficial effect on the health and well being of animals. Because degenerative diseases and neoplasia play such a dominant role in day-to-day veterinary practice, it is important to understand not only

the theory, but also what we practitioners can do to benefit our patients. Can adding these vital nutrients into our patients' daily regime slow the aging process, reduce inflammation, and ultimately affect disease prevention?

As veterinary students we have been taught how to treat disease when it is diagnosed. As practitioners, when dealing with chronic degenerative diseases, we focus upon the signs and symptoms of the disease and upon alleviating our animals' pain and suffering without doing any harm. The inherent issue, however, is that many of the recommended drugs carry long-term side effects that can be counterproductive for the disease and the patient. Take, for example, the treatment of chronic allergic dermatitis with corticosteroids. Although in the short term we are offering our patients the anti-inflammatory and antipruritic effects of the drugs, as well as comfort and self-trauma prevention, we are invariably exposing animals to the long list of inherent side effects that go along with the chronic use of corticosteriods.

One of the important benefits of integrative veterinary medicine is the ability to offer our patients nutritional, herbal, or homeopathic remedies that work alone or in combination with the medical treatment plan that we have selected. These therapies can often help improve the animal's day-to-day quality of life, speed up healing, and add the parameter of preventing future episodes. Although skeptics demand, "Show me the proof," one intent of this book is to compile and document the science and proof of these benefits in an organized format for clinicians.

The unanswered question remains: "What effect do these nutrients, herbs, and homeopathics have on the prevention of degenerative disease and the prevention of neoplasia?"

One possible answer concerns the role of free radicals in the pathogenesis of diseases. The free radical theory of aging, as noted earlier, describes the oxidative damage and altered cellular integrity leading to decreased organ function. This process sets the stage for the initiation of chronic degenerative diseases, such as arthritis, diabetes, heart disease, liver disease, and kidney disease, and of course cancer.

Although many chronic degenerative conditions are reported as "proven cause unknown," there is a mechanism, be it known or unknown, that starts the disease process. More and more scientists, researchers, and practicing doctors believe the disease initiator is this free radical oxidative process. When it occurs in the joints it can lead to arthritis, in the heart it leads to cardiomyopathy, and in the kidneys it may result in chronic renal failure. Although the organ system and disease names may be different, there is a common denominator underlying this initiating process, which if addressed early, can help in preventing degenerative diseases and in maintaining wellness.

The inquiring mind asks, "How does this occur?"

As free radical levels rise and dietary antioxidant levels decrease, the inflammatory process begins and spreads from cells to tissue to organ systems, and cells begin to die. Cellular debris is viewed as being foreign to the body, which responds by sending white blood cells and producing autoantibodies to rid itself of the cellular debris. The continual process of inflammation and immune attack causes organ degeneration, resulting in cellular infiltration, glandular hypofunction or organ hyperfunction, and a flooding of the mesenchyme with byproducts of inflammation.

Although no single theory explains all disease development, free radical damage is intimately involved in many of our most common pathologic processes and deserves attention. Good examples of this process are IBD, hypothyroidism in dogs, and hyperthyroidism in cats. Although these diseases are different, and signs and symptoms are different, the underlying initiating cause remains cellular inflammation, cellular infiltration, cell death, and the interference with normal organ function.

GLAND THERAPY

This book does not spend much time explaining drug therapies and does so only when they are necessary as part of an integrative approach for specific disease protocols. The important distinction made regarding drug therapies is that the medication does not focus upon healing, but rather on controlling the condition. For example, an acute infection treated with antibiotics is not cured by the medication. The antibiotic does destroy the bacteria that cause the infection, but the actual healing mechanism is generated internally by the body itself.

In chapters 6 through 18, which address disease protocols, we present medical therapies in relationship to the definitions and causes of the specific diseases. Most often, drugs address symptoms and signs and do not promote the body's ability to heal. As you read through the nutritional, herbal, and homeopathic sections of the disease protocols, you find that more often these modalities address the body's ability to heal, noting clinical proof substantiating the action that is claimed. It is the collective opinion of the authors of this book that the prudent integration of conventional and alternative therapies to control symptoms and enhance healing is beneficial for the patient's health and maintenance of wellness.

Gland therapy: the precursor to modern pharmaceuticals

Organ therapy, also known as glandular or cellular therapy, is broadly defined as the use of raw glands and organ concentrates to achieve therapeutic results. Glandular extracts possess an affinity for similar tissues and contain many chemical, hormonal, enzyme, and co-factors that exert significant physiological, metabolic, and therapeutic effects on cells and organ systems.

Early examples of this type of therapy include the use of thyroid glands in the treatment of myxedema and the use of dried pancreas extract for the treatment of diabetes; these are well documented in earlier medical literature. More recent medical research discovered quicker-acting, more potent medications. The following quote from Lewis (1995) in *Complementary and Alternative Veterinary Medicine* summarizes this transition from gland therapy to drugs:

> "Analytic methods improved greatly during the middle of this century, and many of the important hormones were discovered and isolated from glandular tissues, such as cortisone from adrenal tissue and thyroxine from thyroid tissue. The biomedical community was quick to ascribe all clinical results of glandular or cellular therapy to the presence of small quantities of hormones, which came to be regarded as the only active constituents of glandular materials. Advanced chemical methods allowed the pharmaceutical industry to produce large quantities of synthetic hormones. The gentle, physiologic action of whole glands or crude extracts was abandoned for the fast, pharmacological action of inexpensive synthetic hormones. This was the age of so-called wonder drugs, when physicians and patients came to expect dramatic and immediate results from medications. These quick results, however, were later associated with problems and side effects, such as the diabetes and immune depression following corticosteroid therapy and the development of antibiotic-resistant strains of bacteria following promiscuous use of antibiotics."

Historical use

Historically, references to gland therapy appear in ancient times, and the use of animal parts in treating diseases of people has been documented. Early physicians such as Aristotle and Pliny the Elder discussed their use, and references exist throughout modern times. In the 1600s, the original theories discussed the workings of gland therapy based upon the principle that "like organs will help cure the same organ." This should not be confused, however, with the underlying principles of "like healing like" that have been defined by classical homeopaths.

The gland therapy theory was introduced by the physician Paracelsus in his "Doctrine of Signatures." This theory rationalized that eating an organ or a specific tissue would heal the same organ in the body. For example, if a person was suffering from a liver disease, eating raw liver would help to cure that disease. Likewise, eating raw heart tissue would help heal a weakened heart, and so on (Harrower 1916).

Although this concept of "like healing like" seems somewhat credible, it also seems scientifically unsound. Skeptics questioned why consuming a particular tissue type in the treatment of corresponding tissues would have any validity at all. They asked, "By what mechanism do these materials act? And where is the evidence to support the claim that they are absorbed and used by the user's body?"

Scientific basis

Historically, there were arguments for and against this unproven theory. Skeptics of gland therapy stated that any tissue that is eaten is digested into its building-block components of proteins, fats, and carbohydrate, which in turn would be exposed to the body's digestive enzymes and therefore completely inactivated. Scientists who supported the theory proposed that the raw glandular tissue, besides being composed of the basic food parts, also contained other factors that were responsible for their activity. It wasn't until the later 1800s and the early 1900s that gland and cellular therapies began to acquire some scientific basis.

First came the understanding that the body is composed of many organs, including specific glands that produce or secrete various chemical compounds (hormones) that have a powerful effect on the functioning of the body and its systems. The use of crude organ extracts began in the early 1900s and was included in day-to-day medical practice. It was also at this time that scientific literature was rapidly expanding with new reports and "miracle cures" from these glandular substances. Harrower reported on the numerous uses and applications of gland therapies in his *Endocrine Handbook* (1939).

The first documented proof of the efficacy of organ therapy came in 1912 when injections of thyroid extract were able to help children suffering from myxedema and cretinism. In 1920, it was documented that thyroid extract could be absorbed from the intestinal tract: "Desiccated thyroid has been found to be absorbed from the gastrointestinal tract with greater regularity than has the sodium salts of thyroxine. At present, we prefer the oral administration of desiccated thyroid standardized on its iodine content" ("The Principles of Internal Secretion" as reported by Cima 1981). Cima continues: "In Addison's disease, there is a definite adrenal deficiency. In some cases, dried adrenal gland produces improvement. Whole gland given in too large an oral dose produces physical and mental weakness, irritability, insomnia, intestinal disturbances and cramps" ("Glandular Therapy" as reported by Cima 1981).

In 1931, Dr. Paul Niehans, considered the father of gland therapy, administered raw parathyroid gland to a patient suffering from serious muscular spasms after a thyroidectomy and accidental destruction of the parathy-

roid glands. The response was immediate and dramatic, and the patient was cured. "The use of purified thyroid hormone and thyroid extracts are compared experimentally. The extracts are safer, and the activity of thyroid extracts is shown to be greater than that of pure synthetic hormone extracted from that amount of gland" ("Internal Secretions" as reported in Cima 1981).

At that time, science and medical research and clinical practice were becoming more sophisticated, as was the ability to document accurate results. One of the pioneers of the organ therapy movement was Dr. Royal Lee, who looked at the use of gland therapy from a different angle. He retraced organ therapy back to its inception, to the originating theory of "like healing like." Many scientists and medical researchers were quick to accept the premise that "If it works, and if it is found to be concentrated in the same organ, then it must function according to the theory of like healing like."

But Lee explored deeper. Lee theorized that as an organ becomes weakened and diseased, the cells are broken, releasing their contents into general circulation of the body. The body's healing system, composed of various organs and chemicals, finds this cellular breakdown debris and immediately reacts by forming an antibody, the body's mechanism to destroy invaders. He further theorized that these antibodies not only attack the cellular debris, they also attack the entire organ via an autoimmune response. The result of this autoiummune reaction is an inflammatory process in which the body inflames its own tissue. The organ weakens and begins to function at less-than-optimum levels, setting the stage for degenerative disease. If, for example, this autoimmune response occurs in the thyroid glands, causing them to function at less-than-optimum levels, the end result could lead to hypothyroidism.

Lee stated that gland extracts work not by "like healing like" but rather in a more straightforward way. The cellular debris contains intrinsic factors that are organ-specific and attracted to the same organ of the body. These factors stimulate production of antibodies that the body perceives as a foreign invader. Gland extracts then help to defend the organ by *neutralizing* the antigen-antibody response and thereby minimizing the autoimmune and inflammatory processes. This results in the organ being protected from the immune system's internal attack, resulting in its ability to rest and heal (Lee 1947.)

Organ specificity

Another area of gland therapy that was rich fodder for the skeptic was and is that of organ specificity, as theorized by Lee. Lee proposed that when a person or animal ingested raw organ tissue such as bovine liver, the macromolecules are absorbed into the system and directed to the liver. The intrinsic factors derived from the ingested

liver would nourish and protect the person's or animal's
own liver by neutralizing any attack from the immune
system, thereby helping to improve the function of the
now-rested and nourished gland.

Farfetched? Maybe not. This theory fits closely with the
modern free radical theory of aging. See Sidebar 2.1 for
further information on this.

Glands: Sources of nutrients, peptides, lipids, enzymes, vitamins, minerals, and precursors of hormones

Glands are generally derived from bovine or porcine
sources. There are several methods of processing gland
extracts, and these usually result in a dry powder extract
of the entire organ or a liquid preparation. It is important
that the source of fresh glands come from non-contami-
nated and disease-free animals that are accepted into the
food chain. The glandulars are ingested and assimilated
from the intestines into the blood and distributed throughout the body. Initially the skeptics of organ therapy
claimed that the glands would be digested and therefore
no beneficial compounds would be available for the body
to use.

The accepted theory regarding absorption from the
intestinal tract claimed that macromolecules would be
reduced to their amino acid components and then
absorbed, and that the intestinal tract itself would be a
barrier to the direct absorption of these proteins. Research
now offers proof that this is not the case, and the evidence
shows that the larger macromolecules (hormones, proteins, enzymes) are absorbed from the gut directly into
the bloodstream and can then have their therapeutic effect
on the body (Ambrus 1966, Baintner 1986, Gardner
1988.)

These ingested, intact macromolecules, which are
similar to the organ from which they came, can neutralize
the autoantibodies that may be attacking that particular
organ. These tissue-specific or physiologically active molecules therefore can be taken up into circulation and may
exert a protective effect on cells and organs. (See tissue
sparing, below.)

THE TISSUE-SPARING EFFECTS OF NUTRACEUTICALS AND PHYTONUTRIENTS

It is believed that gland extracts exert a tissue-sparing
effect on bodily tissues. The mechanism is either neutralizing the autoantibody attack on organ cells or is supplying nutrients and enzymes that allow the specific organ to
rest. Some examples are as follows:

Pancreas extracts

Besides the use of pancreatic enzymes in the digestive
process, research indicates that pancreatic enzymes are
reabsorbed in the lower bowel and returned to the pancreas to be stored for future use (Liebow 1975). It is
believed that administration of pancreas extracts not only
benefits digestion and assimilation, but also increases pancreatic enzyme reserves, thereby resting the pancreas in
its day-to-day functioning. The same could be true for the
adrenal, the gland that is often affected when an animal
or person is under stress. Hans Selye (1976), in one of his
famous books, talks about the direct negative effect of
stress on the adrenal glands.

Adrenal extracts

Advocates of adrenal extract argue that the raw gland
contains many substances and can carry out many metabolic functions that the isolated synthetics such as cortisone cannot. For example, Friedman (1956) reported that
raw adrenal contains enzymes that convert cholesterol
into glucocorticoid, thereby allowing the adrenal glands
to rest. If this premise is true, then other glands and their
intrinsic factors may support other organs and overall
metabolism by supplying the necessary compounds
required for the production of hormones, enzymes, and
other essential body chemicals. In so doing, they can spare
the organ from overworking, thereby promoting its
optimum efficiency.

Liver extracts

A superior, bioavailable source of iron is the liver. When
you compare the absorption rate of inorganic iron
(ferrous sulfate, for example) to that of the iron-bound

hemoglobin (heme iron), the latter is a 30-fold winner. The best source of heme iron is concentrated liver extract. When you couple the iron content with the rich source of B vitamins, including B_{12} and folic acid, liver extract becomes a potent source of nutrients, especially in a chronically degenerating animal. It also has been clinically proven, in double-blind studies, that liver extracts not only improve the functioning and efficiency of the liver but also are helpful in the healing of chronic degenerative liver disease. These studies confirmed that liver extracts can improve circulation; stimulate, regenerate, spare, and protect liver cells; and lower the levels of circulating liver enzymes in the blood (Frykman 1994, Ohbayashi 1972, Fujisawa 1984).

Cartilage extracts

Cartilage extracts are a good source of glycosaminoglycans (GAGS), such as chondroitin sulfate and glucosamine. Several studies have demonstrated the effectiveness of glucosamine and chondroitin in the management of arthritis in dogs (Das 2000, Guastella 2005). Setnikar et al. (1986) described how these compounds actually stimulate the body's own repair mechanism and help in the process of developing new cartilage. There have been numerous double-blind studies comparing the effectiveness of glucosamine and various NSAIDs, and glucosamine has resulted in as good as, or in many cases, even better, pain control and removal of the clinical signs associated with osteoarthritis (Prudden 1974, Brown 1981, Vaz 1982, DeAmbrosia 1982).

Phospholipids

Specialized phospholipids, such as phosphatidyl choline, phosphatidyl serine, and others, have been proposed as therapeutic agents for neurologic and other diseases (Horrocks 1986). These phospholipids are found in glandular brain, liver, and other glands. These glands are sources of highly unsaturated omega-3 fatty acids, which are now thought to play a vital role in the development and maintenance of the central nervous system.

There has been extensive research into the use of phospholipids, particularly phosphatidyl serine, and the positive effects they exert on the brain and central nervous system. Cennacchi (1992), Engle (1992), and Dewaide (1986) have conducted double-blind studies in people with dementia and Alzheimer's disease with positive results. High concentrations of phosphatidyl choline and serine are found in brain tissue. Horrocks (1986) reported on the potential clinical use of these nutrients in chronic neurological conditions.

Heart extracts

The nutraceutical coenzyme Q10 (CoQ10) has been proven to be beneficial as an energy-producing nutrient, with specific applications in heart disease, obesity, and cancer. In heart disease, it has been particularly beneficial in treating congestive heart failure and cardiomyopathy. It has been found to actually increase the levels of oxygen in the blood. Heart tissues contain high levels of CoQ10; therefore, one of the beneficial effects of giving raw heart tissue concentrate to animals with heart disease would be to increase the body's oxygen level (Judy 1984, Gaby 1989).

DO GLAND THERAPIES WORK?

There have been few clinical studies testing gland therapy for the treatment of disease in both animals and humans. Osband et al. (1981) carried out a study on histiocytosis X, published in *The New England Journal of Medicine*, in which 17 patients were injected with bovine thymus extract and 20 patients underwent chemotherapy. This is perhaps the most notable among glandular studies because it is the first controlled U.S. study to test glandulars on humans. Of the 17 patients who received the thymus extract, 10 went into complete remission without being medicated or receiving any chemotherapy. Although this was a preliminary study, the evidence points toward some positive results, especially if an integrative approach were to take the place of using chemotherapy in combination with the thymus therapy.

Clinical trials using thymus extract have shown that it is beneficial in people with hepatitis B (Skotnicki 1989). Additional clinical studies with oral thymus extract showed that blood values related to liver function as well as the blood immune markers all improved. Civereira (1989) showed similar results with hepatitis C (Galli 1985, Bortolotti 1988).

Raw glandular extracts of adrenal, lymph, spleen, bone marrow, and thymus tissue have been clinically shown to be anti-inflammatory, as well as tissue and organ sparing in cancer and other chronic degenerative diseases (Craveri 1971, Hartleb 1997, Singh 1998, Volk 1991, Sing 1985, Kouttab 1989, Schulof 1985).

One of the most powerful, steroid-like hormones is dehydroepiandrosterone (DHEA), which has been proven to have clinical significance for a variety of conditions, such as cognitive dysfunction and aging, diabetes, heart disease, and arthritis. DHEA also may possess anticancer activity. This hormone was left out of the equation when the medical research isolated and synthetically produced cortisone, thereby moving away from the traditional adrenal extract. As it turns out, DHEA's properties are as potent as cortisone itself. One of its properties that can be beneficial for dogs that are cushinoid or have Cushing's disease is its ability to help control and lower cortisol levels (Kroboth 2003). What other yet undiscovered beneficial substances may be found in adrenal extract that are part of the mechanism of action? (Flood 1988, Schwartz 1981, Kalimi 1990.)

THE INTEGRATION OF THERAPEUTIC NUTRITION INTO PRACTICE

Most commonly, when veterinarians graduate, select their desired type of practice, and do an internship, residency, or enter private practice, their focus has been guided toward diagnosis, disease, pathophysiology, and therapy and less toward the underlying cause and prevention. In a typical veterinary practice, prevention and wellness often take a back seat to the treatment of acute, chronic, and neoplastic conditions. Integrative veterinary medicine strives to augment and enhance conventional medicine with therapeutic modalities that inherently address underlying causes and prevention.

Drug therapies are aimed at signs and symptoms and often do not address the underlying cause, nor do they heal. Only the body and its immune and healing systems can promote healing. Drugs are designed to control, suppress, stimulate, quiet, and diminish. Nutritional therapies, on the other hand, are designed to nourish, soothe, reduce inflammation, protect cells and glands, improve metabolism, enhance waste and toxin elimination, and promote homeostasis.

So long as the therapeutic nutrition does not interfere with the intended action of the drug, why would a veterinarian be reluctant to add it to his or her treatment protocol? One of the most common reasons is "I just do not know enough about nutritional therapies to use or recommend them" or "I would use therapeutic nutrition if I could see the evidence or the proof." The purpose of this book is to present to practitioners proven and well-documented protocols that can be used either alone or in combination with needed medical therapies.

This introductory section on therapeutic nutrition explains various nutrients and nutraceuticals, as well as their therapeutic value, and it refers to the scientific clinical documentation. Earlier in this section we presented the science and data behind glandular therapies. Later we present an in-depth discussion of the metabolic, physiological, and biochemical evaluation of routine blood chemistries and complete blood counts. Using routine blood results as a guide for selecting therapeutic nutrients, as well as for supporting weakened, inflamed, or disease organs, places the integrative veterinarian in a knowledgeable position. This knowledge helps veterinarians select the appropriate nutritional remedies that more closely address the specific disease, organ weakness, signs, and

symptoms that the animal is experiencing. The use of diagnostic blood results as a marker for recommending nutritional therapies gives veterinarians the comfort of using accepted clinical data (blood results) as it relates to the AVMA guidelines that "veterinarians extrapolate information when formulating a course of therapy."

THERAPEUTIC NUTRIENTS AND NUTRACEUTICALS

The following is a sampling, rather than an exhaustive list, of some of the more commonly used nutrients and nutraceuticals that are available to practitioners of IVM. In chapters 6 through 18, in the disease protocols sections, additional disease-specific nutrients and nutraceuticals, as well as their use, benefits, and clinical efficacy, may be listed.

Amino acids

Amino acids are defined as the building blocks of proteins. Many amino acids are classified as essential and need to be in the daily diet. Nonessential amino acids can be manufactured by the body or can be produced biochemically from other amino acids. The Association of American Feed Control Officials (AAFCO), in their Nutrient Profiles for Dogs and for Cats, list 10 and 11 essential amino acids for dogs and cats, respectively. They are arginine, histidine, isoleucine, leucine, lysine, methionine, phenylalanine, threonine, tryptophan, and valine; plus taurine for cats. Dogs can manufacture taurine, and cats cannot. A deficiency in any of these amino acids can lead to a disease process (AAFCO official publication).

Amino acids are essential for the health of cells and body tissues, including smooth and striated muscles, as well as for many of the metabolic and physiological processes. They are integral in the production of hormones, enzymes, and immunoglobulins used by the cells and organs to run bodily functions (Brady 1994). Proteins and specific amino acids are also required for the proper functioning of the immune system, the prevention of aging, and the maintenance of health and wellness (Davenport 1998, 2001; Hayek 2001; Lewis 1984; Williams 1998).

Pet food manufacturers spend millions on cutting-edge research design to confirm the importance of proteins and essential fatty acids required by growing, adult, and senior dogs and cats. This research supports the amounts and types of proteins and amino acids that are found in the foods that they produce and offer commercially to pet companions.

Note: *It is important to distinguish the difference between protein and amino acids that are added to dogs' and cats' foods and designed to meet minimum protein* *levels from the therapeutic use of amino acid as part of the treatment for chronic degenerative diseases.*

L-carnitine

L-carnitine is produced from the metabolism of the amino acids lysine and methionine. L-carnitine is a lipotrophic agent and requires vitamin C, thiamin, and pyridoxine to carry out this function. Fatty acids attach to carnitine, which transports them into the cell mitochondria to be converted into energy for the body. Carnitine helps to reduce both the circulating and stored levels of fat in the body. Many human nutraceutical companies tout the benefits of L-carnitine as a "fat buster." L-carnitine is required in the metabolism of fatty acids and for the release of energy by the cells. Supplementing the diet with L-carnitine has a direct lowering effect on blood trigylceride levels (Sachan 1984).

In studies conducted by the Iams Company, the addition of carnitine to the diet of dogs was shown to reduce body weight by 6.4%, compared to 1.8% without supplementation (Sunvold 1998). Similar research in cats also suggests weight loss (Center 1998). Evangeliou (2003) showed that adding carnitine to the diet also helps to lower both cholesterol and triglyceride levels.

Carnitine plays a role in aging. Costell (1989) showed that carnitine levels decreased with aging; however, when animals were fed carnitine, it helped reverse the low levels and reversed the age-related changes in mitochondrial function.

L-carnitine has been proven effective in improving the functioning of the heart, especially when diseased. The heart muscle relies on fatty acids for energy, and L-carnitine is required for the transport of these fatty acids. Research has shown that when oxygen levels in the body are reduced, the cardiac reserves of carnitine are depleted. When L-carnitine is supplemented in the diet, it allows heart muscles to use lower levels of oxygen more efficiently. Cherchi (1985) and Orlando (1986) showed a benefit to heart patients with L-carnitine supplementation, and McEntee (1995) reported on low levels of L-carnitine in a dog with cardiomyopathy. The dog showed clinical improvement after L-carnitine therapy at 50 mg/kg/TID.

In other studies on heart disease, the addition of carnitine to the diet was found to reduce heart damage in animals (Lopaschuk 2000). In human patients with heart disease, it was found that introducing carnitine after the diagnosis of heart disease resulted in a significant improvement over standard drug therapy, in that the mortality rate in the L-carnitine-supplemented group was 1.2% as compared to 12.5% in the group that did not receive supplements (Davini 1992).

Clinical studies in humans show the benefit of L-carnitine on lipid metabolism and conversion to energy.

In diabetics, L-carnitine has been proven to significantly reduce levels of both triglycerides and cholesterol by more than 25% (Abdel-Aziz 1994). In addition, carnitine has been shown to reduce pain in diabetic-associated nerve damage (Onofrj 1995). Acetyl-L-carnitine may slow or reverse mild cognitive impairment and the progression of dementia in Alzheimer's disease in younger patients (Brooks 1998, Sano 1992).

Taurine

Taurine is an amino acid that is nonessential for dogs, but essential for cats (AAFCO Cat Nutrient Profiles 1992, Monson 1989, Morris 1989). Cats, unlike many other mammals, cannot synthesize taurine from other amino acids and require adequate dietary sources. Low levels of taurine have been clinically proven to cause cardiomyopathy and retinal degeneration. Fox (1992), Kramer (1995), Novotny (1994), Ryan (1989), Simpson (1993), Pion (1992), and Wysong (1989) found a direct link between low levels of taurine and cardiac disease. It has been shown that dietary supplementation with taurine leads to clinical improvement in cats with retinal disease and cardiomyopathy. It has also been shown that developmental and platelet abnormalities and reproductive issues that are seen in adult cats and their offspring are related to a corresponding decrease in the taurine levels in mothers' milk (Dieter 1993; NRC 1986; Sturman 1986, 1991; Waltham 1993, 1994).

The health status of these cats is closely aligned with the findings of the Pottenger Cat Experiments that were carried out 60 years ago and that are discussed later in this section (Pottenger 1946).

In addition to the dietary need for taurine, it has been found that the composition and the method of food processing affect taurine requirements. For example, the level of dietary fiber directly affects taurine requirements. Hickman (1990, 1991) and Kim (1996a,b) have shown that the heat processing of food leads to lower plasma levels of taurine. See the sections on clinical nutrition and the biological factor later in this chapter for a more in-depth discussion of the effect of processing on the bioavailability of nutrients and the Pottenger Cat Experiment (NRC 1986; Pottenger 1946, 1995).

Arginine

The amino acid arginine is essential for both dogs and cats. Arginine has been proven beneficial in the healing of naturally occurring and surgical wounds and in the effect of growth hormone on the body. It also improves both gastrointestinal health and immune function (Barbul 1983, 1990; Besset 1982; Buchman 1999; Kirk 1993; Marcell 1999). Double-blind studies in people have also confirmed that arginine is beneficial in the treatment of congestive heart failure and in helping to improve kidney function in these patients (Rector 1996, Watanabe 2000).

In studies of dogs with cancer, it was determined that they had lower plasma levels of arginine and other amino acids, which did not change after the tumor was removed surgically, suggesting that protein metabolism changes in these dogs. It is also felt that the same is true for cats. Hills, in their research for the development of their cancer diet, N/D®, showed that the addition of arginine and essential fatty acids to the daily diet of dogs with cancer can improve the prognosis and remission times (Hills—Canine Cancer, Ogilvie 1990, 2000).

Glutamine

Glutamine is a non-essential and the most abundant amino acid found in dogs and cats. Although it is readily available in food and manufactured by the body, in chronic periods of stress and disease, levels of glutamine can be depleted, negatively impacting health (O'Dwyer 1989). It is during these periods of stress that glutamine becomes so important. It has been shown that when both intracellular and plasma levels of glutamine fall significantly, negative health consequences can occur (Askanazi 1980, Souba 1992).

Glutamine is important for immune system health, especially in critically ill patients (Jones 1999, Griffiths 1997, Klimberg 1990). Besides improving immune function, glutamine is beneficial for the intestinal tract and can improve cellular integrity as well as permeability. This is especially important in immune-mediated disease conditions, such as inflammatory bowel disease (Souba 1985, Windmueller 1982, Yoshimura 1993).

In athletes, glutamine has been proven beneficial in preventing respiratory infections, especially after heavy exercise (Nieman 1998, Castell 1996).

Glutamine is often depleted in cancer cachexia. It has been suggested that supplementation with glutamine decreases tumor growth and improves immune function (Klimberg 1996). Besides being the preferred nutrient of the intestinal cells, research has shown that glutamine is also tissue sparing and cellular regenerative. It is an intermediary for the antioxidant glutathione in its role of protecting against the adverse effects of radiation therapy (Klimberg 1996). When chemotherapy is administered, glutamine helps reduce drug-induced inflammation in the bowel (Rombeau 1990, Fox 1988). In patients receiving chemotherapy, adding dietary glutamine has been shown to enhance the effectiveness of certain chemotherapeutics and to increase patient survival times (Klimberg 1991, 1992).

Enzymes

Metabolically, enzymes are essential in the conversion of nutrients to meet the energy needs of the body. They are also involved as catalysts in many other biochemical processes. Enzyme deficiency is caused either by a specific organ malfunctioning or by a deficiency or lack of availability of the proper nutrients required for enzyme production. Nutrients, such as minerals, amino acids, and fatty acids, are required for the synthesis of various enzymes (Howell 1985).

The commonly known digestive enzymes are:

Amylase: carbohydrate digestion
Protease: protein digestion
Lipase: fat digestion
Cellulase: cellulose digestion

Inadequate or deficient levels of enzymes are caused by excessive free radical load leading to chronic inflammation, chronic disease, and organ malfunction, such as exocrine pancreatic insufficiency (EPI) or secondary to the chronic use of medications such as antibiotics.

Besides their function in the digestive process, which in turn improves the general food absorption and metabolism, enzymes provide the indirect benefit of helping to restore overall health. Given with meals, enzymes assist with digestion. Given separate from meals, they can replenish the body's normal reserves as well as help to process undigested and abnormal protein fragments.

Enzymes are natural protein complexes that digest foods and aid in the assimilation of nutrients. In cancer patients, enzymes can help to destroy immune complexes that are produced by and actually surround the cancer cell. These complexes help deter the immune system from attacking the cancer. Cichoke (1995) and Wrba (1990) talk about the use of enzymes to help contain further cell growth and prevent metastasis of the cancer. Some studies have shown that the ingestion of enzymes reduces the adverse effects of radiation therapy. Dale (2001), Gujral (2001), and Gonzales (1999) reported on increased survival times in patients taking enzyme replacement therapies as part of an overall nutritional support program for the treatment of pancreatic adenocarcinoma. Similarly, a retrospective study by Sakalova (2001) indicated improved quality of life.

Although enzyme replacement therapy is controversial, it is believed that adding enzymes to a sound nutritional program is beneficial, and as such several clinical trials are currently being conducted to establish evidence-based proof for enzyme replacement therapies.

Minerals/essential minerals

Many of the raw ingredients found in pet foods are either mineral deficient because of depleted soils or do not contain adequate levels of the minerals. Therefore, pet food manufacturers add minerals to their products to meet AAFCO label claims. For economic reasons, many minerals used in pet foods are inexpensive, inorganic mineral combinations, such as copper sulfate and ferrous oxide. It has been demonstrated that inorganic combinations of minerals are not as well absorbed, assimilated, and used in the body (Ashmead 1982, 1985).

Metabolically and physiologically, minerals have numerous functions in the body. The osmotic balance that exists between synergistic minerals causes the movement of nutrients in and out of cells as well as throughout the fluid systems. Important mineral ratios include sodium/potassium and calcium/phosphorus, as imbalances can alter physiological balances, leading to deficiencies and disease states.

The following is a short list of minerals and how they are required in the day-to-day metabolic processes.

Calcium

Calcium is the most abundant mineral in the body and is the main mineral in the bones and teeth. Calcium is a catalyst for specific enzyme reactions that are required by various other vitamins and minerals to perform their physiological function. Calcium is required for proper contraction of the muscles of the heart and for the maintenance of blood pressure. It also aids in the metabolism of fat by helping lipoproteins' absorption from the intestines (Jorde 2000, Osborne 1996). Calcium is required for the proper clotting of blood and is needed for vitamin K activation, which is required to stop bleeding (Brody 1999).

The levels of calcium in the blood and tissues are tightly maintained in a range that is monitored closely. The body's physiological mechanisms and the parathyroid glands control calcium levels and if necessary will sacrifice bone to maintain adequate levels. Because of this requirement, adequate amounts of dietary calcium are needed for daily health (Weaver 1999). Calcium helps to mediate blood vessel contraction, constriction, and dilation, as well as nerve impulses and muscle contraction (Food and Nutrition Board 1997).

Studies conducted on animals suggest that adequate calcium levels are required for the prevention of colon cancer (Bostick 2001). Some studies show that diets that are higher in calcium are associated with lower colon cancer risks (Baron 1999, Bostick 1995, Lipkin 1995, Hyman 1998, White 1997).

Studies have shown that dietary essential fatty acids increase intestinal calcium absorption, and along with vitamin D, they help to decrease urinary calcium losses (Hertz-Picciotto 2000). It has also been shown that calcium may decrease the absorption of oxalates and may indirectly reduce the formation of kidney stones in people. Perhaps this is an area for veterinary researchers to study, i.e., the increased incidence of calcium oxalate crystals and stones in dogs and cats (Barilla 1978, Curhan 1993).

Chromium

Chromium assists in the release of sugar from the blood to the muscles and other tissues. It is also involved in helping fatty acids be properly absorbed from the intestines into the blood. Chromium is indicated in the treatment of diabetes mellitus. Early reports show that brewer's yeast, which is rich in chromium, can be helpful in the treatment of diabetes and the improvement of glucose tolerance (Anderson 1998, 2000; Offenbacher 1980).

In people, both type 1 and type 2 diabetes showed improvement with the addition of chromium, and this is believed to be due to improving sensitivity to insulin (Gaby 1996, Evans 1989). Chomium has also been shown to be beneficial in helping to reduce cholesterol and triglyceride levels as they relate to heart disease (Lee 1994, Hermann 1998).

Copper

Copper is an integral part of protein metabolism and in the release of toxins from the body. In veterinary medicine, we are aware of the difficulties animals face when there are higher-than-normal levels of copper (especially in Bedlington Terriers). However, copper deficiencies also present specific problems. Deficiencies can lead to reduced immune functions, less resistance to disease, anemia, and overall physical weakness. Copper can be hepatotoxic; however, the levels of copper in the body, as well as in the food, are important and required for daily health.

Iron

Iron is responsible for the uptake and use of oxygen by the cells. It is essential for life, because it is involved in the formation of hemoglobin and red blood cells. Metabolically, it is required for the proper balance of hydrogen and oxygen in the blood.

Magnesium

Magnesium is essential for the production of amino acids, the formation of RNA and DNA, and in conjunction with calcium, for the regular cardiac rhythm. Magnesium is also involved in the digestion and assimilation of proteins by the cells, by working in concert with and polarizing minerals for uptake through the cell membrane.

Magnesium has been extensively researched in terms of the pathogenesis and treatment of, as well as its beneficial effects in, the treatment of cardiovascular disease in people (Altura 1985; Seelig 1980, 1989; Sjogren 1989). Because of its inverse relationship with calcium, magnesium can act as a calcium channel blocker, helping to reduce blood pressure (Kawano 1998).

Physiologically, magnesium activates adenosine triphosphatase (ATP), which is required for the proper functioning of cell membranes and which fuels the sodium potassium pump. Magnesium deficiencies upset mineral balance required for cardiac muscle contraction and rhythm (Rardon 1990, Whang 1990). Bashir (1993) showed that people taking magnesium supplements had a more than 30% reduction in arrhythmias. In a large population study, Tsuji (1994) associated low serum levels of magnesium with increased rate of arrhythmias. Tzivoni (1990), in a peer-reviewed study, showed that magnesium definitively reduced drug-induced arrhythmias.

Magnesium has also been associated with neuromuscular function and conditions such as muscle cramping, weakness, and neuromuscular dysfunction. Magnesium is recommended for epilepsy therapy and for weakening muscle function (Bibley 1996, Levin, 2002).

Diabetic people have been shown to be traditionally low in magnesium, and this can be corrected with supplementation (Eibl 1995, Paolisso 1990). In addition, magnesium supplementation has been shown to improve the production of insulin in people with type 2 diabetes (Paolisso 1989). It has also been shown that the requirements for insulin in people with type 1 diabetes are lower when supplemented with magnesium and that retinopathy is more likely to occur (McNair 1978, Sjorgren 1988). The American Diabetes Association suggests that there are "strong associations ... between magnesium deficiency and insulin resistance." However, they will not confirm that this is a connection between a deficiency and the risk of developing diabetes (American Diabetes Association 1992).

Manganese

Manganese is an important catalyst and co-factor in many enzymatic and metabolic processes. Along with magnesium, it helps to get protein through the cell membrane. It is found in the pancreas, pituitary, liver, and kidney, and it functions in lipid and cholesterol metabolism as well as in the proper functioning of the pancreas in sugar metabolism. Manganese has also been proven beneficial in the treatment of arthritis in animals (Keen 2000).

Potassium

Potassium is an essential mineral that is found in abundance in the extracellular fluid, and it plays a critical role in the osmotic pressure and water balance. It also plays an important role in acid-base balance as well as in the transmission of electrical impulses in the heart and the regulation and the lowering of blood pressure in people (Whelton 1997). It is important in maintaining a regular heart rhythm, and it is involved in carbohydrate metabolism and assimilation by the cells.

Selenium

Selenium is an important antioxidant, functioning in this capacity along with the enzyme glutathione peroxidase and vitamin E. It is involved in the proper functioning of the pancreas and helps with the absorption of glucose by the cells. It is beneficial in animals with cancer.

Selenium is an essential trace mineral (Burk 1999). There are numerous evidence-based studies that show that the addition of selenium to the diet helps to reduce the incidence of cancer in animals (Rayman 2000).

Sodium

Sodium is responsible for the osmotic balance in the cells and extracellular fluid along with potassium. Sodium is a metabolic indicator of adrenal function, and it is involved in the absorption of proteins and sugars across the cell membrane.

Zinc

Zinc is an essential mineral that is involved in many metabolic and physiological processes, including digestion and the absorption of carbohydrates across cell membranes. It is important in the metabolic processes of the immune system and for reproduction (Prasad 1998). Zinc is particularly beneficial for the metabolism and health of the skin. Zinc can compete with copper for absorption into the blood and therefore can indirectly lower copper levels by reducing its absorption (Broek 1986, King 1999).

Although zinc is required in dog and cat foods, its relative absorption and assimilation can vary depending on the animal and the chemical type of the mineral. A common deficiency disease in animals is zinc-responsive dermatosis, most commonly found in Huskies, Malamutes, and large-breed puppies (Griffin 1993, Werner 2003). Deficiencies occur because of the difficulty of absorbing zinc in certain breeds of animals. Factors that interfere with absorption besides breed predilection are fiber, plant phytates, and calcium, which may bind with zinc and prevent its absorption. Therefore, eating plant-based foods may lead to zinc deficiencies. It is important that dog and cat diets be fortified with zinc. Equally as important is the type of zinc added to the food. Studies indicate that inorganic mineral forms may not be as well absorbed as those bound or chelated to protein (Ashmead 1982, 1985). (See the diet section in this chapter for more details.) In addition, dogs and cats that have chronic intestinal diseases such as IBD may be more prone to zinc deficiencies because of impaired absorption (Lewis 1984, Mosier 1978, Mueller 1989).

Type 1 diabetes in people has been linked to zinc deficiencies, which also may adversely affect general immune function (Nakamura 1991, Mocchegiani 1989). It has also been shown that supplementing the diet with zinc can help to lower blood glucose levels (Rao 1987).

Zinc is related to impaired immune function, and deficiencies can increase susceptibility to various infections (Baum 2000, Shankar 1998). In human HIV patients, low levels of zinc have been associated with higher mortality rates (Lai 2001, Wellinghausen 2000, Mocchegiani 2000).

Essential fatty acids (EFAs)

Much research has been conducted on the importance of essential fatty acids in the daily diet, and on the clinical management of various degenerative diseases (Reinhart 1996, Holub 1995, Herman 1998). The importance of the ratio between omega-3 and omega-6 fatty acids has been substantiated. Research on the use of polyunsaturated fatty acids has shown their beneficial and antipruritic effects on skin (Reinhart 1996, Schick 1996).

Some pet food manufacturers are addressing this important ratio by adding sources of omega-3 and omega-6 fatty acids. Many commercial dog and cat foods contain poultry fat as the primary source of fatty acids. Levels of fat in pet food range from 8% to 20%. Poultry fat contains approximately 20% linoleic acid (omega-6) or 2% to 3% of the total food. There is about 30 times more omega-6 than omega-3 in chicken fat (Erasmus 1993). Therefore, the estimated total amount of omega-3 fatty acids in pet foods that contain poultry fat as the primary fat source is less than 1% (Goldstein 2005).

Kendler (1987) reported that although both linoleic acid (LA) and gamma-linolenic acid (GLA) can be obtained from food, poor-quality ingredients can be low in essential fatty acids and lead to deficiencies. Because many commercially available pet foods obtain their poultry fat from by-products, the chances of EFA deficiencies are even greater (Hilton 1989).

A second important point is that although manufacturers are now adding omega-3 fatty acids to their foods, many of these compounds are easily destroyed by exposure to heat and light (Erasmus 1986). Therefore, it is essential to supplement the diet with a fresh source of omega-3 fatty acids. Good sources include flax, borage, hemp, and fish oil.

Food manufacturers and researchers are focusing on the role of fatty acids in the metabolism of the skin as well as their role in the inflammatory process. The 1998 *Recent Advances in Canine and Feline Nutrition, Vol. II*, sponsored by The Iams Company, focused attention on the role of fatty acids in the inflammatory process, wellness, and disease. Studies demonstrated that fatty acids, such as linoleic (LA) and gamma-linolenic (GLA), promote the formation of eicosinoids, which exert an anti-inflammatory response in the body. Metabolically, these essential fatty acids help to reduce the inflammatory process that predisposes the initiation of many disease processes.

The clinical use of EFAs in medical practice extends beyond the treatment of skin disorders. Other areas of potential use for EFAs include cardiovascular disease (Capron 1993), arthritis (Carmichael 1982), cancer therapy, and renal disease (Holub 1995, Logas et al. 1991, Logas and Kunkle 1994, Herman 1998).

Fish oil

Fish oil contains high levels of eicosapentaenoic acid (EPA), an omega-3 fatty acid that helps to maintain the proper levels of eicosinoids, which in turn help to mediate the body's response to cancer cells. Research has shown that EPA can slow tumor growth and improve the response of the cell to chemotherapeutics (Sagaguchi 1990, Reich 1989). In people with heart disease, there have been reported benefits of fish oil in slowing the progression of arteriosclerosis and in improving disease symptoms (Leaf 1988, von Schacky 1999). Kremer (1995) has shown that fish oil helps reduce inflammation in people with arthritis.

It has been clinically proven that people suffering from colitis and Crohn's disease who supplemented their diet with EPA and DHA, the two omega-3 fatty acids that are found in fish oil, had significantly fewer recurrences over a 1- to 2-year period than those who did not supplement their diets (Belluzzi 1996, Mate 1991).

Flax seed oil

Flax seed oil contains more than 55% linoleic acid (omega-3). Flax seed is considered the "Rolls-Royce" of fatty acids because it contains more omega-3 than any other oil. It has antioxidant, anti-inflammatory, and anticancer effects on the body. Erasmus (1986), Murray (1996), and Budwig (1992) refer to flax seed oil's anticancer effects and its beneficial effects on arthritis.

Evening primrose oil *(Oenothera biennis L.)*

Evening primrose oil (EPO) is a seed oil that contains about 70% gamma-linolenic acid (omega-6), which is essential in the formation of eicosanoids, specifically prostaglandin E1 (PGE1), which has an anti-inflammatory effect. In a double-blind study of people with rheumatoid arthritis, Joe (1993) showed that a number of people had significant benefits from the addition of EPO. Eicosanoids, besides having anti-inflammatory effects, also have anticancer properties. Begin (1986) reported on the ability of omega-6 fatty acids to kill cancer cells. Other studies show that in some cases, patients reported anticancer effects of GLA (Pritchard 1990, Lee 1986, McIllmurray 1987, Naidu 1992, Van der Merwe 1987).

EPO has been proven to have both anti-inflammatory and anti-pruritic effects on skin diseases, and as part of a balanced nutritional program, it can exert a positive effect on animals with dermatological conditions. Studies suggest that EPO is beneficial in people with atopic dermatitis and eczema (Hederos 1996, Humphreys 1994, Morse 1989).

Cotterell (1990), in a double-blind study, showed that more than 50% of the women taking evening primrose oil with menstrually related irritable bowel syndrome improved, while none in the non-EPO group showed any benefit. In another study, Manning (1977) and Hotz (1994) showed improvement with IBS by adding psyllium to the diet.

Borage oil

Derived from the seed of the borage plant (*Borago officinalis*), borage oil, like EPO, is high in gamma-linolenic acid and has similar properties and benefits. Like EPO, borage oil, which contains high levels of GLA, should convert into eicosanoids; however, many factors, such as the quality of food, disease, and vitamin and mineral deficiencies, can influence this conversion to the anti-inflammatory eicosanoids. Therefore, supplementation is recommended to ensure that the adequate amount of GLA is present (Horrobin 1981). Borage oil has also been proven beneficial for skin conditions (Landi 1993, Tolleson 1993) and arthritis (Pullman-Mooar 1990, Leventhal 1993, Zurier 1996).

Seabuckthorne oil

Seabuckthorne oil was therapeutically used and recorded in China more than 1,000 years ago in the Tang Dynasty. In the *Sibu Yidian*, a Tibetan medical book, more than 30 chapters were dedicated to the use of this oil. The *Sibu Yidian* was published in Russia in 1903 (Ma Yingcai 1989). In the 1950s the Sichuan Medical College initiated research into seabuckthorne and its medicinal properties (Xu Zhonglu 1956). It has been discovered that seabuckthorne is rich in essential amino acids, beta carotene, lycopenes, flavonoids, sitosterol, folic acid, and essential fatty acids (Zhang Zhemin 1990). Seabuckthorne oil can be used to treat burns, skin radiation lesions, gastric and duodenal ulcers, and so on (Wu Fuheng 1991).

In animal studies, seabuckthorne oil has been shown to improve cardiac function, contractility, and oxygen utilization (Wu 1994, 1997). In cancer, it has been shown to improve immune function and can inhibit tumor cells. Zhang Peizhen (1989) and Tang Jing (1989) showed that seabuckthorne slowed hepatocyte proliferation in precancerous lesions. Zhong Fei (1989) showed that seabuckthorne could strengthen cellular immunity by improving phogocyte function. Ren Lisa (1992) showed that seabuckthorne oil improves immune and bone marrow function as well as that of natural killer cells. Seabuckthorne oil is clinically approved in Russia for use in circulatory disorders, to reduce inflammation, to protect against radiation damage, and to relax smooth muscles (Yance 2005).

Hemp oil

Hemp oil is a plant-derived oil that is extremely high in both linoleic (LA) and linolenic (LNA) fatty acids. These essential fatty acids are the building blocks for the longer chained eicosapentaenoic (EPA) and docosahexaenoic acid (DHA) that are prevalent in fish oil and have been clinically shown to be beneficial in the treatment of cancer in animals (Ogilvie 2000).

Because the cancer treatment protocols represented in chapter 31 of this book restrict the use of fish and fish oil, hemp oil can be used to supply the required essential fatty acids for these animals. (See the section on diet in chapter 31 for more details about the feeding of fish oil-restricted diets for cancer patients.)

The analysis of hemp oil shows that more than 70% is composed of polyunsaturated fatty acids, while it contains less than 20% saturated fats (Kralovansky 1994, Weil 1993). Because of its high level of gamma-linolenic acid (GLA), it is being investigated for its beneficial effects on immune function and cardiovascular disease (Horrobin 1992).

Nutraceuticals

N,N-Dimethylglycine (DMG)

N,N-dimethylglycine (DMG) is naturally produced by the body and has been clinically proven to support a broad range of immune functions (Graber 1981, Reap 1990). DMG improves circulation and helps the body in the removal of toxins (Kendall 2003). This ability to assist in detoxification is especially important when dealing with chronic and autoimmune conditions of the skin (Verdova 1965).

DMG has been widely researched in both humans and animals. It has been found to increase energy, improve cardiovascular function, and enhance immune function (Barnes 1979, Graber 1981, Walker 1988). Mackenzie (1958) has reported on the biochemistry of DMG. Meduski has called DMG a "metabolic enhancer" because it serves multiple functions, such as improving cellular oxygen use (an important component in cancer therapy) and supporting transmethylation pathways via SAMe, by being an indirect methyl donor.

In cancer treatment, DMG increases tumor necrosis factor (TNF) and interferon production (Graber 1986, Kendall 2003, Reap 1990, Wang 1988). Studies demonstrate that DMG is beneficial in its ability to modulate the immune system and in the prevention and treatment of many types of cancer (Mani 1999). DMG also helps prevent metastasis to other organs (Reap 1988, Kendall 1991). There is indication that DMG is beneficial in repairing DNA and that it helps in the regulation of gene expression and controlled cell division.

Kendall (2003) reports on research that suggests DMG is cellular protective in animals that are receiving radiation therapy. DMG is also indicated as part of an overall therapy program for the prevention and potential treatment of cancer in animals (Balch 1997, Mani 1999). Recent work has shown that DMG is a potent antioxidant and anti-inflammatory agent (Yanez 2007).

DMG has been studied extensively in horses over the past 20 years and has shown a positive effect on stamina and endurance in competing horses (Charles 1982, Jones 1988). Livine (1982) reported on DMG's ability to reduce lactic acid build-up and improve performance. In dogs, Gannon and Kendall (1982) reported improved racing times and stamina, as well as recovery when diets were supplemented with DMG. Seizure activity in dogs can also be reduced by the use of DMG (Kendall 2003).

Lecithin/phosphatidyl choline

Phosphatidyl choline is a phospholipid that is integral to cellular membranes and particularly on nerve and brain cells. It helps to move fats into the cells, and it is involved in neurotransmission and acetylcholine, particularly with cellular integrity. As part of the cell membranes, lecithin is an essential nutrient required by the skin and all the cells of the body for general health and wellness (Hanin 1987).

Studies with lecithin have shown that it can reduce triglyceride and cholesterol levels, because it is an emulsifier of fats (Brook 1986, Spilburg 2003).

Phosphatidyl serine (PS)

Phosphatidyl serine is a phospholipid and an essential ingredient in cellular membranes, particularly of brain cells. It has been studied extensively in people with altered mental functioning and degeneration, with positive results (Crook 1991, Cenacchi 1993). In people with Alzheimer's disease, the addition of PS to the dietary program showed a mild to significant clinical improvement (Delewaide 1986, Engel 1992, Funfgeld 1989).

In studies with PS and cortisol levels, adding PS to the diet significantly reduces both the ACTH and cortisol levels. Reducing cortisol levels is beneficial in cushinoid dogs and in those with overt Cushing's disease (Fahey 1998; Monteleone 1990, 1992).

Medicinal mushrooms (maitake and reishi)

Maitake mushrooms have been used in Eastern herbal medicine for centuries. Studies show that properly extracted mushrooms are rich in beta glucans and help to support and enhance immune function. In stressful conditions, they metabolically support organ systems in maintaining balance and homeostasis. The active ingredient,

beta glucans, is a polysaccharide, which is responsible for the therapeutic action (Nanba 1987).

Numerous studies in Japan and now in the United States confirm their health benefits and immune-enhancing abilities. Recent studies indicate that maitake extracts may also be helpful as adjuncts to chemotherapy, by not only enhancing the drugs' effectiveness but also in the ameliorization of the drugs' potential side effects (Adachi 1987, Nariba 1993, Wagner 1985). Studies have shown the direct anti-tumor effect of an extract of maitake mushrooms called the D-fraction, which has been shown to increase natural killer cell (NK) activity, improves immune function and induces apoptosis. D-fraction extract has been approved for use in dogs and cats (Kodama 2003, Konno 2004, Shimada 2004).

Alpha-lipoic acid (ALA)

Alpha-lipoic acid is classified as an enzyme and is involved in mitochondrial activity. ALA is referred to as the "universal antioxidant" because it is soluble in both water and fat environments. As a potent antioxidant it has been shown to reduce oxidative stress, inflammation, and the mitochondrial decline often associated with the aging process. ALA has also been shown to increase the effectiveness of other antioxidants, such as vitamins C and E, coenzyme Q10, and glutathione, making them more readily available for bodily function (Busse 1992, Lykkesfeldt 1998, Kagan 1990, Scholich 1989).

Clinically, because it is involved metabolically in sugar and fat metabolism, it has been shown to be beneficial in the management and treatment of diabetes mellitus and diabetic neuropathy often found in people (Konrad 1999, Nickander 1996, Packer, 1997). Estrada (1996) has shown ALA to improve glucose uptake in animals. The American Diabetes Association recommends ALA along with vitamin E for helping to prevent diabetic complications such as neuropathy, atherosclerosis, and cataract formation (Ou 1996, Yi 2006).

In the treatment and prevention of glaucoma, Filina (1995) has shown that higher levels of ALA improved clinical parameters associated with open angle glaucoma. Bartter (1980) showed that 67 of 75 patients with mushroom poisoning who took ALA recovered, as compared to the normal, untreated 10% to 50%. Sabeel (1995) showed similar effectiveness with ALA in the treatment of poisonous mushroom toxicity.

In other animal studies, ALA, along with other antioxidants and L-carnitine, was found to improve cognition and memory and to help in preventing cognitive decline (Farr 2003, Hagen 2002, Milgram 2005).

In the treatment of autoimmune encephalomyeletis (a model used in multiple sclerosis research), Marracci (2002) and Morini (2004) found that ALA slowed progression of the autoimmune response and the disease process. It should be noted that free radical inflammation is implicated in initiating many of the disease processes discussed in the book; therefore, ALA and other antioxidants can function to reduce this inflammation, thereby helping to prevent many of these diseases.

One caution with alpha-lipoic acid is the concern of toxicity in cats. Hill (2004) reported that lipoic acid may be 10 times more toxic in cats than reported in dogs and people, so precaution should be used for cats.

Coenzyme Q10 (CoQ10)

Coenzyme Q10 (ubiquinone) is found in the mitochondria and is involved in the cells' energy production, which is required for the daily functioning of the body. CoQ10 is essential for the manufacture of ATP, the energy source for the body's cells and tissues. CoQ10 is a potent antioxidant and helps in the process of neutralizing free radicals and improving cell protection (Thomas 1997, Weber 1994).

Although coenzyme Q10 is produced by the body and is present in many foods, deficiencies can occur. Deficiencies generally affect the heart first, as the heart muscle requires the nutrient and continually uses energy in its functioning. CoQ10 is involved in maintaining the level of oxygen present in the blood and available to the cells.

Being a strong antioxidant and helping to reduce inflammation, CoQ10 has indications in the prevention and treatment of many common diseases, such as gingivitis and periodontal disease, heart disease, arthritis, diabetes, and many types of cancer (Gaby 1998, Shigeta 1966). Regarding periodontal disease, double-blind clinical trials have shown that people supplemented with coenzyme Q10 had improved results over those taking a placebo. Gaby (1998) suggests that periodontal disease is directly linked to a coenzyme Q10 deficiency (Nakamura 1973). In addition, double-blind studies show that taking 50 mg daily for 3 weeks led to a significant reduction in the symptoms of periodontal disease (Wilkinson 1976).

Much of the clinical research on CoQ10 has been in human heart disease. Research has shown that CoQ10 is beneficial in controlling cardiac arrhythmias, congestive heart disease, and cardiomyopathy (Gaby 1996; Giugliano 2000; Greenberg 1990; Folkers 1985, 1986; Harker-Murray 2000; Hofman-Bang 1995; Khatta 2000; Kim 1997; Mortensen 1985; Soja 1997; Morisco 1993; Permanetter 1992). Results of these clinical studies showed an improvement in the related symptoms of heart diseases, such as a reduction in dyspnea and edema, improved blood pressure, and normalized heart rates. Harker-Murray (2000) showed that in dogs, although a deficiency in CoQ10 does not appear to be present with heart disease, supplementation does appear to lessen the resultant hypertrophic response.

In diabetes, Shigeta (1966) and Miyake (1999) have shown that a form of CoQ10 helped to lower blood sugar levels and also showed that diabetic patients had significantly lower levels of CoQ10 in their systems.

In immune system function and cancer, CoQ10 has been proven beneficial as a potent antioxidant and has been proven to be helpful to the available metabolic energy required by the body to heal and prevent disease (Folkers 1982, Lockwood 1995).

Probiotics

The normal flora of the intestines is required for proper assimilation of food and nourishment of the cells. In addition to enhancing digestion, probiotics help to reduce the presence of pathogenic bacteria and increase the general immune response, thereby decreasing the likelihood of infection (De Simone 1993, Kawase 1982, Mel'nikova 1993, Rasic 1983, Smirnov 1993).

The flora balance can be upset or diminished by the following conditions:

- Trauma or injury
- Chronic disease (weak immune system)
- Environmental and/or food toxins
- Pet food ingredients—coloring agents, dyes, digests, chemical additives or preservatives
- Stresses—emotional and physical
- Antibiotics and other medication, such as chemotherapeutics

Adding the proper combination of dietary probiotics can re-establish the population of these beneficial organisms. Common types are *Lactobacillus acidophilus*, *Lactobacillus bifidus*, and *Lactobacillus casei*. Perdigon (1987), Goldin (1984), and Gorbach (1982) have reported on the positive impact probiotics have on the immune system, the intestines, and in the treatment of cancer.

Diarrhea from many different causes diminishes the level of these organisms and thereby leaves the intestines more susceptible to secondary infection from harmful bacteria (Saavedra 1995, 2000). The addition of probiotics to the diet can often prevent diarrhea (Scarpignato 1995). In addition, it has been shown that adding probiotics to the daily diet can help to reduce fungal infections (Hilton 1992, Reid 1994).

In the treatment of inflammatory bowel disease, Washabau (2005) recommends the addition of probiotics, because they can enhance the immune system:

> "The Gram-positive commensal lactic acid bacteria (e.g., Lactobacilli) have many beneficial health effects, including enhanced lymphocyte proliferation, innate and acquired immunity, and anti-inflammatory cytokine production. *Lactobacillus rhamnosus* GG, a bacterium used in the production of yogurt, is effective in preventing and

treating diarrhea, recurrent *Clostridia difficile* infection, primary rotavirus infection, and atopic dermatitis in humans.

Lactobacillus rhamnosus GG has been safely colonized in the canine gastrointestinal tract, although probiotic effects in the canine intestine have not been firmly established. The probiotic organism, *Enterococcus faecium* (SF68), has been safely colonized in the canine gastrointestinal tract, and it has been shown to increase fecal IgA content and circulating mature B (CD21+/MHC class II+) cells in young puppies. It has been suggested that this probiotic may be useful in the prevention or treatment of canine gastrointestinal disease."

Washabau cautions, however, "Two recent studies have shown that many commercial veterinary probiotic preparations are not accurately represented by label claims. Quality control appears to be deficient for many of these formulations. Until these products are more tightly regulated, veterinarians should probably view product claims with some skepticism."

Many veterinarians recommend the addition of probiotics to the diet when animals have a chronic yeast infection of the ears or the skin. One reason for such therapy is that many of these animals are on antibiotics that diminish the levels of normal intestinal bacteria, and secondarily probiotics may have a preventive or therapeutic effect on the overgrowth of various fungi, which can result in such situations.

One important point is that many probiotics are heat sensitive and may be destroyed in processing. One study found that the majority of acidophilus capsules on the market contained no live cultures (Hughes 1990). It is therefore important to understand that the addition of probiotics to pet foods before the high temperatures of the cooking process will more than likely inactivate the effectiveness of friendly bacteria; therefore, additional supplementation with live culture probiotics is essential to create the desired therapeutic effect.

Super oxide dismutase

Super oxide dismutase (SOD) is a potent destroyer of free radicals and can protect cells against oxidative damage (Petkau 1975, Fridovich 1972). McCord (1974) has reported that SOD can protect hyaluronate from free radical damage and that it may also have an anti-inflammatory effect (Salin and McCord 1975).

Quercetin

Quercetin is in the flavonoid family and has potent antioxidant properties (see the phytonutrients section earlier in this chapter.) Quercetin also acts like an antihistamine and has been shown to inhibit cells from releasing histamines (Middleton 1986, Ogasawara 1985). This action is beneficial in the treatment of allergic conditions such as asthma, dermatitis, and eczema.

Quercetin is also a phytoestrogen, which is a plant-derived compound that has estrogenic effects on the body. In this estrogenic category, Miodini (1999) and Shoskes (1999) have demonstrated quercetin's positive effects in inhibiting breast cancer and reducing inflammation in men with prostatitis. Knekt (1997) reported that quercetin has proved beneficial in the inhibition of lung and other cancers.

Vitamins

Vitamins traditionally have been used as supplements when there appears to be a deficiency, or at low levels to help prevent deficiencies. Vitamins, like other nutrients, are required daily for the body's metabolic and physiologic processes. Day-to-day stresses, modern cooking, processing techniques, exposure to chemicals and infectious agents, and treatment with potent and sometimes toxic medications and chemicals all deplete the body's vitamin and antioxidant reserves almost as quickly as they are taken in or manufactured. Therefore, adding vitamins in the proper amount, form, and type is critical for the treatment, maintenance, and restoration of health.

Vitamin A and beta carotene

Vitamin A is a retinoid, a potent antioxidant, and is required for the proper division and growth of cells. It has also been shown to increase immune function and help minimize chemotherapy side effects (Ehrenpreis 2005, McCullough 1999, Michels 2001, Russell 2000, Semba 1998, Thurnham 1999).

Beta carotene is a pigmented phytonutrient and a member of the carotenoid family. Carotenoids have been associated with the reduction of the adverse side effects of chemotherapy and the cancer itself. Although there is some indication that high levels of antioxidants can decrease the effectiveness of chemotherapy, the protocols presented in this book consider dosage of antioxidants (Anon 1994, Baron 2003, Greenberg 1994, Heinonen 1998, Keefe 2001, Lee 2002, Michaud 2002, Toma 2003, Zang 1999).

Vitamin A was first identified in 1913. Research on animals proved that a diet deficient in vitamin A adversely affected growth and weakened the immune system (Olsen 1989). Vitamin A (retinol) and beta carotene (provitamin A) are fat-soluble antioxidants and have proven essential for the proper functioning of the immune system and the health of the skin, eyes, gums, and teeth.

As a free radical scavenger, vitamin A is cell and tissue protective (see the sections on antioxidants and free radicals earlier in this chapter.) It can be therapeutically beneficial in treating chronic degenerative diseases such as cancer, arthritis, autoimmune disorders, and skin disease.

It also can be beneficial for exposure to environmental pollutants (Halliwell 1994).

Recent scientific advances have identified vitamin A as representing a group of compounds known as retinoids that have functional health benefits for the body. The body uses vitamin A in normal cellular division and differentiation processes. Retinoids are particularly important in the differentiation of lymphocytes and the activation of T lymphocytes, the body's prime immune cell regulators (Semba 1998). They are also important for the proper function of the eye and for vision.

Vitamin A plays an integral role in helping the cells of the skin and mucous membranes, which act as the main barrier to protect the body from the environment. It has been shown that retinoids are required to help these cells maintain their integrity.

Vitamin A has proven anticancer properties. In numerous studies, vitamin A and its derivatives have been shown to prevent primary tumor recurrences and spreading. They have been shown to be particularly effective in squamous cell carcinoma and malignant melanoma (Halliwell 1994, Hong 1990, Meyskens 1984, Misckeche 1977, Olsen 1989). In lung and breast cancer in people, Comstock (2001) and Ching (2002) reported a link between the risk of developing the disease and the retinoid levels in the body. The treatment of leukemia with retinoids has led to patient improvement (Thurnham 1999, Ross 1999).

Vitamin A can exert toxicity at high levels, so care must be used to prevent overdosing. Dogs and horses can derive vitamin A activity from beta carotene. Cats, however, cannot convert beta carotene into vitamin A, so adequate amounts must be available in their diet (National Research Council 1989).

Vitamin C

Vitamin C is a water-soluble compound that is the most studied, researched, and controversial of the vitamins (Pauling 1976). Numerous papers, clinical trials, and books have been written about vitamin C's effects as an antioxidant and general stimulant of the immune system, as well as its properties, such as its actions in (1) stimulating the production of interferon, (2) activating natural killer (NK) cells, (3) being cytotoxic to cancer cells, (4) strengthening connective tissue, (5) increasing levels of other antioxidant enzymes, and (6) improving appetite and day-to-day quality of life in terminal cancer patients and others. De la Fuente (1998) and Penn (1991) showed that vitamin C in combination with other vitamins significantly improved immune function, as compared to those people taking placebo.

Vitamin C is required for the synthesis of collagen and is known best for the deficiency disease scurvy. It is a potent antioxidant that is involved in neutralizing free radicals and reactive oxygen species (ROS). Free radicals result from normal metabolism, as well as exposure to chemical and environmental pollutants, and they are believed to be initiators of inflammation and premature aging.

Carr (1999) reports that vitamin C deficiencies can lead to lower levels of L-carnitine, the amino acid that is required for fat metabolism and the proper functioning of the heart. Enstrom (1992) showed that there was a significant reduction in death from heart disease in people who regularly added vitamin C to their daily diet. In addition, Osganian (2003) and Knekt (2004) showed a statistically significant reduction in the risk of heart disease in thousands of patients.

Vitamin C is involved in many of the metabolic and physiological processes of the body. It is accepted that most animals manufacture their own vitamin C, but humans, primates, guinea pigs, and some birds must get vitamin C in their diets. It is now believed that excessive free radicals deplete vitamin C reserves, even in animals that have manufacturing capabilities.

High free radical production can result from:

- Ingestion of chemical additives and preservatives
- Chronic exposure to pesticides, insecticides, herbicides, and environmental pollutants
- Overvaccination
- Chronic use of medications such as antibiotics, corticosteroids, insecticides, and chemotherapeutics

In these situations, antioxidant reserves are depleted and dietary replenishment is either deficient or cannot keep up with the free radical load. This results in secondary inflammation, which can lead to premature aging.

It has been suggested that inferior ingredients used in many pet foods in combinations with chemical additives and preservatives, as well as the high heat of processing, can further reduce and inactivate dietary sources of vitamin C and the necessary nutrients required by the body for its manufacture (Goldstein 2000, 2005; Verde 1986).

Vitamin C has been studied clinically in animals. Brown (1994), Berg (1990), and Newman (1995) reported on the benefits of vitamin C in the treatment of degenerative joint disease and movement in dogs and in horses. Belfield (1981) reported on the beneficial effects of using vitamin C in treatment and prevention of hip dysplasia in dogs.

Vaananen (1993) showed that people who are vitamin C deficient are more prone to periodontal disease. Aurer-Kozelj (1982) showed that increasing the daily dose of vitamin C from 20 to 35 mg to 70 mg showed a significant improvement in periodontal disease.

Vitamin C and cancer

Linus Pauling and his associates, along with numerous other researchers and clinicians, have examined the health and therapy benefits of vitamin C. Vitamin C is the most studied of all vitamins in relationship to its effects on cancer (Bendich 1995, Golde 2003, Hunter 1993, Jacobs 2002, Lee 2002, Michels 2001, Moertel 1985).

Besides its antioxidant and immune-stimulating effects, vitamin C has been clinically proven to be effective in cancer therapy. It stimulates the production of interferon and activates natural killer cells, which can destroy cancer cells.

D. Kromhout (1987) reported a 64% reduction in the risk of lung cancer over a 25-year period in men who took daily doses of vitamin C. In a study in Sweden, women consuming 110 mg/day of vitamin C reported a 39% lower risk of breast cancer (Michels 2001). And Feiz (2002) showed that vitamin C decreases the presence of cancer-causing compounds in the stomach and reduces the risk of stomach cancer.

Linus Pauling was the most well known of the cancer/vitamin C researchers reporting increased survival times in people with cancer. These early studies confirmed that vitamin C, in high doses and given intravenously, helped to extend remission time and improved the day-to-day quality of life (Cameron and Pauling 1976, 1977). Others confirmed these results (Riordan 1995). The Mayo Clinic research, however, has failed to confirm similar results as Pauling and Cameron (Creagan 1979, Moertal 1985).

Recent claims from the American Cancer Society stated that vitamin C may even enhance cancer cell growth by protecting cancer cells from the free radical killing effects of chemotherapy and radiation therapies (Golde 2003). However, findings by Padayatty (2004) at the National Institutes of Health suggest that the IV route achieved much higher blood levels of vitamin C than the oral route that was used in the Mayo Clinic studies and therefore is suggesting that more research be done.

Recent research is now showing that vitamin C inhibits the growth of at least 7 types of cancer and appears to be cytotoxic (Leung 1993). Also, in a more recent study, Gonzales (2005) indicates that this anticancer effect is due to the antioxidant effects of vitamin C.

Intravenous vitamin C is being studied for its cytotoxic effects (Riordan 1995). In one study Riordan et al. (1995) used high-dose IV vitamin C in a person with pancreatic cancer. CT scans 6 months post surgery did not show any tumor progression. However, the cancer did recur when the IV dose of vitamin C was reduced. These studies are encouraging and suggest that more quality research is necessary.

Although there is controversy and questioning of the definitive proof substantiating Pauling's findings, research is continuing. Studies are being conducted to determine if the combination of antioxidant therapies and conventional cancer therapy is beneficial for the quality of life and longevity of treated human breast cancer patients and

dogs with lymphosarcoma and osteosarcoma (Kaegi 1998, Goldstein 2006).

It should be noted that oral use of vitamin C can cause diarrhea. In humans and animals the recommended upper-limit therapeutic dose of vitamin C is at "bowel tolerance." This means the oral dose is increased every other day until the patient's stool loosens. Then the dose is reduced to the next lowest level and maintained. Another approach is to use vitamin C intravenously (in the preservative-free, buffered sodium ascorbate form), especially therapeutically in cancer patients. Veterinarians interested in the therapeutic application of vitamin C should read Belfield (1998).

Vitamin E

Vitamin E is a fat-soluble vitamin and one of the body's main antioxidants, especially in its function of protecting lipids. As a potent antioxidant its primary function is the neutralization of free radicals and reduction of inflammation, particularly as it affects the oxidation and destruction of lipids (Traber 1999). As such, vitamin E is tissue protective for the cellular membranes. Vitamin E has also been found to block the activity of kinase C, which supports the body's cell signaling mechanisms.

Besides its antioxidant functions, vitamin E is involved in the proper functioning of the heart muscle, particularly in improving cardiac output, circulation, and helping to reduce platelet aggregation (Traber 2001). Vitamin E reduces inflammation and improves circulation by helping vessels to dilate and by reducing the agglutination of blood platelets. In cancer, vitamin E has been shown to induce apoptosis (Yu 2003, You 2002). It is also suggested that vitamin E inhibits tumor growth by enhancing tumor necrosis factor (Weber 2002, Malafa 2000, 2002).

Vitamin E is involved in scar tissue formation, and is tissue sparing to many of the glands of the immune system. It works synergistically with selenium, has been shown to have anticancer properties, and has been proven to enhance the effectiveness of specific chemotherapeutics. Also in cancer treatment, vitamin E has been shown to have organ sparing properties when chemotherapy or radiation therapy is being administered (Shklar 1982, 1987; Myers 1976, 1982).

It has been shown that people with lower blood levels of vitamin E are more prone to developing both type 1 and type 2 diabetes (Knekt 1999, Salonen 1995). In addition, it has been shown that vitamin E supplementation has improved glucose tolerance (Paolisso 1993). Vitamin E has also been shown to be beneficial in diabetic side effects, such as retinopathy and nephropathy (Bursell 1999, Ross 1982).

Vitamin B$_{12}$ (cyanocobalamin)

Vitamin B$_{12}$ is essential for the maintenance of the proper levels of red blood cells and nerves, as well as for the manufacture of DNA. In nerve cells, vitamin B_{12} is required for normal function and health.

In studies with people who supplemented their diets with vitamin B_{12}, it was shown that neuropathy and pain associated with diabetes or kidney disease were significantly reduced (Yamane 1995, Kuwabara 1999). Deficiencies of vitamin B_{12} are associated with anemia and decreased function of the immune system. Berlin (1978), Kondo (1998), Lederle (1991), and Tamura (1999) have shown that B_{12} supplementation treats the condition.

Folic acid

Folic acid is a B vitamin that is required for organized cellular division. Folic acid is integral in the synthesis of both DNA and RNA and therefore has an effect on the genetic modeling of the body.

Folic acid, both as a topical rinse and taken systemically, has been clinically proven to be beneficial in reducing inflammation and helping to stop bleeding in people with gingivitis and periodontal disease (Pack 1984; Vogel 1976, 1978).

Folic acid deficiencies affect bone marrow cell division and can lead to a macrocytic anemia (Food Nutrition Board 1998). Low dietary folic acid has been associated with colon cancer prevention in people (Giovannucci 1993). Other studies indicate that low dietary folic acid is associated with the increased risk of cancer in people that have ulcerative colitis (Lashner 1989, 1993, 1997). Freudenheim (1991), in a large population study, showed that decreased dietary folic acid is directly related to increased risk of developing colon cancer.

SUMMARY OF THERAPEUTIC NUTRIENTS AND NUTRACEUTICALS

It is appropriate to finish this discussion on therapeutic nutrients and nutraceuticals with the following quote taken from Roger Kendall's *Complementary and Alternative Veterinary Medicine* (Mosby 1998):

> "Although there are no officially established guidelines for implementing therapeutic nutrition in veterinary practice, many veterinarians are including the aforementioned approaches in their practices. Therapeutic nutrition is based on the idea that if the body is provided with a better nutritional environment, healing will occur at a higher level of efficacy. The rational use of nutritional products and specific nutrients is based on a combination of clinical and nutritional research, clinical experience and the availability of high quality, safe and dependable nutritional products."

It is the author's hope that the material presented in this chapter and in this book on integrative veterinary medicine will give veterinarians the comfort of adding nutritional therapies to their existing medical and surgical protocols.

NUTRITIONAL BLOOD TESTING

Nutritional blood testing (NBT) evaluates blood chemistries physiologically rather than pathologically; i.e., it screens for biochemical changes that often precede overt manifestations of disease. This metabolic interpretation focuses upon organ function rather than the determination of a specific disease process or diagnosis.

Routine blood testing is an important evidence-based diagnostic tool. The chemical analysis of blood identifies levels of enzymes, electrolytes, proteins, and metabolites. These chemicals are indicators of the health or pathology of the organ systems and the mesenchyme that supports these systems. The blood values, along with the clinical picture and other diagnostic procedures (ultrasound, radiographs, cytology, etc), serve as the basis for diagnosis and the recommendation of appropriate medical therapy. The metabolic interpretation of blood results, on the other hand, traces these chemical values toward their underlying physiology, i.e., the biochemical processes that produced these blood chemicals. This type of analysis helps to determine organ functionality and provides an assessment of vitamins, minerals, enzymes, co-factors, and nutrients required to achieve and maintain homeostasis.

The reference range

A reference range for a particular test or measurement is defined as the values into which 95% (or 2 standard deviations) of the population fall (*Science and Technology Dictionary* 2003). This is commonly called the normal range, a term that can be misleading because not all animals outside the range are abnormal, and sick animals may have values inside the range. A good indicator for the diagnosis of a disease clearly delineates between the normal and diseased animals' ranges. Typically, values outside of the reference range are called abnormal.

Blood laboratories set their reference range on this standard deviation of the normal population of animals. Blood results outside the laboratory's reference range furnish veterinarians with the necessary information to localize, confirm, or rule out a specific pathological process or diagnosis and ultimately to recommend the proper therapy.

The physiological range

Another way to evaluate blood test results is to interpret them as a representative of the patient's physiological status. Rather than just identify "normal" or "abnormal," it is possible to examine these tests with the idea that states of health exist as dynamic conditions, which vary between normal ranges. By interpreting blood results along this continuum, decisions regarding organ state can be made, and this information is useful in selecting nutritional programs for patients.

As veterinary students, our training focuses upon an orientation toward pathology and not wellness. As defined above, conventional blood analysis measures organ and tissue health against the normal reference range. Values outside this normal reference range are used to indicate and localize the pathology to a particular organ system.

The physiological range, on the other hand, is a set of values that is used to identify and localize which organs and metabolic processes are functioning well or are beginning to weaken. The underlying theory is based upon a physiological/homeostasis model that says that changes occur in the blood and organ systems and can be identified before pathology occurs and symptoms of disease appear. Results that are outside of the physiological range are not indicative of disease but present an indication that a particular organ system is weak or becoming imbalanced, thereby affecting the overall homeostasis.

The modern medical antiaging movement is focused upon slowing and/or stopping the aging process. The underlying theory is that when the body is in a state of homeostasis, healing occurs. The term "homeostasis" was coined by Walter Cannon, M.D. (1939). In order for homeostasis to be achieved, organ systems and function must remain in balance. This means that the production of function-controlling hormones, the acid-base balance of the blood and body tissue, and the chemicals in the blood must also be in balance. If they are not, then homeostasis is upset, free radicals accumulate, inflammation sets in, and organ degeneration begins.

The blood has a major influence on homeostasis. Nutrients, chemicals, by-products, toxins, and metabolites circulating in the blood, such as glucose, urea nitrogen, minerals, fats, and triglycerides, all play a part in homeostasis (Albrecht 1975, Appleton 2005). Furthermore, the levels of many of these chemicals are influenced by food quality, preservatives, toxins, water, stress levels, and so on. Therefore, observing blood parameters physiologically and looking for early elevations and decreases can be an important pre-disease indicator.

To illustrate this physiological view further, protein and amino acid levels and storage pools are influenced via hormonal control of the pituitary, adrenal, and thyroid glands. Amino acids marked for catabolism are routed to the liver, and via the process of oxidative deamination, they are broken down into keto acids and ammonia, the latter of which is combined with carbon dioxide to form urea, then routed via the blood to the kidneys for excretion. (See pages 84 and 85 for more detail.)

An elevated blood urea nitrogen (BUN) level is one indicator of kidney disease, and the recommendation for therapy is fluid therapy, a low-protein diet, and so on. What is not addressed in this interpretation is the fact that the kidneys are the "metabolic receptacle" for urea nitrogen. The kidneys did not *produce* these wastes but rather function to eliminate them. The conventionally accepted fact is that by the time kidney disease is diagnosed and elevated BUN levels are detected, approximately 75% of the kidney has been damaged. It would be beneficial for the animal if weakening kidneys could be identified, and metabolic waste burden reduced, before the 75% damage occurs and the situation has become critical for the patient.

When viewing the body as a whole, the approach to overburdened and weakening kidneys should take into consideration not only the kidneys and an appropriate diet, but also the organs of protein metabolism, such as the thyroid, pituitary, liver, and adrenal glands. It is these glands, which influence protein catabolism and the metabolic processes, that ultimately result in higher blood urea nitrogen levels, overworking the kidneys and setting the stage for degeneration.

It is therefore important in a preventive approach to disease to ensure that all involved organs (pituitary, thyroid, adrenal, liver, and kidneys) are properly nourished, spared from toxins, that the antioxidant-free radical ratio is monitored, and that the inciting cellular inflammation and resultant degeneration is addressed. This holistic, multiorgan approach to disease prevention and treatment, which focuses upon maintaining homeostasis, can ultimately help prevent degeneration and loss of organ function.

A simpler example is to imagine the sophisticated equipment used by an auto mechanic to diagnose your automobile's malfunction. By testing the exhaust, mechanics can trace back to the malfunctioning parts, which, once replaced, can return your automobile to proper function and performance. Similarly, the metabolic interpretation of blood, by identifying the chemical blood metabolites, serves a similar function of identifying early organ weaknesses that can be nutritionally supported, helping to improve the overall health of the body.

Taking the automobile example one step further, if you add sand to the gas tank and visit your mechanic for repairs, the solution is not just replacement of the sand-clogged carburetor, but also stopping the addition of sand to the gas tank.

The same holds true for the body. Weakened kidneys require a global approach—not only looking at the overloaded kidneys and a restricted protein/phosphorus diet, but also nutritionally addressing the functionality of the organs of protein metabolism (thyroid, adrenals, and the liver). Additionally, supplying antioxidants that reduce free radical-induced inflammation can help to improve organ functionality, as well as slow premature aging and degeneration.

More efficient protein metabolism contributes to lowering the metabolic waste load to an already burdened kidney. Reducing protein input and improving the metabolic efficiency of the liver, adrenals, and thyroid glands, in essence then, takes the "pressure" off the overloaded kidneys, allowing them the ability to rest and improve function (Goldstein 2005).

Lastly, the physiological interpretation of the blood does not conclude with a marker for a specific disease (such as an elevated BUN or ALT as an indicator for kidney or liver disease, respectively). Looking deeper into the underlying cellular physiology and biochemistry helps to determine the nutrients, vitamins, minerals, antioxidants, co-factors, and so on that are required by the cells and organ systems for proper function and the maintenance of homeostasis. Once determined, these nutrients can be added to the diet to ensure their availability when called upon by the cell and can be used for the maintenance of wellness.

Historical perspective

In the 1970s, when the metabolic analysis of animal blood was being clinically evaluated, some interesting concepts relating to animal health surfaced. Many animals with degenerative diseases had medically normal blood values, while perfectly normal animals often showed multiple abnormalities. Referred clients would say, "I know my animal is not well, but my veterinarian cannot find anything wrong, and her blood results are all normal!" We concluded that perhaps the interpretation of "normal values" we were schooled to rely upon for our diagnoses did not represent the complete picture for the early identification of a disease process (Goldstein 1999).

Take Cushing's disease as an example. A negative adrenocorticotropic hormone (ACTH) stimulation or dexamethasone suppression test would rule out hyperadrenocorticism. However, this does not indicate how close an animal is to overt disease requiring treatment. In this "positive" or "negative" approach to disease, there is no medical indicator evaluating compromised adrenal glands that are still functioning within normal medical parameters. There is also no medical data that determine when the degenerative gland will eventually become Cushing's positive. The conventional medical wisdom in this instance is to "wait and see," and if the animals becomes positive for Cushing's, then initiate therapy.

Metabolic blood testing can show early indicators for adrenal dysfunction that may eventually lead to Cushing's

disease. Alkaline phosphatase, for example, is a metabolic indicator of adrenal function. An elevation may indicate an inflamed gland requiring nutritional and/or antioxidant support. If this inflamed, overactive adrenal gland is detected early and supported nutritionally and with antioxidants, it is possible to neutralize free radicals, inflammation, and hyperactivity, and to re-establish normal adrenal function and homeostasis, thereby preventing the disease.

Metabolic blood testing can also help to identify a weakening adrenal gland that could lead to an exhausted adrenal system and eventually Addison's disease. A typical normal range for ALP is 5 to 131. Readings within this range are deemed normal. Readings above 131 are elevated and become suspicious for an active process, neoplasia, or potentially early Cushing's disease. However, what about readings of 6 or 7? These readings are not medically significant; however, they may be an early metabolic indication of a weakening adrenal gland and should be the focus of nutritional support. This is a situation that is not identified with the conventional interpretation of the blood. An animal doesn't close her eyes at night with a healthy adrenal gland and wake up with Addison's. There are progressive weaknesses or stresses that affect the adrenal function and, if detected early, can be addressed and may prevent development of the disease (Cima 2000; Goldstein 1999; Goldstein 2000, 2005).

In this chapter, we refer to free radicals, cellular inflammation, and antiaging science. Research has shown that weakening cells and organs that are inflamed but not yet diseased can be brought back to health and have improved function by antioxidants and phytonutrients. Using the physiological parameters that are representative in the blood as the basis for determining functionality of cells and organs is scientifically sound; however, it is not yet clinically proven. Clinical trials to assess the NBT evaluation and the effect of nutritionally supporting organ systems in animals who have lymphosarcoma and osteosarcoma are currently being carried out (Goldstein 2006) (also see the discussion on evidence-based medicine in chapter 1).

Other indications for blood-based nutritional recommendations

Processed, cooked pet foods are often devoid of organs and glands that are normally consumed by wild canines and felines. Lions, tigers, and wolves regularly eat their entire prey, including all the vital organs (in an uncooked form). Supplementing processed, highly cooked dog and cat foods with vital, unprocessed antioxidant- and phytonutrient-rich nutrients, often omitted from commercially prepared dog and cat foods, is beneficial for the health of the animal.

The standards set by the Association of American Feed Control Officials (AAFCO) are based upon the chemical analysis of the food and certain minimum nutrient requirements. There is no equivalent to the human RDA (recommended daily allowance) or "optimum" nutrient level for dogs and cats. The biochemical, metabolic, and physiological differences inherent in each animal are difficult to address by a "one-size-fits-all" pet food. It is difficult for mass-produced foods to satisfy the needs of all animals. Commercial foods only serve as a "base" diet, offering the basic food and nutrients as set by the AAFCO guidelines.

Feeding a dog or cat based upon his or her individual needs can more closely satisfy the animal's requirements to help maintain wellness.

Disease protocols are presented in chapters 6 through 18 and chapters 32 through 34 of this book. In these protocols, specific nutrients and nutraceuticals are suggested.

These protocols are condition-oriented and may not take into consideration complications of the disease. For example, in the protocol for lymphosarcoma, a concurrent kidney issue and hypercalcemia must be identified and addressed along with the cancer. It is for this reason that when dealing with chronic debilitating diseases such as cancer, the clinician should identify and address all complicating factors. Using physiological blood parameters offers clinicians the ability to identify and specifically support organ complications along with the primary therapy for the condition.

THE GLANDS AND ORGANS (PHYSIOLOGY, METABOLISM, AND RELATED BLOOD TESTS)

The data presented in this section on the physiological and metabolic indications and related blood tests was compiled and summarized from the following sources: Bagnell 1985, Brockman (undated), Cima 2000, Cunningham 1997, Downey 1996, Goldstein 2000, Sodikoff 1995. This data should be viewed as introductory, and the reader is referred to these references for a more in-depth description of the metabolic analysis of blood results.

Adrenal glands

The first recognized report of the use of adrenal extracts was in 1919 when Lucke reported adrenal exhaustion in people who died from the flu epidemic. He reported that the adrenal glands were not infected per se but were exhausted from attempting to restore balance to the body.

In the 1930s and 1940s, adrenal extracts were quite popular and widely used for conditions that were caused by compromised adrenal function, such as fatigue, asthma, diabetes, early Addison's disease, hypoglycemia, and allergies. The extracts were also used to improve resistance to infectious diseases (Harrower 1933, 1939).

Traditionally recognized as the stress glands of "fight or flight," the adrenals are central to many metabolic and physiologic processes and are intricately involved in the functioning of the body's immune system. The adrenal medulla manufactures epinephrine and norepinephrine, which directly affect the sympathetic nervous system and alter both heart rate and respiration. The adrenal cortex manufactures from cholesterol many hormones, such as glucocorticoids, mineralocorticoids, and adrenal androgens (17 ketosteroids, one of which is DHEA). The mineralocorticoids regulate the passage of minerals (primarily sodium and potassium) in the cell and the intercellular space. The glucocorticoids help control blood sugar levels and help in the reduction of inflammation. The adrenal androgens, such as DHEA and many others that have recently been identified, play a role in male and female functions. DHEA is believed to help manufacture other steroid hormones. The introduction of synthetic adrenal hormones such as cortisone replaced the use of adrenal extracts.

A controlled clinical trial has demonstrated that men with determined low levels of DHEA, who were then supplemented, showed a significant increase in immune function. And in a double-blind trial, pregnant women also showed significantly improved immune function (Casson 1993, Khorram 1997).

Pantothenic acid and vitamin C are required for proper action of adrenal hormones and for the metabolic and physiological functioning of the adrenal glands. Because of their central role in the immune system and the body's reaction to stress, the adrenals are more likely to become weakened, inflamed, exhausted, and underactive. The chronic administration of cortisone will also diminish adrenal function, and chronic use of cortisone can cause the gland to underfunction and atrophy.

Adrenal cortex

Glucocorticoids
Glucocorticoids, through the process of gluconeogenesis, are involved in carbohydrate metabolism and help in the maintenance of blood sugar levels. Cortisol is the main glucocorticoid and has primary responsibility for gluconeogenesis and increasing the stored levels of glycogen in the liver. Cortisol also has metabolic functions related to protein and fats: it decreases cellular protein and increases blood and liver protein. Cortisol also increases the rate at which fat is stored in the adipose tissue.

Mineralocorticoids

Aldosterone is the primary mineralocorticoid. It functions by increasing the reabsorption of sodium (and chloride) and by increasing the excretion of potassium. It also works by increasing cellular sodium absorption while transporting potassium out of the cells. In simplified terms, the adrenal cortex directly affects and controls the acid-base balance of the body through mineralocorticoids and glucocorticoids. This is accomplished by controlling the metabolism of minerals (alkaline) and sugars (acid). One of the primary functions of minerals is to transport foods and chemicals throughout the body and across cell membranes. The adrenals function to make sure the minerals are in the proper locations. Proteins, fats, and carbohydrates are osmotically drawn into the cells. Based upon the sodium/potassium balance, chloride shifts at the cell membrane, causing it to open for nutrients to enter.

Adrenal medulla

The adrenal medulla has a direct attachment to the sympathetic nervous system. Sympathetic nerve stimulation directly controls the secretion of epinephrine and norepinephrine.

Epinephrine

Epinephrine does the following:

- Causes glycogenolysis and makes glucose available to the body for rapid metabolism
- Increases the rate of fat metabolism, causing fatty acids to be available to the body
- Neutralizes histamines
- Increases the metabolic rate and is involved in the chloride shift

Norepinephrine

Norepinephrine does the following:

- Is involved in glycogenesis
- Is involved in the chloride shift

Blood tests generally related to the physiology of adrenal function

Chloride

Chloride is one of the controlling minerals of the passage of nutrients through the cell. Chloride levels are influenced by the adrenal medulla.

Sodium

Sodium is influenced by aldosterone and is produced by the adrenal cortex. Lower sodium levels may indicate low aldosterone levels and underactive adrenal gland function.

Table 2.1. Important nutrients related to adrenal function and metabolism.

Elevated	Depressed
Adrenal gland extract	Adrenal gland extract
Gonadal gland extract	Thyroid gland extract
Pantothenic acid	Pituitary gland extract
PABA	Vitamin C (alkaline)
Vitamin C (acid)	Vitamin B complex
	Chloride
	Potassium
	Selenium

Alkaline phosphatase (ALP)

Alkaline phosphatase (ALP) is found in the liver, bone, and intestines. Physiological indications of elevated or depressed ALP levels relate to adrenal function, acid/base balance (alkalinizing effects of minerals), and sugar metabolism (acid effect and pH balance). The enzyme ALP is itself alkaline and affects the pH balance of the blood.

Thyroid hormone (T4)

Low thyroid values may indicate a decrease in deamination related to an underactive adrenal gland. Inefficient adrenal glands lower production of glucocorticoids, which increases protein storage and decreases protein delivered to the liver for deamination and the amount of urea nitrogen routed to the kidney for excretion.

Table 2.1 lists the important nutrients that are related to adrenal function and metabolism.

The heart

The heart, because it is not a secretory endocrine organ, has minimal direct metabolic functions. However, the heart is responsible for the circulation, is vital for life, and it helps to fuel the body's metabolic and physiologic functions. Besides its circulation responsibilities, the heart has its own metabolic needs. Heart muscle contractions require nutrients for their metabolism and produce lactic acid, which is routed through the liver and excreted via the urine.

Blood tests generally related to the physiology of heart function

Potassium

Potassium is involved in the contraction of the muscles and also helps to deliver oxygen to the heart muscles. Heart tissue has the highest level of potassium in the body. Elevated potassium levels may result in increased oxidation and free radical production.

Table 2.2. Important nutrients related to cardiac function and metabolism.

Elevated	Depressed
Heart glandular	Amino acids—taurine, L-carnitine
Vitamin E	Pituitary
Coenzyme Q10	Hypothalamus
L-carnitine	Coenzyme Q10
Magnesium	Lecithin
Calcium	Vitamin B complex
Zinc	Vitamin E
	Potassium

Table 2.3. Important nutrients related to hypothalamic function and metabolism.

Elevated	Depressed
Pituitary glandular	Hypothalamus glandular
Parathyroid glandular	Calcium
Magnesium	Potassium
Lecithin	Lecithin
Inositol	Vitamin B_{12}
Choline	Pancreatin
Vitamin B_6	

Creatine phosphokinase (CPK)

CPK is an enzyme found in striated muscles, the heart, nerves, and the brain. Elevated CPK levels may indicate excessive activity and oxidation in the muscles, nerves, and brain.

Table 2.2 lists important nutrients related to cardiac function and metabolism.

The hypothalamus

The hypothalamus is attached to the pituitary gland by the pituitary infundibulum. The hypothalamus functions as a clearinghouse for nervous impulses (the senses and so forth). It then converts this information into chemicals that direct the pituitary and other glands to produce the hormones required to operate the body's metabolic and physiological processes. The hypothalamus itself is composed of both nervous and endocrine tissue. Several releasing factors are produced by the hypothalamus, which in turn travel to and can cause release of the pituitary hormones.

Blood tests generally related to the physiology of hypothalamic function

Calcium

Calcium acts as catalyst in many metabolic processes. Calcium (along with magnesium) is involved in the transport of fats and proteins across the intestinal wall and is absorbed into the blood. Calcium and the hypothalamus via its pituitary influence are involved in growth, bone and teeth formation, and the intestinal digestion of fats and proteins.

Cholesterol

Cholesterol is a dietary lipid that is derived from animal sources. Cholesterol is used for the manufacture of adrenal steroids. In the process of manufacturing these hormones, fat-soluble vitamins (A, D, E) and proteins are required.

Elevated cholesterol suggests an underactive hypothalamus and pituitary gland.

Potassium

Potassium is found primarily in the intracellular fluid. In the nerve cells, an impulse creates a reciprocal movement of potassium and sodium from intracellular to extracellular, causing movement of the nerve impulse. The hypothalamus, being neurological, requires proper nerve function to operate and is therefore dependent upon proper potassium levels. Low potassium levels can affect hypothalamic function.

Sodium

Sodium must be in balance and is reciprocal with potassium to produce proper nervous impulses. Elevated sodium levels often result in lower potassium levels, which can affect hypothalamic function.

Important nutrients related to hypothalamic function and metabolism are listed in Table 2.3.

The kidneys

The kidneys are the biological filters of metabolic waste removal. Primary kidney wastes include creatinine, urea nitrogen, and uric acid. Urea nitrogen is the primary by-product of protein metabolism. The adrenal and thyroid glands are involved in protein metabolism, and the deamination process occurs in the liver producing urea, which is then transported to the receptacle kidney.

Kidneys are also involved in the maintenance of fluid and mineral levels as well as the proper acid-alkaline balance. These complex metabolic processes are regulated through glandular control of filtration via hormones. For example, the kidney produces renin, which increases the production of angiotensin II, which in turn increases aldosterone levels (synthesized in the adrenal cortex from cholesterol), which in turn decrease the amount of sodium and potassium excreted by the kidneys. This affects the body's total volume of blood. Anti-diuretic hormone

(ADH), which is released by the posterior pituitary gland, also affects urine volume and flow.

Blood tests generally related to the physiology of kidney function

Creatinine
Creatinine is the nonprotein nitrogenous waste product resulting from muscle contractions and metabolism. Besides being a primary kidney function test, creatinine is an indicator of muscle metabolism, which is related to the functioning of the gonadal hormones, the pituitary, and the adrenal glands.

Blood urea nitrogen
Urea is formed in the liver by the deaminization of proteins. The thyroid and iodine are involved in the denitrification process. The process of deaminization and denitrification is under control of the pituitary gland. Metabolically elevated urea nitrogen levels can be related to high-protein diets, as well as pituitary, adrenal, liver, and thyroid functional imbalances. Low levels can be related to low dietary protein as well as hypofunctional liver, thyroid, and pituitary.

Important nutrients related to kidney function and metabolism are listed in Table 2.4.

The liver

The liver is the "seat of the metabolism." It carries out numerous metabolic and physiological processes. The liver is actively involved in the metabolism of proteins, fats, and carbohydrates via such processes as gluconeogenesis, glycolysis, and deamination. The liver is also involved in the production and storage of various compounds, such as: plasma proteins (fibrinogen, prothrombin); lipids (cholesterol and phospholipids); vitamins A, D, and B_{12}; and iron (ferritin).

Detoxification function
The liver's reticuloendothelial system is responsible for filtering toxins from the blood and removing them from the body. Toxins include chemical additives and preservatives, environmental pollutants, pesticides and insecticides, bacteria and viruses, medication and vaccine by-products, and metabolic and physiologic wastes.

Important blood tests related to the physiology of liver function

Alanine transferase (ALT)
ALT (formerly SGPT) is found mainly in cytoplasm of liver cells and is released when there is hepatocyte destruction, both recent and currently occurring. ALT is also found in lesser amounts in muscle and the heart. ALT is an end product of the catabolism of fats and other compounds from cellular membranes, the sinusoids of the liver, and the lymph system. Elevation metabolically indicates liver inflammation and altered function.

Gamma glutamyl transferase (GGTP)
Abnormal levels of GGTP indicate biliary stasis. Metabolically, an elevation can be related to an inflamed liver or overactivity of the adrenal glands and elevated cortisol levels.

Total bilirubin
Bilirubin results from the turnover and breakdown of hemoglobin, which occurs primarily in the bone marrow and spleen. Bilirubin is a bile pigment, which by bacterial action in the intestines gives the feces their color. Elevated blood levels are an indication of liver inflammation or disease. Metabolically it can be interpreted that higher-than-normal levels of metabolic wastes in the blood may increase the body's demand for globulin and involvement of the thymus gland.

Benefits of liver extracts

Liver glandular extracts, besides being a source of protein, provide a biologically available source of iron and vitamin B_{12}. Heme iron has often been used and recommended for anemia. Liver extracts have been clinically tested in people with liver disease and found to be beneficial (Fujisawa 1984, Sanbe 1973).

Table 2.5 lists important nutrients related to liver function and metabolism.

The pancreas

In 1917, William Berkeley read his paper on diabetes to the New York Academy of Medicine, explaining the process of making pancreas extract for medical therapy. It was a simple extract of whole pancreas, taken orally, which dramatically reduced blood-sugar levels within 2 hours of ingestion. It was claimed to work for patients

Table 2.4. Important nutrients related to kidney function and metabolism.

Elevated	Depressed
Kidney glandular	Adrenal glandular
Liver glandular	Pituitary glandular
Adrenal glandular	Magnesium
Thyroid glandular	Lecithin
Vitamin A	Inositol
Vitamin D	Choline
	Vitamin B_6

Table 2.5. Important nutrients related to liver function and metabolism.

Elevated	Depressed
Liver glandular	Thyroid glandular
Spleen glandular	Pituitary glandular
Thymus glandular	Hypothalamus
Iron	glandular
Vitamin B_6	Lecithin
Vitamin B_{12}	Inositol
	Choline

Table 2.6. Important nutrients related to pancreas function and metabolism.

Elevated	Depressed
Pancreas glandular	Vitamin C
Intestine glandular	Folic acid
Stomach glandular	Pancreas glandular
Vitamin B complex	Chromium
Zinc	
Chromium	

with diabetes. In 1922, F.G. Banting published his finding on a substance isolated from the pancreas that addressed the problems of diabetes. He called the substance insulin. He received the Nobel Prize for his work in 1923 (Cima 1981).

The inherent danger of insulin was that if given in too large a dose, it could cause serious side effects and even induce coma and death. The product insert carried the following warning:

> "Insulin, when given too long before a meal, or when given in too large a dose, will cause lowering of blood sugar below the normal level—a hypoglycemia. This is to be avoided, as too great a lowering will cause acute symptoms such as weakness, nervousness, and sweating. These early manifestations may be followed by drowsiness, stupor, and possibly serious results."

The question at the time was "Why was insulin considered so potentially dangerous, whereas whole pancreas or pancreas extract was considered to be generally safe?" In its purified form, insulin is a concentrated medication with a narrow range of safety. By injection, its effects are rapid.

Pancreatic enzymes

The pancreas produces the following enzymes under instructions from the vagus nerve, and the hormones gastrin, cholecystokinin, and secretin: trypsin, chymotrypsin, amylase (digests carbohydrates), lipase, cholesterolesterase (hydrolyzes cholesterol esters), phospholipase (splits fatty acids from phospholipids), and protease.

Minerals involved in pancreas function

Bicarbonate ions (sodium) make up a portion of pancreatic secretions, which alkalize the gastric secretions of the stomach. Bicarbonate is controlled by secretin. Trivalent chromium causes fatty acids to oxidize, dividing fats from sugars. Zinc is used to help balance sugar and water levels. When the extracellular fluid contains higher quantities of zinc in combination with selenium, together they draw sugar out of the blood and into the extracellular fluid. The sugar and water are combusted to form lactic acid, which is then converted back into lactic acid dehydrogenase in the blood.

The islets of Langerhans produce the following hormones:

Insulin—produced by the beta cells (sugar metabolism)
Glucagon—produced by alpha cells (glucogenolysis)
Somatostatin—produced by D cells and decrease pancreatic hormones (insulin and glucagons)

Metabolic note
A glucocorticoid imbalance can result in diabetes mellitus, and an ADH imbalance can result in diabetes insipidus.

Blood tests generally related to the physiology of pancreatic function

Calcium
Calcium bonds with lipoproteins and fatty acids as the intestines absorb it. Improper levels of pancreatic enzymes lead to poor oxidation of fatty acids in the intestines. This increases the need for calcium in the intestines to facilitate absorption and to decrease the optimal levels in the blood.

Lactic acid dehydrogenase (LDH)
LDH is present in the heart, muscles, liver, brain, and kidneys and is medically used as an evaluation of tissue damage, such as in cardiovascular stroke, liver disease, pancreatitis, and anemia. Metabolically, LDH is an enzyme that catalyzes the metabolism of glucose to lactate, which is delivered to the liver, converted back to glucose and picked up by the blood, and delivered to cells and body tissues. The primary organs and cells involved in glucose metabolism are the pancreas, liver, intestines, adrenals, and red blood cells.

Table 2.6 lists important mutrients related to pancreas function and metabolism.

The parathyroid

The parathyroid produces the parathyroid hormone. This hormone, along with calcitonin, is responsible for the regulation of the body's levels of calcium. The parathyroid glands balance calcium and phosphorus levels by working with the kidneys and intestines. The parathyroid also regulates the body's levels of vitamin D. Basic metabolic functions related to calcium and phosphorus levels include:

- Adequate levels of phosphorus are required to maintain stomach hydrochloric acid levels.
- Calcium is required for the absorption of fats and proteins in the gut.

Blood tests generally related to the physiology of parathyroid function

Calcium
Calcium levels are a direct indication of parathyroid activity.

T4
Although the absorption of fat and the resulting blood levels depend on calcium, the release of fat from body tissues is under the control of the thyroid.

Table 2.7 lists important nutrients related to parathyroid function and metabolism.

The pineal gland

The pineal gland is embryonically a vestige of the third eye. It is involved in all the senses, especially vision. The nerve pathway for sight travels from the eyes to the hypothalamus and then to the pineal, activating its hormones. The quantity and type of light that the body is exposed to directly affect the pineal gland.

This gland is thought to be linked to sexual development by inhibiting the hypothalamic releasing factors. It is also believed to be involved in internal balance of water by interacting with the posterior pituitary.

The pineal helps to adjust the overall pH of the body in relationship to external environmental changes of light and sound. This is accomplished by assisting in the balance of sodium (adrenal cortex) and chloride (adrenal medulla).

Table 2.7. Important nutrients related to parathyroid function and metabolism.

Elevated	Depressed
Parathyroid glandular	Pancreatin
Magnesium	Parathyroid glandular
Vitamin B$_6$	Calcium
Taurine	Magnesium
	Vitamin B$_{12}$

Sodium and chloride balances are affected and responsive to the body's exposure to both light and sound.

The pineal gland produces melatonin. Melatonin was discovered in 1958; however, it wasn't until August 7, 1995, that *Newsweek* magazine described melatonin as having the ability to relieve many nagging conditions such as insomnia and jet lag. The article went so far as to report that melatonin boosts the immune system in its fight against certain types of cancer. Although melatonin is still not completely understood, it is believed to be directly involved in the body's internal clock and the regulation and formation of certain hormones at various periods during the day and night.

Similar to the adrenal gland, where scientists focused their attention on corticosteroids and overlooked DHEA, the pineal may contain other yet undiscovered hormones that could have a beneficial effect on the body and its natural balance of glands and hormones. As in the adrenals, this would support using the whole gland extract of the pineal as a legitimate approach, rather than using an isolated hormone such as synthetic melatonin.

Blood tests generally related to the physiology of pineal gland function

Sodium
Sodium is an alkaline mineral that helps to maintain alkaline activity and regulates acid-base balance. This directly affects the balance of the intracellular and extracellular fluid, water levels, and osmotic pressure. Pineal and sodium activity are related with regard to pH balance.

Chloride
Chloride is used to assess pH and electrolyte balance. One purpose of chloride is to block mineral-controlled substances from crossing the cell membrane. Pineal and chloride activity are related with regards to pH balance.

B/C
Urea nitrogen and creatinine are the metabolic by-products and kept in continual balance by the body's level of water. Water and pH balance are controlled by the posterior pituitary, adrenal, pineal, and the kidneys.

Table 2.8 lists important nutrients related to pineal function and metabolism.

The pituitary

Pituitary extracts were used in growth disorders in the 1920s, when gland therapy was enjoying high popularity. Acromegaly was identified as a disease related to an overactive pituitary gland. Evan (1922) discovered that injections of pituitary extracts into rats increased growth and

Table 2.8. Important nutrients related to pineal function and metabolism.

Elevated	Depressed
Kidney glandular	Pineal glandular
Pineal glandular	Pituitary glandular
Acid B vitamins (folic, pantothenic, PABA)	Vitamin B complex
	Potassium

created a condition resembling gigantism. Uhlenhuth (1920) administered pituitary extract to salamanders, and noticed that those which received the substance showed a significantly increased rate of growth.

Since that time, much has been discovered about the pituitary gland, its components, and the physiological and metabolic processes that it, as the master gland, oversees. The pituitary is composed of the anterior and posterior pituitary and the infundibulum (the connector between the pituitary and the hypothalamus). The hypothalamus produces several substances that cause the pituitary to produce its own hormones (See the section on the hypothalamus, above).

Cima said: "The primary purpose of the pituitary is one of anabolism, rather than catabolism. Which means that any catabolic disease that overcomes the human body may have its roots in the anterior pituitary. Needless to say, supplemental pituitary concentrate could support and assist all of the areas in which the organ has activity. The pituitary, in many respects, is a cornerstone endocrine gland, operating in a sophisticated feedback system with other endocrine glands" (Cima 1981, 2000).

The anterior pituitary

The anterior pituitary produces hormones based upon instructions from the hypothalamus gland. The hormones are released into the circulatory system and sent throughout the body to their specific target organs and cells. Because of the numbers of hormones and their relationship to the general metabolism of the body, a well-balanced, optimum-functioning pituitary gland is essential for health and wellness:

- Adrenocorticotrophic stimulating hormone (ACTH): stimulates the adrenal cortex to produce mineralocorticoids and glucocorticoids.
- Follicle stimulating hormone (FSH): stimulates growth of the ovarian follicle.
- Luteinizing hormone (LH): oversees follicle maturation.
- Melanocyte stimulating hormone: stimulates the production of melatonin.

- Somatotrophin (growth hormone): oversees growth and is involved in the metabolism of proteins, fatty acids, and glucose.
- Thyroid stimulating hormone (TSH): stimulates the production of thyroxine.

Blood tests generally related to the physiology of anterior pituitary gland function

Urea nitrogen
Urea nitrogen is formed in the liver by the deamination of protein. Nitrogen is taken from the amino acid under the influence of the thyroid (thyroxine and iodine). The protein part is then used for the production of various hormones, antibodies, etc. This process of converting the protein into various body chemicals is under the control of the adrenal and anterior pituitary glands. The released nitrogen is used in the chemical conversion to urea (ornithine cycle), transported to the kidneys, and released in the urine. (See pages 84 and 85 for more detail.)

Elevated urea nitrogen levels may indicate overactive thyroid glands, increasing the metabolic rate and resulting in an excessive release of nitrogen and the production of higher-than-normal levels of circulating urea produced by the liver. Under this situation, the adrenals and anterior pituitary are overworking in their breakdown function of proteins, hormones, antibodies, etc. Conversely, low urea nitrogen levels may indicate a decrease in the functioning of the adrenal and pituitary, resulting in fewer proteins delivered to the liver for deamination.

Cholesterol
Cholesterol is a by-product of protein metabolism. It is one of the primary building blocks for manufacture of hormones, antibodies, and enzymes. The anterior pituitary, as a result of its role in protein metabolism and the creation of these substances, is linked to the blood levels of cholesterol. Elevated cholesterol levels may indicate an underactive anterior pituitary function while low cholesterol levels may indicate an overactive anterior pituitary.

Calcium
Calcium in the intestines assists in the absorption of lipoproteins across the intestinal wall. Calcium requires magnesium, hydrochloric acid, and vitamin D for optimal metabolism. The amount of calcium present and the level of proteins are directly related. When the ratio of calcium to magnesium is greater than 2:1, fat is drawn through the intestinal wall and cell membrane. This calcium-to-magnesium phenomenon creates an electrical osmotic gradient that draws the calcium and lipoprotein across the membrane of the cell. The anterior pituitary and its hormones are used to control the magnesium and due to

Table 2.9. Important nutrients related to anterior pituitary function and metabolism.

Elevated	Depressed
Kidney glandular	Gonadal glandular
Thyroid glandular	Lecithin
Anterior pituitary glandular	Inositol
Trace minerals	Choline
Magnesium	Calcium
Pancreatin	Vitamin B_{12}

Table 2.10. Important nutrients related to posterior pituitary function and metabolism

Elevated	Depressed
Kidney glandular	Thymus glandular
Whole pituitary glandular	Adrenal glandular
Pancreas glandular	Whole pituitary glandular
Intestine glandular	
Spleen glandular	
Trace and essential minerals	

this "ratio effect," both calcium and anterior pituitary function are required.

Table 2.9 lists important nutrients related to anterior pituitary function and metabolism.

The posterior pituitary

The posterior pituitary's main metabolic function is controlling the body's water levels that indirectly affect the pH balance. This is accomplished by anti-diuretic hormone (ADH) and the presence of intracellular potassium. At the cellular level, potassium (under the control of the posterior pituitary) functions to maintain water balance (intra- and extracellular) and aids in the transport of various substances across the cell membrane. This acid-base balance is also affected by carbohydrate metabolism (acid), the pancreas (sugar digestion and assimilation), and the adrenals (sugar metabolism), all of which are balanced by potassium and other alkaline minerals.

ADH (Vasopressin) controls the retention of water and potassium and the excretion of sodium by the kidneys. This is counteracted and kept in balance by the adrenals and the production of minerals and glucocorticoids, which act to counteract ADH. An ADH imbalance can result in diabetes insipidus. Likewise, a glucocorticoid imbalance can result in diabetes mellitus.

Oxytocin causes contraction of the uterus during the birth process, and causes the contraction of the myo-epithelial cells in the breasts when the baby suckles.

Blood tests generally related to the physiology of posterior pituitary gland function

Potassium

Potassium is an essential mineral used to carry out its physiological and metabolic functions. Potassium is closely involved with the adrenal glands in the proper sodium and acid-base balances via aldosterone. Potassium levels are also involved and closely related to posterior pituitary function.

Triglycerides

Abnormal triglyceride levels metabolically indicate the need for essential fatty acids. Triglycerides are composed of a molecule of glycerol and 3 molecules of fatty acids. The energy necessary for active transport across a cell membrane, via the influence of potassium, is supplied by fatty acids. Primary glands in triglyceride metabolism are the posterior pituitary, adrenals, and pancreas.

Glucose

Glucose, although affected by many other organs and glands, is also affected by the posterior pituitary, as it relates to the proper acid-base balance in the body.

BUN/creatinine ratio (B/C)

Urea, nitrogen, and creatinine ratios are the by-products of protein and muscle metabolism. Metabolism produces their blood levels, while excretion by the kidneys maintains their balance. This excretion is under the control of the posterior pituitary, which is responsible for the body's water balance and acid-base balance.

Important nutrients related to posterior pituitary function and metabolism are listed in Table 2.10.

The spleen

The spleen is the largest of the lymphoid tissue organs and is highly vascular. As the blood passes through the spleen, aged red blood cells are removed and broken down, and the released hemoglobin is routed to the liver. The spleen also contains iron and fat, which are used in the synthesis of new red and white blood cells.

When red blood cells die, they trigger the spleen to start the process of hemopoiesis, which uses the stored iron and fat. This decreases the levels of iron and fat in the blood. Because it is lymphoid-type tissue, the spleen is part of the body's immune system, and has a reticuloendothelial type of cellular system, which contains phagocytes that assist in the removal of foreign material such as bacteria and metabolic wastes.

Blood tests generally related to the physiology of splenic function

Cholesterol
Cholesterol and the spleen are required for the formation of bile salts and many of the immune-modulating hormones.

Hemoglobin
Hemoglobin levels, unless there is anemia, are related to the spleen's efficiency in the storage and breakdown of red blood cells.

Total bilirubin
Bilirubin levels, like hemoglobin levels, are related to the spleen's efficiency in the storage and breakdown of red blood cells.

Important nutrients related to splenic function and metabolism are listed in Table 2.11.

The thymus

Whole thymus extract is one of the most popularly used gland treatments today. Researchers and clinicians believe that the thymus gland is important in immune-boosting function, especially during a challenge from serious chronic degenerative diseases such as cancer and immune-mediated conditions. The thymus produces the hormone thymosin A, which increases the production and activity of the lymphocytes. T Lymphocytes are part of the cellular immune system and destroy invading, foreign, or toxic materials.

Clinical double blind studies with thymus extracts show increased prevention and a reduced rate of respiratory infections in children and adults (Fiocchi 1986, Galli 1990, Vettori 1987, Longo 1988). Thymus extracts have also shown improved immune function in people, some with diabetes (Braga 1994, Wysocki 1992).

Blood tests generally related to the physiology of thymic function

Albumin/globulin ratio (A/G)
The A/G ratio is directly affected by the level of globulin in the blood. When foreign substances (toxins, pathogens, chemicals, etc.) contact the body, the thymus and spleen direct the white blood cell buildup and increase globulin production of thymoglobulin and splenoglobulin to help fight invaders.

Globulin
The thymus gland is directly involved in the production of immuno-proteins, of which globulin is one type. Globulin is a direct assessment of the functioning of the thymus.

Total bilirubin
Immunoglobulin is produced by the destruction of red blood cells by the spleen and liver, which simultaneously release bilirubin. An elevated total bilirubin may also represent the presence of excess toxins in the blood, requiring the thymus to deliver additional globulin. Simultaneously, the spleen stops the production of, and focus on, the destruction of red blood cells.

Table 2.12 lists important nutrients related to thymic function and metabolism.

The thyroid

By the late 1800s, it had been determined that the thyroid gland was responsible for body temperature and for basal metabolism. In 1889, the Clinical Society of London published a report linking the thyroid to myxedema. In the early 1900s the thyroid was a major player in the use of raw organ extracts in the treatment of disease. Cima (1981), in *Biochemical Bloodwork Evaluation*, states the following:

Table 2.11. Important nutrients related to splenic function and metabolism.

Elevated	Depressed
Liver glandular	Iron
Thyroid glandular	Chlorophyll
Thymus glandular	Bone marrow glandular
dl-Methionine	Spleen glandular
Lecithin	Vitamin B (acid)
Inositol	Vitamin B_{12}
Choline	

Table 2.12. Important nutrients related to thymic function and metabolism.

Elevated	Depressed
Thymus glandular	Thymus glandular
Bone marrow glandular	Liver glandular
Adrenal glandular	Spleen glandular
Dimethylglycine	Vitamin B complex
Iron	Vitamin B_{12}
Vitamin C	
Vitamin E	
Vitamin A	
Zinc	
Selenium	

"The well known disease, goiter (a visible enlargement of the thyroid gland, frequently a first step in the development of myxedema) was cured by giving thyroid. Organotherapy won its first triumph with thyroid. This can hardly be disputed, and even now, the generally accepted treatment for myxedema, cretinism and milder forms of hypothyroidism is with thyroid hormone or with whole-desiccated thyroid gland.

"Research into the chemistry of the thyroid hormone showed that iodine was always present in active preparations. By this, iodine itself had been proven to be an effective substance for certain simple goiters. It was later shown that iodine was indispensable to the physiological action of the thyroid gland. In 1917, E.C. Kendall offered his report to the American Chemical Society in Boston. He gave details of the isolation of the active principal of the thyroid gland. Kendall had produced 18 grams of thyroxine after starting with 2 tons of animal gland (not a very good yield). Thyroxine received its name from the fact that it came from the thyroid gland and was found to contain an indol group; hence the name thyroxine.

Thyroxine contained iodine and exerted a very potent effect when injected into laboratory animals. It seemed as though the effects of thyroxine equaled in every way the effects of the desiccated gland. It was stated that 100% positive response was observed. This work was immediately accepted by the medical profession and, in fact, reflects the logical scientific progression, which involves the isolation and purification of physiologically active molecules, and the subsequent clinical and experimental work was with the active hormone or enzyme rather than the tissue or organ from which it came. This became the main theme throughout the development of the field of endocrinology. It is interesting to note that, at that time, thyroxine was believed to be the one and only active principal obtainable from the thyroid; it was only later discovered that two other hormones, tri-iodothyronine (similar to thyroxine) and calcitonin (a plasma-calcium lowering hormone) were also produced by the thyroid."

The thyroid is under the control of the pituitary gland via thyroid stimulating hormone. The thyroid glands are responsible for the metabolic rate and therefore have the following direct effects on organs and metabolic processes:

- Influence fat, carbohydrate, and protein metabolism.
- Influence the levels of enzymes in the body.
- Increase osteoclastic activity.
- Directly affect body weight.
- Direct affect the heart rate, circulation, and pressure.
- Increase the rate of respiration as the demand for oxygen increases.
- Increase the rate of absorption of food from the intestines.

Table 2.13. Important nutrients related to thyroid function and metabolism.

Elevated	Depressed
Thyroid glandular (low dose)	Thyroid glandular (high dose)
Pitutary glandular	Iodine
Kidney glandular	Pituitary glandular
Magnesium	Adrenal glandular
L-Carnitine	Vitamin B complex
Coenzyme Q10	Vitamin C
	Vitamin E

Blood tests generally related to the physiology of thyroid function

T4

T4 is a measurement of the thyroxine circulating in the bloodstream. This is a direct indicator of thyroid function. Too much thyroxine indicates a hyperactive thyroid, and vice versa.

Table 2.13 lists important nutrients related to thyroid function and metabolism.

DIET, NUTRITION, AND THE BIOLOGICAL FACTOR

Hippocrates, in about 400 BC, said, "Let food be your medicine." His writings touted the use of foods and herbs as the basis for the maintenance of health and vigor. The history of food and how it relates to humankind and companion animals is a rich mixture of tradition, fads, panaceas, folklore, and science.

The following is a summary of McCay's (1949) view of the birth of the modern pet food industry:

The modern era of feeding domesticated animals has its roots in home cooking, using the staple foods of the region. American literature from the early to mid 1900s contains references to dogs and cats being fed leftovers from the family table.

These table scraps consisted of boiled grains such as wheat or corn mixed with meat scraps, some ground vegetable parings, and limestone or bone meal. Animals living on farms would be treated to whatever crops or meats were produced, and cats were treated to raw unprocessed milk. As domesticated animals became family members, particularly in more urban and suburban areas, an industry developed around the dietary and health needs of animals. Dog and cat shows became popular, kennel and boarding facilities opened and flourished, and more people looked to adopt or purchase purebred dogs and cats.

Finding a steady supply of quality ingredients was difficult and, even more important, uneconomical since kennels were now a business and needed to make a profit. At the same time, the popularity of dogs and cats as household pets was rising rapidly, adding a second, consumer-driven demand for quality feed.

This also led to another demand on the feed industry, one of convenience, especially in urban areas. Being able to purchase animal food locally in a package that could easily be stored and fed to the animal became important. Packaging and clear instructions were also demanded of manufacturers. The feed industry, recognizing a valuable business opportunity, quickly responded to the growing demands of kennel owners and consumers. Pet food had to fit certain criteria; consistency was at the top of the list. The food had to look the same each time so that kennel and/or pet owners knew that their animals were getting a consistent diet.

The feed industry also had to respond to the economies of operating a business. The search began for a continual supply of raw ingredients. This led to the human food-processing industry, which generated a tremendous amount of leftovers, which at the time were converted into low-profit fertilizers and farm-animal feed. This was the beginning of today's modern pet-food industry.

Pet food raw ingredients

Many pet foods include ingredients taken from leftovers of the human food-processing industry. Meat and chicken meals may contain some ground feathers, nails, claws, cartilage, tendons, bones, blood, and fecal waste, all of which have a low biological and nutritive value. Other components may include indigestible vegetable and grain fillers, such as shells, hulls, and stalks. While they provide bulk and fiber, their nutritive value is low. Other ingredients may be included as additives to make the food look uniform and appealing to the people who buy it. Coloring agents such as dyes, pigments, and minerals are typically added, as are appetite stimulants such as sugar, salt, and animal digests (meat scrap by-products dissolved in an acid to achieve uniformity, then turned into a liquid that is sprayed on the food).

The last decade has seen a strong movement in the pet food industry toward healthier, more nutritious ingredients, including:

- More whole grains such as brown rice, whole wheat, and corn, which replace by-products such as wheat middlings and brewers rice.
- More whole protein sources (chicken, beef, lamb, and turkey) which replace highly processed protein sources such as poultry by-product meal.
- Natural preservative systems using vitamins E and C, and herbs such as rosemary.

This movement is welcomed by many veterinarians and consumers. But change has been slow, hampered in part by pet food guidelines established early on by the National Research Council (NRC) that were based on chemical content assessments (the actual levels of fats, proteins, vitamins, and minerals), and not the biological content (the quality and bio-availability of ingredients used to reach these nutrient levels).

Dr. Mark Morris and the pet food industry

We as veterinarians are familiar with the Guaranteed Analysis chart on the label of all pet foods. In order to qualify as a pet food, the crude protein, crude fat, crude fiber, and moisture categories must be listed on the label. A typical guaranteed analysis required to qualify as a canned pet food would be:

Crude Protein 10%
Crude Fat. 6.5%
Crude Fiber 2.4%
Moisture 68%

Dr. Mark Morris, a pioneer of the American Veterinary Medical Association, put forth to the veterinary and lay communities the following tongue-in-cheek pet-food recipe (Published by Hill's Pet Nutrition, Inc. ®/™):

Blend:

- 1 pail crushed coal (carbohydrates)
- 1 gallon crankcase oil (fat)
- 4 pair old leather work shoes (protein)
- 68 lb water

The caption read, "The ingredient panel and chemical analysis on dog-food labels are not guarantees of nutritional quality." Morris' purpose was to show that the most important consideration in the manufacture of quality dog and cat food is not the chemical composition, but rather the raw ingredients. The government standards for pet food regulations at the time did not address any biological value, and instead were based solely upon chemical analysis. Morris, a true visionary, stated that this reliance on a chemical analysis of pet food was faulty. His recipe mocked the existing regulatory standards by showing that a mixture made of ground, cooked shoes; crankcase oil; and coal would pass the minimum requirements to be called a pet food.

The last item in early pet-food-industry history was the discovery that some pet food manufacturers were unscrupulously trying to increase their profits by using low-grade ingredients. In the early 1940s, the American Veterinary Medical Association, under the active leadership of Morris, set up a committee to certify reliable products. This led to the birth of laboratory and testing facilities and the ultimate standardization of commercially prepared feeds for animals. This laboratory process, however, could only test the feed for its chemical content, i.e., levels of protein, fat, carbohydrates, minerals, water, etc. The only reliable way to test the biological value is to observe it in a living animal and the resulting overall health and well-being of that animal.

The failure of the testing facilities' guidelines and the chemical content assessment is vividly illustrated with the taurine issue. Many cats that were fed a taurine-deficient died from cardiomyopathy. The level of protein in the food was tested and found to be adequate, but the quality was not. The protein used to reach the required levels of crude protein was deficient in taurine. Pet-food manufacturers were slow to respond, but eventually supplemented their feline diets with additional essential amino acid.

The biological aspects of pet foods

There is a second important issue that can be learned from the clinical research carried out on taurine deficiencies in cats, i.e the effect of heat and processing on pet food ingredients. To begin a discussion on the biological aspects of pet food, it is important to present the results of a scientific feeding trial carried out by Dr. Francis M. Pottenger Jr., which clearly demonstrated the debilitating effects of feeding cooked foods to cats.

From 1932 through 1942, Pottenger researched the process of standardizing body tissues and glands to determine their potency. While his focus was a surgical research protocol to set standards for human values, he astutely noticed that his test cats, raised for his procedures, were becoming weaker and more sickly with each successive generation. He believed he was feeding these cats the best possible diet, designed by experts in the field of pet nutrition. The diet consisted of market-grade milk; cod-liver oil; and cooked meat scraps, including cooked liver, beef, tripe, and sweetbreads.

The meat ingredients, obtained from a local sanitarium, were leftovers from what was fed to human patients. Pottenger and the other experts considered this top-notch nutrition for his cats. When they began to show classical signs of nutritional deficiencies, thereby becoming poor surgical risks, Pottenger grew perplexed. The cats were producing fewer kittens, and those that did survive birth had increasing amounts of skeletal deformities, organ malformation, and degenerative diseases. Their life span was also dramatically shortened.

As his program expanded, Pottenger outgrew the supply of cooked sanitarium meats. He approached a local meat packing plant and secured a supply of raw scraps consisting of muscle meat, organs, and bone. This raw meat ration was fed to a segregated group of cats, and in a matter of months, the cats in this group appeared in better health than the cats fed the cooked ration. Furthermore,

their kittens appeared healthier and were less of a surgical risk. The contrast between raw vs. cooked diets was so dramatic that Pottenger designed a formal protocol to study the cats. He published his findings (1946, 1995) on these cat experiments. Over the 10-year period, Pottenger observed the following Pottenger (1983):

Cats fed the raw meat and gland diet looked and felt better, were never sick, and always produced robust, strong kittens.

Cats fed the cooked diets were always sick, died younger, and gave birth to weak and deformed kittens.

After 3 generations of a cooked-food diet, the mother cats could no longer give birth. When cooked-food cats were fed the raw-food diet, their health and reproductive ability was renewed.

It is interesting to note from the study that the degenerative diseases experienced by the cooked-food cats are similar to those that affect modern cats, such as cardiomyopathy, liver and kidney disease, hyperthyroidism, chronic lower urinary tract disease, diabetes, arthritis, and cancer. The question is, are the results that have been reported by Dr. Pottenger the consequences of feeding raw vs. cooked foods or are there other factors that set the stage for deficiencies that may be at play here?

Since Pottenger carried out his clinical trials in the 1940s, he did not have modern testing and instrumentation to confirm the nutrient balance of his diets nor did he know about taurine deficiencies, which could be a factor. Taurine deficiencies in cats was not reported until the 1960s by Jacobsen (1968); they were expanded upon by Huxtable (1992). It was not until 1975 and 1985 that the required importance of taurine in cats was shown. (Hayes 1975a,b in National Research Council 1986, Schaeffer 1985).

We now know that cats lack the ability to manufacture taurine and require that it be added to their diets. We also know that taurine-deficient diets can lead to many disease conditions such as cardiomyopathy, retinal degeneration, and blindness, as well as reproductive issues and musculoskeletal deformities (Dieter 1993; Monson 1989; Morris 1989; Novotny 1994; Pion 1992; Ryan 1989; Sturman 1989, 1991, 1992; Waltham 1993, 1994).

However what is not widely reported is the effect of heating and processing upon taurine deficiencies. Hickmann (1990, 1991) and Kim (1996 a,b) reported that cats that eat cooked and processed foods have lower plasma taurine levels.

It is believed that the issue lies with the Maillard reaction, defined as a reaction between an amino acid and a carbohydrate in a heat condition. The Maillard reaction promotes the growth of intestinal bacteria that degrades the taurine, setting the stage for the deficiency (Hickmann 1990, 1992; Kim 1996). Sturman (1986) presents a link between his modern knowledge and the Pottenger cat experiment from the 1940s. Two groups of cats were fed the same diet except one group's diet was taurine deficient. Sturman reported many malformations that were quite similar to those reported upon by Pottenger: retinal degeneration, a high incidence of still births, and a higher mortality rate in those cats receiving the taurine deficient diets.

This information on taurine serves as the basis to discuss what we call the biological factor in pet foods. The failure of nutritional guidelines to address the biological factor is one of the more serious drawbacks of today's commercial pet foods. Pet foods are required to be cooked at extremely high temperatures to meet government standards which ensure destruction of harmful bacteria and other contaminants. While temperatures well above 212°F are necessary from a bacterial standpoint for canning and cooking pet foods, these high temperatures can alter and inactivate such delicate or vital nutrients as vitamins, enzymes, and cofactors, making them much less effective for maintaining good pet health. Such vital nutrients (termed the "life force" by human nutritionists) are abundant and found in the highest content in raw meat and fresh, raw fruits and vegetables.

Modern pet food formulation, analysis, and regulations

Nutritional claims on pet food labels initially followed the guidelines set forth by the Committee on Animal Nutrition of the National Research Council (NRC). The NRC published the nutrient requirements of dogs in 1974 and of cats in 1978. The Association of American Feed Control Officials (AAFCO) was created to regulate pet food labels based on the guidelines established by the NRC. To simplify the process, AAFCO initially relied upon the NRC standards and the chemical analysis of the food to determine nutritional adequacy.

AAFCO did this despite the fact that experts reported this chemical analysis technique to be flawed. Controversy flared in the pet food industry after the NRC failed to address these known flaws in its guideline revisions of 1985 and 1986. Based upon these later revisions, AAFCO decided, for the interim, to stay with the older recommendations set in 1974 and 1978. In 1990 and 1991, AAFCO put together the canine nutrition expert (CNE) and feline nutrition expert (FNE) subcommittees. Their reports served as the bases for the published AAFCO Dog Food and Cat Food Nutrient Profiles, created to address and correct the flaws in the NRC report.

An unaddressed issue

Today, however, AAFCO profiles unfortunately do not refer to the biological value of the food, i.e., the nutrients that help to create health and maintain wellness. The feeding trials recommended by AAFCO take a step toward biological evaluation by testing some parameters in a living animal, namely proper growth, weight maintenance, gestation, and lactation. But these parameters fall short of a complete definition of health and the prevention of disease.

Living organisms are incredibly complex, and the science of nutrition is still in its infancy. There are many more questions than there are answers regarding proper nutrition. As information increases, consumer and veterinary diets will continue to improve, but for now there are still weaknesses in the production of these products.

The following are some of the attributes related to pet foods and genetic makeup of animals that need further investigation and clarity:

- What effect do the extreme high temperatures of processing (extrusion and retorting) have on the availability and usability of certain nutrients, protein, fat, antioxidants, phytonutrients, and delicate vitamins and enzymes (broadly classified in human health food circles as the "life force" of the food)?
- What cumulative effect does the daily ingestion of small amounts of chemical preservatives and additives, coloring agents, pigments, appetite stimulants, and animal digests (used to color, improve palatability, and extend shelf life) have upon the health of the animal? Does their feeding increase the production of free radicals, leading to inflammation, degeneration, premature aging, and disease?
- What health effect does the feeding of rejected protein (beef, chicken, turkey, lamb, etc.) by-products (such as middlings, hulls, meals, gluten) have upon the long-term health of the animals?
- What effect does the inherent genetic make-up of individuals play in selecting which food substances are most appropriate for a particular animal or breed? (Consider gluten intolerance and other issues related to genetics, which so powerfully impact individual health.)

References

AAFCO Official Publication, Sharon Krebs, AAFCO Assistant Secretary-Treasurer, P.O. Box 478 Oxford, IN 47971, USA

Abdel-Aziz, M.T., Abdou, M.S., Soliman, K., et al. 1984. Effect of carnitine on blood lipid pattern in diabetic patients. *Nutr Rep Int*:29:1071–9.

Adachi, K., Nanba, H., Kuroda, H. 1987. Potentiation of Host-Mediated Antitumor Activity in Mice by Beta-glucan Obtained from Grifola frondosa (Maitake), *Chem. Pharm. Bull*:35;262–270.

Adlercreutz, H., Mazur, W. 1997. Phyto-oestrogens and Western diseases. *Ann Med*:29;95–120.

Agarwal, S., Rao, A.V. 2000 Carotenoids and chronic diseases. *Drug Metab Drug Interact*:17(1-4):189–210.

Albrecht, W.A. 1975. The Albrecht Papers, Kansas City, KS: Acre Publ.

Altura, B.M., Altura, B.T. 1985. New perspectives on the role of magnesium in the pathophysiology of the cardiovascular system. *Magnesium* 4:226–244

Alvarez, R.A., et al. 1994. Plasma lipid changes in PRCD-affected and normal miniature poodles given oral supplements of linseed oil. Indications for the involvement of n-3 fatty acids in inherited retinal degenerations. *Exp. Eye Res*:Feb;58(2): 129–37.

Ambrus, J.L., et al. 1967. Absorption of Exogenous Proteolytic Enzymes. *Clin. Pharmacol. Therap*: 8:362–368.

American Diabetes Association. 1992. Magnesium supplementation in the treatment of diabetes. *Diabetes Care*:15:1065–7.

Ames, B.N., Shigenaga, M.K., Hagen, T.M. 1993. Oxidants, antioxidants and the degenerative diseases of aging. *Proc. Natl. Acad. Sci. U.S.A.*:90:7915–7922.

Anderson R.A. 2000. Chromium in the prevention and control of diabetes. *Diabetes Metab*:26:22–7 [review].

Anderson, R.A. 1998. Chromium, glucose intolerance and diabetes. *J Am Coll Nutr*: 17:548–55 [review].

Anderson, R.A., Polansky, M.M., Bryden, N.A., Canary, J.J. 1991. Supplemental-chromium effects on glucose, insulin, glucagon, and urinary chromium losses in subjects consuming controlled low-chromium diets. *Am J Clin Nutr*:4:909–16.

Anonoymous. 1994. The effect of vitamin E and beta carotene on the incidence of lung cancer and other cancers in male smokers. The Alpha-Tocopherol, Beta Carotene Cancer Prevention Study Group. *N Engl J Med*:330(15):1029–1035.

Appleton, N. 2005. Stopping Inflammation: Relieving the Cause of Degenerative Diseases. New York: Square One Publishers.

Arjmandi, B.H., Khan, D.A., Jurna, S. 1998. Whole flaxseed consumption lowers serum LDL-cholesterol and lipoprotein(a) concentrations in postmenopausal women. *Nutr Res*:18:1203–1214.

Ashmead, H.D., et al. 1985. Intestinal Absorption of Metal Ions. Springfield, IL: Charles C. Thomas.

Ashmead, H.D., et al., 1982. Chelated Mineral Nutrition in Plants, Animals and Man. Springfield, IL: Charles C. Thomas.

Askanazi, J., Carpenter, Y.A., Michelsen, C.B., et al. 1980. Muscle and plasma amino acids following injury: Influence of intercurrent infection. *Ann Surg*:192:78–85.

Aurer-Kozelj, J., Kralj-Klobucar, N., Buzina, R., Bacic, M. 1982. The effect of ascorbic acid supplementation on periodontal tissue ultrastructure in subjects with progressive periodontitis. *Int J Vitam Nutr Res*:52:333–41.

Awad, A. Plant-based fat inhibits growth of breast-cancer cell line, UB researchers show. University of Buffalo press release: April 29, 1999.

Awad, A. Plant-based fat inhibits cancer-cell growth by enhancing cell's signaling system, UB researchers show. University of Buffalo press release: April 29, 1999.

BASF. 1986. Effect of pelleting on the crystal and ethyl-cellulose coated ascorbic acid assay levels of poultry feed. BASF Animal Nutrition Research, RA873. BASF Corporation, Mount Olive, N.J.

BASF. 1983. Vitamins and their stability. No. 7, Animal Nutrition News BASF Corporation, Mount Olive, NJ.

BASF. NSP enzyme stability through pelleting: Product form selection KC 9706, BASF Coroporation, Mount Olive, NJ.

BASF. 1998. The stability of vitamin C in pelleting and storage. Animal Nutrition News No. 48, BASF Coroporation, Mount Olive, NJ.

Bagnell, V.H. 1985. Nutritional Therapy; Energy Industries, Inc.

Baintner, K. 1986. Intestinal Absorption of Macromolecules and Immune Transmission From Mother to Young. Boca Raton, FL: CRC Press.

Balch, J.F., Balch, P.A. 1997. Prescription for Nutritional Healing. New York: Avery Publishing Group.

Barbul, A., Rettura, G., Levenson, S.M., et al. 1983. Wound healing and thymotropic effects of arginine: a pituitary mechanism of action. *Am J Clin Nutr*:37:786–94.

Barbul, A., Lazarou, S.A., Efron, D.T., et al. 1990. Arginine enhances wound healing and lymphocyte immune responses in humans. *Surgery*:108:331–7.

Barbul, A. 1986. Arginine: Biochemistry, physiology, and therapeutic implications. *Journal of Parenteral and Enteral Nutrition*:10:227–238.

Barilla, D.E., Notz, C., Kennedy, D., and Pak, C.Y.C. 1978. Renal oxalate excretion following oral oxalate loads in patients with ileal disease and with renal and absorptive hypercalciurias: effect of calcium and magnesium. *Am J Med*:64: 579–85.

Barnes, L. 1979. B15: The politics of ergogenicity. *Physicians and Sports Medicine*:7(#11):17.

Barnett, Y.A. 1994. Nutrition and the aging process. *Br J Biomed Sci*:51:278–287.

Baron, J.A., Beach, M., Mandel, J.S., et al. 1999. Calcium supplements for the prevention of colorectal adenomas. *N Engl J Med*:340:101–7.

Baron, J.A., Cole, B.F., Mott, L., et al. 2003. Neoplastic and antineoplastic effects of beta-carotene on colorectal adenoma recurrence: results of a randomized trial. *J Natl Cancer Inst*:95(10):717–722.

Bartter, F.C., Berkson, B., Gallelli, J., et al. 1980. Thiotic acid in the treatment of poisoning with alpha-amanitin. In: Faulstich, H., Kommerell, B., Wieland, T., eds. Amanita Toxins and Poisoning. Baden-Baden. *Verlg Gerhard Witzstrock*:197–202.

Bashir, Y., Sneddon, J.F., Staunton, A., et al. 1993. Effects of long-term oral magnesium chloride replacement in congestive heart failure secondary to coronary artery disease. *Am J Cardiol*:72:1156–62.

Bauer, J.E., et al. 1998. Dietary flaxseed in dogs results in differential transport and metabolism of (n-3) poly-unsaturated fatty acids. *J Nutr*:128(Suppl):2641S–4S.

Baum, M.K., Shor-Posner, G., and Campa, A. 2000. Zinc status in human immunodeficiency virus infection. *J Nutr*:130(5S Suppl):1421S–1423S.

Begin, M.E., et al. Differential Killing of Human Carcinoma Cells Supplementing with N-3 and N-6 Poly-unsaturated Fatty Acids *J Natl Cancer Instit*: 77:5 1053–1062, 1986.

Belfield, W.O. 1998. Orthomolecular Medicine: A Practitioners Prospective, in Alternative and Complementary Veterinary Medicine," In: Schoen, A., Wynn, S., St. Louis: Mosby. p 113.

Belfield, W.O., Zucker, M. 1981. How to have a healthy dog; the benefits of vitamin and minerals for your dogs life cycle. New York: New American Library.

Belfield, W.O., 1983. An Orthomolecular Approach to Feline Leukemia Prevention and Control. *J. of Int Acad. of Prev. Med.*, 8(3):40.

Belluzzi, A., Brignola, C., Campieri, M., et al. 1996. Effect of an enteric-coated fish-oil preparation on relapses in Crohn's disease. *N Engl J Med*:334:1557–60.

Bendich, A., Langseth, L. 1995. The health effects of vitamin C supplementation: a review. *J Am Coll Nutr*:14:124–136.

Berg, J., 1990. Polyscorbate (C-Flex): an interesting alternative for problems on the support and movement apparatus in dogs; clinical trial of ester-C ascorbate in dogs, *Norweg Vet J*:102:579.

Berlin, R., Berlin, H., Brante, G., and Pilbrant, A. 1978. Vitamin B$_{12}$ body stores during oral and parenteral treatment of pernicious anaemia. *Acta Med Scand*:204:81–4.

Besset, A., Bonardet, A., Rondouin, G., et al. 1982. Increase in sleep related GH and Prl secretion after chronic arginine aspartate administration in man. *Acta Endocrinol*:99:18–23.

Bilbey, D.L.J., Prabhakaran, V.M. July, 1996. Muscle cramps and magnesium deficiency: case reports. *Canadian Family Physician*:Vol. 42, 1348–51

Blake, G.J., Ridker, P.M. 2003. C-reactive protein and other inflammatory risk markers in acute coronary syndromes. *J Am Coll Cardiol*:41(4 Suppl S):37S–42S.

Block, G., Patterson, B., Subar, A. 1992. Fruit, vegetables and cancer prevention: a review of the epidemiological evidence. *Nutr. Cancer*:18:1–29.

Block, G. 1992. A role for antioxidants in reducing cancer risk. *Nutrition Reviews*:50: 207–213,

Block G. 1992. Vitamin C, Cancer and Aging. *Age* 16:55.

Bohlke, K., Spiegelman, D., Trichopoulou, A., Katsouyanni, K., Trichopoulos, D. 1999. Vitamins A, C and E and the risk of breast cancer: results from a case-control study in Greece. *Br. J. Cancer*:79(1):23–29.

Borreck, S., Hildebrandt, A., Forster, J. Borage seed oil and atopic dermatitis. *Klinische Pediatrie*: 1997;203:100–4.

Bortolotti, F., Cadrobbi, P., Crivellaro, C., et al. 1988. Effect of an orally administered thymic derivative, thymomodulin, in chronic type B hepatitis in children. *Curr Ther Res*:43:67–72.

Bortnick, S.J, Orandle, M.S., Papadi, G.P., Johnson, C.M. 1999. Lymphocyte subsets in neonatal and juvenile cats: comparison of blood and lymphoid tissues. *Lab. Anim. Sci*:44:395–400.

Bostick, R. 2001. Diet and nutrition in the prevention of colon cancer. In: Bendich, A., Deckelbaum, R.J., eds. Preventive Nutrition: The Comprehensive Guide for Health Professionals. 2nd ed. Totowa: Humana Press, Inc:57–95.

Bostick, R.M., Fosdick, L., Wood, J.R., et al. 1995. Calcium and colorectal epithelial cell proliferation in sporadic adenoma patients: a randomized, double-blinded, placebo controlled clinical trial. *J Natl Cancer Inst*:87:1307–15.

Bouic, P.J.D. 1998. Sterols/Sterolins: The natural, nontoxic immuno-modulators and their role in the control of rheumatoid arthritis. *The Arthritis Trust*:Summer:3–6.

Bouic, P.J.D. Sept. 1997. Immunomodulation in HIV/AIDS: The Tygerberg Stellenbosch University experience. AIDS Bulletin published by the Medical Research Council of South Africa:6(3):18–20.

Bouic, P.J.D., Etsebeth, S., Liebenberg, R.W., et al. 1996. Beta-sitosterol and beta-sitosterol glycoside stimulate human peripheral blood lymphocyte proliferation: implications for their use as an immunomodulatory vitamin combination. *Int J Immunopharmacol*:18:693–700.

Bouic, P.J.D. 1999. Plant sterols and sterolins: a review of their immune-modulating properties. *Altern Med Rev*:4:170–177.

Brady, T., 1994. Nutritional Biochemistry. New York: Academic Press.

Braga, P.C., Dal Sasso, M., Maci, S., et al. 1994. Restoration of polymorphonuclear leukocyte function in elderly subjects by thymomodulin. *J Chemother*:6:354–9.

Brennan, L.A., Morris, G.M., Wasson, G.R., Hannigan, B.M., Barnett, Y.V. 2000. The effect of vitamin C or vitamin E supplementation on basal and H$_2$O$_2$-induced DNA damage in human lymphocytes. *Br J Nutr*:84:195–202.

Broadhurst, C.L. 2001. The essential PUFA guide for dogs and cats. *Nutrition Science News*;6(10):366–376.

Brockman, K. Undated. The Use of Serum Venous Analysis to Establish Individual Nutritional Profiles, The Brockman Work.

Brody, T. 1999. Nutritional Biochemistry. 2nd ed. San Diego: Academic Press.

Broek, A., Thoday, K., 1986. Skin Disease in the Dog Associated with Zinc Deficiency: A Report of Five Cases. *J of Small Animal Pract*:27: 313.

Brook, J.G., Linn, S., Aviram, M. 1986. Dietary soya lecithin decreases plasma triglyceride levels and inhibits collagen-and ADP-induced platelet aggregation. *Biochem Med Metab Biol*:35:31–9.

Brooks, J.D., Thompson, L.U. 2005. Mammalian lignans and genistein decrease the activities of aromatase and 17beta-hydroxysteroid dehydrogenase in MCF-7 cells. *J Steroid Biochem Mol Biol*:94(5):461–467.

Brooks, J.O. 3rd, Yesavage, J.A., et al. 1998. Acetyl L-carnitine slows decline in younger patients with Alzheimer's disease: a re-analysis of a double-blind, placebo-controlled study using the trilinear approach. *Int Psychogeriatr*:Jun;10(2):193–203.

Brown, R.A., Weiss, J.B. 1981. Neovascularization and its role in the osteoarthritic process. *Ann. Rheum. Dis*:4.

Brown, L.P. 1994. Ester-C for Joint Discomfort—A Study. *Natural Pet*, Nov–Dec.

Brown, L.P. 1994. Vitamin C (Ascorbic Acid)—New Forms and Uses in Dogs. *Proceeding of the North American Veterinary Conference*, Orlando, FL.

Buchman, A.L., O'Brien, W., Ou, C.N., Rognerud, C., Alvarez, M., Dennis, K., and Ahn. C. 1999. The effect of arginine or glycine supplementation on gastrointestinal function, muscle injury, serum amino acid concentrations and performance during a marathon run. *Int J Sports Med*:Jul;20(5): 315–21.

Budwig, J. 1992. Flax Oil as a True Aid Against Arthritis, Heart Infarction, Cancer and Other Diseases. Vancouver: Apple Publ.

Burger, I. 1993. The Waltham Book of Companion Animal Nutrition. Pergamon Press.

Burk, R.F., Levander, O.A. Selenium. 1999. In: Shils, M., Olson, J.A., Shike, M., Ross, A.C., eds. Nutrition in Health and Disease. 9th ed. Baltimore: Williams and Wilkins:265–276.

Burri, B.J. 2000. Carotenoids and gene expression. *Nutrition* Jul–Aug 31;16(7–8):577–8.

Bursell, S.E., Schlossman, D.K., Clermont, A.C., et al. 1999. High-dose vitamin E supplementation normalizes retinal blood flow and creatinine clearance in patients with type I diabetes. *Diabetes Care*:22:1245–51.

Busse, E., Zimmer, G., Schorpohl, B., et al. 1992. Influence of alpha-lipoic acid on intracellular glutathione in vitro and in vivo. *Arzneimittelforschung*:42:829–31.

Cameron, E., Pauling, L. 1977. Vitamin C and Cancer. *Intl J of Environmental Studies*. 75:4538.

Cameron, E., Pauling, L. 1976. Supplemental ascorbate in the supportive treatment of cancer: Prolongation of survival times in terminal human cancer. *Proc Natl Acad Sci USA*; 73(10):3685–3689.

Campbell, D.J., Rawlings, J.M., Koelsch, S., Wallace, J.M.W., Strain, J.J. and Hannigan, B.M. 2001. Age-related differences in leukocyte populations, lymphocyte subsets, and immunoglobulin (Ig) production in the cat. *Scand J Immunol*. 54 (suppl. 1):1.24–1.59.

Cannon, W.B., 1939. The Wisdom of the Body, 2nd edition. New York: W.W. Norton.

Capron, L. 1993. Marine Oils and Prevention of Cardiovascular Disease. *Revue Practicien*: 43:164.

Carmichael, J. 1982. Use of Nutritional Precursors of Prostaglandin E, in the Management of Rheumatoid Arthritis and Chronic Coxackie Infection. In: Horobin, D., ed., Clinical use of essential fatty acids. Quebec: Eden Press.

Carr, A.C., Frei, B. 1999. Toward a new recommended dietary allowance for vitamin C based on antioxidant and health effects in humans. *Am J Clin Nutr*:69(6):1086–1107.

Casson, P.R., Andersen, R.N., Herrod, H.G., et al. 1993. Oral dehydroepiandrosterone in physiologic doses modulates immune function in postmenopausal women. *Am J Obstet Gynecol*;169:1536–9.

Castell, L.M., Poortmans, J.R., Newsholme, E.A. Does glutamine have a role in reducing infections in athletes? *Eur J Appl Physiol* 1996;73:488–90.

Cator, R.L. 1984. Panhandle Regional Veterinary Clinic, Spearman, Texas, personal communication.

Cenacchi, T., Bertoldin. T., Farina, C., et al. 1993. Cognitive decline in the elderly: a double-blind, placebo-controlled multicenter study on efficacy of phosphatidylserine administration. *Aging*;5:123–33.

Center, S.A. Safe weight loss in cats. 1998. In: Reinhart, G.A., Carey, D.P., eds. Recent Advances in Canine and Feline Nutrition Volume II: Iams Nutrition Symposium Proceedings. Wilmington, Ohio: Orange Frazer Press; 165–181.

Cerutti, P., Ghosh, R., Oya, Y., Amstad, P. 1994. The role of the cellular antioxidant defense in oxidant carcinogenesis. *Environmental Health Perspectives* 102 (suppl 10): 123–130.

Charles, A. 1982. DMG Proving to be a Valuable Aid in Competition. *Horse World*. Oct.:20.

Charlton, C.J., Smith, B.H.E., O'Reilly, J.D., Rock, E., Mazur, A., Treunov, E., Harper, E.J. 2000. Dietary carotenoid absorption in the domestic cat. *FASEB J*:14:363.15.

Cherchi, A., et al. 1985. Effects of L-Carnitine on Exercise Tolerance in Chronic Stable Angina: A Multicenter, Double-blind, Randomized, Placebo-controlled, Crossover Study. *Intl J of Clin Pharm Ther Toxico*: 23:569–72.

Ching, S., Ingram, D., Hahnel, R., Beilby, J., Rossi, E. 2002. Serum levels of micronutrients, antioxidants and total antioxidant status predict risk of breast cancer in a case control study. *J Nutr*;132(2):303–306.

Cichoke, A.J. 1995. The Effect of Systemic Enzyme Therapy on Cancer Cells and the Immune System. Townsend Letter of Doctors and Patients;30–32.

Cima, J., 2000. Biochemical Bloodwork Evaluation, North Palm Beach, FL.

Cima, J., 1981. Biochemical Bloodwork Evaluation, North Palm Beach, FL.

Civeira, M.P., Castilla, A., Morte, S., et al. 1989. A pilot study of thymus extract in chronic non–A, non-B hepatitis. *Aliment Pharmacol Ther*;3:395–401.

Cochrane, C.G., Gimbrone, M.A., Jr. 1992. Biological Oxidants: Generation and Injurious Consequences. San Diego: Academic Press.

Collins, A.R. 1999. Oxidative DNA damage, antioxidants, and cancer. *Bioessays* 21: 238–246.

Committee on Animal Nutrition, SubCommittee on Dogs. 1974. Nutrient Requirements of Dogs, National Research Council. Washington, DC. National Academy of Science. Revised 1985.

Committee on Animal Nutrition, SubCommittee on Cats. 1978. Nutrient Requirements of Cats, National Research Council. Washington, DC. National Academy of Science. Revised 1986.

Comstock, G.W., Helzlsouer, K.J. 2001. Preventive nutrition and lung cancer. In: Bendich, A., Decklebaum, R.J., eds. Preventive Nutrition: The Comprehensive Guide for Health Professionals. 2nd ed. Totowa: Humana Press Inc; 97–129.

Cooper, K.H. 1997. The Antioxidant Revolution. Nashville TN: Thomas Nelson.

Costell, M., O'Connor, J.E., Grisolia, S. 1989. Age-dependent decrease of carnitine content in muscle of mice and humans. *Biochem Biophys Res Commun*;161(3):1135–1143.

Cotterell, C.J., Lee, A.J., Hunter, J.O. 1990. Double-blind crossover trial of evening primrose oil in women with menstrually-related irritable bowel syndrome. In: Omega-6 Essential Fatty

Acids: Pathophysiology and roles in clinical medicine. New York: Alan R Liss; 421–6.

Craveri, F., De Pascale, V. 1971. Activity of orally administered adrenocortical extract. I. Effect on the survival test. *Boll Chim Farm*;110:457–62.

Creagan, E.T., Moertel, C.G., O'Fallon, J.R., et al. 1979. Failure of high-dose vitamin C (ascorbic acid) therapy to benefit patients with advanced cancer. *N Engl J Med*;301(13): 687–690.

Crook, T.H., Tinklenberg, J., Yesavage, J., et al. 1991. Effects of phosphatidylserine in age-associated memory impairment. *Neurology*;41:644–9.

Crook, T., Petrie, W., Wells, C., Massari, D.C. 1992. Effects of phosphatidylserine in Alzheimer's disease. *Psychopharmacol Bull*;28:61–6.

Cunningham, J.G. 1997. Textbook of Veterinary Physiology, Second Edition, Philadelphia, PA.: WB Saunders Company.

Curhan, G.C., Willett, W.C., Rimm, E.B., Stampfer, M.J. 1993. A prospective study of dietary calcium and other nutrients and the risk of symptomatic kidney stones. *N Engl J Med*;328: 833–83.

Dale, P.S., Tamhankar, C.P., George, D., Daftary, G.V. 2001. Co-medication with hydrolytic enzymes in radiation therapy of uterine cervix: evidence of the reduction of acute side effects. *Cancer Chemother Pharmacol*; Jul;47 Suppl:S29–34.

D'Ambrosia, E., Casa, B., Bompani, R., Scali, G., Scali, M. 1982. Glucosamine Sulphate: A Controlled Clinical Investigation in Arthrosis. *Pharmatherapeutica*; 2:504–508.

Das, A.K., Hammad, T.A. 2000. Efficacy of a combination of FCHG49TM glucosamine hydrochloride, TRH122TM low molecular weight sodium chondroitin sulfate and manganese ascorbate in the management of knee osteoarthritis. *Osteoarthritis Cart*;8(5):343–350.

Davenport, G.M., Williams, C.C., Cummins, K.A., Hayek, M. G. 1998. Protein Metabolism and Aging. *Recent Advances in Canine and Feline Nutrition, Volume II, Iams Symposium*. Wilmington, OH: Orange Frazer Press.

Davenport, G., Gaasch, S., Hayek, M.G., Cummins, K.A. 2001. Effect of dietary protein on body composition and metabolic responses of geriatric and young-adult dogs. *J. Vet. Intern. Med.*; 15:306.

Davenport, G.M., Williams, C.C., Cummins, K.A., Hayek, M. G. 1998. Protein Metabolism and Aging. In: Reinhart, G.A., Carey, D.P., eds. Recent Advances in Canine and Feline Nutritional Research, Vol II: 1998 Iams Nutritional Proceeding. Wilmington: Orange Frazier Press; 363–378.

Davies, K.J. 1995. Oxidative stress: the paradox of aerobic life. *Biochem Soc Symp*; 61:1–31.

Davies, K.J.A. 1991. Oxidative Damage and Repair. Chemical, Biological and Medical Aspects. Oxford: Pergamon.

Davini, P., Bigalli, A., Lamanna, F., Boem, A. 1992. Controlled study on L-carnitine therapeutic efficacy in post-infarction. *Drugs Exp Clin Res*; 18(8):355–365.

Dean, G.A., Quackenbush, S.L., Ackley, C.D., Cooper, M.D., Hoover, E.A. 1991. Flow cytometric analysis of T-lymphocyte subsets in cats. *Vet Immunol Immunopathol*:28:327–335.

Deaton, C.M., Marlin, D.J., Smith, N.C., Harris, P.A., Roberts, C.A., Schroter, R.C., Kelly, F.J. 2004. Pulmonary epithelial lining fluid and plasma ascorbic acid concentrations in horses affected by recurrent airway obstruction. *Am J Vet Res*: 65:80–87.

Delgado-Vargas, F., Jimenez, A.R., Paredes-Lopez, O. 2000. Natural pigments: carotenoids, anthocyanins, and betalains—characteristics, biosynthesis, processing, and stability. *Crit Rev Food Sci Nutr*; May;40(3):173–289.

de Kleijn, M.J., van der Schouw, Y.T., Wilson, P.W., Grobbee, D.E., Jacques, P.F. 2002. Dietary intake of phytoestrogens is associated with a favorable metabolic cardiovascular risk profile in postmenopausal U.S. women: the Framingham study. *J Nutr*;132(2):276–282.

de la Fuente, M., Ferrandez, M.D., Burgos, M.S., et al. 1998. Immune function in aged women is improved by ingestion of vitamins C and E. *Can J Physiol Pharmacol*;76:373–80.

Delwaide, P.J., et al. 1986. Double-blind Randomized Controlled Study of Phosphatidylserine in Demented Patients. *Acta Neurol Scand*, 73:136–140.

De Simone, C., Vesely, R., Bianchi, S.B., et al. 1993. The role of probiotics in modulation of the immune system in man and in animals. *Int J Immunother*;9:23–8.

Dieter, J.A, Stewart, D.R., Haggarty, M.A., Stabenfeldt, G.H., Lasley, B.L. 1993. Pregnancy failure in cats associated with long-term dietary taurine insufficiency. *J Reprod Fertil Suppl*;47:457–63.

Divi, R.L., Chang, H.C., Doerge, D.R. 1997. Anti-thyroid isoflavones from soybean: isolation, characterization, and mechanisms of action. *Biochem Pharmacol*;54(10):1087–1096.

Downey, D.S. 1996. Balancing Body Chemistry with Nutrition Seminars for Doctors Licensed in the Healing Arts, 1st Revision. Cannonsburg, MI: Balancing Body Chemistry with Nutrition.

Duke, J. 1992. Handbook of biologically active phytochemicals and their activities. Boca Raton, FL: CRC Press; 131:99.

Duke, J.A. 1992. Handbook of phytochemical constituents of GRAS herbs and other economic plants. Boca Raton, FL: CRC Press;28.

Duthie, S.J., Ma, A.-G., Ross, M.A., Collins, A.R. 1996. Antioxidant supplementation decreases oxidative DNA damage in human lymphocytes. *Cancer Res* 56:1291–1295.

Ehrenpreis, E.D., Jani, A., Levitsky, J., Ahn, J., Hong, J. 2005. A prospective, randomized, double-blind, placebo-controlled trial of retinol palmitate (vitamin A) for symptomatic chronic radiation proctopathy. *Dis.Colon Rectum*;48(1): 1–8.

Eibl, N.L., Schnack, C.J., Kopp, H.-P., et al. 1995. Hypomagnesemia in type II diabetes: effect of a 3-month replacement therapy. *Diabetes Care*;18:188.

Engel, R.R., Satzger, W., Gunther, W., et al. 1992. Double-blind crossover study of phosphatidylserine vs. placebo in patients with early dementia of the Alzheimer type. *Eur Neuropsychopharmacol*;2:149–55.

English, R.V., Nelson, P., Johnson, C.M., Nasisse, M., Tompkins, W.A., Tompkins, M.B. 1994. Development of clinical disease in cats experimentally infected with feline immunodeficiency virus. *J Infect Dis*. 170:543–552.

Enstrom, J.E., Kanim, L.E., Klein, M.A. 1992. Vitamin C intake and mortality among a sample of the United States population. *Epidemiology*;3(3):194–202.

Erasmus, U. 1993. Fats That Heal Fats That Kill; revised and updated edition. Vancouver: Alive Books. The Complete Lecture, www.udoerasmus.com

Erasmus, U., 1986. Fats and Oils. Vancouver: Alive Books.

Erbersdobler, H., et al. 1984. Histopathological studies of rat kidneys following the feeding of heat-damaged proteins. *Z Ernahrungswiss* vol. 23, no. 3 (Sept.), pp. 219–229.

Estrada, D.E., Ewart, H.S., Tsakiridis, T., et al. 1996. Stimulation of glucose uptake by the natural coenzyme alpha-lipoic acid/thioctic acid: participation of elements of the insulin signaling pathway. *Diabetes*;45(12):1798–1804.

Evans, G.W. 1989. The effect of chromium picolinate on insulin controlled parameters in humans. *Int J Biosocial Med Res*;11:163–80.

Evangeliou, A., Vlassopoulos, D. 2003. Carnitine metabolism and deficit—when is supplementation necessary? *Curr Pharm Biotechnol;* Jun;4(3):211–9.

Fahey, T.D., Pearl, M.S. 1998. The hormonal and perceptive effects of phosphatidylserine administration during two weeks of resistive exercise-induced overtraining. *Biol Sport*;15:135–144.

Farr, S.A., Poon, H.F., Dogrukol-Ak, D., et al. 2003. The antioxidants alpha-lipoic acid and N-acetylcysteine reverse memory impairment and brain oxidative stress in aged SAMP8 mice. *J Neurochem*;84(5):1173–1183.

Feiz, H.R., Mobarhan, S. 2002. Does vitamin C intake slow the progression of gastric cancer in Helicobacter pylori-infected populations? *Nutr Rev*;60(1):34–36.

Filina, A.A., Davydova, N.G., Endrikhovskii, S.N., et al. 1995. Lipoic acid as a means of metabolic therapy of open-angle glaucoma. *Vestn Oftalmol*;111:6–8.

Fiocchi, A., Borella, E., Riva, E., et al. 1986. A double-blind clinical trial for the evaluation of the therapeutic effectiveness of a calf thymus derivative (Thymomodulin) in children with recurrent respiratory infections. *Thymus*;8:831–9.

Flood, J.F., Roberts, E. 1988. Dehydroepiandrosterone Sulfate Improves Memory in Aging Mice. *Brain Res;*448:178–181.

Folkers, K., Shizukuishi, S., Takemura, K., et al. 1982. Increase in levels of IgG in serum of patients treated with coenzyme Q10. *Res Commun Pathol Pharmacol*;38:335–8.

Folkers, K., et al. 1985. Biochemical Rationale and Mitochondrial Tissue Data on the Effective Therapy of Cardiomyopathy with Coenzyme Q10. *Proc Natl Acad Sci*;82: 901.

Folkers, K., Yamancria, Y. 1986. Biomedical and Clinical Aspect of Coenzyme Q10. Fifth Edition. New York: Elsevier.

Food and Nutrition Board, Institute of Medicine. 1997. Calcium. Dietary Reference Intakes: Calcium, Phosphorus, Magnesium, Vitamin D, and Fluoride. Washington, DC: National Academy Press;71–145.

Food and Nutrition Board, Institute of Medicine. 2000. Vitamin E. Dietary reference intakes for vitamin C, vitamin E, selenium, and carotenoids. Washington, DC: National Academy Press;186–283.

Fox, P.R., Sturman, J.A. 1992. Myocardial taurine concentrations in cats with cardiac disease and in healthy cats fed taurine-modified diets, *Am J Vet Res*;Feb;53(2):237–41

Fox, A.D., et al. 1988. Effect of glutamine supplemented enteral diet on methotrexate induced enterocolitis, *JPEN*;12:325–331.

Frank, C. 1992. Official Publication of the Association of American Feed Control Officials. Dept of Agriculture. Atlanta, GA. 30334

Freidman, R. 1956. Cholesterol Metabolism. *Ann Rev of Biochem*, 25:613.

Fridovich, I. 1972. Superoxide Radical and Superoxide Dismutase, *Acc Chem Res*;5:321.

Frykman, E., Bystrom, M., Jansson, U., et al. 1994. Side effects of iron supplements in blood donors: superior tolerance of heme iron. *J Lab Clin Med*;123:561–4.

Fujisawa, K., Suzuki, H., Yamamoto, S., et al. 1984. Therapeutic effects of liver hydrolysate preparation on chronic hepatitis—A double-blind, controlled study. *Asian Med J*;26:497–526.

Fünfgeld, E.W., Baggen, M., Nedwidek, P., et al. 1989. Double-blind study with phosphatidylserine (PS) in Parkinsonian patients with senile dementia of Alzheimer's type (SDAT). *Prog Clin Biol Res*;317:123–46.

Gaby, A.R. 1998. Coenzyme Q10. In: Pizzorno, J.E., Murray, M.T., eds. A Textbook of Natural Medicine. Seattle: Bastyr College Publications.

Gaby, A.R., Wright, J.V. 1996. Diabetes. In: Nutritional Therapy in Medical Practice: Reference Manual and Study Guide. Kent, WA: Wright/Gaby Seminars. 54–64 [review].

Gaby, A.R., Wright, J.V. 1996. Nutritional protocols: diabetes mellitus. In: Nutritional Therapy in Medical Practice: Protocols and Supporting Information. Kent, WA: Wright/Gaby Seminars. 10.

Gaby, A.R. 1996. The role of coenzyme Q10 in clinical medicine: part II. Cardiovascular disease, hypertension, diabetes mellitus and infertility. *Altern Med Rev*;1:168–75.

Galli, L., de Martino, M., Azzari, C., et al. 1990. Preventive effect of thymomodulin in recurrent respiratory infections in children. *Pediatr Med Chir*;12:229–32.

Gannon, J., Kendall, R. 1982. A Clinical Evaluation of N,N-Dimethylglycine (DMG) and Disopropylammonium Dichloroacetate (DIPA) on the Performance of Racing Greyhounds. *Canine Practice*;9;7 Nov–Dec.

Gardner, M.J. 1988. Gastrointestinal absorption of intact proteins. *Ann Rev Nutr*;8:329–350.

Gaziano, J.M., et al. 1995. A prospective study of consumption of carotenoids in fruits and vegetables and decreased cardiovascular mortality in the elderly. *Ann Epidemiol*; Jul;5(4):255–60.

Geleijnse, J.M., Launer, L.J., Van der Kuip, D.A., Hofman, A., Witteman, J.C. 2002. Inverse association of tea and flavonoid intakes with incident myocardial infarction: the Rotterdam Study. *Am J Clin Nutr*;75(5):880–886.

Gentile, J.M., et al. 1991. The metabolic activation of 4-nitro-o-phenylenediamine by chlorophyll-containing plant extracts: the relationship between mutagenicity and antimutagenicity. *Mutat Res*;Sep–Oct;250(1–2):79–86.

George, J.W., Pedersen, N.C., Higgins, J. 1993. The effect of age on the course of experimental feline immunodeficiency virus infection in cats. *AIDS Res Hum Retroviruses*;9:897–905.

Gil, M.I., Ferreres, F., Tomas-Barberan, F.A. 1999. Effect of postharvest storage and processing on the antioxidant constituents (flavonoids and vitamin C) of fresh-cut spinach. *J Agric Food Chem*;47(6):2213–7.

Gilchrist, B.A., Bohr, V.A. 1997. Aging processes, DNA damage, and repair. *FASEB J*;11: 322–330.

Giovannucci, E., Stampfer, M.J., Colditz, G.A., et al. 1993. Folate, methionine, and alcohol intake and risk of colorectal adenoma. *J Natl Cancer Inst*;85:875–84.

Giugliano, D. 2000. Dietary antioxidants for cardiovascular prevention. *Nutr Metab Cardiovasc Dis;* Feb;10(1):38–44.

Golde, D.W. 2003. Vitamin C in cancer. *Integr Cancer Ther*;2(2):158–159.

Golden, B.R., Gorbach, S.L. 1984. The Effect of Milk and Lactobacillus Feeding on Human Intestinal Bacteria Activity. *Am J of Clin Nutr*;39:756–61.

Goldstein, R., Goldstein S. 2005. The Goldstein Wellness and Longevity Program, Neptune City, NJ: TFH Publication.

Goldstein R., et al. 2000. The BNA Handbook: A Working Manual for Veterinarians. Westport, CT: Animal Nutrition Technologies.

Goldstein, R., Post, G. 2006. A clinical trial to evaluate chemotherapy in combination with an antioxidant rich nutritional program in the treatment of Lymphosarcoma and Osteosarcoma in dog. Oncology and Hematology Center, Norwalk, CT.

Goldstein, M. 1999. The Nature of Animal Healing. New York: Ballantine Books;106.

Gonzalez, N.J., Isaacs, L.L. 1999. Evaluation of pancreatic proteolytic enzyme treatment of adenocarcinoma of the pancreas, with nutrition and detoxification support. *Nutr Cancer*;33:117–124.

Gonzalez, M.J., Miranda-Massari, J.R., Mora, E.M., et al. 2005. Orthomolecular oncology review: Ascorbic acid and cancer 25 years later. *Integrative Cancer Therapies*;4(1):32–44.

Gorbach, S.L. 1982. The Intestinal Microflora and its Colon Cancer Connection. *Infection*;10(6): 379–384.

Graber, G., Goust. J., Glassman, A., Kendall, R., Loadholt, C. 1981. Immunomodulating Properties of Dimethylglycine in Humans. *Journal of Infectious Disease*;143:101.

Graber, G., Kendall, R. 1986. N,N-Dimethylglycine and Use in Immune Response, US Patent 4,631,189, Dec.

Grant, G., et al. 1982. The effect of heating on the haemagglutinating activity and nutritional properties of bean (*Phaseolus vulgaris*) seeds. *J Sci Food Agric*;vol. 33, no. 12 (Dec.), 1324–1326.

Greeley, E.H., Kealy, R.D., Ballam, J.M., Lawler, D.F., Segre, M. 1996. The influence of age on the canine immune system. *Vet Immunol Immunopathol*;55:1–10.

Greenberg, E.R., Baron, J.A., Tosteson, T.D., et al. 1994. A clinical trial of antioxidant vitamins to prevent colorectal adenoma. Polyp Prevention Study Group. *N Engl J Med*;331(3):141–147.

Greenberg, S., Frishman, W.H. 1990. Co-enzyme Q10: a new drug for cardiovascular disease. *J Clin Pharmacol*;Jul;30(7): 596–608.

Griffin, C.E., Kwochka, K.W., Macdonald, J.M. 1993. Current veterinary dermatology: the science and art of therapy. St. Louis: Mosby.

Griffiths, R.D. 1997. Outcome of critically ill patients after supplementation with glutamine. *Nutrition*;13:752–4 [review].

Guastella, D.B., Cook, J.L., Kuroki, K., et al. 2005. Evaluation of chondroprotective nutriceuticals in an in vitro osteoarthritis model. *Proceedings. 32nd Annual Conference Veterinary Orthopedic Society*;5.

Gujral, M.S., Patnaik, P.M., Kaul, R., Parikh, H.K., Conradt, C., Tamhankar, C.P., Daftary, G.V. 2001. Efficacy of hydrolytic enzymes in preventing radiation therapy-induced side effects in patients with head and neck cancers. *Cancer Chemother Pharmacol*;Jul;47 Suppl:S23–28.

Gupta, M.B., Nath, R., Srivastava, N., et al. 1980. Anti-inflammatory and antipyretic activities of β-sitosterol. *Planta Medica*;39:157–163.

Guyton, A.C. 1961. Textbook of Medical Physiology, Second Edition, Philadelphia: W.B. Saunders Company.

Ha, Y.L., et al. 1987. Anticarcinogens from fried ground beef: heat-altered derivatives of linoleic acid. *Carcinogenesis;* vol. 8, no. 12 (Dec.), 1881–1887.

Hagen, T.M., Liu, J., Lykkesfeldt, J., et al. 2002. Feeding acetyl-L-carnitine and lipoic acid to old rats significantly improves metabolic function while decreasing oxidative stress. *Proc Natl Acad Sci USA*;99(4):1870–1875.

Halliwell, B. 1994. Free radicals and antioxidants: a personal view. *Nutr Rev*;52:253–265.

Halliwell, B., Aruoma, O.I. 1993. DNA and Free Radicals. Chichester, UK: Ellis Horwood.

Halliwell, B., Gutteridge, J.M.C. 1989. Free Radicals in Biology and Medicine. Oxford, UK: Clarendon Press.

Halliwell, B. 1997. Antioxidants and human disease: a general introduction *Nutr Rev*;55:S49–S52.

Halliwell, B. 1999. Establishing the significance and optimal intake of dietary antioxidants: the biomarker concept. *Nutr Rev*;57:104–113.

Hand, M., Thatcher, C., Remillard, R., Roudorbush, R. 2000. Small Animal Nutrition, 4th Edition, Topeka, KS: Mark Morris Institute.

Hanin, I., Ansell, G.B. 1987. Lecithin: Technological, Biological, and Therapeutic Aspects. New York: Plenum Press, 180, 181.

Hanioka, T., Tanaka, M., Ojima, M., et al. 1994. Effect of topical application of coenzyme Q10 on adult periodontitis. *Mol Aspects Med*;15(Suppl):S241–8.

Hariganesh, K., Prathiba, J. 2000. Effects of DMG on Gastric Ulcers in Rats. *J Pharm Pharmacol*;52:1519.

Harker-Murray, A.K., Tajik, A.J., Ishikura, F., Meyer, D., Burnett, J.C., Redfield, M.M. 2000. The role of coenzyme Q10 in the pathophysiology and therapy of experimental congestive heart failure in the dog. *J Card Fail*;Sep;6(3):233–42.

Harman, D. 1992. Free radical theory of aging. In: Emerit, I., Chance, B., eds. Free Radicals and Aging. Basel: Birkhauser Verlag.

Harman, D. 1994. Free-radical theory of aging: increasing the functional life span. *Ann NY Acad Sci*;717:1–15.

Harman, D. 1955. Aging: A theory based on free radical and radiation chemistry. *Univ Calif Rad Lab Report No. 3078*, July 14.

Harman, D., Miller, R.W. 1986. Effects of vitamin E on the immune response to influenza virus vaccine and the incidence of infectious disease in man. *Age*;9:21–23.

Harrower, H., et al. 1939. Endocrine Handbook, The Harrower Laboratory, Inc., Glendale, CA.

Harrower, H.B. 1916. Practical Hormone Therapy—A Manual of Ongoing Therapy. NY.

Harrower, H.R. 1933. Endocrine Pointers. The Harrower Laboratory, Inc. Glendale, CA. 205p.

Harrower, H.L. 1913. *Lancet*;1:524.

Hartleb, M., Leuschner, J. 1997. Toxicological profile of a low molecular weight spleen peptide formulation used in supportive cancer therapy. *Arzneimittelforschung*;47:1047–51.

Harttig, U., et al. 1998. Chemoprotection by natural chlorophylls in vivo: inhibition of dibenzo[a,l]pyrene-DNA adducts in rainbow trout liver. *Carcinogenesis* Jul;19(7): 1323–6.

Hayek, M.G., Massimino, S.P., Burr, J.R., Kearns, R.J. 2000. Dietary vitamin E improves immune function in cats. In: Reinhart, G.A. Carey, D.P., eds. Recent Advances in Canine and Feline Nutrition, Iams Nutrition Symposium Proceedings III:555–563 Wilmington, OH: Orange Frazer Press.

Hayek, M.G., Davenport, G.M. 1998. Nutrition and aging in companion animals. *J Anti-Aging Med*;1:117–123.

Hayek, M.G., Reinhart, G.A. 1998. Utilization of w3 fatty acids in companion animal nutrition. *World Rev Nutr Diet*;83:176–85.

Head, K.A. 1999. Ipriflavone: an important bone-building isoflavone. *Altern Med Rev*;Feb;4(1):10–22.

Heaton, P.R., Ransley, R., Charlton, C.J., Mann, S.J., Stevenson, J., Smith, B.H., Rawlings, J.M., Harper, E.J. 2002. Application of single-cell gel electrophoresis (comet) assay for assessing levels of DNA damage in canine and feline leukocytes. *J Nutr*;132:1598S–1603S.

Heaton, P.R., Blount, D.G., Devlin, P., Koelsch, S., Mann, S.J., Smith, B.H.E., Stevenson, J., Harper, E.J. 2002. Assessing age-related changes in peripheral blood leukocyte phenotypes in Labrador retriever dogs using flow cytometry. *J Nutr*; 132:1655S–1657S,June.

Heaton, P.R., Reed, C.F., Mann, S.J., Ransley, R., Stevenson, J., Charlton, C.J., Smith, B.H., Harper, E.J., Rawlings, J.M. 2002. Role of dietary antioxidants to protect against DNA damage in adult dogs. *J Nutr*;132:1720S–1724S.

Hederos, C.A., Berg, A. 1996. Epogam evening primrose oil treatment in atopic dermatitis and asthma. *Arch Dis Child*; 75(6):494–497.

Heinonen, O.P., Albanes, D., Virtamo, J., et al. 1998. Prostate cancer and supplementation with alpha-tocopherol and beta-carotene: incidence and mortality in a controlled trial. *J Natl Cancer Inst*;90(6):440–446.

Helzlsouer, K.J., Huang, H.Y., Alberg, A.J., et al. 2000. Association between alpha-tocopherol, gamma-tocopherol, selenium, and subsequent prostate cancer. *J Natl Cancer Inst*;92(24): 2018–2023.

Hermann, J., Chung, H., Arquitt, A., et al. 1998. Effects of chromium or copper supplementation on plasma lipids, plasma glucose and serum insulin in adults over age fifty. *J Nutr Elderly*;18:27–45.

Herman, H.A., et al. 1998. The Influence of Dietary Omega-6: Omega-3 Ratio in Lameness in Dogs with Osteoarthrosis of the Elbow Joint Recent Advances in Canine and Feline Nutrition, Volume II. Iams Proceedings; p 325.

Hertog, M.G., Feskens, E.J., Kromhout, D. 1997. Antioxidant flavonols and coronary heart disease risk. *Lancet*;349(9053): 699.

Hertz-Picciotto, I., Schramm, M., Watt-Morse, M., Chantala, K., Anderson, J., Osterloh, J. 2000. Patterns and determinants of blood lead during pregnancy. *Am J Epidemiol*;152(9): 829–837.

Hickman, M.A., et al. 1990. Effect of processing on fate of dietary [14C]taurine in cats. *J Nutr*;vol. 120, no. 9 (Sept.), pp. 995–1000.

Hickman, M.A., et al. 1992. Intestinal taurine and the enterohepatic circulation of taurocholic acid in the cat. In: Lombardini, J.B., et al., eds. Taurine: Nutritional Values and Mechanisms of Action. New York: Plenum.

Hill, A.S., Werner, J.A., Rogers, Q.R., et al. 2004. Lipoic acid is 10 times more toxic in cats than reported in humans, dogs, or rats. *Journal of Animal Physiology and Animal Nutrition*;88:150–156

Hills Company. Canine Cancer Topeka KS.

Hilton, J.W. 1989. Potential Nutrient Deficiencies in Pet Food. *Can Vet J*;30(7):599–601,Jul.

Hilton, E., Isenberg, H.D., Alperstein, P., et al. 1992. Ingestion of yogurt containing Lactobacillus acidophilus as prophylaxis for candidal vaginitis. *Ann Intern Med*;116: 353–7.

Hofman-Bang, C., Rehnqvist, N., Swedberg, K., Wiklund, I., Astrom, H. 1995. Coenzyme Q10 as an adjunctive in the treatment of chronic congestive heart failure. The Q10 Study Group. *J Card Fail*;Mar;1(2):101–7.

Hoffman-Goetz, L., Pedersen, B.K. 1994. Exercise and the immune system: A model of the stress response. *Immunology Today*;15:382–387.

Holub, B. 1995. The Role of Omega-3 Fatty Acids in Health and Disease. *Proceeding of the 13th Annual Conference, American College of Veterinary Medicine.*

Hong, W.K., et al. 1990. Prevention of Second Primary Tumors with Isoreninoin in Squamous Cell Carcinoma of the Head and Neck. *N. England J. of Med*;323:795–801.

Horrocks, L.A., et al. 1986. Phosphatidyl Research and the Nervous System, Berlin: Springer Verlach.

Horrobin, D.F. 1981. The importance of gamma-linolenic acid and prostaglandin E1 in human nutrition and medicine. *J Holistic Med*;3:118–39.

Horrobin, D.F. 1992. Nutritional and medical importance of gamma-linolenic acid. *Prog Lipid Res*;31(2):163–94.

Hotz, J., Plein, K. 1994. Effectiveness of plantago seed husks in comparison with wheat bran on stool frequency and manifestations of irritable colon syndrome with constipation. *Med Klin*;89:645–51.

Howell, E. 1985. Enzyme Nutrition, The Food Enzyme Concept. Garden City, NY: Avery Publ.

Huber, L.G., N.D., 2003. Green tea catechins and L-theonine in integrative cancer care. *Focus*;May,p.4.

Hughes, V.L. 1990. Microbiologic characteristics of Lactobacillus products used for colonization of the vagina. *Obstet Gynecol*;75:244–248.

Humphreys, F., Symons, J., Brown, H., et al. 1994. The effects of gamolenic acid on adult atopic eczema and premenstrual exacerbation of eczema. *Eur J Dermatol*;4(598):603.

Hunter, D.J., Manson, J.E., Colditz, G.A., et al. 1993. A prospective study of the intake of vitamins C, E, and A and the risk of breast cancer. *N Engl J Med*; 329:234–240.

Huxtable, R.J. 1992. Physiological actions of taurine. *Physiological Reviews*;vol.72, pp. 101–163.

Hyman, J., Baron, J.A., Dain, B.J., et al. 1998. Dietary and supplemental calcium and the recurrence of colorectal adenomas. *Cancer Epidemiol Biomarkers Prev*;7:291–5.

Hyson, R.D. 2002. The Health Benefits of Fruits and Vegetables, A Scientific Overview for Health Professionals. Better Health Foundation, p16

International Agency for Research on Cancer. 1998. IARC Handbooks of Cancer Prevention: Carotenoids, Lyon.

Ioku, K., Aoyama, Y., Tokuno, A., et al. 2001. Various cooking methods and the flavonoid content in onion. *J Nutr Sci Vitaminol*(Tokyo);41(7):78–83.

Ito, Y., et al. 1999. A study of serum carotenoids levels in breast cancer in Indian women in Chenni, India. *J Epidemiol*; Nov:9(5):306–14.

Jacobs, E.J., Connell, C.J., McCullough, M.L., et al. 2002. Vitamin C, vitamin E, and multivitamin supplement use and stomach cancer mortality in the Cancer Prevention Study II cohort. *Cancer Epidemiol Biomarkers Prev*;11:35–41.

Jacobsen, J.G., Smith, L.H. 1968. Biochemistry and physiology of taurine and taurine derivatives. *Physiological Reviews*;vol. 48, pp. 424–511.

Jenkins, D.J., Kendall, C.W., Vidgen, E., et al. 1999. Health aspects of partially defatted flaxseed, including effects on serum lipids, oxidative measures, and ex vivo androgen and progestin activity: a controlled crossover trial. *Am J Clin Nutr*;69(3):395–402.

Jenkinson, A. McE., Collins, A.R., Duthie, S.J., Wahle, K.W.J., and Duthie, G.G. 1999. The effect of increased intakes of polyunsaturated fatty acids and vitamin E on DNA damage in human lymphocytes. *FASEB J*;13:2138–2142.

Joe, L.A., Hart, L.L. 1993. Evening primrose oil in rheumatoid arthritis. *Ann Pharmacother*;27:1475–7 [review].

Jones, P.J., Raieini-Sarjaz, M. 2001. Plant sterols and their erivatives: the current spread of results. *Nutr. Rev*;59: 21–4.

Jones, C., Palmer, T.E., Griffiths, R.D. 1999. Randomized clinical outcome study of critically ill patients given glutamine-supplemented enteral nutrition. *Nutrition*;15:108–15.

Jorde, R., Sundsfjord, J., Haug, E., Bønaa, K.H. 2000. Relation between low calcium intake, parathyroid hormone, and blood pressure. *Hypertension*;35:1154–9.

Jones, W. 1988. Lactic Acid and DMG. *The Quarter Racing Journal*;46, June.

Judy, W.V., et al. 1984. Myocardial Effects of Coenzyme Q10 in Primary Heart Failure. Biomedical and Clinical Aspects of Coenzyme Q10. Vol. 4. In: Folkers, K., Yamamura, Y., eds. Amsterdam: Elsevier Science Publishers, pp.353–357.

Kaegi, E. 1998. Task Force on Alternative Therapeutics of the Canadian Breast Cancer Research Initiative. Unconventional therapies for cancer: 5. Vitamins A, C, and E. *CMAJ*;158(11): 1483–1488.

Kagan, V., Serbinova, E., Packer, L. 1990. Antioxidant effects of ubiquinones in microsomes and mitochondria are mediated by tocopherol recycling. *Biochem Biophys Res Commun*;169: 851–7.

Kalimi, M., Regelsen, W. 1990. The Biological Role of Dehydroepiandrosterone. NY: de Gruter.

Kang, S.D., Lee, B.H., Yang, J.H., Lee, C.Y. 1985. The effects of calf-thymus extract on recovery of bone marrow function in anticancer chemotherapy. *New Med J*;28:11–5.

Kawano, Y., Matsuoka, H., Takishita, S., Omae, T. 1998. Effects of magnesium supplementation in hypertensive patients. *Hypertension*;32:260–5.

Kawase, K. 1982. Effects of nutrients on the intestinal microflora of infants. *Jpn J Dairy Food Sci*;31:A241–3.

Keefe, K.A., Schell, M.J., Brewer, C., et al. 2001. A randomized, double blind, Phase III trial using oral beta-carotene supplementation for women with high-grade cervical intraepithelial neoplasia. *Cancer Epidemiol Biomarkers Prev*;10(10): 1029–1035.

Keen, C.L., Ensunsa, J.L., Clegg, M.S. 2000. Manganese metabolism in animals and humans including the toxicity of manganese. *Met Ions Biol Syst*;37:89–121.

Keli, S.O., Hertog, G.L., Feskens, E.J.M., Kromhout, D. 1996. Dietary flavanoids, antioxidant vitamins, and the incidence of stroke. *Arch Int Med*;154:637–642.

Kendall, R., Lawson, J.W. 2000. Recent Findings on N,N-Dimethylglycine (DMG): A Nutrient for the New Millennium, *Townsend Letter for Doctors and Patients*;May.

Kendall, R.V., 2003. Building Wellness with DMG. Topanga, CA: Freedom Press.

Kendall, R., Lawson, J. 1991. Treatment of Melanoma Using N,N-Dimethylglycine, US Patent 4,994,492, Feb.

Kendall, R. 1998. Therapeutic Nutrition for the Cat, Dog and Horse. In: Schoen, A.M., Wynn, S.G., editors. Complementary and Alternative Veterinary Medicine: Principles and Practice. St Louis: Mosby. p.69.

Kendler, B. 1987. Gamma Linolenic Acid: Physiological Effects and Potential Medical Applications. *J of Appl. Nutr*;39:79.

Khatta, M., Alexander, B.S., Krichten, C.M., Fisher, M.L., Freudenberger, R., Robinson, S.W., Gottlieb S.S. 2000. The effect of coenzyme Q10 in patients with congestive heart failure. *Ann Intern Med*;Apr 18;132(8):636–40.

Khorram, O., Vu, L., Yen, S.S. 1997. Activation of immune function by dehydroepiandrosterone (DHEA) in age-advanced men. *J Gerontol A Biol Sci Med Sci*;52: M1–7.

Kim, S.W., et al. 1996a. Dietary antibiotics decrease taurine loss in cats fed a canned heat-processed diet. *J Nutr*;vol. 126, no. 2 (Feb.), pp. 509–515.

Kim, S.W., et al. 1996b. Maillard reaction products in purified diets induce taurine depletion in cats which is reversed by antibiotics. *J Nutr*;vol. 126, no. 1 (Jan.) pp. 195–201.

Kim, Y., Sawada, Y., Fujiwara, G., Chiba, H., Nishimura, T. 1997. Therapeutic effect of co–enzyme Q10 on idiopathic dilated cardiomyopathy: assessment by iodine-123 labelled 15-(p-iodophenyl)3(R,S)-methylpentadecanoic acid myocardial single-photon emission tomography. *Eur J Nucl Med*; Jun;24(6):629–34.

King, J.C., Keen, C.L. Zinc. 1999. In: Shils, M., Olson, J.A., Shike, M., Ross, A.C., eds. Nutrition in health and disease. 9th ed. Baltimore: Williams and Wilkins. 223–239.

Kirk, S.J., Hurson, M., Regan, M.C., et al. 1993. Arginine stimulates wound healing and immune function in elderly human beings. *Surgery*;114:155–60.

Kirschvink, N., Art, T., Smith, N., Lekeux, P. 1999. Effect of exercise and COPD crisis on isoprostane concentration in plasma and bronchoalveolar lavage fluid in horses. *Equine Vet J Supp*;30:88–91.

Kirschvink, N., Smith, N., Fievez, L., Bougnet, V., Art, T., Degand, G., Marlin, D., Roberts, C., Genicot, B., et al. 2002. Effect of chronic airway inflammation and exercise on pulmonary and systemic antioxidant status of healthy and heaves-affected horses. *Equine Vet J*;34:563–571.

Kirschvink, N., Fievez, L., Bougnet, V., Art, T., Degand, G., Smith, N., Marlin, D., Roberts, C., Harris, P., Lekeux, P. 2002. Effect of nutritional antioxidant supplementation on systemic and pulmonary antioxidant status, airway inflammation and lung function in heaves-affected horses. *Equine Vet J*;34:705–712.

Kleinsmith, L.J., Kerrigan, D., Kelly, J. 2003. Science Behind the News: Understanding Estrogen Receptors, Tamoxifen and Raloxifene. National Cancer Institute [Web site]. January. Available at: http://press2.nci.nih.gov/sciencebehind/estrogen/estrogen01.htm. Accessed April 5, 2004.

Klimberg, V.S., et al. 1991. Does glutamine facilitate chemotherapy while reducing toxicity? *Surg Forum*;42:16–18.

Klimberg, V.S. 1990. Glutamine: A key factor in establishing and maintaining intestinal health. Symposium Proceedings, October.

Klimberg, V.S., et al. 1992. Effect of supplemental dietary glutamine on methotrexate concentration in tumors. *Arch Surg*;127:1317–1322.

Klimberg, V.S., et al. 1996. Glutamine, cancer, and its therapy. *Am J Surg*;172:418–424.

Klimberg, V.S. 1996. How glutamine protects the gut during irradiation. *ICCN*;3:21.

Klimberg, V.S., et al. 1996. Glutamine, cancer, and its therapy. *Am J Surg*;172:418–424.

Kment, A. 1967. The Objective Demonstration of the Revitalization Effect After Cell Injections. In: Schmidt, F., ed. Cell Research and Cellular Therapy. Thoune, Switzerland.

Knekt, P., Kumpulainen, J., Jarvinen, R., et al. 2002. Flavonoid intake and risk of chronic diseases. *Am J Clin Nutr*;76(3): 560–568.

Knekt, P., Jarvinen, R., Seppanen, R., et al. 1997. Dietary flavonoids and the risk of lung cancer and other malignant neoplasms. *Am J Epidemiol*;146:223–30.

Knekt, P., Ritz, J., Pereira, M.A., et al. 2004. Antioxidant vitamins and coronary heart disease risk: a pooled analysis of 9 cohorts. *Am J Clin Nutr*;80(6):1508–1520.

Knekt, P., Reunanen, A., Marniumi, J., et al. 1999. Low vitamin E status is a potential risk factor for insulin-dependent diabetes mellitus. *J Intern Med*;245:99–102.

Kodama, N., Komuta, K., Nanba, H. 2003. Effect of Maitake (Grifola fondosa) D-Fraction on the Activation of NK Cells in Cancer Patients, *J of Medicinal Foods*;6(4),371–377.

Kondo, H. 1998. Haematological effects of oral cobalamin preparations on patients with megaloblastic anaemia. *Acta Haematol*;9:200–5.

Konno, S. 2004. Potential Anticancer Effect of Maitake D-Fraction on Canine Cancers. Companion Animal Practice. *Vet Ther*;Winter;5(4):263–71.

Konrad, T., Vicini, P., Kusterer, K., Hoflich, A., Assadkhani, A., Bohles, H.J., Sewell, A., Tritschler, H.J., Cobelli, C., Usadel, K.H. 1999. alpha-Lipoic acid treatment decreases serum lactate and pyruvate concentrations and improves glucose effectiveness in lean and obese patients with type 2 diabetes. *Diabetes Care*;Feb;22(2):280–7.

Kouttab, N.M., Prada, M., Cazzola, P. 1989. Thymomodulin: biological properties and clinical applications. *Med Oncol Tumor Pharmacother*;6:5–9 [review].

Kralovansky, U.P., Marthné-Schill, J. 1994. Data composition and use value of hemp seed (Hungarian with English summary). *Novenytermeles*;43(5):439–446.

Kramer, G.A., Kittleson, M.D., Fox, P.R., Lewis, J., Pion, P.D. 1995. Plasma taurine concentrations in normal dogs and in dogs with heart disease. *J Vet Intern Med*;9(4):253–258.

Kremer, J.M., Lawrence, D.A., Petrillow, G.F., et al. 1995. Effects of high-dose fish oil on rheumatoid arthritis after stopping nonsteroidal anti-inflammatory drugs. *Arthritis Rheum*;38:1107–14.

Kroboth, P.D., Amico, J.A., Stone, R.A., et al. 2003. Influence of DHEA administration on 24-hour cortisol concentrations. *J Clin Psychopharmacol*; Feb;23(1):96–9.

Kromhout, D. 1987. Essential micronutrients in relation to carcinogenesis. *Am J Clin Nutr*;45(5 Suppl):1361–1367.

Kuwabara, S., Nakazawa, R., Azuma, N., et al. 1999. Intravenous methylcobalamin treatment for uremic and diabetic neuropathy in chronic hemodialysis patients. *Intern Med*; 38:472–5.

Lai, H., Lai, S., Shor-Posner, G., Ma, F., Trapido, E., Baum, M.K. 2001. Plasma zinc, copper, copper:zinc ratio, and survival in a cohort of HIV-1-infected homosexual men. *J Acquir Immune Defic Syndr*;27(1):56–62.

Landi, G. 1993. Oral administration of borage oil in atopic dermatitis. *J Appl Cosmetology*;11:115–20.

Lashner, B.A., Heidenreich, P.A., Su, G.L., et al. 1989. Effect of folate supplementation on the incidence of dysplasia and cancer in chronic ulcerative colitis. A case-control study. *Gastroenterology*;97:255–9.

Lashner, B.A. 1993. Red blood cell folate is associated with the development of dysplasia and cancer in ulcerative colitis. *J Cancer Res Clin Oncol*;119:549–54.

Lashner, B.A., Provencher, K.S., Seidner, D.L., et al. 1997. The effect of folic acid supplementation on the risk for cancer or dysplasia in ulcerative colitis. *Gastroenterology*;112: 29–32.

Lavoie, J. 1997. Chronic obstructive pulmonary disease. In: Robinson, N.E. Current Therapy in Equine Medicine. Philadelphia: W.B. Saunders. pp. 79–127.

Leaf, A., Weber, P.C. 1988. Cardiovascular effects of n-3 fatty acids. *N Engl J Med*;318:549–57.

Lederle, F.A. 1991. Oral cobalamin for pernicious anemia. Medicine's best kept secret? *JAMA*;265(1):94–5.

Lee, I.M., Cook, N.R., Manson, J.E., et al. 2002. Randomized beta-carotene supplementation and incidence of cancer and cardiovascular disease in women: is the association modified by baseline plasma level? *Br J Cancer*;86(5):698–701.

Lee, J.H., Sugano, M. 1986. Effects of linoleic and gamma-linolenic acid on 7,12-dimethylbenz(a)anthracene-induced rat mammary tumors. *Nutr Rep Int*;34:1041.

Lee, K.W., Lee, H.J., Kang, K.S. et al. 2002. Preventive effects of vitamin C on carcinogenesis. *Lancet*;359:172.

Lee, N.A., Reasner, C.A. 1994. Beneficial effect of chromium supplementation on serum triglyceride levels in NIDDM. *Diabetes Care*;17:1449–52.

Lee, R., Hanson, W. 1947. Protomorphology, The Principles of Cell Auto-Regeneration. Lee Foundation for Nutritional Research, Milwaukee, WI.

Le Marchand, L., Murphy, S.P., Hankin, J.H., et al. 2000. Intake of flavonoids and lung cancer. *J Natl Cancer Inst*;92:154–60.

Leung, P.Y., Miyashita, K., Young, M., Tsao, C.S. 1993. Cytotoxic effect of ascorbate and its derivative on cultured malignant and non-malignant cell lines. *Anticancer Research*;13: 47–80.

Leventhal, L.J., Boyce, E.G., Zurier, R.B. 1993. Treatment of rheumatoid arthritis with gammalinolenic acid. *Ann Intern Med*;119:867–73.

Levin, C. 2002. Canine Epilepsy. Oregon City, Oregon: Lantern Publication. pp. 18–19.

Lewis, E.L., Schoen, A.M. 1995. Glandular Therapy, Cell Therapy and Oral Tolerance. In: Schoen, A.M., Wynn, S., eds. Complementary and Alternative Medicine. St. Louis: Mosby. p 81.

Lewis, L., Morris, M. 1984. Small Animal Clinical Nutrition. Mark Morris Associates. Topeka, KS.

Liebow, C., Rothman, S.S. 1975. Enteropancreatic Circulation of Digestive Enzymes. *Science*;189:472–474.

Lindley, M.G. 1998. The impact of food processing on antioxidants in vegetable oils, fruits and vegetables. *Trends Food Sci Technol*; 9:336–40.

Lipkin, M., Newmark, H. 1995. Calcium and the prevention of colon cancer. *J Cell Biochem Suppl*;22:65–73 [review].

Lisoni, P., et al. 1991. Clinical results with the pineal hormone melatonin in advanced cancer resistant to standard anti-tumor therapies. *Oncology*;48:448–450.

Livine, S., Myhre, G., Smith, G., Burns, J. 1982. Effect of a Nutritional Supplement Containing N,N-Dimethylglycine (DMG) on the Racing Standard Bred. *Equine Practice*;4: March.

Lloyd, D. 1990. Essential fatty acids in dermatological disorders of dogs and cats. In: Horrobin, D., ed. Omega-6 essential fatty acids: pathophysiology and roles in clinical medicine. NY: LNAn R. Liss Inc. p 113–20.

Lockwood, K., Moesgaard, S., Yamamoto, T., Folkers, K. 1995. Progress on therapy of breast cancer with vitamin Q10 and the regression of metastases. *Biochem Biophys Res Commun*;212:172–7.

Logas, D., Beale, K.M., Bauer, J.E. 1991. Potential Clinical Benefits of Dietary Supplementation of Marine Liver Oil. *JAVMA*;99:1631.

Logas, G., Kunkle, G.A. 1994. Double-blind Crossover Study with Marine Oil Supplementation Containing High-dose Eicosapentaenoic Acid for the Treatment of Canine Prurutic Skin Disease. *Vet. Derm*;5:99.

Longo, F., Lepore, L., Agosti, E., Panizon, F. 1988. Evaluation of the effectiveness of thymomodulin in children with recurrent respiratory infections. *Pediatr Med Chir*;10:603–7.

Lopaschuk, G. 2000. Regulation of carbohydrate metabolism in ischemia and reperfusion. *Am Heart J*;139(2 Pt 3):S115–119.

Lovell, C.R., Burton, J.L., Horrobin, D.F. 1981. Treatment of atopic eczema with evening primrose oil. *Lancet*;I:278.

Loveridge, G. 1994. Provision of environmentally enriched housing for dogs. *Anim. Technol*;45:1–19.

Lykkesfeldt, J., Hagen, T.M., Vinarsky, V., Ames, B.N. 1998. Age-associated decline in ascorbic acid concentration, recycling, and biosynthesis in rat hepatocytes—reversal with (R)-alpha-lipoic acid supplementation. *FASEB J*;12:1183–9.

Ma, Y. 1989. Thesis Collection of International Academic Exchange Meeting on Seabuckthorn. Wugong Centre For Agricultural Science Research, Xi'an.

MacKenzie, C., Frisell, W. 1958. Metabolism of Dimethylglycine by Liver Mitochondria. *Journal of Biology and Chemistry*; 232:417.

Malafa, M.P., Fokum, F.D., Mowlavi, A., Abusief, M., King, M. 2002. Vitamin E inhibits melanoma growth in mice. *Surgery*;131(1):85–91.

Malafa, M.P., Neitzel, L.T. 2000. Vitamin E succinate promotes breast cancer tumor dormancy. *J Surg Res*;93(1):163–170.

Malanin, K., et al. 1995. Anaphylactic reaction caused by n eoallergens in heated pecan nut. *Allergy*;vol. 50;pp. 998–991.

Mani, S., Lawson, J.W. 1999. Partial fractionation of Perna and the effect of Perna and Dimethylglycine on immune cell function and melanoma cells. South Carolina Statewide research conference, Charleston, SC. Jan;3–5.

Mani, S., Whitesides, J.F., Lawson, J.W. 1999.Role of Perna and Dimethylglycine (DMG) in modulating cytokine response and their impact on melanoma cells. 99th General Meeting of the American Society for Microbiology, Chicago, IL May 30–June 3.

Mani, S., Whitesides, J. Lawson, J. 1999. Role of Dimethylglycine in Melanoma Inhibition—Abstract from Nutrition and

Cancer Prevention: American Institute for Cancer Research, Sept.

Mani, S., Whitesides, J.F., Lawson, J.W. In Press. Use of Perna and Dimethylglycine (DMG) as immunotherapeutic agents in autoimmune disease and melanoma. *Critical Reviews in Biomedical Engineering.*

Manku, M.S., Horrobin, D.F., Morse, N.L., et al. 1984. Essential fatty acids in the plasma phospholipids of patients with atopic eczema. *Br J Dermatol*;110:643–8.

Manning, A.P., Heaton, K.W., Harvey, R.F., Uglow, P. 1977. Wheat fibre and irritable bowel syndrome. *Lancet*;ii:417–8.

Marcell, T.J., Taaffe, D.R., Hawkins, S.A., et al. 1999. Oral arginine does not stimulate basal or augment exercise-induced GH secretion in either young or old adults. *J Gerontol A Biol Sci Med Sci*;54:M395–9.

Marlin, D.J., Fenn, K., Smith, N., Deaton, C.D., Roberts, C.A., Harris, P.A., Dunster, C., Kelly, F.J. 2002. Changes in circulatory antioxidant status in horses during prolonged exercise. *J. Nutr*;132:1622S–1627S.

Marr, K.A., Foster, A.P., Lees, P., Cunningham, F.M., Page, C.P. 1997. Effect of antigen challenge on the activation of peripheral blood neutrophils from horses with chronic obstructive pulmonary disease. *Res. Vet. Sci*;62:253–260.

Marracci, G.H., Jones, R.E., McKeon, G.P., Bourdette, D.N. 2002. Alpha lipoic acid inhibits T cell migration into the spinal cord and suppresses and treats experimental autoimmune encephalomyelitis. *J Neuroimmunol*;131(1–2):104–114.

Martin, T., Uhder, K., Kurek, R., Roeddiger, S., Schneider, L., Vogt, H.G., Heyd, R., Zamboglou, N. 2002. Does prophylactic treatment with proteolytic enzymes reduce acute toxicity of adjuvant pelvic irradiation? Results of a double-blind randomized trial. *Radiother Oncol*;Oct;65(1):17–22.

Masoro, E.J. Theories of aging. 1993. In: Yu, B.Y. (ed.) Free Radicals in Aging. Boca Raton, FL: CRC Press, Inc.

LJ. Mate, J., Castanos, R., Garcia-Samaniego, J., Pajares, J.M. 1991. Does dietary fish oil maintain the remission of Crohn's disease: a case control study. *Gastroenterology*;100:A228.

McCay, C.M. 1949. The Nutrition of the Dog. Ithaca, NY: Comstock Publishing Company, Inc.

McCord, J. 1974. Free Radicals and Inflammations: Protection of Synovial Fluid by Superoxide Dismutase. *Science*;185,529.

McCullough, F., Northrop-Clewes, C.A., Thurnham, D.I. 1999. The effect of vitamin A on epithelial integrity. *Proc.Nutr. Soc*;58(2):289–293.

McCullough, F. et al. 1999. The effect of vitamin A on epithelial integrity. *Proceedings of the Nutrition Society*;volume 58: p 289–293.

McEntee, K., Clercx, C., Snaps, F., Henroteaux, M. 1995. Clinical, Electrocardiographic, and Echocardiographic Improvements After L-Carnitine Supplementation in a Cardiomyopathic Labrador. *Canine Practice*;20:12–15.

McIllmurray, M.B., Turkie, W. 1987. Controlled trial of gamma linolenic in Duke's C colorectal cancer. *Br Med J*;294: 1260.

McNair, P., Christiansen, C., Madsbad, S., et al. 1978. Hypomagnesemia, a risk factor in diabetic retinopathy. *Diabetes*;27:1075–7.

Meduski, J., Hyman, S., Kilz, R., Kim, K., Thein, P. and Yoshimoto, T. 1980. Pacific Slope Biochemical Conference. Abst. July 7–9 University of California, San Diego.

Mel'nikova, V.M., Gracheva, N.M., Belikov, G.P., et al. 1993. The chemoprophylaxis and chemotherapy of opportunistic infections. *Antibiotiki i Khimioterapiia*;38:44–8.

Meydani, S.N., Meydani, M., Blumberg, J.B., Leka, L.S., Siber, G., Loszewski, R., Thompson, C., Pedrosa, M.C., Diamond, R.D., Stoller, B.D. 1997. Vitamin E supplementation and in vivo immune response in healthy elderly subjects. A randomised controlled trial. *JAMA*; 227:1380–1386.

Meydani, S.K., Beharka, A.A. 1996. Recent developments in vitamin E and immune response. *Nutr. Rev*;56:S49–S58.

Meyskens, F.L. 1984. Prevention and Treatment of Cancer with Vitamin A and the Retinoids, Vitamins, Nutrition and Cancer. Prosad, K.N., ed. Basil, Switzerland: Karger.

Michaud, D.S., Pietinen, P., Taylor, P.R., et al. 2002. Intakes of fruits and vegetables, carotenoids and vitamins A, E, C in relation to the risk of bladder cancer in the ATBC cohort study. *Br J Cancer*;87(9):960–965.

Michels, K.B., Holmberg, L., Bergkvist, L., Ljung, H., Bruce, A., Wolk, A. 2001. Dietary antioxidant vitamins, retinol, and breast cancer incidence in a cohort of Swedish women. *Int. J.Cancer*;2–15;91(4):563–567.

Middleton Jr., E., Kandaswami, C. 1993.The impact of plant flavonoids on mammalian biology: implications for immunity, inflammation and cancer. Chapter 15. In: Harbourne, J.B., ed. The flavonoids: advances in research since 1986. London: Chapman and Hall. 619–652.

Middleton, E., Kandaswami, C. 1992. Effects of flavonoids on immune and inflammatory cell functions. *Biochem Pharmacol*;43(6):1167–1179.

Middleton Jr., E. 1986. Effect of flavonoids on basophil histamine release and other secretory systems. *Prog Clin Biol Res.*;213:493–506.

Milgram, N.W., Head, E., Zicker, S.C., et al. 2005. Learning ability in aged beagle dogs is preserved by behavioral enrichment and dietary fortification: a two-year longitudinal study. *Neurobiol Aging*;26(1):77–90.

Miodini, P., Fioravanti, L., di Fronzo, G., Capelletti, V. 1999. The two phyto-oestrogens genistein and quercetin exert different effects on oestrogen receptor function. *Br J Cancer*; 80:1150–5.

Misckesche, M., et al. 1977. Vitamin A in the Treatment of Metastatic, Unresectable, Squamous Cell Carcinoma of the Lung. *Oncology*;34:234,

Miyake, Y., Shouzu, A., Nishikawa, M., et al. 1999. Effect of treatment of 3-hydroxy-3-methylglutaryl coenzyme I reductase inhibitors on serum coenzyme Q10 in diabetic patients. *Arzneimittelforschung*;49:324–9.

Mo, H., Elson, C.E. 1999. Apoptosis and cell-cycle arrest in human and murine tumor cells are initiated by isoprenoids. *J Nutr Apr*;129(4):804–13.

Mobarhan, S. 1994. Micronutrient supplementation trials and the reduction of cancer and cerebrovascular incidence and mortality. *Nutrition Reviews*;52:102–105.

Mocchegiani, E., Muzzioli, M. 2000. Therapeutic application of zinc in human immunodeficiency virus against opportunistic infections. *J Nutr*;;130(5S Suppl):1424S–1431S.

Mocchegiani, E., Boemi, M., Fumelli, P., Fabris, N. 1989. Zinc-dependent low thymic hormone level in type I diabetes. *Diabetes*;12:932–7.

Moertel, C.G., Fleming, T.R., Creagan, E.T., Rubin, J., O'Connell, M.J., Ames, M.M. 1985. High-dose vitamin C versus placebo in the treatment of patients with advanced cancer who have had no prior chemotherapy. A randomized double-blind comparison. *N Engl J Med*;312(3):137–141.

Monson, W. 1989. Taurine's Role in the Health of Cats. *Vet. Med*;84(10):1013–105, Oct.

Monteleone, P., Beinat, L., Tanzillo, C., Maj, M., Kemali, D. 1990. Effects of phosphatidylserine on the neuroendocrine response to physical stress in humans. *Neuroendocrin*;Sep;52(3):243–8.

Monteleone, P., Maj, M., Beinat, L., Natale, M., Kemali, D. 1992. Blunting by chronic phosphatidylserine administration of the stress-induced activation of the hypothalamo-pituitary-adrenal axis in healthy men. *Eur J Clin Pharmacol*;42(4):385–8.

Morini, M., Roccatagliata, L., Dell'Eva, R., et al. 2004. Alpha-lipoic acid is effective in prevention and treatment of experimental autoimmune encephalomyelitis. *J Neuroimmunol*; 148(1–2):146–153.

Morisco, C., Trimarco, B., Condorelli, M. 1993. Effect of coenzyme Q10 in patients with congestive heart failure: a long-term multicenter randomized study. *Clin Investig*;71:S134–6.

Morris, J.G., Rogers, Q.R., and Pacioretty, L.M. 1989. Taurine: An Essential Nutrient for Cats. *J Sm Anim Practice*; 108:773.

Morse, P.F., Horrobin, D.F., Manku, M.S., et al. 1989. Meta-analysis of placebo-controlled studies of the efficacy of Epogam in the treatment of atopic eczema: relationship between plasma essential fatty acid changes and clinical response. *Br J Dermatol*;121(1):75–90.

Mortensen, S.A., Vadhanavikit, S., Baandrup, U., Folkers, K. 1985. Long-term coenzyme Q10 therapy: a major advance in the management of resistant myocardial failure. *Drug Exptl Clin Res*;11:581–93.

Mosier, J.E. 1978. Relationships of Nutrition and Skin Problems. *Mod Vet Pract*;59:105–109.

Muller, G.H., Kirk, R.W., Scott, D.W. 1989. Small Animal Dermatology,4th ed. Philadelphia: W.B. Saunders. 1–48.

Murray, M.T. 1996. Encyclopedia of Nutritional Supplements. Prima Publ. p 267.

Myers, C., McQuire, W., Young, R. 1976. Adriamycin amelioration of toxicity by alpha-tocopherol. *Cancer Treat Rep*; Jul;60(7):961–962.

Myers, C.E., et al. 1982. Effect of Tocopherol and Selenium on Defenses Against Reactive Oxygen Species and their Effect on Radiation Sensitivity. *Annals of the NY Acad of Sci*;393: 419–425.

Myhrstad, M.C., Carlsen, H., Nordstrom, O., et al. 2002. Flavonoids increase the intracellular glutathione level by transactivation of the gamma-glutamylcysteine synthetase catalytical subunit promoter. *Free Radic Biol Med Mar*; 1;32(5):386–93.

Naguib, Y. 2003. Carotenoids come of age. *Functional Foods and Nutraceuticals*;Mar.,p. 68.

Naidu, M.R.C., Das, U.N., Kshan, A. 1992. Intratumoral gamma-linolenic acid therapy of human gliomas. *Prostaglandins Leukot Essent Fatty Acids*;45:181–4.

Nair, P.P., Turjman, N., Kessie, G., Calkins, C., Goodman, G. T., Davidovitz, H., Nimmagadda, G. 1984. Diet, nutrition intake, and metabolism in populations at high and low risk for colon cancer. Dietary cholesterol, beta-sitosterol, and stigmasterol. *American Journal of Clinical Nutrition*;40(4 Suppl):927–30,Oct.

Nakamura, Y., et al. 1996. Inhibitory effect of pheophorbide a, a chlorophyll-related compound, on skin tumor promotion in ICR mouse. *Cancer Lett*;Nov 29;108(2):247–55.

Nakamura, T., Higashi, A., Nishiyama, S., et al. 1991. Kinetics of zinc status in children with IDDM. *Diabetes Care*;14: 553–7.

Nakamura, R., Littarru, G.P., Folkers, K. 1973. Deficiency of coenzyme Q in gingiva of patients with periodontal disease. *Int J Vitam Nutr Res*;43:84–92.

Nanba, H., Hamaguchi, A.M., Kuroda, H. 1987. The chemical structure of an antitumor polysaccharide in fruit bodies of *Grifola frondosa* (maitake). *Chem Pharm Bull*;35: 1162–8.

Nariba, H. 1993. Antitumor Activity of Orally Administered 'D-Fraction' from Maitake mushroom (*Grifola frondosa*). *J of Nat Med*;1(4):10–15.

National Research Council.1986. Nutritional Requirements of Cats, Revised Edition. Washington, D.C.: National Academy Press.

Neumann, K.H. 1967. The influence of tissue injections on experimental liver damage. In Schmid, F., ed: Cell Research and Cellular Therapy. Switzerland:Thoune.

Neuzil, J., Weber, T., Schroder, A., et al. 2001. Induction of cancer cell apoptosis by alpha-tocopheryl succinate: molecular pathways and structural requirements. *FASEB J*;15(2):403–415.

Newman, N.L. 1995. Equine Degenerative Joint Disease. *Natural Pet*;March, April,p. 56.

Nickander, K.K., McPhee, B.R., Low, P.A., Tritschler, H. 1996. Alpha-lipoic acid: antioxidant potency against lipid peroxidation of neural tissues in vitro and implications for diabetic neuropathy. *Free Radic Biol Med.*;21(5):631–9.

Nicoli, C., et al. 1999. Influence of processing on the antioxidant properties of fruit and vegetables. *Trends Food Sci Technol*; 10(3):94–100.

Nicoli, M.C., et al. 1997. Loss and/or formation of antioxidants during food processing and storage. *Cancer Lett*;vol. 114,no.1–(Mar. 19),71–74.

Nieman, D.C. 1998. Exercise and resistance to infection. *Can J Physiol Pharmacol*;76:573–80 [review].

Niehans, P. Introduction to cellular therapy, Pagent Books, New York, 1960.

Nishino, H. et al. 2000. Cancer prevention by carotenoids. *Biofactors*;13:89.

Novotny, M.J., Hogan, P.M., Flannigan, G. 1994. Echocardiographic evidence for myocardial failure induced by taurine deficiency in domestic cats. *Can J Vet Res*;Jan;58(1):6–12.

O'Dwyer, S., et al, 1989. Maintenance of small bowel mucosa with glutamine-enriched parenteral nutrition, *Journal of Parenteral and Enteral Nutrtion*;13:579.

Offenbacher, E.G., Pi-Sunyer, F.X. 1980. Beneficial effect of chromium-rich yeast on glucose tolerance and blood lipids in elderly subjects. *Diabetes*;29:919–25.

Ogasawara, H., Middleton Jr., E. 1985. Effect of selected flavonoids on histamine release (HR) and hydrogen peroxide (H2O2) generation by human leukocytes [abstract]. *J Allergy Clin Immunol.*;75(suppl):184.

Ohbayashi, A., Akioka, T., Tasaki, H. 1972. A Study of the Effects of Liver Hydrolysate on Hepatic Circulation. *J. Therapy*;54:1582–1585.

Ogilvie, G.K., Fettman, M.J., Mallinckrodt, C., et al. 2000. Effect of fish oil and arginine on remission and survival in dogs with lymphoma: A double-blind, randomized placebo controlled study. *Cancer*;88[8]:1916–28.

Ogilvie, G.K., Vail, D.M. 1990. Advances in nutritional therapy for the cancer patient. Veterinary Clinics of North America: *Small Animal Practice*;0:969–985.

Okuda, T., Yoshida, T., Hatano, T. 1993. Antioxidant phenolics in oriental medicine. In: Yagi, K., ed. Active oxygens, lipid peroxides, and antioxidants. Tokyo: Japan Sci Soc Press. 333–346.

O'Leary, K.A., de Pascual-Tereasa, S., Needs, P.W., Bao, Y.P., O'Brien, N.M., Williamson, G. 2004. Effect of flavonoids and vitamin E on cyclooxygenase-2 (COX–2) transcription. *Mutat Res*;551(1–2):245–254.

Olsen, R., 1989. Nutrition Reviews: Present Knowledge in Nutrition, 6th Edition. Washington, DC: Nutrition Foundation. pp 96–107.

Omenn, G.S., Goodman, G.E., Thornquist, M.D., Balmes, J., Cullen, M.R., Glass, A., Keogh, J.P., Meyskens, F.L., Valanis, B., Williams, J.H., Barnhart, S., Hammar, S. 1996. Effects of a combination of beta carotene and vitamin A on lung cancer and cardiovascular disease. *N Engl J Med*;334(18):1150–1155.

Onofrj, M., Fulgente, T., Mechionda, D., et al. 1995. L-acetylcarnitine as a new therapeutic approach for peripheral neuropathies with pain. *Int J Clin Pharmacol Res*;15:9–15.

Opara, E.C. 1997. Antioxidants—The latest weapon in the war on smoking. *VRP Nutritional News*;Vol 11 (July).

Opara, E., 2002. Oxygen Free Radicals and Aging: Part III, presented at Vitamin Research Products. (http://www.vrp.com), November 17.

Orlando, G., Rusconi, C. 1986. Oral L-Carnitine in the Treatment of Chronic Cardiac Ischemia in Elderly Patients. *Clin Trials J*;23:238–244.

Osband, M., Lipton, J., et al. 1981. Histiocytosis-X: Demonstration of abnormal immunity T-cell histamine H2 receptor deficiency, and successful treatment with thymic extract. *N Engl J Med*;304: 146–53.

Osborne, C.G., McTyre, R.B., Dudek, J., et al. 1996. Evidence for the relationship of calcium to blood pressure. *Nutr Rev*;54:365–81.

Osganian, S.K., Stampfer, M.J., Rimm, E., et al. 2003. Vitamin C and risk of coronary heart disease in women. *J Am Coll Cardiol*;42(2):246–252.

Ou, P., Nourooz-Zadeh, J. Tritschler, H.J., Wolff, S.P. 1996. Activation of aldose reductase in rat lens and metal-ion chelation by aldose reductase inhibitors and lipoic acid. *Free Radic Res*;25:337–346.

Pack, A.R.C. 1984. Folate mouthwash: effects on established gingivitis in periodontal patients. *J Clin Periodontol*;11: 619–28.

Packer, L., Tritschler, H.J., Wessel, K. 1997. Neuroprotection by the metabolic antioxidant alpha-lipoic acid. *Free Radic Biol Med*;22(1–2):359–78.

Padayatty, S.J., Sun, H., Wang, Y., et al. 2004. Vitamin C pharmacokinetics: implications for oral and intravenous use. *Ann Intern Med*;140(7):533–537.

Panthong, A., Kanjanapothi, D., Tuntiwachwuttikul, P., et al. 1994. Anti-inflammatory activity of flavonoids. *Phytomedicine*;1:141–144.

Paolisso, G., D'Amore, A., Giugliano, D., et al. 1993. Pharmacologic doses of vitamin E improve insulin action in healthy subjects and non-insulin dependent diabetic patients. *Am J Clin Nutr*;57:650–6.

Paolisso, G., Scheen, A., D'Onofrio, F.D., Lefebvre, P. 1990. Magnesium and glucose homeostasis. *Diabetologia*;33:511–4 [review].

Paolisso, G., Sgambato, S., Pizza, G., et al. 1989. Improved insulin response and action by chronic magnesium administration in aged NIDDM subjects. *Diabetes Care*;12:265–9.

Paolisso, G., Sgambato, S., Gambardella, A., et al. 1992. Daily magnesium supplements improve glucose handling in elderly subjects. *Am J Clin Nutr*;55:1161–7.

Pauling, L. 1976. Vitamin C: The common cold and the flu. San Francisco: W.H. Freeman.

Pegel, K.H. 1997. The importance of sitosterol and sitosterolin in human and animal nutrition. *South African Journal of Science* 93:263–268, June.

Penn, N.D., Purkins, L., Kelleher, J., et al. 1991. The effect of dietary supplementation with vitamins A, C and E on cell-mediated immune function in elderly long-stay patients: a randomized controlled trial. *Age Ageing*;20:169–74.

Perdigon, G.N., de Masius, N., Alvarez, S., et al., 1987. Enhancement of Immune Response in Mice fed with S. Thermophilus and L. Acidophilus. *J of Dairy Sci*;70: 919–926.

Permanetter, B., Rossy, W., Klein, G., et al. 1992. Ubiquinone (coenzyme Q10) in the long-term treatment of idiopathic dilated cardiomyopathy. *Eur Heart J*;13:1528–33.

Petkau, A., Chelack, W., Pleskach, S., Meeker, B., and Brady, C. 1975. Radioprotection of Mice by Superoxide Dismutase. *Biochem Biophys Res Commun*;65,886.

Pion, P.D., Kittleson, M.D., Skiles, M.L., Morris, J.G. 1992. Dilated Cardiomyopathy Associated with Taurine Deficiencies in the Domestic Cat: Relationship of Diet and Myocardial Taurine Content. *Advances in Experimental Medicine and Biology*; 315:63–73.

Pion, P.D., Kittleson, M.D., Thomas, W.P., Skiles, M.L., Rogers, Q.R. 1992. Clinical findings in cats with dilated cardiomyopathy and relationship of findings to taurine deficiency. *J Am Vet Med Assoc*;Jul 15;201(2):267–74.

Pion, P.D., Kittleson, M.D., Thomas, W.P., Delellis, L.A., Rogers, Q.R. 1992. Response of cats with dilated cardiomyopathy to taurine supplementation, *J Am Vet Med Assoc*;Jul 15;201(2):275–84.

Pitcairn, R., Pitcairn, S. 1995. *Natural Health for Dogs and Cats*. Emmaus, PA: Rodale Press.

Poli, G., Albano, E., Diazani, M.U. 1993. Free Radicals: from Basic Science to Medicine. Basel: Birkhäuser Verlag.

Popov, I.M., 1977. Cell therapy. *J of Internatl Acad. of Preventive Medicine*;3:74.

Pottenger, F.M. 1946. The effect of heat-processed foods and metabolized vitamin D milk on the dentofacial structures of experimental animals. *American Journal of Orthodontics and Oral Surgery*;vol. 32, pp. 467–485.

Pottenger, F.M. 1995. Pottenger's Cats—A Study in Nutrition. The Price Pottenger Nutrition Foundation, Inc., PO Box 2614, La Mesa, CA 92041.

Prasad, K. 1997. Dietary flax seed in prevention of hypercholesterolemic atherosclerosis. *Atherosclerosis*;132:69–76.

Prasad, A.S. 1998. Zinc deficiency in humans: a neglected problem. *J Am Coll Nutr*;17(6):542–543.

Price, et al. 1998. Composition and content of flavonol glycosides in broccoli florets (*Brassica olearacea*) and their fate during cooking. *J Sci Food Agric*;77(4):468–72.

Pritchard, G.A., Mansel, R.E. 1990. The effects of essential fatty acids on the growth of breast cancer and melanoma. In: Horrobin, D.F., ed. Omega–6 Essential Fatty Acids: Pathophysiology and Roles in Clinical Medicine. New York: Alan R. Liss. 379–90.

Prudden, J.F., Balassa, L.L. 1974. The Biological Activity of Bovine Cartilage Preparations. *Semin Arthrit Rheum*, 4:287–321.

Pullman-Mooar, S., Laposata, M., Lem, D., et al. 1990. Alteration of the cellular fatty acid profile and the production of eicosanoids in human monocytes by gamma-linolenic acid. *Arthritis Rheum*;33:1526–33.

Puotinen, C.J. 1998. The Encyclopedia of Natural Pet Care. Keats Publ.

Rao, K.V.R., Seshiah, V., Kumar, T.V. 1987. Effect of zinc sulfate therapy on control and lipids in type I diabetes. *J Assoc Physicians India*;35:52 [abstract].

Rardon, D.P., Fisch, C. 1990. Electrolytes and the Heart. In The Heart, 7th edition. Hurst, J.W., ed. New York: McGraw-Hill Book Co. 1567.

Rasic, J.L. 1983. The role of dairy foods containing bifido and acidophilus bacteria in nutrition and health. *N Eur Dairy J*;4:80–8.

Rayman, M.P., Clark, L.C. 2000. Selenium in cancer prevention. In: Roussel, A.M., ed. Trace elements in man and animals. 10th ed. New York: Plenum Press;575–580.

Reap, E., Lawson, J. 1990. Stimulation of the Immune Response by Dimethylglycine, a non-toxic metabolite. *Journal of Laboratory and Clinical Medicine*;115:481.

Reap, E., Lawson, J. 1988. The Effects of Dimethylglycine on B-16 Melanoma in Mice. Annual Meeting of the American Soc. of Microbiology, Oct.

Rector, T.S., Bank, A., Mullen, K.A., et al. 1996. Randomized, double-blind, placebo controlled study of supplemental oral L-arginine in patients with heart failure. *Circulation*;93: 2135–41.

Reich, R., et al. 1989. Eicosapentanoic Acid Reduces the Invasive and Metastatic Activities of Malignant Tumor Cells. *Biochemical and Biophysical Res Comm*;160:2,59.

Reid, G., Millsap, K., Bruce, A.W. 1994. Implantation of Lactobacillus casei var rhamnosus into vagina. *Lancet*;344: 1229.

Reinhart, G.A. 1996. A Controlled Dietary Omega-6: Omega-3 Ratio Reduces Pruritus in Nonfood Allergic Atopic Dogs. Recent Advances in Canine and Feline Nutritional Research: Iams Proceedings. p 277.

Ren, L., et al. 1992. Positive effects of seabuckthorn seed oil on induced mutation and suppressed immunity. *Hippophae*;5(4): 23–26.

Rimm, E.B., Katan, M.B., Ascherio, A., Stampfer, M.J., Willett, W.C. 1996. Relation between intake of flavonoids and risk for coronary heart disease in male health professionals. *Ann Intern Med*;125(5):384–389.

Riordan, N.H., et al. 1995. Nutrition Therapy for Cancer Patients. Adjuvant nutrition in cancer treatment symposium. Tampa, FL. Sept. 30.

Riordan N.H., et al. 1995. Intravenous Ascorbate as a Tumor Cytotoxic Chemotherapeutic Agent. *Medical Hypothesis*;44:3 p 205.

Riordan, N.H., Riordan, H.D., Meng, X., Li, Y., Jackson, J.A., 1995. Intravenous Ascorbate as a Tumor Cytotoxic Chemotherapeutic Agent. *Medical Hypotheses*;Volume 44, Number 3, March, pp. 207–213.

Riso, P., Pinder, A., Santangelo, A., Porrini, M. 1999. Does tomato consumption effectively increase the resistance of lymphocyte DNA to oxidative damage? *Am J Clin Nutr*;69: 712–718.

Roger, C.R. 1988. The nutritional incidence of flavonoids: some physiologic and metabolic considerations. *Experientia*; 44(9):725–804.

Rombeau, A. 1990. A review of the effects of glutamine-enriched diets on experimentally induced enterocolitis. *JPEN*;14 supplement 100S–105S.

Roodberg, A.J., et al. 2000. Amount of fat in the diet affects lutein esters but not of alpha carotene, beta carotene, and vitamin E in humans. *Am J Clin Nutr* May;71(5):1187–93.

Ross, A.C. 1999. Vitamin A and retinoids. In: Shils, M., ed. Nutrition in Health and Disease. 9th ed. Baltimore: Williams and Wilkins. 305–327.

Ross, J.A., Kasum, C.M. 2002. Dietary flavonoids: bioavailability, metabolic effects, and safety. *Annu Rev Nutr*;22:19–34.

Ross, W.M., Stewart-DeHaan, P.J., et al. 1982. Modelling cortical cataractogenesis: 3. In vivo effects of vitamin E on cataractogenesis in diabetic rats. *Can J Ophthalmol*;17:61.

Ruan, E.A., Simbasiva, R., Burdick, S., Stryker, S.J., Telford, G.L., Otterson, M.F., Opara, E.C., Koch, T.R. 1997. Glutathione levels in chronic inflammatory disorders of the human colon. *Nutrition Research*;17:463–473.

Russell, R.M. 2000. The vitamin A spectrum: from deficiency to toxicity. *Am J Clin Nutr*;71(4):878–884.

Ryan, J.A. 1989. Taurine Deficiency in Cats. *Comp Anim Pract*;19(4and5):28–31, Apr/May.

Saavedra, J. 2000. Probiotics and infectious diarrhea. *Am J Gastroenterol*;95:S16–8 [review].

Saavedra, J.M., Bauman, N.A., Oung, I., et al. 1994. Feeding of Bifidobacterium bifidum and Streptococcus thermophilus to infants in hospital for prevention of diarrhoea and shedding of rotavirus. *Lancet*;344:1046–9.

Sabeel, A.I., Kurkus, J., Lindholm, T. 1995. Intensive hemodialysis and hemoperfusion treatment of Amanita mushroom poisoning. *Mycopathologia*;131:107–114.

Sachan, D.H., Rhew, T.H., Ruark, R.A. 1984. Ameliorating Effects of Carnitine and its Precursers on Alcohol-Induced Fatty Liver. *Amer J of Clin Nut*;38,738–744.

Sakaguchi, M., et al. 1990. Reduced Tumor Growth of Human Colonic Cancer Cell Lines COLO-320 and HT29-in Vivo by Dietary n-3 Lipids. *British J of Cancer*;62:5,742–747.

Sakalova, A., Bock, P.R., Dedik, L., Hanisch, J., Schiess, W., Gazova, S., Chabronova, I., Holomanova, D., Mistrik, M., Hrubisko, M. 2001. Retrolective cohort study of an additive therapy with an oral enzyme preparation in patients with multiple myeloma. *Cancer Chemother Pharmacol*;Jul;47 Suppl:S38–44.

Salin, M., McCord, J. 1975. Free Radicals and Inflammation. Protection of Phagocytosing Leukocytes by Superoxide Dismutase. *J Clin Invest*;56,1319.

Salonen, J.T., Nyssonen, K., Tuomainen, T.-P., et al. 1995. Increased risk of non-insulin dependent diabetes mellitus at low plasma vitamin E concentrations: a four year follow up study in men. *BMJ*;311:1124–7.

Sanbe, K., Murata, T., Fujisawa, K., et al. 1973. Treatment of liver disease—with particular reference to liver hydrolysates. *Jap J Clin Exp Med*;50:2665–76.

Sano, M., Bell, K., Cote, L., et al. 1992. Double-blind parallel design pilot study of acetyl levocarnitine in patients with Alzheimer's disease. *Arch Neurol*;Nov;49(11):1137–41.

Scarpignato, C., Rampal, P. 1995. Prevention and treatment of traveler's diarrhea: a clinical pharmacological approach. *Chemotherapy*;41:48–81.

Schaeffer, M.C., Rogers, Q.R., Morris, J.G. 1985. Protein in the nutrition of dogs and cats. In: Burger, I.H., Rivers, J.P.W., eds. Nutrition of the Dog and Cat, Waltham Symposium Number 7. Cambridge University Press.

Schalin-Karrila, M., Mattila, L., Jansen, C.T., et al. 1987. Evening primrose oil in the treatment of atopic eczema: effect on clinical status, plasma phospholipid fatty acids and circulating blood prostaglandins. *Br J Dermatol*;117:11–9.

Schick, M.P., Schick, R., Reinhart, G. 1996. The Role of Polyunsaturated Fatty Acids in the Canine Epidermis. Recent Advances in Canine and Feline Nutritional Research: Iams Proceedings, p 267.

Scholich, H., Murphy, M.E., Sies, H. 1989. Antioxidant activity of dihydrolipoate against microsomal lipid peroxidation and its dependence on alpha-tocopherol. *Biochem Biophys Acta*; 1001:256–61.

Schulof, R.S. 1985. Thymic peptide hormones: basic properties and clinical applications in cancer. *Crit Rev in Oncol Hematol*;3:309–76.

Schwartz, A.G, et al. 1981. Dehydroepiandrosterone: Anti-Obesity and Anti-Carcinogenic Agent. *Nutr Cancer*;3:46.

Science and Technology Dictionary, copyright 2003, 1994, 1989, 1984, 1978, 1976, 1974. McGraw-Hill Dictionary of Scientific and Technical Terms. McGraw-Hill Companies, Inc.

Seddon, J.M., et al. 1994. Dietary carotenoids, vitamin A, C, and E, and advanced age-related macular degeneration: eye disease case-control study group. *JAMA*;Nov 9;272(18):1413–20.

Seelig, M.S. 1980. Magnesium Deficiency in the Pathogenesis of Disease: Early Roots of Cardiovascular Skeletal, and Renal Abnormalities. New York: Plenum Medical Book Company. 1–24,141–266.

Seelig, M. 1989. Cardiovascular consequences of magnesium deficiency and loss: Pathogenesis, prevalence and manifestations—magnesium and chloride loss in refractory potassium repletion. *Am J Cardiol*;63, 4G–21G.

Sellmayer, A., Witzgall, H., Lorenz, R.L., Weber, P.C. 1995. Effects of dietary fish oil on ventricular premature complexes. *Am J Cardiol*;76:974–7.

Sellon, R.K., Levy, J.K., Jordan, H.L., Gebhard, D.H., Tompkins, M.B., Tompkins, W.A. 1996. Changes in lymphocyte subsets with age in perinatal cats: late gestation through eight weeks. *Vet Immunol Immunopathol*;53:105–113.

Selye, H. 1976. Stress in Health and Disease. London: Butersworth.

Semba, R.D. 1998. The role of vitamin A and related retinoids in immune function. *Nutr Rev*;56(1 Pt 2):S38–S48.

Semba, R.D. 2001. Impact of vitamin A on immunity and infection in developing countries. In: Bendich, A., Deckebaum, R.J., eds. Preventive Nutrition: The Comprehensive Guide for Health Professionals. 2nd ed. Totowa: Humana Press Inc. 329–346.

Serraino, M., Thompson, L.U. 1992. The effect of flaxseed supplementation on the initiation and promotional stages of mammary tumorigenesis. *Nutr Cancer*;17:153–159.

Sesso, H.D., Gaziano, J.M., Liu, S., Buring, J.E. 2003. Flavonoid intake and the risk of cardiovascular disease in women. *Am J Clin Nutr*;77(6):1400–1408.

Setnikar, I., Giachetti, C., Zanolo, G. 1986. Pharmacokinetics of Glucosamine in the Dog and in Man. *Arzneimittelforschung*;36:729–735.

Shahidi, et al. 1997. Changes in edible fats and oils during processing. *J Food Lipids*;4:199–231.

Shankar, A.H., Prasad, A.S. 1998. Zinc and immune function: the biological basis of altered resistance to infection. *American Journal of Clinical Nutrition*;volume 68:pages 447S–463S.

Shigeta, Y., Izumi, K., Abe, H. 1966. Effect of coenzyme Q7 treatment on blood sugar and ketone bodies of diabetics. *J Vitaminol*;12:293–8.

Shils, M., Olsen, J., Moshe, S., 1992. Modern Nutrition in Health and Disease. 8th ed. Philadelphia: Lea and Febiger.

Shils, M.E., et al. 1994. Modern nutrition in health and disease, 8th ed. Philadelphia: Lea and Febiger. p 290.

Shimada, T., Schnidman, E., Shirota, M. 2004. Usefulness of Anti-cancer Complementary Immune Therapy with DVM Fraction. *JAHVMA*;Volume 23, 2, P 17.

Shklar, G. 1982. Oral Mucosal Carcinogenesis in Hamsters: Inhibition by Vitamin E. *J Natl Cancer Inst*; 68:791–797.

Shklar, G. Schwartz, J., Trickler, D., Niukian, K. 1987. Regression by Vitamin E of Experimental Oral Cancer. *J Natl Cancer Inst*;78:987–992.

Shoskes, D.A., Zeitlin, S.I., Shahed, A., Rajfer, J. 1999. Quercetin in men with category III chronic prostatitis: a preliminary prospective, double-blind, placebo-controlled trial. *Urology*; 54:960–3.

Sies, H. 1985. Oxidative Stress. London: Academic Press.

Sies, H. 1991. Oxidative Stress: Oxidants and Antioxidants. London: Academic Press.

Simond, J., 1996. The Antioxidant Defense System. *Natural Pet*;Jan–Feb, p 15.

Singh, V.K., Biswas, S., Mathur, K.B., et al. 1998. Thymopentin and splenopentin as immunomodulators. Current status. *Immunol Res*;17:345–68.

Simpson, J., Anderson, R., Markwell, P. 1993. Clinical Nutrition of the Dog and Cat. London: Blackwell Scientific.

Simpson, J.W., et al. 1993. Clinical Nutrition of the Dog and Cat. Santa Barbara: Veterinary Practice Publ. Co.

Sjogren, A., Edvinsson, L., Fallgren, B. 1989. Magnesium deficiency in coronary artery disease and cardiac arrhythmias. *J Int Med*;226, 213–222.

Skotnicki, A.B. 1989. Therapeutic application of calf thymus extract (TFX). *Med Oncol Tumor Pharmacother*;6:31–43.

Sketris, I.S., Farmer, P.S., Fraser A. 1984. Effect of vitamin C on the excretion of methotrexate. *Cancer Treat Rep*; 68:446–447.

Skinner, N.D., Martin, D.J., Harper, E.J. 1999. Effect of a vitamin C supplement on plasma status in healthy adult cats. FASEB Congress Abstracts 671.17:A892.

Slattery, M.L., et.al. 2000. Carotenoids and colon cancer. *Am J Clin Nutr*;Feb:71(2),575–82.

Smellie, W.S., O'Reilly, D.S., Martin, B.J., Santamaria, J. 1993. Magnesium replacement and glucose tolerance in elderly subjects. *Am J Clin Nutr*;57:594–6 [letter].

Smirnov, V.V., Reznik, S.R., V'iunitskaia, V.A., et al. 1993. The current concepts of the mechanisms of the therapeutic prophylactic action of probiotics from bacteria in the genus bacillus. *Mikrobiolohichnyi Zhurnal*;55:92–112.

Smith, N.C., Dunnett, M., Mills, P.C. 1995. Simultaneous quantitation of oxidised and reduced glutathione in equine biological fluids by reversed-phase high-performance liquid chromatography using electrochemical detection. *J Chromatogr B Biomed Appl*;673:35–41.

Sodikoff, C.H. 1995. Laboratory Profile of Small Animal Diseases, 2nd Edition. St. Louis: Mosby.

Soja, A.M., Mortensen, S.A. 1997. Treatment of chronic cardiac insufficiency with coenzyme Q10, results of meta-analysis in controlled clinical trials. *Ugeskr Laeger*;159:7302–8.

Souba, W.W. 1992. Glutamine physiology, biochemistry, and nutrition in critical illness. Austin, TX: R.G. Landes Co.

Souba, W., et al. 1985. Glutamine metabolism in the intestinal tract: invited review. *JPEN*;9:608–617.

Spatz, L., Bloom, A.D. 1992. Biological Consequences of Oxidative Stress. Implications for Cardiovascular Disease and Carcinogenesis. New York: Oxford University Press.

Spilburg, C.A., Goldberg, A.C., McGill, J.B., Stenson, W.F., Racette, S.B., Bateman, J., McPherson, T.B., Ostlund Jr., R.E. 2003. Fat-free foods supplemented with soy stanol-lecithin powder reduce cholesterol absorption and LDL cholesterol. *J Am Diet Assoc*;103:577–81.

Starzyl, T., et al. 1979. Growth Stimulating Factors in Regenerating Canine Liver. *Lancet*;1:127.

Stein, J. 1967. Objective Demonstration of the Organ-Specific Effectiveness of Cellular Preparations. In: Schmidt, F., ed. Cell Research and Cellular Therapy. Thoune, Switzerland.

Stein, J. 1967. Specific effects of implanted endocrine tissue. In: Schmidt, F., ed. Cell Research and Cellular Therapy. Thoune, Switzerland.

Steinmetz, K.A., Potter, J.D. 1996. Vegetables, fruit and cancer prevention: a review. *J Am Diet Assoc*;Dec;96(10):1027–39.

Strasser, A., Teltscher, A., May, B., Sanders, C., Niedermuller, H. 2000. Age-associated changes in the immune system of German Shepherd dogs. *J Vet Med*;47:181–192.

Sturman, J.A., Gargano, A.D., Messing, J., Imaki, H. 1986. Feline maternal taurine deficiency: effect on mother and offspring. *Journal of Nutrition*; vol.116, pp. 655–667.

Sturman, J.A. 1991. Dietary taurine and feline reproduction and development. *J Nutr*;vol.121(11 suppl)(Nov.)S166–170.

Sturman, J.A., Messing, J.M. 1992. High dietary taurine effects on feline tissue taurine concentrations and reproductive performance. *J Nutr*;Jan;122(1):82–8.

Sugimura, T., et al. 1990. Mutagens and carcinogens formed by cooking meat and fish: heterocyclic amines. In: Finot, P.A., et al., eds. The Maillard Reaction in Food Processing, Human Nutrition and Physiology. Basel; Boston: Birkhäuser Verlag. pp. 323–334.

Sung, M.K., Lautens, M., Thompson, L.U. 1998. Mammalian lignans inhibit the growth of estrogen-independent human colon tumor cells. *Anticancer Res*;18:1405–1408.

Sunvold, G.D., Tetrick, M.A., Davenport, G.M., Bouchard, G. F. 1998. Carnitine supplementation promotes weight loss and decreased adiposity in the canine. Proceedings of the XXIII World Small Animal Veterinary Association. p.746. October.

Tamura, J., Kubota, K., Murakami, H., et al. 1999. Immunomodulation by vitamin B12: augmentation of CD8+ T lymphocytes and natural killer (NK) cell activity in vitamin B12-deficient patients by methyl-B$_{12}$ treatment. *Clin Exp Immunol*;116:28–32.

Tang, J., et al. 1989. Effects of seabuckthorn leaf on the hepatocarcinogenesis of aflatoxin B1. Proceedings of the International Symposium on Seabuckthorn, Xi'an, China. 384–386.

Tarayre, J.P., Lauressergues, H. 1977. Advantages of a combination of proteolytic enzymes, flavonoids, and ascorbic acid in comparison with non-steroidal anti-inflammatory agents. *Arznein-Forsch*;27:1144–1149.

The Iams Co. 1998. Recent Advances in Canine and Feline Nutrition, Vol. II. Dayton, Ohio.

Thomas, S.R., Neuzil, J., Stocker, R. 1997. Inhibition of LDL oxidation by ubiquinol-10. A protective mechanism for coenzyme Q in atherogenesis? *Mol Aspects Med*;18:S85–103.

Thompson, L.U. 1998. Experimental studies on lignans and cancer. *Baillieres Clin Endocrinol Metab*;12:691–705.

Thompson, L.U., Rickard, S.E., Orcheson, L.J., et al. 1996. Flaxseed and its lignan and oil components reduce mammary tumor growth at a late stage of carcinogenesis. *Carcinogenesis*;17:1373–1376.

Thurnham, D.I., Northrop-Clewes, C.A. 1999. Optimal nutrition: vitamin A and the carotenoids. *Proc Nutr Soc*;58(2):449–457.

Tolleson, A., Frithz, A. 1993. Borage oil, an effective new treatment for infantile seborrhoeic dermatitis. *Br J Dermatol*; 25:95.

Toma, S., Bonelli, L., Sartoris, A., et al. 2003. Betacarotene supplementation in patients radically treated for stage I-II head and neck cancer: results of a randomized trial. *Oncol Rep*;10(6):1895–1901.

Tompkins, M.B., Nelson, P.D., English, R.V., Novotney, C. 1991. Early events in the immunopathogenesis of feline retrovirus infections. *J Am Vet Med Assoc*;199:1311–1315.

Traber, M.G. 2001. Does vitamin E decrease heart attack risk? Summary and implications with respect to dietary recommendations. *J Nutr*;131(2):395S–397S.

Traber, M.G. 1999. Vitamin E. In: Shils, M., Olson, J.A., Shike, M., Ross, A.C., eds. Nutrition in Health and Disease. 9th ed. Baltimore: Williams and Wilkins. 347–362.

Tschetter, L. et al., 1983. A Community-based Study of Vitamin C (Ascorbic Acid) Therapy in Patients with Advanced Cancer. *Proc of the American Society of Clinical Oncology*; 2:92.

Tsuji, H., Venditti, F.J., Evans, J.C., et al. 1994. The associations of levels of serum potassium and magnesium with ventricular premature complexes (the Framingham Heart Study). *Am J Cardiol*;74:232–5.

Tzivoni, D., Keren, A. 1990. Suppression of ventricular arrhythmias by magnesium. *Am J Cardiol*;65:1397–9 [review].

Uhlenhuth, K. 1920. *J. of Gen. Physiol*;3;347.

Vaananen, M.K., Markkanen, H.A., Tuovinen, V.J., et al. 1993. Periodontal health related to plasma ascorbic acid. *Proc Finn Dent Soc*;89:51–9.

Vahlquist, A. 1985. Clinical use of vitamin A and its derivatives—physiological and pharmacological aspects. *Clin Exp Dermatol*;10(2):133–143.

Vanderhaeghe, L.R., Bouic, P.J.D. 1999. The Immune System Cure: Optimize Your Immune System in 30 Days—The Natural Way! New York: Kensington Books. p. 205.

Van der Merwe, C.F., Booyens, J. 1987. Oral gamma-linolenic acid in 21 patients with untreatable malignancy. An ongoing pilot open clinical trial. *Br J Clin Pract*;41:907–15.

Vanharanta, M., Voutilainen, S., Rissanen, T.H., Adlercreutz, H., Salonen, J.T. 2003. Risk of cardiovascular disease-related and all-cause death according to serum concentrations of entero-lactone: Kuopio Ischaemic Heart Disease Risk Factor Study. *Arch Intern Med*;163(9):1099–1104.

Vaz, A.L., 1982. Double-blind Clinical Evaluation of the Relative Efficacy of Ibuprofen and Glucosamine Sulfate in the Management of Osteoarthritis of the Knee in Outpatients. *Curr Med Re. Opin*;8:145–149.

Verde, M., Piquer, J. 1986. Effects of stress on the corticosteroid and ascorbic acid content of the plasma of rabbits. *J Appl Rabbit*;9:181.

Verdova, I., Chamaganova, A. 1965. Use of vitamin B₁₅ for the treatment of certain skin conditions. Vitamin B₁₅ (Pangamic Acid) Properties, Functions and Use. Naooka, Moscow: Science Publishing.

Vettori, G., Lazzaro, A., Mazzanti, P., Cazzola, P. 1987. Prevention of recurrent respiratory infections in adults. *Minerva Med*;78:1281–9.

Vina, J., Sastre, J., Anton, V., Bruseghini, L., Esteras, A., Aseni, M. 1992. Effect of aging on glutathione metabolism. Protection by antioxidants. In: Emerit, I., Chance, B., eds. Free Radicals and Aging. 136–144.

Vogel, R.I., Fink, R.A., Frank, O., Baker, H. 1978. The effect of topical application of folic acid on gingival health. *J Oral Med*;33(1):20–2.

Vogel, R.I., Fink, R.A., Schneider, L.C., et al. 1976. The effect of folic acid on gingival health. *J Periodontol*;47:667–8.

Volk, H.D., Eckert, R., Diamantstein, T., Schmitz, H. 1991. Immunorestitution by a bovine spleen hydrosylate and ultrafiltrate. *Arzneimittelforschung*;41:1281–5.

von Schacky, C., Angerer, P., Kothny, W., et al. 1999. The effect of dietary omega-3 fatty acids on coronary atherosclerosis. A randomized, double-blind, placebo-controlled trial. *Ann Intern Med*;130:554–62.

Wagner, H., Proksch, A. 1985. Immunostimulatory Drugs of Fungi and Higher Plants, Ecorpomic and Medical Plant Research. New York: Academic Press.

Walker, M. 1988. Some Nutri-Clinical Applications of N,N-Dimethylglycine. *Townsend Letter for Doctors*. June.

Wang, C., Lawson, J. 1988. The Effects on the Enhancement of Monoclonal Antibody Production. Annual Meeting of the American Soc. of Microbiology, Oct.

Wang, L.Q. 2002. Mammalian phytoestrogens: enterodiol and enterolactone. *J Chromatogr B Analyt Technol Biomed Life Sci*.777(1–2):289–309.

Washabau, R.J. 2005. G.I. and Liver Disease, presented at the District of Columbia Academy of Veterinary Medicine.

Watanabe, G., Tomiyama, H., Doba, N. 2000. Effects of oral administration of L-arginine on renal function in patients with heart failure. *J Hypertens*;18:229–34.

Weaver, C.M., Heaney, R.P. 1999. Calcium. In: Shils, M., Olson, J.A., Shike, M., Ross, A.C., eds. Nutrition in Health and Disease. 9th ed. Baltimore: Williams and Wilkins. 141–155.

Weber, C., Jakobsen, T.S., Mortensen, S.A., et al. 1994. Antioxidative effect of dietary coenzyme Q10 in human blood plasma. *Int J Vitam Nutr* Res;64:311–5.

Weber, T., Lu, M., Andera, L., et al. 2002. Vitamin E succinate is a potent novel antineoplastic agent with high selectivity and cooperatively with tumor necrosis factor-related apoptosis-inducing ligand (Apo2 ligand) in vivo. *Clin Cancer Res*;8(3):863–869.

Weil, A. 1993. Therapeutic hemp oil. *Natural Health*; March/April; 10–12.

Weihrauch, J.L., Gardner, J.M. 1978. Sterol content of foods of plant origin. *J Am Diabetes Assoc*;73:39–47.

Wellinghausen, N., Kern, W.V., Jochle, W., Kern, P. Zinc serum level in human immunodeficiency virus-infected patients in relation to immunological status. *Biol Trace Elem Res* 2000;73(2):139–149.

Werner, A.H. 2003. Dermatosis, Exfoliative, In: Tilley, L., Smith, F., eds. The 5-Minute Veterinary Consult: Canine and Feline, Blackwell Publishing.

Whang, R., Ryder, K.W. 1990. Frequency of hypomagnesemia and hypermagnesemia: Requested vs. routine. *J Am Med Assoc;263*, 3063–3064.

Whelton, P.K., He, J., Cutler, J.A., et al. 1997. Effects of oral potassium on blood pressure: meta-analysis of randomized controlled clinical trials. *JAMA;277*:1624–32.

White, E., Shannon, J.S., Patterson, R.E. 1997. Relationship between vitamin and calcium supplement use and colon cancer. *Cancer Epidemiol Biomarkers Prev;6*:769–74.

Wilkinson, E.G., Arnold, R.M., Folkers, K. 1976. Bioenergetics in clinical medicine. VI. Adjunctive treatment of periodontal disease with coenzyme Q10. *Res Commun Chem Pathol Pharmacol;14*:715–9.

Williams, C., Cummins, K., Hayek, M., Davenport, G. 2001. Effect of dietary protein on whole-body protein turnover and endocrine function in young-adult and aging dogs, *J Anim Sci;79*:3128–3136.

Wills, J., Simpson, K.W. The Waltham Book of Clinical Nutrition of the Dog and Cat. 1994. Pergamon Press.

Windmueller, H.G. 1982. Glutamine utilization by the small intestine. *Adv Enzymol;53*:201–237.

Wrba, H., 1990. New Approaches in Treatment of Cancer. Lecture at the First International Conference on Systemic Enzyme Therapy. Sept.

Wright, S., Burton, J.L. 1982. Oral evening-primrose oil improves atopic eczema. *Lancet;ii*:1120–2.

Wu, F. 1991. Seabuckthorn medicine in Russia. *Hippophae;* 4(2):38–41.

Wu, J., Yu, X.J., Ma, X., Li, X.G., Liu, D. 1994. Electrophysiologic effects of total flavones of Hippophae rhamnoides L on guinea pig papillary muscles and cultured rat myocardial cells. *Chung Kuo Yao Li Hsueh Pao;*Jul;15(4):341–3.

Wu, Y., Wang, Y., Wang, B., Lei, H., Yang, Y. 1997. Effects of total flavones of fructus Hippophae (TFH) on cardiac function and hemodynamics of anesthetized open-chest dogs with acute heart failure. *Chung Kuo Chung Yao Tsa Chih;*Jul;22(7):429–31,448.

Wysocki, J., Wierusz-Wysocka, B., Wykretowicz, A., Wysocki, H. 1992. The influence of thymus extracts on the chemotaxis of polymorphonuclear neutrophils (PMN) from patients with insulin-dependent diabetes mellitus (IDD). *Thymus;20:* 63–7.

Wysong, R. 1989. Taurine and Arterial Thromboembolism in Cats. *JAVMA;*195(11):1463–1464, Dec. 1.

Xu, Z. et al. 1956. Preliminary research on acetylsalicylic sea-buckthorn juice. *J Nutrition;*(1):333.

Yamada, Y., Nanba, H., Kuroda, H. 1990. Antitumor effect of orally administered extracts from fruit body of *Grifola frondosa* (maitake). *Chemotherapy;*38:790–6.

Yamane, K., Usui, T., Yamamoto, T., et al. 1995. Clinical efficacy of intravenous plus oral mecobalamin in patients with peripheral neuropathy using vibration perception thresholds as an indicator of improvement. *Curr Ther Res;*56:656–70.

Yance, D., 2005. Reported at http://www.naturahealthproducts.com/. Natura Health Products, Ashland, OR.

Yanez, J., et al. 2007. Pharmacological evaluation of Glycoflex III and its ingredients on canine chondrocytes. Washington State University, North American Veterinary Conference, Orlando FL.

Yang, J. et al. 1989. Preliminary studies on the effects of oil from fruit residues of seabuckthorn upon anti-tumor. Proceedings of International Symposium on Seabuckthorn, Xi'an, China. 382–386.

Yi, X., Maeda, N., 2006. Alpha-Lipoic Acid Prevents the Increase in Atherosclerosis Induced by Diabetes in Apolipoprotein E-Deficient Mice Fed High-Fat/Low-Cholesterol Diet. *Diabetes;* 55(8):2238–44.

Yoshimura, K., et al. 1993. Effects of enteral glutamine administration on experimental inflammatory bowel disease. *JPEN;*17:235.

You, H., Yu, W., Munoz-Medellin, D., Brown, P.H., Sanders, B.G., Kline, K. 2002. Role of extracellular signal-regulated kinase pathway in RRR-alpha-tocopheryl succinate-induced differentiation of human MDA-MB-435 breast cancer cells. *Mol Carcinog;*33(4):228–236.

Yu, W., Sanders, B.G., Kline, K. 2003. RRR-alpha-tocopheryl succinate-induced apoptosis of human breast cancer cells involves Bax translocation to mitochondria. *Cancer Res;* 63(10):2483–2491.

Yu, S.H., Reiter, R.G. 1993. Melatonin Biosynthesis, Physiological Effects and Clinical Applications. Boca Raton, FL: CRC Press.

Zeegers, M.P. 2001. Are retinol, vitamin C, vitamin E, folate and carotenoids intake associated with bladder cancer risk? Results from the Netherlands Cohort Study. *Br J Cancer;*Sep 28:85(7):977–83.

Zhang, R., et al. 1997. Enhancement of immune function in mice fed with high doses of soy daidzein. *Nutr Cancer;*29:24–8.

Zhang, P., et al. 1989. Anti-cancer activities of seabuckthorn seed oil and its effect on the weight of the immune organs. *Hippophae;*2(3):31–34.

Zhang, S., Hunter, D.J., Forman, M.R., et al. 1999. Dietary carotenoids and vitamins A, C, and E and risk of breast cancer. *J Natl Cancer Inst;*91(6):547–556.

Zhang, Z. 1990. Advance and counter-measure on research and use of seabuckthorn in Russia. *Hippophae* 3(3):42–46.

Zhang, Z. 1990. Advance and counter-measure on research and use of seabuckthorn in Russia. *Hippophae;*3(3):42–46.

Zhong, F. et al. 1989. Study on the immunopharmacology of the components extracted from *Hippophas rhamnoides* L. Proceedings of the International Symposium on Seabuckthorn. Xi'an, China 368–370.

Ziegler, J. 1995. It's not easy being green: chlorophyll being tested. *J Natl Cancer Inst;*Jan4;87(1):11.

Zurier, R.B., Rossetti, R.G., Jacobson, E.W. et al. 1996. Gamma-linolenic acid treatment of rheumatoid arthritis. A randomized, placebo-controlled trial. *Arthritis Rheum;*39:1808–17.

Chapter Three

The Modern Approach to the Integration of Chinese Herbal Medicine

TRADITIONAL CHINESE MEDICINE THEORY AND PRACTICE

The Chinese theory of medicine has a long history. This theory has developed and been modified over 4,000 years. It is an organized health system based heavily upon patterns observed by the ancient Chinese scholars and is a body of science that uses a combination of herbs, physical therapy, mental medicine (meditation techniques), and dietary therapy to restore a patient to a healthy state. This chapter gives a brief overview of Traditional Chinese Medicine from the Eastern perspective to serve as background for those interested in the theories and TCM terminology. In the following sections, only a brief TCM explanation will be given; the authors then provide a Western interpretation for the TCM diagnosis.

YIN AND YANG AND CHI—A BRIEF OVERVIEW OF TCM

A brief history of Traditional Chinese Medicine and an explanation of basic concepts are presented to facilitate the use of the herbs. However, it is not the intent of this book to make the reader a master herbologist. Those with a background in TCM will find the following text basic and incomplete. To try to put the background, history, and herbal therapy and acupuncture in one book would be equivalent to writing "the book" of veterinary medicine. It is simply not possible to encompass an entire course of study into 1 book. For further information, one may take courses at various colleges around the country or see the texts in the appendix.

Traditional Chinese Medicine is based upon patterns observed by the ancient Chinese. They noticed that all things consisted of 2 opposing and complementary facets, termed Yin and Yang. The Chinese character for Yang means the sunny side of a hill, whereas the character for Yin means the shaded side. The concept of Yang was then expanded to mean positive, strong, male, upwards, external, hot, energetic, bright. Yin is used to indicate passive, female, internal, restive, dark, moist, and cool aspects of

life. Yin and Yang must co-exist. Without dark, one cannot appreciate light. Neither one is better or worse than the other. They must be in balance. For example, the active, energetic Yang aspects of a being must be interrupted by peaceful, restful Yin aspects. Consider a person who is always active. Without a quiet "Yin" period, the person would be manic, unable to rest or enjoy the completion of a task.

Yang and Yin evolve into each other. For example, day is Yang and night is Yin. Night and day flow into each other as Yin and Yang do. Everything has both a Yin and a Yang component. In the example of the day, there is a very Yang aspect, that being noon. It is the brightest time of the day. Yet the day has a Yin component within it. After noon, the evening approaches. The evening is Yin within Yang or night within the day. Yin and Yang nourish, support, oppose, and evolve into one another.

A second basic tenet of Traditional Chinese Medicine is the existence of vital substances. There are 4 vital substances—Qi (also spelled Chi), Blood, Essence, and Body Fluids. Qi is an ineffable concept. It can be described as force, life force, movement, breath, energy, material force, mater-energy and vital power. It can be said that where there is Qi, there is life, where there is no Qi, there is no life. Qi flows throughout the body in meridians, or channels, in the body. Qi performs various functions within the body. It warms, defends, holds, activates, transforms, and contains. Qi activates all processes within the body. Without Qi, the organism would die.

Blood is similar to the Western concept of blood, but extends beyond our concept of the red liquid that flows in veins and carries oxygen, hormones, nutrients, and waste products. In the Chinese understanding, Blood also functions to nourish the mind, moisten the tissues of the body, and serve as a vessel to carry Qi around the body.

Essence, or "Jing," is the substance that forms the basis for birth, development, and reproduction. It determines our basic constitution. It is responsible for our basic tendency to be healthy or subject to chronic illness. Essence influences fertility, the tendency toward degenerative diseases, and aging. In Western terms it may be considered our genetic potential.

Body Fluids are all other liquids in the body, including sweat, tears, urine, saliva, mucus, and so on. This is also called yin. In this case, however, the Chinese do not use the term yin to contrast Yang. This yin is a separate concept. Unfortunately, since most Chinese words are composed of 1 to 2 syllables, there is a great deal of repetition in the Chinese language. Often a capital "Y" is used for the Yin that is the complement of Yang and a small "y" is used for the yin indicating fluids.

PATHOGENS

Pathogens such as viruses, bacteria, and fungi are not recognized in TCM. This is not surprising, given the fact that microscopes were not invented until 1590 (by Zaccharias and Hans Janssen) or 1674 (by Anthony Leeuwenhoek), depending upon one's definition of the term "microscope" (Parker 1991). The ancient Chinese described 6 external pathogens based upon what they saw in nature: Heat or Fire, Wind, Damp, Cold, Summerheat, and Dry. Wise people observed that during windy, colder weather people developed nasal discharge and coughs. Not knowing about viruses and bacteria, they theorized that Wind and Cold entered the body to cause illness.

When studied, the pathogens make sense. Cold causes stagnation and pain in the body. Think of how it feels to put your hand in a glass of ice water for a prolonged period. If Cold gets into the digestive system it will cause a watery diarrhea with undigested food. This is due to the fact that there is not enough heat to digest the food. Discharges caused by Cold are usually clear or white.

The opposite of Cold is Heat or Fire. The translation into modern medicine would be inflammation or infection. Fever is an obvious sign of Heat invasion. A red, sore throat with purulent plaques would be Fire or Heat. The skin may show red, hot rashes. Discharges are yellow and commonly thick. In Western terms this makes sense because if Heat is translated into the term infection, the associated discharges consist of purulent debris. Purulent discharges are yellow. The heat of the disease evaporates the fluids, making the discharges less watery than a cold condition. Diarrhea due to Heat is usually foul smelling and fully digested. Again, in Western terms, fever in the body helps to speed the digestive enzymes so the food is completely broken down.

Wind is an interesting pathogen. On its own it can cause movement. Seizures and tremors are a sign of Wind. Think of wind blowing through trees causing them to sway. Wind can assist other pathogens to enter the body. It can, in effect, blow the pathogen into the body. A Western-trained physician may consider this to be airborne transmission. As wind is motion, a shifting joint pain is a sign of Wind. Wind, therefore, could be the Western equivalent of migratory pain.

Damp is a heavy, thick pathogen. It disrupts the smooth flow of Qi and leads to stagnation. Damp is sticky and hard to treat. It tends to cause a feeling of heaviness or fullness. The Western equivalents are discharge, leukorrhea, and similar symptoms. Discharges due to Damp tend to be sticky. They may be white if combined with Cold or yellow if combined with Heat. For example, a cough with thick yellow sputum is attributed to Damp Heat in the lungs; whereas thin, copious, white sputum is a sign of Damp Cold in the Lungs.

Untreated Dampness can lead to Phlegm. Phlegm is created in the body, as opposed to an external pathogen. It can have the same meaning as it has in Western medicine, i.e. sputum. In addition, practitioners of TCM state that it can form nodules or masses. Lipomas and tumors are also considered Phlegm.

Dryness is the pathogen that tends to damage the body fluids. It can cause dry eyes and skin, constipation, and a dry throat. This is a broad term that is subdivided in Western medicine. Depending upon the location of the dryness, Western equivalents include dehydration, xerostoma, keratoconjunctivitis sicca, and so forth.

Summerheat is the only pathogen restricted to a season—it is only seen in the summer. It causes sweating, thirst, headache, oligouria, and a rapid pulse. This is similar to heat stroke in Western medicine.

THE ORGANS ACCORDING TO TRADITIONAL CHINESE MEDICINE

There are 6 basic organ system pairs in TCM.[1] Each pair consists of a Yin and a Yang organ, also called zang and fu organs. Zang and fu are both translated as organ in English. Zang organs are considered storage organs. They are the Yin aspect of the organ pair and are concerned with the storage of vital substances. The Yang organs are called the fu organs. These are considered to be hollow and function to move substances within the body. The following organ pairs are recognized:

Yin organs	Yang organs
Lungs	Large intestine
Spleen	Stomach
Heart	Small intestine
Kidney	Bladder
Pericardium	Triple heater
Liver	Gall bladder

The functions of these organs are not necessarily those learned in Western medical schools. The Chinese assigned additional or different functions to the various organs based upon their interpretation of how the body was affected in different states of pathology. It is a system that is intrinsically true to itself. If one allows one's mind to accept an altered perception for a while, one will come to realize that their theories were consistent, but the language we use to describe the observations is different.

We can modify these ideas to fit our research. For example, the Chinese called mental illness a shen disturbance and assigned shen to the Heart. We now know that mental illness is a disorder of the brain. However, the Chinese use the acupuncture point they have designated as PC 6 (pericardium 6) effectively to calm agitated patients. Perhaps if we had discovered this point today, we would have named this point meninges 6 to keep in line with our understanding of the body.

A brief overview of each organ system and its assigned function is given below. The name of each organ is capitalized according to convention to indicate that the traditional Chinese theory of organ systems is being discussed.

Lung

The Lungs function in respiration. They bring the Qi from the environment (oxygen, in Western parlance) into the body. The Chinese physicians also recognize that dyspnea and coughing are related to the Lungs. In TCM they have an expanded role. They also are in charge water and sweat. To a certain sense we do agree that the Lungs have a role in fluid homeostasis. Much of the insensible water loss from the body is via respiration. The Lungs control the skin in Traditional Chinese Medicine theory. Rashes are a sign that the Lungs have some pathologic condition occurring. Again, this is not so farfetched. Think of an atopic animal. The offending allergen enters the body via the lungs and the allergic reaction is manifested by the skin.

Large Intestine

The Large Intestine reabsorbs water and sends it to the Kidneys. The impure water is sent to the Bladder for voiding. We recognize the absorption function of the large intestine in Western medicine and the role of the bladder in voiding liquid wastes.

Stomach

The Stomach is involved in the transportation of food. It prepares the food for the action of the Spleen. This is similar to what we now know of the biological function of the stomach. It indeed transports the food, but we are now aware that it also produces digestive enzymes and that the food is prepared for digestion in the small intestines, not by splenic enzymes, but rather pancreatic and hepatic substances.

Spleen

The main function of the Spleen is the extraction of the "food essence" or nutrients in Western thought. This role is now given to the pancreas and liver in modern medicine. The Spleen also has the function of "holding" in TCM theory. For example, the Spleen holds the blood in the vessels. If the Spleen is weak, petechiae, ecchymoses, and frank hemorrhage occur. If it cannot hold organs in place the patient may experience prolapses. An additional function assigned to the Spleen is the control of the flesh (muscles), so a weak Spleen can lead to a feeling of weakness.

Heart

The Heart governs the blood and circulation. This is self-explanatory to Western-trained practitioners. However, the Chinese believe that the Heart is also the house of the Shen, or mind. They do not recognize the brain as performing this function the way that Western-trained doctors do. Disturbances in this function of the Heart lead to abnormal behaviors much as we would recognize that disturbances in the brain's function can cause altered behavior.

Small Intestine

The Small Intestine is involved in fluid (think chyme) transformation. It separates clear from turbid fluid and sends the clear fluid into the body and the turbid fluid into the Large Intestine. The turbid fluid can be thought of as the chyme sent to the large intestine according to Western thought. The clear fluid is really the nutrients that the body absorbs. The functions of the Small Intestine are therefore basically identical in both systems.

Bladder

The Bladder takes fluids and combines them with toxins to make urine. Toxins can be translated into metabolic waste products, i.e. ammonia. The fluids are the water needed to excrete the toxins.

Kidney

The function of the Kidney does not correlate at all with Western thought. In TCM it does not play a role in the production of urine. The Kidneys store the body's Essence. The Kidneys control the fundamental substance for birth, growth, and reproduction. They provide the motive force for all physiological functions. Therefore, the Kidneys are the basic organs for providing the warmth for all of the functions in the body, i.e., oxidizing food to provide energy. They also guide our birth and development and produce the Marrow that fills the bones.

Pericardium

In Chinese, the character for pericardium can be translated as heart bag or mind enclosure. It surrounds and protects the Heart and is often the target of herbal formulas used to treat emotional problems because the Heart is the home of the shen or mind.

Triple Heater

This is a concept that is not present in Western medicine. It is not truly an organ, per se, but a depiction of the 3 divisions of the body—the upper (head to diaphragm), middle (diaphragm to navel), and lower (navel to foot) sections. The upper section of the body is concerned with respiration and circulation. The middle part is concerned with digestion and the lower part is charged with the function of excretion.

Liver

The Liver performs many functions in Western thought. However, the Chinese did not assign to this organ any of the digestive, detoxification, or storage functions that we now recognize. In TCM, the Liver ensures the smooth flow of Qi throughout the body. It also stores Blood and controls the joints and tendons. Ensuring the smooth flow of Qi can be thought of as making certain that all parts of the body have the required energy and blood flow. The Liver's function of Blood storage allows it to regulate the volume of Blood in circulation and regulate the menses. In TCM terms, the ability of the animal to ambulate normally may be compromised if there is Liver dysfunction because it controls the joints and sinews.

Gall Bladder

The Gall Bladder stores bile. Its role in digestion is easily comprehended by those with a Western background. In addition, in TCM theory, it stores Blood and cleans the Blood at night. We know that the gall bladder does not actually store blood, but it is closely associated with the liver in Western thought. The liver has the function of "cleaning the blood" by neutralizing toxic metabolites, providing proteins to encapsulate and transport the lipids in the blood, and so on. A final function of the Gall Bladder is to assist the Liver in controlling the sinews.

Each of these organs has a meridian associated with it that is used for acupuncture. A meridian is defined as a pathway through which energy (Qi) can flow. The meridian connects the internal organ with the surface of the body, allowing the insertion of acupuncture needles to affect the organs.

CHINESE HERBAL REMEDIES

Traditional Chinese herbal therapy has a long history. The Huang di Nei Jing—the Yellow Emperor's Inner Classic—was written during the period of the Warring States (475 to 221 BC) (Bensky 1990). The theory behind Traditional Chinese Medicine was discussed In this text. Later, during the Han Dynasty (25 to 200 CE), the Shen Nong Ben Cao Jing—Divine Husbandman's Classic of Materia Medica—was written. This is the earliest book of Chinese material medica (Chen 2001). It contained 364 entries, 1 for every day of the year, as the Chinese interwove health and nature to create their system of health care. Throughout the years, more experimentation has led to the discovery of more substances with useful effects on the body. The current Chinese Materia Medica, published in 2002, contains almost 9,000 different herbs, minerals, and animal-based materials (Bensky 2004). Many of these are used locally, while about 600 are commonly used throughout the world.

To facilitate the reading of this chapter, all substances, whether plant-based, mineral, or of animal origin, will be referred to as "herbs."

Herbs are assigned several properties, the most important of which are taste and temperature. Taste does not always conform to what the taste bud on a tongue would register; rather, it is more an effect on the body. Herbs are classified as:

Sour: Sour herbs have the action of astringing abnormal leakage of fluids such as diarrhea, excess sweating, or polyuria.
Salty: Salty herbs soften masses. They may have the additional effects of treating constipation or tonifying the Kidney.
Acrid/pungent: These herbs promote the circulation of Qi and Blood and act as diaphoretics.
Bitter: These herbs dry and clear Heat and Damp.
Sweet: Sweet herbs are tonifying and moistening. They can also harmonize or decrease toxicity of other herbs in a formula.
Bland: These herbs promote urination.

Herbs are also described as hot, cold, cool, warm, and neutral in temperature. Again, this does not necessarily correspond to the feel in the mouth, but rather to the action on the body. Cool and cold herbs tend to clear pathological Heat and nourish fluids. Warm and hot herbs are used to counteract Cold conditions in the body.

Throughout the years herbalists have combined single herbs into formulas to modify or broaden their actions or to decrease toxicity of any one single herb. When combined, herbs may have one of several interactions as follows:

Potentiation/accentuation: This occurs when herbs of similar taste or nature are added together to increase the effect upon the body. For example a formula may use anemarrhena rhizome (Zhi mu) with phellodendron bark (Huang bai) because both are bitter and cold when treating a very hot condition.

Enhancement: In this case, a primary herb is used with a secondary herb that enhances the effect of the primary herb. Sophora root (Ku shen) is a very good itch reliever. In some formulas, cypress (Di fu zi) is added to enhance the relief of pruritis.

Counteraction: This is the concept of using a second herb to decrease or eliminate the toxicity of a primary herb. Pinellia (Zhi ban xia) can irritate the gastrointestinal tract. If one wanted to use this herb for its action of drying Damp with moist coughs, but did not want to experience adverse gastrointestinal effects, one might combine it with fresh ginger (Sheng jiang).

Antagonism: In this case, each herb decreases the curative effect of the other. For example, Scutellaria root (Huang qin) is bitter and cold and clears heat. Fresh ginger (Sheng jiang) is warm. Added together, scutellaria root (Huang qin) would be less effective at clearing heat.

Incompatibility: When herbs that are incompatible are added together severe side effects can be seen that would not occur if the herbs were used alone. For this reason, Sechuan aconite root (Wu tou) is not used with tendrilled fritillary bulb (Bei mu).

Single effect: In this method, a single herb, rather than a mixture, is used to treat a patient.

Mixing herbal formulas is complex and takes years of study so most veterinarians use described formulas. A brief overview is given for those interested in the theory.

The ancient Chinese described their formulas in the form of feudal hierarchy. Herbs were assigned roles, much as members of the courts were. The king (jun) herb is the main ingredient in the formula. It is the herb prescribed to treat the main symptoms of the illness. It is assisted by deputy herbs (chen) that increase or enhance the action of the king herb. Assistant or adjutant herbs (zuo) are then added to the formula to treat less bothersome symptoms or decrease the toxicity or side effects of the primary herbs. Finally, there may be envoy herbs (shi), which may be used to direct the action of the formula to one part of the body or harmonize the body (see following definitions). Thus, the direction of Chinese herbal therapy is very different than the Western view.

TCM uses a combination of substances to enhance, modulate the activity, or decrease the toxicity of the formula. In Western medicine the trend is toward single substances at a specific concentration, i.e., 325 mg of acetylsalicylic acid per adult strength aspirin. Both systems have their merits and neither one should be considered inferior to the other. The Western-trained practitioner must become comfortable with the concept that the strengths of the various ingredients in an herbal formula may vary a bit from season to season as the growing seasons vary.

This is not a bad thing, but rather a natural occurrence. We assign a nutrition profile to our foods and vegetables. For example, a medium carrot has 26 calories, 1.83 g of fiber, 0.63 g of protein, and 17,158 IU of vitamin A (http://www.truestarhealth.com/Notes/1691007.html Accessed 11/05/2006). Common sense tells us that this is just an average. Carrots come in different sizes. Storage affects the nutritional content, and so on. To become comfortable with TCM the practitioner must accept variation as normal.

Some Western practitioners are uncomfortable with the number of different ingredients in herbal formulas. It is precisely the interactions between ingredients that make the formulas so safe and effective. We know side effects occur with single-ingredient medicines. Aspirin, a wonder drug, can cause ulcers, bleeding tendencies, Reye's syndrome, and so much more. We now realize that anesthesia and analgesia protocols are safer if combinations of opioids and dissociative, inhalant, and nonsteroidal medications are mixed so we can lower the dose of any one single medicament. With this trend in Western medicine, it will be easier for practitioners to become comfortable with TCM.

Diet and herbal therapy

Herbs work best if given on an empty stomach or with a small amount of food to facilitate administration. Large meals tend to delay the absorption of the herbs and decrease efficacy. There is also the possibility that the animal may not consume a large meal and then the dose of the herb becomes insufficient. (For diet related to cancer, please see the introduction to the cancer section).

ACUPUNCTURE

Acupuncture comes from the Latin words *acus*, which means needle, and *pungare*, which means to pierce (Schoen 1994). In its simplest form acupuncture is the introduction of a needle into a specific point on the body to cause a desired reaction in the body.

The Chinese word for acupuncture point is *shu xue*. *Shu* means communication and *xue* is hole. Together, the term *shu xue* denotes a hole in the body that communicates with the internal organs. The point is connected to the organs via the *jing luo*. The term *jing* can be translated into weave, warp (the straight threads of a weaving), pathway, channel, or meridian. *Luo* means woof (the curved part of a weaving), connect, collateral, link, or interweave. Together, the term *jing luo* denotes a blanket of channels connecting the entire body—the surface to the interior, one organ to another, the upper part to the lower part, the left side of the body to the right. The meridians and collaterals are a set of imaginary lines through which Qi flows. The channel system forms a closed circuit of energy throughout the entire body.

Meridians serve multiple purposes. In addition to carrying Qi, they also coordinate the action of the Zang fu organs and can be used diagnostically to locate the site of disease. For example, the eyes are connected to the Liver by the Liver meridian. If the eyes are inflamed, the doctor trained in TCM may diagnose Heat in the Liver. They can be used therapeutically by transmitting the effect of acupuncture and herb.

There are 14 main meridians. Each of the 12 Zang fu organs has its own meridian; these 12 are the regular meridians. There are 2 other major meridians—the Conception vessel, which runs along the ventral midline, and the Governing vessel, which runs along the dorsal midline. Finally, there are 6 additional extraordinary meridians that are large branches of the 12 regular meridians. The 6 extraordinary meridians crosslink the left side of the body to the right and the back of the body to the front. These 6 meridians share points with the other meridians. There are many points on the body that do not belong to a meridian, yet can exert an influence on the physiology of the individual.

We still do not understand how acupuncture exerts an effect on the body. In all likelihood, acupuncture has multiple effects via multiple mechanisms. There are anatomical explanations for efficacy. In general, acupuncture points are located in areas of the body with a higher concentration of free nerve endings, arterioles, lymphatic vessels, and mast cells. For example, some meridians run along the radial or median nerves. On the head, points are often located where nerves emerge through foramina. There are 4 acupuncture point types based upon their location in relation to nerves and muscles. Type I are classified as motor points. These are located at sites where nerves enter a muscle. Type II are located on the dorsal or ventral midline where superficial nerves meet. Type III are located on superficial nerves or nerve plexi. Type IV are located at the junctions between muscles and tendons (Schoen 1994).

Electrical conductance has been measured at acupuncture points and along meridians. In general, 70% to 80% of the acupuncture points studied have been demonstrated to be positively charged compared to their surroundings and some studies have demonstrated lower alternating current impedance along meridians (Reichmanis 1976). Because the body depends upon ionic charges for all nervous system function, muscle contraction, and cellular activity, it is apparent that one can alter the actions in the body by manipulating charges.

There are also physiological explanations for efficacy. It has been demonstrated that acupuncture incites a local inflammation. Hageman factor XII, bradykinin, histamine, heparin, and kinin protease are all released (Kendall 1989). These chemicals result in activation of the coagulation cascade, production of prostaglandins, vasodilation, increased vascular permeability, and activation of the complement system.

The neural segmental gate theory states that acupuncture stimulates the afferent A-delta fibers (Melzack 1965). These nerves carry non-painful sensory stimulation up to the substantia gelatinosa where they connect with inhibitory interneurons. These inhibitory neurons then close the "gate," preventing the pain-stimulating impulse traveling along the more slowly conducting C fibers from reaching the higher nervous system and preventing the recognition of pain by the brain. This may explain some, but not all, of the effects of acupuncture.

A somatovisceral reflex can be incited by stimulating acupoints (Chang 1996). Sensory and somatic fibers connect in the central nervous system so stimulation of a sensory nerve can cause firing of somatic fibers. Somatic pain can cause visceral reactions. Pain may increase heart rate and blood pressure and cause an individual to vomit, depending upon the severity. Therefore, it is understandable that manipulation of somatic nerves by acupuncture needles can cause a reaction in a body organ.

Opioids also seem to play a role in the effect of acupuncture. Acupuncture increases the circulating levels of b-endorphin (Abenyakar 1994). In the CNS, levels of met-enkephalin, leu-enkephalin, and NAGA increase after treatment with acupuncture (Wang 1989, Pan 1984). In many cases, naloxone can reverse the analgesic effects of acupuncture (Pert 1982). Experiments have demonstrated that dexamethasone can decrease b-endorphine levels and decrease the analgesic effect of acupuncture (Han 1982).

Acupuncture is becoming more accepted for the treatment of musculoskeletal conditions; some insurance companies even cover treatment. It has been demonstrated to relieve pain and increase mobility without the harmful side effects of nonsteroidal anti-inflammatories and steroids and without the possible threat of addiction that opioids pose. Its applications are far more numerous, however.

Acupuncture can be used to reduce fever, stimulate the immune system, decrease blood pressure, relieve diarrhea, regulate the reproductive system, and so on. In fact, in most every disease condition, acupuncture can be part of the therapy protocol.

The how to's

The authors strongly discourage veterinarians with no formal training from attempting acupuncture. This section is provided as a quick review for those who have been trained. Suggested points are mentioned in each disease section.

There are 10 basic methods of acupuncture:

1. Dry needling: using very thin needles in the specific acupuncture point.
2. Aquapuncture: injecting a liquid such as a vitamin solution, Adequan©, or another solution into the specific site (Schoen 1994).
3. Electroacupuncture: attaching electric leads to the needles after they are inserted into the acupoint. The frequency and amplitude are then adjusted to achieve the desired response (Schoen 1994).
4. Hemoacupuncture: inserting needles into a blood vessel to promote bleeding. Common acupuncture needles may be used, but often the practitioner uses cutting edge or hollow needles to allow more blood to flow from the point.
5. Moxibustion: burning Artemisia vulgaris directly over the acupuncture point or on a needle which has been inserted into the point (Schoen 1994).
6. Laser therapy: applying low intensity lasers to the acupuncture points (Schoen 1994).
7. Acupressure: applying pressure, usually digital, to the acupuncture point.
8. Gold bead implants: placing sterile gold beads into the site to prolong the effect once the practitioner is certain that the animal is responding to the therapy. Less common.
9. Magnetic acupuncture: applying magnetic waves to the acupoints. Rarely used.
10. Ear or auricular acupuncture: using only acupuncture points on the ear.

The decision to select a certain number of points depends upon the condition of the patient, the disorder to be treated, and the preference of the practitioner. Most practitioners use 4 to 8 points per treatment, but some conditions respond to a single point and some acupuncturists use as many as 30 needles per session. A general rule is that debilitated patients do not receive high numbers of needles because they may be too weak. When treating a single condition, fewer needles may be required than would be needed for more complex cases.

An acupuncture session usually lasts 10 to 30 minutes. Very rarely, a session may last 3 hours. This is generally only when severe pain or conditions such as status epilepticus are being treated. Some practitioners assign special significance to the number 12 because there are 12 organs in the 6 Zang-fu pairs, 12 major channels on the body, and 12 periods in the day, each associated with a specific organ. These acupuncturists feel that acupuncture sessions should last for 12 or 24 minutes.

Patients are generally treated daily to weekly for the first 3 to 6 weeks. Once the patient responds, treatment may be decreased to once a week or every other week for up to 6 months. Depending upon the condition, therapy may be lifelong. For example, an elderly German Shepherd with severe hip dysplasia is likely to require acupuncture for the rest of its life. A young dog with paralysis secondary to spinal injury may recover completely and therapy may be discontinued.

Depth of insertion varies from point to point. Obviously, there is very little soft tissue on the digits so deep insertion to the points around the nail bed is impossible. When using points around the eyes, it is important to angle the needle such that the globe is not entered. CV8, the umbilicus, is not needled. Instead, this point is only treated with moxibustion. Needles are never inserted directly into ulcerated or infected skin, tumors, or scar tissue.

Needle size also varies. In general, 0.30-gauge needles are used in large animals and 0.22-gauge needles are used in small animals. The most common length used in cats is 13 mm. Depending upon the size of the dog and the site chosen, 13- to 50-mm needles are used. In a horse, 13-mm needles are used in the extremities, but a 100-mm needle may be used in the hip area.

Further exploration of the basic techniques

Dry needling

With dry needling, the practitioner may use a cotton ball with alcohol to move fur out of the way. Clients often expect this because they see their physician wipe the inoculation site with alcohol prior to an injection. In reality, an alcohol wipe probably has little effect on infection prevention. Of course, if the site selected is visibly soiled, it should be cleaned prior to use. Once the needle is inserted, the animal usually relaxes. Many even go to sleep. If the animal seems distressed by the needle, you may wish to remove it and either re-insert or select a different point. Because there are so many points with overlapping functions, and the body is interconnected by meridians such that by treating the left side the right also benefits, it is rare that you must use a point that causes obvious distress.

Some form of stimulation is often performed once the needle is inserted. The needle is manipulated periodically by twisting, thrusting, or scraping the handle with the practitioner's fingernail. (Schoen 1994). Many practitioners manipulate the needle in a very specific manner to achieve the desired response.

Tonification versus sedation

In general, practitioners tonify weak or deficient patients. On the other hand, those patients suffering from excess conditions require sedation. The desired effect may be achieved by manipulating needles as follows:

- To tonify the patient, the practitioner may twist the needle rapidly for a short burst; whereas to sedate the patient he or she may twist the needle more slowly and for a longer period of time.
- Thrusting and lifting techniques may be used. In general, the needle is lifted partially out of the site forcefully and rapidly, then slowly and gently re-inserted—the effect is to tonify the patient. Conversely, slowly and gently lifting the needle and then rapidly and forcefully re-inserting it is said to sedate the patient.
- Insertion of the needle may be timed to the patient's breath. If the needle is inserted as the patient inhales it theoretically brings Qi into the body with the needle and tonifies the patient. If the needle is inserted as the patient exhales, the opposite effect is seen and the patient is sedated.
- The Qi in a meridian flows in a specific direction. Insertion of a needle with the flow of the Qi is tonifying, whereas insertion counter to the flow has a sedative effect.
- Points can be "closed" or "opened" upon withdrawal of the needle. If the patient is to be tonified, the acupuncturist may immediately press his or her finger over the site for a minute or so after withdrawing the needle. The idea is that this prevents Qi from escaping. To sedate the patient, the practitioner may twirl the needle at a slight angle to enlarge the hole prior to withdrawal. This "opens" the point to allow the pathogenic factor to leave the body.

Many people feel that you do not need to follow the guidelines above. These practitioners twist at moderate speeds and evenly to the left and right or thrust up and down gently with no dominant direction. The theory is that this allows the body to decide whether it requires tonification or sedation. This method is also used if the patient has a mixed condition—one with some signs of deficiency and some of excess.

Warming versus clearing

It may be desirable to warm patients with cold conditions such as Yang deficiency. This can be done by moxibustion of the points or by a technique known as Shao Shan Huo, or setting the mountain on fire. In this method, the acu-

puncture point is assigned 3 levels of depth. The most superficial level is called Heaven. Deep to this is Human and the deepest extent of the point is called Earth. To "set the mountain on fire" or warm the patient, the needle is slowly inserted to the first level, Heaven. It is then lifted and thrusted shallowly or rotated 9 times. Next, the needle is advanced to the Human level and the manipulation process repeated. Finally, the needle is placed in the Earth level and the 9 thrusts or rotations are performed. The needle is then quickly withdrawn back to Heaven. The sequence is begun again. It is repeated 3, 5, 7, or 9 times, until the point feels warm. Once this point is reached, the needle is quickly withdrawn completely and the point is pressed.

A clearing technique may be employed in patients with excess Heat patterns. This is essentially the opposite of setting the mountain on fire. The clearing method is called Qing fa. In this approach, the needle is quickly inserted to the level of Earth; then it is rotated or lifted and inserted in small increments 6 times. The needle is then backed out to the Human level, where the needle is manipulated for another 6 times. Finally, the needle is brought to the Heaven level. After manipulating the needle at this level, it is rapidly thrust back to the Earth level. This process is repeated 2, 4, 6, or 8 times, until the point feels cool. At this point the needle is slowly withdrawn.

Aquapunture

Some animals will not sit for dry needling. Birds, for example, resist being restrained for prolonged periods of time. Some animals are quite aggressive in hospital settings and need to be muzzled during treatment. Some cats will not relax in a hospital setting. Finally, some points, such as those near the nail bed, are often very sensitive, so many animals do not tolerate prolonged needling of these areas. In these cases, aquapuncture is often the preferred modality. Very small amounts of liquid can be injected into the site. Commonly employed substances include vitamin B, vitamin C, Adequan©, or saline. Only small volumes are needed. Vitamin C is most commonly used in the author's practice, because vitamin B may be too irritating. Most practitioners who use the vitamin B solution dilute it. Volumes as low as 0.15 to 0.25 cc can be used, even in large dogs.

Electroacupuncture

Electroacupuncture is performed by attaching wires to the needles after insertion. The frequency and amplitude should be set at zero prior to turning the electroacupuncture machine on. The frequency is set first. There are 2 commonly used frequencies. Low frequency is 4 or fewer Hz, and this is more commonly used. The authors use 1 to 2 Hz. High frequency is above 100 Hz. This high frequency is used for surgical analgesia, which is not frequently employed in veterinary medicine. Once the frequency is selected, the amplitude is slowly increased until the muscles just start to twitch. Most animals tolerate this well. If the animal seems uncomfortable, decrease the amplitude until the animal relaxes. After 5 to 10 minutes, the amplitude may be increased slightly.

Hemoacupuncture

Hemoacupuncture is used for excess conditions. The most common indications in veterinary medicine are high fever and laminitis. In febrile conditions such as heatstroke, a 25-gauge needle may be inserted into the appropriate acupoint and a few drops of blood are allowed to drip from the body. The tip of the ear is frequently used for this purpose in veterinary medicine. One must be careful if the patient is debilitated and febrile. It is important to avoid hypovolemia, so large amounts of blood are not taken. In addition, care must be taken if a bloodborne disease is causing fever. Anthrax is considered to be a febrile disease not treated by hemoacupuncture because this could spread disease.

In horses, laminitis is commonly treated by hemoacupuncture, especially when acute. This is one instance in which large amounts of blood may be removed. It is important to warn the owner of this so he will not become upset.

Moxibustion

Moxibustion is limited by the fact that veterinary patients tend to have fur or feathers, which may catch fire. The herb also has a strong marijuana-like odor when burned. Animals may object to the burning odor and the clinic will smell like moxa. One must also be sure clients do not think marijuana is used in the clinic or a visit by authorities may result.

Laser therapy

Some people feel that laser therapy is most useful for musculoskeletal disorders. Others claim that the energy does not penetrate deep enough to have a physiological effect.

Acupuressure

Acupressure is generally quite safe. Practitioners may wish to show clients the acupuncture points selected and have them press their fingers into the sites between clinic visits. In general, the pressure can be applied for 5 to 10 minutes; animals tolerate this quite well.

Gold bead implants

It is best to ensure that the patient will respond to the selected acupuncture point by dry needling, aquapuncture, or electroacupuncture before going to the expense of gold bead implants.

The patient is usually sedated and the area around the acupuncture point clipped and scrubbed as for surgery. A hypodermic needle can be introduced to the point and the implant passed down into the site. If necessary, a small needle can be used as a stylet to push the bead through the larger needle. After situating the bead, the needle is withdrawn. No sutures or glue should be needed to close the site.

Auricular acupuncture

Dry needling techniques may be used in auricular acupuncture. Alternatively, beads may be placed on acupuncture points by adhesive tape. These are left in place and manipulated by hand periodically.

INTEGRATNG CHINESE HERBAL MEDICINE INTO MODERN VETERINARY PRACTICE

Many feel that traditional Chinese herbal medicine is a pure art. That is, you must have a Traditional Chinese Medicine diagnosis to properly select an herbal formula or proper acupuncture points. In Western medicine, people with a sore throat due to overgrowth of Streptococcus bacteria are given amoxicillin for 10 days. It does not matter if one person has a fever and sore throat and another has swollen lymph nodes and a sore throat. The therapeutic regimen is the same for both. The Chinese treated symptoms rather than etiology. In TCM, both may be diagnosed as having Fire in the throat (redness). However, the doctor for the second patient may say that the Heat has boiled away body fluids, leaving masses of thick phlegm (enlarged lymph nodes). These two patients would receive different herbal prescriptions.

In addition, a single patient may receive different prescriptions depending upon the stage of the disease. With influenza, the patient initially experiences fever, muscle and body aches, and sweating. These symptoms later recede, leaving a patient tired and pale, sometimes for weeks, depending upon her constitution. A doctor trained in TCM would treat the patient for an excess condition initially, then a deficiency condition later in the course of disease. A Western-trained physician does not change antibiotics for a patient with a streptococcal sore throat after the fever subsides. The course of antibiotics is finished in the prescribed time period.

As we accumulate knowledge we find that we can combine the two modalities. Ancient Chinese doctors used the only tools available to them at that point in history—the 4-point diagnosis. This consisted of asking, observing, hearing and smelling, and palpating. Asking is basically the equivalent of anamnesis. Observing involved looking at the person's overall appearance. This would included an assessment of a person's color—pale, flushed, or normal? Are the eyes bright or dull? Is the posture upright or hunched? Is there a limp? Hearing was used to detect unusual breath or heart sounds. Palpating is similar to our understanding of the word. Masses were palpated and musculoskeletal structures examined.

The ancient Chinese took this concept further when feeling the pulse. There is a whole school of study on pulse diagnositics. Pulses were palpated not only to assess the state of the cardiovascular system as they are today, but to give information about the entire body. The Chinese recognized 28 separate pulse qualities using terms such as wiry, choppy, full, scattered, and such.[2]

By contrast, today we are blessed with incredible diagnostic power. We can literally see into the body using ultrasound waves, X-rays, and magnetic resonance. Simple blood tests tell us about the chemical state of the body. Immunology tests such as fluorescent antibody and enzyme-linked immunofluorescence assays tell us about exposure to pathogens. Using cultures, we can grow pathogens in the laboratory. It does not make sense to ignore all the information we can glean from these modern modalities when treating a person or animal with herbs and acupuncture. The ancient Chinese masters would certainly have used any method at their disposal to cure their patients, just as we are bound to do professionally.

One must be open-minded and critical to incorporate herbal medicine and acupuncture into Western practice. We must be able to judge whether patients respond to a treatment or not, not stubbornly remain attached to what we were told in school. Neither Western nor Eastern medicine can cure all ills, but using them wisely improves the quality of care our patients receive.

Purists have stated that in order to use herbs and acupuncture, a doctor must be able to make a TCM diagnosis. However, it is illogical to say that one cannot apply Chinese herbal medicine to a Western diagnosis. Both a doctor trained in TCM and another trained in Western medicine can treat a given patient, despite using different terms to describe the patient's state of health. The patient can be given a modern drug by one doctor or a traditional herbal preparation by the other and improve either way. Given this, why can one not use herbal medicines with a Western diagnosis? It merely requires that individuals trained in both modalities guide the process and make it understandable to both schools of thought.

There has been some apprehension expressed about long-term use of herbal supplements. This is an interesting concern because many people in this country are on chronic medications for arthritis, high blood pressure, high cholesterol, and so on. Many women remain on birth control pills for 15 years or more. When properly balanced, herbal supplements are safe and effective. This is the idea behind using combinations rather than single herbs in traditional Chinese practice.

Recent research has begun to assign Western indications to herbs. Not surprisingly, the Western and Eastern indications tend to match. In TCM, ginseng (ren shen) is used for "wasting and thirsting disorder," which is a syndrome of polydipsia and weight loss. In Western medicine we find that it improves clinical signs and lowers blood glucose levels (Chavez 2001). It is also known to benefit Heart Qi in TCM. Modern research has demonstrated that it has inotropic effects similar to cardiac glycosides in dogs, cats, and rabbits (CA, 1992). It is indicated for calming the spirit and palpitations with anxiety due to Qi and Blood deficiency (Bensky 2004). It is clear that although the terminology differs between the two modalities, both describe the same effect upon the body.

Purists may also state that a patient must be treated with herbal supplements or Western medications. They worry about interactions between the herbs and the drugs. These interactions can and do occur, of course. But we must also admit that interactions, both beneficial and detrimental, occur between various drug classes in Western medication. We have all been warned against combining corticosteroids and nonsteroidal anti-inflammatories. We often augment the action of one antibiotic by combining it with another, i.e. enrofloxacin with amoxicillin/clavulanic acid. When combining herbs with drugs, the same relationships occur. Occasionally there may be counteraction, i.e. it is not wise to combine St. John's wort with warfarin because this may increase the chance of bleeding (Yue 2000). However, in general, interactions between herbs and Western drugs are much less severe than interactions between two Western medications.

Combining the 2 modalities may expand therapeutic options. Take borreliosis, for example. It is common medical practice to treat seropositive dogs with clinical signs compatible with Lyme disease with antibiotics. These can be combined effectively with herbal supplements to protect joints and minimize the formation of arthritis. Veterinary oncologists who have treated patients on herbal supplements have been pleasantly surprised to see that these patients have much less severe neutropenia than animals not given herbs. This allows the oncologists to give the full dose of chemotherapy at the prescribed intervals and improves the efficacy of the chemotherapy. To restrict oneself to one modality is to miss the opportunity to improve the life of one's patient.

The final stumbling block for acceptance by "modern" practitioners is the often mentioned lack of scientific studies concerning herbs. Throughout this book, references are cited to demonstrate the use of herbs for each specific condition.

Traditionally, professional journals have been reluctant to publish articles about herbs, preferring a more progressive image. Just recently have veterinarians who use herbs been given columns in professional journals. *Veterinary Forum*, the *Journal of the American Veterinary Medical Association*, and *Veterinary Practice News* have published articles concerning herbal medicine and acupuncture.

There are now entire publications directed toward practitioners that carry studies about herbal and homeopathic medicine and acupuncture. For example, *Alternative Therapies in Health and Medicine* is a peer-reviewed journal that has been available at the National Library of Medicine since 1996. Books devoted to acupuncture and herbal medicine are being published in record numbers. Universities and governmental agencies are beginning to conduct research into the use and abuse of herbs. With this increase in research comes a greater understanding of the efficacy and safety of herbal therapy.

Estimates vary according to the source, but between 11% and 80% of Americans take herbal supplements on a daily basis. For this reason alone, it is important for doctors to be familiar with herbs. Even if a physician is not prescribing the herbs, she is seeing patients that use them. Many people extend their use of herbs to animals. A veterinarian who is interested in providing optimal care for his patients has an obligation to become familiar with herbs. People will seek more herbal therapies as research demonstrates the efficacy of herbs and as more lawsuits are published highlighting the potentially serious side effects of Western medications.

Western medicine and herbal supplements should not be considered antagonistic modalities, but rather different sites along a spectrum of therapeutic options. They can and should be combined as needed to treat the patient in the most safe, efficacious, and cost-effective manner. Herbal therapies have become more popular as people find the positive effects of these supplements. As doctors and veterinarians become more familiar with the supplements, we will be able to use them along with Western medications to provide the safest, most comprehensive, and most efficacious therapy for our patients. Then we can truly fulfill our oath to protect animal health and relieve animal suffering.

REFERENCES

Abenyakar, S., Boneval, F. 1994. Increased Plasma B-endorphin Concentration after Acupuncture: Comparison of Electroacupuncature, Traditional Chinese Acupuncture, TENS and Placebo Tens. *Acup in Med*; May vol 12(1) p 21–23.

Bensky, D., Clavey, S., Stoger E. 2004. Material Medica 3rd edition. Seattle: Eastland Press, Inc. p. xv, 711

Bensky, D., Barolet R. 1990. Chinese Herbal Medicine Formulas and Strategies. Seattle: Eastland Press Inc.

CA, A. *Cancer Journal for Clinicians* 1992;116: 34223d.

Chang, F.Y., Chey, W.Y., Ouyang, A. 1996. Effect of transcutaneous nerve stimulation on esophageal function in normal subjects: Evidence for a somatovisceral reflex. *Am. J. Chin. Med.*; vol. 24(2), pp. 185–192.

Chavez, M. 2001. *Journal of Herbal Pharmacotherapy*, volume 1 Number 2: 99–113.

Chen, J., Chen T. 2001. Chinese Medical Herbology and Pharmacology. Art of Medicine Press, California p1.

Han, J.S., Terenius, I. 1982. Neurochemical basis of acupuncture analgesia. *Ann Rev Pharmacol Toxicol*; 22:193–220.

Journal of Herbal Pharmacotherapy, volume 1 Number 2 2001: 99–113 http://www.truestarhealth.com/Notes/1691007.html Accessed 11/05/2006

Kendall, D.E. 1989. Part I: A scientific model of acupuncture. *Am J Acupuncture*; 17(3):251–268.

Melzack, R., Wall, P.D. 1965. Pain Mechanisms: a new theory. *Science* 150:971.

Pan, X.P., et al. 1984. Electroacupuncture analgesia and analgesic action of NAGA. *J Trad Chin Med*; 4(4): 273–278.

Parker, S. 1991. How Things Work. New York: Random House Inc.

Pert, A. 1982. Mechanisms of opiate analgesia and role of endorphins in pain suppression. *Adv Neurol*; 33:107–122.

Reichmanis, M., Marino, A.A., Becker, R.O. 1976. D.C. skin conductance variation at acupuncture loci. *Am J Chin Med.*; 4:69–72.

Schoen, A. 1994. Veterinary Acupuncture: Ancient Art to Modern Medicine. Goleta, CA: American Veterinary Publications, Inc. p6, 24.

Wang, Y.J., Wang, S.K. 1989. Effects of phentolamine and propranolol on the changes of pain threshold and contents of Med and Lek in rat brain after EA. *J Trad Chin Med*; 9(3):210–214

Yue, Q.Y., Bergquist, C., Gerden, B. 2000. Safety of St John's Wort (*Hypericum perforatum*). *Lancet*; 355:576–577.

Notes

1. Some clinicians disparaged Traditional Chinese Medicine because of the lack of specificity in assigning functions in the body to the proper organ. This occurred because it was not considered proper to perform autopsies in ancient Chinese culture. For this reason, it was difficult to assign a function to a particular organ. However, despite the dearth of information gleaned from autopsies, the ancient Chinese physicians did fairly well assigning various functions to the organs. They correctly surmised that the heart was related to circulation and the stomach and intestines to digestion. They did, however, assign various functions to organs that we now know are incorrect. For example, the spleen was believed to play a major role in digestion. We have

discovered that the pancreas and liver are responsible for the digestive roles the Chinese assigned the spleen. This does not, however, render Traditional Chinese Medicine incorrect. We merely need to change our vocabulary somewhat and we can recognize the inherent consistency in their theories. Perhaps when one substitutes liver/pancreas in one's mind when reading the Chinese concept of spleen, it will make the theory more palatable to those of us trained in modern medicine.

2. It is not possible to become proficient in pulse diagnosis by reading books. The interested reader is referred to courses listed in the appendix for further information.

Chapter Four

Homotoxicology—The Modern Approach to Homeopathy

Hans-Heinrich Reckeweg was born in 1905 and became a physician in pre-war Germany. At 18 years of age and following the cure of his father's degenerative kidney condition by homeopathy, Reckeweg declared that he would meld the disciplines of allopathic medicine and homeopathy. As a young medical practitioner, well schooled in the discipline of homeopathy, he noted patterns of disease and therapy emerging. Dr. Reckeweg combined frequently used remedies based upon symptom pictures, and developed an extensive formulary geared at modern scientific Western medical diagnoses.

Seeking to meld the gentler healing potential of homeopathic medicines with the diagnostic capabilities of Western medicine, Dr. Reckeweg spent his life in the pursuit of uniting the unexplained but often very successful art of homeopathy with the science and technology of allopathic medicine. In doing so, he engaged the known principles of both disciplines in a truly brilliant scheme for tracing the ebb and flow of biological systems.

He borrowed freely from the work of Hans Eppinger (1879–1946) and Alfred Pischinger (1899–1983) who were convinced that the body's health was vastly dependent upon the workings of the connective tissue. This opinion was in contrast to the more popular theories of Rudolf Virchow (1821–1902), a contemporary whose theories were based on cellular changes, and though scientific in its observations, were based on the static "photograph" of images seen transfixed on a microscope slide. Virchow's cell theory was the path upon which medical research and theory progressed. However, the fascinating, ever-changing life of the connective tissue ground substance, which constitutes the majority of body tissues, was incorrectly reduced to the importance of a mere sponge or sieve, with no bearing on the health of the organism.

Reckeweg recognized the importance of the intracellular space and developed therapies to affect its actions. As veterinary medicine moves into the next phase of integration, it will become readily evident that we must consider and make use of knowledge involving both the cell and the matrix surrounding it.

Dr. Hartmut Heine of the Institute of Antihomotoxic Medicine and Ground Regulation Research in Baden-Baden, Germany, continues the work of Eppinger and Pischinger today. Regulatory medicine seeks to understand complex metabolic interrelationships and enzymatic systems. The ultimate purpose of this effort is to bring about healing through attempts to gently shift the organism's own biological balance back toward homeostatic optimums through the use of Reckeweg's complex, biologically friendly formulas.

The resulting field known as homotoxicology is that branch of medicine which seeks to identify the toxins in the body, and then aid the organism's natural defense mechanisms in mobilizing the homotoxins, thereby rendering the fluids, intercellular spaces, and cells free of toxic debris. This chapter offers an introduction to this new field.

INTRODUCTION

Homotoxicology is the study of agents toxic or destructive to biological systems, and the organism's biological response to those toxins in the manifestation of disease and pathologic processes. Originally coined by its founder, German physician Hans-Heinrich Reckeweg, the term homotoxicology originates from "Homo sapiens" and "toxicology."

Dr. Reckeweg studied these reactions, made fundamental observations, and developed therapeutic formulas which gently stimulate the natural defense mechanism of mammalian systems toward healing (Homeopathia 2006). Originally designed for humans, homotoxicology has clinically shown promise in many mammalian species and is being used in veterinary practices around the world. (Heel 2005; Reinhart, Broadfoot, Hanover 2005). Reckeweg was a man of science, trained in conventional, scientific medicine. His primary concern was the rapid and complete resolution of his patient's healthcare issues. Reckeweg's homeopathic training and his clinical familiarity made him acutely aware of the often-miraculous results inherent in the field of low-dose therapy. He reasoned that since both methods of treatment yielded improvement in a patient's health, there must be some connection in the broader field of biology, which, when used, would permit a better understanding of healing processes and pathologies. Homotoxicology evolved from this strong intention to unite fields of healing, and has proven to be a very helpful modality in both human and veterinary clinical practice.

In this chapter the reader will be introduced to the subject of homotoxicology, become familiar with a brief history of the science, learn the terms and fundamental concepts necessary to understand and practice homotoxicology in a clinical setting, and gain an initial understanding of low-dose pharmacology and homeopathy. Scientific evidence supporting this modality is contained at the chapter's end. Many veterinarians will quickly recognize and find attractive the fact that homotoxicology aligns nicely with other subjects studied on the path to becoming an effective veterinary practitioner, a fact that supports the validity of homotoxicology theories. Terminology is minimal and aligns with other biological and physical sciences.

The general field of medicine grew out of our mutual desire to help others recover from illness and ultimately live longer, more successful lives. Medicine is a rapidly expanding field, and the advent of a technology which gently stimulates the natural processes of a patient in his path to survival, allows for less invasive forms of treatment, and reduces the toxic side effects of other medical modalities should be readily welcomed.

The main barrier to learning this subject, like any other specialty, is in the definition of words and understanding the concepts that make homotoxicology cohesive with the entire fields of biology, chemistry, and physics. Because this is a rapidly developing field, this is a most exciting time to become involved. It is the author's sincere intent to assist the veterinary practitioner in becoming familiar and competent in the application of biological therapies in clinical practice. This text should not be considered an end to inquiry into the subject of homotoxicology. Interested students should pursue the subject further and will find that as their understanding increases, so will their clinical outcomes improve. As with all medical modalities, the science and technology combine with astute clinical skills to make this a most useful healing art in the hands of one properly trained.

TERMINOLOGY OF HOMOTOXICOLOGY

Every subject has its special terminology. Studies have shown that a major barrier to learning lies in misunderstanding the definitions of words (Hubbard 1992). A student should make a particular effort to duplicate correctly the basic words of any new subject. Because homotoxicology integrates and unites other fields of scientific study, it contains many specialized terms. Most of these terms are identical to the allied field's usage. Fortunately for the student, there are only a few very simple and basic terms and concepts necessary to begin study and practice in homotoxicology.

In studying these terms, keep in mind that homotoxicology is the examination of the relationship of toxins to disease manifestations, and views those disease manifestations as healing. Disease is the body's effort to recover. Biological therapy works with this natural flow of processes to assist the organism's goal of recovery and improvement of its homeostatic condition. When properly managed, pathology is the organism's friend. This concept will become much clearer as the student progresses in his or her study. Reckeweg (2000) defined this first tenet of homotoxicology as:

> "According to homotoxicology all of those processes, syndromes, and manifestations, which we designate as diseases, are the expression, thereof that the body is combating poisons and that it wants to neutralize and excrete these poisons. The body either wins or loses the fight thereby. Those processes, which we designate as diseases, are always biological, that is natural teleological processes, which serve poison defense and detoxification."

NOTE: *This is the principle or theory from which all of homotoxicology proceeds. It is the center point of biological therapy.*

In examining this tenet we can easily see that there are toxic substances. Reckeweg (2000) called these **homotoxins**, from "Homo sapiens" and "toxin." Homotoxins are properly defined as "all those substances (chemical/biochemical) and non-material influences (physical, psychical) which can cause ill health in humans. Their appearance results in regulation disorders in the organism. Every illness is due therefore to the effects of homotoxins. Homotoxins can be introduced from exterior (exogenic homotoxins) or originate in the body itself (endogenic homotoxins)."

By convention, veterinary homotoxicologists have adopted this term to apply to animals as well. Clinical observation has shown that the concept is applicable in diverse species, including mammals, reptiles, and birds, and while the remedies or specific formulas needed by a particular species may vary, the concept is still quite appropriate. While some veterinarians may be tempted to coin terms such as "canitoxin," "felitoxin," "equitoxin," "bovitoxin," or the broader term "zootoxin" in an attempt to differentiate veterinary homotoxicology from its human field, at this time we do not commonly distinguish verbally between toxins damaging to humans or other species. All such substances are currently simply called homotoxins by convention.

In this definition of a homotoxin we perceive the broad scope contained within homotoxicology and we can begin to see why it has such a powerful unifying effect on the subjects upon which it interacts. When we study the interaction of homotoxins upon organisms, we literally are considering all the data concerning disease, all of data regarding pathology, and all of physiology and psychology involved as well. Homotoxicology becomes the center spoke in the wheel of medicine, at once involving and aligning other fields of healing. For this alone Reckeweg deserves great accolade.

Homotoxins can originate from the environment; these exogenic or **exogenous homotoxins** can harm the body and lead to pathologic response. As an example, if air quality is poor, then the body must react to the noxious stimuli. One physiologic reaction is to secrete more tears and mucus to flush the toxic components away and buffer the extreme pH caused by air pollutants. The disease symptom of epiphora is actually the body's attempt to handle the noxious stimuli by elimination and dilution, and thereby regain homeostasis. The body handles these exogenic homotoxins by dilution, excretion, conjugation, and sequestration. Tears physically wash material away, dilute the toxins to lower dilutions, interact with the toxic material chemically through enzymes, and adjust the pH of the resultant area to reduce injury to local tissues. Conventional medicine terms this as irritant conjunctivitis, a quite accurate description. In all three spheres of life, the organism's physiology, conventional Western medical thinking, and homotoxicology, successful treatment begins by removing the organism from the noxious material. If the exposure to the toxin continues, or if the concentration is too high, then more severe damage can ensue and the organism must recruit other methods of handling the situation in its attempt to maintain homeostasis.

Because chemical and physical laws apply to the organism's body, we readily observe that chemical toxins introduced into the system must remain within the system, be altered, or be excreted. These chemical agents can react further with other chemicals within the body and generate new compounds that may be useful or harmful to the organism in its attempt to maintain homeostasis. A practical example of this is heavy metal poisoning in which the toxic metal combines with bodily proteins and alters their function, leading to decreased viability. The body's particular handling of these agents gives us vast fields of

biochemistry, pharmacology, enzymology, and toxicology, to name but a few.

It is important to note that homotoxins are NOT necessarily just chemical poisons. Factually, there are many things that can negatively affect living systems. Anything in excess can become a homotoxin. Take, for example, excess carbohydrates in the diet, which are processed into glucose and used for available energy needs. If biological energy needs are satisfied, then the excess glucose is converted and stored as fatty tissue in adipocytes. These adipocytes require circulatory exchange and energy to continue to function. As fatty tissue accumulates, the organism must supply blood to the area. This takes energy away from the body and is part of the reason why obese patients have less energy and feel tired. In felines, we know that continual exposure of the pancreatic tissue to excess glucose leads to secretion of amyloid and deposition of this material eventually is part of the onset of diabetes mellitus. Excess quantities of glucose in the diet can lead to disease states, and for those interested in disease pathology, that means that seemingly nontoxic items can be homotoxins and contribute to the development of disease.

Radiation and other forms of energetic injury can occur exogenously. These homotoxins lead to coagulation of proteins, DNA alteration, and subsequent loss of structural elements and cellular function, which leads to a decline in organismal integrity. Homeostasis is interrupted and negatively affected by these agents.

Homotoxins originating from within the organism are termed endogenic, or **endogenous homotoxins**. There are many examples of such homotoxins. One metabolic byproduct, ammonia, which results from the metabolism of protein, is a reactive and damaging compound. Raising ammonia levels only slightly leads rapidly to altered central nervous system activity. The body has developed a pathway to reduce the levels of toxic ammonia to maintain proper balance. This system, well known by physiology students, takes place in the hepatocyte, and involves a very powerful but simple biological process whereby enzymes take two toxic ammonia molecules and combine them into a less toxic molecule of urea (Figure 4.1) (Wikipedia 2006).

The resultant urea molecule can be excreted or used in metabolic processes, most notably the conservation of water by the renal medulla (Figure 4.2) ((Nicholson 2002). The nontoxic substance which results from the conjugation of homotoxins is called a **homotoxone**. In this example the homotoxin (ammonia) is conjugated into the homotoxone (urea).

Free radicals are another category of endogenous homotoxin. Free radicals are essential components of cellular metabolism, but if they accumulate to levels in excess of the body's compensatory mechanisms, then cellular

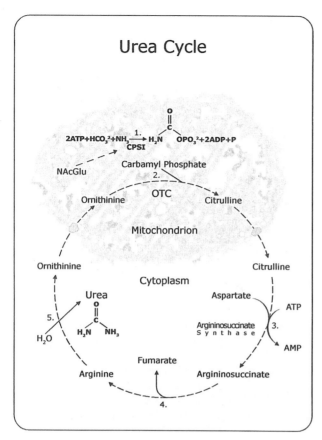

Urea Cycle

$$NH3 + NH3 + CO_2 + 4ATP + Aspartate$$
$$\rightarrow Urea + fumarate + 4ADP\ 4P_i$$

Figure 4.1. In the hepatocyte, toxic ammonia molecules (homotoxins) are combined through enzymatic action to yield nontoxic urea (homotoxone), which is useful for maintaining water balance and can be excreted easily by the kidney. (Modified from Wikipedia courtesy of Alyx MacKenzie.)

injury can result. This appears to be a strong component in the aging sequence. Free radicals can cause direct oxidative damage and alter other molecules and allow for new reactive compounds to be produced. These steps are part of disease pathogenesis (Harman 1998).

On a slightly more abstract level, psychological stress, such as self-created worry, fear, or frustration, can promote tissue damage. It can become a philosophical exercise to determine whether these are actually intrinsic or exogenous homotoxins. One may argue the point either way regarding whether such emotional states are exogenic or intrinsic, but for the purpose of this discussion, it is unnecessary to make this distinction. The more important point is that these stressful states contribute to disease (Kendall 1998). Besides just creating altered circulation patterns, such emotional distress can result in altered nutritional requirements, allow for toxic compounds to accumulate, and alter energy metabolism.

Veterinarians are familiar with protracted states of anxiety or stress leading to increased cortisol levels and a corresponding increase in the frequency of infections and gastric ulcers. In human patients, there is evidence that many emotional states, particularly excessive fear, grief, anger, or worry, can generate specific particles, which act negatively on the organism. (Birnbaum, et al. 2004) As veterinarians, we do not usually deal directly with these psychological issues, but we are well informed about the negative effects of stress on the health of our livestock and pets. Some agents produced by the body in stressful conditions are directly harmful, such as excess hormonal secretion of epinephrine, insulin, and cortisone, while other mechanisms involved in chronically negative emotional states lead to altered mucosal function, diminished circulation, and decreased immune status, and subsequently lead to an increased potentiality for disease to manifest in a patient's overall condition.

Modern human and veterinary medicine are only beginning to scratch the surface of these complex and very important factors in the pathogenesis of disease conditions in living organisms. Oriental medical doctors have long seen a relationship between excessive or prolonged emotional states and specific organ disease. The following emotional relationships are commonly discussed in Oriental medicine: Anger affects liver and gallbladder, joy and love affect heart, worry affects lungs and spleen, pensiveness affects spleen, sadness and grief affect lungs, fear affects kidneys, shock affects kidneys and heart, hatred affects heart and liver, craving affects heart, and guilt affects kidneys and heart (Maciocia 1994). Homotoxicologists view these as biological states, which allow for homotoxin accumulation with resulting damage to the biological system, and corresponding tissue compromise.

It is fascinating to note the improved mental status of patients undergoing detoxification and organ-building therapies in homotoxicology. Patients frequently look brighter and act happier in relatively short periods of time. In one study, 78% of human patients older than 65 and suffering from a wide variety of ailments were found to feel better after just 30 days of treatment with 1 homotoxicology remedy called Galium Heel (Weiser, Gottwald 2000). With the aforementioned information in mind, we can now continue with the discussion of basic terminology and concepts.

In chronic conditions, homotoxins can become deposited with endogenous substances, which cannot be eliminated via normal excretion pathways or through irritation/inflammation. These residual toxins are known as **retoxins** (Reckeweg 2000). Reckeweg coined this term because a significant disease can persist or recur as a result of these agents. A commonly seen retoxin is represented in the nonenzymatic glucosilization of tissues and cell membranes in cases of glucose excess in poorly controlled diabetes mellitus. This

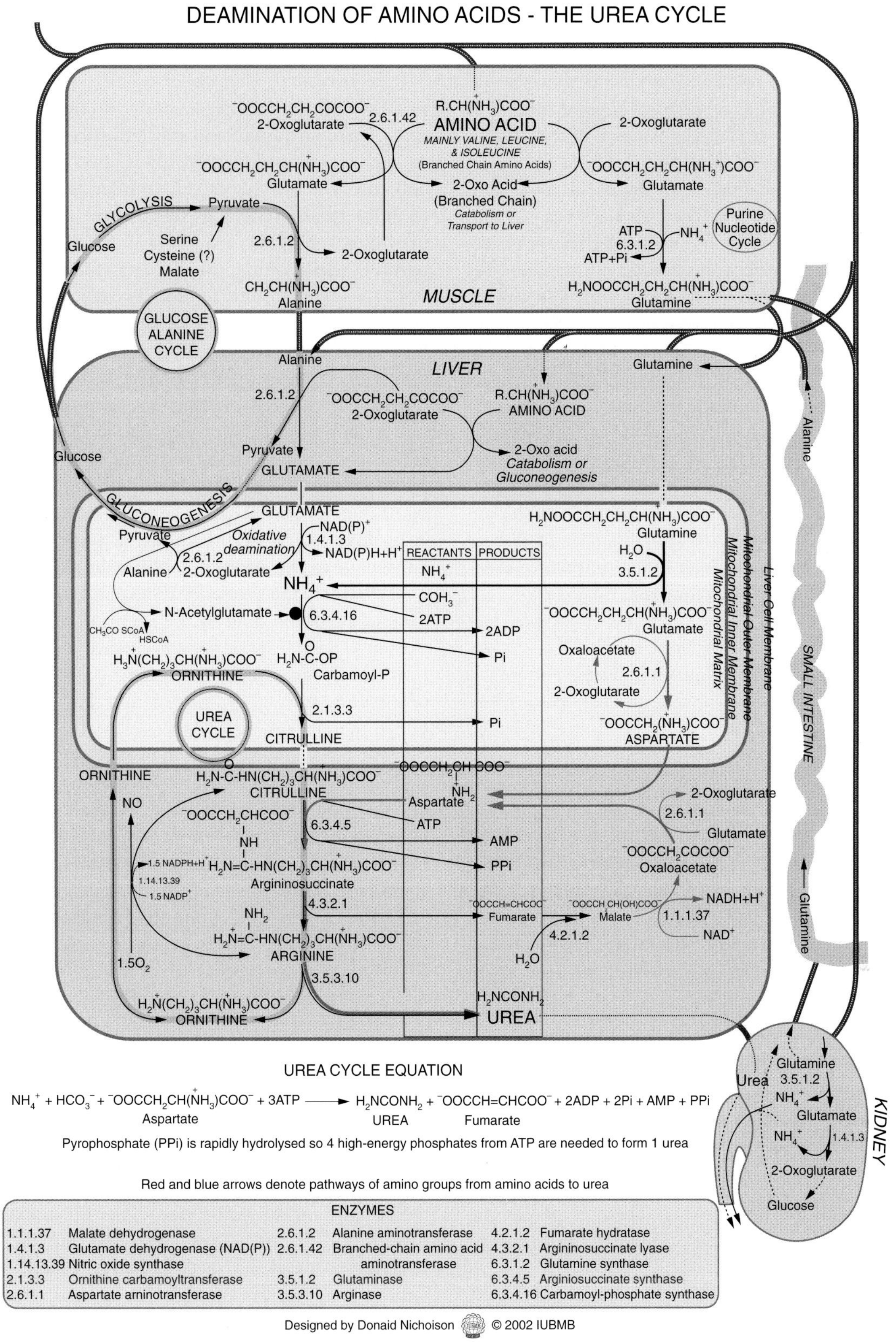

DEAMINATION OF AMINO ACIDS - THE UREA CYCLE

Figure 4.2. Deamination of amino acids leads to toxic ammonia formation. Multiple organ systems reduce this toxic material and excrete it as part of the basic metabolic process. Mitochondria are a major contributor to this important cellular function. (Image used courtesy of IUBMB, all rights reserved.)

glucosilization leads to cellular components that are less flexible and less available to perform their duties. This further leads to progression and worsening of the organic pathology manifested by the patient.

Homotoxicosis is the concept of disease according to homotoxicologists. This is defined by Reckeweg (2000) as "A non-physiological condition which arises after reaction of a homotoxin on cells and tissues. A homotoxicosis occurs as a humeral or cellular appearance and can be followed by morphological changes on tissues. The homotoxicosis leads to defensive measures of the organism whose goal is to eliminate the homotoxins and to restore the physiological conditions when possible."

A homotoxicologist is concerned with both the patient's medical diagnosis and the historical progression of disease signs. These relate to the state of homotoxicosis in a particular case. The medical diagnosis determines which remedies are selected, but the case progression and disease history allow the clinician to determine if a homotoxicosis is worsening or improving. From this information, the homotoxicologist works to alter the state of homotoxicosis present in the particular patient.

This dynamic process of monitoring disease patterns to properly prescribe for a patient requires a frame of reference, and in homotoxicology that reference is called "phase theory." Reckeweg noted that homotoxicoses have chronological progressions and present the practitioner with varied clinical symptoms dependent upon the response of the "ground regulation" of the organism's defense system. Ground regulation simply refers to the local regulation processes as well as the responses coordinated within the neurological, endocrine, humeral, and cellular immune responses. The so-called ground substance is monitored by the fibrocyte, and consists of proteoglycans and glycosaminoglycans as well as the structural and messaging glycoproteins. This connective tissue is also referred to as the "matrix."

The Six-Phase Table of Homotoxicology

The response by the ground system results in a disease pattern indicative of the degree of penetration and damage done to the body by homotoxins. These responses are divided into 6 phases of activity (Figure 4.3) (Reckeweg 2000b):

Phase 1—Excretion Phase
Phase 2—Inflammation/Reaction Phase
Phase 3—Deposition Phase
Phase 4—Impregnation Phase
Phase 5—Degeneration Phase
Phase 6—Dedifferentiation Phase

The final basic concept of homotoxicology is the idea of vicariation, which can be progressive or regressive.

It is critical to our understanding that we see these phases as the natural progression of illness under specific sets of circumstances and the influences of toxins, both exogenous and endogenous. As we begin to recognize the ebb and flow of body defense mechanisms, we can begin to enlist these systems to the benefit of our patients by providing guidance to the regulatory reactions with natural, gentle stimulatory biotherapeutics.

The Six-Phase Table of Homotoxicology is both a conceptual and clinical tool. As students first approach the field of homotoxicology, they are directed to the conceptual tools contained therein. The Six-Phase Table maps disease pathologies resulting from exposure to homotoxins. As homotoxins approach the body, they act on specific tissues and the body responds in specific ways. The resulting signs, symptoms, and pathologies create a recognizable homotoxicosis. The first phases of a homotoxicosis take place in the humeral system and are less dangerous to the survival goals of the organism.

In Phase 1, the Excretion Phase, the body attempts to excrete the homotoxin by the action of various glandular elements. Saliva, tears, sebum, mucus, and sweat all lead to increased flow of material out of the body. Exposure of the body to cigarette smoke, and the homotoxins contained therein, provide a practical example of this principle. The eye and nose respond by secreting more tears and slightly more mucus. Such responses simply wash the area clean of homotoxins. This natural method of removal of homotoxins is extremely important to the maintenance of health in the organism. Generally speaking, such reactions should not be inhibited, and certain agents which decrease secretion of tears and body fluids make the body more susceptible to side effects caused by the body's inability to properly clean itself. An example is increased gum disease seen in psychiatric patients placed on certain medications known to cause xerostomia. Inhibition of salivation leads to increased dental calculus deposition and worsening of periodontal disease.

If the body fails to properly excrete a homotoxin, or if the homotoxin penetrates past the epithelial barrier, then the bioregulatory defense mechanisms can trigger the inflammatory cascade in the continued attempt to remove the homotoxin through Phase 2, the Inflammation/Reaction Phase. In this phase, through the inflammatory cascade, humeral and cell-mediated responses serve to remove homotoxins through the actions of antibodies, cellular responses, phagocytosis, proteolytic enzymes, and increased blood flow to the affected area. Inflammatory exudates move to the surfaces of epithelial surfaces and are eventually excreted to the outside or absorbed by the bloodstream and processed by the lymphoreticular system. These immune system components exist to detoxify inflammatory material and remove it from the body, while simultaneously obtaining vital biological

SIX-PHASE TABLE

	HUMORAL PHASES		MATRIX PHASES		CELLULAR PHASES	
Organ system	Excretion Phases	Inflammation Phases	Deposition Phases	Impregnation Phases	Degeneration Phases	Dedifferentiation Phases
Skin	Episodes of sweating	Acne	Naevi	Allergy	Scleroderma	Melanoma
Nervous system	Difficulty concentrating	Meningitis	Cerebrosclerosis	Migraine	Alzheimer's disease	Gliosarcoma
Sensory System	Tears, otorrhea	Conjunctivitis, otitis media	Chalazion, cholesteatoma	Iridocyclitis, tinnitus	Macular degeneration, anosmia	Amaurosis, malignant tumor
Locomotor System	Joint pains	Epicondylitis	Exostosis	Chronic rheumatoid arthritis	Spondylosis	Sarcoma, chondroma
Respiratory Tract	Cough, expectoration	Bronchitis, acute	Silicosis, smoker's lung	Chronic (obstructive) bronchitis	Bronchiectasia, emphysema	Bronchial carcinoma
Cardiovascular System	Functional heart complaint	Endocarditis, pericarditis, myocarditis	Coronary heart disease	Heart failure	Myocardial infarction	Endothelioma
Gastrointestinal System	Heartburn	Gastroenteritis, gastritis	Hyperplastic gastritis	Chronic gastritis, malabsorption	Atrophic gastritis, liver cirrhosis	Stomach cancer, colon cancer
Urogenital System	Polyuria	Urinary tract infection	Bladder stones, kidney stones	Chronic urinary tract infection	Renal atrophy	Cancer
Blood	Reticulocytosis	Leucocytosis, suppuration	Polycythaemia, thrombocytosis	Aggregation disturbance	Anemia, thrombocytopenia	Leukemia
Lymph System	Lymphedema	Lymphangitis, tonsillitis, lymphadenitis	Lymph-node swelling	Insufficiency of the lymph system	Fibrosis	Lymphoma, Hodgkin-/non-Hodgkin-lymphoma
Metabolism	Electrolyte shift	Lipid metabolism disturbance	Gout, obesity	Metabolic syndrome	Diabetes mellitus	Slow reactions
Hormone System	Globus sensation	Thyroiditis	Goitre, adenoma	Hyperthyroidism, glucose intolerance	Menopausal symptoms	Thyroid cancer
Immune System	Susceptibility to infection	Weak immune system, acute infection	Weak reactions	Autoimmune disease, immunodeficiency, chronic infections	AIDS	Slow reactions
	Alteration*	Reaction*	Fixation*	Chronic Forms*	Deficits*	Decoupling*
Psyche	Functional psychological disturbance, "nervousness"	Reactive depressive syndromes, hyperkinetic syndrome	Psychosomatic manifestation, neuroses, phobias, neurotic depression	Endogenous depression, psychosis, anxiety neurosis, organic psychosyndrome	Schizophrenic defective states, mental deficiency	Mania, catatonia

BIOLOGICAL DIVISION

The six-phase table is a field matrix reflecting medical experience based on careful observation and empirical learning. It is a phase-by-phase arrangement of disorders with no direct relationship between them. No causal pathogenetic link between disorders can be inferred.
The structure of the table makes it suitable for developing a prediction system giving a better assessment of the possibilities for a vicariation effect.
* Phase nomenclature in psychology.

Figure 4.3. As homotoxins accumulate, the greater host defenses of the body respond in an attempt to remove or reduce their damaging nature. These responses can be placed on a descriptive table, which aids clinicians in understanding a particular patient's pathology. Understanding the phase of disease assists clinicians in selecting specific therapy and predicting patient response as well. (© Biologische Heilmittel Heel GmbH, all rights reserved. The Six-Phase Table is copyrighted under German laws protecting intellectual property. Users may download, print, and copy the Six-Phase Table only for personal, non-commercial use. All other intended usage requires the prior written permission of Biologische Heilmittel Heel GmbH. Information contained in the Six-Phase Table has been reviewed and checked with great care. Biologische Heilmittel Heel GmbH, however, makes no representations or warranties about the accuracy or completeness of the Six-Phase Table's content and assumes no liability for its use. All users must agree to use the Six-Phase Table at their own risk. Biologische Heilmittel Heel GmbH reserves the right to delete, alter, or add to the contents of the Six-Phase Table at any time without prior announcement and will incur no liability for doing so.)

Table 4.1. Selected Phase 2 (Inflammation Phase) disorders.

Acne	Cellulitis	Eczema	Otitis	Ranula
Arthritis	Meningitis	Endocarditis	Gastritis	Subluxation
Blepharitis	Cholangitis	Fistula	Polyarthritis	Ulcers
Bronchitis	Dermatitis	Folliculitis	Pyometra	Wounds

Table 4.2. Selected Phase 3 (Deposition Phase) disorders.

Adiposis	Bacterial Overgrowth	Cholesterol Elevations	Fibroma	Hypertension
Arthritis	Chalazion	Constipation	Hematoma	Flatulence
Ascites	Cysts	Exostosis	Helminthiasis	Ostealgia

information necessary for the protection of the body's form and function. Table 4.1 demonstrates the wide variety of pathologies represented by the Inflammatory Phase.

Inflammation literally "burns" certain homotoxins, through enzymatic action, much the same way that a homeowner might burn leaves which have accumulated on his property in the winter. Realize that homotoxins are chemicals and are guided by chemical laws. Once they exist in the body they cannot simply disappear. The body's defense mechanisms must expend energy to excrete, transform, isolate, or neutralize the homotoxin before it does further damage to the body. Inflammation is a major process for the destruction and elimination of homotoxins.

There are many fascinating aspects to the inflammatory reactions of the body. The science of inflammation has advanced tremendously in recent years, and this chapter contains a more in-depth view of inflammation and its relationship to healing in a latter section. Modern veterinary medicine has a mixed relationship with inflammation: On one hand, understanding that inflammation is necessary for proper immune function, and on the other hand, battling and suppressing the signs of inflammation by blocking essential enzyme systems, the result of which can result in devastatingly serious side effects. One example is the recent withdrawal of several prominent nonsteroidal anti-inflammatory drugs in the human medical field. Inflammation has been found to be absolutely necessary in disease recovery and it should not be interfered with unless no other options are available.

In many chronic disease states, the first major sign of true healing is activation of rather remarkable inflammatory signs. Patients may experience reddened eyes, mucus discharges, coughing, vomiting or diarrhea, and skin irritation as they begin to heal. The biological therapist, being properly informed about the importance of inflammation, welcomes these reactions because they signal healing. Fortunately, as we shall see later in this chapter, homotoxicology contains several novel methods of dealing with inflammation, which do not require suppression and enzyme blockages to occur. In many cases, biological therapy can actually speed up the completion of the inflammatory reaction and so resolve the condition rather than simply suppress it.

The third phase is the Deposition Phase, in which the body experiences the effects of toxins depositing deeper into the tissue matrix. The homotoxins enter the matrix and the alterations seen, such as pigmentation, are the result of this infiltration. The excretory mechanisms of the body are overwhelmed and the homotoxin gains access to deeper portions of the tissue. Many disorders that occur in the Deposition Phase are not obvious, because the body compensates sufficiently that the biological reaction is not obvious to either patient or doctor. This phase is particularly difficult due to the occult nature of many of these changes. Table 4.2 shows some commonly encountered Deposition Phase disorders.

The **biological division or biological divide** is an imaginary, conceptual notion of a demarcation, which when crossed over, consists of sufficient damage that the organism is unlikely to recover when left to its own mechanisms. It is a biological point of no return. This imaginary line occurs at the precise moment when the homotoxins make the transition from simply residing in the connective tissue matrix to actually destroying its structure and function. To the right of the biological divide, homotoxicoses have resulted in severe damage and alteration, resulting in dysfunction and predilection to pathological processes. The biological division occurs midway in the matrix phases between the Deposition Phase and the next phase of disease.

If the homotoxins are not handled in Phase 3, or if the insult is severe enough to result in deeper damage, then their deposition and accumulation results in Phase 4, the Impregnation Phase disease. This is the final disease in the matrix phases and is to the right of the biological divide. The name of this phase describes the exact nature of the

Table 4.3. Selected Phase 4 (Impregnation Phase) disorders.

Diabetes mellitus	Inflammatory bowel disease	Heavy metal poisoning	Chronic hepatitis	Myasthenia gravis
Dyspnea	Neuralgia	Nephrosis	Polyneuritis	Asthma
Emaciation	Colic	Ostealgia	Snake bite	Viruses

disorder as homotoxins enter the tissue matrix and are incorporated into the connective tissue, thus compromising its functionality by loss of structural and functional elements such as collagen and enzymes. The progressive worsening of symptoms in this phase results from the alteration in structure and function caused by the homotoxins, and the body's often failed attempts to eradicate them. Symptoms or signs of pain, discomfort, and fatigue frequently accompany these disease states. Allergies or viral infections are classic examples of Impregnation Phase diseases. Impregnation disorders tend to be chronic forms of diseases. Some other common diseases represented by this phase are included in Table 4.3.

The last 2 phases of the Six-Phase Table consist of cellular responses. In these phases the homotoxins enter the cellular sphere and compromise cellular function and structure. In the first phase of cellular disease we have Phase 5, or Degeneration Phase diseases. In this phase homotoxins cause more serious damage and even destruction of larger groups of cells in the tissue or organ. Severe compromise of the body's homeostatic systems leads to progressive, persistent disease. In some cases even these can be reversed through biological means, but in many instances the damage is too thorough for cure, and palliation of symptoms is often all that can be done.

With proper biological therapy and care not to exacerbate the homotoxicosis, such patients can often live long and very pleasant lives. However, all patients to the right of the biological division are prone to acute exacerbation and worsening from minor exposures to homotoxins. Drugs, food additives, environmental toxins or allergens, or even minor viral infections may cause a patient to worsen precipitously and move toward death. When handling these cases the therapist must be extremely careful not to increase the toxin load of the patient or compromise the immune system in any way.

The final phase is Phase 6, the Dedifferentiation Phase, which was formerly known as the Neoplastic Phase. The nomenclature was recently corrected to reflect the fact that not all cases in this phase develop clinical neoplasia. Dedifferentiation homotoxicoses result when homotoxins have penetrated the nucleus of the cell and have altered and damaged the cellular control and repair mechanisms, i.e. decoupling of the DNA strand, enzyme blockage, gene alteration, and gene blocking leading to an inability of

cellular repair. As oncogenes are activated and apoptosis is interrupted we see an increase in tumorgenesis (Bellavite, Signorini 2002).

Accumulated toxic material leads to a cytosol, which is not conducive to basic life processes. The cell, in an attempt to survive a bit longer in an acid environment deficient in oxygen, "de-evolves" and manifests more primitive metabolic pathways (Jordan, et al. 2002). These alterations in the cell population allow for prolonged survival of individual cells, but ultimately bring about a fatal stage of pathology. Even at this late phase, we see the organism creating a response intended to promote the isolation of homotoxins for the purpose of extending organismal survival. Examine the Six-Phase Table below and notice the relationships to clinical entities that are commonly presented to practicing veterinarians (Figure 4.4).

Vicariation, which considers the dynamic course of the patient's condition, is the final basic concept of homotoxicology. It was defined by Reckeweg (2000) as "The transition of the indicating signs of an illness within one phase to another organ system, or the change of the fundamental symptoms and signs into another phase, with or without a change of the organ system."

A veterinarian practicing homotoxicology is concerned with:

1. The homotoxins present
2. Their location
3. The level of penetration and damage to the organism
4. The response of the organism in terms of the phase represented by that response

Patients are found to progress either to the left or right of the Six-Phase Table in their disease patterns. Progression from left to right on the Six-Phase Table means that the homotoxins are doing further damage to the organism and its greater defenses are failing to reverse these effects (Reckeweg 1983).

The term **progressive vicariation** refers to this progression in the disease severity, wherein the patient's condition moves down and to the right of the Six-Phase Table. It means that therapy must be radically altered because the patient is moving closer to death. The desired effect of therapy is for a patient's signs and symptoms to move up and to the left of the Six-Phase Table of

Recovery and Self Healing ⟵   ⟶ Chronic Disease

Embryonic Tissue	Excretion Phase	Inflammation Phase	Deposition Phase		Impregnation Phase	Degeneration Phase	Dedifferentiation Phase
Ectodermal 1. Epidermal	Sebum, cerumen	Pyoderma, erythema	Keratosis, pigmentation		Chronic pigmentation	Dermatosis	Basal cell neophasia, squamous cell tumor
2. Orodermal	Saliva	Stomatitis	Nasal polyps		Chronic stomatitis	Chronic atrophic rhinitis	Oral and nasal neoplasia
3. Neurodermal	Neuro-homones	Feline herpes dermatitis	Neuralgia, neuroma		Viral infection	Paresis, nerve atrophy	Neuroma
4. Sympathico-dermal	Neuro-hormones	Feline herpes dermatitis	Neuralgia, neuroma		Viral infection	Paresis, nerve atrophy	Neuroma
Entodermal 1. Mucodermal	GI secretion	Pharyngitis, enterocolitis	Constipation		Asthma, duodenal ulcers	Chronic bronchial disease, COPD	Cancer of stomach, small & lg intestines
2. Organodermal	Pancreatic secretions	Hepatitis, pneumonia	Gall stones		Chronic hepatitis, viral diseases	Liver cirrhosis, hyperthyroidism	Cancer liver, lung, gall bladder, pancreas
Mesenchymal 1. Interstitiodermal	Hyaluronic acid, GAGs	Abscess, deep pyoderma	Edema, adiposis		Influenza virus infection	Cachexia	Varrious fibrosarcomas
2. Osteodermal	WBC production	Osteomyelitis	Exostoses		Osteomalacia	Spondylitis deformans	Osteosarcoma
3. Hemodermal	RBC, lymph production	Embolism, sepsis	Thrombus		Endocardiosis	Anemia	Leukemia, hemangiosarcoma
4. Lymphodermal	Antibodies, lymph	Tonsilitis	Swollen lymph nodes		Lymphatism	Lymphogranulo-matosis	Lymphosarcoma
5. Cavodermal	Synovial fluid	Polyarthritis	Dropsy		Hydrocephalus	Coxarthrosis	Chondrosarcoma, synoviosarcoma
Mesodermal 1. Nephrodermal	Urine	Nephritis, cystitis	Nephroliths, BPH		Hydronephrosis, albuminuria	Polycystic kidney disease	Renal carcinoma
2. Serodermal	Serous secretions	Pericarditis, peritonitis	Ascites		Preliminary tumor phase	Tuberculosis of the serosa	Serous membrane neoplasia
4. Germinodermal	Ovary, sperm	Prostatitis	Ovarian cysts		Preliminary tumor phase	Sterility	Ovaries, testes, and uterine neoplasia
5. Musculodermal	Lactate	Myositis	Myogelosis		Myositis	Musc dystrophy	Myosarcoma

(Biological Divide)

Figure 4.4. Patterns of disease relationships and the development of pathological states; disease patterns, known as homotoxicoses, can be tracked as they progress or regress in severity using this table. GAG (glycoaminoglycan), WBC (white blood cell), RBC (red blood cell), BPH (benign prostatic hypertrophy), COPD (chronic obstructive pulmonary disease).

Homotoxicology; this movement to the left is termed **regressive vicariation** and is highly desirable. Regressive vicariation indicates that a patient's greater defense mechanisms are activating to remove or neutralize homotoxins. By using the Six-Phase Table of Homotoxicology while monitoring the patient's condition, the homotoxicologist can make therapeutic decisions.

As an example of the concept of vicariation, an aged, canine, pug patient is treated for pigmentary keratitis of both eyes. While supporting hepatic detoxification, the eyes suddenly become red and begin to discharge massive amounts of mucus. The dog feels better but continues to discharge mucus. Biologically, a homotoxicologist's approach to this case is to note that the pigmentation indicates a Deposition Phase disease (Phase 3). Upon starting detoxification, the dog begins to have inflammation and excrete mucus copiously (Phase 2). A well-trained homotoxicologist recognizes this as a shift on the Six-Phase Table and records this as a regressive vicariation in the medical record. He advises the owner that this was critical to the pet's recovery and advises rechecking the case in a few weeks. On the recheck examination the doctor notes reduced pigmentation and reduced inflammation, and the Schirmer tear test reveals increased tear film. Also, closer examination demonstrates the mucus secretion has faded and now the dog is secreting more normal tears. These positive findings indicate healing in action. Therapy should be continued and monitored.

In a similar example, the owner fails to follow the instructions, becomes nervous, and seeks out a conventional veterinarian who prescribes suppressive cortisone eye drops. These reduced the symptom of pigmentation, but the dog later develops kerato-conjuntivitis sicca. This progression of the disease to a more serious and nonreversible disease is an example of progressive vicariation, and serves to demonstrate the importance of proper biological therapy whenever possible.

Understanding the aforementioned simple fundamentals and terminology allows for a nearly infinite number of approaches to a patient's treatment. For the student who spends time comprehending these basics, the application of biological therapy becomes as exciting as it is effective. It is rewarding to assist patients in their own efforts to recover. If, however, a student experiences confusion or difficulty at this point it is best to return to the beginning of this chapter and restudy, paying particular attention to the definition of words. The authors cannot emphasize enough how important these fundamentals are to becoming a successful homotoxicologist.

THE GREATER DEFENSE MECHANISMS

A complex treatise on the immune system is beyond the scope of this text. The authors assume a basic understanding obtained from training in professional schools when addressing basic sciences. Suffice it to say that the better a practitioner understands pathology, biochemistry, cytology, and immunology, the more she will appreciate the subtle workings of biological therapies. Fortunately, we do not have to become master immunologists to use homotoxicology, and in the future much will likely be discovered to explain the precise mechanisms of actions of many of these treatment formulas. It is useful, though, to have a basic understanding of the immune system, and particularly the ground regulation system, and its interactions with antihomotoxic medicines.

Each organism takes up a defined area of space and organizes it for the production of life activities. In the case of animals, these organisms take in physical chemicals and obtain energy through complex metabolic processes we call metabolism. Literally, every body is a mass of cells and control systems, which allow for chemicals (energy) to flow through the system and be organized as is necessary to maintain homeostasis. Hundreds of billions of reactions occur at any moment in a body at rest. Energy flows into the animal body as food and is converted and transported by a wide variety of mechanisms. Undesirable energy, commonly called waste products, must be eliminated. Disorders in energy production or transport negatively affect the ability of the organism to regulate itself. The very processes of life depend upon the organism's ability to maintain the appearance of a steady state in an open energy system, which the laws of entropy constantly attempt to disorganize and disperse. This is the state of health available to an organism as it pursues its course of survival.

Biochemistry teaches us that organisms maintain their reactions at relatively low temperatures, and to do this they require the activity of catalysts called enzymes. These bioactive substances assist in forwarding chemical reactions at these low temperatures. Enzymes require assistance in terms of proper temperature, pH, and co-factors, and agents such as vitamins and minerals.

Most professionals are well versed in the cellular activities of life; however, many professionals know little about the activities that take place in the extracellular spaces of the body. The regulation of physiology in this area is what we are referring to when we talk about the ground regulation system. The extracellular space is filled with a wide variety of substances and acts as a sieve for materials leaving the circulatory system and progressing to the cell. It also contains waste products actively excreted by the cell, as well as through the process of osmosis. Structural proteins such as elastin and collagen provide form and support to a gel-like matrix composed of sugar protein complexes including proteoglycans and glycosaminoglycans. The latter are electrostatically charged in such a way that they bind water and regulate the volume of the connective tissue state. Through their actions the osmotic and ionic state of the tissue is maintained and regulated. We see the basic structural components, which coordinate their functions to maintain the ground regulation system, in the diagram below (Figure 4.5).

Axons contained in the ground substance convey information to the central nervous system, while capillaries carry substrates to the endocrine system and return hormonal substances to the ground substance for action on target cells. The fibrocyte reacts to local conditions and to control center instructions, and maintains proper conditions of the ground substance. Products of the fibrocyte maintain the proper sieve-like state of the ground substance. Note that improper pH or clogging of the matrix by other molecules detrimentally affects the functioning of the ground substance and can lead to deficiencies or excesses of substances needed by the cells that reside there. "Clogging" of the matrix is undesirable and leads to altered flows of waste and nutritional substances in the system.

The ground system maintains a balance of pH by alternating through fluctuating conditions of acidity and alkalinity. Work by Heine, et al. (1997) shows that the matrix's pH alters predictably in human subjects and these swings through pH extremes allow the remaking and maintenance of the structural collagen fibers. During the acid period the collagen molecules become softer and thinner and the matrix becomes more liquid. During the

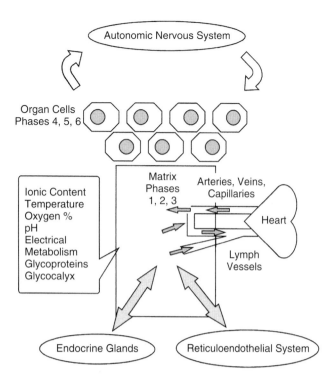

Figure 4.5. The ground regulation system. Note the reciprocal relationships of the components of tissue shown in this figure. Every cell the the body is in contact with the ground substance, which acts like the Internet for bodily information collection, transmission, and evaluation. The functional control cell of the ground substance is the fibroblast, which is the metabolically active center, and controls the activities occurring there. The entire neuroendocrine system works through the ground substance to coordinate bodily functions. (Reckeweg 1983) (Image modified and used courtesy of Corazon Ibara 1983).

alkaline phase the matrix gels and collagen swells (Broadfoot 2004). Pathological pH excesses, particularly acidosis, and the corresponding increase in free radicals, are very damaging to the ground substance and eventually to the cells that reside within. While work of this type has not been done in animals, it makes sense that such a system exists in all higher level, multicellular species. Pain fibers and other inflammatory substances are activated under such circumstances, and can result in immune system overactivity and tissue damage from inflammatory mediators. This may be one of the mechanisms present in autoimmune syndromes. A practitioner can use low-dose antihomotoxic formulas to activate the fibrocyte and other aspects of the autoregulation system to assist the organism in recovery from homotoxin exposure.

The immune system responds to material in the ground substance in several ways. Homotoxicology formulas, also called antihomotoxic drugs, rely on a portion of the immune system for their effects. The immunological bystander reaction is one theory explaining the effects of

these medicines (Reckeweg 2000). When a macrophage contacts an antihomotoxic medicine and/or an antigen, it phagocytizes the material. Macrophages can also be exposed by contact with lympocytes, which have patrolled mucous membrane surfaces and had contact with the material. After phagocytosis, the macrophage processes the material and adds it to an amino acid motif, which consists of the material conjugated to an amino acid chain of 9 to 15 amino acids. This amino acid motif is placed on the surface of the macrophage. Naïve Th0 lymphocytes are presented with these motifs and become recognizable. After accepting the amino acid motif, these Th0 lymphocytes become regulatory Th3 cells, which form motivated clones. After wandering through the lymphatic system and encountering a lymph node, these motivated clones migrate through the circulatory system and distribute to the entire body.

Motivated clones are attracted into areas by a wide variety of chemotactic agents (complement, chemokines), especially those resulting from inflammation. Upon entering the dysregulated area, they can react with other inflammatory lymphocytes (Th4 cells and their subtypes: T-Helper 1 and T-Helper 2 cells). A similarity between amino acid motifs of the lymphocytes allows the production of anti-inflammatory cytokines such as tissue growth factor-beta (TGF-b) and interleukins 4 and 10. TGF-b is a powerful anti-inflammatory cytokine and results in the suppression of the Th4 and other helper cells. Th-2 cells also release TGF-b and inactivate themselves by releasing IL-4 and IL-10, a reaction furthered by TGF-b. This reaction naturally ends or reduces the inflammatory reaction and results in the production of antibodies by B-cell lymphocytes, which have been stimulated by the processes at hand. In this way, antigen insult leads to inflammation, which results in antibody production and body-wide control of the offending agent (Heine 1997b).

Note that the amino acid motif presented does not have to be identical. When a similar agent is present on the amino acid motif, this leads to a reduction of the severity of inflammation and down regulation of the area to a more normal state (Brandtzaeg 1996). It is as if the body is saying, "We have seen this and responded to it already. Please, relax and handle the situation more calmly." We address this circumstance by using homotoxicology formulas that are similar to the disease-causing homotoxin. These much-diluted, low-potency agents stimulate the body into getting well more quickly. Interestingly and importantly, it appears that this reaction can ONLY occur with antigens at very low dosing. The calculated range for the immunological bystander reaction to take place is with antigen dosing of 1ug to a maximum of 1 gram per day per body (Reckeweg 2000). This mechanism provides homotoxicology formulas with several decided advantages. First, the practitioner does not have to know the

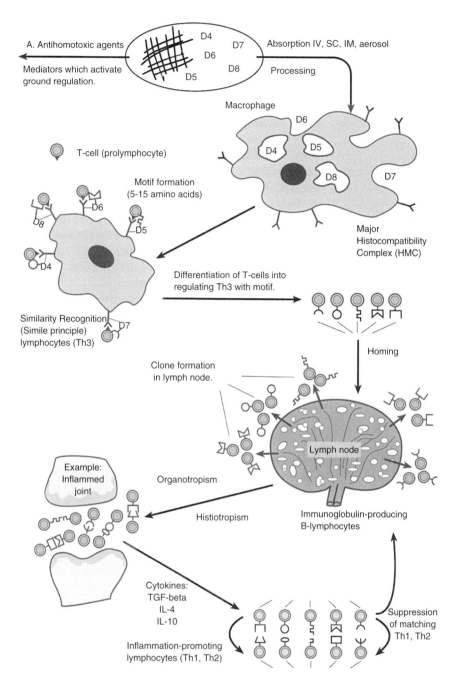

A. Antihomotoxic agents

Mediators which activate ground regulation.

D4 D7 D6 D8 D5

Absorption IV, SC, IM, aerosol

Processing

Macrophage

T-cell (prolymphocyte)

D6 D4 D5 D8 D7

Major Histocompatibility Complex (HMC)

Motif formation (5-15 amino acids)

D6 D8 D5 D4

Differentiation of T-cells into regulating Th3 with motif.

Similarity Recognition (Simile principle) lymphocytes (Th3) D7

Homing

Clone formation in lymph node.

Lymph node

Example: Inflamed joint

Organotropism

Histiotropism

Immunoglobulin-producing B-lymphocytes

Suppression of matching Th1, Th2

Cytokines: TGF-beta IL-4 IL-10

Inflammation-promoting lymphocytes (Th1, Th2)

Figure 4.6. The immunological bystander reaction and its relationship to low-dose antihomotoxic formulas (A). Macrophages are stimulated by low-potency homeopathic dilutions in the D1 to D14 dilution range. These agents can be presented by administration via several routes including subcutaneous (SC), intravenous (IV), intramuscular (IM), and across respiratory mucosal membranes (aerosol). Upon uptake of these antihomotoxic agents, the macrophages form antigen motifs, which are prerequisites for the response by lymphocytes (Th3). These Th3 lymphocytes find chemotactically phlogogenic lymphocytes (T4, Th1, Th2) with similar antigen motifs and suppress these by releasing cytokines. (Image used courtesy of Prof Heine, all rights reserved 1997).

specific offending antigen, but can select one similar to treat a specific organ disease (Reckeweg 2000). Second, the bystander reaction is initiated by oral, subcutaneous, intramuscular, or intravenous routes of administration, a fact that provides the homotoxicologist greater latitude in therapeutic planning (Reckeweg 2000).

The bystander reaction works by further bioregulation and not by suppression, thereby keeping the patient's immune system intact and reducing the chances of further toxicity from higher drug dosages. As a summation, the immunological bystander reaction is illustrated above in Figure 4.6 (Heine 1997b).

WHAT ARE THE DANGERS OF HOMOTOXICOLOGY?

Since the inception of homotoxicology in the early 1950s, millions of doses of antihomotoxic medicines have been administered by a wide variety of dosing routes. According to Heel, 300,000 injections are given daily. Life-threatening adverse reactions so common to pharmaceutical agents have not been observed or reported. In examining injectable antihomotoxic agents the low rate of complication is remarkable, and most commonly involves some minor pain, redness, or swelling at the injections site.

Veterinarians have observed similar statistics (Broadfoot, Demers, Palmquist 2004). Properly used, these agents do not cause severe harmful side effects.

The main danger in practicing homotoxicology is failing to recognize disease patterns that have moved across the biological divide in either direction. Because diseases on the right side of the Six-Phase Table may not improve, patients may receive symptomatic or suppressive therapies to alleviate their immediate symptoms.

Another danger is the confusion that can result if clients and professionals are not properly educated about vicariation reactions. If a patient has begun healing and is involved in inflammatory reactions, some clients may become startled and seek out unnecessary allopathic therapy, which can slow patient recovery. While homotoxicology remedies can be used along with standard pharmacologic agents, caution should be used when choosing suppressive medications during a period of regressive vicariation. Patients who are on the right side of the biological divide can suddenly decompensate and even die after exposure to any toxic agent, including pharmaceutical ones. While this is not the fault of homotoxicology, it can lead to confusion involving those who do not understand biological therapeutic principles. Often this takes the form of a professional administering a standard drug that then gives an unusual reaction caused by the sudden weakening of an already compromised regulatory system. While a patient is receiving biological therapy it is important to avoid unnecessary drugs or chemicals that could cause progressive vicariation to occur.

THE SCIENCE OF LOW-DOSE THERAPY: A NEW FIELD

Nanopharmacology, which literally means small drug study, involves understanding the effects of extremely low doses of substances on the physiology of the body, (Bellavite, Signorini 2002). Until recently, modern medicine has concerned itself mostly with researching agents for pharmaceutical use in the traditional drug marketplace. New data is emerging and our understanding of low-dose therapy is expanding. Dr. Reckeweg and his homotoxicology formulas have provided strong evidence for the effectiveness of such therapy. In 1796, the German doctor Samuel Hahnemann was the first professional to discover the surprising effects of miniscule doses of individual substances and publish a body of empirical research based upon individual case responses. He discovered that when people took very small doses of substances, which in larger doses caused toxic reactions similar to their current disease symptomology, they would often recover from disease states. He called his new form of healing "homeopathy" from the principle "similia

similibus curentur," which in Latin means "Like may be cured by like."

From this practice, the Austrian veterinarian Wilhelm Lux further developed the science of vaccines in the 1830s by manufacturing the first vaccine for canine distemper, as well as anthrax. Hahnemann's clinical practice became wildly successful and excitement spread throughout the world. Constantine Hering established the first homeopathic medical school in the United States in 1835, in Pennsylvania, where it remains today as an orthodox medical school, the Hahnemann Medical College and Hospital. It is unfortunate that, of the many medicines introduced by Hering, only nitroglycerine, a homeopathic medicine commonly used in conventional cardiology, remains in medical practice as a tribute to his medical genius.

Tremendous results from homeopathic therapies in several epidemic diseases helped homeopathy grow in the United States, so much so that by the turn of the 20th century, there were 22 homeopathic medical schools, including Boston University, University of Michigan, New York (Homeopathic) Medical College, and University of Minnesota. Approximately 15% of American doctors considered themselves homeopathic physicians, and there were more than 100 homeopathic hospitals. Homeopathy's popularity declined sharply after the turn of the century, primarily due to the active efforts of the American Medical Association and its collaboration with American drug companies following the Flexner Report.

Because homeopathy had no hard scientific explanation for how these agents worked, and because of Hahnemann's often invalidative, disdainful, and venomous attitude toward conventional medicine, newer doctors who were more interested in a Western scientific explanation fell away from studying homeopathy. The biggest problem with homeopathy has been the inability of anyone to truly explain how it actually works and the difficulty of arranging scientific trials to validate the practice. This remains a stumbling block to this day. Nevertheless, homeopathy has survived into the present time and still is a very valid field of healing thanks to its success in treating patients. Interested readers may find further data about homeopathy and research supporting the field in *The Emerging Science of Homeopathy: Complexity, Biodynamics and Nanopharmacology* by Paolo Bellavite, MD, and Andrea Signorini, MD (North Atlantic Books 1995).

In the late 1800s Dr. Rudolf Arndt and Hugo Schulz, a pharmacist, observed the Arndt-Schulz Principle, which states:

- Weak stimuli stimulate life functions.
- Moderately strong stimuli accelerate them.
- Strong stimuli act as inhibitors.
- The strongest stimuli suspend life functions.

In other words, low dilutions of agents stimulate the body. Moderate doses act as a stimulus to life functions while even higher levels lead to suppression and ultimately death. Take, for example, caffeine in coffee. A cup of coffee wakes a person up and prepares him for the day. Two cups makes him hyper, while 10 cups makes him lethargic. An overdose of coffee of more than 5 cups per day has a direct dose-related effect on the central nervous system, and may affect the heart and its rhythm, blood vessel diameter, and coronary circulation, and increase blood pressure, urine volume, and gastric secretions. These effects are capable of producing bizarre signs and symptoms, which are very baffling, i.e.: high fever or low-grade fever unresponsive to persistent antibiotic treatment, psychoneurosis (anxiety) unresponsive to diazepam, and paroxysmal atrial tachycardia (Flynn 1970).

Modern medical practitioners make use of this principle every day in clinical practice, and pharmaceutical companies have grown very wealthy and powerful using the higher doses of substances and stimulants and/or inhibitors. Most modern drugs, and many herbal preparations, fit this category of the Arndt-Schulz Principle. The lower dilution principles are used but less often appreciated by conventional clinicians.

Nitroglycerine, for instance, is a potent high explosive, but when used in low dilutions acts as a cardiovascular stimulant and vasodilator highly prized by cardiologists. Herbalists naturally use agents in the lower doses and this approach has been discussed in the herbal sections of this text. As scientific knowledge expands, we will no doubt gain information that explains the oftentimes miraculous results which can occur from application of low-dose therapy. The safety and efficacy of these remedies have given birth to a new field and nanopharmacology offers new frontiers for research and development with great potentials for those interested in healing human and veterinary patients.

THE DIFFICULTY OF THE INTEGRATION OF CLASSICAL HOMEOPATHY—A COMPARISON OF MODERN HOMEOPATHY AND MODERN HOMOTOXICOLOGY

While homeopathy dates back to Hippocrates, the founder of what is now modern homeopathy a German doctor, Samuel Hahnemann, who practiced in the late 1700s to mid 1800s. His original theory is based upon the principle of "similia similibus curentur" or "like cures like." Simplified, when a large amount of a toxin is ingested, it can cause death. On the other hand, when this toxic substance is highly diluted, it can often reverse the effects of the toxin. Veterinarians may be familiar with this from the use of phenobarbital. In high doses this barbiturate can cause death. If small amounts of the drug are placed in the body, the liver responds by increasing enzyme-based metabolism, thus reducing the toxicity of the drug.

In homeopathy, highly diluted mixtures of plant, animal, or mineral substances are administered to the patient. Since these remedies are designed to cause the symptoms of the disease they are intended to cure, they actually work with the body's own innate processes. This process is unlike the use of standard medications, which are designed to either block or cover up symptoms. In contrast, a homeopathic treatment is designed to stimulate the innate healing power of the body so that all systems function at their optimum levels.

The symptoms, not pathological signs, of the sick patient are thus the most important guide to the choice of the correct remedy. Classical homeopaths view the animal as having one disease that shows several symptoms. Based upon their level of training and expertise, homeopaths select a single homeopathic remedy that most closely mimics all the symptoms. If the selected remedy is correct, it will cause a healthy animal to react with all the symptoms of the disease. This automatically boosts the body's natural defenses, resulting in healing.

Classical homeopathy (single remedy)

The classical use of homeopathy as espoused by Hahnemann relies on a specific set of symptoms and circumstances occurring in the animal's body. These are the very symptoms that result from the body's inherent defense. The suppression of these symptoms usually inhibits the body in its healing process. Suppose, for example, that an animal has an upper respiratory infection with an ocular and nasal discharge. From the homeopathic point of view, the discharge is proper and beneficial to the body's efforts to heal. The discharge is a combination of body wastes and the local infective bacteria (that are really secondary invaders). If this animal is given an antihistamine and an antibiotic, which dries and removes the inflammation in the mucous membranes, these medications will stop or hinder the process of the body ridding itself of these wastes, and homotoxins can accumulate, causing further damage to local tissues.

Homeopathically, the body is not efficient in discharging the wastes. The body wastes are then retained, which eventually may lead to a more serious condition such as chronic bronchitis or pneumonia. Inflammation and fevers literally burn off trapped homotoxins. They can be necessary to proper and full recovery.

What emerges from this example is a different perspective of the approach to disease and the healing process.

Instead of focusing on the suppression or removal of symptoms, the homeopathic approach is to support and augment the immune system and the cleansing effect of the eliminative processes so the body moves itself toward healing.

While classical homeopathy is a proven science and form of medicine and is supported by numerous medical and healthcare professionals, it also has a divisive side. In the 19th and early 20th centuries, it served as the catalyst in the development of modern medicine as the allopathic professionals left no stone unturned to discredit the science and art of homeopathy. While veterinary homeopathy is much more acceptable now, it still has an unintentionally divisive side with regards to integrative veterinary medicine. A veterinarian who steps away from the classical homeopathic model and focuses the homeopathic remedies instead of relying on the classical method of practice is derogatorily labeled an "allopathic homeopath" who uses a buffet type of approach to the treatment of the animal, bringing out the difficulty of integrating classical homeopathy within the holistic veterinary arena. Frankly, this difficulty may not be a bad thing, as classical homeopathy works best when done according to Dr. Hahnemann's research findings. For the time being it appears that classical homeopaths get their best results when they maintain their separate status.

Classical versus combination homeopathy

Based upon the very nature and philosophy embodied by classical homeopathy, the use of other remedies and certainly any medications during treatment is not recommended and is, in fact, counterproductive. This is because the classical homeopathic approach uses a single remedy to achieve the same symptoms as the disease. Other medications and remedies that could alter these symptoms give the homeopath a false read and interfere with the treatment. Therefore, classical homeopathy does not lend itself to integration into veterinary practice.

Professionals who use combinations of homeopathic remedies differ from those who use classical, single remedies in their approach to a condition. The theory behind combinations is that several low-dilution remedies are mixed together with the purpose of addressing a specific symptom, supporting an organ or tissue, or helping set the stage for regeneration and healing. Good examples are combinations that are used in arthritic animals. Some individual ingredients may address inflammation, and others pain, while still others may support the body in the elimination of excess minerals and toxins. The overall result is that the remedy works with the body's metabolic processes to reduce the symptoms at their origins and promote healing. In this regard, the homotoxicologist is

kin to the herbalist and this approach is found to be successful in both fields.

Homotoxicology—a more modern approach

Homotoxicology, founded by Dr. Hans-Heinrich Reckeweg in 1952, is a branch of medicine which combines classical homeopathy with conventional medicine to achieve the benefits of both art forms of practice. Dr. Reckeweg's tenet of homotoxicology is that all signs, symptoms, and syndromes which we classify as disease processes are an expression of the organism in its active effort to combat homotoxins. The anti-homotoxic therapy uses low-potency combination homeopathic remedies in an indication-based approach to help the body to rid itself of toxic debris by supporting the natural defense mechanisms, thereby setting the stage for healing. Because homotoxicology uses conventional medical indications along with combination homeopathic solutions, it serves as the connecting link and basis for the integration of alternative therapies into conventional practice.

Homotoxicology works by engaging a complex set of bioregulatory feedback loops and improving the enzymatic and energy-producing activities of the cells, which regulate the relationship between anabolic and catabolic processes. The working principles of such a biological medicine use the body's own self-regulating processes (autoregulation) to achieve self-healing. Dr. Reckeweg, in 1948, devised a brilliant concept for tracking the flow of disease, in what is called the Six-Phase Table of Homotoxicology. It is, in effect, a road map of the biological system's response to the presence of toxins in the system, and it provides a logical sequence of events for the veterinary practitioner to evaluate therapeutic efficacy. One of the advantages of this modality is that a deep understanding of the principles is not required for a practitioner to find success in therapy. The remedies have such broad and deep activity, that even a superficial knowledge of the combinations produces startlingly good results.

Unlike the incredible fields of traditional Oriental medicine, Ayurveda, and other ancient healing arts, which can be nearly incomprehensible to novice practitioners, homotoxicology diagnosis and case programming is based upon symptom pictures and clinical diagnoses which are easily recognized by doctors trained in Western medicine. It is a "take home" kind of therapy. Armed with a few anti-homotoxic remedies and a desire to learn a gentler medicine, one can have a positive impact on the quality of life of his or her patients.

The following table illustrates how homotoxicology is a link between conventional and alternative practices and sets the stage for true integration by combining medical and diagnostic procedures along with the more natural healing techniques of homeopathy (Table 4.4).

Table 4.4.   A comparison of homotoxicology with classical homeopathy and allopathic medicine.

	Allopathy	Homotoxicology	Classical homeopathy
Diagnosis	Using clinical findings	Using clinical findings	Using mental and somatic/constitutional findings
Therapy	To treat local symptoms	To create general well-being	To create general well-being
Remedy	Clinical preparations	Homeopathic combination preparations	Homeopathic single remedies

CLINICAL APPROACHES USING HOMOTOXICOLOGY AND NANOPHARMACOLOGY

We now have a basic understanding of the progression and pathogenesis of disease states according to basic homotoxicology theory. We have also seen how the immune system regulates itself and how low-dose agents appear to assist in regulating the greater defense mechanisms by gently stimulating the normal bioregulatory functions of the organism. In this next section, we examine the clinical approach to viewing a patient's particular conditions and the biological therapy steps which can be taken to assist the organism in its pursuit of better states of survival. As we move toward specific therapy, it is useful to gain some familiarity with the basic formulas available for use in the clinical environment.

Homotoxicology formulations

Homotoxicology contains a myriad of formulas designed by Dr. Reckeweg and distributed by a German company (with United States distribution) called HEEL, which stands for "herba est ex luce," or "herbs are from light" (Heel Web site). HEEL (usually written Heel) and Heel USA produce more than 200 separate formulas.

The clinical use of these particular remedies is detailed in the publication entitled *Biotherapeutic Index: Ordinatio Antihomotoxica et Materia Medica*. Serious use of homotoxicology requires an understanding of this text and it is highly recommended that readers obtain a copy as soon as possible in their study of homotoxicology. It has been observed that individual success in the subject depends upon having this text available in the clinical setting. Readers are also referred to *Materia Medica* by Hans-Heinrich Reckeweg and *Homeopathic Homotoxicological Repertory* by Ivo Bianchi for more detailed reading about individual ingredients and indications for use of these antihomotoxic formulas. Students greedy for knowledge will find a tremendous amount of useful material contained in these basic clinical references. A nearly infinite number of treatment options can be produced once a practitioner becomes familiar with their basic purposes and functions. Homotoxicology is well described as an art or applied science for this reason.

Other companies besides Heel produce combinations of low-dose agents, but few, if any, have produced the volume of agents and the research and support of practitioners seen at Heel. Therefore, this text deals extensively with Heel-produced remedies. This is not due to corporate sponsorship, but rather the experience of the authors with their products. Without doubt there are many products on the marketplace for clinicians and researchers to evaluate, and the Heel line is only one such product line. As this field develops, further research will no doubt expand our formulary of useful antihomotoxic medicines.

Examination of individual remedies is too extensive for this brief treatise. In the following paragraphs we peruse a few major remedies and provide some understanding on their applications. We also provide some literature citations for interested students to use as a springboard into their improved understanding and use of homotoxicology. Antihomotoxic formulas produced by Heel come in several forms:

Homaccords, so called because they contain one or more agents originating from mineral, plant, or animal sources, which have been prepared homeopathically in several different homeopathic dilutions. Examples of these are *Nux vomica homaccord*, *Cocculus homaccord*, *Phosphor homaccord*, and a host of others.

Compositae, which represent a unique development by Dr. Reckeweg. These agents contain a wide range of mineral, plant, and animal products that are at low-dilution strengths. These low-dilution substances gently strengthen particular organs or tissues. They assist the healing of specific organ syndromes and are extremely useful, especially in more chronic forms of pathology. The agents theoretically assist healing by many mechanisms including organ trophism, toxin drainage, inflammation moderation, and activation of fibroblast activity in the repair of tissue. These include, among many others, *Echinacea compositum*, *Apis compositum*, and *Placenta compositum*.

One of the most remarkable categories of antihomotoxic medicines is the remedy group known as catalysts. Dr. Reckeweg made a major contribution to medical therapy with these agents, which gently stimulate the basic metabolic processes and rehabilitate mitochondrial function. This allows for improved energy metabolism, a requirement of nearly all chronically diseased patients. Three commonly used catalysts are *Ubichinon compositum*, *Coenzyme compositum*, and *Glyoxal compositum*. *BHI Enzyme* is another product with catalyst activity. In addition, many of the combination remedies in the compositae group contain catalysts for cellular and mitochondrial function (e.g. *Hepar compositum*, *Thyroidea compositum*).

Injeels, which are single-agent homeopathic preparations in a wide variety of dilutions. The word injeel comes from "<u>inj</u>ection-remedy H<u>eel</u>." For readers in the United States, many of the injeel products are not readily available. European markets do provide these agents, which can be of great assistance in handling cases. Hopefully, in the future, more of these will become available to practices in the United States. This text does not deal with these products because they are not available in the United States, but basically they are applied according to their indications in classical homeopathy. Injection of these agents, as well as other antihomotoxic drugs, into acupuncture points is known as biopuncture, and it has many intriguing applications in human and veterinary medical practice (Kersschot 2002).

Symptom-based therapeutic formulas contain a wide variety of therapeutic agents and are designed to address specific clinical syndromes. Table 4.5 contains a list of important symptom remedy formulas. There are many of these formulas; those listed below are simply the most commonly used in veterinary practice. In a recent survey of active veterinary homotoxicologists, these formulas were listed in the top 25 antihomotoxic medications currently in use in the United States (Broadfoot 2004).

Table 4.5. Common antihomotoxic symptom remedies and their uses.

Remedy formula	Clinical application
Cralonin	Cardiac disease
Engystol-N	Influenza, viral infections, allergy, immune stimulation
Gripp-Heel	Influenza-like infections
Lymphomyosot	Lymphoedema, immune suppression
Rheuma-Heel	Non-articular rheumatism syndrome
Spascupreel	Colic, migraine-spastic, myogelosis
Spigelon	Headache
Traumeel S	Arthritis, traumatic injury
Vertigoheel	Vestibular syndromes
Viburcol	Fever, mild infection, excitation
Ypsiloheel	Central control
Zeel/Zeel compositum	Arthritis

One of the most researched and best-known homotoxicology remedies is *Traumeel*-S, which is formulated to decrease the severity of inflammatory reactions. It is a nonsteroidal, anti-inflammatory combination antihomotoxic remedy that does not inhibit necessary enzyme systems. *Traumeel*-S assists in ending the inflammatory reaction by accelerating the body through the Inflammatory Phase into the healing phase, as outlined previously in the section on immunological bystander reaction. It is one of the most used and recognized complementary medicines in the world. It has practically no listed side effects, other than some very rare minor reactions in individuals who are sensitive to its ingredients. Excretion and minor inflammatory reactions may occur as the body mobilizes and begins clearing homotoxins, and this is usually a desirable result as opposed to an adverse reaction. *Traumeel* is supplied as a tablet, oral vial, injectable vial, ointment, and gel. It is useful in many clinical syndromes, a partial list of which includes:

Soft tissue trauma of any kind
Inflammation of any kind
Postoperative pain
Arthritis, especially of the hip, knee, and small joints
Arthralgia
Regulation rigidity, type 1
Pyoderma
Otitis externa
Otitis media
Pruritic dermatitis
Peridontitis
Gingivitis
As an adjunct post radiation
Abscess and furunculosis
Intervertebral disc disorders

Traumeel's exact mechanism of action is not known, but it decreases inflammation, stabilizes blood vessels, modulates pain, and stimulates regeneration (Reckeweg 2000). Further discussion of this remedy occurs in the evidentiary section of this chapter.

If a student of homotoxicology progresses no further than to include one remedy, it should be *Traumeel*-S. Applying this remedy to the common issues seen each day in veterinary practice rapidly gives a new homotoxicologist the confidence needed to pursue other remedies. The authors use this preparation in nearly every surgery case for pain control as well as modulation and stimulation of the greater defense mechanisms, which are essential for rapid and proper healing. The results from using one vial of *Traumeel*-S in a bottle of IV fluids during routine treatment for shock can be very rewarding.

Another commonly used symptom remedy formula is *Zeel*, which comes as an oral drop, tablets, injection, and

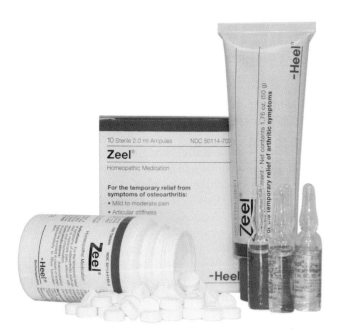

Figure 4.7. Zeel is a commonly used antihomotoxic formula for treatment of osteoarthritis. (Image courtesy of Heel USA. All rights reserved.)

ointment. (Figure 4.7). *Zeel* contains a wide variety of low-dilution herbal, animal tissue, mineral, and organic molecular ingredients, which improve tissue function, reduce pain and inflammation, and fuel metabolism of cellular elements. This formula was recently evaluated in a double-blind placebo study and was compared against the NSAID drug Diclofenac. (Marrona, Weiser, Klein 2000). The study revealed that *Zeel* worked as well as the pharmaceutical NSAID in relieving arthritis pain of the knee in human patients, and has no dangerous side effects. Another study examined the effectiveness of *Zeel* versus Celebrex and yielded similar results (Birnesser, Klein, Weiser 2003). The onset of effect can be rapid but in most cases takes 4 to 5 weeks to become evident (Weiser 2003). *Zeel* has been demonstrated in vivo to effectively inhibit serine proteinases and metalloproteinases (Heine 1997, Stancikova 1999). The fact that *Zeel* has been shown to act on both the LOX and COX system explains its observed clinical effect as well as its increased safety (Jaggi et al. 2004).

Many acute cases of arthritis can be improved with of a combination of *Zeel* for long-term use, *Traumeel* for short-term pain management, nutraceuticals (glycoaminoglycans, MSM, SAMe, omega-3 fatty acids, etc.), and herbs. More details on these combinations appear in the clinical protocol section of this text. Because of its safety and the widespread incidence of various forms of arthritis in elderly patients, *Zeel* is a popular formula in both human and veterinary medicine. It often gives a patient her first exposure to natural medicine. It is not unusual

for a client to begin her pet on a course of *Zeel* and then develop further interest in pursuing biological therapy for her pet and herself.

Cralonin is a useful formula for management of geriatric cardiac conditions, both minor and more serious (Schroder, Weiser, Klein 2003). It contains homeopathic dilutions of Crataegus, commonly known as whitethorn or hawthorne. This herb and its homeopathic preparation is well known for its supportive effects on cardiac function, and hawthorne is used globally for this purpose. It is thought to increase blood flow to the heart and act as an antioxidant, thereby strengthening weakened cardiac tissues. Homotoxicologists frequently prescribe this formula to assist general cardiac issues, as well as strengthen geriatric patients whose examinations suggest decreased circulation. A case report demonstrates reversal of symptoms and echocardiographic lesions in a cat with hypertrophic cardiomyopathy. (Palmquist 2005, 2006). It will be some time before such reports can be substantiated through repetition and scientific study, but the prospects are exciting. In the meanwhile, use of *Cralonin* often yields excellent results and it should be readily considered in both early cardiac cases, as well as adjunctive therapy for more advanced cases. This particular formula is frequently prescribed for long-term use. As with all cardiac patients, regular re-evaluation of patients with heart disease is recommended.

The purpose of this section is to give a basic understanding of the types of symptomatic remedies available to the homotoxicologist and to provide the reader with some comfort in using these agents. Further clinical and scientific evidence is contained in the evidentiary section, which follows later in this chapter. By now the reader has a good foundation with which to approach cases, so now we embark on a clinical case that serves to illustrate how the theory of homotoxicology becomes an applied technology for healing.

Proceeding toward a treatment plan

We have reviewed the basic concepts and terms, discussed remedies briefly, and given the reader some familiarity with homotoxicology theory. In this section we begin to assemble what is needed for a student to apply this field to patients seen in clinical practice. As we proceed, please do not lose sight of the fact that all legitimate forms of healing can be considered in the development of a treatment plan. It is not our purpose to develop rote methods of application, because a competent practitioner will readily recognize that each patient's disease is a unique expression of his biological response. It is totally possible to have two patients share signs, symptoms, and pathological diagnoses that appear identical, but require vastly different treatment methods to get positive responses. The application of theoretical principles and established technologies by an informed professional is what makes this the art of practice. Just as an artist uses many different media to convey his message, so may a doctor practicing biological therapy find a wide variety of valid pathways in her search for healing. Any methods which lead to regressive vicariation and an increase in ability for a patient are valid therapy. There are, though, predictable ways to approach patient programming and that is the purpose of this current discussion.

When presented with a patient, just as in regular veterinary practice, it is prudent to begin with a thorough medical history. If multiple doctors have been involved, it is a good idea to obtain copies of all medical records, laboratory tests, imaging, and other diagnostic testing, and review these with emphasis on the following items:

Environmental history: Where a patient has lived. Any stressful situations involving people or other animals (e.g., abuse, drug dependency, family strife, etc.). Known exposure to environmental chemicals (e.g. herbicides, pesticides, construction materials, tobacco smoke, incense, aromatherapy, etc.).

Disease history: Make a list of all diseases or problems in the medical record in order of appearance. Seasonality can be a major clue in many cases.

Therapeutic history: Make a list of all drugs, vaccines, topicals, supplements, and prescription diets.

Dietary history: Knowing which foods are eaten can give great assistance in evaluating a patient's disease evolution.

Current symptoms/diseases and their duration: Acute cases are often phases one through three, while more chronic cases fall in the last three phases of homotoxicoses.

Client's disagreements, upsets, or problems: Issues with past therapy, as well as client's current goals of therapy.

Complete physical examination: This is no different than any routine examination, and should include all body systems. Biological therapists pay particular attention to changes, which give a clue as to phase of disease. Some common clues can be seen as follows:

- **Discharges in excretion and reaction phases.** Generally, watery discharges locate a lesion more to the left of the phase table. Suppurative discharges usually occur in the Inflammation Phase, but can be observed in other phases and in particular the Impregnation Phase. As a homotoxicosis shifts phases, the clinician frequently notices the discharge will begin as solid or firm, then change to waxy or thick, and then finally become more oily or serous. Such changes indicate better prognosis. Because many of our common diseases, such as allergies, occur in the Impregnation Phase, it is common that these patients have little or no obvious signs and then after beginning biological therapy develop copious discharges. These are greeted with excitement by skilled homotoxicologists because they signal the body's attempt to improve its status and health.

- **Pigmentation variations.** Pigment occurs when a chronic change has been in effect. It often signals a Deposition Phase disorder. If the pigment has been there chronically, then often these cases are in Impregnation or Degeneration phases. As they undergo regressive vicariation, patients with pigment commonly become intensely itchy and then develop inflammatory changes, which eventually discharge waxy or greasy material. If the clinician is aware, he or she will note that the pigmentation is thinning, often even developing small foci of normal or slightly pink coloring in the pigmented area. This is a very good prognostic sign and should NOT be interfered with or suppressed. Clients need to be advised regarding this for the best results to occur. Normally pigmented body parts losing pigment is a sign of serious homotoxicoses, which usually represent Degeneration Phase disorders. Diseases such as discoid lupus erythematosis (DLE) are marked by nasal depigmentation and represent autoimmunity aggravated by solar exposure and subsequent tissue degeneration. They can signal a patient's movement toward the neoplastic state.

- **Thickened or less flexible muscles, skin, tendons, or ligaments.** Thickening indicates a compensatory deposition of connective tissue fibers. These commonly occur in the Impregnation, Degeneration, and Dedifferentiation phases. Any veterinarian who has treated chronic cocker spaniel otitis or chronic anterior cruciate ligament tears (medial buttress) is familiar with these changes. Such alterations rapidly lead to a Degeneration Phase if left untreated. Upon activating the greater defense mechanism, affected patients frequently develop productive otitis. Chronic proliferative otitis shifts upon healing into an inflammatory condition, which represents a Phase 2 inflammatory reaction. If these cases are supported biologically and not suppressed, they can improve and reduce canal scarring and pinnal thickness, but the alteration in structure usually fails to resolve in its entirety. The clinician should expect a long course of healing and advise the caregiver accordingly. Not all clients agree to continue therapy, and their decision must be taken into account when approaching chronic cases. If a client is not willing to pursue a long course of therapy and the chronic inflammatory and exudative actions of the case as it heals, it may be more appropriate to resort to medical drugs and simply manage the symptoms.

- **Corneal and lenticular clarity.** The eyes become cloudier as homotoxins are deposited into connective tissue. Clients commonly report better corneal or lenticular clarity while undergoing detoxification therapy. Cataracts are generally in the Degeneration Phase and are irreversible in most patients. Detoxification of the liver frequently results in mucoid ocular discharge. During such periods the eyes can turn red as well. It is routinely noted that as the liver recovers this discharge declines and becomes more fluid. Chinese medicine has long realized this relationship between liver disorders and ocular changes and it is fascinating to see this connection appear in patients as they recover. This is a normal and good prognostic sign to an aware homotoxicologist.
- **Nails and hair coat characteristics.** Vital patients have adequate resources to produce healthy hair coats and nails. If the body is deficient or diseased, then the coat or nails are often dry or less vital. As a patient moves on the phase table, the coat and nails can serve as a clue as to whether the changes are regressive or progressive vicariation. Alopecia resulting from rabies vaccination has been reversed using antihomotoxic medications and biological therapy in the author's practice.
- **Mobility, vitality, and awareness.** These indicate the level of energy and assist in evaluating a patient's progress on the current treatment plan. It is often observed that a patient with discharges or showing other signs of disease such as coughing, vomiting, or fever demonstrates improving mental status. In cases where the patient's vitality is increasing, the clinician frequently finds that the disease signs actually represent active regressive vicariation. This can be extremely useful in determining when to intervene and when to allow the body the freedom and support to accomplish its reparative efforts. Many such exacerbations improve within 3 days of their appearance. When improvement of the condition is observed in this time period, the clinician can be reasonably certain that regressive vicariation is occurring and should reassure the client as continued patient monitoring occurs.
- **Oral health and breath.** Oral disease and conditions of the tongue, teeth, and gums can be very helpful in location and correct treatment. This is not unique to biological therapy, but the mouth is often overlooked, especially in fractious patients. Traditional Oriental medicine has much to say about diagnosis through evaluation of the tongue (Maciocia 1995). This is a useful modality for biological therapists in determining remedy selection and the efficacy of a treatment plan. Most courses in Oriental medicine include a section on tongue and pulse diagnosis.

The reader will recognize the aforementioned as common steps in conventional examination and diagnosis. Interpretation of signs can vary when one adds on understanding of homotoxicoses and the Six-Phase Table of Homotoxicology, but good medicine is the hallmark of good biological therapy. The best results in any medical scene occur with professionals who are well trained, effective observers, and who involve their clients in the process.

Upon completing and evaluating the examination, the doctor proceeds by listing conditions to rule out. A diagnostic plan is constructed and carried out with the client's understanding and consent. Once again, this is no different than conventional practice; however, by now the clinician should be forming some ideas about the phase of the patient's condition. Tests are completed and examined and a working diagnosis is developed. If the diagnosis is unclear, then the homotoxicologist can proceed to assist the patient by prescribing symptom- and phase-based remedies, while the process of diagnosis continues. One or more phase remedies can be selected from the table below (Figure 4.8).

The phase remedy or remedies selected are combined with a symptom remedy and the owner is instructed to administer the combination twice daily according to the dose schedule below (Table 4.6) (Broadfoot 2002).

Detoxification

Detoxifying the body involves draining the homotoxins from the area, and there are many remedies that assist in performing this action. For superficial cases—those in the Excretion or Inflammation phases—simple drainage and detoxification using the *Detox Kit*, which consists of *Berberis homaccord* (drains kidney and liver and supports adrenal function), *Lymphomyosot* (immune stimulation and lymphatic drainage), and *Nux vomica homaccord* (supports liver and drains the gastrointestinal system) is an excellent choice. For medium cases—those in the Inflammatory Phase more chronically or those in the Deposition Phase—a mixture of *Solidago compositum* (kidney support and drainage), *Hepar compositum* (liver support and drainage), *Galium-Heel* (cellular detoxification and drainage and organelle repair), and *Lymphomyosot* (lymphatic drainage and immune support) are selected.

For deeper cases—those in the Impregnation to Dedifferentiation phases—the detoxification formula is customized to the specific needs of the patient. Generally, this formula includes *Galium-Heel, Lymphomyosot, Thyroidea compositum, Solidago compositum, Hepar compositum* and/or *Hepeel*, and especially catalysts such as *Ubichinon compositum, Coenzyme compositum,* and *Glyoxal compositum*. These are dosed depending upon

Excretion Phase	Inflammation Phase	Deposition Phase	Biological Divide	Impregnation Phase	Degeneration Phase	Dedifferentiation Phase
Remedies	*Remedies*	*Remedies*		*Remedies*	*Remedies*	*Remedies*
Nux vomica Homaccord	Traumeel	Galium-Heel		Thyroidea Compositum Rx	Mucosa Compositum	Tonsilla Compositum
Lymphomyosot	Belladonna Homaccord	Lymphomyosot		Tonsilla Compositum	Molybdan Compositum	Galium-Heel
Berberis Homaccord	Aconitum Homaccord	Solidago Compositum		Psorinoheel Rx	Coenzyme Compositum	Lymphmyosot
Hepeel	Echinacea Compositum	Placenta Compositum		Echinacea Compositum	Ubichinon Compositum	Viscum Compositum
Reneel Rx		Pulsatilla Compositum			Galium-Heel	Glyoxal Compositum
Psorinoheel Rx					Lymphomyosot	
					Glyoxal Compositum	
					Placenta Compositum	
Alteration	**Reaction**	**Fixation**		**Chronic Forms**	**Deficits**	**Decoupling**

Figure 4.8. Phase remedies address the specific nature and location of pathology being manifested in a particular disease state. In treating with homotoxicology, the doctor selects 1 or more phase remedies to begin the process of homotoxin mobilization and excretion. These remedies are continued as long as the patient's status continues to change. As homotoxicoses shift, the practitioner alters the phase remedies selected. When used properly, these formulas lead to a regressive vicariation and patient improvement.

Table 4.6. Dosing schedule for oral antihomotoxic formulas in common veterinary practices.

Species and dose	Tablets	Tinctures	Ampoules 5ml	Oral vials/ampules	Ear drops	Ointment/ gel
Horse/cow	4—5 tabs 2—3X	10—20 drops 2—3X	1 vial 2—3X	1—3 vials 2—3X	1 vial 2—3X	Apply
Large dogs	1—2 tabs 2—3X	10—15 drops 2—3X	1/4—1/2 vial 2X	1/2—1 vial 2—3X	1 vial 2—3X	topically
Medium dogs	1 tab 2—3X	8—10 drops 2—3X	1/4 vial 2—3X	1/2—1 vial 2—3X	1/2—1 vial 2—3X	Apply as
Small dogs/cats	1/2—1 tab 2—3X	5—8 drops 2—3X		1/4—1/2 vial 2—3X	1/2 vial 2—3X	needed
Puppies/ kittens	1/2—1 tab 2—3X	5 drops 2—3X		1/4—1/2 vial 2—3X	1/2 vial 2—3X	
Pocket pets	1/2 tab 2—3X	2—5 drops 2—3X		1/4 vial 2—3X	1/4 vial 2—3X	

patient response. They can be given as infrequently as twice per week and as often as several times daily. Most often they are given twice daily unless detoxification signs are too intense or uncomfortable, in which case the dosage is reduced so that the patient's system is not overwhelmed by excessive levels of homotoxins.

Because the process of biological therapy is dynamic, it is vital to note things clearly in the record and then recheck the case regularly. The authors use the following schedule for many cases:

1. Initial consultation. History, examination, diagnostics, phase and symptom picture; begin treatment program.
2. Recheck in two weeks. If good progress, then recheck in 30 days. If no progress or problems, re-evaluate

the case and make changes necessary to allow the case to move.

3. Recheck cases every 1 to 3 months as needed. Instruct owners on the Six-Phase Table of Homotoxicology and have them contact the clinic if changes occur.

4. In healthy-appearing pets, or those that have successfully completed a course of biological therapy, it can be very helpful to do routine detoxification twice a year with a formula of *Berberis homaccord*, *Lymphomyosot*, *Nux vomica homaccord*, and possibly *BHI-Body Pure* (eliminates common toxins such as tobacco and petroleum byproducts). Using this mixture in the spring and fall for 30 days helps make pets more energetic and happy.

Demonstration case: a roadmap to biological therapy

Name: Sid Jones

Breed: Pug, male intact

Age: 24 Weeks

Vaccine History: DHPP 8, 12 weeks; Bordatella 12 weeks (dog park frequently); rabies 1 yr, 16 weeks

Drug History: Drontal Plus 8, 12, 16 weeks; Albon dose unknown 6 weeks of age

Environmental History: Private breeder until 7 weeks of age; owner home since then.

Disease History: Coccidiosis treated at 6 weeks of age; roundworms treated 8, 12, 16 weeks of age

Dietary History: Innova EVO puppy food and home-prepared scraps of meat and veggies (no raisins, grapes, onions, garlic, or chocolate verified)

Current Signs: Erythema on pinnae and multifocal small folliculitis lesions on abdomen

Rule-Outs: Staph pyoderma, demodex, sarcoptes, fungal, vaccination regressive vicariation

Phase: Inflammation Phase; Phase 2

Diagnostic Plan: Skin scrape→negative; Wood's lamp→ negative

Client Decision: Owner declines fungal culture as lesions not typical. Advise owner fungal infections zoonotic can appear in many ways. If lesions spread or if people develop lesions call the office.

Treatment Plan: Phase remedy: *Echinacea compositum* 1 tablet BID PO 10 minutes before meals

Symptom Remedy: *Traumeel* 5 drops BID PO

Detoxification: *Detox Kit* 5 drops BID X 30days PO

Diet: Maintain present diet.

Recheck in Two Weeks

Recheck 7 Days: Lesions gone and dog doing well. Owner reports he began itching for several days and then developed a runny nose and eyes, which cleared in a week. Soft stools for 3 days but better now.

Assessment: Phase shifted from inflammation to excretion and to normal! Successful clearing of homotoxins, espe-

cially other viruses. Note: Advised owner that viral infections are usually Impregnation Phase disorders so be prepared if other conditions arise.

New Plan: Advise owner to avoid unnecessary chemicals or vaccinations, and consider titer testing next year instead of routine annual or triannual DHPP vaccinations, which may cause progressive vicariation.

The above example gives a basic roadmap to those new to biological therapy. New practitioners would be wise to make a standard form they could use in their clinics as they learn this subject. Taking an organized approach greatly assists the student in learning the craft as well as in evaluating cases when they seem to be slowing their response. Figure 4.9 presents an example of such a worksheet from the author's hospital (Palmquist 2000).

AUTOSANGUIS THERAPY

There are a host of other subjects for consideration in homotoxicology, and autosanguis (self plus blood) therapy is of great benefit in many different case presentations. Use of patient blood has long been promoted in healing arts, but only recently has it become evident why this practice can cause such startlingly effects. This advanced form of treatment involves taking patient blood and mixing it with various antihomotoxic remedies, thereby exposing the cellular arm of the immune system to a mixture of biological therapy agents in tandem with the current antigens in dilution. This mixture is presented to the patient by injection or oral routes, whereby the patient's immune system responds according to the immunological bystander principle discussed earlier in this chapter. The patient's own blood contains specific homotoxins associated with the present disease state, and when diluted in this manner, local macrophages can pick up this information and process it into data usable by local lymphocytes. Biological information specific and unique to the patient's form of homotoxicosis is made available to begin various immune cascades (Broadfoot 2005).

There are several methods commonly used to perform autosanguis therapy. The following method is commonly performed in the United States (Broadfoot 2002, 2005). Many modifications that can be made to individualize therapy for a particular patient or situation, but this basic technique is extremely workable and gives good results. Patients have a drop of blood drawn and then this blood is mixed in a sterile syringe with remedies from four categories:

1. Stage one. Symptom remedy or remedies are selected to match the present situation. Examples include *Traumeel-S*, *Belladona homaccord*, *Engystol-N*, or *Apis homaccord*.

New Case History Form

Date: _____   Veterinarian: _____

Client Name: _____

Name: _____   Patient

Breed: _____   Sex: F, M, Altered, Intact

Age: _____

Chief Complaint/Duration: _____

Vaccine History: Vaccination reaction? Y   N
_____

Puppy/Kitten Series _____

FVRCP _____ Rabies _____ FeLV _____

FIV _____

DHPP _____ Rabies _____ Lepto _____

Lymes _____

Other vaccines?

Drug History:

Environmental History:

Disease History:

Dietary History: (include supplements)

Current Signs/Physical Exam:

Temp	Pulse	Eyes	Urogenital	Neuro
Weight	Cardiac	Oral/Dental/MM	Abdomen	Lymph Nodes
Mentation	Respiration	Hair/Skin/Nils	Musculoskeletal	GI/Stool

OD   OS

Tongue

Phase? (circle estimated phase area)

| Excretion   Inflammation   Deposition   []   Impregnation   Degeneration   Dedifferentiation |

Diagnostic Plan:

Treatment Plan:

Client Education: (list handouts or data to cover)

Next Visit: _____ . Appointed? Y   N

Reminder?   Y   N

Figure 4.9. Use of an organized method of admitting new cases can greatly assist the biological therapist in properly diagnosing and treating patients

2. Stage two. Drainage remedy or remedies are selected to drain the affected terrain. Examples include *Lymphomyosot, Galium-Heel*, or *Engystol N*.
3. Stage three. Organ preparation or preparations including such remedies as *Hepar compositum, Solidago compositum, Mucosa compositum, Tonsilla compositum, Thyroidea compositum*, etc.
4. Stage four. Nosode preparation or preparations such as *Echinacea compositum* and *Psorinoheel*. Catalysts such as *Ubichinon compositum, Glyoxal compositum*, and *Coenzyme compositum* are frequently given in this stage.

The first drop of blood is drawn into the syringe and then mixed with the first stage remedy/remedies. Mixing is accomplished by a practice known as succussion. The mixture is strongly struck against the palm of the opposite hand 10 times. In homeopathic practice, succussion is believed to activate the formulas. Conventionally speaking, this strong impact may provide more intimate contact between cellular elements and homotoxins present. This mixture is given to the patient, and then the second stage remedy/remedies are drawn into the same syringe, succussed and then administered. This is continued through stages three and four using the same syringe.

Where allowed by law, autosanguis functions best when given by injection. While these injections may be given subcutaneously, or intramuscularly anywhere on the body, the clinician will find that using specific acupuncture points gives even better and more remarkable results. This practice is called biopuncture. The remedies can be given orally where the law does not allow such practices. It is common practice to mix at least a portion of each stage in a bottle of oral antihomotoxic medications to be taken home and given orally to the patient for an extended period of time. It is advisable to refrigerate these mixtures.

More on autosanguis appears in this text under the subject of cancer therapy; however, it has been found that often-miraculous results can be obtained following application of this sophisticated form of immune therapy. Autosanguis can be used in any phase of homotoxicosis, and its application is appropriate in nearly all cases from Deposition Phase to the right on the Six-Phase Table. Factually, many chronic and deep homotoxicoses do not respond until they are approached with autosanguis therapy, as developed by Dr Reckeweg and others (Broadfoot, Demers, Palmquist 2004).

WHAT IS THE SCIENTIFIC PROOF OF THE EFFICACY OF HOMOTOXICOLOGY?

Numerous scientific studies support the clinical use of antihomotoxic agents in human medicine. Efforts to document these results in veterinary medicine are just beginning.

Many conversations regarding homotoxicology begin by questioning homeopathy as a valid science. Researching classical homeopathy is difficult, because no two identical patients exist. The allopathic method of diagnosis is not valid in homeopathy, since remedies are selected based upon symptoms and not classical Western pathological or etiological diagnosis. This makes it most challenging to design double-blind, controlled studies involving classical homeopathy.

In 1991, Kleijnen, et al. reviewed the literature and performed a meta-analysis of studies involving homeopathy. They examined 105 clinical trials involving homeopathic medicines and found positive results in 81 of the studies. Strong responses were identified in the treatment of respiratory disease (13 out of 19 studies showed positive response) and trauma and pain management (18 out of 20 studies indicated positive responses). Such a study is far from a final answer, but indicates why clients seek out homeopathic doctors for their healthcare needs. Something is working in these patients, and bearing in mind that homeopathic remedies are nontoxic and have no life-threatening side effects, using nanopharmacologic modalities, particularly in the field of pain management, becomes a very tempting impulse. Clients are well informed about the risks of NSAID drugs and actively pursue alternatives.

As research is done, more and more evidence exists to support the practice of homeopathy (Bellavite, Sinorini 2002). Many clients seek out homeopathic doctors as their first choice because they feel they recover faster, better, and more naturally using this form of medicine and the findings of research involving animals makes the likelihood of a placebo effect much less plausible (Reckeweg 2000). Since homotoxicology and conventional medicine share common diagnostic criteria, research is easier to perform and an active research arm involved in exploring homotoxicology and regulation medicines is emerging.

By actual fact, the most common way that conventional veterinarians enter upon the field of CAVM is in search of safer, more effective ways to manage their patient's pain. This is another example of how truth spreads through good results, even in the absence of concrete understanding of a modality's method of action. This is good medicine, using a field with some clinical evidence and improved safety before using a method that is known to be potentially damaging and dangerous. While classical homeopathy might not easily integrate with conventional allopathic medical practice, such studies should serve to indicate that homeopaths deserve respect as healers and medical professionals. They should also serve to interest medical practitioners in finding out more about these modalities, and statistics show more veterinarians are trained in homeopathy than at any time in modern history.

Because of the obvious effectiveness of homeopathy, and out of respect for the infinite value of scientific diagnostic processes, the field of homotoxicology has evolved. The founder of homotoxicology, Dr. Hans-Heinrich Reckeweg, sought to integrate the field of homoeopathy and Western, scientific medicine. Through direct clinical observation and trial and error, he developed a series of formulas from mineral, plant, and animal components, which assisted his patients in their recoveries. Homotoxicology contains a very active clinical research structure. Sadly, Dr. Reckeweg was a German and so much of his writing and clinical research was not widely known in the United States. Recently, though, English material has become more available and the work that is ongoing in Baden-Baden, Germany, continues to demonstrate the effectiveness and usefulness of homotoxicology remedies. The presence of clinical research and the results of these studies have led many medical doctors and veterinarians, and a large number of patients to move toward homotoxicology remedies.

Once again, we see the pattern of a single person who observed irregularities, created a theory explaining these irregularities, and then hypothesized a solution based on the theory. His clinical success led to the creation of a company to market his materials, and this company is the largest one of its type worldwide because its products are so helpful to those who use them. More and more homotoxicology data is emerging that can be integrated nicely into conventional veterinary practices. Furthermore, these practices gain new tools to examine disease pathogenesis as well as offer therapy. The authors, who began their journey from a skeptical view, now see this fact daily and hope that readers may benefit to the same degree from use of these gentle biological therapies.

It is only natural that veterinarians' interest is growing in this category of biological therapies. Only a few years ago, all seminars in homotoxicology were sponsored by the parent company, Heel, but homotoxicology is now taught at American Veterinary Medical Association and American Holistic Veterinary Medical Association meetings, as well as a rapidly expanding number of local meetings such as the North American Veterinary Medical Conference and the Annual Homotoxicology Conference of the American Holistic Veterinary Medical Association.

Positive clinical results fuel this interest, but there are evidence-based reasons for selecting homotoxicology, as well. While the majority of high-quality research in homotoxicology involves human medicine, which is logical considering that a human practitioner initially developed this field for human patients, the veterinary clinician often finds excellent results in the application of human proto-

cols. Veterinary research in Europe has been more active in recent years than in the United States, with veterinary data beginning to accumulate. This supports this statement from the *Biotherapeutic Index* (Reckeweg 2000):

> "Animal diseases react to Heel biotherapeutical and antihomotoxic agents with visible success, the objections occasionally raised being invalidated, i.e. that in the application of high dilution medicaments the effect is based predominantly on suggestion. The indications and methods of administration are the same as in human medicine."

In this section, due to the relatively small size of the veterinary literature on homotoxicology, most of the sources quoted are from human literature.

The most famous homotoxicology formula is *Traumeel*-S, and is properly classified as a nonsteroidal anti-inflammatory and is listed in the *Physician's Desk Reference* (Thompson 2005). This antihomotoxic formula contains 12 botanical and 2 mineral substances and is officially classified as a homeopathic remedy. The package insert carries this information (Heel unpublished):

> "While its precise mechanism of action is not known, *Traumeel* does not seem to work as a result of cyclooxygenase (COX) or lipoxygenase (LOX) enzyme inhibition as is the case with many of the NSAID agents currently receiving such negative press for dangerous side effects. It does not inhibit aracadonic acid or prostaglandin pathways, either. *Traumeel* appears to work by modulation of the release of oxygen radicals from activated neutrophils, and the inhibition of the release of inflammatory mediators (possibly interleukin 1 from activated macrophages) and neuropeptides."

In vitro studies show the ingredients of *Traumeel* are noncytotoxic to granulocytes, lymphocytes, platelets, and endothelia, which indicates that the defensive functions of these cells are preserved during treatment with *Traumeel* (Comforti, et al. 1995).

Traumeel is one of the best-researched homeopathic agents in the world today, with its use supported in more than 2 dozen scientific articles and clinical studies (Broadfoot 2003). It carries an indication for inflammation of all kinds. Porosov, et al. recently found another cue to its mechanism of action in a study indicating that *Traumeel* affects immune system cell function related to inflammation by inhibiting, in a dose dependant fashion, the secretion of pro-inflammatory cytokines from both gut epithelium and leucocytes. The observed inhibition is inversely dose dependent, with no evidence of pro-inflammatory activity at any dose examined. Only extremely low dilutions of this mixture were found to have this effect, a finding that further supports the observations made by homeopathic doctors for more than 200 years. This study postulated that *Traumeel*-S might work by interference with specific intracellular signal transduction pathways (Porosov, et al. 2004).

Zell, et al. showed substantial results in the treatment of sprains in a placebo-controlled, randomized double-blinded study published in 1989 (Zell, et al. 1989). Athletes all over the world are familiar with *Traumeel* in its various forms of gel, ointment, tablet, and oral liquid, and many Olympic teams regularly use it in their training and competition programs. Demonstrating the wide variety of clinical applications in which *Traumeel* has proven efficacious, Oberbaum, et al. demonstrated the usefulness of *Traumeel*-S in the treatment of chemotherapy-induced stomatitis in children undergoing stem cell therapy (Oberbaum, et al. 2001). This study was also a randomized, controlled clinical trial and showed clear improvement in the stomatitis parameters measured in the group which received *Traumeel*. The study, published in 2001 in the prestigious journal of the American Cancer Society, *Cancer*, concluded that *Traumeel*-S may significantly reduce the severity and duration of chemotherapy-induced stomatitis in children undergoing bone marrow transplantation. Stomatitis is a significant complication of this procedure in children, and in this study 33% of the *Traumeel*-S-treated group did not develop stomatitis, while 97% of the placebo group did. This represents a significant advancement in patient comfort. Currently there is little effective or safe therapy for children with stomatitis of this type. Local anesthetics have unpleasant tastes and the risk of absorption limits the frequency at which these agents may be given. *Traumeel*-S was found to be nearly free of adverse side effects, and has a relatively low cost per patient, making it a highly desirable therapeutic agent.

Examination of *Traumeel*-S and other homotoxicology remedies may prove equally helpful for veterinary oncology patients. In one new study, comparisons of canine mammary patients receiving homotoxicology remedies after surgery were encouraging (Kurth, Neumann, Reinhart 2000). Patients receiving *Coenzyme compositum* were found to have increased survival times and reduced metastasis when compared to the expected results published in current veterinary literature. These findings coupled with clinically observed improvement in veterinary oncology patients' level of comfort provide some exciting possibilities for research.

The story of science's progression in this instance is equally fascinating and illustrates our points regarding evidentiary medicine. *Traumeel*-S has been widely used in Europe for nearly 80 years. Medical doctors, athletes, arthritis suffers, and a wide variety of other users have observed excellent results from *Traumeel*-S and with minimal side effects. Clinicians using *Traumeel*-S frequently observe near miraculous results in a wide variety

of applications. These anecdotal reports have collected quietly for 8 decades. After patients undergoing chemotherapy reported some benefit, an interested doctor did a preliminary open study in 20 patients and compared the results with 7 untreated patients who were selected randomly. The results of this preliminary study were favorable and published in the *Biomedical Therapy* journal by Heel in 1998.

Finally, in 2001, the full study was completed and published by the American Cancer Society (Oberbaum, et al. 2001). Now that the data is in the mainstream American medical literature, it will take some time for the material to be disseminated widely, accepted, and put into use by oncologists. This clearly shows the long runway that data must undergo before being proven scientifically to be effective. If the medical doctors involved in this case had waited to use *Traumeel*-S until it was proven, we might never have known about this data. Because *Traumeel*-S is so safe, it seems prudent to attempt its use where there is no safe or truly effective option. Those patients lucky enough to receive *Traumeel* prior to 2001 benefited greatly even though no double-blind randomized study had been completed. Ethically, this was an acceptable activity because it improved patient comfort and did no harm.

Observing a single fact, accumulating a bit more data in support of that observation, and finally, when the results are nearly certain, designing an experiment to clearly demonstrate the desirable effect illustrate an ideal research pathway. Pain management is a massive issue and the present pharmaceutical agents subject patients to a wide variety of undesirable and dangerous risks including decreased fibroplasia and wound healing, skin eruptions, pulmonary complications, gastrointestinal ulceration and hemorrhage, drug-induced hepatitis, renal disease, bone marrow dyscrasias, keratoconjunctivitis sicca, myocardial infarction, and sudden death syndromes; therefore, homotoxicology remedies may prove extremely helpful to our profession in reducing pain as well as reducing iatrogenic damage to patients.

A human study examined the antihomotoxic formula known as *Zeel*, which is commonly used in clinical practice for treatment of oseoarthritis pain, especially arthritis of the knee. The paired cohort study compared Vioxx and Celebrex to *Zeel* and found that the NSAID drugs reduced pain and increased mobility slightly faster, but by 6 weeks there was no difference in efficacy. *Zeel* took longer to create a biological effect, but had NO adverse side effects (Birnesser, Klein, Weiser 2003). In a post marketing drug survey of human patients by Heel, which involved 190 orthopedists who administered 1 ampule of *Zeel* intra-articularly twice weekly for 4 to 5 weeks, it was found that 93.1% of clients reported positive results and only 0.45% reported adverse side effects, which all consisted of local irritation at the injection site. Similar veterinary studies have not been conducted, but clinical responses appear to parallel this data and it seems prudent to pay attention to findings in the human medical field as we consider therapies for the veterinary profession.

When a clinician is faced with an agent that achieves the desired goals of therapy and knows that it has no major side effects, it seems prudent to select such therapies as initial treatments for patients seen in the clinic. If patients fail to respond to these treatments, then the clinician could consider other, more potentially dangerous or expensive agents for use in that patient's treatment program. At a minimum, clinicians need to advise their clients of these side effects and allow the client the freedom to choose the risk factors that they are most comfortable facing. Just making this minor change in practice could reduce the number of adverse drug reactions and the major problem with drug-related deaths and hospitalizations in the United States. The savings in costs associated with hospitalization, lost productivity, medical litigation, and bad public relations are substantial and well worth consideration in managing medical protocols.

In a human study involving *Cralonin*, the Crataegus-containing antihomotoxic symptom formula for cardiac patients was compared to the usual therapies for mild phase II heart failure. The study found no statistical difference between therapy groups, and concluded that (Schroder, Weiser, Klein 2003):

> "The Crataegus-based preparation *Cralonin* is non-inferior to usual ACE inhibitor/diuretics treatment for mild cardiac insufficiency on all parameters except BP reduction."

It is interesting to note that 15 variables were examined. Both treatment protocols were well tolerated by patients. In the author's practice, we frequently use both conventional cardiac drugs as well as homotoxicology formulas with excellent outcomes (Palmquist 2005). It will likely be some time before studies are done to compare the results of such integrative protocols. These results are not really a surprise to those familiar with use of Crataegus in treating cardiac disease, which has been well known since the 17th century. The herb and homeopathic preparation is known to affect several cardiac parameters including increasing heart stroke volume, contractility, and coronary blood flow. Such changes are greatly appreciated by many geriatric patients and their caregivers.

Engystol-N, a common and extremely useful antihomotoxic preparation for activating the nonspecific defensive mechanisms of organisms, is indicated for a wide variety of uses including viral infections, allergies, vague feverish conditions, eczema, furunculosis, neurodermatitis, urticaria, asthma, migraine, diseases of the kidney, liver, and central nervous system, and experimentally in toxo-

plasmosis cases treated concurrently with *Traumeel* (Reckeweg 2000). The active ingredient is postulated to be Vincetoxicum hirundinaria, which is commonly called "shallowwort." *Engystol-N* is not thought to be directly antiviral. Heel awarded the Hans-Heinrich Reckeweg Prize for outstanding research to Professor Ryszard Matusiewicz of the Department of Internal Medicine of Gorchowski Hospital in Warsaw for his double-blind, placebo-controlled study of 40 human asthmatic patients. These patients had all required corticosteroid use prior to the study. The *Engystol* group experienced improvements in pulmonary function and were able to reduce corticosteroid use by significant levels (Malave, Manialavori, and Matusiewicz 1991).

In another study, Fimiani, et al. demonstrated an immunomodulatory effect of *Engystol* on some activities of isolated human leukocytes in whole blood (Fimiani, et al. 2000). The study demonstrated increased superoxide anion generation by leukocytes and increased cytokine production by T lymphocytes. This strongly supports the powerful effect of *Engystol* when used in autosanguis therapy and easily explains why *Engystol* appears to strengthen the immune system of patients suffering from viral infections. Finally, a European veterinary study showed reduced somatic cell counts in dairy cows receiving *Engystol* biopuncture (Ben-Yakir 2004).

Every veterinary practitioner has wished for weapons in the war against viruses, and homotoxicology has several powerful tools for the arsenal against viral infections. *Engystol* is certainly one such weapon, but research has also demonstrated antiviral activity in *Euphorbium nasal spray*. In one in vitro study the nasal spray demonstrated clear antiviral activity by itself and by 2 of its 3 ingredients (Glatthaar-Saalmuller, Fallier-Becker 2001). In another study, *Euphorbium nasal spray* was found to work as well as xylometazoline for nasal and sinus congestion in human patients (Ammerschlager et al. 2005).

Another remedy which strongly appeared to assist recovery of human patients with influenza is *Gripp-Heel* (Rabe, Weiser, Klein 2004). At the conclusion of one multicenter study comparing *Gripp-Heel* with conventional therapy, 67.9% of the *Gripp-Heel* group was asymptomatic versus 47.9% of the control group, which received conventional therapy. While tolerability and compliance were similar in both groups, treatment results were rated "very good" in 88.9% of those receiving *Gripp-Heel* versus 38.8% of those receiving conventional therapy.

Vertigoheel is another common homotoxicology remedy that is indicated for vestibular signs. This antihomotoxic drug has been evaluated in a randomized clinical trial and found to be equivalent to betahistadine in assisting human patients with attacks of vertigo (Weiser, et al. 1998). Both treatment groups had significantly reduced frequency, duration, and intensity of the vertigo attacks. In a double-blinded, randomized controlled clinical study researchers found *Vertigoheel* noninferior to Ginkgo biloba in humans with atherosclerosis-related vertigo (Issing, Klein, Weiser 2005).

Klop, et al. examined the microcirculatory effects of *Vertigoheel* in human patients suffering from mild vertigo and documented marked alterations in microcirculation in patients following 12 weeks of therapy (Klopp, Niemer, Weiser 2005). None of the control patients experienced these changes, a fact indicating that this particular remedy has physiological effects on microcirculation. Increased partial oxygen pressures and increased levels of adhesion molecules ICAM-1 as well as increased levels of cell-wall adhering leukocytes were observed to occur in the *Vertigoheel*-treated group but not the controls. This documentation of altered microcirculation supports the activity and observed results claimed by Dr. Reckeweg, and indicates biological activity induced by use of the medicant. This agent is ripe for research in veterinary medicine and may also have a place in the treatment of vestibular disorders in veterinary patients.

Following the theories of homotoxicology, it would be nearly axiomatic that providing increased drainage of the lymph system would assist in removing homotoxins and lead to improvement in a wide variety of homotoxocoses. Dr. Reckeweg developed a formula known as *Lymphomyosot* to drain the lymph system and stimulate the greater defense system. This agent is recommended for a wide variety of disorders including hypertrophy of the lymph glands, edema, increased susceptibility to infection, glandular swelling, tonsillar swelling, and chronic tonsillitis. It is also a phase remedy for Excretion, Deposition, Degeneration, and Dedifferentiation phase conditions.

Recently, an additional indication for diabetic polyneuropathy in people has been added (Dietz 2000). A 2000 study found *Lymphomyosot* superior to α-lipoic acid in treatment of human type II diabetic polyneuropathy. This study involved 90 patients followed over an 8-month period. Three groups received *Lymphomyosot* or *Lymphomyosot* and α-lipoic acid. Nuclear magnetic angiography and color sonography were used to examine vascular lesions and edema and sensitivity to pain were measured and monitored. Seventy-five percent of *Lymphomysot*-treated patients experienced a reduction of pain and edema and *Lymphomyosot* treatment was found to be superior to α-lipoic acid treatment.

Lymphomyosot and α-lipoic acid together worked synergistically to further improve patient conditions and the study rightly concludes that *Lymphomyosot* should become a standard agent in treating human diabetes type II patients. This agent seems ready-made for combination therapy wherein differing antihomotoxic agents are combined further to support various organ systems or tissue

needs during detoxification and repair. *Lymphomyosot* is a truly integrative biological agent. Broadfoot (2002)has reported success in using *Lymphomyosot* combined with *Apis homaccord* in treatment of insect bite hypersensitivity. *Lymphomyosot* research promises to yield helpful facts in many different conditions.

Veterinary homotoxicology research, while nearly nonexistent in the United States, is beginning to accelerate in European countries. One veterinary study in Israel demonstrated clear results in cows treated with a homeopathic agent over placebos and controls treated with saline. The number of animals in this study is low, but the groups had clearly different results. Significantly reduced somatic cell counts resulted from use of the homeopathic agent. The antihomotoxic medicine selected, *Engystol*, is promoted by Heel for its ability to increase the greater defenses, and this new research supports that by showing a biological response associated with increased immune cell activity. Because livestock producers are severely limited in the drugs they can use, the option of treating with gentle antihomotoxic medicines that do not require withdrawal periods is enticing and exciting indeed (Ben-Yakir 2004).

Clinical observations support that homotoxicology improves patient comfort, which is worthwhile. There also is evidence that antihomotoxic medicines may improve survival of veterinary cancer patients. A German study examining survival of dogs with mammary neoplasia demonstrated that the group receiving homeopathic medicines had prolonged survival rates over dogs receiving conventional surgery and chemotherapy alone. While all the dogs in this study received homotoxicology and the resultant survival times were compared with survival times as determined by the existing veterinary literature, this finding is reason enough to further examine the use of antihomotoxic medicines in treatment of cancer in veterinary patients (Reinhart, Broadfoot, Hanover 2005). The field of oncology would welcome nontoxic and effective means to reduce nausea and discomfort associated with chemotherapy and other cancer therapies. The idea that survival could be increased with gentle, nontoxic, antihomotoxic agents is welcome news to the field. Such statements are not strongly supported by sufficient scientific evidence but the possibilities make this research highly desirable.

The prior studies in this section should serve to demonstrate that something beneficial is happening through the application of homotoxicology principles and antihomotoxic agents. The question, "Does homotoxicology work?" would seem to be answered, at least superficially, in the affirmative. Evidence does exist that homotoxicology and other low-dose therapies can and do improve physiological states and disease recovery in people and animals. Further research and clinical application will continue, and in the author's opinion such research will continue to demonstrate the usefulness of biological therapy to those with an inclination to assist their patients through this fascinating modality.

New biological practitioners should keep records of their results, and by sharing this information with other professionals our patients can benefit from newly acquired information. Through such actions the science of homotoxicology can expand even more quickly and better serve our clients and patients. The future appears bright for integrative veterinarians using this new modality.

REFERENCE SOURCES FOR HOMOTOXICOLOGY

Homotoxicology is a vast subject and requires continued and diligent study. This chapter is intended to provide some basic information and create interest in this wonderful form of healing technology. This text can never hope to contain the full subject, because it is simply too large, but it is a seminal effort to move integrative veterinary medicine forward on its search for better and safer therapeutic plans for our patients. As with any form of medicine, it is essential that the practitioner obtain a set of texts and references to adequately practice homotoxicology. Through the process of study, increased competence, and further handling of clinical cases, the veterinarian can find homotoxicology to be an exciting tool to add to the clinic's healthcare toolbox.

A recommended list of invaluable references for further study includes:

The Biotherapeutic Journal. This non-refereed publication is published by Heel. While it is a company-controlled publication, it contains the earliest and most complete history of literature in homotoxicology. Because the majority of homotoxicology research is currently done in Europe at this time, this journal is a significant source of information for both human and veterinary practitioners.

Biotherapeutic Index: Ordanatio Antihomotoxica et Materia Medica. Available from Heel. This text includes detailed descriptions of the 200 distinct homotoxicology formulations produced by Heel.

Veterinary Materia Medica. Available from Heel. This rather limited text includes commonly used veterinary applications of the remedies.

Journal of the American Holistic Veterinary Association. This journal contains frequent articles and comments regarding homotoxicology. Information is available at www.ahvma.org.

Obtaining and studying these texts will greatly assist any practitioner interested in biological therapy.

Professional organizations, which forward the art and science of homotoxicology, include:

The International Society of Homotoxicology. PO Box 100 264, 76483 Baden-Baden, Germany. info@homotox.de. Phone +49-7221-63252. Fax +49-7221-501-490.

The Society of Homotoxicology of North America. PO Box 2698, Edgewood, NM 87015.

The American Holistic Veterinary Medical Association. Dr. Carvel G. Tiekert, Executive Director, 2218 Old Emmorton Road, Bel Air, MD. 21015. Phone (410) 569-0795, fax (410)569-2346. www.ahvma.org. Annual meeting on homotoxicology in Denver, CO; annual complementary-alternative veterinary medicine multimodality conference, and journal.

REFERENCES

Ammerschlager H, Klein P, Weiser M, Oberbaum M. 2005. Treatment of inflammatory diseases of the upper respiratory tract—Comparison of a homeopathic complex remedy with xylometazoline. *Forsch Komplementarmed Klass Naturheilkd*, 12(1):pp 24–31.

Bellavite P, Signorini A. 2002. The Emerging Science of Homeopathy: Complexity, Biodynamics and Nanpharmacology. Berkeley: North Atlantic Books, pp preface, 2, 56–83, 111–39.

Ben-Yakir S. 2004. Primary evaluation of homeopathic remedies injected via acupuncture points to reduce chronic high somatic cell counts in modern dairy farms. *Veterinary Acupuncture Newsletter*, (27)1:pp 19–21.

Birnbaum S, et al. 2004. Protein Kinase C Overactivity Impairs Prefrontal Cortical Regulation of Behavior. *Science*, (306):5697, 882–884.

Birnesser H, Klein P, Weiser M. 2003. A modern homeopathic medication works as well as COX2 inhibitors for treating osteoarthritis of the knee. *Der Allgemeinarzt*, 25(4):pp 261–4.

Brandtzaeg, P. 1996. History of Oral Tolerance and Mucosal Immunity. In Oral Tolerance: Mechanisms and Applications, Weiner HW, Mayer, LF, eds. *Ann New York Acad Sci*; 778: pp 1–27.

Broadfoot P. 2002. Personal communication.

Broadfoot P. 2005. Autosanguis Therapy: New Insights Into an Ancient Therapeutic Tool, proceedings from 1st Veterinary Congress, Memphis, TN. May 11–13. Heel USA.

Broadfoot, P. 2003. Traumeel and Zeel in Veterinary Medicine. Seminar Notes. Heel.

Broadfoot, P. 2004. Inflammation—Homotoxicology and Healing. Homotoxicology Seminar. American Holistic Veterinary Medical Association. May 15, Denver, CO, p.30.

Broadfoot, P. 2004. Inflammation: Homotoxicology and Healing, Lecture during AHVMA Homotoxicology Seminar, Denver, CO, May 15, p.6.

Broadfoot P, Demers J, Palmquist R. Unpublished personal communication. Denver, CO. May 2004.

Conforti, A et al. 1995. In Vitro and In Vivo Studies on the Anti-Inflammatory Activity of Traumeel S. Unpublished report on file. Heel GmbH, Baden-Baden, Germany.

Dietz A. 2000. Possibilities for a lymph therapy with Diabetic Polyneuropathy. Reprint translated from *Biologische Medzin.* 29(1):pp 4–9.

Fimiani V, Cavarello A, Ainis O, Bottari C. 2000. Immunomodulatory effect of the homoeopathic drug Engystol-N on some activities of isolated human leukocytes and in whole blood. *Immunopharmacol Immunotoxicol*, 22(1):pp 103–15.

Flynn J. 1970. Arrhythmias related to coffee and tea, *JAMA*, 211: p. 663.

Glatthaar-Saalmuller B, Fallier-Becker P. 2001. Antiviral action of Euphorbium compositum and its components (English translation). *Forsch Komplementarmed Klass Naturheilkd*, 8: pp 207–212.

Harman J. 1998. Holistic Approach to Equine Practice. In: Complementary and Alternative Veterinary Medicine: Principles and Practice, Schoen AM and Wynn SG, eds. St Louis: Mosby, p. 606.

Heel. 2005. Homotoxicology in Veterinary Practice. http://www.heel.com/products/?smid=3.

Heel. The Story of Heel. http://heelusa.com/about_story_of_heel.html

Heel. Unpublished data on file. GmbH, Baden-Baden, Germany.

Heine H. 1997. *Lehrbuch der Biologischen Medizin.* Auflage Stuttgart: Hippokrates, pp. 39–41.

Heine H. 1997b. Neurogene Entzundung als Basis Chronischer Schmerzen. *Beziehungen zur Antihomotoxischen Therapie. (31)* Med. Woche Baden-Baden, (Biol Medizin, in German) diagram of bystander.

Hellemans A, Bunch B. 1988. The Timetables of Science: A Chronology of the Most Important People and Events in the History of Science. New York: Simon and Schuster, p vii.

HOMOEOPATHIA—ANTIHOMOTOXICA publié par: Aurelia-Verlag, Postfach 10 00 45, D-76481 Baden-Baden, Germany. PHOTOTHÈQUE HOMÉOPATHIQUE:présentée par Homéopathe International: Dr Hans-Heinrich RECKEWEG (1905–1985). http://www.homeoint.org/photo/r/reckeweghh.htm. Accessed January 2006.

Hubbard L. 1992. Learning How to Learn. Los Angeles: Effective Education Publishing, pp 101–155.

Issing W, Klein P, Weiser M. 2005. The homeopathic preparation Vertigoheel versus Ginkgo biloba in the treatment of vertigo in an elderly population: a double-blinded, randomized, controlled clinical trial. *J Altern Complement Med.* 11(1):pp 155–60.

Jaggi R et al. 2004. Dual inhibition of 5-lipoxygenase/cyclooxygenase by a reconstituted homeopathic remedy; possible explanation for clinical efficacy and favorable gastrointestinal tolerability. *Inflamm Res.* 53(4): pp 150–7.

Jordan B et al. 2002. Insulin increases the sensitivity of tumors to irradiation: Involvement of an increase in tumor oxygenation mediated by a nitric oxide-dependent decrease of the tumor cell's oxygen consumption. *Cancer Research*, 15(62): pp 3555–6.

Kendall, R. 1998. Basic and Preventative Nutrition for the Cat, Dog, and Horse. In: Complementary and Alternative Veterinary Medicine: Principles and Practice, Schoen AM and Wynn SG, eds. St Louis: Mosby. p. 31.

Kersschot, J. 2002. Biopuncture and Antihomotoxic Medicine: The Extra Dimension in Medicine, 3rd edition. Belgium. http://users.skynet.be/inspiration/biopuncture.htm.

Klopp R, Niemer W, Weiser M. 2005. Microcirculatory effects of a homeopathic preparation in patients with mild vertigo: an intravital microscopic study. *Microvasc Res.* 69(1–2):pp 10–6.

Kurth T, Neumann S, Reinhart E. 2000. Homeopathic remedies prolong the lives of dogs that have undergone cancer surgery. *Der praktische Tierarzt.* 81(4):pp 276–91.

Maciocia G. 1994. The Practice of Chinese Medicine: The Treatment of Diseases with Acupuncture and Chinese Herbs. Singapore: Longman Singapore Publishers, p 211.

Maciocia G. 1995. Tongue Diagnosis in Chinese Medicine. Seattle, WA: Eastland Press, Inc, p. 1.

Malave E, Manialavori M, Matusiewicz R. 1991. Mixed modality outcome study of adult and pediatric asthma. *J Naturopath Med*, 2(1):pp 43–44.

Marrona U, Weiser M, Klein P. 2000. Orale Behandlung der Gonarthrose mit Zeel© comp. Orthopädische Praxis;(5): pp 285–91.

Nicholson D. 2002. Deamination of Amino Acids—The Urea Cycle. International Union of Biochemistry and Molecular Biology. http://www.tcd.ie/Biochemistry/IUBMB-Nicholson/gif/18.gif.

Oberbaum Y et al. 2001. Randomized, controlled clinical trial of the homeopathic medication Traumeel S in the treatment of chemotherapy-induced stomatitis in children undergoing stem cell transplantation. *Cancer.* (92)3:pp 684–690.

Palmquist R. 2000. New Patient Worksheet in Centinela Animal Hospital Doctor's Policy Manual. Centinela Animal Hospital, Inc.

Palmquist R. 2005. Case Studies of Heart Patients. Lecture notes of the AHVMA and BHI/Heel 2nd Annual Veterinary Homotoxicology Seminar. Denver, CO. May 29.

Porosov C et al. 2004. Inhibition of IL-1beta and TNF-alpha secretion from resting and activated human immunocytes by the homeopathic medication Traumeel S. *Clin Dev Immunol.* 11(2):pp 1–7.

Rabe A, Weiser M, Klein P. 2004. Effectiveness and tolerability of a homoeopathic remedy compared with conventional therapy for mild viral infections. *Int J Clin Pract.* 58(9):pp 827–32.

Reckeweg H. 1983. Homotoxicosis: The conception of disease. *Biotherapeutic Journal*, 1(4):p 62.

Reckeweg H. 2000. Biotherapeutic Index: Ordinatio Antihomotoxica et Materia Medica, 5th ed. Baden-Baden, Germany: Biologische Heilmittel Heel GMBH, pp 9, 10, 12, 14, 15, 279, 333, 420–3.

Reckeweg H. 2000b. Table of Homotoxicoses (Six Phase Table), Abridged Version. International Society of Homotoxicology. Baden-Baden: Biologische Heilmittel Heel GMBH.

Reilly D, Taylor M, McSharry C, Aitchison T. 1986. Is homeopathy a placebo response? Controlled trial of homeopathic potency, with pollen in hayfever, a model. *Lancet*, i:pp 881–5.

Reinhart E, Broadfoot P, Hanover J. 2005. First Annual Veterinary Congress. Lecture Proceedings November 11–13. Memphis, TN, USA.

Schroder D, Weiser M, Klein P. 2003. Efficacy of a homeopathic *Crataegus* preparation compared with usual therapy for mild (NYHA II) cardiac insufficiency: results of an observational cohort study. *Eur J Heart Fail*, 5(3):pp 319–26.

Stancikova M. 1999. Hemmung der Leukozytenelastase-Aktivität in vitro mit Zeel T, Zeel comp. und ihren verschiedenen Bestandteilen. *Biol Med* 28(2): pp 83–4.

Thompson. 2005. Physicians' Desk Reference, 59th ed. Montvale, NJ: Thompson PDR, pp 1709–10.

Weiser M, Gottwald R. 2000. Treatment with an immune stimulating homeopathic preparation: Results of a drug-monitoring study. *Biotherapeutic Journal*, 18(2).

Weiser M. 2003. A Modern Homeopathic Medication Works As Well As COX 2 Inhibitors for Treating Osteoarthritis of the Knee. Reprinted in English in *J Biomed Ther* Fall 2003; p9.

Weiser M et al. 1998. Homeopathic versus conventional treatment of vertigo: a randomized double-blind controlled clinical study. *Arch Otolaryngol Head Neck Surg*, 124(8):pp 879–85.

Wikipedia. Urea Cycle. 2006. http://en.wikipedia.org/wiki/Urea_cycle.

Zell J, Connert WD, Mau J, Feuerstake G. 1989. Treatment of acute sprains of the ankle: A controlled double-blind trial to test the effectiveness of a homeopathic ointment. *Biological Therapy*, 8(1):pp 1–6.

Chapter Five

A Practical Approach to the Integration of Western Herbal Medicine into Veterinary Practice

WESTERN VETERINARY HERBAL MEDICINE THEORY AND PRACTICE

The use of herbal treatments within veterinary medicine is not a new phenomenon, nor has it always been considered alternative! Ever since veterinary medicine as a discipline began in Europe in the 17th and 18th centuries, plants have been an important part of veterinary herbal medicine. In fact, many herbs were considered orthodox within the veterinary profession until at least the 1960s.

Contemporary veterinary herbal medicine is both a science and a tradition. It represents the synthesis of many fields, including botany, pharmacology, philosophy, history, pathology, ethnoveterinary medicine, research, clinical practice, and monograph study. Why use an herb when we have well-researched, established medicines for many veterinary conditions? We believe that where a conventional medicine is both safe and effective, it makes sense to use it. However for many conditions, drug use isn't safe and it's not always effective; chronic diseases are chronic because the medicine does not restore health (albeit relieving symptoms). And while we currently have good treatment options for patients with infections or parasite burdens, for example, we are challenged by diseases like cancer and allergic and degenerative diseases in animals.

For these conditions, if for no other reason, the traditions of herbal medicine deserve consideration. Herbs can simply represent another pharmacy toolkit; we have herbs to treat diarrhea or hepatitis, for example. We also have herbs (such as adaptogens and alteratives) that have properties that we simply don't have in conventional medicine. We can use herbs as pharmaceutical substitutes or we can undertake to use herbal medicine as a discipline in its own right. This means changing the way we think about medicine, from using drugs or herbs to relieve symptoms to using herbs to fundamentally alter the physiology of our patients toward health (Wynn 2006).

HISTORY OF WESTERN VETERINARY HERBAL MEDICINE

There are herbs for nearly every disease or symptom known and herbal medicine is currently used by 80% of the world's human population (Farnsworth 1985). This is not surprising, considering that for many centuries plants have formed the basis of every system of medicine in the world, including the Indian Ayurvedic system and Traditional Chinese Medicine. Even our Western system of pharmacology has its origins rooted in plant medicine. Despite a relative lack of modern research into the use of herbs in animals in the West, they are used extensively in many countries right now and have been throughout history.

These herbal traditions are even less familiar to scientifically trained modern veterinarians than human doctors. For the most part these traditions are completely ignored by veterinary colleges. However, there is no excuse for ignoring herbal possibilities when our orthodox medicine fails to serve our patients. Herbal tradition offers a long history of empirical experience and new avenues for scientific investigation. Veterinary herbalists can learn a lot from tradition as well as the plethora of emerging science (Wynn 2006).

We can also learn from the grandfathers of veterinary medicine. Any antiquarian veterinary textbook discusses the use of herbal medicines. In *The Illustrated Stock Doctor* (1883), Russell Mannings, MDVS, wrote that to treat "nasal gleat" (rhinitis) of horses, one should "inject the nasal passages thoroughly with the following: 1 oz bayberry bark, 1 pint boiling water. When cool, strain through a close linen or white flannel cloth and inject daily." The text also advises, that for simple colic in horses "If there is griping give the following: 15 to 20 drops of oil of peppermint, 1 oz laudanum." For early colic: "6 Drachms powdered aloes, 1 oz syrup of buckthorn, 1 oz tincture of ginger. Dissolve the aloes in a pint of warm water, add the buckthorn and ginger and give as a drench."

In 1895, Finlay Dun, a respected lecturer at the Edinburgh Veterinary College and an examiner in chemistry at the Royal College of Veterinary Surgeons, published the 9th edition of his popular textbook *Veterinary Medicines, Their Actions and Uses*. He details the use of remedies such as gentian as a bitter tonic "useful in treating atonic digestion" and dissolved linseed tea or ale together with nitre and Epsom salts for treating "simple catarrh in the horse." Juniper is described as a topical irritant, a mild stimulant, a carminative, and diuretic "of use in treating indigestion and flatulence, diminishing the evil effects of bad fodder and marshy pastures."

Herbs were still prominent in the veterinary literature into the 1900s. In Harold Leeney's (1929) *Home Doctoring of Animals*, fennel, aniseed, gentian, fenugreek, ginger, opium, cassia bark, cinnamon, caraway, peppermint, cumin, aloes, thymol, male fern, digitalis leaves, elm bark, camphor, capsicum, belladonna, Peruvian bark, linseed, quassia, oak bark, licorice, cinchona, and other herbs were featured in standard powders, ball and drench recipes.

Even into the 1960s in P.W. Daykin's *Veterinary Applied Pharmacology and Therapeutics*, a textbook used in veterinary schools throughout the UK, Australia, and United States, male fern, acacia, podophyllum, camphor, buchu, cascara, senna, peppermint, betel nut, calabar, kamala, licorice, aniseed, belladonna, ginger, and nux vomica among others still featured highly as contemporary medicines among vaccines, antibiotics, corticosteroids, and hormone treatments now available.

Unfortunately, however, human herbal medicine suffered a demise with the rise of "scientific" medicine, veterinary medicine also began to turn away from these traditional medicines. Many of the patented remedies used in veterinary medicine at the time had become associated with the use of inorganic substances such as mercury and arsenic. It is therefore not surprising that the use of such remedies came into some disrepute with the advent of "modern" pharmaceuticals. Perhaps paralleling the contemporary story of Western herbal medicine, as pharmaceuticals and the double-blind placebo controlled trial become the modern standard of medicine (including veterinary), within a decade the study of herbs all but disappeared from the curriculum of veterinary schools (Griggs 1981). Instead, plants as treatments were replaced with the study of plant toxicology.

Veterinary botanical medicine renaissance

Because the fundamental principles of modern herbal medicine, which are based on science and tradition, are sound, and because there has been a resurging interest in herbal medicine for people since the 1960s, it is not surprising that there has been a corresponding increase in demand for herbal medicine for animals. "Clearly a new opportunity had surfaced to improve the quality of practicing veterinary medicine by using herbal plants and their extracts to improve health, increase energy, facilitate healing, modify symptoms, help the immune system function and improve quality and longevity of patients lives" (Basko 2002).

The first international veterinary herbal organization, the Veterinary Botanical Medicine Association, (www.vbma.org) was formed in 2000 to develop responsible herbal practice by encouraging research and education, strengthening industry relations, keeping herbal tradition alive as a valid information source, and increasing professional acceptance of herbal medicine for animals. A growth in interest and use is expected to continue as we reflect on the various traditions and scientific applications of herbal medicines and find their place within the context of veterinary medicine. Research needs to continue into the safety, efficacy, and appropriate applications of herbal medicines and comparative costs and benefits in veterinary practice.

Sidebar 5.1   Global Warming's Effect on Sustainable Herbal Medicine

The global environment is changing rapidly with global warming, deforestation, and pollution. Many plant species are threatened with extinction or are becoming poisoned with chemicals and pesticides. Herbs incorporate what is in their environment as they grow. What is taken in the roots will be part of that plant forever.

Veterinary herbalists are concerned about herb sustainability and plant conservation. Organic sustainable cropping and harvesting of medicinal herbs needs to be supported to ensure the safety, efficacy, and integrity of the herbs that we use. We need to care about our herbs as much as our patients in this emerging field of veterinary herbal medicine, and consider "sustainable" medicine as the interconnectedness and dependency between animal health and ecosystem health. This must be understood, embraced, and respected.

INTEGRATING WESTERN HERBAL MEDICINE INTO VETERINARY PRACTICE

Veterinarians are using herbal medicine again. A recent survey of 2,675 veterinarians in Austria, Germany, and Switzerland showed that approximately three-quarters of veterinarians in those countries are using herbal medicine, especially for chronic diseases and as adjunct therapy (Hahn 2005).

Herbal medicine is used differently from the ways pharmacologic drugs are used. Herbs are complex compounds with nutritional elements and multiple pharmacological elements that interact both synergistically and antagonistically within the same plant and with other herbal medicines within a formula. At first, this polypharmacy seems a weakness and contrary to what we are philosophically taught in veterinary school; however, this is also an incredible strength. Once the practitioner becomes familiar with herbal medicines and their actions, constituents, and indications, the clinical effects of using numerous properties are more profound than those seen in drug therapy. Patient prescriptions are based on both the pharmacology AND the traditional indications for the herbs; they do not just treat the symptoms, but also the physiology of the affected tissues (Wynn 2006).

There is no reason why herbal medicine cannot be used concurrently with conventional medicine, except to say that careful monitoring and attention to drug doses are needed, because these frequently need to be reduced as the patient's health improves. This is how many veterinary herbalists begin, covering all bases. As confidence improves, it becomes a strategy to withdraw conventional medications over time, while still working on various aspects of the patient.

The use of herbal medicines in veterinary practice offers an extremely rewarding expansion of therapeutic options, especially for chronic disease. However, like any medicine, a good working knowledge is important, and it behooves the veterinary practitioner seeking to integrate herbal medicine into practice to study and learn herbal medicine as a professional rather than as a dabbler. The efficacy of herbal medicine is increased by experience and knowledge, and if it doesn't work, it is more likely a fault of the practitioner than the medicine!

NOTE: *A veterinary herbalist's goal is to restore a patient's vitality and well-being by addressing the underlying and perpetuating causes of the disease. The practitioner works to improve physiology at an organ and cellular level as well as relieve symptoms.*

MODERN WESTERN HERBAL MEDICINE—UNDERSTANDING THE TERMINOLOGY

Alteratives, anodynes, adaptogens, galactogogues, and other seemingly old-fashioned herbal terms appear in our veterinary textbooks of yesteryear. They were words in common use to the orthodox veterinary practitioner, and are becoming increasingly more common again in the contemporary veterinary herbal literature. One of the most common ways herbs are discussed is by their action,

or their effect, on an organ, tissue, or system. By understanding the actions of herbs and knowing the pathophysiology of a particular condition we can strategize the selection and use of particular herbs for individual patients.

Many actions are completely understandable to veterinarians; there are antacid, anthelmintic, anti-inflammatory, and antimicrobial herbs, for example. However, based on individual symptoms, an herb might be chosen for its breadth of action for one patient with multiple systems involved, or for a single, particularly strong action for another patient. This is the beauty and art of herbal medicine—the herbs have appropriate actions and yet are tailored to the whole health of the individual patient. A complete review of an herb's actions, traditional use, doses, and other pertinent information is called an herbal monograph. The *Veterinary Herbal Medicine* (Wynn, Fougere 2006) reviews more than 120 herbs from a veterinary perspective and is a useful guide for new veterinary herbalists. The following section outlines some less familiar herbal terminology that is used to describe the actions of some herbs. This is by no means complete, and there are differences in the potency of the actions of individual herbs.

Alteratives

The alterative classification was used in veterinary herbal medicine literature until the 1950s. These herbs tend to stimulate metabolism so that all functions of the body are enhanced. They have a role in stimulating the elimination of wastes from tissues and organs and are often referred to as blood cleansers or depuratives. Although there are different alteratives for each body system, alteratives are most commonly applied to the skin, lymphatics, GIT (liver and large intestine), and kidneys.

Traditional alteratives used to cleanse the skin include Iris versicolor, Scrophularia nodosa, Fumaria officinalis, Mahonia aquifolium, Urtica dioica, Trifolium pratense and Rumex crispus. Those that cleanse the lymphatic system include Gallium aparine, Phytolacca decandra, and Thuja spp.

Traditional alteratives that cleanse the liver and large intestine include Arctium lappa, Mahonia aquifolium, Taraxacum officinalis root, and Sanguinaria canadensis. Those that cleanse the kidneys: Apium graveolens, Betula alba, Urtica dioica, and Fucus vesiculosis.

Adaptogens

Adaptogens help regulate and balance the body's response to stress, i.e., adaptation. They support adrenal function, and often affect the immune and nervous systems. The original definition of adaptogen is (Panossian, 1999):

1. The adaptogenic effect is non-specific in that the adaptogen increases resistance to a very broad spectrum of harmful factors ("stressors") of different physical, chemical and biological natures;
2. an adaptogen is to have a normalizing effect, that is, it counteracts or prevents disturbances brought about by stressors and
3. an adaptogen must be innocuous to have a broad range of therapeutical effects without causing any disturbance (other than very marginally) to the normal functioning of the organism.

Herbalists believe that in addition to those criteria, adaptogens must work through the hypothalamic-pituitary-adrenal access, which differentiates them from other function-regulators such as immunostimulants. Adaptogenic herbs are especially useful for mitigating the effects of stress in overworked horses and dogs, run-down production animals such as dairy cows, and perhaps chronically stressed dogs and cats exhibiting anxiety-related behaviors. They also help elderly or chronically ill animals counteract lethargy and weakness. These herbs have been investigated for use in enhancing performance in healthy athletes; early clinical trials in humans suggested the effect but more recent high-quality studies do not support this.

Some of the major adaptogenic herbs are *Panax ginseng*, *Panax quinquefolium*, *Eleuthrococcus senticosus*, and *Withania somnifera*. *Centella asiatica*, *Ganoderma lucidum*, *Avena sativa*, *Verbena officinalis*, and *Glycyrrhiza glabra* also have adaptogenic activity.

Amphoterics

Amphoterics normalize organ or system dysfunction. If deficient, the herb stimulates activity, and if excessive, the herb normalizes or even blunts the activity. In other words, they "know what to do."

Anodynes

Anodynes herbs that relieve pain by topical application.

Anthelmintics

Intestinal worms have been and continue to be of the most common problems of domesticated animals. Many plants were used to expel infestations and are still used in ethnoveterinary medicine today. Areca compounds, extract of male fern, kamala, and santonin (from Artemesia spp.) were used in different animals to varying effect in veterinary medicine. A common procedure was to follow administration of these plant compounds with a purgative. The difficulty in killing intestinal worms without harming the patient meant that skill was always required in administering these anthelmintics (Mills 1989).

Antiemetics

Antiemetics, which suppress emesis, include demulcents which coat, protect, lubricate, and soothe the gastric mucosa. Local gastric sedatives (antacids and alkaline stomachics) act by acid neutralization (coating the gastric mucosa) or by local nerve sedation. Central gastric sedatives depress the vomiting center.

Aperients

Aperients are mild laxatives which help to promote natural movement of the bowels, rather than provoking them forcibly. Examples include bulk laxatives such as psyllium and linseed and dietary fiber and plant remedies such as *Articum lappa* (burdock), *Berberis aquifolium* (Oregon grape), and *Berberis vulgaris* (barberry).

Bitter tonics

The taste of bitterness is an extremely common feature of many herbs, and it is important to note that this taste has a major pharmacological action. The bitter principles are a range of chemicals with the common ability to stimulate the bitter receptors inside the mouth, which in turn send signals via the gustatory nerve (Mills 1989) and stimulate the release of gastrointestinal hormones. They also affect other physiological functions. Bitters traditionally have been used for liver and digestive complaints, poor appetite, debility, and a wide range of other conditions.

In traditional medicine this property was highly regarded as leading to a real tonic improvement in health. Bitters were seen as "cooling," or reducing fever by switching blood flow to the breakdown of food and reducing toxin resorption in such conditions, and even more generally by improving nourishment at the expense of "circulatory heat." Bitters were therefore prescribed in "hot" conditions, or those in which the patient felt the heat, were thirsty, had a dry tongue, red tongue, or that experienced nervous agitation, restlessness, and tension. The bitter option still remains one of the most central choices facing the herbalist (Mills 1989). See also Sialagogues, below.

Carminatives

Carminative herbs cause the expulsion of gases from the stomach and large intestine. They are mainly volatile compounds in oils from herbs such as aniseed, ginger, and peppermint. They cause mild irritation of the gastrointestinal mucosa, which results in vasodilation. This is probably responsible for the well-known "warm feeling" which follows the swallowing of these compounds. These herbs also cause the relaxation of the gastrointestinal musculature, but particularly the cardiac sphincter, for a period of up to 30 minutes, which probably plays a large part in releasing gases from the stomach. The rhythm and tone of peristalsis may be initially increased, but this is often followed by a decrease of movement, which helps to relax colic spasms (Daykin 1960).

Cholagogues

Cholagogues stimulate the release and flow of bile already formed in the liver. They are generally a property of bitters, but are also produced by other plant constituents. Cholagogues are used to improve the cleansing of the liver and to aid it in removing material as excretion in bile. They are often combined with laxatives, and formerly emetics, and make up an important part of the eliminative regime and in the treatment of liver disease and wider liver dysfunction (Mills 1989).

Choleretics

Choleretics stimulate bile production by hepatocytes and most have effective cholagogue properties as well. There is very little interest in choleretic and cholagogue treatments in conventional veterinary medicine. Interestingly, NSAIDS, especially aspirin, (in one study at a level of 100 mg/kg) caused choleresis in animals. Magnesium sulphate (Epsom salts) sometimes used for constipation, has been shown at doses of 500 mg to exert a direct effect on the motor activity of the gallbladder in dogs (Mills, Bone 2002).

Contraindications for choleretic and cholagogues include obstructed bile ducts (e.g., cancer of bile duct or pancreas), jaundice following hemolytic diseases, acute or severe hepatocellular disease (e.g. viral hepatitis), septic cholecystitis, intestinal spasm or ileus, and liver cancer.

Demulcents

Demulcents are used to lubricate, soothe, and protect mucous membranes, but the term is usually applied only to those that affect the mouth, pharyngeal, oesophageal, and gastric mucosa. Demulcents can be used to protect the mucous membranes prior to and during administration of irritants to allay irritation and inflammation already caused by chemical or bacterial action. They also can act as bulking agents for other drugs/herbs. Examples of demulcents include honey, treacle, malt extracts, linseed mucilages, and licorice powder.

Diuretics

Diuretic herbs promote the flow of urine, but not necessarily in the same way as conventional diuretic drugs.

They treat urinary tract infections and conditions in which the body retains water. Traditionally, these herbs were given as teas; with the increased water consumption there was a natural increase in urine output. Herbal diuretics work in three basic ways: by increasing renal circulation and therefore the glomerular filtration rate (e.g. *Crataegus oxycanthoides*), by decreasing reabsorption of salts or sugars (e.g., *Agropyron repens* or *Zea mays*), or by irritating the kidneys (eg., *Juniperus communis*).

Laxatives

Many laxatives contain anthraquinone glycosides and bitter constituents. They are classified into four groups, from the mild aperients to the powerful purgatives:

Aperients: e.g., *Taraxacum officinale* root, *Arctium lappa*, *Mahonia aquifolium*, and *Rumex crispus*
Bulk Laxatives: e.g., *Linum usitatissimum* seed, *Plantago psyllium* seed, and *Cannabis sativa* seed
Cathartics: e.g., *Rheum palmatum*, *Cassia angustifolia*
Purgatives: *Aloe barbadensis*, *Phytolacca decandra*

Astringents

Astringent are compounds which precipitate protein, whether intracellular or extracellular. The precipitate of protein covering the surface of the cell or tissue is relatively impermeable to the passage of fluids in either direction. It also acts as a barrier between tissue and irritant and the underlying tissue is therefore soothed and protected from further damage so that healing can take place. The protecting and soothing effect is enhanced by an astringent action on any exposed nerve ending so that pain is lessened; the toxins and histamine-like substances released in damaged tissues are not absorbed. Local and generalized shock are both reduced while the recovery rate is speeded up (Daykin 1960).

An example is tannic acid, found in most plants in small quantities. Stewed tea is very high in tannic acid, as are rhubarb and oak gall. It is suggested that these be used for a limited time (no longer than about 2 weeks). Herbs that are high in tannins can interact or limit absorption of some alkaline drugs.

Sialagogues

The aim of sialagogues is to improve a patient's digestion and appetite through increasing saliva production. They may also increase gastric secretion (such as gentian), so they may be classed as stomachics or gastric stimulants, as well. Gentiana is a reflex sialagogue; it initiates a reflex by stimulating the taste buds on the tongue, which results in salivation.

Sialagogues are also referred to as "bitters." The bitter principles vary considerably and may contain alkaloids. "Simple bitters" can be divided into aromatic simple bitters, such as orange and lemon peel, and non-aromatic simple bitters, such as gentian. Because sialagogues act locally on the taste buds, they must be administered in the form of a powder or tincture. Tablets, pills, and capsules bypass the taste buds. They should be administered 5 to 15 minutes before feeding or be mixed in with food. Dogs and cats usually object to the taste, so meat or meat extracts are probably more useful as salivary or gastric stimulants. Gentian can be mixed with bran mashes for convalescing cattle and horses (Daykin 1960).

Tonics

In Western herbal medicine "tonic" refers to herbs that increase the tone of a tissue or an organ. Tonics might also be taken for their nourishing and supportive effect—what traditional herbalists more clearly referred to as "trophorestoratives." They can be classified according to the tissues or organs upon which they act.

Cardiovascular tonics: e.g., Crataegus oxycanthoides, Convallaria majalis, Leonurus cardiaca, Achillea millefolium, Aesculus hippocastanum, Vaccinium spp., Vitis vinifera, Salvia miltorrhiza, and Polygonum multiflorum

Nervous tonics: e.g., Avena sativa, Scutellaria lateriflora, Verbena officinalis, Turnera diffusa, Ganoderma lucidum, Panax spp., Centella asiatica, Withania somnifera, and Hypericum perforatum

Upper gastrointestinal tonics: e.g., Agrimonia eupatoria, Mahonia aquifolium, Hydrastis canadensis, and Gentiana luteum

Lower gastrointestinal tonics: e.g., Myrica cerifera, Rhamnus purshiana, and Terminalia chebula

Mucous membrane tonics: e.g., Hydrastis canadensis, Mahonia aquifolium, Myrica cerifera, Vaccinium spp., Plantago lanceolata, and Calendula officinalis

Liver tonics: e.g., Cynara scolymus, Silybum marianum, Berberis vulgaris, Andrographis paniculata, Schizandra chinensis, Curcuma longa, and Taraxacum officinalis root

Reproductive tonics: e.g., Turnera diffusa, Serenoa serrulata, Withania somnifera, Panax quinquefolium, Chamaelirium luteum, Rubus ideaus, Angelica sinensis, and Cimicifuga racemosa

Urinary tonics: e.g., Rehmannia glutinosa, Urtica dioica seed, Tribulus terrestris, Althaea offininalis, Solidago virgaurea, and Plantago lanceolata

Respiratory tonics: e.g., Equisetum arvensis, Inula helenium, Glycyrrhiza glabra, Panax quinquefolium, Plantago lanceolata, Astragalus membranaceus, Adhatoda vasica, and Bryonia alba

Immune tonics: e.g., Echinacea spp., Astragalus membranaceus, Ganodernma lucidum, Picrorrhiza kurroa, Andrographis paniculata, Atractylodes macrocephala, Withania somnifera and Codonopsis pilosula

WHAT IS THE SCIENTIFIC PROOF OF THE EFFICACY OF WESTERN HERBAL MEDICINE?

The gold standard for research is the double-blinded placebo controlled trial, which reduces variability and compares the test agent with a placebo. Contrary to what many veterinarians may imagine, there are many rigorous clinical studies on herbs in the literature. These are primarily in human medicine, but a small yet growing number are in veterinary herbal medicine. These, combined with an enormous number of laboratory studies both in vivo and in vitro on herbs and herbal extracts, explain the mechanisms of action and efficacy for a large number of herbs. There have been a surprising number of research studies performed on cats, dogs, and some large animals, and thousands on rats, mice, rabbits, and guinea pigs, which are outlined further in this text.

Many of the published efficacy studies are available on PubMed (www.ncbi.nlm.nih.gov/entrez) or Medline (www.medline.cos.com). Authorative reviews of herbal efficacy can be accessed in the Cochrane reports (www.update-software.com/publications/cochrane) and the European Scientific Cooperative on Phytotherapy (www.escop.com). ESCOP is an international network of scientists and physicians who have published material submitted to the central European medicines regulatory authorities. Another database that ranks herbal efficacy according to the rigor of the studies is available on www. phytotherapy.info. Many of these studies confirm that whole plant extracts have more than a dietary supplement effect, that they can have efficacy on a particular disease and set of symptoms. However, it is likely that the efficacy of herbal medicine is still underrated, and problems with clinical research in herbal medicine can include using doses that are much smaller than in traditional herbal medicine. The use of Echinacea for colds is one example in which research doses are much smaller than those used by herbalists. Another problem is the use of the same herb or herbal combination for a particular disease when the philosophy of herbal medicine is to treat the individual patient; in other words, aiming to improve overall physiology rather than to treat the disease as such.

MODES OF ACTION AND EFFICACY OF WESTERN HERBAL REMEDIES

It is necessary to know something about herbs' active constituents and their effectiveness to understand their uses and modes of action. Herbalists think of plants as more than the sum of their constituents, and avoid considering a researched "active constituent" as being the reason for a plant's efficacy. While it is important to know that research confirms a particular activity, herbalists use the whole plant rather than a single constituent. Dr. Duke's Phytochemical and Ethnobotanical Database (www.ars-grin.gov/duke) states which nutritional and other constituents occur within any given herb and which herbs contain a particular constituent. Plants produce a vast range of chemical constituents, which can have important physiological effects on animals. Several of the most common constituent categories are listed below, along with research that supports their traditional and modern uses.

Flavonoids

Flavonoid compounds are found in many plants; high levels are found in hawthorn, grapes, elderflower, and bilberry. Flavonoids and proanthocyanidins, which are oligomers of flavonoids, are almost universally antioxidant (Moreira 2004, Fremont 1998, Ferrali 1997, Hu 1995). Most are anti-inflammatory (Pelzer 1998, Robak 1996, Pathal 1991) antineoplastic (Vayalil 2004, Hou 2004), and anti-allergic (Lee, et al. 2004), and they reduce capillary permeability and fragility (Roger 1988, Keli 1996, Knekt 1996).

Anthraquinones

Anthraquinones are red or yellow pigments found in well-known laxative herbs, including aloe vera, senna, yellow dock, turkey rhubarb, and cascara. Their laxative effects have been supported by pharmacological research (Leng-Peschlow 1993, Mascolo 1998). They also have anti-inflammatory action (Anton 1980, Spencer 1997).

Coumarins

Coumarin compounds are found in many plants, including lavender, horse chestnut, dandelion, solanaceous plants, poppies, sweet clover, parsley, and angelica. Their fermentation product, dicoumarol, is a potent anticlotting agent and forms the basis of warfarin. Several coumarin derivatives have been used as anticoagulants, but other coumarins do not have this property. Their actions are antibacterial (de Souza, et al. 2005), spasmolytic (Khadzhaĭ, et al. 1966), vasodilative (Chen, et al. 2005), and antiedema (Kontogiorgis, et al. 2006). As medical herbs they have use as venous and lymphatic vessel tonics.

Oxalic acid and oxalates

Oxalates and oxalic acid tend to be found in leaves of yellow dock and rhubarb. They have a mild laxative effect but can precipitate calcium ions under certain circumstances, leading to the formation of stones. The use of oxalate-containing herbs should be limited in quantity and duration of treatment.

Alkaloids

Alkaloids are derived from amino acids and tend to taste bitter (thus acting on the digestive system). They are precipitated by tannins, so should not be mixed together (tannins can therefore be used to treat acute alkaloid toxicity). Pyrrolizidine alkaloids as a subgroup are important for their potential toxicity; for example, in comfrey. Another group, isoquinolone alkaloids, include berberine, hydrastine, and sanguinarine, which are found in herbs such as barberry, Oregon grape root, goldenseal, and bloodroot. Among the actions of these alkaloids: antimicrobial (Cernakova 2002, Sun 1988), antioxidant (Ju 1990), anti-inflammatory (Akiba 1995), ionotropic (Zeng 2003), and antineoplastic (Eun 2004, Kuo 1995).

Salicylates

Salicylic acid is classified with simple phenols as a carboxylated phenol. It occurs naturally as salicylic glycoside precursors (such as salicin, spiraein, salicortin, and populin), esters (such as methyl salicylate), and salts in many fruits and vegetables, processed cheese, nuts, and herbs. The best known are plants including *Salix* species, willow (*Salix spp.*), wintergreen (*Gaultheria procumbens*), black cohosh root (*Cimicifuga racemosa*), poplar tree bark (*Populus* spp.), sweet birch tree bark (*Betula lenta*), silver birch (*Betula pendula*), marshmallow (*Althaea officinalis*), red clover (*Trifolium pratense*), black haw (*Viburnum prunifolium*), cramp bark (*Viburnum opulus*), oak (*Quercus robar*), and meadowsweet (*Filipendula ulmaria*). Salicylates are antiseptic (ESCOP 1997), analgesic (Scmid 2001), antipyretic, anticoagulant, and anti-inflammatory (Hardman 1996, Weissmann 1991).

Saponins

Saponins generally have a sweet taste and they lather in water. They are found in herbs such as wild yam, panax ginseng, astragalaus, licorice, and ivy. They tend to have steroidal molecules that can modulate effects on steroidal receptors (Baker 1995, Rao 1992). They have demonstrated anti-inflammatory, antiviral effects (Davis 1991). They increase mucous production in the lungs and act as expectorants (Shin 2002, Boyd 1946) and reduce cholesterol (Oakenfull 1990). Saponin glycosides can cause hemolysis in large amounts, but are extremely safe when used normally.

Sterols and sterolins

Sterols and sterolins, also known as phytosterols, are present in all plants, fruits, and vegetables, and are chemically similar to cholesterol. Betasitosterol is the major phytosterol in higher plants and beta sitosterolin is its glycoside. Animal studies have demonstrated that phytosterols have anti-inflammatory and antipyretic (Gupta 1980), antineoplastic (Bouic 1997), glucose-lowering (Ivorra 1988), and immune-modulating activity (Bouic 1996).

Tannins

Tannins are generally astringent in nature due to their ability to bind protein molecules. They are found in many herbs including oak bark, black tea, blackberry, witch hazel, and galls. Tannins are used as astringents for wounds and have styptic activity (Rot-Bernstein 1982, Akah 1988), anti-inflammatory and antiulcer action (Maity 1995, Ezaki 1985, Murakami 1991) in the gastrointestinal tract, and are valuable in the treatment of diarrhea (Lamaison 1990). They also have antioxidant activity (Haslam 1996, Okuda 1991).

Volatile oils

Volatile oils are found in aromatic herbs and include the common kitchen herbs such as peppermint, lemon balm, fennel, rosemary, cardamon, and cinnamon. They are used variously to stimulate digestion and reduce flatulence (carminatives) (Giachetti 1988), and have shown spasmolytic activity on tracheal and gastrointestinal smooth muscles (Reiter 1985, Sparks 1995), expectorant activity affecting mucociliary clearance (Dorow 1987), anti-inflammatory activity (Albring 1983), and antiseptic activity (Moleyar 1992, Pattnaik 1997, Janssen 1987).

VETERINARY HERBAL MEDICINE— THE PRACTICE

Veterinarians who choose to incorporate herbal medicine into their practice should obtain a good understanding of both the traditional and scientific aspects of herbal medicine and gain qualifications in this form of medicine to provide the most appropriate individualized treatment for patients. Each herb must be studied and its full range of therapeutic activity, contraindications, and dose should be known. When clients want their veterinarian to use herbs or when a veterinarian elects to treat with herbs without this education, these guidelines apply:

Patients should be monitored carefully when using herbs for the first time. Ensure that the client is able to give the herbs without stressing the patient to increase compliance. Some improvement should be observed within 2 weeks or sooner. Herbs generally take longer to work, although some can work within hours. If no improvement is seen, reassess the case and prescription and possibly increase the dose.

Use good-quality herbs that state the species and potency and are from reputable companies. Most herbs are available for purchase as teas, tinctures, tablets, capsules, salves, and ointments. Sending clients to health food stores is risky because they may not be able to make these assessments.

Ideally, choose companies that demonstrate ethical harvesting of herbs and concern for conservation. Organic products are ideal.

Use up to 5 herbs at a time if making formulas to enable pharmacological dosing. Dilution occurs with multiple herbs and each dose will have to be increased accordingly or herbs will have more of a physiological rather than therapeutic effect.

Choose a main herb that provides the general thrust of the formula. Consider the predisposing and perpetuating factors that keep the patient in a chronic state and deal with those. Pay special attention to the digestive system. If this isn't working, bioavailability of herbal constituents may be compromised.

Start with small doses and increase if you are inexperienced. Adjust on a weekly basis until a therapeutic effect is observed, then hold.

For long-term use give the client and patient a break on weekends or a week off once a month by stopping herbs during these times.

HERB FORMS AND DOSES

Forms

Fresh herbs: Many fresh garden herbs such as parsley, thyme, and rosemary can be added to food, although palatability can be affected by adding too much! Alternatively, make a tea from fresh herbs and mix it with food. Avoid picking wild herbs unless you are trained to identify and harvest ethically.

Dried herbs: Dried herbs are frequently used in capsules or tablets. Dried herbs without further processing are not as potent as herbs that have undergone extraction processes, but they are still useful and relatively easy to add to food. Ensure they are free of mold.

Tablets or capsules: Tablets or capsules may contain dried herbs or dried herbs that have been extracted and concentrated, which affects dosing. Sometimes extracted dried herbs are 5 to 10 times more potent that their dried forms. They are often easy for clients to give because they are familiar with tablets and capsules. Lubricate them with butter, sardines, pate, cheese, mashed sweet potato, or peanut butter to help them down.

Infusions and decoctions: Infusions are teas made by pouring 1 cup of boiling water over 1 teaspoon of an herb (usually fresh leaves and flowers) in a glass or china cup. Infuse for 3 to 15 minutes; the tea may become more bitter with time. Strain and add to food or administer with syringe by mouth. Add honey or chicken broth if needed. A decoction is simply made by simmering hard herbal materials such as roots, wood, and barks. Place 1 teaspoon in 1 cup of cold water in a glass or ceramic vessel. Bring to a boil, and then simmer, cool, and strain. Make the infusion or decoction daily and discard leftovers.

Tinctures: Tinctures are generally made by placing dried herbs in varying proportions of alcohol, depending on the nature of the constituents. After a period of time the alcohol is strained from the plant material and bottled. Each herb is prepared specifically according to prescribed methods as a quality control measure. Sometimes the alcohol is evaporated or removed and replaced by glycerin, producing potent but sweet-tasting herbs. Herbs also may be placed directly in glycerin for extraction of particular constituents. Alcohol tinctures are very stable, and are particularly useful in acute conditions because the alcohol promotes the absorption of the herb across the mucous membranes and the skin. The major disadvantage is that most dogs and cats hate the taste of alcohol but this can be dealt with by disguising the taste in food, or evaporating the alcohol as much as possible by allowing the herb liquid to sit over warm water (or add warm water). These are best given diluted in water, or in food. Milk, glycerin, or honey can be added to them.

Glycetract glycerine tinctures: Glycetract glycerine tinctures have a sweet and warming taste and are readily accepted by dogs and cats. They are suitable to give to diabetic dogs, when monitored. They are less potent in general than alcohol tinctures, so more is required. They can be given directly or added to food. They may need to be refrigerated.

Fresh plant creams: Chickweed, calendula, comfrey, Echinacea, and other herbs can be made into creams by juicing the fresh plant, then filtering the juice through a coffee filter. Combine 10 ml of the juice with 100 grams of vitamin E cream, sorbelene, or olive oil. Many commercial skin preparations can be purchased. Remember that whatever is applied is likely to be licked off, so check the ingredients and safety before applying.

Doses

One of the major difficulties in veterinary herbalism has been the lack of research to provide the most appropriate dosage of specific herbs and formulations for dogs. The variable concentration of different products containing the same herb further complicates dosing. The active compounds also can vary in potency, depending on when and where herbs are harvested. As a result, it is much easier to administer correct dosages of conventional drugs than herbs.

Herbs are best used in formulas to exploit synergies while minimizing the potential for side effects. Human herb doses are better established due to traditional use and published research. The following list contains very general guidelines. Ideally, more specific dose rates are available for veterinary use (Fougere, Wynn 2006).

Single herbs per 10 kg/20 pounds:

Capsules or tablets: 1 to 3 twice daily. The actual dose depends upon whether the herbs are concentrated, extracted forms (low dose) or dried powder herbs (high dose).

Dried herbs: 1 to 2 teaspoons daily in divided doses mixed with food.

Infusion: One-fourth cup of infusion or decoction up to 3 times daily.

Tinctures: 0.5 to 1 ml tincture daily (in divided doses) up to 3 ml daily for very safe herbs; 1 to 2 ml glycetract daily (in divided doses) up to 4 ml daily for very safe herbs. Note that the dose is for individual herbs with a potency of 1:2 or 1:3. If more herbs are added the total volume increases proportionally. For example, a 10-pound cat would receive 0.5 to 1 ml of a glycetract of marshmallow: 0.25 to 0.5 ml in the morning and 0.25 ml to 0.5 ml in the evening.

Multiple herbs (for 10 kg/20 pounds): 0.5 ml to 1 ml of each tincture (up to 5 tinctures) in divided doses. For example, a 5-kg cat would receive 0.25 to 0.5 ml of each herb daily. A total dose of 5 herbs would equal 1.25 to 2.5 ml daily, with 1 ml given at morning and night.

SAFETY AND HERB-DRUG INTERACTIONS

It is important to note that some herbs (for example, yellow jasmine, pokeroot, and comfrey) are very toxic, and even lethal in very small doses. Likewise, even the safer herbs can be potentially dangerous if used inappropriately. There have been many reports of toxicities in people, ranging from allergic reactions to the plants themselves to side effects such as vomiting, diarrhea, and liver damage caused by the actives in the herbs, to death, although this is rare. Herbs work best and are safest when prescribed by a veterinary herbalist who can tailor the most appropriate herbs at the most effective doses. It behooves us as responsible practitioners to have a working knowledge of the herbs, their actions, clinical uses, contraindications, and doses. These are potent plant medicines.

The issue of herb-drug interactions is important and serious, but perhaps overemphasized by the published literature. Herb-drug interactions are less about the chemical interaction between a drug and an herb and more about 1 herb constituent causing an increase or decrease in the amount of drug in the bloodstream. For example, frequently cited herb-drug concerns center on warfarin, in which the impact of the herb on warfarin, an anticoagulant, leads to a bleeding episode or formation of a dangerous clot. Other concerns often stem from pharmacology studies rather than actual clinical experience, such as those about the impact of valerian, which may increase the effects of certain anti-seizure medications or prolong the effects of anesthetic agents.

One review consolidated the clinical and pharmacologic aspects of drug-herb interactions by searching databases from 1966 to 2002; 162 citations were identified. Only 22 citations met the inclusion criteria of being adequately reported. Most interactions were pharmacokinetic; most actually or theoretically affected the metabolism of the affected product by way of the cytochrome P450 enzymes. In this review, warfarin was the most common drug and St. John's wort was the most common herbal product reported in drug-herb interactions (Brazier 2003).

In an earlier review, an intensive search of the literature and evaluation of reports of herb-drug interactions yielded the following: "108 cases of suspected interactions were found: 68.5% were classified as 'unable to be evaluated,' 13% as 'well-documented,' and 18.5% as 'possible' interactions.' Warfarin was the most common drug (18 cases) and St. John's Wort the most common herb (54 cases) involved." Thus, 14 cases were well-documented in this report published about 2 years earlier than the new report, which found 22 reasonably supported cases (Fugh-Berman 2001). So perhaps drug-herb interactions are overstated but no doubt many other instances occur and go unreported. None the less, in this author's experience herb-drug interactions have not been detrimental. Rather, they have been beneficial to the patient and lower doses of drugs such as prednisolone or non-steroidals have been achieved. If an herb-drug interaction is suspected, or to check the literature to see if it has been reported, access Entrez-PubMed on http://www.ncbi.nlm.nih.gov/PubMed/ or use a search engine to locate PubMed. The procedure for checking herb-drug interactions is to type in: (name of the drug), herb-drug interactions.

Adverse events associated with herbs and potential herb-drug interactions can be reported on the Web site of the Veterinary Botanical Medicine Association: www.vbma.org

REFERENCES

Akah PA. Haemostatic activity of aqueous leaf extract of Ageratum conyzoides L. *International Journal of Crude Drug Research* 1988; 26(2): 97–101.

Akiba S, Nagatomo R, Ishimoto T, Sato T (1995) Effect of berbamine on cytosolic phospholipase A2 activation in rabbit platelets. *Eur J Pharmacol* 291:343–50.

Albring M, Albrecht H, Alcorn G, Lücker PW. The measuring of the antiinflammatory effect of a compound on the skin of volunteers. *Meth Find Exp Clin Pharmacol* 1983;5:575–7.

Anton R, Haag-Berrurier M. Therapeutic use of natural anthraquinone for other than laxative actions. *Pharmacology* 1980; 20 (supp 1): 104–112.

Baker ME. Endocrine activity of plant-derived compounds: an evolutionary perspective. Proceedings of the Society for Experimental Biology and Medicine 1995; 208: 131–138.

Basko I. Introduction to Veterinary Western Herbology. Proceedings of the 17th Annual Conference of the American Holistic Veterinary Medical Association; September 28–October 1, 2002; Eugene, OR.

Bouic PJ, Etsebeth S, Liebenberg RW, et al. Beta sitosterol and beta–sitosterol glycoside stimulate human peripheral blood lymphocyte proliferation: implications for their use as immunomodulatory vitamin combination. *Int J Immunopharmacol* 1996:18; 693–700.

Bouic PJ. Plant sterols and sterolins. *Alt Med Rv* 2001 Vol 6:2 203: 206.

Boyd EM, Palmer ME. The effect of quillaia, senega, squill, grindelia, sanguinaria, chionanthus and dioscorea upon the output of respiratory tract fluid. *Acta Pharmacologica* 1946; 2: 235–246.

Brazier NC, Levine MA. Drug-herb interaction among commonly used conventional medicines: a compendium for health care professionals. *Am J Ther.* 2003 May-Jun;10(3): 163–9.

Cernakova M, Kostalova D. Antimicrobial activity of berberine—a constituent of *Mahonia aquifolium. Folia Microbiol.* 2002:47:375–8.

Chen YL, Lu CM, Lee SJ, Kuo DH, Chen IL, Wang TC, Tzeng CC. Synthesis, antiproliferative, and vasorelaxing evaluations of coumarin alpha-methylene-gamma-butyrolactones. *Bioorg Med Chem.* 2005 Oct 15;13(20):5710–6.

Davis EA, Morris DJ. Medicinal uses of licorice through the millennia: The good and plenty of it. *Molec Cell Endocrinol.* 1991. 78:1–6.

Daykin PW. Veterinary and Applied Pharmacology and Therapeutics. Bailliere, Tindall and Cox. 1960 p 70–72.

de Souza SM, Delle Monache F, Smania A Jr. Antibacterial activity of coumarins. *Z Naturforsch* [C]. 2005 Sep-Oct; 60(9–10):693–700.

Dorow P, Weiss T, Felix R, et al. Effect of a secretolytic and a combination of pinene, limonene and cineole on mucociliary clearance in patients with chronic pulmonary obstruction. *Arzneimittel-Forschung* 1987; 37(12): 1378–1381.

Eun JP, Koh GY. Suppression of angiogenesis by the plant alkaloid, sanguinarine. *Biochem Biophys Res Commun,* 2004: 317:618–24.

Ezaki N, Kato M, Takizawa N et al. Pharmacological studies on Linderae umbellatae Ramus, IV. Effects of condensed tannin related compounds on peptic activity and stress-induced gastric lesions in mice. *Planta Medica* 1985; 34–38.

Farnsworth N, et al. Medicinal plants in therapy. *Bull World Health Org* 1985, 63 pp 965–981.

Ferrali M, Signorini C, Caciotti B, et al. Protection against oxidative damage of erythrocyte membrane by the flavonoid quercetin and its relation to iron chelating activity. *FEBS Letters* 1997; 416(2): 123–129.

Fremont L, Gozzelino MT , Franchi MP, et al. Dietary flavonoids reduce lipid peroxidation in rats fed polyunsaturated or monounsaturated fat diets. *Journal of Nutrition* 1998; 128(9): 1495–1502.

Fugh-Berman A, Ernst E. Herb-drug interactions: review and assessment of report reliability, *British Journal of Clinical Pharmacology* 2001, 52(5): 587–595.

Giachetti D, Taddei E, Taddei I. Pharmacological activity of essential oils on Oddi's Sphincter. *Planta Medica* 1988; 389–392.

Griggs B. Green Pharmacy: A History of Herbal Medicine. New York: Viking Press; 1981.

Gupta MB, Nath R, Srivastava N, et al. Antiinflammatory and antipyretic activities of Beta sitosterol. *Planta Medica* 1980; 39: 157–163.

Hahn I, Zitterl-Eglseer K, Franz CH. Phytomedizin bei Hund und Katze: Internetumfrage bei Tierärzten und Tierärztinnen in Österreich, Deutschland und der Schweiz. *Schweiz Arch Tierheilk* 2005;147:135–141.

Hardman J, et al. The pharmacological basis of therapeutics, 9th ed. New York: McGraw-Hill;1996:1,905.

Haslam E. Natural polyphenols (vegetable tannins) as drugs: possible modes of action. *Journal of Natural Products* 1996; 59: 205–215.

Hou DX, Fujii M, Terahara N, Yoshimoto M. Molecular Mechanisms Behind the Chemopreventive Effects of Anthocyanidins. *J Biomed Biotechnol* 2004(5):321–325.

Hu JP, Calomme M, Lasure A, et al. Structure-activity relationship of flavonoids with superoxide scavenging activity. *Biological Trace Element Research* 1995; 47(1–3): 327–331.

Ivorra MD, D'Ocon MP, Paya M, Villar A. Antihyperglycaemic and insulin releasing effects of Beta sitosterol 3-B-D Glucoside and its aglycone B-sitosterol. *Arch Int Pharmacodyn Ther* 1988; 296; 224–231.

Janssen AM, Scheffer JJC, Baerheim Svendsen A. Antimicrobial activity of essential oils: A 1976–1986 literature review. Aspects of the test methods. *Planta Medica* 1987; 395–398.

Ju HS, Li XJ, Zhao BL, et al. Scavenging effect of berbamine on active oxygen radicals in phorbol ester-stimulated human polymorphonuclear leukocytes. *Biochem Pharmacol.* 1990: 39:1673–8.

Keli SO, Hertog MG, Feskens EJ. Dietary flavonoids, antioxidant vitamins, and incidence of stroke: the Zutphen study. *Archives of Internal Medicine.* 1996; 156(6): 637–642.

Khadzhaĭ IaI, Obolentseva GV, Prokopenko AP. On the relation between the structure and spasmolytic activity in a series of derivatives of coumarin and furocoumarins. *Farmakol Toksikol.* 1966 Mar-Apr;29(2):156–63.

Knekt P, Jarvinen R, Reunanen A, et al. Flavonoid intake and coronary mortality in Finland: a cohort study. *British Medical Journal* 1996; 312(7029): 478–481.

Kontogiorgis CA, Savvoglou K, Hadjipavlou-Litina DJ. Anti-inflammatory and antioxidant evaluation of novel coumarin derivatives. *J Enzyme Inhib Med Chem.* 2006 Feb; 21(1):21–9.

Kuo CL, Chou CC, Yung BY. Berberine complexes with DNA in the berberine-induced apoptosis in human leukemic HL-60 cells. *Cancer Lett.* 1995; 93(2):193–200.

Lamaison JL, Carnat A, Petitjean-Freytet C. Teneur en tanins et activité inhibitrice de l'élastase chez les Rosacae. *Annales de Pharmaceutiques Françaises* 1990; 48(6): 335–340.

Lee NK, Choi SH, Park SH, Park EK, Kim DH. Antiallergic activity of hesperidin is activated by intestinal microflora. *Pharmacology.* 2004: 71(4):174–80.

Leeney H. MRCVS Home Doctoring for Animals. London: Macdonald and Martin; 1929.

Leeney H. MRCVS Home Doctoring for Animals. London: Macdonald and Martin; 1921.

Leng-Peschlow E. Sennoside-induced secretion is not caused by changes in mucosal permeability or Na+,K(+)-ATPase activity. *Journal of Pharmacy and Pharmacology* 1993; 45(11): 951–954.

Maity S, Vedasiromoni JR, Ganguly DK. Anti-ulcer effect of the hot water extract of black tea (Camellia sinensis). *Journal of Ethnopharmacology* 1995; 46: 167–174.

Mascolo N, Capasso R, Capasso F. Senna. A safe and effective drug. *Phytotherapy Research* 1998; 12: S143–S145.

Mills S. The Complete Guide to Modern Herbalism. London: Thorsons 1989 p22.

Mills S. Acupharmacology: A fundamental approach to herbal therapeutics Part 2. *Modern Phytotherapist* Vol 3 No 3.

Mills S, Bone K. Principles and Practice of Phytotherapy. New York: Churchill Livingstone, 2000.

Moleyar V, Narasimham P. Antibacterial activity of essential oil components. *International Journal of Food Microbiology* 1992; 16(4): 337–342.

Moreira AJ, Fraga C, Alonso M, et al. Quercetin prevents oxidative stress and NF-kappaB activation in gastric mucosa of portal hypertensive rats. *Biochem Pharmacol* 2004: 68(10):1939–46.

Murakami S, Isobe Y, Kijima H, et al. Inhibition of gastric H+,K+-ATPase and acid secretion by ellagic acid. *Planta Medica* 1991; 57: 305–308.

Oakenfull D, Sidhu GS. Could saponins be a useful treatment for hypercholesterolaemia? *European Journal of Clinical Nutrition* 1990; 44: 79–88.

Okuda T, Yoshida T, Hatano T. Chemistry and biological activity of tannins in medicinal plants. In: Wagner N, Farnsworth NR. Economic and medicinal plant research. Volume 5. London: Academic Press, 1991; pp 130–165.

Panossian A, Wikman G, Wagner H. Plant adaptogens. III. Earlier and more recent aspects and concepts on their mode of action. *Phytomedicine* 1999 Oct;6(4):287–300.

Pathak D, Pathak K, Singla AK. Flavonoids as medicinal agents—recent advances. *Fitoterapia* 1991; LXII(5): 1991

Pattnaik S, Subramanyam VR, Bapaji M, et al. Antibacterial and antifungal activity of aromatic constituents of essential oils. *Microbios* 1997; 89(358): 39–46.

Pelzer LE, Guardia T, Osvaldo JA, et al. Acute and chronic antiinflammatory effects of plant flavonoids. *Farmaco* 1998; 53(6): 421–424.

Rao AR, Kale RK. Diosgenin—a growth stimulator of mammary gland of ovariectomized mouse. *Indian Journal of Experimental Biology* 1992; 30: 367–370.

Reiter M, Brandt W. Relaxant effects on tracheal and ileal smooth muscles of the guinea pig. *Arzneimittel-Forschung* 1985; 35(1A): 408–414.

Robak J, Gryglewski RJ. Bioactivity of flavonoids. *Polish Journal of Pharmacology* 1996; 48(6): 555–564.

Roger CR. The nutritional incidence of flavonoids: some physiological and metabolic considerations. *Experientia* 1988: 44(9):725–33.

Root-Bernstein RS. Tannic acid, semipermeable membranes and burn treatment. *The Lancet* 1982; 2: 1168.

Schmid B, Kotter I, Heide L. Pharmacokinetics of salicin after oral administration of a standardised willow bark extract. *Eur J Clin Pharmacol* 2001 Aug;57(5):387–91.

Shin CY, Lee WJ, Lee EB, et al. Platycodin D and D3 increase airway mucin release in vivo and in vitro in rats and hamsters. *Planta Med* 2002: 68(3):221–5.

Sparks MJ, O'Sullivan P, Herrington AA, et al. Does peppermint oil relieve spasm during barium enema? *British Journal of Radiology* 1995; 68(812): 841–843.

Spencer CM, Wilde MI. Diacerein. *Drugs* 1997; 53(1): 98–106

Sun D, Courtney HS, Beachey EH. Berberine sulfate blocks adherence of *Streptococcus pyogenes* to epithelial cells, fibronectin, and hexadecane. *Antimicrob Agents Chemother* 1988: 32(9):1370–4.

Vayalil PK, Mittal A, Katiyar SK. Proanthocyanidins from grape seeds inhibit expression of matrix metalloproteinases in human prostate carcinoma cells, which is associated with the inhibition of activation of MAPK and NF kappa B. *Carcinogenesis* 2004: 25(6):987–95.

Weissmann G. Aspirin. *Sci Am* 1991;264(1):84–90.

Wynn S, Fougere B. Veterinary Herbal Medicine. Oxford, UK: Elsevier, 2006.

Zeng XH, Zeng XJ, Li YY. Efficacy and safety of berberine for congestive heart failure secondary to ischemic or idiopathic dilated cardiomyopathy. *Am J Cardiol* 2003: 92:173–6.

SECTION 2

Integrative Therapy Protocols by Organ System

In the "Author's Suggested Protocol" section of each disease, the authors recommend products and dose schedules used in their practices. The author may have an affiliation with the company producing such products. These specific products are listed because of the author's clinical experience and use patterns. No author has experience with all products available and it was deemed prudent to recommend those products for which we had clinical experience. When applicable, the authors have included alternative product recommendations in some protocols. In the case of homotoxicology and Chinese herbal formulations, there are often few or no alternatives. When determining the remedies recommended for any condition, combination formulas of nutraceuticals, herbs, or homotoxicology agents often have enhanced, synergistic activity when compared to their individual components.

It is important for veterinarians to understand that natural, herbal, and nutritional products can differ dramatically from each other, even if the listed ingredients are the same. Practitioners should not assume any government regulation of these products. Also, practitioners who are accustomed to the standardization of pharmaceuticals should realize that these natural products are impossible to compare without extensive clinical testing of each product. Pharmaceuticals are chemical products produced under stringent standardized regulation and can usually be reliably compared to each other. For most suggested therapies recommended in this book, the rationale for use of the strongest indicated components are outlined within the text. It is beyond the scope of this text to deal with each ingredient individually, and the reader is referred to the list of supportive texts in the reference and resource sections of this book for further information and study.

Chapter Six

Autoimmune Disease

AUTOIMMUNE ANEMIA AND THROMBOCYTOPENIA

Definition and cause

Autoimmune anemia and thrombocytopenia are the result of increased destruction or decreased production of red blood cells or platelets. While the literature cites many causes for both diseases, such as destruction by antibodies, infectious agents, exposure to antigens, neoplasia and tick borne diseases, the basic mechanism of action is an exaggerated immune response against its own tissue (RBCs, thrombocytes) or a decreased production by the bone marrow (Calia 2003, Lewis 1996, Regan 1995, Stewart 1993, Thompson 1995, Bucheler 1995). Some research has suggested that combination vaccinations may be associated with a higher incidence of these diseases (Duval 1996).

Medical therapy rationale, drug(s) of choice, and nutritional recommendations

In the majority of instances, the rationale for treatment is direct suppression of the exaggerated immune response with cortisone (prednisone or dexamethasone) or chemotherapeutics (azothiaprine and cyclophosphamide) along with supportive care (Calia 2003). Nutritionally, the dietary addition of essential fatty acids such as eicosapentaenoic acid has been shown to be beneficial (Harbige 1998).

Anticipated prognosis

It is estimated that one-third of animals will be nonresponsive to therapy and will die from either disease (Calia 2003, Williams 1984).

Integrative veterinary therapies

In addition to proper medical therapy, IVM focuses on the imbalanced immune system and its exaggerated response toward its own tissue. The removal of the offending cause is important for long-term remission. One underlying principle of alternative therapies focuses upon the inflammatory process that results from oxidation and an excessive free radical load. A local, cellular autoimmune response progresses and the target tissue (the red blood cells or thrombocytes) begin to be destroyed. The goal of integrative therapies is to quiet or neutralize this autoimmune pathogenesis and help to prevent further cellular destruction and the initiation of a chronic disease process.

Nutrition
General considerations/rationale

An imbalanced immune system, one that has an exaggerated response against its own tissue, requires nutritional supplementation, reduction of oxidative damage, and cell or organ sparing. In addition to addressing the autoimmune response, the nutritional support program should also supply nutrients required by other target cell or organ.

Appropriate nutrients

Gland therapy: Glandular bone marrow, liver, spleen, and thymus support supply intrinsic nutrients and can help protect target organs. One of the most bioavailable sources of iron is liver. Comparing of the absorption rate of inorganic iron (for example, ferrous sulfate versus heme-iron), the latter is 30 times more effective. The best source of heme-iron is concentrated liver extract (Frykman 1994). Liver is also a superior source of vitamin B_{12} and folic acid.

Note that autoimmune anemia and thrombocytopenia are serious diseases and can involve multiple organs. It is recommended that blood be analyzed both medically and physiologically to determine associated organ involvement and disease. This will allow for a more specific gland and nutritional support protocol (see Chapter 2, Nutritional Blood Testing, for more information).

Betasitosterol: Plant-derived sterols such as betasitosterol show anti-inflammatory properties that appear to be similar to corticosteriods (Gupta 1980). A cortisone-like effect without the associated immune suppressing effects is beneficial in immune-mediated anemia. Bouic (1996) reports on the immune-enhancing and -balancing effect of plant sterols, which can be beneficial to an animal with immune-mediated anemia.

Vitamin B$_{12}$: Essential for the maintenance of the proper levels of red blood cells. Deficiencies of vitamin B$_{12}$ are associated with anemia and decreased function of the immune system. Supplementation with vitamin B$_{12}$ often addresses the condition (Berlin 1978, Kondo 1998, Lederle 1991).

Folic acid: A B vitamin that is required for organized cellular division. Folic acid is integral in the synthesis of both DNA and RNA, and therefore has an effect of the genetic modeling of the body. Folic acid deficiencies affect bone marrow cell division and can lead to a macrocytic anemia (Food Nutrition Board 1998).

Chinese herbal medicine
General considerations/rationale

Autoimmune hemolytic anemia: Practitioners of TCM define autoimmune hemolytic anemia as a Yin deficiency and internal heat. The Heat leads to toxin formation. The Western interpretation is that the Heat is the immune reaction that destroys the blood. Toxins, in this case substances such as bilirubin, build up in the blood. Because Blood is part of Yin, the fluids of the body, one can translate the concept of Yin deficiency into blood deficiency (anemia).

Immune-mediated thrombocytopenia (ITP): In traditional Chinese medicine, ITP is considered to be a result of Blood, Yin, and Spleen Qi deficiency with internal Heat. For the Western interpretation, the authors translate this etiology as follows: Again, Heat can be translated as the inflammation or excessive immune reactivity of the body. This inflammation is directed toward the blood components, the thrombocytes in this situation. In TCM theory, one function of the Spleen is to use its energy to keep blood in the vessels. When the Spleen energy is too weak, blood can leave the vessels. The result is the petechiae seen in ITP. Blood deficiency is the anemia and thrombocytopenia is seen in this condition. Yin is the fluids of the body. Because Blood is a component of Yin, when there is a Blood deficiency, there must be a Yin deficiency.

Appropriate Chinese herbs
Immune-mediated hemolytic anemia (IMHA)

Immuneregulator: Contains Astragalus (Huang qi), which has been shown to increase the production of blood cells in the bone marrow (Nan Jing Zhong Ye Xue Yuan Xue Bao 1989), and Ligustrum (Nu zhen zi), which stimulates the production of blood cells in mice (Zhong Yao Tong Bao 1983).

Immune-mediated thrombocytopenia (ITP)

H13: Contains Astragalus (Huang qi), which has been shown to increase the production of blood cells in the bone marrow (Nan Jing Zhong Ye Xue Yuan Xue Bao 1989).

Agrimony (Xian he cao): Increases the platelet count in dogs and rabbits (Zhong Yao Yao Li Yu Ying Yong 1983).

Eclipta (Han lian cao): Extremely effective at stopping hemorrhage (Zhe Jiang Zhong Yi Za Zhi 1988).

Litospermum root (Zi cao gen): Has been used to treat patients with purpura (Zhong Hua Nei Ke Za Zhi 1976).

Madder (Qian cao): Decreases bleeding time in rabbits (Zhong Yi Yao Yan Jiu 1991).

Moutan (Mu dan pi): Has been used successfully to treat humans with anemic purpura (Zhong Xi Yi Jie He Za Zhi, 1985).

Notoginseng (San qi): Used topically, decreased bleeding time in transected rat tails by 30% compared to controls that were treated with wheat flour (Fan 2005).

Rehmannia (Sheng di huang): Improves hemostasis (Zhong Yao Xue 1998). Also increases the plasma levels of adrenocortical hormone (Zhong Yao Xue 1998). By increasing the ACTH level it may increase the corticosterone levels in the body. This would have a similar effect to administration of prednisone on decreasing the immune response.

Acupuncture

Acupuncture has been shown to increase the hematocrit and platelet count in various pathologies. One case study reported increased platelet and red blood cell numbers in a 69-year-old man with aplastic anemia. The patient had been treated with prednisone, which caused compressive spinal fractures, and cyclosporine, which caused toxicity. Still his counts remained low. Treatment with electroacupuncture was begun at various locations depending upon his presenting signs. Both the platelet number and red blood cell count returned to normal parameters (Lu 2002). Some practitioners claim that acupuncture should be avoided due to potential hemorrhage problems.

Homotoxicology
General considerations/rationale

Autoimmune hemolytic anemia and immune-mediated thrombocytopenia represent Impregnation and Degeneration Phase disorders. Homotoxins have altered normal structure and function to the degree that dangerous imbalances occur and cellular damage leads to life threatening circumstances.

Conventional therapy is needed to block inappropriate savage attempts by the organism's immune system, which, left unchecked, would tip the biological balance toward death. Intensive medical monitoring and support are recommended and biological therapy is initiated to assist in normalizing responses, supporting injured tissues, removing homotoxins that are responsible for initiation of the imbalance, and re-establishing normal autoregulation (Reckeweg 2000). Extreme care must be taken to avoid progressive vicariation in these patients. Vaccinations, which can alter red cell or thrombocyte surface antigens, and use of drugs that are not directly indicated should be avoided in these patients unless vital (Duval 1996, Dodds, 2005).

Appropriate homotoxicology formulas

Due to the severe nature of these homotoxicoses, many systems may be involved. The practitioner using biological therapies must be well versed to program these long-term cases (Smit 2004). Exact treatment programs depend upon the precise cause of the condition, which is usually difficult if not impossible to elucidate. The practitioner must evaluate the state of vicariation currently being manifested by a specific, individual patient, and use this data to direct therapy. Compositae antihomotoxic formulas are vital for success in these patients, and autosanguis therapy should be considered (Broadfoot 2004). In initial phases of therapy, where immunosuppression is desired, avoid use of immune stimulating antihomotoxic medicines such as Echinacea compositum, Engystol-N, and Tonsilla compositum. Once the condition is under control, such formulas may prove helpful in repairing damage, normalizing immune function, and leading to regressive vicariation.

Please note the following convention throughout this book: (1) Italicized and capitalized terms are Heel product names; (2) Capitalized, nonitalicized names involve product constituents. Agents are selected for therapeutic use which match the present symptoms or signs of the patient.

The following agents may be useful in approaching anemia and thrombocytopenia:

Aletris heel: Exhaustion, anemias.

BHI-Exhaustion: The ingredient Cinchona officinalis 4X assists in cases of exhaustion resulting from loss of blood (Heel 2002).

China homaccord: Exhaustion, weakness, and collapse after blood or fluid loss.

Coenzyme compositum: Support of cellular energy metabolism.

Ferrum homaccord: A main remedy in cases of secondary anemia, anemia of iron deficiency, or anemia of chronic disorder wherein iron sequestration has occurred. May be used in inflammatory or febrile conditions, particularly after infectious disease (Bianchi 1995).

Galium-Heel: Important phase remedy for both Impregnation and Degeneration phase homotoxicoses. Activates the nonspecific defense mechanisms in cellular phases. This is a main remedy in all anemia cases.

Glyoxal compositum: Decouples polymers, which block enzyme systems.

Graphites homaccord: Exudative diatheses, petechial hemorrhages.

Hepar compositum: Support of hepatic detoxification, drainage, and repair, as well as support for iatrogenic damage caused by corticosteroid therapy.

Lymphomyosot: Support of endocrine and lymphatic function.

Mucosa compositum: Support of mucous membranes, particularly related to damage from corticosteroid therapy. Phase remedy for Degeneration Phase disorders.

Phosphor homaccord: Tendencies toward hemorrhage or bleeding (Reckeweg 2002).

Pulsatilla compositum: Regulation rigidity cases and to reverse the iatrogenic damage from corticoids.

Solidago compositum: Support of renal function and detoxification.

Thryoidea compositum: Matrix drainage and endocrine support.

Tonsilla compositum: Supports bone marrow, spleen, and immune function, and assists in repair in Impregnation Phase diseases. Broadfoot (2005) recommends tonsilla and *Traumeel-S* as a mixed autosanguis, with Lymphomyosot. In cases of acute chronic inflammation it is useful in preventing a trend toward Degeneration (Bianchi 1989).

Traumeel S: Activation of inactive sulfur-containing enzyme systems, nonsteroidal anti-inflammatory effects, modulation of the inflammatory system.

Ubichinon compositum: Support of cellular energy metabolism and mitochondrial repair. Para-benzoquinone should be considered in conditions with damage to the spleen and changes in the blood composition, and in states arising from removal of the spleen and in which auto-antigens (wild peptides) are involved, such as auto-immune diseases (Reckeweg 2002).

Authors' suggested protocols

Nutrition

Glandular therapy: Blood, bone marrow, and immune support formulas at 1 tablet for each 25 pounds of body weight BID.

Energizing iron (liver extract plus iron): 1 capsule for every 25 pounds of body weight, maximum 4 capsules daily.

Betathyme: 1 capsule for each 35 pounds of body weight BID, maximum 6 capsules daily.

Folic acid: 50 micrograms for every 35 pounds of body weight

Fishoil: 1 tsp for each 20 pounds of body weight with meals.

Chinese herbal medicine

Immune-mediated hemolytic anemia (IMHA): The authors recommend Immuneregulator at 1 capsule per 10 to 20 pounds twice daily. In addition to the herbs cited above, Immuneregulator also contains bamboo leaves (Zhu ye), coix (Yi yi ren), dendrobium (Shi hu), light wheat (Fu xiao mai), lotus seed (Lian zi xin), ophiopogon (Mai men dong), and poria (Fu ling). These herbs increase the efficacy of the cited herbs.

Immune-mediated thrombocytopenia (ITP): The authors recommend H13 at 1 capsule per 10 to 20 pounds twice daily. In addition to the herbs listed above, this supplement contains angelica root (Dang gui), donkey skin gelatin (E jiao), fleece flower root (He shou wu), gardenia (Zhi zi), red peony (Chi shao), and spatholobus (Ji xue teng). These additional herbs enhance the formula's effectiveness.

Typically the authors try to avoid acupuncture treatments due to potential complications of hemorrhage. The combination of herbs and Western therapy is the usual approach to critical cases.

Homotoxicology (Dose: 10 drops for 50-pound dog; 5 drops for cat or small dog)

Symptom formula: *Galium-heel, Ferrum homaccord, Phosphor homaccord, China homaccord, Traumeel, BHI Exhaustion*, PO BID.

Deep detoxification formula: *Lymphomyosot, Thyroidea compositum, Hepar compositum, Solidago com-positum, Mucosa compositum, Coenzyme compositum, Ubichinon compositum*; PO EOD. *Glyoxal compositum* weekly.

Product sources

Nutrition

Blood, bone marrow, and immune support formulas: Animal Nutrition Technologies. **Alternatives:** Immune System Support-Standard Process Veterinary Formulas; Immuno Support—Rx Vitamins for Pets; Immugen—Thorne Veterinary Products.

Energizing iron (contains vitamin B$_{12}$): PhytoPharmica, Inc.

Betathyme—Best for Your Pet. **Alternative:** Moducare—Thorne Veterinary Products.

Folic acid: Progressive Labs.

Eskimo Fish oil: tyler Encapsulations

Chinese herbal medicine

Formula Immuneregulator and H13 (immune-mediated thrombocytopenia): Natural Solutions Inc.

Homotoxicology remedies

BHI/Heel Corporation

REFERENCES

Western medicine references

Bucheler J, Cotter S. Canine immune mediated hemolytic anemia. In: Bonagura J, Kirk R, eds. Current veterinary therapy XII, Philadelphia: Saunders, 1995:152–157.

Calia CM. Anemia, Immune Mediated. In: Tilley, L., Smith, F., The 5-Minute Veterinary Consult: Canine and Feline, Blackwell Publishing, 2003.

Duval D, Giger U. Vaccine-associated immune-mediated hemolytic anemia in the dog, *J Vet Intern Med*, 1996 Sep-Oct;10(5):290–5.

Harbige LS. Dietary n-6 and n-3 fatty acids in immunity and autoimmune disease, 1998, *Proc. Nutr. Soc.* 57 (4), 555–562.

Lewis DC, Myers KM. Canine idiopathic thrombocytopenia purpura. *J Vet Int Med* 1996;10:207–218.

Reagan WJ, Rebar AH. Platelet disorders. In: Ettinger SL, Feldman EC, eds. Textbook of veterinary internal medicine. 4th ed. Philadelphia: Saunders, 1995:1964–1976.

Stewart A, Feldman B. Immune-mediated hemolytic anemia. Part I. An overview. *Comp Cont Ed Pract Vet*, 1993;15:372–381.

Stewart A, Feldman B. Immune-mediated hemolytic anemia. Part II. Clinical entity, diagnosis, and treatment theory. *Comp Cont Ed Pract Vet*, 1993;15:1479–1491.

Thompson JP. Immunologic diseases. In: Ettinger SL, Feldman EC, eds. Textbook of veterinary internal medicine. 4th ed. Philadelphia: Saunders, 1995:2002–2029

Williams DA, Maggio-Price L. Canine idiopathic thrombocytopenia: clinical observations and long-term follow-up in 54 cases. *J Am Vet Med Assoc*, 1984;185:660–663.

Nutrition references

Berlin R, Berlin H, Brante G, Pilbrant A. Vitamin B$_{12}$ body stores during oral and parenteral treatment of pernicious anaemia. *Acta Med Scand*, 1978;204:81–4.

Bouic, PJD, et al. Beta-sitosterol and beta-sitosterol glucoside stimulate human peripheral blood lymphocyte proliferation: Implications for their use as an immunomodulatory vitamin combination. *International Journal of Immunopharmacology*, 1996; 18:693–700.

Food and Nutrition Board, Institute of Medicine. Folic Acid. Dietary Reference Intakes: Thiamin, Riboflavin, Niacin, Vitamin B$_6$, Vitamin B$_{12}$, Pantothenic Acid, Biotin, and Choline. Washington, D.C.: National Academy Press; 1998:193–305.

Frykman E, Bystrom M, Jansson U, et al. Side effects of iron supplements in blood donors: superior tolerance of heme iron. *J Lab Clin Med* 1994;123:561–4.

Gupta MB, Nath R, Srivastava N, et al. Anti-inflammatory and antipyretic activities of β-sitosterol. *Planta Medica* 1980;39:157–163.

Kondo H. Haematological effects of oral cobalamin preparations on patients with megaloblastic anaemia. *Acta Haematol* 1998;9:200–5.

Lederle FA. Oral cobalamin for pernicious anemia: medicine's best kept secret? *JAMA* 1991;265:94–5.

Chinese herbal medicine references

Fan C, Song, J, White, MC. A Comparison of the Hemostatic Effects of Notoginseng and Yun Nan Bai Yao to Placebo Control. *Journal of Herbal Pharmacotherapy* 2005, vol. 5 no. 2.

Lu, TV. Treatment of aplastic anemia with acupuncture. *Med Acup* 2002; volume 15 number 1:23–32

Nan Jing Zhong Ye Xue Yuan Xue Bao. *Journal of Nanjing University of Traditional Chinese Medicine*, 1989;1:43.

Zhe Jiang Zhong Yi Za Zhi. *Zheijiang Journal of Chinese Medicine*, 1988; 2:55.

Zhong Hua Nei Ke Za Zhi. *Chinese Journal of Internal Medicine*, 1976; 6: 339.

Zhong Xi Yi Jie He Za Zhi. *Journal of Integrated Chinese and Western Medicine*, 1985; 4: 245.

Zhong Yao Tong Bao. *Journal of Chinese Herbology*, 1983; 8(6):35.

Zhong Yao Xue. *Chinese Herbology*, 1998; 156:158.

Zhong Yao Yao Li Yu Ying Yong. *Pharmacology and Application of Chinese Herbs*, 1983:323.

Zhong Yi Yao Yan Jiu. *Research of Chinese Medicine and Herbology*, 1991;(3):54.

Homotoxicology references

Bianchi I. Principles of Homotoxicology Vol. 1, First English Edition, 1989 Aurelia-Verlag Baden-Baden.

Bianchi I. Homeopathic Homotoxicological Repertory. Aurelia Verlag Baden-Baden, 1995. p 370, 390–392.

Broadfoot P. Autosanguis Therapy: A brief overview of an ancient therapeutic tool, in proceedings AHVMA and Heel Homotoxicology Seminar, 2004. Denver, CO, pp 1–6.

Broadfoot P. Personal unpublished communication. 2005.

Dodds W. Adverse Vaccine Reactions. Handout Hemopet, 2005. Santa Monica, CA.

Duval D, Giger U. Vaccine-associated immune-mediated hemolytic anemia in the dog. *J Vet Int Med* 1996;10: 290–295.

Heel. BHI Homeopathic Therapy. 2002. Heel Inc./Albuquerque, NM.

Reckeweg H. *Biotherapeutic Index: Ordinatio Antihomotoxica et Materia Medica*, 5th ed. 2000. Baden-Baden, Germany: Biologische Heilmittel Heel GMBH, p. 19.

Reckeweg H. *Homeopathia Antihomotoxica Materia Medica* 4th Completely Revised Edition. Aurelia-Verlag Baden-Baden, Germany 2002p. 177, 490.

Smit A. Cancer and Chronic Disease, on lecture proceedings CD. 2004. Heel.

IMMUNE-MEDIATED ARTHRITIS

Definition and cause

Immune-mediated arthritis (rheumatoid) is an inflammatory, non-infectious polyarthritis. It occurs mainly in dogs 2 to 8 years of age, and less commonly in cats. Its basic form is defined as an exaggerated response of the immune system resulting in destruction of the joint via erosion or inflammation. The two forms, erosive and non-erosive, have the common underlying cause of an antigen/antibody reaction similar to rheumatoid arthritis (RA) in people. The underlying cause is a cellular and humeral exaggerated response from the immune system toward the joint tissue (Beale 1998, 2003; Goring 1993; Pederson 1976, 1983; Tizard 2004; Zvaifler 1979).

Immune-mediated arthritis affects the synovial tissue, as opposed to degenerative joint disease, which is categorized as inflammation and destruction of the cartilage. There are specific stages of classification of rheumatoid arthritis in people, which relate to dogs only because of the similarity of RA and immune-mediated arthritis. In cats, progressive polyarthritis is linked to feline leukemia (Pederson 1980).

Medical therapy rationale, drug(s) of choice, and nutritional recommendations

Once the immune-mediated process begins, it is reported that there is no cure. The goal of medical therapy, therefore, is to improve the animal's day-to-day quality of life by reducing pain and inflammation and helping to prevent the immune destruction of joint tissues. Besides immunosupressive drugs such as cortisone, azathioprine, and cyclophosphamide, NSAIDS such as aspirin, carprofen (Rimadyl), and other Cox2 inhibitors such as Metacam and Previcox are indicated. There has been some recent research regarding the use of essential fatty acids and their benefit in reducing inflammation and improving healing. As a result, some veterinarians are recommending the use of fatty-acid-rich oils in the treatment of arthritis (Campbell 1992, Darlington 2001, DeGroot 1998, Goring 1993, Levinthal 1994).

Anticipated prognosis

Because the etiology of immune-mediated arthritis is unknown, conventional treatment is directed toward suppressing the immune response and controlling pain. Because the medical approach does not address the underlying cause, the prognosis is poor and the disease will continue to progress and worsen (Beale 2003, Goring 1993, Pederson 1989).

Integrative veterinary therapies

While synovial tissue is the target tissue and the surface diagnosis is arthritis, the underlying mechanism is an exaggerated response via the immune system against its own tissue. The use of immune-suppressing drugs such as cortisone and chemotherapeutics, along with anti-inflammatory drugs such as NSAIDs, pays little attention to this underlying cause. An integrated approach to immune-mediated arthritis considers the immune system and the resultant inflammation and destruction of tissue.

Nutrients, nutraceuticals, medicinal herbs, and combination homeopathics that have anti-inflammatory, tissue-sparing, and regenerative effects on the cells of the synovial tissue can often control the clinical signs, improve the day-to-day level of comfort, reduce pain, protect against the ongoing assault on the synovial cells, and in many cases reduce the need for and reliance on drugs that may have long-range, undesirable side effects (Little 2001).

Nutrition
General considerations/rationale
Immune-mediated arthritis is not a disease of the joints, but rather the cartilage, joint capsule, and synovium are the target organs of the immune attack. While medical therapy is focused upon the joints, nutritional therapies should focus upon reducing free-radical-incited inflammation, helping balance the glands of the immune system, and supplying the required nutrients for repairing damaged cells (Goldstein 2000, 2005).

Appropriate nutrients
Gland therapies: Glandular adrenal and thymus, glucosamine and chondroitin, and other intrinsic nutrients that can help reduce inflammation and protect target organs. The adrenal and thymus glands are integral to the immune response and are important in all autoimmune diseases (Goldstein 2000).

Betasitosterol: Plant-derived sterols that show anti-inflammatory and antipyretic properties and appear to be similar to corticosteriods and aspirin (Gupta 1980). In addition, sterols can enhance immune function. Sterols have been found to be able to enhance T-lymphocyte production and moderate B-cell activity, thereby helping to balance the immune response and indirectly reducing the risk of an autoimmune reaction (Bouic 1996).

Vitamin C: Required for the synthesis of collagen and a potent antioxidant that is involved in the free radical and reactive oxygen species (see free radicals in Chapter 2), which result from normal metabolism as well as exposure to chemical and environmental chemicals and pollutants (Carr 1999). Vitamin C has been studied clinically in animals. Brown (1994), Berg (1990), and Newman (1995) reported on the benefits of vitamin C in the treatment of degenerative joint disease and movement in dogs and horses.

Super oxide dismutase (SOD): A potent destroyer of free radicals; can protect cells against oxidative damage (Petkau 1975, Fridovich 1972). McCord (1974) has reported that SOD can protect hyaluronate from free radical damage and may also have an anti-inflammatory effect (Salin and McCord 1975).

Glucosamine and chondroitin: Glycosaminoglycans (GAGS) such as chondroitin sulfate and glucosamine are beneficial for cartilage repair. Clinical studies have demonstrated the effectiveness of glucosamine and chondroitin in the management of arthritis in dogs (Das 2000, Gaskell 2005). Stinker, et al. (1986) have described how these compounds stimulate the body's own repair mechanism and help in the process of developing new cartilage. Numerous double-blind studies have compared the effectiveness of glucosamine against various NAIADs, with glucosamine resulting in as good as, or in many cases, better pain control and improved symptoms associated with osteoarthritis (Prudden 1974, Brown 1981, Vaz 1982, DeAmbrosia 1982).

Chinese herbal medicine
General considerations/rationale
Arthritis is due to a combination of Wind, Damp, and Cold or Heat affecting the Kidneys. This leads to Qi and Blood stagnation. In the later stages there is Qi and Blood deficiency. The Chinese thought that Wind blew the pathogen into the body. It is also considered to be the reason why some patients experience migrating joint pain: it was as though the Wind was blowing the pathogen from place to place. The target organ was considered to be the Kidney because this organ is given the function of controlling bones in TCM.

In terms of traditional Chinese medicine, immune-mediated arthritis is a result of the accumulation of fluid (Damp) and inflammatory mediators in the joints. This manifests as swelling of the joints. The inflammatory mediators generate Heat in the joints, making them painful and even warm to the touch in some cases. Later on, the joint cools off and becomes stiff, yet still painful. Application of external heat to the joint often provides relief. At this stage, the ancient practitioners believed there was stagnation of the Qi and Blood. The treatment goals are to decrease inflammation, stop pain, and improve motility.

Appropriate Chinese herbs
Achyranthes (Niu xi): Has been found to have significant analgesic and anti-inflammatory effects in a variety of animals (Zhong Yao Tong Bao 1988).

Aconite (Chuan wu): Has anti-inflammatory and analgesic properties and seems to have a centrally mediated analgesic effect. In mice it was shown to be effective for decreasing inflammation and pain. It is stronger than aspirin in reducing inflammation (Xian Dai Zhong Yao Yao Li Xue 1997). Aconite controlled the signs in 92% of 150 human patients with arthritis when given in combination with Cao wu, Qiang huo, Du hua, Fu zi, Mo yao, Ru xiang, Dang gui, Chuan niu xi, Ma huang, Gui zhi, Wu gong, Chuan xiong, and Ma qian zi (Nei Meng Gu Zhong Yi Yao 1986).

Artemesia (Yin chen hao): Contains capillarin. This compound has been shown to have analgesic properties in mice and anti-inflammatory and antipyretic effects in rats (Wan 1987, Shan 1982).

Citrus (Chen pi): Has anti-inflammatory effects and has been shown to decrease vascular permeability and reduce inflammation in mice (Zhong Yao Yao Li Yu Ying Yong 1983).

Cyperus, processed (Xiang fu zi): Has analgesic effects (Gui Yang Yi Xue Yuan Xue Bao 1959) and is 6 times stronger than aspirin at relieving fever in rats (Gupta 1971).

Frankincense (Ru xiang): Has boswellic acids that have demonstrated anti-inflammatory effects both in vivo and in vitro. These decrease capillary permeability and stabilize mast cells (Roy 2006, Pungle 2003). Frankincense also has analgesic properties (Zhong Yao Xue 1998, 539:540). It decreases signs of arthritis in dogs and humans (Reichling 2004, Kimmatkar 2003).

Milettia (ji xue teng): Helps to regulate the immune system. It inhibits the cell-mediated immunity by inhibiting T-lymphocyte blastogenesis and decreasing interleukin-2 activity (Yang 1997, Xu 1993).

Myrrh (Mo yao): A very good analgesic, especially when combined with ru xiang (Zhong Yao Xue 1998, 541:542).

White peony (Bai shao): Has been shown to have analgesic effects (Shang Hai Zhong Yi Yao Za Zhi 1983). It contains paeoniflorin, which is a strong antipyretic and anti-inflammatory (Zhong Yao Zhi 1993).

Acupuncture

Relief of musculoskeletal disorders is one of the most common reasons why humans seek acupuncture. The World Health Organization has placed musculoskeletal disorders on their list of conditions responsive to acupuncture (World Health Organization 2006).

Homotoxicology
General considerations/rationale

Acute polyarthritis is an Inflammation Phase disorder. More chronic immune-mediated arthritides are Impregnation Phase to Degeneration Phase homotoxicoses. Alteration of matrix elements leads to improper host immune responses, which damage rather than protect tissues. Basic biological therapy can be very rewarding in many of these cases. Dietary therapy can yield remarkable results in cases involving adverse reactions to food or true food allergy. Vaccination can be associated with polyarthritis syndromes, and if recent vaccination is in the medical history, then steps should be taken to address their presence.

Autosanguis may present a perfect modality in such cases. Careful search for occult infections can be impor-

tant to successful outcomes. In many cases a complete dental evaluation yields chronic dental disease with periapical or periodontal abscessation. Proper treatment of these lesions can lead to total resolution of the autoimmune disorder, but caution should be exercised following such a circumstance so that other agents are not given which could aggravate the patient and shift them to progressive vicariation.

Compositae remedies play largely in homotoxicoses right of the biological divide. Autosanguis therapy is particularly useful in these cases because blood elements may be present that are actively associated with the disease process. The author has several cases of polyarthritis associated with recent vaccination, which resolved quickly using autogenous blood therapy (Palmquist 2003).

Appropriate homotoxicology formulas

Aconitum Homaccord: Acute cases, particularly if they are accompanied by fever or generalized erythema.

Arsuraneel: In severely ill patients, in marked regressive vicariations.

Berberis homaccord: Detoxification and support of urinary and hepatic systems.

BHI-Arthritis: Arthritic support alternated with *Zeel* (for joint repair, joint pain relief).

Bryaconeel: Rheumatic pain, inflammation, influenza-like conditions, myalgia/neuralgia, tearing pains (e.g. after a sports injury) with damage to synovial and fibrous tissue and muscles, intercostal pains (Reckeweg 2002).

Causticum compositum: Weakness, paresis, neuralgias. Suited for Impregnation Phase with arthrosis, cracking of joints, and stiffness (Reckeweg 2002).

Coenzyme compositum: Energy metabolism support.

Colocynthis homaccord: Pain from arthrosis or neuritis, particularly lumbosacral location.

Cruroheel: Soft tissue pain and inflammation, particularly in hind limb, tarsal region issues.

Discus compositum: Widely useful for musculoskeletal ailments of varying descriptions (Broadfoot 2003). Contains berberis vulgaris(joint pain, heaviness of limbs, drawing and tightness of muscles), Cartilago suis (rheumatoid: intra- or peri-articular) (Reckeweg 2002).

Echinacea compositum: Fever, bacterial infections.

Engystol N: Matrix drainage and immunostimulation, particularly in viral infections or allergies.

Ferrum homaccord: Shoulder pain, anemia, rheumatism.

Galium-Heel: Cellular detoxification and repair, activation of the nonspecific host defenses, support in vaccine reactions, renal tubular support. Phase remedy in Deposition and Degeneration Phase conditions.

Gelsemium homaccord: Rear leg weakness and pain (Demers 2005).

Graphites homaccord: Rheumatism with joint deformities.

Hepar compositum: Hepatic drainage and support, relief of iatrogenic damage from corticosteroid therapy.

Lymphomyosot: Detoxification, drainage, and immune support of lymphoreticular system.

Neuralgo-rheum: Rheumatism and neuralgia, particularly in cold weather.

Nux vomica homaccord: Detoxification and support of liver and gastrointestinal systems.

Rheuma-Heel: Soft tissue and periarticular conditions.

Rhododendroneel: Extremity arthritic pain. Contains benzoic acid for shifting pains, periodically and at rest, sleep disturbed between 2 and 4 a.m. (Reckeweg 2002).

Solidago compositum: Urinary tract support and drainage.

Spascupreel: Muscle spasms and associated pain.

Tonsilla compositum: Activation of reticuloendothelial elements in deeper homotoxicoses.

Thuja forte: Vaccination-related disorders. (Thuja is also present in Galium-heel).

Thyroidea compositum: Deep matrix drainage and detoxification and hormonal support. Contains funiculus umbilicalis suis, which is indicated for autoimmune problems.

Traumeel S: This remedy is indicated in all cases because it relieves pain and reduces inflammation and corresponding joint injury while modulating the inflammatory reaction. In acute cases it can be given by injection, IV, IM, or subcutaneously, and then followed every 15 minutes orally as an oral drop or tablet. It is available in a topical cream and gel, which is well tolerated by veterinary patients.

Ubichinon compositum: Mitochondrial energy production/autoimmune issues.

Authors' suggested protocols

Nutrition

Gland therapy: Cartilage and immune support formulas at 1 tablet for 25 pounds of body weight BID.

SOD: Follow manufacturers suggested dosage.

Vitamin C: 100 mgs per 10 pounds of body weight BID.

Betathyme: 1 capsule for each 35 lbs of body weight BID (maximum 3 capsules BID).

Chinese herbal medicine

Rheumatoidin: 1 capsule for each 10 to 20 pounds of body weight BID. In severe cases the dose may be increased to effect. Rheumatoidin also contains aconite (Cao wu), astragalus (Huang qi), atractylodes (Bai zhu), aurantium

fruit (Zhi qiao), centipede (Wu gong), eupolyphaga (Di bie chong), hornet's nest (Feng fang), poria (Fu ling), saussurea (Mu xiang), and scorpion (Quan xie). These herbs help balance the formula and increase the efficacy of the herbs mentioned above.

The authors recommend the following acupoints: GV20, Baihui, LI11, PC6, GB30, ST36, SP6, BL20, BL22 and BL23 as generalized points. The patient may also benefit from local treatment of local points.

Homotoxicology (Dose: 10 drops for 50-pound dog; 5 drops for small dog or cat)

Acute case symptom formula: *Traumeel, Zeel,* or *BHI arthritis, Aconitum homaccord, Rhododendroneel* (polyarthritis of extremities), *Colocynthis homaccord* (if severely painful particularly lumbar pain), *Echinacea compositum* (if infection or vaccination suspected), *Engystol N* (if viral suspected). Give PO every 15 to 30 minutes until relief, then BID to TID as needed.

Acute case detoxification formula: *Lymphomyosot, Nux vomica homaccord, Berberis homaccord.* Give PO BID 30 to 60 days.

Chronic case symptom formula: *Traumeel, Galium-heel, Zeel, Bryaconeel, Rhododendroneel* (polyarthritis of extremities), *Colocynthis homaccord* (if severely painful particularly lumbar pain), *Echinacea compositum* (if infection or vaccination suspected), *Engystol N* (if viral suspected). Give PO every 15 to 30 minutes until relief, then BID to TID as needed.

Chronic case deep detoxification formula: *Lymphmyosot, Hepar compositum, Thyroidea compositum, Solidago compositum, Tonsilla compositum, Coenzyme compositum, Ubichinon compositum.* Give PO EOD to E3D for 60 to 120 days.

Product sources

Nutrition

Cartilage and immune support formula: Animal Nutrition Technologies. **Alternatives:** Cosequin, Nutramaxx Lab. Glycoflex, Vetri Science; Nutriflex—Rx Vitamins for Pets; Liquid Glucosamine—K9 Liquid Health; Immune System Support Standard Process Veterinary Formulas; Immuno Support—Rx Vitamins for Pets; Immugen—Thorne Veterinary Products.

SOD: Cell Advance—Vetri Science, NaturVet SOD, BioPet International, N-Zymes.com.

Betathyme: Best for Your Pet. **Alternative:** Moducare—Thorne Veterinary Products.

Vitamin C: Over the counter.

Chinese herbal medicine

Rheumatoidin—Natural Solutions Inc.

Homotoxicology remedies
BHI/Heel Corporation

REFERENCES

Western medical references

Beale BS. Arthropathies. In: Bloomberg MS, Taylor RT, Dee J, eds. Canine sports medicine and surgery. Philadelphia: Saunders, 1998:517–532.

Beale, BS. Polyarthritis, Nonerosive, Immune-mediated, In: Tilley L, Smith F. The 5-Minute Veterinary Consult: Canine and Feline, 2003. Blackwell Publishing.

Campbell KL. Therapeutic indications for dietary lipids. In Kirk RW, ed. Current Veterinary Therapy XI. Philadelphia: W.B. Saunders Co. 1992;36–39.

Darlington LG, Stone TW. Antioxidants and fatty acids in the amelioration of rheumatoid arthritis and related disorders. *Br J Nutr.* 2001;85(3):251–269.

DeGroot, JE. Veterinary medical uses and sources of omega-3 fatty acids. *Veterinary Forum.* 1998; May:42–48.

Goring RL, Beale BS. Immune mediated arthritides. In: Bojrab MJ, ed. Disease mechanisms in small animal surgery. Philadelphia: Lea and Febiger, 1993:742–750.

Leventhal LJ, Boyce EG, Zurier RB. Treatment of rheumatoid arthritis with black currant seed oil. *Br J Rheumatol.* 1994;33(9):847–852.

Pedersen NC, Pool RR, O'Brien T. Feline chronic progressive polyarthritis. *Am J Vet Res* 41:522, 1980.

Pedersen NC, Weisner K, Castles, JJ, et al: Noninfectious canine arthritis: The inflammatory, nonerosive arthritides. *J Am Vet Med Assoc,* 1976, 169:304.

Pedersen NC. Joint diseases of dogs and cats. In: Ettinger SJ, ed. Textbook of veterinary internal medicine. 3rd ed. Philadelphia: Saunders, 1989:2329–2377.

Tizard, IR. Veterinary Immunology, An Introduction, 7th ed. Philadelphia: W.B. Saunders Co., 2004, pp.405–408.

Zvaifler NJ. Etiology and pathogenesis of rheumatoid arthritis. In: McCarty DJ, ed. Arthritis and Allied Conditions, 9th ed. 1979, Philadelphia: Lea and Febiger.

Intergrative/nutritional references

Berg J. Polyscorbate (C-Flex): an interesting alternative for problems on the support and movement apparatus in dogs; clinical trial of ester-C ascorbate in dogs, *Norweg Vet J,* 102:579, 1990.

Bouic, PJD, et al. Beta-sitosterol and beta-sitosterol glucoside stimulate human peripheral blood lymphocyte proliferation: Implications for their use as an immunomodulatory vitamin combination. *International Journal of Immunopharmacology* 1996; 18:693–700.

Brown LP. Ester-C for Joint Discomfort—A Study. *Natural Pet,* 1994, Nov.-Dec.

Brown LP. Vitamin C (Ascorbic Acid)—New Forms and Uses in Dogs. Proceeding of the North American Veterinary Conference, 1994, Orlando, FL.

Brown RA, Weiss JB. Neovascularization and its Role in the Osteoarthritic Process. *Ann. Rheum. Dis.,* 1981; 4.

Carr AC, Frei B. Toward a new recommended dietary allowance for vitamin C based on antioxidant and health effects in humans. *Am J Clin Nutr.* 1999;69(6):1086–1107.

Das AK, Hammad TA. Efficacy of a combination of FCH-G49TM glucosamine hydrochloride, TRH122TM low molecular weight sodium chondroitin sulfate and manganese ascorbate in the management of knee osteoarthritis. *Osteoarthritis Cart* 2000;8(5):343–350.

D'Ambrosia E, Casa, B, Bompani R, Scali G, Scali M. Glucosamine Sulphate: A Controlled Clinical Investigation in Arthrosis. *Pharmatherapeutica.* 1982, 2:504–508.

Fridovich I. Superoxide Radical and Superoxide Dismutase, *Acc Chem Res* 1972; 5, 321.

Goldstein R, Goldstein S. The Goldstein Wellness and Longevity Program. 2005. Neptune City, NJ: TFH Publication.

Goldstein R, et al. The BNA Handbook: A Working Manual for Veterinarians. 2000. Westport, CT: Animal Nutrition Technologies.

Gupta MB, Nath R, Srivastava N, et al. Anti-inflammatory and antipyretic activities of β-sitosterol. *Planta Medica* 1980;39: 157–163.

Guastella DB, Cook JL, Kuroki K, et al. Evaluation of chondroprotective nutriceuticals in an in vitro osteoarthritis model. Proceedings of the 32nd Annual Conference Veterinary Orthopedic Society 2005;5.

Little C, Parsons T. Herbal therapy for treating rheumatoid arthritis. *Cochrane Database Syst Rev.* 2001;(1):CD002948.

McCord J. Free Radicals and Inflammations: Protection of Synovial Fluid by Superoxide Dismutase, *Science* 185, 529, 1974.

Newman NL. Equine Degenerative Joint Disease, *Natural Pet.* 1995 March, April, p. 56.

Petkau A, Chelack W, Pleskach S, Meeker B, Brady C. Radioprotection of Mice by Superoxide Dismutase. *Biochem Biophys Res Commun.* 1975; 65, 886.

Prudden JF, Balassa LL. The Biological Activity of Bovine Cartilage Preparations. *Semin. Arthrit. Rheum.,* 1974; 4: 287–321.

Salin M, McCord J. Free Radicals and Inflammation. Protection of Phagocytosing Leukocytes by Superoxide Dismutase, *J Clin Invest,* 1975; 56, 1319.

Setnikar I, Giachetti C, Zanolo G. Pharmacokinetics of Glucosamine in the Dog and in Man. *Arzneimittelforschung,* 1986; 36:729–735.

Vaz AL. Double-blind Clinical Evaluation of the Relative Efficacy of Ibuprofen and Glucosamine Sulfate in the Management of Osteoarthritis of the Knee in Outpatients. *Curr. Med. Res. Opin.,* 1982; 8:145–149.

Chinese herbal medicine references

Gui Yang Yi Xue Yuan Xue Bao. *Journal of Guiyang Medical University,* 1959:113.

Gupta MB, Palit TK, Singh N, Bhargava KP. Pharmacological studies to isolate the active constituents from Cyperus rotundus possessing anti-inflammatory, anti-pyretic and analgesic activities. *Indian J Med Res* 1971 Jan;59(1):76–82.

Kimmatkar N, Thawani V, Hingorani L, et al. Efficacy and tolerability of Boswellia serrata extract in treatment of osteoarthritis of knee—a randomized double-blind placebo controlled trial. *Phytomedicine.* 2003;10:3–7.

Nei Meng Gu Zhong Yi Yao. Traditional Chinese Medicine and Medicinals of Inner Magnolia, 1986;(3):7.

Pungle P, Banayalikar M, Suthar A, et al. Immunomodulatory activity of boswellic acids of Boswellia serrata Roxb. *Indian Journal of Experimental Biology.* 2003;41:1460–1462.

Reichling J, Schmokel H, Fitzi J, et al. Dietary support with Boswellia resin in canine inflammatory joint and spinal disease. *Schweiz Arch Tierheilkd.* 2004;146(2):71–9.

Roy S, Khanna S, Krishnaraju AV et al. Regulation of vascular responses to inflammation: inducible matrix metalloproteinase-3 expression in human microvascular endothelial cells is sensitive to anti-inflammatory Boswellia. *Antioxidants and Redox Signaling.* 2006;8(3 and 4):653–660.

Shan Yuan Tiao Er, et al. *Journal of Pharmacy.* Japan. 1982;102(3):285.

Shang Hai Zhong Yi Yao Za Zhi. *Shanghai Journal of Chinese Medicine and Herbology,* 1983; 4:14.

Wan Yao De. The antipyretic effects of capillarin. *Pharmacy Bulletin.* 1987;(10):590–593.

World Health Organization. List of common conditions treatable by Chinese medicine and acupuncture. Available at: http://tcm.health-info.org/WHO-treatment-list.htm. Accessed 10/18/2006.

Xian Dai Zhong Yao Yao Li Xue. Contemporary Pharmacology of Chinese Herbs. 1997;425.

Xu Qiang, et al. *Journal of Pharmacology and Clinical Application of TCM.* 1993;9(4):30–33.

Yang Feng, et al. *China Journal of Experimental Clinical Immunology.* 1997;9(1):49–52.

Zhong Yao Tong Bao. *Journal of Chinese Herbology,* 1988;13(7):43.

Zhong Yao Xue. Chinese Herbology, 1998; 539:540.

Zhong Yao Xue. Chinese Herbology, 1998; 541:542.

Zhong Yao Yao Li Yu Ying Yong. Pharmacology and Application of Chinese Herbs, 1983:567.

Zhong Yao Zhi. *Chinese Herbology Journal,* 1993:183.

Homotoxicology references

Broadfoot P. Homotoxicology for Musculoskeletal Problems. Heel/AHVMA Homotoxicology Seminar. 2003. May, Denver, CO. CD.

Demers J. Inflammation, Lameness, Pain and Homotoxicology, Vol 20, Small Animal and Exotics. Proceedings North American Veterinary Conference, 2005,Orlando, FL, p 35.

Palmquist R. Two Rottweilers Suffering Severe Polyarthritis and Multiple Pathologies Following Rabies Vaccination: Resolution with Autosanguis Therapy. 2003. Unpublished case data on file.

Reckeweg H. *Biotherapeutic Index: Ordinatio Antihomotoxica et Materia Medica,* 5th ed. Baden-Baden, Germany: Biologische Heilmittel Heel GMBH, 2000, p 92.

Reckeweg H. *Homeopathia Antihomotoxica Materia Medica,* Part II Index of Symptoms and Modalities, 4th edition. Aurelia-Verlag, Baden-Baden, Germany, 2002. pp 179–80, 187, 213, 219.

SYSTEMIC AND CUTANEOUS (DISCOID) LUPUS

Definition and cause

Systemic lupus erythematosus is an autoimmune disease that can affect many organ systems and result in many signs and conditions such as those of the skin, joints, kidneys, blood etc. Both systemic lupus erythematosus (SLE) and the less severe cutaneous lupus erythematosus (CLE or discoid) result from an exaggerated immune response. Commonly affected breeds are Labradors, Collies, Shetland Sheepdogs, and German Shepherds. Lupus is less common in cats (Halliwell 1989; Lewis 1989; Friberg 2006; Jackson 2004, 2006; Peterson 1991; Rosenkrantz 1993).

Medical therapy rationale, drug(s) of choice, and nutritional recommendations

As an immune-mediated disease, SLE is treated with cortisone and when necessary with chemotherapeutics such as azathioprine, cyclophosphamide or chlorambucil. CLE is much more responsive to lower doses of cortisone along with adequate levels of essential fatty acids and vitamin E. More care must be taken in cats due to their susceptibility to drug side effects (Scott 1995).

Anticipated prognosis

Systemic lupus offers a poor prognosis because of either the direct side effects of the immunosuppressive drugs or secondary complications such as glomerular nephritis or anemia. CLE can usually be brought under control with less likelihood of secondary organ complications (Scott 1995, Halliwell 1989).

Integrative veterinary therapies

As is common with many autoimmune diseases, the medical approach focuses on suppression of the immune response, and in the case of SLE, support of secondary organ disease such as kidney disease or anemia. Integrative veterinary therapies expand the approach to support and help balance the glands of the immune system as well as the animal's emotional well-being. In addition, the focus is on neutralizing the antibody attack upon the target organs (skin, kidneys, blood) to help achieve remission; however, the prognosis is still guarded for SLE (Bardana 1982, Cooke 1985, Gershwin 1984, Newbold 1976, Segal 2004, Simopoulos 2002, Vien 1988).

Nutrition
General considerations/rationale

The nutritional approach is aimed at reducing inflammation and supporting associated organs that have been affected by the autoimmune attack. Support of bone marrow, liver, heart, skin, and kidney is often indicated. In addition, the nutritional support of the organs of elimination, such as the liver and kidneys, helps the body eliminate accumulated toxins that can increase free radical load and propagate inflammation.

Appropriate nutrients

Glandular therapy in support of immune system organs: Adrenal, thymus, lymph and bone marrow. In addition, based upon disease presence, other organ support such as for the skin, liver, kidney, and heart may be indicated.

Note: Lupus can be severe and involve multiple organs. It is recommended that blood be analyzed both medically and physiologically to determine associated organ involvement and disease. This allows for a more specific gland and nutritional support protocol (See Chapter 2, Nutritional Blood Testing, for more information).

Betasitosterol: Plant-derived sterols show anti-inflammatory and antipyretic properties that appear to be similar to corticosteriods and aspirin (Gupta 1980). In addition, sterols can enhance immune function. Sterols have been found to be able to enhance T-lymphocyte production and moderate B cell activity, thereby helping to balance the immune response and indirectly reducing the risk of an autoimmune reaction (Bouic 1996).

Quercetin: Functions like an antihistamine as well as a potent antioxidant. It has been shown to inhibit cells from releasing histamines (Middleton 1986, Ogasawara 1985). This, therefore, is beneficial in the treatment of allergic conditions.

Vitamin C: Has been confirmed via clinical trials to be a potent antioxidant and a balancer of immune function. Regarding immune function, vitamin C has been shown to stimulate production of interferon and natural killer cells (NK) and to increase production of other antioxidant enzymes (Bendich 1995, Carr 1999, Padayatty 2004).

Vitamin A: Has been shown to be beneficial to the skin, helps balance and improve immune function, and helps minimize chemotherapy side effects (McCullough 1999, Semba 1998). As a potent antioxidant, vitamin A is also cell and tissue protective in that it acts as a free radical scavenger (See free radicals in Chapter 2). In this area of free radical scavenger and inflammation reduction, vitamin A can be therapeutically beneficial in treating chronic degenerative diseases such as cancer, arthritis, and autoimmune and skin disease. It also can be beneficial for exposure to environmental pollutants (Halliwell 1994).

Vitamin E: As a potent antioxidant, vitamin E's primary function is to neutralize free radicals and reduce inflammation, particularly as it affects the oxidation and destruction of lipids (Traber 1999).

Chinese herbal medicine
General considerations/rationale

Lupus is a combination of Wind, Heat, and Toxins invading the body. TCM treats the various manifestations of systemic lupus as separate diseases. In general, the signs are caused by inflammation and toxins in the body. The toxins in this case are the inflammatory mediators released by the immune system of the affected animal. These inflammatory toxins cause rashes in the dermatological presentation or accumulation of fluids or swelling in the joints. The renal presentation is due to accumulation of the immune complexes in the kidney. The resultant renal failure leads to further toxin accumulation in the body.

Treatment is aimed at decreasing the inflammation and controlling secondary effects such as anemia and hypertension from renal disease and skin infections from secondary invaders.

Appropriate Chinese herbs

For dermatological manifestations, the following herbs may be useful:

Bupleurum (Chai hu): Decreases dimethyl benzene-induced auricular concha inflammation in mice (Liu 1998). It may help to decrease skin inflammation in lupus.

Dandelion (Pu gong ying): Inhibits various bacteria including Staphylococcus aureus and B-hemolytic streptococci (Zhong Yi Yao Xue Bao 1991). It may help prevent secondary bacterial infections of dermal lesions.

Earthworm (Di long): Enhances the growth of fibroblasts, capillaries, and collagenous fibers in the skin. This promotes wound healing (Zhang 1999).

Fleece flower root (He shou wu): Increases the hormonal secretion by the adrenal gland (Zhong Yao Yao Li Yu Lin Chuang 1989). This may mimic the administration of corticosteroids.

Honeysuckle (Jin yin hua): Contains chlorogenic acid and isochlorogenic acid, both of which have strong antibacterial properties. Among the bacteria inhibited are Staphylococcus aureus and b-hemolytic streptococci (Xin Yi Xue 1975, Jiang Xi Xin Yi Yao 1960). This may help to reduce secondary infections.

Kochia (Di fu zi): Has been shown to inhibit the growth of some dermatophytes (Yun Nan Zhong Yao Zhi 1990).

Licorice (Gan cao): Contains glycyrrhizin and glycyrrhetinic acid. These compounds have approximately 10% of the corticosteroid activity of cortisone (Zhong Cao Yao 1991).

Moutan (Dan pi): Inhibits various bacteria including Staphylococcus aureus and b-hemolytic streptococci (Zhong Yao Cai 1991). It contains paeonol, which has decreased the mass of immune organs and prevented splenic lymphocyte proliferation in mice. It also inhibited delayed hypersensitivity reactions in the mice (Wang 1992). These properties suggest that it may be useful in immune-mediated diseases. It may be able to down regulate the immune system.

Poria (Fu ling): Has antibacterial efficacy and has been shown to inhibit Staphylococcus aureus (Nanjing College of Pharmacy 1976).

Rehmannia (Sheng di huang): Increases the plasma levels of adrenocortical hormone (Zhong Yao Xue 1998). This may have the effect of increasing serum corticosterone levels and calming the excessive immune response.

Scutellaria (Huang qin): Contains biacalin which has antibiotic activity against Stapylococcus aureus and b-hemolytic streptococcus and some dermatophytes (Zhong Yao Xue 1988, Liu 2000). This may help prevent secondary infection of the dermal lesions.

Siegesbeckia (Xi xian cao): Decreases both humoral and cellular immunity in mice (Zhong Guo Zhong Yao Za Zhi 1989).

White peony (Bai shao): Inhibits a variety of bacteria including Staphylococcus aureus and b-hemolytic streptococci. It also has activity against some dermatophytes (Xin Zhong Yi 1989).

For renal manifestations the following herbs may be useful:

Achyranthes (Niu xi): Has anti-inflammatory effects. It decreases egg white-induced foot swelling in rats (Xong 1963).

Angelica root (Dang gui): As strong as aspirin in decreasing inflammation (Yao Xue Za Zhi 1971).

Astragalus (Huang qi): Can increase serum albumin and decrease proteinuria, which in turn helps to preserve amino acids, and improves the dysfunctional protein metabolism in glomerulopathy (Zhou 1999). Renal failure is often associated with hypertension. Astragalus has demonstrated ability to lower the blood pressure of cats, dogs, and rats under anesthesia (Modern TCM Pharmacology 1997, Xu 1999, Luo 1999).

Cnidium (Chuan xiong): Dilates blood vessels and reduces blood pressure (Zhong Yao Yao Li Yu Ying Yong 1989). It also inhibits blood platelet aggregation induced by ADP, collagen, and thrombase (Pharmaceutical Industry Research Institute of Beijing 1977).

Codonopsis (Dang shen): Can increase the hematocrit and lower blood pressure (Zhong Yao Xue 1998).

Corn silk (Yu mi xu): Has been shown to lower blood pressure in dogs (Zhong Yao Da Chi Dien 1037). In a trial involving 9 people with chronic nephritis, 3 recovered completely and 2 improved after 2 weeks to 6 months. Kidney function improved, edema was reduced, and proteinuria decreased (Zhong Hua Yi Xue Za Zhi 1956).

Eucommia bark (Du Zhong): Lowers blood pressure. The zinc:copper ratio in RBC is elevated in hypertensive people as compared to individuals with normal blood pressure. Eucommia can lower the zinc:copper ratio and the blood pressure (Wang 1997).

Giant knotweed root (Hu zhang): Lowers blood pressure (Xi An Yi Ke Da Xue Xue Bao 1982). It also has anti-inflammatory properties (Zhong Guo Yi Yuan Yao Xue Za Zhi 1988).

Honeysuckle (Jin yin hua): Has demonstrated anti-inflammatory effects in mice and rabbits (Shan Xi Yi Kan 1960).

Imperata (Bai mao gen): Has been used to treat renal inflammation. In one trial 11 children with acute nephritis were treated with imperata. Nine recovered completely and 2 showed moderate improvement. Edema and hypertension resolved and hematuria and proteinuria cleared (Guang Dong Yi Xue 1965).

Leonurus (Yi mu cao): May protect the kidney. In one experiment it was shown to decrease renal damage in gentamicin-induced acute renal failure in rats (Xia 1997).

Moutan (Mu dan pi): Possesses anti-inflammatory properties. In mice, it can prevent dimethylbenzene-induced ear inflammation and carrageenin-, formaldehyde-, or egg white-induced foot swelling (Wu 1990). Moutan can decrease blood pressure (Liao Ning Yi Xue Za Zhi 1960).

Phellodendron (Huang bai): Decreases blood pressure (Zhong Guo Yao Li Xue Tong Bao 1989).

Rehmannia (Sheng di huang): Lowers blood pressure (Zhong Yao Xue 1998).

Salvia (Dan shen): Controlled the signs of 70% of 48 patients with chronic nephritis in one study (Shang Hai Yi Yao Za Zhi 1981). It also reduces blood pressure (Guo Wai Yi Xue Zhong Yi Zhong Yao Fen Ce 1991).

Scrophularia (Xuan shen): Can lower blood pressure (Gong 1981).

White atractylodes (Bai zhu): Can increase the proliferation rate of CFU-E and BFU-E colonies (Hou 1999). This may make it useful for treating anemia associated with kidney failure. It also decreases the degeneration rate of the kidney (Jing 1997). This effect may help protect the kidney from damage from the immune complex deposition.

Wolfberry (Gou qi zi): Has several functions in an herbal supplement designed for renal disease. It increases the production of red blood (Zhong Yao Xue 1998) and decreases blood pressure (Zhong Yao Zhi 1984).

For skeletal manifestations the following herbs may be of use:

Achyranthes (Niu xi): Has demonstrated analgesic effects in experiments using hot plates in mice (Li 1999).

Aconite (Chuan wu): Has a centrally mediated analgesic effect. In mice it was shown to be effective for decreasing inflammation and pain. It is stronger than aspirin at reducing inflammation (Xian 1997) and has been used successfully for arthritis pain. It controlled the signs in 92% of 150 human patients with arthritis when given in combination with Cao wu, Qiang huo, Du hua, Fu zi, Mo yao, Ru xiang, Dang gui, Chuan niu xi, Ma huang, Gui zhi, Wu gong, Chuan xiong, and Ma qian zi (Nei Meng Gu Zhong Yi Yao 1986).

Citrus (Chen pi): Was shown to have bidirectional effects on the immune system of guinea pigs. It increased serum lysozyme levels and the number of cardiac blood T-lymphocytes but also inhibited the T-lymphocyte transformation rate (Jin 1992). This indicates that it may have the ability to regulate the abnormal immune system, possibly decreasing excessive action while enhancing suppression.

Cyperus (Xiang fu zhi): Has been shown to have analgesic effects in mice (Gui Yang Yi Xue Yuan Xue Bao 1959).

Mastic (Ru xiang): Contains boswellic acids which have anti-inflammatory effects (Roy 2006). It has been used to decrease signs of arthritis in dogs (Reichling 2004) and humans (Kimmatkar 2003).

Milettia (Ji xue teng): Depresses cellular immunity. It inhibits T-lymphocyte blastogenesis and interleukin-2 activity (Yang 1997, Xu 1993). This may help decrease the hyperactive immune activity seen in lupus.

Myrrh (Mo yao): A very good analgesic, especially when combined with mastictis (Ru xiang) (Zhong Yao Xue 1998).

Oriental wormwood (Yin chen hao): Has analgesic and anti-inflammatory effects. It contains 6, 7-dimethoxy coumarin which has shown analgesic effects on acetic acid-induced body twisting and anti-inflammatory effects on carrageenin-induced foot swelling in rats (Wan 1987, Shan 1982).

White atracylodes (Bai zhu): Has been shown to be effective in humans in treating chronic back and leg pain (Hu Bei Zhong Yi Za Zhi 1982).

White peony (Bai shao): Contains paeoniflorin which is a strong anti-inflammatory (Zhong Yao Zhi 1993). This may help decrease pain.

Acupuncture

Some patients with lupus seem to respond to a combination of herbal formula and acupuncture. Thirty-two people with a diagnosis of SLE were treated with a formula containing aconite (Cao wu),buck grass (Shen jin cao), cinnamon (Gui zhi), epimedium (Xian lin pi), licorice (Gan cao), schizonepeta (Jing jie), scrophularia (Xuan shen), and siler (Fang feng) along with acupuncture. The points chosen included GV 20, GB 20, GV 14, LI 11, LI 4, BL 23, ST 36, SP 1, and Liv 3. More than half of the patients reported significant decreases in the signs,

and another 28% reported some improvement (Wang 1998).

Homotoxicology
General considerations/rationale
These are Degeneration Phase disorders wherein the tissue undergoes significant damage associated with autoaggressive attack by the host immune system (Reckeweg 2000). Multiple tissues and organ systems may be involved and treatment must be individualized for each case. Care should be taken to thoroughly diagnose these cases so that occult infections are detected and resolved. Dental disease or kidney infections can potentiate autoaggression (Emily 1982). Efforts are made to rehabilitate energy metabolism, drain the matrix, and allow for oscillation between inflammation and repair stages.

Appropriate homotoxicology remedies
Numerous antihomotoxic formulas may be needed because these patients move through their disease cycles. There are no canine or feline studies from which a protocol can be designed. One successfully managed case of canine discoid lupus involved use of the deep detoxification formula listed below in conjunction with niacinamide and vitamin E. In that case both vitamin and homotoxicology formulas were needed to resolve the symptoms (Palmquist 2005).

Major remedies that have theoretical usefulness are listed below:

Abropernol: Hyperkeratosis, hyperhydrosis, pigmented skin, vascular disease, swollen glands.

Aesculus compositum: Assists with peripheral circulation.

Arsuraneel: Contains Condurango indicated for cracks and ulcers on lips.

BHI stramonium complex: contains Aurum iodatum and sulphur.

Causticum compositum: Burns or burn-like lesions on the skin. This is helpful for some cases of discoid lupus, particularly as they are worsened in UV light.

Coenzyme compositum: Cytosol energy metabolism. Contains nicotinamidum indicated for pigmentary disturbances and stomatitis.

Cruroheel: Used intermittently to preserve tendon health.

Cutis compositum: Repair and detoxification of the skin.

Galium-Heel: Main formula for cellular phase diseases. Drains the cell and deep matrix, and stimulates repair mechanisms. Supports kidney tubules. Contains Thuja occidentalis, which is helpful in many cases of vaccine-associated disease.

Hepar compositum: Liver support and drainage.

Lamioflur: In cases involving gastrointestinal or urogenital mucocutaneous junctures.

Lymphomyosot: Lymph drainage and immune system support.

Hormeel: Normalization of hormonal patterns.

Mucosa compositum: Support and drainage of mucosal elements. Contains Condurango indicated for cracks and ulcers on lips.

Placenta compositum: Promotes vascular repair. See Vitiligo protocol (Heel 2003).

Psorinoheel: Drainage of dermatological homotoxins and in deep cases of constitutional disease. Cracked, peeling lips, nodules, vesicles, diffuse red patches, internal soreness and dryness of nose (Reckeweg 2000).

Traumeel: Anti-inflammatory.

Ubichinon compositum: Mitochondrial rehabilitation. Contains nicotinamidum indicated for pigmentary disturbances, and stomatitis.

Thyroidea compositum: Matrix drainage as regressive vicariation begins. Support of thyroid and thymus glands and metabolism.

Solidago compositum: Renal support, glomerulonephritis.

Zeel: Joint pain.

Authors' suggested protocols

Nutrition

Nutrition/glandular therapy: Immune and Lymph support formulas at 1 tablet for 25 pounds of body weight BID. In addition Liver, Kidney, Skin, Heart or Bone Marrow support formulas may be indicated.

Quercetin tablets: 35 mg for each 10 pounds of body weight daily.

Betathyme: 1 capsule for each 35 pounds of body weight BID (maximum 2 capsules BID).

Fishoil: 1 tsp for every 20 pounds of body weight.

Chinese herbal medicine

In TCM, the presentation of the disorder is treated, not the etiology. In disease processes such as lupus, where multiple organ systems are affected, multiple formulas may be used. The authors use 1, 2 or all 3 of these formulas simultaneously depending upon the presenting signs.

For cutaneous manifestations, the authors recommend ImmunoDerm at a dose of 1 capsule per 10 to 20 pounds twice daily. In addition to the herbs cited above, ImmunoDerm contains angelica root (Dang gui), atractylodes (Cang zhu), buffalo horn shavings (Shui niu jiao), oldenlandia (Bai hua she cao), tokoro (Bi xie), and xanthium fruit (Cang er zi) to help improve efficacy of the formulation.

For renal manifestations, the authors recommend H87 Shar pei fever at a dose of 1 capsule per 10 to 20 pounds twice daily. This supplement is designed for renal disease with an immune component. In addition to the herbs

above, H87 contains areca peel (Da fu pi), ciborium (Gou ji), fleece flower root (He shou wu), fossil bones (Long gu), isatis root (Ban lan gen), oldenlandia (Bai hua she cao), ophiopogon (Mai dong), oyster shell (Mu li), poria (Fu ling), pyrola (Lu xian cao), and tortoise plastron (Gui ban) and carapace (Bie jia).

For skeletal manifestations, the authors recommend Rheumatoid arthritis at a dose of 1 capsule per 10 to 20 pounds twice daily. Rheumatoid arthritis contains aconite (Cao wu), astragalua (Huang qi), aurantium fruit (Zhi qiao), centipede (Wu gong), eupolyphaga (Di bie cong), hornet's nest (Feng fang), poria (Fu ling), saussurea (Mu xiang), and scorpion (Quan xie). These herbs complete the formula.

Homotoxicology (Dose: 10 drops or 1 pill for 50-pound dog; 5 drops for 10-pound dog or cat)

Symptom Formula: *Galium-Heel, Lymphomyosot, Psorinoheel, Aesculus compositum, Abropernol, Causticum compositum* (if ulcerated) PO BID.

Deep detoxification formula: *Lymphomyosot, Hepar compositum, Solidago compositum, Thyroidea compositum, Ubichinon compositum,* used for 60 to 120 days or longer as indicated by patient response.

Cutis compositum intermittently PO Q3D as needed.

Coenzyme compositum, Ubichinon compositum, Placenta compositum, Testes compositum, OR *Ovarium compositum* (use gender appropriate formula). PO or injected SQ or IM Q3D.

In discoid lupus, depigmented areas on the nose can be treated with a mixture of *Lymphomyosot* gel and *Traumeel* gel, applied sparingly to small areas every other day (Broadfoot 2003). NOTE: This can trigger regressive vicariation. If a patient so treated becomes lethargic do not repeat until recovery is noted. This is not an adverse reaction but signals major clearance of homotoxins. Do NOT treat ulcerated or large areas with this mixture because excessive homotoxins can be released. Discoid lupus cases should receive vitamin E, niacinamide, Standard Process Veterinary Formulas Hepatic Support (or other liver support formula), and tetracycline may be required as well as immunosuppressive agents, depending upon case response.

Product sources

Nutrition

Immune, Lymph, Liver, Kidney, Heart or Bone Marrow support formulas: Animal Nutrition Technologies. **Alternatives:** Immune System Support Standard Process Veterinary Formulas; Immuno Support—Rx Vitamins for Pets; Immugen—Thorne Veterinary Products.

Quercetin: Source Naturals, Quercitone—Thorne Veterinary Products.

Betathyme: Best for Your Pet. Alternative: Moducare—Thorne veterinary products. Eskimo Fishoil—Tyler Encapsulation.

Chinese herbal medicine
Natural Solutions, Inc.: ImmunoDerm, Sharpei Fever, and Rheumatoid Arthritis.

Homotoxicology remedies
BHI/Heel Corporation

REFERENCES

Western medicine references
Krum SH, Cardinet GH, 3rd, Anderson BC, et al. Polymyositis and polyarthritis associated with systemic lupus erythematosus in a dog. *J Am Vet Med Assoc* 1977; 170:61–64.

Friberg C. Feline facial dermatoses. *Vet Clin N A: Small Anim Pract* 2006;36:115–140.

Halliwell REW, Gorman NT. Veterinary clinical immunology, 1989, Philadelphia: Saunders.

Jackson HA. Vesicular cutaneous lupus. *Vet Clin N A: Small Anim Pract* 2006;36:251–255.

Jackson HA. Eleven cases of vesicular cutaneous lupus erythematosus in Shetland sheepdogs and rough collies: clinical management and prognosis. *Vet Dermatol* 2004;15:37–41.

Lewis RM, Picut CA. Veterinary clinical immunology, 1989, Philadelphia: Lea and Febiger.

Pedersen NC, Barlough JE. Systemic lupus erythematosus in the cat. *Feline Pract* 1991;19:5–13.

Rosenkrantz WS. Discoid lupus erythematosus: current veterinary dermatology, 1993. St. Louis: Mosby.

Scott DW, Miller WH, Griffin CE. Immunologic Skin Diseases. *In:* Muller and Kirk's Small Animal Dermatology. Toronto: W.B. Saunders Co. 1995, p. 578–588.

IVM references
Bardana EJ Jr, et al. Diet-induced systemic lupus erythematosus (SLE) in primates. *Am J Kidney Dis.* May, 1982; 1(6):345–352.

Cooke HM, Reading CM. Dietary intervention in systemic lupus erythematosus: 4 cases of clinical remission and reversal of abnormal pathology. *Intl Clin Nutr Rev.* 1985;5(4):166–76.

Gershwin ME, et al. Nutritional factors and autoimmunity. IV. Dietary vitamin A deprivation induces a selective increase in IgM autoantibodies and hypergammaglobulinemia in New Zealand black mice. *J Immunol.* July1984;133(1):222–6.

Newbold PCH. Beta-carotene in the treatment of discoid lupus erythematosus. *Br J Dermatol.* 1976;95:100–101.

Segal R, et al. Anemia, serum vitamin B$_{12}$, and folic acid in patients with rheumatoid arthritis, psoriatic arthritis, and systemic lupus erythematosus. *Rheumatol Int.* 2004;24:14–19.

Simopoulos AP. Omega-3 fatty acids in inflammation and autoimmune diseases. *J Am Coll Nutr.* 2002;21(6):495–505.

Vien CV, et al. Effect of vitamin A treatment on the immune reactivity of patients with systemic lupus erythematosus. *J Clin Lab Immunol.* May, 1988;26:33–35

Yell JA, Burge S, Wojnarowska F. Vitamin E and discoid lupus erythematosus. *Lupus* 1992;1:303–5.

Nutrition references
Bendich A, Langseth L. The health effects of vitamin C supplementation: a review. *J Am Coll Nutr* 1995; 14:124–136.

Bouic PJD, et al. Beta-sitosterol and beta-sitosterol glucoside stimulate human peripheral blood lymphocyte proliferation: Implications for their use as an immunomodulatory vitamin combination. *International Journal of Immunopharmacology* 199618:693–700.

Carr AC, Frei B. Toward a new recommended dietary allowance for vitamin C based on antioxidant and health effects in humans. *Am J Clin Nutr.* 1999; 69(6):1086–1107.

Gupta MB, Nath R, Srivastava N, et al. Anti-inflammatory and antipyretic activities of β-sitosterol. *Planta Medica* 1980; 39:157–163.

Halliwell B. Free Radicals and Antioxidants: a Personal View. *Nutr. Rev.*, 1994; 52:253.

McCullough F, et al. The effect of vitamin A on epithelial integrity. Proceedings of the Nutrition Society. 1999; volume 58: p 289–293.

Middleton E Jr. Effect of flavonoids on basophil histamine release and other secretory systems. *Prog Clin Biol Res.* 1986;213:493–506.

Ogasawara H, Middleton E Jr. Effect of selected flavonoids on histamine release (HR) and hydrogen peroxide (H2O2) generation by human leukocytes (abstract). *J Allergy Clin Immunol.* 1985; 75(suppl):184.

Padayatty SJ, Sun H, Wang Y, et al. Vitamin C pharmacokinetics: implications for oral and intravenous use. *Ann Intern Med.* 2004;140(7):533–537.

Semba RD. The role of vitamin A and related retinoids in immune function. *Nutr.Rev.* 1998;56(1 Pt 2):S38–S48.

Traber MG. Vitamin E. In: Shils M, Olson JA, Shike M, Ross AC, eds. Nutrition in Health and Disease. 9th ed. Baltimore: Williams and Wilkins; 1999:347–362.

Chinese herbal medicine for dermatology references
Jiang Xi Xin Yi Yao. Jiangxi New Medicine and Herbology, 1960 (1):34.

Liao Ning Yi Xue Za Zhi. Liaoning Journal of Medicine. 1960;(7):48.

Liu IX, Durham DG, Richards RM. Baicalin synergy with beta-lactam antibiotics against methicillin-resistant Staphylococcus aureus and other beta-lactam-resistant strains of S. aureus. *J Pharm Pharmacol.* 2000 Mar;52(3):361–6.

Liu Wei, et al. *Henan Journal of TCM Pharmacy.* 1998;13(4): 10–12.

Nanjing College of Pharmacy. *Materia Medica*, vol. 2. 1976. Jiangsu: People's Press.

Xin Yi Xue. New Medicine, 1975; 6(3): 155.

Xin Zhong Yi. New Chinese Medicine, 1989; 21(3):51.

Wang Xing Wang, et al. Journal of Pharmacology and Clinical Application of TCM. 1992;8(2):29–30.

Yun Nan Zhong Yao Zhi Yunnan. *Journal of Chinese Herbal Medicine*, 1990;244.

Zhang Feng Chun, et al. Research into Di Long's mechanism in its recovery effects on rabbit back injury. *China Journal of Pharmacy.* 1999;34(2):93–96.

Zhong Cao Yao. Chinese Herbal Medicine 1991;22 (10):452.

Zhong Guo Zhong Yao Za Zhi. *People's Republic of China Journal of Chinese Herbology*, 1989; 14(3):44.

Zhong Yao Cai. Study of Chinese Herbal Material, 1991; 14(2):41.

Zhong Yao Xue. Chinese Herbology, 1998, 156:158.

Zhong Yao Yao Li Yu Lin Chuang. Pharmacology and Clinical Applications of Chinese Herbs, 1989; 5(1):24.

Zhong Yi Yao Xue Bao. Report of Chinese Medicine and Herbology, 1991;(1):41.

Chinese herbal medicine for renal references

Gong Wei Gui, et al. *Zhejiang Journal of Medicine.* 1981;3(1): 11.

Guang Dong Yi Xue. Guangdong Medicine, 1965; 3:28.

Guo Wai Yi Xue Zhong Yi Zhong Yao Fen Ce. *Monograph of Chinese Herbology from Foreign Medicine*, 1991; 13(3): 41.

Hou Dun, et al. *Journal of Jiangxi College of TCM.* 1999; 11(1):28.

Jing Wei Zhe, et al. *China Journal of Geriatrics.* 1997;17(6): 365–367.

Luo Xin Ping, et al. *China Journal of Pathology and Physiology.* 1999;15(7):639–643.

Modern TCM Pharmacology. 1997. Tianjin: Science and Technology Press.

Pharmaceutical Industry Research Institute of Beijing. *China Journal of Medicine.* 1977;57(8):464.

Shan Xi Yi Kan Shanxi. *Journal of Medicine*, 1960; (10):32.

Shang Hai Yi Yao Za Zhi. *Shanghai Journal of Medicine and Herbology*, 1981; 1:17.

Wang Cai Lan, et al. *Journal of Trace Elements and Health Research.* 1997;14(4):33–34.

Wu Guan Zhong, et al. *Journal of University of Pharmacology of China.* 1990;21(4).

Xi An Yi Ke Da Xue Xue Bao. *Journal of Xian University School of Medicine*, 1982; 3(4):941.

Xia Xiao Hong, et al. *China Journal of Pathology and Physiology.* 1997;13(2):183–187.

Xong Zheng Yu, et al. *Journal of Pharmacology.* 1963; 10(12):708.

Xu Shi An, et al. *China Journal of Pharmacy.* 1999; 34(10)663–665.

Yao Xue Za Zhi. *Journal of Medicinals*, 1971;(91):1098.

Yao Xue Xue Bao. *Journal of Herbology*, 8 (6):250.

Zhong Guo Yao Li Xue Tong Bao. *Journal of Chinese Herbal Pharmacology*, 1989; 10(5):385.

Zhong Guo Yi Yuan Yao Xue Za Zhi. *Chinese Hospital Journal of Herbology*, 1988; 8(5):214.

Zhong Hua Yi Xue Za Zhi. *Chinese Journal of Medicine*, 1956; 10:922.

Zhong Yao Da Chi Dien. Dictionary of Chinese Herbs, 1037.

Zhong Yao Xue Chinese. Herbology, 1998; 156:158.

Zhong Yao Xue Chinese. Herbology, 1998; 739:741.

Zhong Yao Xue. Chinese Herbology, 1998; 860:862.

Zhong Yao Yao Li Yu Ying Yong. Pharmacology and Applications of Chinese Herbs, 1989; (2):40.

Zhong Yao Zhi. *Chinese Herbology Journal*, 1984:484.

Zhou Qin. *Journal of Chinese Materia Medica.* 1999;30(5): 386–388.

Chinese herbal medicine for skeletal manifestation references

Gui Yang Yi Xue Yuan Xue Bao. *Journal of Guiyang Medical University*, 1959:113.

Hu Bei Zhong Yi Za Zhi Hubei. *Journal of Chinese Medicine*, 1982; 6:57.

Jin Zhi Cui, et al. *Journal of Chinese Materia Medica.* 1992;23(11):612.

Kimmatkar N, Thawani V, Hingorani L, et al. Efficacy and tolerability of *Boswellia serrata* extract in treatment of osteoarthritis of knee—a randomized double-blind placebo controlled trial. *Phytomedicine.* 2003;10:3–7.

Li Xiao Chuan, et al. *Shannxi Journal of Medicine.* 1999; 28(12):735–736.

Nei Meng Gu Zhong Yi Yao. Traditional Chinese Medicine and Medicinals of Inner Magnolia, 1986;(3):7.

Reichling J, Schmokel H, Fitzi J, et al. Dietary support with Boswellia resin in canine inflammatory joint and spinal disease *Schweiz Arch Tierheilkd.* 2004;146(2):71–9.

Roy S, Khanna S, Krishnaraju AV, et al. Regulation of vascular responses to inflammation: inducible matrix metalloproteinase-3 expression in human microvascular endothelial cells is sensitive to anti-inflammatory *Boswellia.* *Antioxidants and Redox Signaling.* 2006; 8(3and4):653–660.

Shan Yuan Tiao Er, et al. *Journal of Pharmacy.* Japan. 1982; 102(3):285.

Wan Yao De. The antipyretic effects of capillarin. *Pharmacy Bulletin.* 1987;(10):590–593.

Xian Dai Zhong Yao Yao Li Xue. Contemporary Pharmacology of Chinese Herbs, 1997;425.

Xu Qiang, et al. *Journal of Pharmacology and Clinical Application of TCM.* 1993;9(4):30–33.

Yang Feng, et al. *China Journal of Experimental Clinical Immunology.* 1997;9(1):49–52.

Zhong Yao Xue. Chinese Herbology, 1998; 541:542.

Zhong Yao Zhi. *Chinese Herbology Journal*, 1993:183.

Acupuncture reference

Wang Hong Liang, et al. *Shanxi Journal of TCM.* 1998; 14(2):11–13.

Homotoxicology references

Broadfoot P. Unpublished communication. 2003.

Emily P. Veterinary Dentistry Elective, notes on the lectures from Colorado State University School of Veterinary Medicine professional course. Unpublished. 1982.

Heel. Practitioners Handbook of Homotoxicology, 1st edition. 2003. Heel Inc, p 114.

Palmquist R. Discoid lupus successfully maintained on nutraceutical and antihomotoxic treatment. Unpublished case report on file. 2005.

Reckeweg H. *Biotherapeutic Index: Ordinatio Antihomotoxica et Materia Medica*, 5th ed. Baden-Baden, Germany: Biologische Heilmittel Heel, GMBH, 2000. p 180.

Reckeweg H. *Homeopathia Antihomotoxica Materia Medica*, 4th edition. Aurelia-Verlag, Baden-Baden, Germany 2002. pp. 254, 310, 456, 558–560.

PEMPHIGUS

Definition and cause

The pemphigus complex, consisting of pemphigus vulgaris, foliaceus, erythematosus, and vegetans, all have a common underlying autoimmune cause and the formation of antibodies that attack the outer layers of the skin, resulting in blisters, sores, pustules, crusting, and ulcerations. The different forms are usually diagnosed via histopathology. The complex is common in Chows, Newfoundland, Dachshunds, Collies, and Dobermans; it occurs much less commonly in cats (Halliwell 1989, Muller 1989, Swartout 2003).

Medical therapy rationale, drug(s) of choice, and nutritional recommendations

Medical treatment for pemphigus is usually lifelong use of immune-suppressing drugs such as corticosteroids, many times in combination with chemotherapeutics, such as azothiaprine, chlorambucil, cyclophosphamide or cyclosporine, along with topical applications of shampoos and medicated salves (Halliwell 1991, Swartout 2003, Thompson 1989).

Anticipated prognosis

The prognosis is related to the pemphigus type. Erythematosus and vegetans are controllable with low-dose cortisone, whereas vulgaris and foliaceus are potentially more serious and likely to become systemic. There are also more chances of serious secondary side effects due to prolonged use of immunosuppressing drugs. It has been reported that approximately 50% of all pemphigus animals respond well to cortisone alone, while others require additional chemotherapeutics or immunosuppressants (Scott 1995, Muller 1989).

Integrative veterinary therapies

Generally with autoimmune diseases, the medical approach focuses on immune suppression and secondary complications. In most cases, lifelong medication is required. Integrative veterinary therapies consider all aspects of the animal, including the skin (target organ) and the glands of the immune system, and help to balance the emotions (sense of well-being). Helping to balance and nourish the immune system, which includes helping to neutralize antibody attack of the target organ, can often help prevent recurrences of the disease and other system autoimmune signs (Cargill 1993; Dodd 1992, 1993).

Nutrition
General considerations/rationale

Therapeutic nutrition focuses on reducing of inflammation and preventing secondary skin infections, which helps to counteract and protect the organ systems from the long-term use of antimicrobials and immune-suppressing drugs and supports and balances the compromised immune system glands.

Appropriate nutrients

Nutrition/gland therapy: Glandular adrenal, thymus, and lymph supply intrinsic nutrients required by these organs. These nutrients help to neutralize a cellular immune attack, thereby sparing these organs from ongoing inflammation and eventual degeneration (See Chapter 2, Gland Therapy, for more details).

Lecithin/phosphatidyl choline: Phosphatidyl choline is a phospholipid that is integral to cellular membranes. Lecithin, as a part of the cell membranes, is an essential nutrient required by the skin and all of the body's cells for general health and wellness (Hanin 1987).

Alpha lipoic acid (ALA): Involved in mitochondrial activity and referred to as the "universal antioxidant." As a potent antioxidant it has been proven to reduce oxidative stress and inflammation. It has also been shown to increase the effectiveness of other antioxidants, such as vitamins C and E, Coenzyme Q10, and glutathione, making them more readily available for bodily function (Busse 1992, Scholich 1989).

In the treatment of autoimmune encephalomyelitis (a model used in multiple sclerosis research), Marracci (2002) and Morini (2004) found that ALA slowed progression of the autoimmune response and the disease process. Free radical inflammation is implicated as the initiator of many disease processes that are discussed in the book. ALA and other antioxidants have been proven to reduce this initiation of inflammation, and therefore are indicated in the prevention of many of these disease conditions.

Dimethylglycine: N,N-Dimethylglycine (DMG) is naturally produced by the body and has been clinically proven to support and enhance immune function. It has also been found to improve cellular oxygenation and circulation, and it helps remove toxins. The latter is quite important in dealing with chronic and autoimmune skin conditions (Verdova 1965). DMG has immune-modulating ability and has been clinically proven to increase both tumor necrosis factor (TNF) and interferon production (Graber 1986, Kendall 2003, Reap 1990, Wang 1988).

Chinese herbal medicine
General considerations/rationale
In TCM terms, pemphigus is caused by Wind, Heat, and Toxins invading the body. This leads to Qi and Blood stagnation in Liver and Qi and Yin deficiency. The Western translation of the etiology of pemphigus uses the term inflammation in the skin to mean Heat. Toxins are the inflammatory mediators from immune cells. These chemicals act on the skin to cause the typical signs of blisters, ulcers, and crusting. These lesions can then become infected with bacteria or fungi.

The ancient Chinese believed that Wind helped blow the disease into the body and spread it around. The protective Qi or Wei Qi keeps the individual healthy. This can be translated into the proper function of the immune system in protecting the individual. In the case of pemphigus, the Wei Qi or protective Qi is deficient. In Western terms, the underlying cause of the lesions is the disregulation of the immune system. Blood and Qi stagnation can lead to pain, and many patients have painful skin lesions. In addition, the stagnation of the Blood leads to the discoloration of the skin seen in these patients.

Yin deficiency meant lack of fluids to cool the patient to the ancient Chinese. Yin-deficient patients could have dry skin. There may be a low-grade fever due to lack of fluids to cool the body. To treat the patient the doctor must regulate the immune system (Wei Qi) and decrease the toxicity from the inflammatory mediators and the secondary invaders.

Appropriate Chinese herbs
Atractylodes (Cang zhu): Has activity against Staphylococcus aureus and some dermatophytes (Zhong Yao Xue), 1998).

Angelica radix (Dang gui): Has been used to treat a variety of dermatological disorders with excellent results (Shan Xi Yi Yao Za Zhi, 1975).

Bupleurum (Chai hu): Has anti-inflammatory effects (Zhong Yao Yao Li Yu Ying Yong 1983 Liu Wei 1998).

Dandelion (Pu gong ying): Has antibacterial effects against Staphylococcus aureus, B-hemolytic streptococci, and pseudomonas aeruginosa (Zhong Yi Yao Xue 1991).

Earthworm (Di long): Enhances the healing rate of skin lesions (Zhang Feng Chun 1999).

Honeysuckle (Jin yin hua): Contains many compounds with antibacterial activity. The strongest among these are chlorogenic acid and isochlorogenic acid. This herb can help to control secondary bacterial infections by Staphylococcus aureus, b-hemolytic streptococci, E. coli, and Pseudomonas aeruginosa (Xin Yi Xue 1975, Jiang Xi Xin Yi Yao 1960).

Licorice (Gan cao): Can inhibit the immune system. Glycyrrhizin and glycyrrhetinic acid have anti-inflammatory effects. They have approximately 10% of the corticosteroid activity of cortisone (Zhong Yao Xue 1991).

Poria (Fu ling): Inhibits Staphylococcus aureus, a common skin inhabitant, and can help prevent secondary infections (Nanjing College of Pharmacy 1976).

Rehmannia (Sheng di huang): Has anti-inflammatory effects. Both water and alcohol extracts decrease inflammation in mice (Zhong Yao Yao Li Yu Ying Yong 1983).

Scutellaria (Huang qin): Contains flavones, which have an anti-inflammatory action (Cao Zhi Sheng 1999).

White peony (Bai shao): Contains paeoniflorin, a strong anti-inflammatory compound (Zhong Yao Zhi, 1993).

Homotoxicology
General considerations/rationale
These are Degeneration Phase homotoxicoses, and as such, may not be clinically reversible. Several approaches can be taken, depending upon the treatment goals. Simply detoxifying and supporting these patients may make them feel better and assist with managing side effects of immunosuppressive, chronic allopathic drug therapy. In cases in which it is desirable to attempt cure, the owners must be well advised that this may not be possible and will entail long periods of itching, discharge, and other biological processes which occur during tissue repair. Such treatment is purely experimental; there are no cases of cure in the veterinary literature. The use of other medications may well interfere with necessary biological processes and can cause progressive vicariation. In one case it was observed that a canine patient lived comfortably while under biological therapy, and deteriorated rapidly once placed on immunosuppressive drugs. The protocol listed below is based on this single case (Palmquist 2005). All these circumstances need to be thoroughly discussed with the owner before a course of therapy is chosen.

Appropriate homotoxicology remedies
Because of the wide variety of other signs that can occur, many possible remedies may be used to manage pemphigus vulgaris. While no published veterinary cures exist, applications of basic biological therapy principles apply. Autosanguis therapy should be considered where allowed by law. Several commonly used remedies are listed below:

Abropernol: Eczema, erythema multiforme, hyperkeratosis, hyperhidrosis.

Aesculus compositum: Apis and Dulcamara address swelling and itching, and this formula promotes healthier vascular functions.

BHI Skin: Blisters, eczema, rashes, and hives (Heel 2002).

Causticum compositum: Ulcerated or burned appearing lesions.

Coenzyme compositum: Supports cellular energy metabolism.

Cutis compositum: Support and drains skin in all phases.

Echinacea compositum: Bacterial infections and immune modulation, particularly in regressive vicariation stages.

Engystol N: Sulfur-containing formula that is indicated in allergic skin conditions and to increase immune function, particularly in viral disorders.

Galium-Heel: Important phase remedy for both Impregnation and Degeneration Phase homotoxicoses. Activates the nonspecific defense mechanisms in cellular phases. Contains Caltha palustris, which has a favorable action in cellulitis and is indicated in pemphigus vulgaris with bullae surrounded by a ring accompanied by pruritis. This is a main remedy in all anemia cases (Reckeweg 2002).

Glyoxal compositum: Decouples polymers, which block enzyme systems.

Graphites homaccord: Exudative diatheses; greasy, hyperpigmented hair coat.

Hepar compositum: Supports hepatic detoxification, drainage, and repair, as well as iatrogenic damage caused by corticosteroid therapy. Hepar suis is indicated for skin with popular or blotchy eruptions which itch (Riley 1995). This remedy is valuable for those patients with liver damage and deficient detoxifying action of liver that may manifest in chronic eczemas, neurodermatitis, psoriatic conditions, erythema, dermatomycoses, and pemphigus (Reckeweg 2002).

Histaminum: As a single remedy, is suggested for Impregnation Phases and retoxications of all kinds, including eczemas and other skin diseases such as neurodermatitis, pyoderma, and pemphigus. It is frequently indicated as an intermediate remedy in all cellular phases, and is preferably combined with the intermediary acids of the citric acid cycle and other intermediary catalysts (Reckeweg 2002). It is found in the aforementioned combinations of *Hepar compositum* and *Ubichinon compositum*.

Lymphomyosot: Supports endocrine and lymphatic function.

Molybdan compositum: Trace mineral support.

Mucosa compositum: Support mucous membranes, particularly related to damage from corticosteroid therapy. Phase remedy for Degeneration Phase disorders.

Psorinoheel: Deep remedy for constitutional issues. The German Monograph-Preparation Commission lists Bufo rana, contained in *Psorinoheel*, for purulent blisters (pemphigus) on the skin and mucosa and dermal inflamma-

tions with a tendency toward suppuration (Reckeweg 2002).

Pulsatilla compositum: Regulates rigidity cases and reverses the iatrogenic damage from corticoids.

Solidago compositum: Supports renal function and detoxification.

Thyreoidea compositum: Matrix drainage and endocrine support.

Tonsilla compositum: Supports bone marrow, spleen, and immune function, and assists in repair in Impregnation Phase diseases. Broadfoot (2005) recommends *Tonsilla compositum* and *Traumeel-S* as a mixed autosanguis, with Lymphomyosot. According to Bianchi, it is useful in preventing a trend toward degeneration in cases of acute chronic inflammation.

Traumeel S: Activates inactive sulfur-containing enzyme systems and nonsteroidal anti-inflammatory effects, and modulates the inflammatory system.

Ubichinon compositum: Supports cellular energy metabolism and mitochondrial repair.

Authors' suggested protocols

Nutrition
Nutrition/glandular therapy: Skin and immune support formulas at 1 tablet for 25 pounds of body weight BID

Alpha-lipoic acid: 10 mg per 15 pounds of body weight daily; maximum of 100 mgs

DMG: 5 mg per pound of body weight daily

Lecithin/phosphatidyl choline: One-fourth teaspoon for every 25 pounds of body weight BID

Chinese herbal medicine
Formula ImmunoDerm: 1 capsule per 10 to 20 pounds twice daily. In addition to the herbs listed above, ImmunoDerm contains buffalo horn shavings (Shui niu jiao),fleece flower root(He shou wu), fructus xanthii (Cang er zi), kochia (Di fu zi), moutan (Mu dan pi), oldenlandia (Bai hua she cao), siegesbeckia (Xi xian cao), and tokoro (Bi xie). These herbs help increase the efficacy of the herbs above in treating pemphigus.

Homotoxicology formulas (Dose: 10 drops for 50-pound dog; 5 drops for cat or small dog)
Autosanguis: *Causticum compositum, Hepar compositum* plus *Solidago compositum, Thyroidea compositum, Ubichinon compositum*. Inject half into patient where allowed by law and combine the remaining material into the oral cocktail below.

Oral cocktail: *Galium-heel, Lymphomyosot, Berberis homaccord, Nux vomica homaccord, Mucosa compositum*, plus autosanguis therapy mixture. Refrigerate. Administer PO BID. Reduce the frequency of dosing to every three days if signs of detoxification are too strong.

Also consider adding *Aesculus compositum* TID orally if nonresponsive. *Psorinoheel* may be helpful as well.

Administer with nutritional support of vitamin E, niacinamide, Standard Process Veterinary Formula Hepatic Support. Consider oral tetracycline (not given in successful case report).

Product sources

Nutrition
Skin and immune support formulas: Animal Nutrition Technologies. **Alternatives:** Immune System Support—Standard Process Veterinary Formulas; Immuno Support—Rx Vitamins for Pets; Immugen—Thorne Veterinary Products; Derma-Strength—Vetri Science Laboratories; Canine Dermal Support—Standard Process Veterinary Formulas.

DMG: Vetri Science.
Alpha-lipioic acid: Source Naturals.
Lecithin/phosphatidyl choline: Designs for Health.

Chinese herbal medicine
Formula ImmunoDerm: Natural Solutions, Inc.

Homotoxicology
BHI/Heel Inc.

REFERENCES

Western medicine references
Halliwell REW, Gorman, NT. Autoimmune and other immune-mediated skin diseases. In: Veterinary clinical immunology, Philadelphia: W.B. Saunders, 1989. pp. 285–307.
Halliwell REW. Rational use of shampoos in veterinary dermatology. *J. Small Anim. Pract.* 1991. 32: 401–407.
Muller GH, Kirk RW, Scott DW. Immunologic diseases. In: Small animal dermatology, 4th ed. Philadelphia: W.B. Saunders, 1989. pp. 427–574.
Scott DW, Miller WH, Griffin CE. Immunologic Skin Diseases. *In* Muller and Kirk's Small Animal Dermatology. Toronto: W.B. Saunders Co., 1995 p. 500–518.
Swartout MS, Pemphigus, In: Tilley L, Smith F, The 5-Minute Veterinary Consult: Canine and Feline, 2003. Blackwell Publishing.
Thompson JP. Immunologic diseases. In: Ettinger SJ, ed. Textbook of veterinary internal medicine. Diseases of the dog and cat, 3rd ed. Vol 2., 1989. Philadelphia: WB Saunders pp. 2297–2328.

Integrative references
Cargill J, Thorpe-Vargas S. Feed that dog. Parts IV–VI. *Dog World*, 1993; 78 (10–12): 36–42, 28–31, 36–41.
Dodds WJ. Autoimmune thyroid disease. *Dog World*, 77 (4): 3640, 1992.

Dodds WJ, Donoghue S. Interactions of clinical nutrition with genetics. Chapter 8. In: The Waltham Book of Clinical Nutrition of the Dog and Cat. 1993. Oxford: Pergamon Press Ltd. (In Press).

Nutrition references
Busse E, Zimmer G, Schorpohl B, et al. Influence of alpha-lipoic acid on intracellular glutathione in vitro and in vivo. *Arzneimittelforschung*, 1992; 42:829–31.
Graber G, Kendall R. N,N-Dimethylglycine and Use in Immune Response, US Patent 4,631,189, Dec 1986.
Hanin I, Ansell GB. Lecithin: Technological, Biological, and Therapeutic Aspects, 1987, New York: Plenum Press, 180, 181.
Kendall RV. Building Wellness with DMG, 2003, Topanga, CA: Freedom Press.
Marracci GH, Jones RE, McKeon GP, Bourdette DN. Alpha lipoic acid inhibits T cell migration into the spinal cord and suppresses and treats experimental autoimmune encephalomyelitis. *J Neuroimmunol.* 2002;131(1–2):104–114.
Morini M, Roccatagliata L, Dell'Eva R, et al. Alpha-lipoic acid is effective in prevention and treatment of experimental autoimmune encephalomyelitis. *J Neuroimmunol.* 2004;148(1–2):146–153.
Reap E, Lawson J. Stimulation of the Immune Response by Dimethylglycine, a Non-toxic Metabolite. *Journal of Laboratory and Clinical Medicine.* 1990; 115:481.
Scholich H, Murphy ME, Sies H. Antioxidant activity of dihydrolipoate against microsomal lipid peroxidation and its dependence on alpha-tocopherol. *Biochem Biophys Acta* 1989;1001:256–61.
Verdova I, Chamaganova A. Use of vitamin B_{15} for the treatment of certain skin conditions, Vitamin B_{15} (Pangamic Acid) Properties, Functions and Use. 1965. Naooka, Moscow, Science Publishing.

Chinese herbal medicine references
Cao Zhi Sheng, et al. *Strait Journal of Pharmacology.* 1999;11(3):53–54
Jiang Xi Xin Yi Yao. Jiangxi New Medicine and Herbology, 1960 (1):34.
Liu Wei, et al. *Henan Journal of TCM Pharmacy.* 1998; 13(4):10–12.
Nanjing College of Pharmacy. *Materia Medica,* vol. 2. Jiangsu: People's Press; 1976.
Shan Xi Yi Yao Za Zhi. *Shanxi Journal of Medicine and Herbology,* 1975.
Xin Yi Xue. New Medicine, 1975; 6(3): 155.
Zhang Feng Chun, et al. Research into Di Long's mechanism in its recovery effects on rabbit back injury. *China Journal of Pharmacy.* 1999;34(2):93–96.
Zhong Yao Xue. Chinese Herbology, 1991; 22 (10):452.
Zhong Yao Xue. Chinese Herbology, 1998; 318:320.
Zhong Yao Yao Li Yu Ying Yong. Pharmacology and Applications of Chinese Herbs, 1983:400.
Zhong Yao Yao Li Yu Ying Yong. Pharmacology and Applications of Chinese Herbs, 1983;888.
Zhong Yao Zhi. *Chinese Herbology Journal,* 1993:183.

Zhong Yi Yao Xue Bao. Report of Chinese Medicine and Herbology, 1991;(1):41.

Homotoxicology references
Broadfoot P. Unpublished personal communication. 2005.
Heel. 2002. BHI Homeopathic Therapy. Heel Inc/Albuquerque, NM, p 96.
Palmquist R. 2005. Pemphigus vulgaris diagnosed by biopsy and treated biologically. Unpublished case data on file.
Reckeweg H. 2000. *Biotherapeutic Index: Ordinatio Antihomotoxica et Materia Medica*, 5th ed. Baden-Baden, Germany: Biologische Heilmittel Heel GMBH, p. 19.
Reckeweg H. 2002 Homeopathia *Antihomotoxica Materia Medica 4th Completely Revised Edition*. Aurelia-Verlag Baden-Baden, Germany pp. 190–1, 201, 269, 338–340.
Riley D. 1995. Drug Proving for Hepar Suis. Santa Fe, New Mexico, July.

MYASTHENIA GRAVIS

Definition and cause

Myasthenia gravis is an autoimmune disease that targets the neuromuscular junction, resulting in poor nerve impulses and weakness and atrophy of the muscles. The mechanism is a blocking of acetylcholine receptors on striated muscles so that muscular function does not occur. It is common in Jack Russell terriers, Akitas, and Fox terriers, and rare in cats. The disease is more commonly acquired than congenital (Cuddon 1989; Hopkins 1992; Pedroia 1992; Shelton 1992, 2002, 2004; Melmed 2004).

Medical therapy rationale, drug(s) of choice, and nutritional recommendations

The common therapy is the anticholinesterase drug pyridostigmine bromide syrup (Mestinon syrup). A second option involves corticosteroids and immunosuppressive drugs, such as azothiaprine, if there is little response to the anticholinergics.

Anticipated prognosis

The prognosis for acquired myasthenia gravis is often good, with proper and supportive care. The primary concern is the prevention of aspiration pneumonia, so feeding from an elevated position is important (Shelton 2001).

Integrative veterinary therapies

While the target of the exaggerated immune response is the acetylcholine receptors, the underlying mechanism is an imbalanced immune system. The fact that the literature reports spontaneous remissions with myasthenia gravis suggests that it is possible to balance the immune system's response. The addition of nutraceuticals, medicinal herbs, and combination homeopathics that have anti-inflammatory, regenerative, and balancing effects on the organs of the immune system can help to augment the process of healing. At the same time, medications such as the pyridostigmine bromide syrup can act to bridge the gap and strengthen muscle activity while underlying healing takes place (Shelton 2001).

Nutrition
General considerations/rationale

The nutritional approach to myasthenia involves support of the nervous system and its ability to conduct impulses. Simultaneously, supporting weakened immune system organs and protecting the body from potential adverse side effects of antiocholinergic or immune suppressing medication is beneficial for the animal.

Appropriate nutrients

Gland therapy: Involves nutritionally supporting the nerves and brain with intrinsic factors and vital nutrients that improves the metabolism of the nerve cells. In addition, supporting the immune system glands of the thymus, adrenal, and spleen help to facilitate balance and the reduction of inflammation.

Lecithin/phosphatidyl choline: Phosphatidyl choline is a phospholipid that is integral to cellular membranes and particularly the nerve and brain cells. It helps to move fats into the cells and is involved in acetylcholine uptake, neurotransmission, and cellular integrity. As a part of the cell membranes, lecithin is an essential nutrient required by the nerves and all of the body's cells for general health and wellness (Hanin 1987).

Phosphatidyl serine (PS): A phospholipid that is essential for the integrity of cell membranes, particularly of the nerve and brain cells. It has been studied extensively in people with impaired mental functioning and degeneration with positive results (Cenacchi 1993). People with Alzheimer's disease who had PS added to the program showed a mild to significant clinical improvement (Funfgeld 1989).

Coenzyme Q10 (ubiquinone): Found in the mitochondria and is involved in the cell's energy production; it is required for the daily functioning of the body. It is essential in the manufacture of ATP, the energy source for all the body's cells and tissues. CoQ10 is also a potent antioxidant and helps in the process of neutralizing free radicals and cell protection (Thomas 1997, Weber 1994).

Betasitosterol: A plant-derived sterol which has anti-inflammatory properties similar to corticosteriods and aspirin (Gupta 1980). In addition, sterols have been proven to enhance immune function (Bouic 1996). Sterols have been found to be able to enhance T-lymphocyte production and moderate B-cell activity, thereby helping to balance the immune response and indirectly reducing the risk of an autoimmune reaction (Bouic 1996).

Magnesium: Physiologically, magnesium activates adenosine triphosphatase, which is required for the proper functioning of the nerve cell membranes, and it fuels the sodium potassium pump. Magnesium deficiencies can upset the proper mineral balance required for cardiac muscle contraction and rhythm (Rardon 1990, Whang 1990). Magnesium is associated with neuromuscular function and conditions such as muscle cramping, weakness, and neuromuscular dysfunction. Magnesium is recommended for therapy for epilepsy and weakening muscle function (Bibley 1996, Levin 2002).

Chinese herbal medicine
General considerations/rationale
According to TCM, myasthenia gravis is the result of Qi deficiency and stagnation with phlegm accumulation in the middle burner, affecting the Stomach and Spleen. According to Western interpretation, myasthenia gravis is a deficiency of energy or strength (Qi). In terms of gastrointestinal signs, the animal does not have the strength to digest food, leading to the accumulation of Phlegm. In this case the term Phlegm refers to the liquid ingesta in the gastrointestinal tract as well as the interference with normal digestion. According to the traditional Chinese medicine system, the Stomach and Spleen are both involved with digestion. The Spleen is easily obstructed by excess liquid (or Phlegm) and becomes unable to function correctly. The normal flow of ingesta through the gastrointestinal tract is disrupted, resulting in vomiting. In addition, because an additional function of the Spleen is to control the muscles, there is the potential for weakness when a Spleen deficiency exists. The energy (or Qi) deficiency affects the nervous system, leading to further weakness.

Appropriate Chinese herbs
The following herbs may be useful for the esophageal weakness leading to regurgitation:

Cyperus seeds (Xiang fu zi): Stops stomach cramping (Zhong Cao Yao Fang Ji De Ying Yong 1976).

Licorice (Gan cao): Contains glycyrrhizin and glycyrrhetinic acid which have anti-inflammatory effects. They have approximately 10% of the corticosteroid activity of cortisone (Zhong Cao Yao 1991). This may be equivalent to using low-dose steroid therapy.

The following herbs are helpful for the muscle weakness secondary to myasthenia gravis:

Atractylodes (Bai zhu): Has been shown experimentally to increase swimming endurance in mice (Xin Yi Yao Xue Za Zhi 1974). That same effect could help with muscular weakness seen in myasthenia gravis.

Cuscata (Tu si zi): Modulates the immune system. Depending on the dose it can either increase or decrease the transformation of lymphocytes. It can either enhance or depress IL-2 production (Li 1997). This property of moderating the immune system may be useful in a condition such as myasthenia gravis, in which the body seems to lose the ability to regulate its own function.

Deer horn gelatin (Lu jiao jiao): Has a general strengthening effect on the body (Zhong Yao Da Ci Dian 1977).

Gastrodia (Tian ma): Increases strength. In one experiment it enhanced the subjects' swimming endurance (Bai 1996).

Homotoxicology
General considerations/rationale
Myasthenia gravis is an Impregnation Phase disorder early in the disease course, which progresses to a Degeneration Phase disorder. Many cases of myasthenia gravis go into spontaneous remission (Brooks 2003). Myasthenia gravis associated with thymoma is a Dedifferentiation Phase disorder. Because it is on the right side of the biological divide, this condition may not be reversed to the point of cure. Vaccination has been shown to exacerbate active myasthenia gravis, and should be delayed or avoided in such cases (Brooks 2003). The *Veterinary Guide* contains no protocols for this disease, but Reckeweg formulated treatment recommendations for human patients (Reckeweg 2000). These have been updated and are in clinical use in Europe (Smit 2006). Clients should be so advised prior to beginning therapy.

Appropriate homotoxicology remedies
Aesculus compositum: Provides support for circulatory disturbances.

Aletris homaccord: Contains Cocculus, which is indicated for CNS disorders, primarily vagotonous states and symptoms of exhaustion to the point of paralysis or unconsciousness. Also indicated for weakness of the neck muscles and in the legs (Reckeweg 2002).

Arsuraneel: Severe illness, loss of body condition, hopelessness, and weakness.

Causticum compositum: A high degree of weakness, often associated with trembling and an unsteady gait, so that the patient stumbles easily. Weakness associated with trembling, and with unsteadiness while walking, possibly to the point of paralysis, especially localized on the right side. Local pareses, e.g. of the vocal cords, muscles of deglutition, the eyelids, the bladder sphincter, musculature of the extremities, and Bell's palsy (Reckeweg 2002).

Cerebrum compositum: Dahlke describes Kali phosphoricum as a universal nerve remedy, which may at times be used simply on the basis of nervous weakness. Magnesium phosphoricum is indicated in rheumatic pains in the limbs, associated with weakness in the arms and hands and stiffness and possible numbness in the fingers, with general muscular weakness. Also contains cocculus, conium, and gelsemium (Reckeweg 2002).

Coenzyme compositum: Energy metabolism.

Galium-Heel: Cellular phase support in all cases, at least intermittently.

Gelsemium homaccord: Support of cranium and posterior limb strength. The most prominent symptom is the complete relaxation and exhaustion of the entire muscular system, with partial or complete paralysis of the motor nerves, as though the muscles no longer obey the will (Reckeweg 2002).

Ginseng compositum: Weakness and exhaustion. Conium for increasing paralysis and weakness, Hydrastis canadensis for severe muscular weakness and emaciation, and Ginseng for general weakness and debilitation (Reckeweg 2002).

Glyoxal compositum: Used intermittently and not repeated until recovery wanes.

Ovarium compositum: Female gonadal support.

Phosphor homaccord: Weakness and tremor with exertion.

Placenta compositum: Revitalizing connective tissue support and recirculation.

Testes compositum: Male gonadal support. Also has a revitalizing effect, and good for paretic, weakness syndromes.

Thyroidea compositum: Hormonal support and matrix drainage. This remedy contains Thymus suis for regulation via the thymus, and Funiculus umbicalis suis for revitalization (Smit 2006).

Traumeel: Enzyme activation and anti-inflammatory characteristics.

Ubichinon compositum: Mitochondrial support, general weakness (ubiquinone, which is Coenzyme Q10), and Hydrastis canadensis for severe muscular weakness and emaciation (Reckeweg 2002).

Authors' suggested protocols

Nutrition

Glandular therapy: Brain, nerve support and immune support formulas at 1 tablet per 25 pounds of body weight BID.

Lecithin/phosphatidyl choline: one-fourth teaspoon for every 25 pounds of body weight BID.

Phosphatidyl serine: 25 mg for every 25 pounds of body weight BID.

Coenzyme Q10: 25 mg for every 10 pounds of body weight SID.

Betathyme: 1 capsule for each 35 pounds of body weight BID (maximum 2 capsules BID).

Magnesium: 10 mg for every 10 pounds of body weight SID.

Chinese herbal medicine

Ding chen rou ge tang: This patent formula may be used for regurgitation. In addition to the herbs cited above, this formula contains agaste (Huo xiang), amomum fruit (Sha ren), aquilaria (Chen xiang), astragalus (Huang qi), atractylodes (Bai zhu), blue citrus (Qing pi), Chinese eaglewood (Chen xiang), citrus (Chen pi), cloves (Ding xiang), ginseng (Ren shen), leaven (Shen qu), lindera (Wu yao), magnolia bark (Hou po), malt (Mai ya), massa fermentata (Shen qu), nutmeg seeds (Rou dou kou), ophiopogon (Mai men dong), pinellia (Ban xia), poria (Fu ling), pueraria (Ge gen), round cardamon (Bai dou kou), tsaoko fruit (Cao guo), and white peony (Bai shao). These additional herbs increase the efficacy of the formula. The supplement is dosed to the supplier's directions.

Qi wei fang: This patent formula is indicated for the muscle weakness secondary to myasthenia gravis. In addition to the herbs cited above, it contains aconite (Fu zi), angelica root (Dang gui), astragalus (Huang qi), Chinese quince fruit (Mu gua), codonopsis (Dang shen), epimedium (Yin yang huo), and rehmannia (Shu di huang). The addition of these herbs improves efficacy. This supplement is dosed according to the supplier's directions.

Acupuncture points: The authors are not aware of any well-controlled studies to evaluate the efficacy of acupuncture. The following points are suggested points based upon TCM theory: PC 6, BL 17, CV 22, CV 23, and CV17.

Homotoxicology (Dose: 10 drops for 50-pound dog; 5 drops for cat or small dog)

Symptom formula: *Aletris homaccord, Gelsemium homaccord, Gallium-heel, Arsuraneel, Traumeel, Neuralgo-Rheum,* and *Circuloheel,* PO BID to TID. Use TID dosage until progress is made and then reduce to BID.

Deep detoxification formula: *Lymphomyosot, Hepar compositum, Solidago compositum, Thyroidea compositum, Coenzyme compositum, Ubichinon compositum, Testis compositum,* OR *Ovarium compositum,* PO EOD.

Cerebrum compositum: Twice weekly.

Glyoxal compositum: One injection and do not repeat until recovery wanes.

Product sources

Nutrition

Brain, nerve support and immune support formulas: Animal Nutrition Technologies. Alternatives: Immune System Support Standard—Process Veterinary Formulas; Immuno Support—Rx Vitamins for Pets; Immugen—Thorne Veterinary Products.

Lecithin/phosphatidyl choline: Designs for Health.
Phosphatidyl serine: Integrative Therapeutics.
Betathyme: Best for Your Pet. **Alternative:** Moducare—Thorne Veterinary Products.
Coenzyme Q10: Vetri Science—Thorne Veterinary Products.
Magnesium: Over the counter.

Chinese herbal medicine
Ding Chen Tou Ge Tang and Qi Wei Fang: Can be special ordered from herbal distributors such as Mayway and Blue Light, Inc.

Homotoxicology remedies
BHI/Heel Corporation.

REFERENCES

Western medical references
Cuddon PA. Acquired immune-mediated myasthenia gravis in a cat. *J. Small Anim. Pract.*, 1989; 30, 511–516.
Hopkins AI. Canine myasthenia gravis. *J. Small Anim. Pract.*, 1992, 33, 477–484.
Shelton GD, Barton C, Bergman R., Melmed C. Masticatory muscle myositis: Pathogenesis, diagnosis, and treatment. *Compend Cont Ed Prac Vet. Small Animal.* 26:590–605, 2004.
Pedroia V. Disorders of the skeletal muscles. In: Ettinger SJ: Textbook of Veterinary Internal Medicine, Vol. I, 3rd ed., 1989, Philadelphia: W.B. Saunders Corp. 733–744.
Shelton GD. Canine myasthenia gravis. In: Kirk RW, Bonagura JD (eds.) Current Veterinary Therapy XI. 1992. Philadelphia: W.B. Saunders Co., 1039–1042.
Shelton GD. Megaesophagus secondary to acquired myasthenia gravis. In: Kirk RW, Bonagura JD (eds.) Current Veterinary Therapy XI, W.B. 1992. Philadelphia: Saunders Co. 580–583.
Shelton GD. Neuromuscular Diseases. *The Veterinary Clinics of North America. Small Animal Practice.* 2002. 32: January.
Shelton GD. Neuromuscular Diseases II. The *Veterinary Clinics of North America. Small Animal Practice,* 2004. 34: November.
Shelton GD, Lindstrom JM. Spontaneous remission in canine myasthenia gravis: Implications for assessing human MG therapies. *Neurology.* 2001 Dec 11;57(11):2139–2141.

Nutrition references
Bilbey DLJ, Prabhakaran VM. Muscle cramps and magnesium deficiency: case reports. *Canadian Family Physician*, Vol. 42, July 1996, pp. 1348–51.
Bouic PJD, et al. Beta-sitosterol and beta-sitosterol glucoside stimulate human peripheral blood lymphocyte proliferation: Implications for their use as an immunomodulatory vitamin combination. *International Journal of Immunopharmacology* 1996. 18:693–700.

Cenacchi T, Bertoldin T, Farina C, et al. Cognitive decline in the elderly: a double-blind, placebo-controlled multicenter study on efficacy of phosphatidylserine administration. *Aging (Milano)* 1993;5:123–33.
Fünfgeld EW, Baggen M, Nedwidek P, et al. Double-blind study with phosphatidylserine (PS) in Parkinsonian patients with senile dementia of Alzheimer's type (SDAT). *Prog Clin Biol Res* 1989;317:1235–46.
Gupta MB, Nath R, Srivastava N, et al. Anti-inflammatory and antipyretic activities of β-sitosterol. *Planta Medica* 1980;39: 157–163.
Hanin I, Ansell GB. Lecithin: Technological, Biological, and Therapeutic Aspects, 1987, Plenum Press, NY, 180, 181.
Levin C. Canine Epilepsy, Oregon City, OR: Lantern Publication, 2002 p 18–19.
Rardon DP, Fisch C. Electrolytes and the Heart. In The Heart, 7th edition. Hurst, JW (ed). 1990. New York: McGraw-Hill Book Co. 1567
Thomas SR, Neuzil J, Stocker R. Inhibition of LDL oxidation by ubiquinol-10. A protective mechanism for coenzyme Q in atherogenesis? *Mol Aspects Med* 1997;18:S85–103.
Weber C, Jakobsen TS, Mortensen SA, et al. Antioxidative effect of dietary coenzyme Q10 in human blood plasma. *Int J Vitam Nutr Res* 1994;64:311–5.
Whang R, Ryder KW. Frequency of hypomagnesemia and hypermagnesemia: Requested vs. routine. *J Am Med Assoc* 1990;263, 3063–3064.

Chinese herbal medicine references
Bai Xiu Rong, et al. *Journal of Mathematical Medicine.* 1996;9(2):180–182.
Li Geng Sheng, et al. The immunological activity of Tu Si Zi's water-soluble components. *China Journal of TCM Science and Technology.* 1997;4(4):256–258.
Xin Yi Yao Xue Za Zhi. *New Journal of Medicine and Herbology,* 1974; 8:13.
Zhong Cao Yao Fang Ji De Ying Yong. Applications of Chinese Herbal Formulas, 1976;101.
Zhong Cao Yao. Chinese Herbal Medicine 1991;22 (10):452.
Zhong Yao Da Ci Dian. Dictionary of Chinese Herbs, 1977: 2232

Homotoxicology references
Brooks W. Myasthenia gravis. The Pet Health Library. 2003. Website: http://www.veterinarypartner.com/Content.plx?P=A&S=0&C=0&A=1544/.
Dahlke R. *Malattia linguaggio dell'anima,* Ed. 1996. Mediterranee.
Heel. 2003. Veterinary Guide, 3rd English edition. Baden-Baden, Germany: Biologische Heilmittel Heel GMBH.
Reckeweg H. *Biotherapeutic Index: Ordinatio Antihomotoxica et Materia Medica,* 5th ed. 2000. Baden-Baden, Germany: Biologische Heilmittel Heel GMBH, p. 191–2.
Reckeweg H. *Homeopathia Antihomotoxica Materia Medica* 4th ed. 2002. Aurelia-Verlag, Baden-Baden, Germany, pp 218–19, 244, 254, 255, 310–11, 315–16, 344–45.
Smit A. Personal communication. Medicine and Research Biologische Heilmittel Heel GmbH, February 2006.

Chapter Seven

Diseases of the Blood and Lymph

ANEMIA

Definition and cause

Anemia is caused by many different conditions and classified into many different types, including: regenerative, non-regenerative, aplastic, autoimmune, iron deficiency, anemia of chronic disease (such as renal failure), babesia, parasites (fleas, hookworms, or whipworms), vaccine-induced, secondary to onion ingestion, and neoplasia. In all instances it is imperative to diagnose the underlying cause and initiate corrective medical measures (Birkenheuer 1999, Cowgill 1992, Duval 1996, Knoll 2003, Kristensen 1995, Morgan 1999, Rebar 1981, Yamato 1998, Young 1997).

Medical therapy rationale, drug(s) of choice, and nutritional recommendations

Medical therapy focus not only on replacing blood, but also on the underlying cause. This includes stabilizing the azotemia, blocking the immune attack of the RBCs, stimulating the production of RBC with eryhthropoeitin, augmenting the diet with hematinic nutrients such as iron and folic acid, and correcting the bleeding, such as in a bleeding gastric ulcer or cystitis (Knoll 2003, Rogers 1995).

Anticipated prognosis

The anticipated course of anemia depends on the underlying cause, which, if diagnosed and addressed, often sets the stage for a good prognosis (Knoll 2003, Rogers 1995).

Integrative veterinary therapies

After the cause of the anemia is established and addressed, it is prudent to integrate nutrition, homeopathy, and herbal remedies to support the body's organ system and the bone marrow's production of red blood cells, and to supply the nutrients required for the formation of red blood cells.

Nutrition
General considerations/rationale

After the cause of the anemia is established, nutritional support focuses upon the bone marrow, liver, and spleen, along with the required nutrients for the manufacture of red blood cells.

Appropriate nutrients

Nutrition/gland therapy: Glandular bone marrow, liver, and spleen supply the intrinsic nutrients for these organs. One of the most bioavailable sources of iron is the liver. Comparing the absorption rate of inorganic iron (for example, ferrous sulfate versus heme-iron), the latter is 30 times more effective. The best source of heme-iron is concentrated liver extract (Frykman 1994). Liver is also a superior source of vitamin B_{12} and folic acid.

Vitamin B_{12}: Essential for the maintenance of the proper levels of red blood cells. Deficiencies of vitamin B_{12} are associated with anemia and decreased function of the immune system; supplementation with vitamin B_{12} often addresses the condition (Berlin 1978, Kondo 1998, Lederle 1991).

Folic acid: A B vitamin that is required for organized cellular division. Folic acid is integral in the synthesis of both DNA and RNA and therefore affects the genetic modeling of the body. Folic acid deficiencies affect bone marrow cell division and can lead to a macrocytic anemia with fewer but larger red blood cells (Food Nutrition Board 1998).

Chinese herbal medicine
General considerations/rationale

According to Traditional Chinese Medicine theory, anemia is a combination of Yin and Blood deficiency in the Liver, Kidney, and Spleen. This leads to secondary Qi and Yang deficiency. According to the Western interpretation, Yin is fluid and blood is a component of fluid, so

when there is a blood deficiency there is also a Yin deficiency. The Liver stores the Blood, and the Kidney and
Spleen play a role in making the blood. Secondary to the
loss of blood, there is Qi and Yang deficiency. Basically,
Qi deficiency refers to the weakness that an anemic patient
might feel. As red blood cells carry the oxygen, anemic
patients may have oxygen-deprived tissues. Many anemic
people report feeling cold. This corresponds to the TCM
concept of Yang deficiency. In order to treat anemia, it is
necessary to discover and treat the underlying cause. If
there is chronic blood loss or destruction or underlying
nutritional deficiencies, these must also be addressed.

Appropriate Chinese herbs

Astragalus (Huang qi): Stimulates the production and
maturation of cells in the bone marrow (Nan Jing Zhong
Yi Xue Yuan Xue Bao 1989).

Atractyoldes (Bai zhu): Promotes the proliferation rate
of colony-forming units (CFU-E) and erythroid burst-
forming units (BFU-E), thereby increasing the red blood
cell count (Hou 1999).

Codonopsis (Dang shen): Increases the red blood cell
count and hemoglobin levels (Zhong Yao Xue 1998).

Cuscuta (Tu si zi): Increases resistance to hypoxia
(Chang Yong Zhong Yao Cheng Fen Yu Yao Li Shou Ce
1994).

Donkey skin gelatin (E jiao): In one experiment in
which anemia was induced in dogs via hemorrhage, e jiao
increased the red blood cell count and hemoglobin level
more than iron treatment (Zhong Cheng Yao Yan Jiu
1981).

Fleece flower root (He shou wu): Promotes hematopoi-
etic stem cells (Zhou 1991).

Scrophularia (Xuan shen): Significantly increases the
ability of healthy mice to tolerate oxygen deprivation
(Zhang Bao Heng 1959, Gong 1981).

Wolfberry (Gou qi zi): Increases the production of red
blood cells in mice (Zhong Yao Xue 1998).

Homotoxicology
General considerations/rationale
Anemia can originate from many different causes and the
phase of disease depends upon the precise cause in each
case. Most cases represent Impregnation or Degeneration
Phase homotoxicoses. Each case should receive a standard
medical and historical approach so that all predisposing
factors are uncovered. Many cases are so-called "anemia
of chronic disorder," and taking steps to improve general
health can also improve the patient's anemia. Monitoring
these patients over time gives valuable information about
treatment response as well as the potential to uncover
further unknown pathology. Autoimmune hemolytic
anemia requires extensive support (see Chapter 6, Autoimmune Disease).

Appropriate homotoxicology
Any antihomotoxic medicine that improves general health
may assist these patients. The following list consists of
major remedies only:

Aletris-Heel: An important remedy for anemia because
Aletris is indicated for anemia and weakness, as is Chininum arsenicosum, which serves as a tonic remedy. Helo-
nius also has indications for weakness. Other constituents
support debility, weakness, and exhaustion.

BHI-Bleeding: Contains Aceticum acidum for edematous swellings, which have a waxy appearance and may
be associated with anemia. Rapid emaciation with fainting, despondency, irritability, attacks of anxiety and great
debility, weakness, confusion of thoughts and a kind of
stupor may occur, and there may be steatorrhea and
intestinal bleeding (Reckeweg 2002). *Bursa pastoris*
(shepherd's purse), which was introduced for hemostatic
purposes because of a shortage of *Secale* during World
War I (Reckeweg 2002), is also of critical value in this
combination. The main indications for *Bursa pastrois* are
hemorrhages, metrorrhagia, menorrhagia, hematuria, epistaxis, bloody diarrhea, hemorrhoidal bleeding, etc.

Crotalus horridus (rattlesnake venom) is another very
powerful component of this remedy. Indications for its
use include: hemorrhages from eyes, ears, nose, and any
organ of dark, fluid blood. Aggravation is in the spring.
Other indications include inflammations with gangrene
and sepsis and purpura, toxic icterus, and viral hepatitis.
Typical of Crotalus is the great lassitude and exhaustion
and the rapid dwindling of energy, which can occur with
fainting, trembling all over, and convulsions. In chronic
conditions there is apathy, despondency, and anxiety,
with restlessness and unsociability. There may be hemorrhages from orifices of the body, and general jaundiced
skin discoloration and hemorrhages from the capillary
network of the skin, and possible ecchymoses (Reckeweg
2002).

BHI-Enzyme: Adjunctive agent that supports metabolism (Heel 2002). Of primary importance is succinic acid,
which is related to blood formation and should therefore
be used in cases of anemia and leukemia, anemic headaches, nutritional disturbances of vegetarians (human; in
which there is the typical pale appearance), after the consequences of antibiotic treatment for frequent catarrhal
affections, and possibly for pulmonary hemorrhage and
epistaxis. There may also be signs of vitamin deficiency,
nerve-pain (trigeminal, sciatic), and lumbago. There is
always a characteristic disturbance of the red blood cells
and there may be nervous irritation of the stomach, hypo-
chlorhydria, dyspepsia with flatulence, duodenal ulcers
which do not heal, enteritis, and colitis with diarrhea at
the slightest excitement. It is used as a subsidiary remedy
in intestinal bleeding (Reckeweg 2002). This component
is also found in *Coenzyme compositum.*

BHI-Exhaustion: Contains *Cinchona officinalis* for exhaustion following blood loss or fluid loss (nursing). Citricum acidum supports the citric acid cycle and improves oxygen use (Heel 2002).

China homaccord: Weakness following blood loss. It takes its name from China Peruvian bark (*Cinchona officianalis*), (and not the country of same spelling), from which quinine is obtained. It was formerly used as a specific against malaria. China is used less as a fever-remedy, and more in states of weakness and anemia after substantial loss of blood or losses of vital fluids of all kinds. China symptoms are characterized by a pale, yellowish face with sunken eyes and dark rings around them, anemic headache with air, hunger, pulsation of the carotid arteries, and possibly edema. "There is also a tendency to profuse haemorrhage of dark blood from various organs. If these have been temporarily treated with some haemostatic, then after a dose of China has been given they may reappear if China is given in too low a dosage. Thus it has generally proved expedient, where haemorrhage is present, first of all to treat the haemorrhage symptomatically (e.g. with preparations of Cinnamomum), and only to use China later on in order to remove the secondary anaemia" (Reckeweg 2002).

Icterus may occur as well. The fevers, which respond to China, are extraordinarily characteristic, with the fever worsening day by day. The liver and spleen may be swollen and sensitive. There is a tendency for profuse hemorrhages (Reckeweg 2002). This remedy is one that fits the disease picture of many tick borne diseases such as *Ehrlichia canis*, et. al. Cinchona is also common to *Arsuraneel*, *Hepar compositum*, and *Hepeel*.

Cinnamomum homaccord: Active hemorrhage, epistaxis, etc. (Reckeweg 2000).

Duodenoheel: Support of gastrointestinal tissues, especially in ulcerative disease.

Ferrum homaccord: Iron deficiency and iron sequestration anemias. Contains a group of several ferrum (iron-containing) compounds: ferrum metallicum, muriaticum, phosphoricum, and sulphuricum. These are broadly used for anemias, splenomegaly, and general weakness (Reckeweg 2002).

Galium-Heel: Cellular detoxification and repair.

Gastricumeel: Support of the stomach during nausea and ulceration disorders.

Graphites homaccord: Petechial eruptions; constitutional remedy for tendency toward obesity, chronic constipation, and eczema with honey-colored crusts.

Molybdan compositum: Used as a donor for rebuilding blood cells. Zincum gluconicum is one of the many components of this combination. Zinc compounds influences important enzyme functions, e.g. in anemia, diabetes mellitus, liver damage, kidney diseases, degeneration phases, and particularly neoplasm phases. Cobaltum gluconicum,

another component, is important because the anti-anemic principle in vitamin B_{12} is a complex compound of Co^{++}. Cobalt deficiency causes a serious degenerative disease of sheep in Australia, "coast disease," which is distinguished by progressive emaciation, weakness, loss of appetite, and apathy, leading to severe anemia. Niccolum metallicum (nickel) is another component, with the following pertinent indications: hoarseness, spasmodic coughing, and nosebleeds. It stimulates blood coagulation (Reckeweg 2000).

Mucosa compositum: Support of mucosal barriers in Degeneration Phase disorders or in repair following other mucosal defects; support of mucosal elements after iatrogenic damage (NSAIDs, corticosteroid therapy, etc). *Mucosa compositum* owes some of its value to the Lachesis (bushmaster venom) component; it is suitable in widely varying illnesses, of both a functional and an organic kind. It is particularly suitable to septic illnesses and decomposition of the blood, thrombocytopenic purpura, hemorrhagic diathesis, gangrene, malaria, and kidney diseases with edematous swelling. *Lachesis* is often indicated in serious blood dyscrasias and in disorders of hormonal function, particularly at menopause, but also in catarrhs of the mucosa, hemorrhoids, suppurations, inflammations with the development of sepsis, and malignant infectious diseases. It usually works particularly well in the form of injections, since this is most similar to the natural toxic action of snake venoms (Reckeweg 2002).

Phosphor homaccord: In cases of petechial hemorrhage, tendency toward hemorrhages or bruising, laryngitis (Heel 2003). Also used for purpura, thrombocytopenia, bleeding hemorrhoids, protracted hemorrhages, and hematoma without obvious injuries. Higher potencies must be used when there is a hemorrhagic tendency. Phosphorus is indicated in other kinds of Impregnation and Degeneration phases, e.g. myocardial damage, endocarditis and fatty degeneration of the heart, and typhoid anemia, and in suppurations of connective tissues and glands. Clear states of exhaustion require phosphorus in low potency (Reckeweg 2002). This remedy is also found in *Galium-heel*, *Hepeel*, *Mucosa compositum*, et al.

Solidago compositum: Support of urogenital tissues, renal failure.

Tonsilla compositum: Trophic function on spleen and bone marrow. Contains homeopathically potentized cortisone (*Cortisonum aceticum*) that is indicated for damage to the adrenal cortex and pituitary and connective tissue. May also be tried for inflammation, ulceration, and bleeding of the mucosa of the alimentary tract; bone decalcification; disorders of the skin, blood, and vascular systems; and behavioral disorders and emotional discord or upset (Reckeweg 2002). There are consequences for cortisone abuse of cortisone and other iatrogenic damage. Cortisone is also found in *Thyroidea compositum* along with

Medulla ossis suis (bone marrow). The main indications are: anemia, leukemia, agranulocytosis and other iatrogenic conditions, and radiation damage. (This formula is particularly suitable after radiation therapy, given its therapeutic range).

Authors' suggested protocols

Nutrition
Blood/bone marrow support formula: 1 tablet for each 25 pounds of body weight BID.

Energizing iron (liver extract plus iron): 1 capsule for every 25 pounds of body weight, maximum 4 capsules SID.

Vitamin B$_{12}$: 50 micrograms for every 25 pounds; maximum 200 micrograms.

Folic acid: 50 micrograms for every 35 pounds of body weight, maximum 200 micrograms.

Chinese herbal medicine
H28 anemia: Recommended by the authors at 1 capsule per 10 to 20 pounds twice daily as needed. In addition to the herbs mentioned above, H28 also contains aconite (Fu zi), amomum fruit (Sha ren), angelica root (Dang gui), antler powder (Lu jiao jiao), cordyceps (Dong chong xia cao), cornus (Zhu yu), licorice (Gan cao), moutan (Mu dan pi), poria (Fu ling), and rehmannia (Shu di huang). These herbs help to increase the efficacy and decrease potential side effects of the formula.

It is also important to address the underlying cause of the anemia.

Homotoxicology (Dose 10 drops for 50-pound dog; 5 drops for small dog or cat)
Select the symptom remedy or remedies that best match the case and then select the Detoxification formula which is applicable based upon the case's location on the Six-Phase Table of Homotoxicology.

Symptom formula (anemia of chronic disorder): *Galium-heel, Phosphor homaccord, Ferrum compositum* BID PO.

Symptom formula (blood loss): *Traumeel, Cinnamomum compositum, China homaccord.*

Deep detoxification formula: *Lymphomyosot, Hepar compositum, Solidago compositum, Thyroidea compositum* E3D PO.

Product sources

Nutrition
Blood and bone marrow support formulas: Animal Nutrition Technologies
Energizing iron: PhytoPharmica, Inc.
Folic acid: Progressive Labs

Chinese herbal medicine
H28 anemia: Natural Solutions Inc.

Homotoxicology
BHI/Heel Inc.

REFERENCES

Western medicine references
Birkenheuer AJ, Levy MG, Savary KC, Gager RB, Breitschwerdt EB. Babesia gibsoni infections in dogs from North Carolina, J Am Anim Hosp Assoc, 1999, Mar-Apr; 35(2):125–8.

Cowgill LD. Pathophysiology and management of anemia in chronic progressive renal failure. Semin Vet Med Surg, 1992; 7:175–182.

Duval D, Giger U. Vaccine-associated immune-mediated hemolytic anemia in the dog. J Vet Intern Med 1996 Sep-Oct; 10(5):290–5.

Knoll JS. Anemia (Regenerative and Non-Regenerative). In: Tilley L, Smith F, The 5-Minute Veterinary Consult: Canine and Feline, 2003 Blackwell Publishing.

Kristensen AT, Feldman BF. Blood banking and transfusion medicine. In: Ettinger SJ, Feldman EC, eds. Textbook of veterinary internal medicine: diseases of the dog and cat. Vol. 1. 4th ed. Philadelphia: Saunders, 1995:347–360.

Morgan LW, McConnell J. Cobalamin deficiency associated with erythroblastic anemia and methylmalonic aciduria in a border collie. J Am Anim Hosp Assoc 1999 Sep-Oct; 35(5):392–5.

Rebar AH, Lewis HB, DeNicola DB, Halliwell WH, Boon GD. Red blood cell fragmentation in the dog: an editorial review. Vet Pathol 1981;18:415–426.

Rogers K. Anemia. In: Ettinger SJ, Feldman EC, eds. Textbook of veterinary internal medicine: diseases of the dog and cat. Vol. 1. 4th ed. Philadelphia: Saunders, 1995:187–191.

Weiser EG. Erythrocyte responses and disorders. In: Ettinger SJ, Feldman EC, eds. Textbook of veterinary internal medicine. 4th ed. Philadelphia: Saunders, 1995:1864–1891.

Yamato O, Hayashi M, Yamasaki M, Maede Y. Induction of onion-induced haemolytic anaemia in dogs with sodium n-propylthiosulphate. Vet Rec 1998 Feb 28;142(9):216–9.

Young NS, Maciejewski J. The Pathophysiology of acquired aplastic anemia. New Engl J Med 1997;336:1365–1372.

Nutrition references
Berlin R, Berlin H, Brante G, Pilbrant A. Vitamin B$_{12}$ body stores during oral and parenteral treatment of pernicious anaemia. Acta Med Scand 1978;204:81–4.

Food and Nutrition Board, Institute of Medicine. Folic Acid. Dietary Reference Intakes: Thiamin, Riboflavin, Niacin, Vitamin B$_6$, Vitamin B$_{12}$, Pantothenic Acid, Biotin, and Choline. Washington, D.C.: National Academy Press; 1998: 193–305.

Frykman E, Bystrom M, Jansson U, et al. Side effects of iron supplements in blood donors: superior tolerance of heme iron. J Lab Clin Med 1994;123:561–4.

Kondo H. Haematological effects of oral cobalamin preparations on patients with megaloblastic anaemia. *Acta Haematol* 1998;9:200–5.

Lederle FA. Oral cobalamin for pernicious anemia: medicine's best kept secret? *JAMA* 1991;265:94–5.

Chinese herbal medicine references

Chang Yong Zhong Yao Cheng Fen Yu Yao Li Shou Ce. A Handbook of the Composition and Pharmacology of Common Chinese Drugs, 1994;1563:1564.

Gong Wei Gui, et al. Zhejiang *Journal of Medicine.* 1981;3(1):11.

Hou Dun, et al. *Journal of Jiangxi College of TCM.* 1999;11(1):28.

Nan Jing Zhong Yi Xue Yuan Xue Bao (*Journal of Nanjing University of Traditional Chinese Medicine*), 1989;1:43.

Zhang Bao Heng. *Journal of Beijing Medical College.* 1959; (1):59.

Zhong Cheng Yao Yan Jiu (Research of Chinese Patent Medicine), 1981;(5):31.

Zhong Yao Xue (Chinese Herbology), 1998;739:741.

Zhong Yao Xue (Chinese Herbology), 1998;860:862.

Zhou Zhi Wen, et al. *Journal of TCM Pharmacology and Clinical Application.* 1991;7(5):19.

Homotoxicology references

Heel. 2002. BHI Homeopathic Therapy. Heel, Inc, Albuquerque, New Mexico, pp 8, 54–55.

Heel. 2003. Veterinary Guide, 3rd edition. Biologische Heilmettel Heel GmbH:Baden-Baden, Germany, pp 104–5.

Reckeweg H. 2000. Biotherapeutic Index: Ordinatio Antihomotoxica et Materia Medica, 5th ed. Baden-Baden, Germany: Biologische Heilmittel Heel GMBH, p 312.

Reckeweg H. 2002. Homeopathia Antihomotoxica Materia Medica, 4th edition. Aurelia-Verlag, Baden-Baden, Germany, pp 177, 191. 228–30, 244, 259, 263–4, 296–9, 410, 456, 489–90, 542, 553, 610.

CHYLOTHORAX

Definition and cause

The accumulation of thoracic fluid that is high in chylomicrons. Initially, chylothorax was believed to be secondary to injury or a rupture of the thoracic duct such as is found in a diaphragmatic hernia. Because the thoracic duct was found to be unaltered in most animals with chylothorax, it is now believed that any process that interferes or inhibits normal lymph flow can lead to chylothorax. These processes include high venous pressure, dilated lymph vessels, heart disease such as cardiomyopathy or heartworm disease, and hyperplastic or neoplasia of the mediastinal lymph nodes. (Birchard 1998; Fossum 1986, 1994, 2003; Kerpsack 1994; Meadows 1994).

Medical therapy rationale, drug(s) of choice, and nutritional recommendations

All cases should receive a complete work-up and the client should be advised that the prognosis is guarded. Chylothorax cases can respond to basic therapy with thoracocentesis, and rutin therapy may be beneficial (Fossum 2003, Thompson 1999). Surgical repair of thoracic duct ligation is indicated where possible, but many cases have nonsurgical disease (Kerpsack 1994, Fossum 2001). Patients may develop fibrosing pleuritis from scar tissue deposition caused by any thoracic exudates such as chylothorax or pyothorax. The recommended dietary support is a low-fat diet which helps to decrease fat in the pleural effusion (Fossum 2003).

Anticipated prognosis

May resolve spontaneously. Surgery is indicated if medical therapy and thorocentesis do not control the condition. A continual requirement for thoracentesis or secondary complications such as dyspnea or fibrosing plueritis often lead to the decision to euthanize.(Fossum 1986, 1991, 2001).

Integrative veterinary therapies

Besides direct injury to the thoracic duct, chylothorax is a result of circulatory and lymphatic stasis secondary to a blockage or an inflammatory process within the system, or is related to associated organ conditions such as enlarged lymph nodes or heart disease.

An integrated approach considers the reduction of inflammation and improvement of fluid stasis. The use of nutraceuticals, medicinal herbs, and combination homeopathics that have anti-inflammatory, tissue-sparing, and regenerative effects on the organs and vessels and can help improve circulation.

Nutrition
General considerations/rationale

After the cause(s) of chylothorax has been established and medical or surgical therapy is initiated to control the condition, nutritional support focuses on the heart, lung, and lymphatic systems. Support is also directed toward reducing free radical load and associated inflammation inside vessels or in perfused organs.

Appropriate nutrients

Nutritional/gland therapy: Glandular heart, lung, and lymph supply intrinsic nutrients that help neutralize a cellular immune inflammatory process. This helps spare the organ from cascading inflammation and eventual degeneration. (See Gland Therapy in Chapter 2 for a more detailed explanation).

Betasitosterol: Plant-derived sterols have been shown to have anti-inflammatory and antipyretic properties that appear to be similar to corticosteroids and aspirin (Gupta 1980). In addition, sterols have been proven to enhance immune function (Bouic 1996). Sterols have been shown to enhance T-lymphocyte production and moderate B-cell activity, thereby helping to balance the immune response and indirectly reducing the risk of an autoimmune reaction (Bouic 1996).

Vitamin A: Is an antioxidant, cell and tissue protector, and free radical scavenger (See Antioxidants and Free Radicals, Chapter 2). By reducing inflammation, vitamin A is therapeutically beneficial in treating chronic degenerative diseases (Halliwell 1994).

Vitamin E: Reduces inflammation and improves circulation by helping vessels to dilate and reducing the agglutination of blood platelets (Traber 1999, 2001). Vitamin E also has organ-sparing properties that help to reduce scarring (Meyers 1982).

Lecithin/phosphatidyl choline: Studies with phosphatidyl choline have shown that it can reduce triglyceride and cholesterol levels because it emulsifies fats (Brook 1986, Spilburg 2003).

Chinese herbal medicine/acupuncture
General considerations/rationale
Chylothorax is the result of Qi and Blood deficiency in the Spleen and Lung, with Qi and Water stagnation. Spleen Qi deficiency leads to Spleen Blood deficiency (insufficient Spleen Qi leads to the inability to produce Blood). The Spleen can't produce adequate Qi without adequate Blood. As a result, a circular pattern of progressive deficiency occurs.

In the Western interpretation, the spleen holds fluids in the correct location. When the spleen is Qi-deficient it lacks the energy to do this and fluid can leak into abnormal compartments. In this disease process, the plasma and chylomicrons, which should be held in the blood vessels, leak into the thoracic cavity. The lung is responsible for helping to distribute fluid. When it is Qi-deficient, fluids can accumulate in abnormal places because the Lung does not have the energy to function normally. The term "water stagnation" refers to the fluid in the chest. Treatment is aimed at decreasing fluid in the chest and addressing lipid abnormalities.

Appropriate Chinese herbs
Apricot seed (Xing Ren): Can increase serum HDL levels while lowering the total cholesterol (Dilinuer 1999); also lowers blood pressure (Zhong Cao Yao Xue 1976).

Bupleurum (Chai hu): Contains saikosaponin A and D which decrease triglyceride levels and to a lesser extent cholesterol levels (Zhong Yao Xue 1988). This may decrease the lipid content of the effusion.

Lepidium (Ting li zi): Has diuretic actions (Zhong Yao Zhi 1984) and may help drain fluid from the chest.

Imperata (Bai mao gen): Has diuretic properties (Ren Min Wei Sheng Chu Ban She 1983), which may help to decrease thoracic fluid.

Platycodon (Jie geng): Decreases blood lipid levels (Chang Yong Zhong Yao Cheng Fen Yu Yao Li Shou Ce 1994). It also decreases blood pressure (Zhong Yao Yao Li Yu Ying Yong 1983).

Poria (Fu ling) also has diuretic effects on the body; this was shown in rabbits after 5 days of treatment with 500 mg poria/kg/day (Lu 1987, Lu 1988).

Homotoxicology
General considerations/rationale
Chylothorax represents serious deterioration of the body's ability to maintain normal structure and function, and represents a Degeneration Phase disorder. It can be associated with a wide variety of predisposing issues including trauma, cranial vena caval thrombosis, granuloma, right heart failure, neoplasia, lymphangiectasia, and any issue that alters the flow of lymph through the thoracic duct. The prognosis is guarded and many cases are found to have undiagnosed neoplasia. This connection makes it appropriate to address these cases as Dedifferentiation Phase homotoxicoses if they fail to respond to traditional therapies.

Appropriate homotoxicology formulas
There are no known published case reports or studies of successful handling of chylothorax in veterinary patients with homotoxicology. Basic homotoxicology phase theory should guide practitioners wishing to use such therapies in their practice. Palmquist (2006) was recently successful in handling a case of chylothorax which initially presented with no signs of other concurrent illness. This patient resolved its thoracic fluid accumulation, but ultimately developed pancreatic carcinoma and was euthanized a few months later.

Abropernol: Contains Abrotanum, which can be useful in chronic pleurisy with effusion and other exudative processes, including the after effects of chest surgery for hydrothorax or empyema. Difficult respiration and a dry, persistent cough, plus a sensitivity to cold air, are characteristic of this remedy. Nitricum acidum is also included for mucosal and respiratory conditions (Reckeweg 2002).

Aesculus compositum: A peripheral circulatory remedy that contains Colchicum, which, according to Heinigke, acts upon individual areas of the mucosa and the serous membranes (pleura, peritoneum, and pericardium), and the muscle fibers (especially of the intercostal muscles and the diaphragm), where inflammatory processes predominate. It is thus useful in endocarditis and edema (pleura, pericardium, peritoneum) with effusions into body cavities (Reckweg 2002). Colchicum compositum S. is a remedy that is not available in the U.S. but can be obtained from Europe. This remedy is also common to *Ginseng compositum* (see below).

Antimonium arsenicosum: A single remedy with excellent properties for this type of condition. It has indications for bronchiolitis with weakness of the heart and symptoms of dyspnea, cyanosis, and capillary congestion. It has been used for pulmonary emphysema, pulmonary edema, and bronchial asthma with circulatory weakness and myocarditis. A strong indication for this remedy is extreme dyspnea, and effusion, which occurs in pleurisy and pericarditis (Reckeweg 2002). The remedy can be ordered from Europe.

Apis homaccord: Used for mobilizing fluid accumulations and for edema, by way of Apis mellifica (bee venom). Also indicated for pleural effusions and ascites, diseases of the serosa, edematous swellings with formations that resemble water-filled sacs, and infiltration of the cellular tissues (Reckeweg 2002). Also contains Scilla for laryngeal and bronchial catarrhs with difficult expectoration, pleurisy with effusion, and edema in heart and kidney disease (Reckeweg 2002). This remedy also contains Antimonium tartaricum and has strong indications for inflammations of the lower respiratory passages with circulatory insufficiency, accumulation of mucus on the chest with rales and inability to raise the mucus, pneumonia and pulmonary catarrhs, and consolidation of the lungs persisting after the use of antibiotics (Reckeweg 2002).

Cor compositum: Contains many remedies that are useful for pulmonary and cardiac complaints, and supports the strained cardiovascular system. The pulmonary remedies include Arsenicum album, Naja, Carbo vegetalis, Kali carbonicum, and Ranunculus, for shortness of breath, chest constriction, pleurisy with serous effusion, and consequent adhesions and diseases of the parietal pleura (Reckeweg 2002).

Ginseng compositum: Has several indications in the pulmonary sphere and is a good regulating agent for accompanying exhaustion. It contains Colchicum, Galium aparine, Kreosotum, Natrum oxalaceticum, and Sulfur, which figures heavily into the cellular respiration cycles and in deep diseases, particularly with retoxic damage.

Hepar compositum: Contains several useful remedies for the disposition of toxins and edema, including Calcium carbonicum or effusions. The functioning of the lymphatic system is generally disturbed in the Calcium carbonicum patient. Carduus marianus has indications for coughing and congestive states of the pleura and peritoneum. Chelidonium is used for inflammation of the respiratory organ and pleuritic conditions. Cynara scolymus has tonic, resolvent, and diuretic action by way of an enzyme, which converts insulin into levulose. This is a deep-acting, effective liver remedy and is useful in edema to stimulate the detoxifying function of the liver (Reckeweg 2002).

Lymphomyosot: Lymphatic drainage.

Mucosa compositum: Broad support of mucosal elements throughout the body and useful in Degeneration Phase disorders.

Placenta compositum: Assists in healing of vessels; contains stem cell components.

Tonsilla compositum: in Traditional Chinese Medicine the spleen helps hold fluids in, which makes *Tonsilla compositum* (Spleen suis) a viable item for experimentation. Response was noted in one unpublished clinical case with this remedy (Palmquist 2006). It is indicated in Dedifferentiation and Impregnation phases.

Traumeel S: Indicated in all potentially traumatic cases and as an initial agent for many other conditions. May function through its nonsteroidal anti-inflammatory actions in all phases of homotoxicosis per the Six-Phase Table of Homotoxicology. Indicated in nonresponsive cases as a therapy that addresses regulation rigidity.

Ubichinon compositum: Contains Anthracinon, which has strong indications in affections of the lungs, pleurisy, pneumonia, and respiratory illness, where there is usually effusion (Reckeweg 2002).

Authors' suggested protocols

Nutrition
Cardiac and lymph support formulas: 1 tablet for every pounds of body weight BID.

Lecithin/phosphatidyl choline: One-fourth teaspoon for every 25 pounds of body weight BID.

Betathyme: 1 capsule for every 35 pounds of body weight BID, (maximum 2 capsules BID). **Alternative Choice**: Moducare—follow manufacturer's directions.

Vitamin A: 2,500 IU for every 35 pounds of body weight SID.

Vitamin E: 50 IU for every 20 pounds of body weight SID.

Chinese herbal medicine/acupuncture
Formula H61 chylothorax: 1 capsule per 10 to 20 pounds twice daily, depending upon severity. It may still be necessary to drain the thoracic fluid of some animals periodically, however the frequency of drainage should be lower. In addition to the herbs discussed above, H61 contains aurantium (Zhi qiao), benincasa seed (Dong gua ren), coix (Yi yi ren), phragmites (Lu gen), talc (Hua shi), and trichosanthes (Gua lou).

Homotoxicology (Dose 10 drops for 50-pound dog PO; 5 drops for small dog or cat PO)

Select the symptom remedy or remedies that best match the case and then select the Detoxification formula which is applicable based upon the case's location on the Six-Phase Table of Homotoxicology.

Usage is in addition to proper medical care (also see cancer, chapters 31 through 34).

Symptom formula: Because every case of chylothorax is caused by differing pathogenesis, no protocol can address this adequately, but consider starting by mixing the following agents together and giving orally BID for 5 to 7 days: *Traumeel S, Abropernol, Aesculus compositum, Lymphomyosot, Apis* and *Ginseng compositum.*

Tonsilla compositum: 1 to 3 times weekly.

Cor compositum: 1 to 3 times weekly.

Deep detoxification formula: *Thyroidea compositum, Hepar compositum, Solidago compositum, Ubichinon compositum, Coenzyme compositum, Testes compositum* OR *Ovarium compositum* mixed together and given orally every 2 to 3 days.

Product sources

Nutrition

Cardiac and Lymph support formulas: Animal Nutrition Technologies. **Alternatives:** Formula CV—Rx Vitamins for Pets, Cardiac Support Formula—Standard Process Veterinary Formulas, Cardio-Strength—Vetri Science Laboratories, Bio-Cardio—Thorne Veterinary Products.

Lecithin/phosphatidyl choline: Designs for Health

Betathyme: Best for Your Pets, Moducare—Thorne Veterinary Products

Vitamin A: Over the counter

Vitamin E: Over the counter

Chinese herbal medicine

H61 Chylothorax: Natural Solutions, Inc.

Homotoxicology remedies

BHI/Heel Corporation

REFERENCES

Western medicine references

Birchard SJ, Smeak DD, McLoughlin MA. Treatment of idiopathic chylothorax in dogs and cats. *J Am Vet Med Assoc* 1998;212:652–657.

Breznock EM. Management of chylothorax: Aggressive medical and surgical approach. *Vet Med Report* 1987;1:380,382–384.

Fossum TW. In: Tilley L, Smith F. The 5-Minute Veterinary Consult: Canine and Feline, 2003, Blackwell Publishing.

Fossum TW, Birchard SJ, Jacobs RM. Chylothorax in thirty-four dogs. *J Am Vet Med Assoc* 1986;188:1315–1318.

Fossum TW, Forrester SD, Swenson CL, Miller MW, Cohen ND, Boothe HW, Birchard SJ. Chylothorax in cats: 37 cases (1969–1989). *J Am Vet Med Assoc* 1991;198:672–678.

Fossum TW, Miller MW, Rogers KS, et al. Chylothorax associated with right-sided heart failure in 5 cats. *J Am Vet Med Assoc* 1994;204:84–89.

Fossum T. Chylothorax in cats: Is there a role for surgery? *J Feline Med Surg*, 2001;3: pp 73–79.

Fossum TW. The characteristics and treatments of feline chylothorax. *Comp on Cont Ed Sept* 1998;914–928.

Kerpsack SJ, McLoughlin MA, Birchard SJ, et al. Evaluation of mesenteric lymphangiography and thoracic duct ligation in cats with chylothorax: 19 cases (1987–1992). *J Am Vet Med Assoc* 1994;205:711–715.

Meadows RL, MacWilliams PS. Chylous effusions revisited. *Vet Clin Pathol* 1994;23:54–62.

Thompson MS, Cohn LA, Jordan RC. Use of rutin for medical management of idiopathic chylothorax in four cats. *J Am Vet Med Assoc* 1999;15:345–348.

Nutrition references

Bouic PJD, et al. Beta-sitosterol and beta-sitosterol glucoside stimulate human peripheral blood lymphocyte proliferation: Implications for their use as an immunomodulatory vitamin combination. *International Journal of Immunopharmacology* 1996;18:693–700.

Brook JG, Linn S, Aviram M. Dietary soya lecithin decreases plasma triglyceride levels and inhibits collagen- and ADP-induced platelet aggregation. *Biochem Med Metab Biol* 1986;35:31–9.

Gupta MB, Nath R, Srivastava N, et al. Anti-inflammatory and antipyretic activities of β-sitosterol. *Planta Medica* 1980; 39:157–163.

Halliwell B. Free Radicals and Antioxidants: a Personal View. *Nutr. Rev.*, 1994;52:253.

Myers CE, et al. Effect of Tocopherol and Selenium on Defenses Against Reactive Oxygen Species and their Effect on Radiation Sensitivity. *Annals of the N.Y. Acad. of Sci.*, 393:1982;419–425.

Spilburg CA, Goldberg AC, McGill JB, Stenson WF, Racette SB, Bateman J, McPherson TB, Ostlund RE Jr. Fat-free foods supplemented with soy stanol-lecithin powder reduce cholesterol absorption and LDL cholesterol. *J Am Diet Assoc* 2003; 103:577–581.

Traber MG. Does vitamin E decrease heart attack risk? Summary and implications with respect to dietary recommendations. *J Nutr.* 2001;131(2):395S–397S.

Traber MG, Vitamin E. In: Shils M, Olson JA, Shike M, Ross AC, eds. Nutrition in Health and Disease. 9th ed. Baltimore: Williams and Wilkins; 1999;347–362.

Chinese herbal medicine/acupuncture references

Chang Yong Zhong Yao Cheng Fen Yu Yao Li Shou Ce (A Handbook of the Composition and Pharmacology of Common Chinese Drugs), 1994;1488;1491.

Dilinuer Taji, et al. Xing Ren's effect on serum SOD and MDA levels in quails of experimental hyperlipidemia. *Journal of Xinjiang University of Medicine.* 1999;22(3):178–179.

Lu Ding, et al. *Journal of China Medical Academy*. 1987;9(6): 433.

Lu Ding, et al. *Journal of China Medical Academy*. 1988;10(4): 294.

Ren Min Wei Sheng Chu Ban She (*Journal of People's Public Health*), 1983;327.

Zhong Cao Yao Xue (*Study of Chinese Herbal Medicine*), 1976;411.

Zhong Yao Xue (*Chinese Herbology*), 1988;103:106.

Zhong Yao Yao Li Yu Ying Yong (*Pharmacology and Applications of Chinese Herbs*); 1983;866.

Zhong Yao Zhi (*Chinese Herbology Journal*), 1984;625.

Homotoxicology references

Palmquist R. A case of chylothorax treated integratively using rutin, periodic thoracocentesis, and homotoxicology. 2006. Unpublished data on file.

Reckeweg H. Homoeopathia Antihomotoxica Materia Medica, 4th edition. Aurelia-Verlag GMBH, Baden-Baden, 2002. pp. 115–6, 136–138, 137–39, 141–2, 195–6, 213, 227, 250, 270, 508, 525, 566–7.

Thompson M, Cohn L, Jordan R. Use of rutin for medical management of idiopathic chylothorax in four cats. *J Am Vet Med Assoc*. 215: pp 345–348, 1999.

HEMOBARTONELLA/FELINE INFECTIOUS ANEMIA/FELINE HEMOTROPIC MYCOPLASMOSIS

Definition and cause

Hemobatonella felis, recently renamed *Mycoplasma haemophilus*, is a parasitic organism which resides on the surface of the red blood cell. Infection is thought to occur from exposure to bloodsucking parasites such as fleas and ticks. Once the organism gains access to the bloodstream it attaches to red blood cells, rapidly reproduces, and feeds upon the substrate of the blood. The host antibody is produced and directed against the organism and becomes deposited on the red blood cell membrane. The reticuloendothelial elements of the spleen and liver phagocytize sections of the red blood cell membrane, leading to a form of hemolytic anemia. Immunosuppression by agents such as FeLV and FIV make clinical disease more likely, but normal cats can be infected as well. Cats may be diagnosed by direct observation of the parasite, but such observation can be difficult and the development of PCR testing specific for this agent has greatly assisted veterinarians in accurate diagnosis (Carney 1993, Eberhardt 2006).

Medical therapy rationale, drug(s) of choice, and nutritional recommendations

Treatment involves an antibiotic (usually doxycycline or a quinolone) for 3 weeks. Hemolytic anemic cats are usually given immunosuppressive doses of corticosteroid, such as prednisone, so that the immune-mediated hemolysis is decreased sufficiently for the patient to recover. A blood transfusion may be required (Greene 1998).

Anticipated prognosis

Prognosis if fair for most cats that are diagnosed early and properly treated. Ectoparasite control is recommended (Greene 1998).

Integrative veterinary therapies

Integrating nutrition and medicinal herbal and biological therapies can help counteract the side effects of medications designed to destroy the parasite and suppress the immune system. These therapies also support immune function and red blood cell regeneration.

Nutrition
General considerations/rationale
Nutritional support supplies the nutrients required for the production of new red blood cells. In addition, immune system organs receive nutrient support to help balance the immune response.

Appropriate nutrients
Nutritional/gland therapy: Bone marrow, liver, adrenal, thymus, and spleen supply the intrinsic nutrients to support these organs and produce new red blood cells. The most bioavailable source of iron is the liver. Comparing the absorption rate of inorganic iron (for example, ferrous sulfate versus heme-iron), the latter is 30 times more effective. The best source of heme-iron is concentrated liver extract (Frykman 1994). Liver is also a superior source of vitamin B_{12} and folic acid.

Vitamin B_{12}: Essential for maintaining the proper levels of red blood cells. Deficiencies of vitamin B_{12} are associated with anemia and decreased immune function. Supplementation with vitamin B_{12} often addresses the condition (Berlin 1978, Kondo 1998, Lederle 1991).

Folic acid: A B vitamin that is required for organized cellular division. Folic acid is integral in the synthesis of both DNA and RNA and therefore affects the genetic modeling of the body. Folic acid deficiencies affect bone marrow cell division and can lead to macrocytic anemia with fewer but larger red blood cells (Food Nutrition Board 1998).

Chinese herbal medicine/acupuncture
General considerations/rationale
Hemobartonella is a disorder caused by parasites. It leads to Qi, Blood, and Yin deficiency in the Kidney and Spleen.

Author's interpretation

Both schools of thought consider hemobartonella to be a parasitic disease. The Kidney is the main immune organ in TCM theory. If the Kidney is deficient, it is hard for the body to eliminate the parasite. The Spleen produces the Blood, so if the Spleen is deficient, anemia may result, leading to weakness, a manifestation of Qi deficiency. Treatment is aimed at eliminating the organism and treating secondary effects such as anemia and pyrexia.

Appropriate Chinese herbs

Angelica root (Dan gui): Increases phagocytic activity of macrophages (Zhong Hua Yi Xue Za Zhi 1978) and has some antibiotic effects (Hou Xue Hua Yu Yan Jia 1981). It may help clear the organism.

Astragalus (Huang qi): Has antibiotic activity (Zhong Yao Zhi 1994) and may help clear infection. It is also an immunostimulant. Astragalus contains astragalan, which increases phagocytic activity of macrophages and the production of antibodies (Jiao 1999), which may help the body clear the infection.

Atractyloides (Cang zhu): Has shown efficacy against some bacteria (Zhong Yao Xue 1998). It is possible that atractyloides may help eliminate the organism.

Bupleurum (Chai hu): Stimulates both humoral and cellular immunity in mice (Shang Hai Yi Ke Da Xue Xue Bao 1986). It also has antibiotic effect (Zhong Yao Xue 1988), which may inhibit the microorganism.

Codonopsis (Dang shen): Increases the hematocrit (Zhong Yao Xue 1998) and stimulates the immune system. It not only increases the number of leukocytes, but was shown to counteract the reduction in the white blood cell count induced by hydrocortisone (Huang 1994). This may indicate that it can be used with prednisone to support an immune system yet prevent autoimmune destruction of the red blood cells.

Coptis (Huang lian): Reduces fevers (Zhong Guo Bing Li Sheng Li Za Zhi 1991). In vitro experiments have shown that coptis has antibacterial properties (Chen 1996).

Dandelion (Pu gong ying): Has antibiotic properties (Zhong Yi Yao Xue Bao 1991) and is an immunostimulant (Zhong Yao Xue 1988). It may help the body clear the infection.

Forsythia fruit (Lian qiao): Inhibits a variety of bacteria and has antipyretic effects (Ma 1982).

Honeysuckle (Jin yin hua): Contains chlorogenic acid and isochlorogenic acid, which have antibacterial properties (Xin Yi Xue 1975, Jiang Xi Xin Yi Yao 1960). It also has antipyretic effects (Shan Xi Yi Kan 1960).

Licorice (Gan cao): Contains glycyrrhizin and glycyrrhetinic acid. These compounds have approximately 10% of the corticosteroid activity of cortisone (Zhong Cao Yao 1991) and may help decrease immune-mediated destruction of red blood cells. Licorice also has antibiotic properties (Zhong Yao Zhi 1993).

Phellodendron bark (Huang bai): Has antibiotic efficacy (Zhong Yao Xue 1998, Zhong Yao Da Ci Dien 1977).

Poria (fu ling): Has antibacterial effects (Nanjing College of Pharmacy 1976). Poria contains pachman, which enhances the phagocytic ability of macrophages (Lu 1990).

Scrophularia (Xuan shen): Inhibits various bacteria and reduces fevers (Zhong Yao Yao Li Yu Ying Yong 1983).

Scutellaria (Huang qin): Contains biacalin, which has antibiotic activity (Zhong Yao Xue 1988). Both biacalin and another compound found in scutellaria, biacalein, suppress inflammation (Kubo 1984). Scutellaria enhances cellular immunity (Pan 1991) and has antipyretic effects (Xu 1999).

Homotoxicology
General considerations/rationale

This is an infectious disease and it progresses rapidly from Inflammation phase (phagocytosis and immune processing by macrophages and antibody production) to Deposition phase (red blood cell attachment) to Impregnation phase (antibody attachment), and becomes a Degeneration phase homotoxicosis upon cell destruction by the reticuloendothelial system. Bear in mind that the blood is considered to be an active connective tissue and so access into the blood is a matrix phase. There are no proven veterinary homotoxicology protocols that have evidence sufficient to recommend them over conventional therapy, which is indicated in all overt clinical cases. Treatment programs may be augmented with biological therapies aimed at improving immune status, eliminating organisms, supporting production of new red blood cells, and enhancing the removal of homotoxins and damaged tissue elements. Antihomotoxic drugs may also assist the patient's recovery by reducing iatrogenic damage caused by pharmaceutical agents such as tissue deposition, impaired intestinal mucosal health, altered flora, enzyme blockage, and mitochondrial injury.

Appropriate homotoxicology formulas

Also see Tick Borne Diseases in Chapter 18; Chapter 6, Autoimmune Diseases; and Chapter 11, Chronic Active Hepatitis. The following agents are theoretically indicated for this type of issue:

China homaccord: For exhaustion and collapse.

Coenzyme compositum: Metabolic support following antibiotic therapy and in Degeneration phase disorders.

Echinacea compositum: Inflammation and Impregnation phases. Supports the immune system and encourages elimination of the organism. An antihomotoxic antibiotic.

Ferrum homaccord: For anemia.

Galium-Heel: Assists in cases of anemia and in detoxification following antibiotic therapy.

Ginseng compositum: For collapse, weakness, and exhaustion.

Hepar compositum: Reversal of damage to the liver from hemolysis and anemia, as well as iatrogenic damage from pharmaceutical agents used to control the disease.

Lymphomyosot: Lymph drainage and immune support.

Solidago compositum: Support of urinary tissues in deep detoxification and in Deposition Phase regressive vicariations following this disease.

Thyroidea compositum: Hormonal support and deep matrix clearing.

Tonsilla compositum: Degeneration Phase cases to normalize immune function and support splenic, adrenal, hepatic, bone marrow, lymphoreticular, and hypothalamic defense systems.

Ubichinon compositum: Metabolic support following antibiotic therapy and in Degeneration Phase disorders.

Authors' suggested protocols

Nutrition
Blood, bone marrow, and immune support formulas: 1 tablet for every 25 pounds of body weight BID.

Energizing iron (liver extract plus iron): 1 capsule for every 25 pounds of body weight, maximum 4 capsules.

Vitamin B_{12}: 50 micrograms for every 25 pounds, maximum 200 micrograms.

Folic acid: 50 micrograms for every 35 pounds of body weight, maximum 200 micrograms.

Chinese herbal medicine/acupuncture
The author recommends the following formulation: astragalus (Huang qi), 50 g; codonopsis (Dang shen), 50 g; atractyloides, 50 g; poria (Fu ling), 50 g; dandelion (Pu gong ying), 50 g; honeysuckle (Jin yin hua), 50 g; forsythia fruit (Lian qiao), 50 g; raw rehmannia (Sheng di huang), 40 g; scrophularia (Xuan shen), 40 g; phellodendron bark (Huang bai), 40 g; licorice (Gan cao), 40 g; angelica root, 40 g; coptis (Huang lian), 50 g; scutellaria (Huang qin), 50 g; bupleurum (Chai hu), 50 g; and lithospermum (Zi cao gen), 50 g (Cong 1986). It is dosed according to the manufacturer's recommendations.

Homotoxicology
Symptom formula: Tonsilla compositum given every 3 days during acute phase of hemolysis. Galium-heel and Lymphomyosot mixed together and given orally at 5 drops BID PO.

Deep detoxification formula: Galium-heel, Lymphomyosot, Hepar compositum, Solidago compositum, Thyroidea compositum, Coenzyme compositum, and Ubichinon compositum given every 3 days for 60 to 120 days following recovery.

Also see Autoimmune Diseases (Chapter 6) and Tick Borne Diseases (Chapter 18).

Product sources

Nutrition
Immune and blood bone marrow support formula: Animal Nutrition Technologies. **Alternative:** Immune system support—Standard Process Veterinary Formulas, Immugen—Thorne Veterinary Products.

Energizing iron: PhytoPharmica, Inc.
Folic acid: Progressive Labs.

Chinese herbal medicine
This formula can be mixed by the practitioner or ordered through Mayway Company.

Homotoxicology remedies
BHI/Heel Corporation

REFERENCES

Western medicine references
Carney HC, England JJ. Feline hemobartonellosis. *Vet Clin North Am Small Anim Pract* 1993;23:79–90.
Eberhardt J, Neal K, Shackelford T, Lappin M. Prevalence of selected infectious disease agents in cats from Arizona. *J Feline Med Surg.* 2006;Jan 26; [Epub ahead of print].
Greene CE. Infectious Diseases of the Dog and Cat. WB Saunders Company, Philadelphia, 1998, pp. 166–171.

Integrative veterinary medicine/nutrition references
Berlin R, Berlin H, Brante G, Pilbrant A. Vitamin B_{12} body stores during oral and parenteral treatment of pernicious anaemia. *Acta Med Scand* 1978;204:81–4.
Food and Nutrition Board, Institute of Medicine. Folic Acid. Dietary Reference Intakes: Thiamin, Riboflavin, Niacin, Vitamin B_6, Vitamin B_{12}, Pantothenic Acid, Biotin, and Choline. Washington, D.C.: National Academy Press; 1998;193–305.
Frykman E, Bystrom M, Jansson U, et al. Side effects of iron supplements in blood donors: superior tolerance of heme iron. *J Lab Clin Med* 1994;123:561–4.
Kondo H. Haematological effects of oral cobalamin preparations on patients with megaloblastic anaemia. *Acta Haematol* 1998;9:200–5.
Lederle FA. Oral cobalamin for pernicious anemia: medicine's best kept secret? *JAMA* 1991;265:94–5.

Chinese herbal medicine/acupuncture references
Chen Zhi Yun, et al. Experimental research on 100 Chinese herbs' antibacterial effects on helicobacteria. *Journal of Shizhen Medicinal Material Research.* 1996;7(1):25–26.

Cong, Yu. Handbook of new practical veterinary practitioners. Chinese Agricultural Science and Technology Press. Oct. 1986. p 987.

Hou Xue Hua Yu Yan Jia (*Research on Blood-Activating and Stasis-Eliminating Herbs*), 1981;335.

Huang Tai Kang, et al. Pharmacology research on Ming Dang Shen decoction solution and polysaccharides. *Journal of Chinese Patented Medicine*. 1994;16(7):31–33.

Jiang Xi Xin Yi Yao (*Jiangxi New Medicine and Herbology*), 1960;(1):34.

Jiao Yan, et al. *China Journal of Integrated Medicine*. 1999; 19(6):356–358.

Kubo M, Matsuda H, Tanaka M, Kimura Y, Okuda H, Higashino M, Tani T, Namba K, Arichi S. Studies on Scutellariae radix. VII. Anti-arthritic and anti-inflammatory actions of methanolic extract and flavonoid components from Scutellariae radix. *Chem Pharm Bull*, 1984;32(7):2724–9.

Lu Su Cheng, et al. *Journal of No. 1 Military Academy*. 1990;10(3):267.

Ma Zhen Ya. *Shannxi Journal of Traditional Chinese Medicine and Herbs*. 1982;(4):58.

Nanjing College of Pharmacy. Materia Medica, vol. 2. Jiangsu: People's Press; 1976.

Pan Ju Fen, et al. *Tianjin Journal of Medicine*. 1991;19(8): 468–470.

Shan Xi Yi Kan (*Shanxi Journal of Medicine*), 1960;(10):32.

Shang Hai Yi Ke Da Xue Xue Bao (*Journal of Shanghai University of Medicine*), 1986;13(1):20.

Xin Yi Xue (*New Medicine*), 1975;6(3):155.

Xu Gang, et al. *China Journal of TCM Science and Technology*. 1999;6(4):254–255.

Zhong Cao Yao (*Chinese Herbal Medicine*) 1991;22(10):452.

Zhong Guo Bing Li Sheng Li Za Zhi (*Chinese Journal of Pathology and Biology*), 1991;7(3):264.

Zhong Hua Yi Xue Za Zhi (*Chinese Journal of Medicine*), 1978;17(8):87.

Zhong Yao Da Ci Dien (*Dictionary of Chinese Herbs*), 1977:2032.

Zhong Yao Xue (*Chinese Herbology*). 1988;103:106.

Zhong Yao Xue (*Chinese Herbology*), 1988;137:140.

Zhong Yao Xue (*Chinese Herbology*), 1988;171:172.

Zhong Yao Xue (*Chinese Herbology*), 1998;144:146.

Zhong Yao Xue (*Chinese Herbology*), 1998;318:320.

Zhong Yao Xue (*Chinese Herbology*), 1998;739:741.

Zhong Yao Yao Li Du Li Yu Lin Chuan (*Pharmacology and Applications of Chinese Herbs*), 1983;370.

Zhong Yao Zhi (*Chinese Herbology Journal*), 1994;(12):648.

Zhong Yao Zhi (*Chinese Herbology Journal*), 1993;358.

Zhong Yi Yao Xue Bao (*Report of Chinese Medicine and Herbology*), 1991;(1):41.

HYPERLIPIDEMIA

Definition and cause

Hyperlipidemia can be primary (idiopathic) or secondary (diet, or to a disease such as liver disease, diabetes, Cushing's disease). The disease is found in cats and dogs. It is common in miniature Schnauzers, where it is often associated with hypertension. While post-prandial hyperlipidemia is normal, some animals have a difficult time metabolically clearing fat from the blood. The primary underlying cause is either genetic or secondary to another condition, which affects lipid metabolism such as diabetes mellitus (Armstrong 1989; Greco 2003, 1997).

Medical therapy rationale, drug(s) of choice, and nutritional recommendations

Treatment is to feed a fat-restricted diet (reducing the fat to the 7% to 10% range) such as Hills W/D or Science Diet Lite and re-check the blood in 4 to 5 weeks. This confirms dietary hyperlipedemia. Other recommended therapies include the addition of fish oil (omega-3-fatty-acid rich) along with vitamin B_2 (niacin) to help bring the triglyceride levels down. Medication such as Gemfibrozil (to increase levels of lipoprotein lipase) and cholesterol-lowering drugs have also been recommended (Armstrong 1989, Bauer 1995, Ford 1994, Greco 2003, Jones 1994).

Anticipated prognosis

Animals that respond to the dietary adjustments, including the addition of fish oils, have a much improved prognosis. The prognosis is less positive when elevated fat levels persist, primarily because of secondary disease complications such as diabetes, fatty liver, pancreatitis, and Cushing's disease.

Integrative veterinary therapies

The integrative approach closely follows the medical approach of dietary fat restriction, paying particular attention to ensure that sources of ingredients are biologically correct, in addition to being chemically correct. The recommended ingredients should be highly bio-available, contain lower levels of saturated fats, contain beneficial fiber, and produce lower levels of metabolic wastes.

Nutrition
General considerations/rationale
Nutritionally, the approach includes feeding a diet that is higher in protein and soluble and insoluble fiber, recommending food that is lower in saturated fats and higher in omega-3 and beneficial omega-6 fatty acids, a supplement program that contain support nutrients for intestinal and pancreatic digestion while protecting the liver from inflammation and fatty infiltration. With client compliance, the diet should contain higher levels of

fresh meat or poultry, more omega-3- and omega-6-rich vegetable oils, and fiber from vegetable or whole grain sources. Home-prepared raw or cooked foods are recommended (see Product Sources) (Goldstein 2005).

Appropriate nutrients

Nutritional/gland therapy: The liver, pancreas, and intestines are the key organs in the metabolic processes of digestion and assimilation. The supply of intrinsic nutrients and the control of free radical build-up help reduce cellular inflammation, which improves organ function and helps to prevent the body's infiltrative process and fat deposition.

Lecithin/phosphatidyl choline: Studies have shown that lecithin reduces trigylceride and cholesterol levels. Lecithin is an emulsifier of fats and helps to improve overall lipid metabolism (Brooks 1986, Spilburg 2003).

Enzymes: Pancreatic lipase is essential for lipid metabolism and assimilation. Enzyme deficiencies caused by organ underproduction or excessive dietary fats (especially saturated types) contribute to hyperlipedemia (Howell 1985).

Probiotics: The normal flora of the intestines is required for proper assimilation of food and nourishment of the body's cells (De Simone 1993, Smirnov 1993).

Oils: Many commercial dog and cat foods contain high levels of poultry by-product fat as the primary source of fatty acids. Levels of fat in many pet foods generally range from 8% to 20%. Poultry fat contains approximately 20% linoleic acid (omega-6) or about 2% to 3% of the total food (Goldstein 2000, 2005). Erasmus (1986) reports that there is about 30 times more omega-6 than omega-3 in chicken fat, equaling less than 1% omega-3 fatty acids. This imbalance can adversely affect lipid metabolism in general. Kendler (1987) reported that while both linoleic acid (LA) and gamma-linolenic acid (GLA) can be obtained from food, poor-quality foods can be low in essential fatty acids, leading to deficiencies.

L-carnitine: A lipotrophic agent known in human circles as a "fat buster." L-carnitine is required in the metabolism of fatty acids for the release of energy by the cells. Supplementing the diet with L-carnitine has a direct lowering effect on the blood trigylceride levels (Sachan 1984). In studies conducted by the Iams Company, the addition of carnitine to the diet of dogs was shown to reduce body weight by 6.4% compared to 1.8% without supplementation (Sunvold 1998). Similar research in cats suggests weight loss (Center 1998). Evangeliou (2003) showed that the addition of carintine to the diet helps to lower both cholesterol and triglyceride levels.

Vitamin E: A fat-soluble vitamin and is one of the body's main antioxidants, especially in its function of protecting lipids. As a potent antioxidant its primary function is the neutralization of free radicals and reduc-

tion of inflammation, particularly as it affects the oxidation and destruction of lipids (Traber 1999).

Chinese herbal medicine
General considerations/rationale
Based upon TCM theory, hyperlipidemia is a matter of Qi deficiency, Blood stagnation, and Phlegm and Damp accumulation.

Phlegm and Damp are thick liquid substances in the Western interpretation. Hyperlipidemia causes lipemic blood. Many people with hyperlipidemia feel heavy and fatigued. Some have shortness of breath due to arteriosclerosis. The plaques in the vessels are accumulations of Phlegm. The blood flow may be slow due to sludging when there are very high levels of lipids. This is described as Blood stagnation in Eastern terms. The Qi deficiency is manifested by fatigue.

Appropriate Chinese herbs
Alisma (Ze xie): Has several uses in cases of hyperlipidemia. It has been proven to lower blood cholesterol and triglyceride levels in humans. Half of the subjects in one study had a decrease of 10% or more (He 1981). In experiments on hamsters, alisma decreases the levels of total cholesterol and LDL-cholesterol in the serum. In addition, it protects the liver from lipidosis in animals that consume high-fat diets (Institute of Pharmacy 1976). This may help prevent the development of hepatic disease in patients with chronic hyperlipidemia.

Cinnamon (Gui zhi): Dilates blood vessels and promotes blood circulation (Zhong Yao Xue 1998).

Crataegus (Shan zha): Was used experimentally in quails with high blood cholesterol levels. Blood cholesterol levels were decreased by 34% to 63%. In addition, it decreased the formation of arterial atheromatous plaque in the quails, preventing the development of experimental atherosclerosis (Chu 1988). It was also shown to have the potential to prevent the deposition of lipids on vascular walls in rats (Cai 2000).

Fleece flower root (He sou wu): Normalizes the blood lipid profile. It has been shown to increase the levels of HDL while simultaneously lowering the total cholesterol and triglyceride levels (Zhong Cao Yao 1991). In humans with high cholesterol, 5 g/kg can lower cholesterol to the normal level. In one experiment taking fleece flower root for 1 week lowered the total cholesterol level in the treatment group to 88 ± 11 mg. Untreated control subjects had blood levels of 188 ± 12 mg (Zhao 1984, Mei 1979).

Pinellia (Ban xia): Can prevent the development of dietary hyperlipidemia in rats. It lowers both total cholesterol and LDL levels (Hong 1995).

Pueraria (Ge gen): Contains daidzein, formononetin, and genistein. These compounds lower blood lipids (Modern TCM Pharmacology 1997).

Homotoxicology
General considerations/rationale

Hyperlipidemia has many causes; in some breeds, a constitutional predisposition exists. Most hyperlipidemias benefit from a low-fat diet with higher fiber levels. Weight loss and exercise may also help. Support of liver function is recommended for this Deposition phase disorder and monitoring appropriate laboratory data is recommended (Reckeweg 2000).

Appropriate homotoxicology formulas

No studies document the use of homotoxicology for hyperlipidemia in veterinary medicine. Extrapolation from human practice is appropriate, but should be considered as experimental. Useful remedies may include:

Aesculus compositum: Regulates peripheral blood flow and vascular health, improves cerebral blood flow, tones the arterial system, and eliminates homotoxins from the lymph system (*Baptisia*). Hamamelis assists in venous stasis and venous hemorrhages. Ateria suis supports repair of structures.

Barijodeel: In arteriosclerosis, and lymphatism, for altered cerebral blood flow. This is a major remedy with common use in human geriatric patients. Because arteriosclerosis is not as severe an issue for animals, *Aesculus compositum* may prove stronger in assisting veterinary patients.

Cerebrum compositum: Acts on the central nervous system and after stroke.

Cor compositum: Reinforces cardiac functions.

Berberis homaccord: Drains the kidney and lower urinary tract in prostatic disease, supports the adrenal in stressful conditions and support of liver. Use intermittently in cases with pigmentation in the axillary region.

Galium-Heel: Provides cellular detoxification, renal support, and anticancer effects. Indicated for vaccine reactions and allergies, and is a phase remedy for Deposition Phase disorders (Palmquist 2006).

Hepeel: Used intermittently for liver support, drainage, and detoxification. May be combined with *Coenzyme compositum* for powerful action on the liver and can be useful in allergy therapy as well.

Hepar compositum: Used for liver detoxification and support, metabolic support.

Lymphomyosot: Provides lymph drainage, and is a phase remedy for Deposition phase disorders.

Nux vomica homaccord: Acts on hepatic and gastrointestinal function.

Placenta compositum: Provides peripheral vascular support and helps with cold extremities, and is a phase remedy for Deposition phase disorders.

Psorinoheel: A constitutional remedy for cases that may have genetic causes, and a phase remedy for Deposition phase disorders.

Solidago compositum: Provides urogenital support, and is a phase remedy for Deposition phase disorders.

Veratrum homaccord: Used in cases of collapse, weakness, and/or diarrhea.

Authors' suggested protocols
Nutrition

Pancreatic and intestinal support formulas: 1 tablet for 25 lbs of body weight BID.

Megaliptrophic: 1 capsule for every 20 pounds of body weight; give with food.

L-Carnitine: 100 mg for every 20 pounds of body weight; give with food.

Eskimo fish oil: One-half to 1 teaspoon per meal for cats. 1 teaspoon for every 35 pounds of body weight per meal for dogs.

Lecithin/phosphatidyl choline: One-fourth teaspoon for every 25 pounds of body weight BID.

Probiotic MPF: $\frac{1}{2}$ capsule per 25 pounds of body weight with food.

Chinese herbal medicine-3

Formula lipidemia: 1 capsule per 10 to 20 pounds twice daily to start. The dose is modified based upon serial blood monitoring.

In addition the herbs listed above, lipidemia also contains astragalus (Huang qi), notoginseng (San qi), poria (Fu ling), rhubarb (Da huang), salvia (Dan shen), trichosanthes (Gua lou), and white atractylodes (Bai zhu).

Homotoxicology (Dose: 10 drops PO for 50-pound dog, 5 drops PO for small dog or cat)

Symptom remedy: *Nux vomica homaccord, Aesculus compositum, Lymphomyosot,* and *Barijodeel* mixed together and given BID to TID.

Detoxification remedy: *Galium-Heel, Hepar compositum,* and *Solidago compositum* mixed together and given twice weekly PO. *Hepeel* and *BHI-Enzyme:* 1 tablet each evening for general liver support.

Product sources
Nutrition

Pancreatic and intestinal support formulas: Animal Nutrition Technologies. **Alternatives:** Enteric Support—Standard Process Veterinary Formulas, NutriGest—Rx Vitamins for Pets.

Megaliptrophic: Best For Your Pet.

L-Carnitine: Over the counter.

Eskimo fish oil: Tyler Encapsulations.

Lecithin/phosphatidyl choline: Designs for Health.

Probiotic MPF: Progressive Labs.

Chinese herbal medicine
Formula Lipidemia: Natural Solutions, Inc.

Homotoxicology remedies
BHI/Heel Corporation

REFERENCES

Western medicine references
Armstrong PJ, Ford RB. Hyperlipidemia. In: Kirk RW, ed. Current veterinary therapy X. Philadelphia: Saunders, 1989;1046–1050.
Bauer JE. Evaluation and dietary considerations in idiopathic hyperlipidemia in dogs. *J Am Vet Med Assoc.* June 1995; 206(11):1684–8.
Ford R. Canine hyperlipidemias. In: Ettinger ST, Feldman EC, eds. Textbooks of veterinary internal medicine. 4th ed. Philadelphia: Saunders 1994;1414–1418.
Greco DS. Lipids, Hyperlipidemia. In: Tilley L, Smith F. The 5-Minute Veterinary Consult: Canine and Feline, Blackwell Publishing, 2003.
Jones B. Feline hyperlipidemias. In: Ettinger ST, Feldman EC, eds. Textbook of veterinary internal medicine. 4th ed. Philadelphia: Saunders, 1994;1410–1413.

Nutrition references
Brook JG, Linn S, Aviram M. Dietary soya lecithin decreases plasma triglyceride levels and inhibits collagen- and ADP-induced platelet aggregation. *Biochem Med Metab Biol* 1986;35:31–9.
Center SA. Safe weight loss in cats. In: Reinhart GA, Carey DP, eds. Recent Advances in Canine and Feline Nutrition Volume II: 1998 Iams Nutrition Symposium Proceedings. Wilmington, OH: Orange Frazer Press, 1998;165–181.
De Simone C, Vesely R, Bianchi SB, et al. The role of probiotics in modulation of the immune system in man and in animals. *Int J Immunother* 1993;9:23–8.
Erasmus U. Fats and Oils. Vancouver, BC: Alive Books, 1986.
Evangeliou A, Vlassopoulos D. Carnitine metabolism and deficit—when supplementation is necessary? *Curr Pharm Biotechnol.* 2003 Jun;4(3):211–9.
Goldstein RS. The BNA Veterinary Handbook: A Working Manual for Veterinarians, BioNutritional Diagnostics, 2000.
Goldstein RS, Goldstein SJ. The Goldsteins' Wellness and Longevity Program, Neptune City, NJ: TFH Publication, 2005.
Howell E. Enzyme Nutrition, The Food Enzyme Concept. Garden City, NY. Avery Publ., 1985.
Kendler B. Gamma Linolenic Acid: Physiological Effects and Potential Medical Applications. *J. of Appl. Nutr,* 1987;39:79.
Sachan DH, Rhew TH, Ruark RA. Ameliorating Effects of Carnitine and its Precursors on Alcohol-Induced Fatty Liver. *Amer. J. of Clin. Nut.,* 1984;38:738–744.
Smirnov VV, Reznik SR, V'iunitskaia VA, et al. The current concepts of the mechanisms of the therapeutic prophylactic action of probiotics from bacteria in the genus bacillus. *Mikrobiolohichnyi Zhurnal* 1993;55:92–112.
Spilburg CA, Goldberg AC, McGill JB, Stenson WF, Racette SB, Bateman J, McPherson TB, Ostlund RE Jr. Fat-free foods supplemented with soy stanol-lecithin powder reduce choles-

terol absorption and LDL cholesterol. *J Am Diet Assoc* 2003; 103:577–81.
Sunvold GD, Tetrick MA, Davenport GM, Bouchard GF. Carnitine supplementation promotes weight loss and decreased adiposity in the canine. Proceedings of the XXIII World Small Animal Veterinary Association. October, 1998, p.746.
Traber MG. Does vitamin E decrease heart attack risk? Summary and implications with respect to dietary recommendations. *J Nutr.* 2001;131(2):395S–397S.

Chinese herbal medicine references
Cai Lei, et al. Research on the therapeutic effects and mechanisms of exercise and Shan Zha on rat hyperlipidemia. *China Journal of Sports Medicine.* 2000;19(1):29–32.
Chu Yan Fang, et al. Effects of Shan Zha core alcohol soluble extracts on quail blood serum and cholesterol level on artery walls. *Journal of Chinese Materia Medica.* 1988;19(1): 25–27.
He XY. Effects of alisma Plantago 1 on hyperlipidemia, arteriosclerosis and fatty liver. *Chinese Journal of Modern Developments in Traditional Medicine.* 1(2):114–7, Oct. 1981.
Hong Xing Qiu, et al. *Journal of Zhejiang College of TCM.* 1995;19(2):28–29.
Institute of Pharmacy. People's Experiment Hospital of Zhejiang. Chinese Materia Medica Bulletin. 1976;(7):26–30.
Mei Mei Zhen, et al. *Journal of Pharmacy.* 1979;14(1):8.
Modern TCM Pharmacology. Tianjin: Science and Technology Press; 1997.
Zhao Bin, et al. *Journal of Chinese Patent Medicine Research.* 1984;(10):6.
Zhong Cao Yao (*Chinese Herbal Medicine*). 1991;22(3):117.
Zhong Yao Xue (*Chinese Herbology*) 1998;65:67.

Homotoxicology references
Palmquist R. A case of chylothorax treated integratively using rutin, periodic thoracocentesis, and homotoxicology. 2006. Unpublished data on file.
Reckeweg H. Biotherapeutic Index: Ordinatio Antihomotoxica et Materia Medica, 5th ed. 2000. Baden-Baden, Germany: Biologische Heilmittel Heel GMBH, p 299.

LEUKOPENIA

Definition and cause

Leukopenia simply refers to a reduction in the number of circulating leukocytes; this descriptive term is not a diagnosis. The clinician should do appropriate testing to determine the underlying cause of the reduced leukocyte numbers and address that specific cause wherever possible. Generally speaking, reduced white blood cell numbers come from increased loss, decreased production, or a combination of these circumstances. Causes include corticosteroid administration (secondary effect), systemic viral infection such as parvovirus in dogs and FeLV, FIP, or panleukopenia in cats; as well as neoplasia. Leukopenia is often seen in lymphoma (Aiello, Merck Manual 2006).

Medical therapy rationale, drug(s) of choice, and nutritional recommendations

Medical therapy depends on the determination of and subsequent addressing of the underlying cause or causes. For example, leukocytosis secondary to corticosteroid administration requires stopping the medication. Leukocytosis secondary to parvo, panleukopenia, or FeLV requires intensive medical therapies.

Anticipated prognosis

The prognosis depends upon finding and addressing the underlying cause.

Integrative veterinary therapies

Once the underlying cause has been determined, integrative therapies can be selected as an adjunct to medical therapy or as a stand-alone treatment plan, depending upon the diagnosis and the choice of the clinician. The use of nutraceuticals, medicinal herbs, and combination homeopathics that have regenerative and nutritive effects on the organs of white blood cell can help resolve the leukopenia.

General considerations/rationale

Addressing leukopenia nutritionally requires a determination of the underlying cause(s). Nutritional therapies are directed at nourishing the bone marrow and spleen, supplying the vital nutrients required for production of white blood cells, and supporting the organs of the immune system such as the adrenal, thymus, and lymph glands.

Appropriate nutrients

Nutrition/glandular therapy: Bone marrow, adrenal, thymus and spleen add specific vital nutrients required by these organs for their metabolic and biochemical processes. If these organs are compromised secondary to a free-radical-induced process or a disease, the addition of dietary glandulars can help to neutralize an immune attack and reduce secondary inflammation (Goldstein 2000) (Also see also Gland Therapy in Chapter 2).

N,N-Dimethylglycine (DMG): Has been shown to support immune function and improve removal of toxins (Verdova 1965). DMG has immune-modulating ability and has been clinically proven to increase both tumor necrosis factor (TNF) and interferon production (Graber 1986, Kendall 2003, Reap 1990, Wang 1988).

Maitake mushrooms: Rich in beta-glucans, which help to support and enhance immune function and can stimulate the production of natural killer cells (NK) (Kodama 2003, Nanba 1987).

Chinese herbal medicine/acupuncture
General considerations/rationale

Leukopenia is due to Qi and Yin deficiency in the Spleen and Kidney. Heat and toxins build up and Qi and Blood stagnate. According to the author's interpretation, the Kidney controls the bones and marrow. If the Kidney is too weak (Qi deficiency) or lacks nourishment (Yin deficiency) it cannot nourish the marrow, and blood cell proliferation and maturation are disrupted. The Spleen is too deficient in Yin and Qi to send nutrients to the Kidney to correct this organ's insufficiencies. This closely reflects the Western idea of using iron and vitamin B supplements to treat anemia. Both Western and Eastern medicines recognize that proper nutrition is necessary for normal bone marrow function.

When the marrow is deficient, Heat and Toxins can build up. This is the Eastern description for the immunosuppression and secondary infections seen with bone marrow suppression. Qi and Blood stagnation cause pain. Some conditions causing leucopenia, i.e. neoplasia, can be quite painful. Treatment involves increasing the white blood cell count, preventing secondary infections during the leukopenic period, and treating the underlying cause of the leucopenia.

Appropriate Chinese herbs

Arisaema pulvis (Dan nan xing): Has anticancer properties (Zhong Yao Yao Li Yu Ying Yong 1983). It may treat neoplastic causes of leucopenia.

Astragalus (Huang qi): Enhances both the cellular and humoral immune system. It contains astragalan, which increases the phagocytic action of macrophages and increases antibody production (Jiao Yan 1999). This may help protect the body from secondary infections. Astragalus also promotes the production and maturation of leukocytes in the bone marrow (Nan Jing Zhong Yi Xue Yuan Xue Bao 1989).

Atractylodes (Bai zhu): Can increase the T helper count (Xu 1994). It also increases the weight of the thymus gland and the spleen (Tang 1998).

Barbat skullcap (Ban zhi lian): Has shown the ability to inhibit various bacteria (Sato 2000). It may treat underlying bacterial causes of leucopenia or prevent secondary infections. It also has antineoplastic properties (Ren Min Wei Sheng Chu Ban She 1988). It may treat neoplastic causes of neoplasia.

Burreed tuber (San leng): Has demonstrated antineoplastic effects (Zhong Yao Xue 1988).

Centipede (Wu gong): Has both antineoplastic and antibacterial properties (Chang Yong Zhong Yao Cheng Fen Yu Yao Li Shou Ce 1994). It may treat the underlying etiology of the leucopenia or prevent secondary infections.

Codonopsis (Dang shen): Has been shown to increase the weight of the spleen and thymus and raise the white blood cell count (Huang 1994).

Coix (Yi yi ren): Helps inhibit the growth of neoplastic cells and increases the phagocytic abilities of macrophages (Li 2000). It may help reverse immunosuppression and treat some of the causes or secondary pathogens involved in leucopenia.

Cornus (Shan zhu yu): Has antibacterial properties (Shang 1994). It may help treat underlying bacterial etiologies of leucopenia and prevent secondary bacterial complications.

Dioscorea (Shan yao): Stimulates both humoral and cellular immunity (Miao 1996). This may help prevent secondary pathogens from invading while the patient is immunosuppressed.

Forsythia (Lian qiao): Inhibits multiple strains of bacteria (Ma 1982). It contains rengynic acid, which has been shown to inhibit RSV in vitro (Zhang 2002). It may help to control viral and bacterial etiologies and prevent secondary invasion of pathogens.

Hornet's nest (Feng fang): Has anti-neoplastic properties (Li Li 1999). It may help treat leucopenia secondary to neoplasia.

Mastic (Ru xiang): Contains boswellic acids, which have anti-neoplastic effects (Shao 1998). It may help control neoplastic etiologies.

Oldenlandia (Bai hua she cao): Prevents the growth of cancer cells (Gupta 2004, Wong 1996). This may treat neoplastic causes of leucopenia.

Poria (Fu ling): Contains pachman, which has been shown to increase the phagocytic activity of macrophages (Lu 1990). This may help decrease the immunosuppression associated with leucopenia.

Prunella (Xia ku cao): Has demonstrated inhibitory effects against several bacteria and some dermatophytes (Zhong Cao Yao 1989).

Sage tangle (Kun bu): Contains iodine and therefore can kill a number of bacteria and viruses (Kong 1994).

Salvia (Dan shen): Has some anti-cancer effects (Li Xu Fen 1999). Salvia may be of use in neoplastic etiologies.

Sargassum (Hai Zao): Increases phagocytic activity of macrophages (Zhong Guo Yao Ke Da Xue Xue Bao 1988). It may help treat underlying infectious causes of the leucopenia or prevent secondary infections.

Scorpion (Quan xie): Has inhibitory effects on cancer cells (Jiang Su Yi Yao 1990).

Silkworm (Jiang can): Has been shown to inhibit the growth of bacteria (Zhong Yao Xue 1998).

White peony (Bai shao): Has shown efficacy against several bacteria and some dermatophytes (Xin Zhong Yi 1989). It may prevent secondary infections while the white blood cell count is low.

Wolfberry (Gou qi zi): Has been shown to prevent cyclophosphamide-induced leucopenia experimentally (Pu 1998). It promotes lymphocyte transformation and improves the phagocytic abilities of macrophages (Geng 1988).

Zedoaria (E zhu): Has antineoplastic activity (Xin Yi Yao Xue Za Zhi 1976).

Homotoxicology
General considerations/rationale
Homotoxicologists view leukopenia as a hemodermal pathology in the Impregnation or Degeneration phase.

Appropriate homotoxicology formulas
Because a wide variety of factors may be involved, the following list is only a superficial consideration of major remedies:

BHI-Echinacea PC: Supports the immune system in minor infections.

Aletris-Heel: Combination well suited for cases manifesting exhaustion, anemia, and metabolic fatigue. Contains Natrium muriaticum, and is recommended for drug-induced leukopenias (Bianchi 1995).

BHI-Infection: Immune supportive; also given for fever, inflammation.

BHI-Inflammation: Similar to a combination of *Traumeel* and *Echinacea compositum*, this remedy contains Staph and Strep nosodes for immune stimulation and direction. Useful for arthritis, fever, inflammation, acne, and minor injuries.

Coenzyme compositum: Provides metabolic support. A primary constituent in this condition is Cysteinum, a sulfydryl group (SH-group) containing factor of redox potentials (e.g. Glutathione). It is useful in retoxic and iatrogenic damage of all kinds, e.g. leukemia, pre-cancerous states, and neoplastic diseases (Reckeweg 2002).

Echinacea compositum: Functioning as a natural antibiotic and immune-supporting formula, this remedy is helpful in all cases of infection. It is particularly indicated in the Inflammation and Impregnation phases. *Echinacea angustfolia* is listed for pancytopenic conditions in the Degeneration phase (Bianchi 2005). Zinc is critical to immune function, according to a number of studies (Kirsteen, et al. 2001). Because Zincum metallicum is no longer available as an injeel in the United States, the remedies *Echinacea compositum* and *Testis compositum* are both sources of Zinc, which is critical because DNA makes RNA, which in turn makes proteins that further drive biological function. Trace minerals work as catalysts in enzyme complexes and alter reactions and stability of proteins. Zinc acts as an anti-oxidant, and in addition, studies have shown that Zinc must be present for lymphocyte maturation and is a lymphocyte mitogen. Additionally, zinc is a necessary co-factor in activation of serum thymic factor (Clark). Thymocytes undergo rapid apoptosis and changes in the susceptibility of cells to undergo apoptosis when high levels of exogenous zinc are provided, which may explain resistance of cells to certain toxic agents after exposure to various agents, including glucocorticoids, ionizing radiation, and environmental agents. Cellular zinc content is an important factor in the propensity of thymocytes to undergo apoptosis. Changes in the susceptibility of cells to undergo apoptosis when high levels of exogenous zinc are provided may explain the resistance of cells to certain toxic agents (Kirsteen 2001).

Engystol N: Increases white blood cell numbers. Commonly used in viral infections and allergies. Along with *Coenzyme compositum* and *Ubichinon compositum*, it has been recommended for agranulocytosis and bone marrow deficiencies. It also is used for iatrogenic damage to bone marrow due to antibiotics and for leukopenias in general (Bianchi 2005).

Euphorbium compositum: Due to its antiviral activity this remedy may assist in cases of leukopenia caused by to viral infection and replication.

Galium-heel: Cellular detoxification in anemia and leukopenia. It is immune supportive.

Glyoxal compositum: A cellular phase remedy directed at improving metabolism and cellular functioning by removal of homotoxin "polymers" that act to block enzyme systems.

Hepar compositum: Used to drain, detoxify, and repair liver tissue, and support pancreas and gastrointestinal tissues.

Lymphomyosot: Drains lymphatics and may reduce toxin levels at the site of pathology. It contains thyroxine, which provides immune and endocrine support.

Molybdan compositum: A trace mineral donor. Contains copper and molybdan, among many others. These trace minerals are involved in many biochemical processes such as cellular respiration, cellular use of oxygen, DNA and RNA reproduction, maintenance of cell membrane integrity, and sequestration of free radicals, which helps to maintain the integrity of membranes, reduces the risk of cancer, and slows the aging process (Chan 1998). It has been recommended for bone marrow deficiencies resulting in agranulocytosis (Bianchi 2005). Clients need to keep this particular medicine out of the reach of their pets and children because accidental ingestion can lead to toxicity. At normal dosing it is quite safe, but caution is indicated in allowing access to the product.

Solidago compositum: Provides renal support and detoxification.

Testis compositum: Contains factors for regeneration of blood and lymphoid tissue. It also contains factors for other metabolic dysfunctions, such as exhaustion issues, including: Zincum (see *Echinacea compositum*), Embryo

suis (a gland therapy source of stem cells and stem cell associated micromolecules), Glandula suprarenalis suis for adrenal dysfunction, and Ginseng for exhaustion. Cortisonum, as cortisone, can have immensely damaging effects on the production of immune cells, because it induces leukopenia, lymphopenia, eosinopenia, and thymic and adrenal atrophy (Committee for Veterinary Medical Products 1999). The effects of corticosterone and hydrocortisone on the thymus and the pituitary-adrenal axis have been studied. Short-term effects within 48 hours after 1 or 2 corticoid injections and late effects 7 days after a regimen of 4 corticoid injections were discerned, with an induction of leukopenia and monocytopenia being quantified from the parenteral administration of glucocorticoids (Van Dijk 1979).

Thyroidea compositum: Provides endocrine support and activation, as well as deep matrix drainage. Contains Thymus suis, a glandular extract of the thymus, which is intimately involved in the signaling pathways of leukocytes (Clark). The thymus involutes early in life, and corresponds to decline in function of the hypothalamic-pituitary-endocrine axis and cellular immune deficiencies of aging. The pituitary, pineal gland autonomic nervous system, thyroid, gonads, and adrenals all factor into thymic integrity and function. An important endocrine function of the thymus is to package zinc in zinc-thymulin for delivery to the periphery. There have been recent efforts to treat immune deficiency in aged and cancer-bearing patients (Hadden 1998). Listed in the spectrum of activity for Splen suis (also in *Tonsilla compositum*) are leukemia and anemia, as well as action for general revitalization and in weakness of old age in order to enhance the resistance to infection (Reckeweg 2002). It is recommended for agranulocytosis, particularly when due to a bone marrow deficit (Bianchi 1995). Medulla ossis suis (also in *Tonsilla compositum*) has indications in anemia, leukemia, agranulocytosis, and other iatrogenic conditions (Reckeweg 2002).

Tonsilla compositum: By virtue of its effect on bone marrow and blood development this remedy should be considered in all cases of leukopenia, especially those deeper homotoxicoses to the right of the Biological Division on the Six-Phase Table. It has deep acting effects on the endocrine system and central controls. Stem cell activity may stimulate repair or cellular activation.

Ubichinon compositum: Provides mitochondrial support of metabolism. In particular, help is sourced via para-Benzochinonum, which helps with regenerative action on cell respiration and also in cases of genetic mutations. It is indicated in all cellular phases, leukemia, neoplasm phases, and other conditions. It can have protective functions against viral infections, and is useful after damage to the spleen with changes in the blood composition. It can have a positive effect on all illnesses, which could be connected with auto-immune disease (Reckeweg 2002).

Authors suggested protocols

Nutrition
Immune support and blood bone marrow support formulas: 1 tablet for every 25 pounds of body weight BID.

Maitake DMG: 1 ml per 25 pounds of body weight BID.

Chinese herbal medicine/acupuncture
The authors recommend formula H98 Lymph "K" at a dose of 1 capsule per 10 to 20 pounds twice daily as needed. In some cases conventional drugs are given in conjunction with the herbs to increase their efficacy. In addition to the herbs mentioned above, H98 Lymph "K" also contains eupolyphaga (Tu bie cong), fritillaria (Bei mu), house lizard (Bi hu), myrrh (Mo yao), rehmannia (Shu di huang), Selaginellae doederleini (Shi shang bai), and Typhonium gigantium rhizome (Bai fu zi). These additional herbs help increase the efficacy of the formula.

Homotoxicology (Dose: 10 drops PO for 50-pound dog, 5 drops PO for small dog or cat)
Symptom formula In Phases 1 through 3: *Echinacea compositum, Engystol N* plus *Galium-Heel*, preferably as an autosanguis. The action of these are reinforced by activation of intermediary metabolism through administration of *Coenzyme compositum* and *Ubichinon compositum*. The entire therapy is complemented by the activation of the mesenchyme, an indispensable step of therapy made possible by application of the preparation *Lymphomyosot* (see detoxification formula below), rounded off by nosode therapy, such as *Psorinoheel. Molybdan compositum* and *Causticum compositum* may also be of value in refractory cases.

Detoxification formula in Phases 1 through 3: *Berberis homaccord, Nux homaccord,* and *Lymphomyosot* mixed together and given BID for 30 to 90 days.

Symptom formula in Phases 4 through 6: *Tonsilla compositum* every 3 days and *Echinacea compositum* daily until main infection has ceased. *Galium-heel* BID.

Deep detoxification formula in Phases 4 through 6: *Lymphomyosot, Hepar compositum, Thyroidea compositum, Solidago compositum, Coenzyme compositum,* and *Ubichinon compositum* mixed together and given every 3 days.

Product Sources

Nutrition
Immune and blood/bone marrow support formulas: Animal Nutrition Technologies. Alternatives: Immune System Support Standard Process Veterinary Formulas, Immuno Support—Rx Vitamins for Pets, Immugen—Thorne Veterinary Products.

Maitake DMG Vetri Science.

Chinese herbal medicine
Formula H98 Lymph "K": Natural Solutions, Inc.

Homotoxicology remedies
BHI/Heel Corporation

REFERENCES

Western medicine references
Duncan JR, Prasse KW, Mahaffey EA. Veterinary Laboratory Medicine, ed 3. Ames, IA: Iowa State University, 1994, pp 37–62.
Merck Veterinary Manual, 9th edition. Kahn CM, Line S, Aiello S, eds. 2006. Merck and Co., Merial Ltd., New Jersey.
Meyer DT, Coles EH, Rich LJ. Veterinary Laboratory Medicine: Interpretation and Diagnosis. Philadelphia: WB Saunders, 1992, pp 27–41.

Nutrition references
Goldstein R, et al. The BNA Handbook: A Working Manual for Veterinarians, 2000. Westport, CT: Animal Nutrition Technologies.
Graber G, Goust J, Glassman A, Kendall R, Loadholt, C. Immunomodulating Properties of Dimethylglycine in Humans. *Journal of Infectious Disease.* 1981;143:101.
Graber G, Kendall R. N,N-Dimethylglycine and Use in Immune Response, US Patent 4,631,189, Dec 1986.
Kendall RV. Building Wellness with DMG. 2003: Topanga, CA: Freedom Press.
Kodama N, Komuta K, Nanba H. Effect of Maitake (Grifola fondosa) D-Fraction on the Activation of NK Cells in Cancer Patients, *J of Medicinal Foods,* 6(4) 2003, 371–377.
Nanba H, Hamaguchi AM, Kuroda H. The chemical structure of an antitumor polysaccharide in fruit bodies of Grifola frondosa (maitake). *Chem Pharm Bull* 1987;35:1162–8.
Reap E, Lawson J. Stimulation of the Immune Response by Dimethylglycine, a non-toxic metabolite. *Journal of Laboratory and Clinical Medicine.* 1990;115:481.

Chinese herbal medicine/acupuncture references
Chang Yong Zhong Yao Cheng Fen Yu Yao Li Shou Ce (A Handbook of the Composition and Pharmacology of Common Chinese Drugs), 1994;1725:1728.
Geng C, Wang G, Lin Y, et al. Effects on Mouse Lymphocyte and T Cells from Lycium Barbarum Polysaccharide (LBP). Zhong Cao Yao (Chinese Herbs). 1988,19(7):25.
Gupta S, Zhang D, Yi J, Shao. J Anticancer Activities of Oldenlandia diffusa. *Journal of Herbal Pharmacotherapy,* 2004 volume 4(1):21–33.
Huang Tai Kang, et al. Pharmacology research on Ming Dang Shen decoction solution and polysaccharides. *Journal of Chinese Patented Medicine.* 1994;16(7):31–33.

Jiang Su Yi Yao (*Jiang Su Journal of Medicine and Herbology*), 1990;16(9):513.

Jiao Yan, et al. *China Journal of Integrated Medicine.* 1999; 19(6):356–358.

Kong Li Jun, et al. *Journal of Dalian Medical College.* Sep1994;16(3):212–213.

Li Feng Yun, et al. Yi Yi Ren's synergistic effects with cisplatin and mitomycin. *Journal of Traditional Chinese Medicine and Herbs.* Apr2000;28(2):44–45.

Li Li, et al. *Journal of Beijing Medical University.* 1999;22(3): 38–40.

Li Xu Fen, et al. In vitro anti-tumor effects of Dan Shen and Dan Shen compound injection. *Zhejiang Journal of Integrated Medicine.* 1999;9(5):291–292.

Lu Su Cheng, et al. *Journal of No. 1 Military Academy.* 1990; 10(3):267.

Ma Zhen Ya. *Shannxi Journal of Traditional Chinese Medicine and Herbs.* 1982;(4):58.

Miao Ming San. *Henan Journal of TCM.* 1996;16(6):349–50.

Nan Jing Zhong Yi Xue Yuan Xue Bao (*Journal of Nanjing University of Traditional Chinese Medicine*), 1989;1:43.

Pu Shuan Jin, et al. The pharmacodynamics of Gou Qi Zi of Hebei origin. *Journal of Chinese Materia Medica.* 1998; 29(7):472–474.

Ren Min Wei Sheng Chu Ban She (*Journal of People's Public Health*), 1988;302.

Sato Y, Suzaki S, et al. Phytochemical flavones isolated from Scutellaria barbata and antibacterial activity against methicillin-resistant Staphylococcus aureus. *J Ethnopharmacol* 2000 Oct;72(3):483–8.

Shang Sui Cun, et al. *Henan Journal of TCM Pharmacy.* 1994;(6):21–22.

Shao Y, Ho C-T, Chin C-K, et al. Inhibitory activity of boswellic acids from *Boswellia serrata* against human leukemia HL-60 cells in culture. *Planta Medica.* 1998;64:328–331.

Tang Xin Hui. *Journal of Research in Traditional Chinese Medicine.* 1998;11(2):7–9.

Wong BY, et al. *Oldenlandia diffusa* and *scutellaria barbata* augment macrophage oxidative burst and inhibit tumor growth. *Cancer Biotherapy and Radiopharmacology* 1996; 11(1):51–56.

Xin Zhong Yi (*New Chinese Medicine*), 1989;21(3):51.

Xu Shang Cai, et al. *Shanghai Journal of Immunology.* 1994;14(1):12–13.

Zhang G, Song S, Ren J, Xu S. A New Compound from Forsythia suspense (Thunb.) Vahl with Antiviral Effect on RSV. *J of Herbal Pharmacotherapy.* 2002;2(3):35–39.

Zhong Cao Yao (*Chinese Herbal Medicine*), 1989;20(6):22.

Zhong Guo Yao Ke Da Xue Xue Bao (*Journal of University of Chinese Herbology*), 1988;19(4):279.

Zhong Yao Xue (*Chinese Herbology*), 1988;549:550.

Zhong Yao Xue (*Chinese Herbology*), 1998;706:708.

Zhong Yao Yao Li Yu Ying Yong (*Pharmacology and Applications of Chinese Herbs*), 1983;162.

Homotoxicology references
Bianchi I. 1995. Homeopathic Homotoxicological Repertory. Arelia Publishers, Ltd: Baden-Baden, Germany, pp 210–11.

Chan S, Gerson B, Subramaniam S. 1998. The role of copper, molybdenum, selenium, and zinc in nutrition and health. *Clin Lab Med.* Dec;18(4):pp 673–85.

Clark D. BioProtein+Plus—Biologically Active Thymus Proteins plus Zinc Balances Immune System Function. www.bioproteinplus.com

Committee for Veterinary Medical Products. Betamethasone Summary Report: The European Agency for the Evaluation of Medical Products. 1999. June:No 605. http://www.emea.eu.int/pdfs/vet/mrls/060599en.pdf

Van Dijk H, Bloksma N, Rademaker PM, Schouten WJ, Willers JM. Differential potencies of corticosterone and hydrocortisone in immune and immune-related processes in the mouse. *Int J Immunopharmacol.* 1979;1(4):pp 285–92.

Hadden JW. Thymic endocrinology; Neuroimmunomodulation: Molecular Aspects, Integrative Systems, and Clinical Advances. *Ann NY Acad Sci.* 1998;May:840:p 352.

Kirsteen H, Maclean J, Cleveland L, Porter J. Cellular zinc content is a major determinant of iron chelator-induced apoptosis of thymocytes. *Blood.* 2001;15 December, 98(13):pp 3831–9.

Reckeweg, H. *Homeopathia Antihomotoxica Materia Medica,* 4th edition. 2002. Aurelia-Verlag GMBH, Baden-Baden, pp. 177–9, 271, 542.

Ricken K-H. Chronic polyarthritis and other immunological diseases: A field for antihomotoxic therapy. Reprinted from *Biologische Medizin,* 1995. 3:pp. 142–149.

LYMPHADENOPATHY/TONSILLITIS

Definition and cause

Lymphadenopathy/tonsillitis is defined as enlarged lymph nodes and glands. Causes can range from generalized inflammation with or without hyperplasia to infectious with white blood cell component infiltration to neoplasia—either primary as lymphoma or secondary to metastatic diseases. Lymphadenitits or hyperplasia can be local as in tonsillitis or local lymphadenopathy, or generalized throughout the peripheral and internal nodes.

Medical therapy rationale, drug(s) of choice, and nutritional recommendations

The medical and or nutritional recommendations for treatment depend upon the diagnosis. In this section we address tonsillitis, lymphadenopathy, and lymph hyperplasia. For lymphoma please see Chapters 31 through 34, which address cancer. Generally, treatment focuses upon the reduction of inflammation and prevention of cellular infiltration using corticosteroids and antibiotics.

Anticipated prognosis

The prognosis is generally good for tonsillitis, lymphadenopathy, and lymph hyperplasia as primary conditions.

The prognosis changes based upon secondary involvement of the lymph system. Surgical removal of the tonsils is often recommended when there are associated signs of gagging, excessive salivation, and vomiting.

Integrative veterinary therapies

The cause of lymph inflammation, hyperplasia, and WBC infiltration begins secondary to local, cellular inflammation leading to hyperplasia and cellular infiltration. Treatment with corticosteroids and antibiotics suppresses the inflammatory process and resultant infiltration and hyperplasia but does not address the underlying causes. Examples include: the inciting cause of the inflammation such as excessive free radical production; the reaction to and the removal of specific allergens, toxins, vaccinations, environmental chemicals, pesticides, herbicides etc.; the organ elimination of foreign materials; the balancing of the immune response and the quieting of an exaggerated response (Appleton 2005).

Nutrition
General considerations/rationale
The lymph system is one of the body's primary immune defense mechanisms and as a result is a primary location for a free radical cascade and resulting inflammation. Early lymph system inflammation results in swelling and stasis of lymph flow. More chronic, unaddressed inflammation can result in cellular infiltration and gland enlargement. The integrative use of therapeutic nutrition can help address and neutralize free radical production, inflammation, and cellular infiltration.

Appropriate nutrients
Nutrition/gland therapy: Oral administration of glandular lymph, thymus, adrenal, and bone marrow can neutralize a cellular autoimmune attack and help prevent secondary cellular infiltration (Goldstein 2000) (See Gland Therapy in Chapter 2 for more detailed information).

Vitamin A: A retinoid and a potent antioxidant that is required for the proper division and growth of cells. As a potent antioxidant, vitamin A is cell and tissue protective in that it acts as a free radical scavenger (See Antioxidants and Free Radicals, Chapter 2). In this area of free radical scavenger and the reduction of inflammation, vitamin A can be therapeutically beneficial in treating early inflammatory disease conditions such as lymphoid hyperplasia (Halliwell 1994).

Vitamin C: An effective antioxidant, which helps to reduce tissue and cellular inflammation. It has also been shown to increase the levels of other antioxidant enzymes. Vitamin C is involved in the free radical and reactive oxygen species (See free radicals in Section 1) which result from normal metabolism as well as exposure to chemical and environmental pollutants (Bendich 1995, Carr 1999, Pauling 1976).

Vitamin E: A fat-soluble vitamin and one of the body's main antioxidants, especially in its function of protecting lipids. As a potent antioxidant, its primary function is the neutralization of free radicals and reduction of inflammation, particularly as it affects the oxidation and destruction of lipids (Traber 1999). As such, it is tissue protective for the cell membranes.

Betasitosterol: A phytosterol found in higher plants; betasitosterolin is its glycoside. Animal studies have demonstrated that phytosterols have anti-inflammatory, antipyretic (Gupta 1980), and immune-modulating activity (Bouic 1996).

Chinese herbal medicine
General considerations/rationale
Tonsillitis is due to Wind and Heat affecting the Lung and Stomach. According to the Western interpretation, wind blows the pathogen into the body. Heat refers to the inflammation seen in the throat. The Stomach opens to the mouth so inflammation in the Stomach can be evidenced by oral pathology. The Lung controls the airways. The treatment goals are to cool the inflammation and repel the pathogen causing the inflammation. In the acute phase there may also be fever, which must be addressed.

Appropriate herbs
Acute tonsillitis

Arctium (Niu bang zi): Has anti-inflammatory and antipyretic effects (Zhong Yao Xue 1998; 91:92). It also has antibacterial efficacy (Group of Virology 1973).

Coptis (Huang lian): Has antibiotic and antiviral effects (The Merck Index 2000). It contains berberine which has demonstrated anti-inflammatory actions in rats (Yao Xue Za Zhi 1981). Coptis also has antipyretic effects (Zhong Guo Bing Li Sheng Li Za Zhi 1991).

Forsythia (Lian qiao): Contains rengynic acid, which has been shown to inhibit RSV in vitro (Zhang 2002). It also inhibits multiple bacteria and has anti-inflammatory, analgesic, and anti-pyretic effects (Ma 1982).

Gardenia fruit (Zhi zi): An anti-inflammatory (Zhang 1994). It contains geniposide, which has analgesic properties (Zhong Yao Zhi 1984). It has demonstrated efficacy against several types of bacteria (Zhong Yao Zhi 1984).

Honeysuckle (Jin yin hua): Has chlorogenic acid and iso-chlorogenic acid. These compounds have strong antibacterial properties (Xin Yi Xue 1975, Jiang Xi Xin Yi Yao 1960). Anti-inflammatory and antipyretic actions have been demonstrated in rabbits and mice (Shan Xi Yi Kan 1960).

Licorice (Gan cao): Has analgesic properties (Zhong Yao Xue 1998). It contains glycyrrhizin and glycyrrhetinic acid which have anti-inflammatory effects (Zhong Cao Yao 1991). Glycyrrhizin has been shown in vitro to inhibit a number of viruses (Zhu 1996). Licorice also has antibacterial effects (Zhong Yao Zhi 1993).

Mint (Bo he): Decreases fevers and has anti-inflammatory effects (Zhong Yao Xue 1998). It has shown efficacy against viruses and bacteria (Wang 1983).

Platycodon root (Jie geng): Contains platycodin, an antipyretic compound (Li 1984, Zhang 1984). It causes anti-inflammatory effects by promoting the secretion of corticosterone (Li 1984, Zhang 1984, Zhou 1979).

Rhubarb (Da huang): Contains emodin, rhein, and aloe-emodin which have antibiotic effects (Zhong Yao Xue 1998). Rhubarb has also been shown to inhibit viruses (Xie 1996). It has antipyretic, analgesic, and anti-inflammatory properties (Chang Yong Zhong Yao Cheng Fen Yu Yao Li Shou Ce 1994). Finally, it can enhance immunity (Zhang 1997), which may help the patient recover more quickly.

Schizonepeta stem (Jing jie): Has analgesic effects (Zhong Yao Cai 1989), which may help soothe sore throats.

Scrophularia (Xuan shen): Has antibacterial action against various bacteria (Chen 1986). It also reduces fevers (Zhong Yao Yao Li Yu Ying Yong 1983).

Scutellaria (Huang qin): Contains biacalin, which has antibiotic activity (Zhong Yao Xue 1988, Liu 2000). Both baicalin and a second ingredient, biacalein, have been shown to suppress inflammation in mice (Kubo 1984). It seems to act on the central nervous system to reduce fevers (Xu 1999).

Siler (Fang feng): Has been shown to decrease fevers (Zhong Yi Yao Xin Xi 1990). It also has demonstrated antibacterial and antiviral effects (Zhong Yao Tong Bao 1988).

Chronic tonsillitis

Licorice (Gan cao): See above.

Loquat leaf (Pi pa ye): Has antibiotic properties (Chang Yong Zhong Yao Cheng Fen Yu Yao Li Shou Ce 1994).

Ophiopogon (Mai men dong): Was shown to increase mucociliary transport and decrease respiratory tract mucus secretion (Tai 2002). This may decrease congestion in the throat and help sweep pathogens out of the pharynx. It has antibiotic actions (Zhong Yao Xue 1998).

Oriental wormwood (Yin chen hao): has shown antibiotic activity against a variety of bacteria and some viruses (Zhong Yao Yao Li Yu Ying Yong 1990). It has analgesic and anti-inflammatory effects (Wan 1987, Shan 1982).

Rehmannia (Shu di huang): When cooked, increases the plasma levels of adrenocortical hormone (Zhong Yao Xue 1998). This in turn may increase the plasma cor-

tisone level and decrease inflammation. Raw rehmannia (Sheng di huang) reduces swelling and inflammation (Zhong Yao Yao Li Yu Ying Yong 1983).

Scutellaria (Huang qin): See above.

Acupuncture

The World Health Organization placed tonsillitis on the list of conditions responsive to acupuncture in 1979 (World Health Organization Accessed 10/20/2006). In a study involving 220 people, Chen (1987) showed that tonsillitis symptoms could be decreased by acupuncture.

General considerations/rationale

Generalized lymphadenopathy: Lymphadenopathy is due to Heat and Toxins affecting the Lung, which leads to blockage of the meridians. There is also Qi and Blood stagnation with Ying Qi and Wei Qi disharmony.

According to the Western interpretation, Heat and Toxin refer to inflammation and the cause of that inflammation. Just as swelling can lead to blockage of vessels in Western medicine, swelling can block the meridians in TCM. The blockage leads to Blood and Qi stagnation as the normal flow is disrupted. Stagnation can lead to swelling—of the lymph nodes in this case.

Wei Qi is translated as protective Qi. It can be thought of as the immune system. The Ying level is the muscle layer and when the Ying Qi and Wei Qi are in disharmony it means that the immune system is battling the pathogen. The pathogen is stuck in the muscle layer, but is prevented from getting deeper into the body by the immune system. Treatment is aimed at decreasing the swelling and eliminating the cause of the lymphadenopathy.

Appropriate Chinese herbs

Anemarrhena root (Zhi mu): Has anti-inflammatory effects. It has been found to raise the plasma corticosterone level in mice (Chen 1999), which suggests it may be of use in decreasing the inflammation in lymph nodes.

Dandelion (Pu gong yin): Has antibiotic properties (Zhong Yi Yao Xue Bao 1991). It may possess anti-inflammatory actions (Mascolo 1987).

Forsythia fruit (Lian qiao): Contains rengynic acid, which has been shown to have antiviral properties (Zhang 2002). In addition it has antibacterial effects (Ma 1982). These actions may be of use in infectious lymphadenopathy.

Honeysuckle (Jin yin hua): Has chlorogenic acid and isochlorogenic acid, which have very strong antibacterial functions (Xin Yi Xue 1975, Jiang Xi Xin Yi Yao 1960).

Licorice (Gan cao): Contains glycyrrhizin and glycyrrhetinic acid, which have approximately 10% of the corticosteroid activity of cortisone (Zhong Cao Yao 1991).

This may help in inflammatory lymphadenopathy. In addition, licorice has antiviral and antibacterial properties (Zhu 1996, Zhong Yao Zhi 1993).

Phellodendron bark (Huang bai): Has antimicrobial effects (Zhong Yao Xue 1998).

Rehmannia (Sheng di huang): Reduces swelling and inflammation (Zhong Yao Yao Li Yu Ying Yong 1983). This may help decrease the inflammation in the nodes.

Scutellaria (Huang qin): Contains biacalin which has antibiotic activity against multiple strains of bacteria fungi and viruses (Zhong Yao Xue 1988, Liu 2000). Baicalein, another component of Huang qin, causes apoptosis of human myeloma cells in vitro (Zi 2005). The flavone component decreases inflammation (Cao 1999). This may be useful to decrease inflammation in the lymph nodes.

Siler (Fang feng): Has some antibacterial and antiviral effect (Zhong Yao Tong Bao 1988). It was shown experimentally to inhibit the development of solid tumors in mice (Li 1999). It may help to inhibit neoplastic causes of lymphadenopathy.

White peony (Bai shao): Has antibacterial and antifungal properties (Xin Zhong Yi 1989). It contains paeoniflorin which is a strong antipyretic and anti-inflammatory (Zhong Yao Zhi 1993).

Homotoxicology
General considerations/rationale
Tonsillitis and lymphadenopathy are Inflammation Phase disorders. As disease processes continue they can progress to Impregnation Phase disorders. In acute cases it is desirable to determine the aggravating factors present, but there is some indication that the pathogenic bacteria, viruses, or fungi might not be capable of causing infection if the matrix was healthy. In cases of homotoxicoses there may well be phenomena at work, making the immune system more susceptible to infection. In the extreme, it is possible that infectious agents may actually be involved in devouring and processing homotoxins into less dangerous material. Of course, pathogens may produce or release other toxic agents into the milieu and further the progression of the homotoxicosis. Therapy is aimed at supporting detoxification, promoting lymph drainage, and improving immune function. Providing adequate rest and improved environmental conditions (proper temperature, reduced stress, adequate fluid intake and proper diet), along with gentle massage or movement to mobilize lymph is also helpful.

Antibiotics can cause bacterial death and release of homotoxins that become deposited in tissues. They can further accumulate and there is an observed link in humans between the treatment of tonsillitis and the onset of agranulocytosis or even further, into the neoplastic phase of leukemia. This represents an undesirable progressive vicariation (Reckeweg 1989). Antibiotics may be needed in these cases, but if they present early it is advisable to attempt treatment biologically and avoid further damage.

Appropriate homotoxicology formulas
Special note: The combination of *Lymphomyosot* and *Apis homaccord* provides a powerful weapon against both swelling and pain.

Apis homaccord: Used for pain and swelling. Apisinum and Apis have edematous swellings with formations like water-filled sacs, infiltration of the cellular tissues, and right-sided tonsillitis with edematous swelling of uvula (Reckeweg 2002) as indications. Apis is also found in *Arnica Heel*, below.

Arnica-Heel: Used for tonsillitis with pain. Significant remedies include *Eucalyptus*, with its main indications: influenza and influenzal catarrhs, tracheitis, laryngitis, bronchiolitis, swollen lymph nodes, rheumatic pains with a pricking sensation in the muscles and joints with nocturnal aggravation, tiredness, and stiffness of the limbs (Reckeweg 2002).

Belladonna homaccord: Treats acute inflammatory issues. Belladonna's list of complaints includes typical engorgement and swelling of mucosa, the mucous membranes of the oral cavity, and a dry, red tongue, a catarrh of the soft palate with inflammatory swelling, extending from the tonsils, linked with overwhelming thirst. Usually this is accompanied by difficulty and pain in swallowing, and on attempting to drink (Reckeweg 2002). This is also a component of Mercurius Heel, Mucosa compositum, and Traumeel.

BHI-Infection: Used for sharp, splinter-like pain, sensitivity to being touched, minor infections.

BHI-Lymphatic Rx: Used to treat swollen glands, bronchial cough, eczema, rhinitis, and sensitivity to weather changes. It contains nosodes to improve immune function (Currently unavailable).

BHI-Throat: Used for sore throat. It contains Calcium carbonicum with indications for swellings of the lymphnodes, tonsils, hilar glands, and mesenteric glands (Reckeweg 2002). It is used with Hyoscyamus, whose range includes parotitis and tonsillitis. Hyoscyamus should also always be indicated by the symptom of grinding the teeth in sleep. Acute tonsillitis reacts mostly, but not only, to Belladonna, but also to Hyoscyamus, when there is the sensation of great dryness, scratching and burning in the palate and the esophagus, with swallowing difficulties caused by the inflamed swelling of the tonsils (Reckeweg 2002).

Echinacea compositum: Immune support in infections. This remedy contains Hepar sulphuris calcareum, which is often used for chronic catarrhs of the respiratory organs with expectoration of purulent sputum and croupy cough.

Because of its action in suppurations, Hepar sulph is the main remedy for abscesses of the lung and in the tonsils (Reckeweg 2002). It is also found in *Traumeel*.

Engystol N: Used for viral infections. This seemingly simple remedy contains Vincetoxicum, which is used in acute febrile reaction phases. It is used for mononucleosis (glandular fever), lymphadenitis, and viral diseases. The other component is Sulphur, which figures into chronic diseases, particularly in the context of retoxic Impregnation phases and cellular phases that show a tendency toward regressive vicariation but are unable to complete the process. Also used for viral illnesses (Reckeweg 2002).

Galium-Heel: Used in Deposition Phase cases and to the right on the Six-Phase Table. It also is used as a cellular detoxification and repair agent with immune stimulation. This contains *Thuja*, which has in its remedy picture swollen gums as well as ulcers in the mouth and throat and possibly swellings of the tonsils and glands. It also contains Clematis erecta for very sensitive pustular eruptions, characterized by burning, stinging pains, and also pustules, which often proceed with inflammatory swellings of the neighboring lymph nodes. Another valuable component is Saponaria, which is almost exclusively used in the treatment of acute colds, coryza and throat pains, tonsillitis, pharyngitis, and laryngitis. Saponaria is used in combination remedies because of a certain blood cleansing action by which it facilitates the elimination of homotoxins which have been freed through harmless catarrhal symptoms such as an acute cold or, in serious cases, tonsillitis. "Saponaria then compensates for this by inhibiting inflammation in a biological way by changing the homotoxic 'soil'" (Reckeweg 2002).

Lymphomyosot: Used for lymphatic drainage, fever, and immune and hormonal support. This complex includes Juglans, whose prime indication is lymphadenopathy and lymphadenitis (Reckeweg 2002).

Mercurius-Heel S: An antiviral and antibacterial for very red and inflamed, painful tonsils. This wide-ranging remedy has Mercurius solubilis, (see Tonsilla compositum), Belladonna (see Belladonna compositum), and Phytolacca, whose main indications include tonsillitis. It is characterized by violent inflammation of the whole pharyngeal area and the throat is swollen and dark red (Reckeweg 2002).

Tonsilla compositum: Used in Degeneration Phase, Impregnation Phase, and Dedifferentiation Phase cases for immune support. It primarily takes its name from Tonsilla suis, which is indicated for hypertrophy of the tonsils. It is also used for chronic tonsillitis, enlarged lymph glands, tubercular glands, and exudative diathesis. May also be tried experimentally in lymphogranulomatosis and reticulosis. It also contains Calcium phosphoricum, a constitutional remedy for status lymphaticus, and

is also found in *Lymphomyosot*. *Tonsilla compositum* also contains *Dulcamara*, which has proved its worth in chronic sore throats that are worsened in wet weather, particularly if they are suppurative (Reckeweg 2002). Glandula lymphatica suis is another valuable component with the following indications: lymphadenopathy, exudative diathesis, vague swellings of the lymph nodes from other causes, agranulocytosis, chronic tonsillitis, and hypertrophy of the tonsils (Reckeweg 2002). Mercurius solubilis Hahnemanni (Merc. Sol), another component, is useful in patients that have a tendency toward suppurations of all kinds, including tonsillitis, sinusitis, empyema, or of the thorax (Reckeweg 2002). Merc. Sol. is also a component common to *Traumeel*.

Traumeel S: An anti-inflammatory used in acutely painful cases and in regulation rigidity cases to activate sulfur-containing enzymes. Calendula, which is homeopathically characterized by great irritability with a tendency to choke and rheumatoid pains everywhere, has a beneficial effect on vesicular eruptions and on inflammatory swelling of the submaxillary gland, tonsils, parotid glands, and various lymph glands. It could also be used for mononucleosis—also known as glandular fever—along with Vincetoxicum or *Engystol* (Reckeweg 2002). Many recurrent tonsillar issues may be based in viral impregnation diseases.

Ubichinon compositum: Includes Napthaquinone in its remedy list. A shortage of oxygen in the tissues is expressed as cyanosis of the lips, conjunctiva, and nails. In severe cases of cancer, lymphatic congestion may also be present. Since Naphthoquinone has particular affinities for the tonsils and the appendix, i.e. for the secondary defenses of the lymphatic mechanism, it should also be used after tonsillectomy or appendectomy (human).

Authors' suggested protocols

Nutrition
Immune and Lymph support formulas: 1 tablet for every 25 pounds of body weight BID.

Betathyme: 1 capsule for every 35 pounds of body weight BID (maximum, 2 capsules BID).

Chinese herbal medicine
Tonsillitis

Acute stage: Use patent formula "Qing Yan Li Ge Tang" at the recommended dose (Yu 2000). In addition to the herbs cited above, Qing Yan Li Ge Tang also contains mirabilite (Mang xiao).

Chronic stage: Use patent formula "Gan Lu Yin" at the recommended dose (Yu 2000). In addition to the herbs cited above it also contains asparagus tuber (Tian men dong), bitter orange (Zhi ke), and dendrobium (Shi hu).

Recommended acupuncture points: GB4, LI11, LU5 and TH1 (Handbook of TCM Practitioner 1987).

Generalized lymphadenopathy
Use patent formula "Ji Yin Tang." In addition to the herbs discussed above, Ji Yin Tang also contains angelica radix (Bai zhi), cyperus(Xiang fu), fritillaria (Bei mu) and orange peel (Chen pi) as part of the patent formula. Dose according to manufacturer's recommendations (Yu 2000).

Homotoxicology (Dose: 10 drops for 50-pound dog, 5 drops for cat or small dog)
Lymphomyosot, Mercurius, Apis homaccord, Belladonna homaccord: Mixed together and given every 15 minutes in acute cases and then BID to TID PO. Antibiotic therapy is appropriate if patient response fails to appear rapidly.
BHI-Lymphatic Rx tablets: An option; give TID PO.

Product sources

Nutrition
Immune and Lymph support formulas: Animal Nutrition Technologies. **Alternative:** Immune System Support Standard Process Veterinary Formulas, Immuno Support—Rx Vitamins for Pets, Immugen—Thorne Veterinary Products.

Betathyme: Best for Your Pet. **Alternative:** Moducare—Thorne Veterinary Products, follow manufacturers directions.

Chinese herbal medicine
Gan lu Yin: Bluelight Company.

Qing Yan Li: Ge Tang and Ji Yin Tang—Mayway Company.

Homotoxicology remedies
BHI/Heel Inc.

REFERENCES

Western medicine references
Day MJ, Whitbread TJ. Pathological diagnoses in dogs with lymph node enlargement. *Vet Rec* 1988;136:72–73.
Duncan JR. The lymph nodes. In: Cowell RL, Tyler RD, eds. Diagnostic cytology of the dog and cat. Goleta, CA: American Veterinary, 1989:93–8.
Rogers KS, Barton CL, Landis M. Canine and feline lymph nodes. II. Diagnostic evaluation of lymphadenopathy. *Compend Contin Ed Pract Vet* 1993;15:1493–1503.

Integrative veterinary medicine references
Appleton N. Stopping Inflammation: Relieving the Cause of degenerative Diseases, 2005. Garden City Park, NY: Square One Publishing.

Goldstein R, et al. The BNA Handbook: A Working Manual for Veterinarians. 2000. Westport, CT: Animal Nutrition Technologies.

Nutrition references
Bendich A, Langseth L. The health effects of vitamin C supplementation: a review. *J Am Coll Nutr* 1995;14:124–136.
Bouic PJD. Plant sterols and sterolins: a review of their immune-modulating properties. *Altern Med Rev* 1999;4:170–177.
Carr AC, Frei B. Toward a new recommended dietary allowance for vitamin C based on antioxidant and health effects in humans. *Am J Clin Nutr.* 1999;69(6):1086–1107.
Gupta MB, Nath R, Srivastava N et al. Anti-inflammatory and antipyretic activies of Beta sitosterol Planta Medica 1980; 39:157–163.
Halliwell B. Free Radicals and Antioxidants: a Personal View. *Nutr. Rev.*, 1994;52:253.
Pauling L. Vitamin C: The common cold and the flu. 1976. San Francisco: WH Freeman.
Traber MG. Does vitamin E decrease heart attack risk? Summary and implications with respect to dietary recommendations. *J Nutr.* 2001;131(2):395S–397S.

Chinese herbal medicine references for acute tonsillitis
Chang Yong Zhong Yao Cheng Fen Yu Yao Li Shou Ce (A Handbook of the Composition and Pharmacology of Common Chinese Drugs), 1994;226:323.
Chen Shao Ying, et al. *Fujian Journal of Chinese Medicine.* 1986;17(4):57.
Group of Virology. Institute of Pharmacy. Academy of Traditional Chinese Medicine. *Journal of Modern Medicine and Pharmacology.* 1973;(12):38.
Jiang Xi Xin Yi Yao (Jiangxi New Medicine and Herbology), 1960;(1):34.
Kubo M, Matsuda H, Tanaka M, Kimura Y, Okuda H, Higashino M, Tani T, Namba K, Arichi S. Studies on Scutellariae radix. VII. Anti-arthritic and anti-inflammatory actions of methanolic extract and flavonoid components from Scutellariae radix. *Chem Pharm Bull*, 1984;32(7):2724–9.
Li Yin Fang (translator). Foreign Medicine, vol. of CM. 1984;6(1):15–18.
Liu IX, Durham DG, Richards RM. Baicalin synergy with beta-lactam antibiotics against methicillin-resistant Staphylococcus aureus and other beta-lactam-resistant strains of S. aureus. *J Pharm Pharmacol.* 2000 Mar;52(3):361–6.
Ma Zhen Ya. *Shannxi Journal of Traditional Chinese Medicine and Herbs.* 1982;(4):58.
Shan Xi Yi Kan (*Shanxi Journal of Medicine*), 1960;(10):32.
The Merck Index 12th edition, Chapman and Hall/ CRCnet-BASE/Merck, 2000.
Wang Yu Sheng. Application and Pharmacology of TCM. 1983. Beijing: People's Health Press.
Xie Yan Ying, et al. *Journal of Shandong Medical University.* 1996;34(2):166–169.
Xin Yi Xue (New Medicine), 1975;6(3):155.
Xu Gang, et al. *China Journal of TCM Science and Technology.* 1999;6(4):254–255.
Yao Xue Za Zhi (*Journal of Medicinals*), 1981;101(10):883.

Yu Chuan, Chen Zi Bin. Modern Complete Works of Traditional Chinese Veterinary Medicine. Guanxi Science and Technology Press, March 2000.

Zhang Bing Sheng, et al. *Journal of Traditional Chinese Medicine Material.* 1997;20(2):85–88.

Zhang G, Song S, Ren J, Xu S. A New Compound from Forsythia suspense (Thunb.) Vahl with Antiviral Effect on RSV. *J of Herbal Pharmacotherapy.* 2002;2(3):35–39.

Zhang Shu Chen, et al. *Journal of Chinese Patent Medicine Research.* 1984;(2):37.

Zhang Xue Lan, et al. *Journal of Shandong College of TCM.* 1994;18(6):416–417.

Zhong Cao Yao (Chinese Herbal Medicine) 1991;22(10):452.

Zhong Guo Bing Li Sheng Li Za Zhi (*Chinese Journal of Pathology and Biology*), 1991;7(3):264.

Zhong Yao Cai (*Study of Chinese Herbal Material*), 1989;12(6):37.

Zhong Yao Tong Bao (*Journal of Chinese Herbology*), 1988:13(6):364.

Zhong Yao Xue (*Chinese Herbology*), 1988;137:140.

Zhong Yao Xue (*Chinese Herbology*), 1998;89:91.

Zhong Yao Xue (*Chinese Herbology*), 1998;91:92.

Zhong Yao Xue (*Chinese Herbology*), 1998;251:256.

Zhong Yao Xue (*Chinese Herbology*), 1998;759:765.

Zhong Yao Yao Li Yu Ying Yong (Pharmacology and Applications of Chinese Herbs), 1983;370.

Zhong Yao Zhi (Chinese Herbology Journal), 1984;578.

Zhong Yao Zhi (Chinese Herbology Journal), 1993;358.

Zhong Yi Yao Xin Xi (Information on Chinese Medicine and Herbology), 1990;(4):39.

Zhou Wen Zheng, et al. *Pharmacy Bulletin.* 1979;14(5):202–203.

Zhu Li Hong. *China Journal of TCM Information.* 1996;3(3):17–20.

Chinese herbal medicine references for chronic tonsillitis

Chang Yong Zhong Yao Cheng Fen Yu Yao Li Shou Ce (A Handbook of the Composition and Pharmacology of Common Chinese Drugs), 1994;1970:10.

Shan Yuan Tiao Er, et al. *Journal of Pharmacy.* Japan. 1982;102(3):285.

Tai S, Sun F, O'Brien D, Lee M, Zayaz J, King M. Evaluation of a Mucoactive Herbal Drug, Radix Ophiopogonis, in a Pathogenic Quail Model. *J of Herbal Pharmacotherapy* 2002;2(4):49–56.

Wan Yao De. The antipyretic effects of capillarin. *Pharmacy Bulletin.* 1987;(10):590–593.

Zhong Yao Xue (*Chinese Herbology*), 1998;156:158.

Zhong Yao Xue (*Chinese Herbology*), 1998;845:848.

Zhong Yao Yao Li Yu Ying Yong (*Pharmacology and Applications of Chinese Herbs*), 1983;400.

Zhong Yao Yao Li Yu Ying Yong (*Pharmacology and Applications of Chinese Herbs*), 1990;15(6):52.

Acupuncture references

Chen RH. Acupuncture treatment of 220 cases of acute tonsillitis. *Chinese Acupuncture and Moxibustion,* 1987;7(3):54 [in Chinese].

Handbook of TCM practitioner. Shanghai Science and Technology Press. Hunan College of TCM, Oct. 1987.

World Health Organization. List of common conditions treatable by Chinese Medicine and Acupuncture. Available at: http://tcm.health-info.org/WHO-treatment-list.htm. Accessed 10/20/2006.

Yu Chuan and Chen Zi Bin. Modern Complete Works of Traditional Chinese Veterinary Medicine. Guanxi Science and Technology Press, March 2000.

Chinese herbal medicine references for general lymphadenopathy

Cao Zhi Sheng, et al. *Strait Journal of Pharmacology.* 1999;11(3):53–54.

Chen Wan Sheng, et al. *Journal of Second Military Medical College.* 1999;20(10):758–760.

Jiang Xi Xin Yi Yao (*Jiangxi New Medicine and Herbology*), 1960;(1):34.

Li Li, et al. *Journal of Beijing Medical University.* 1999;22(3):38–40.

Liu IX, Durham DG, Richards RM. Baicalin synergy with beta-lactam antibiotics against methicillin-resistant Staphylococcus aureus and other beta-lactam-resistant strains of S. aureus. *J Pharm Pharmacol.* 2000 Mar;52(3):361–6.

Ma Zhen Ya. *Shannxi Journal of Traditional Chinese Medicine and Herbs.* 1982;(4):58.

Mascolo N, Autore G, Capasso F, et al. Biological screening of Italian medicinal plants for anti-inflammatory activity. Phytotherapy Res 1987;1(1):28–31.

Xin Yi Xue (*New Medicine*), 1975;6(3):155.

Xin Zhong Yi (*New Chinese Medicine*), 1989;21(3):51.

Zhang G, Song S, Ren J, Xu S. A New Compound from Forsythia suspense (Thunb.) Vahl with Antiviral Effect on RSV. *J of Herbal Pharmacotherapy.* 2002;2(3):35–39.

Zhong Cao Yao (*Chinese Herbal Medicine*) 1991;22 (10):452.

Zhong Yao Tong Bao (*Journal of Chinese Herbology*), 1988:13(6):364.

Zhong Yao Xue (*Chinese Herbology*), 1988;137:140.

Zhong Yao Xue (*Chinese Herbology*), 1998;144:146.

Zhong Yao Yao Li Yu Ying Yong (*Pharmacology and Applications of Chinese Herbs*), 1983;400.

Zhong Yao Zhi (*Chinese Herbology Journal*), 1993;183.

Zhong Yao Zhi (*Chinese Herbology Journal*), 1993;358.

Zhong Yi Yao Xue Bao (*Report of Chinese Medicine and Herbology*), 1991;(1):41.

Zhu Li Hong. *China Journal of TCM Information.* 1996;3(3):17–20.

Zi Ma, Ken-ichiro Otsuyama, Shangqin Liu, Saeid Abroun, Hideaki Ishikawa, Naohiro Tsuyama, Masanori Obata, Fu-Jun Li, Xu Zheng, Yasuko Maki, Koji Miyamoto, Michio M. Kawano. Baicalein, a component of *Scutellaria* radix from Huang-Lian-Jie-Du-Tang (HLJDT), leads to suppression of proliferation and induction of apoptosis in human myeloma cells. *Blood.* 2005;105:3312–3318.

Homotoxicology references

Reckeweg H. *Biotherapeutic Index: Ordinatio Antihomotoxica et Materia Medica, 5th ed.* 2000. Baden-Baden, Germany: Biologische Heilmittel Heel GMBH, p 180, 266–7.

Reckeweg H. *Homotoxicology, Illness and Healing through Anti-homotoxic Therapy*, 3rd edition. 1989. Menaco Publishing Co: Albuquerque, NM, pp 23–25.

Reckeweg H. *Homeopathica Antihomotoxica Materia Medica*, 4th ed. 2002. Aurelia-Verlag, Baden-Baden, Germany, pp. 141–2, 174, 197, 199, 200, 243, 283, 292, 321, 350–1, 363, 438, 490, 523–4, 560, 577, 597.

Chapter Eight

Behavior and Emotional Conditions

AGGRESSION

Aggressive behavior often originates from anxiety and generally represents a biological response to the environment. It may represent a wide variety of conditions (Beata 2006a). There has been a tremendous amount of study, observation, and explanation of aggression in both dogs and cats in relation to their ancestry and domestication. Classifications of aggression are based upon a number of factors, such as the following, which have been well described: (a) lack of socialization; (b) play, fear, or pain; (c) predatory; (d) territorial; and (e) idiopathic aggression. For more information, see Beata (2001).

Medical therapy rationale, drug(s) of choice, and nutritional recommendations

The important point is that medical therapy will not cure any behavior problem. Due to the large amount of research that has been done, the response to drugs can be predicted and often dogs or cats improve for periods of time. However, medications do not cure the condition. The current veterinary approach to aggression in dogs and cats is a combination of behavior modification techniques along with appropriate and predicable drug therapy. The rationale for the use of psychotropic drugs is that if they are not used, then the number of aggression-related euthanasias will rise dramatically (Beata 2001, Houpt 1998, Overall 1994, 1997).

Typical drug therapies are: sedatives such as acepromazine or risperidone, thymoregulators such as carbamazepine, antidepressants such as fluoxetine, and anti-anxiety medications such as amitriptyline or buspirone. Besides the inherent side effects associated with the drugs, the more important point again is that drugs alone, without behavior modification, simply are not effective (Beata 2001, Houpt 1998).

Anticipated prognosis

Aggression can be a real problem for people as well as the animal, and therefore the prognosis is individualized.

Veterinarians should play an integral part in the treatment decisions and instruct clients when the prognosis is poor and danger exists (Beata 2001).

Integrative veterinary therapies

Neither drug nor behavior modification approaches consider internal, physiological, biochemical, nutritional, and autoimmune reactions, such as those to vaccines. When integrative therapies—including nutrition, medicinal herbs, and homotoxicology remedies—are used with drugs and behavior modification or as a free-standing protocol, the day-to-day quality of life as well as the cessation and control of the aggression can be improved.

In addition, the authors recommend liver support in nearly all cases of aggression; this can take the form of nutritional or herbal support, acupuncture, biopuncture, or antihomotoxic medicines.

Nutrition
General considerations/rationale
The nutritional approach to aggression is often multifaceted, consisting of nutrient support of the brain and nervous system; detoxification and elimination of chemicals, toxins, and prior vaccinations; removal of chemical additives, preservatives, coloring agent, dyes, and other unnatural ingredients from the diet; and the addition of behavior modifying natural remedies.

Appropriate nutrients
Nutrition/gland therapies: Glandular brain and liver supply intrinsic nutrients and can help improve circulation and reduce inflammation in the brain, central nervous system, and liver (Goldstein 2000) (see Chapter 2, Gland Therapy, for more detailed information).

Specialized phospholipids, such as phosphatidylcholine, phosphatidylserine, and others, have been proposed as therapeutic agents for neurologic and other diseases (Horrocks 1986). These phospholipids are found in high concentrations in the brain, liver, and other glands. These glands are also sources of unsaturated omega-3 fatty acids, which are thought to play a vital role in the development and maintenance of the central nervous system. Horrocks (1986) reported on the potential clinical use of these nutrients in chronic neurological conditions.

Lecithin/phosphatidyl choline: Phosphatidyl choline is a phospholipid that is integral to cellular membranes, particularly of nerve and brain cells. It helps to move fats into the cells and is involved in acetylcholine uptake, neurotransmission, and cellular integrity. As part of the cell membranes, lecithin is an essential nutrient required by the nerves and all of the cells of the body for general health and wellness (Hanin 1987).

Phosphatidyl serine (PS): A phospholipid that is an essential ingredient in cellular membranes, particularly of brain cells. It has been studied in people with altered mental functioning and degeneration with positive results (Crook 1991, Cenacchi 1993). In people with Alzheimer's disease the addition of PS to the program showed a mild to a significant clinical improvement (Delewaide 1986, Engel 1992, Funfgeld 1989).

Blue-green algae: Blue-green algae have been observed to create a generalized feeling of well being in humans taking the product and may prove helpful in veterinary patients. This may be due in part to their content of natural antihistaminic compounds or their levels of omega-3 fatty acids (Bruno 2001). Many studies in recent years have confirmed the beneficial results from these critical fatty acids. Aphanizomenon flos aquae, a blue-green algae, has been shown in clinical settings to have positive effects on brain function. In addition to omega-3 fatty acids, it contains a full spectrum of essential amino acids, a broad-based mineral content, a rapidly assimilable glyolipoprotein cell wall, and a wide variety of vitamins. It has mild chelating properties, and therefore can be of value in heavy metal toxicoses. It is an asset as a micronutrient resource and figures prominently in many treatment programs (Broadfoot 1997).

Chinese herbal medicine
General considerations/rationale

According to TCM theory, aggression is a result of excessive Yang and Fire in the Liver and Heart. In the Western interpretation, Yang can be thought of as energy and Fire as heat. In Western parlance one might say an aggressive person is hot-headed. The ancient Chinese believed that the Heart housed the Shen, or spirit. When the Shen is disturbed, a patient is unable to relax. He is easily upset. The Liver ensures a smooth flow of blood to the mind, according to TCM. When the Liver is hot, the smooth flow is disrupted, leading to irritability. The image conveyed by the TCM terms is an individual who is hyper-reactive, easily angered. In order to treat such a patient it is necessary to soothe or sedate the psyche. In

Western parlance this means sedating the central nervous system.

Appropriate chinese herbs

Albizzia flower (He huan hua): Has sedative effects (Zhong Yao Xue 1998).

Bupleurum (Chai hu): Contains saikosaponins, which have sedative effects (Zhong Yao Yao Li Yu Ying Yong 1983).

Curcuma root (Yu jin): Contains curdione, a compound that sedates the central nervous system. Experiments on cats showed that the effect of curcuma root on sleep patterns indicates that it inhibits the central nervous system (Hao 1994).

Grass-leaf sweet-flag root (Shi chang pu): A central nervous system suppressant (Zhong Yao Xue 1998). Grass-leaf sweet-flag root was used along with Shu di huang, Shan zhu yu, Fu ling, Tai zi shen, Suan zao ren, Hu po, Dang gui, Gou qi zi, Wu wei zi, and Zhi gan cao in 48 people with anxiety disorders. Seventy-five percent showed significant improvement and 22% had some improvement (Wang 1998).

Polygala root (Yuan zhi): Causes sedation (Zhong Yao Yao Li Yu Ying Yong 1983). It contains a high level of bromine, and therefore a tranquilizing effect (Ou 1990).

Polygonum (Ye jiao teng): A tranquilizer. Experiments in mice showed that it can decrease the amount of pentobarbital needed to sedate animals (Chen 1999).

White peony (Bai shao): Causes sedation, as has been shown experimentally in mice (Zhong Yao Tong Bao 1985).

Zizyphus (Suan zao ren): Has demonstrated sedative effects in various animals (Chang Yong Zhong Yao Xian Dai Yan Jiu Yu Lin Chuan 1995).

Homotoxicology
General considerations/rationale

From a homotoxicologic viewpoint, aggression represents homotoxicoses typical of the neurodermal Inflammation Phase (Heel 2003). As homotoxins accumulate or do further damage, these cases may deteriorate to involve any phase to the right (Deposition, Impregnation, Degeneration, and Dedifferentiation) (Palmquist 2005). Proper diagnosis is critical and every case should have a complete history, physical examination, dietary consultation, and full laboratory testing including CBC, chemistry, and thyroid or other endocrine tests as appropriate (Beaver 2003).

Toxins play a large part in aggression and properly dealing with homotoxins can lead to remarkable results. One homotoxicologist feels there is a connection between canine distemper and aggression in some cases (Palmquist 2003). Rabies vaccination has been associated with aggression, but this assertion is not widely accepted by conventional veterinarians at this time. The evidence in support of this is the response of some of these cases to the homeopathic remedy *Lyssin*, which comes from rabies virus. Vaccines may contain heavy metals and other agents, which can negatively affect the nervous system. Products now exist which contain no added thimerosol and are recommended for routine use in veterinary practice. It should be remembered that negative emotions, thoughts, and treatments are all categories of homotoxins (see Chapter 4), and that these can aggravate neurological tissue.

Traditional Oriental medicine has instructed students for years that anger and aggression are related to the Liver (Maciocia 1989). Certainly it is noted that excessive anger subjects the organism to increased quantities of toxic substances that must be handled by the liver (i.e., histamine, serotonin, epinephrine, corticoids). Support of the liver in aggressive patients can yield many remarkably improved cases, as can elimination diets (Palmquist 2003). The exact mechanics of this is not currently quantified in the literature, but CAVM practitioners have long observed this and recommended support of the liver in these cases.

Classical homeopathy may yield surprising responses in some cases of aggressive behavior, and should be considered (Day 1990). This subject is beyond the scope of this text, but it is important to note that aggression can be a manifestation of many different emotional states (anxiety, fear, anger, frustration, resentment, and antagonism, to name just a few), and each of these require separate consideration in developing a classical homeopathic approach (Kent 1921). Seeking a trained homoeopathic practitioner with experience in behavioral cases is advised in such situations (Pitcairn 2006).

Another area of CAVM anecdotally reported to assist with aggression involves the use of Bach flower essences. They are used primarily when there are disturbances of a mental, emotional, or behavioral nature. *Rescue Remedy* is the most well-known flower essence combination. It consists of five different flower essences: Cherry plum, clematis, impatiens, rock rose, and star of Bethlehem. *Rescue Remedy* is used in situations of high stress and anxiety. It is important to note that *Rescue Remedy* does not have conventional tranquilizing properties but simply a calming effect that reduces or relieves the sense of stress and anxiety. Many practitioners use *Rescue Remedy* in their practices to settle fractious dogs and cats and its use is much appreciated by patients, clients, and technicians alike. Today there are hundreds of other regional flower essences besides Dr. Bach's original 38 English essences. Each individual flower essence has its particular area of mental, emotional, or behavioral use. For example, Aspen helps in situations of apprehension or fear, but not of a known entity—rather, the fear of an unknown. Mimulus, on the other hand, is useful for fears of known things.

Holly is used in the strong and aggressive emotions of outright anger and jealousy (Wright 2006).

Of course, a discussion of appropriate handling and treatment of these patients must include consideration of consultation with a qualified behavioral specialist, and use of pharmaceutical agents should be considered as experimental. Psychiatric drugs should be reserved for only the most severe cases because they may cause further, as yet unknown, damage to the liver and nervous system of the affected animals. No amount of drugs, whips, shocks, or other treatment can substitute for proper, compassionate handling in these cases, and improper treatment of aggressive patients can do far more damage than good.

The client should always be informed that such treatment is not without risks. Aggressive patients treated with any modality may suddenly and unpredictably aggress and cause injury to themselves or others. Risk should always be assessed properly, because aggression may recur at unpredictable times (Beata 2006). Proper handling of such patients is critical to success. It should be recognized that patients with impregnated homotoxins may develop Inflammatory Phase changes, and when this occurs intracranially, the resultant neurological swelling and inflammation can cause changes in emotion and behavior, and lead to physical signs such as cranial pressure/headache, altered sensation, photosensitivity, altered perceptions, seizures, weakness, tremors, and a host of other phenomena, which when approached biologically often lead to improved patient condition. This is especially common in heavy metal and viral homotoxicoses (Palmquist 2004).

The professional and client must remember that regressive vicariation is desirable and must work with the patient's own autoregulatory system in this fashion. Similarly, when treating patients with homotoxicology, it may be observed that mental changes occur during detoxification. These are usually mild and should be supported because most disappear in 1 to 3 days. These signs may cycle in and out of clinical significance as tissue repair occurs.

Appropriate homotoxicology formulas

An unpublished clinical report shows that homotoxicology formulas were used to treat a case of feline aggression of two months' duration involving housemate cats. The formula consisted of *Nervoheel* (1 tablet), *Neuroheel* (1 tablet), *Ypsiloheel* (1 tablet), *Berberis homaccord* (15 drops), and *Valerianaheel* (15 drops), mixed with water to make 1 ounce (Roach 2006). A 90% reduction in aggressive incidents was reported within 14 days and owner satisfaction was high. Long-term follow-up is not currently available due to the recent nature of the report.

Appropriate antihotomotixic medicines include:

Aconitum homaccord: Used for nervous conditions involving irritation with great agitation, pain, paralysis, restlessness, fear of death, and consequences of fright, which are made much worse by the slightest contact. Also used in cases involving violent, acute complaints of red skin, fever, and fear aggression (Palmquist 2006).

Belladona homaccord: Used when patient strikes out to bite suddenly and ferociously when afraid.

Berberis homaccord: Provides support of liver and adrenal gland function.

BHI-Calming: Used more for anxiety, but used in humans in cases of swearing mad and mania (Heel 2002).

Cerebrum compositum: Combination remedy that supports cerebral tissues and blood flow. It contains Hyoscyamus for states of excitement with great restlessness, mobility, vehemence, jealousy, raving, and attacks of fury. At the other end of the scale, this formula may be indicated when there is depression to the point of melancholia, and dull apathy (in chronic poisoning). The eyes may have a glazed stare and an unusual sheen (Reckeweg 2002). This description may partially fit those animals with rage syndromes.

Cerebrum compositum also contains Anacardium with indications for retoxic impregnations after suppressed skin eruptions, in particular cerebral and emotional symptoms with irritability, timidity, and fearfulness of misfortune and danger. This is also indicated for mental exhaustion, emotional discord or upset, and delusions. A human patient may feel as if he has two wills, each driving him to do opposing things, such as is found in schizophrenia (Reckeweg 2002). The remedy also contains Embryo suis with notes of anxiety on waking, an aversion to or a desire for company, and fears that something bad will happen. Patients who need this combination may be irascible or irresolute. They may be irritable with a changeable mood or be sensitive to music and noise. They also may be sensitive to touch and so aggravated by contact (Reckeweg 2002).

Chelidonium homaccord: Used for patients that manifest bilious anger, gallbladder pain, or pain at alarm point for gallbladder; also used in cases with elevated serum alkaline phosphatase values.

Gastricumheel: Used for the behavioral trait of "bites when nervous" (Heel 2003).

Gelsemium homaccord: Indicated for headaches, rear leg weakness, anxiety.

Glyoxal compositum: Provides enzyme activation. Has been used in human medicine at the outset of schizophrenia (Reckeweg 2000).

Hepar compositum: Drains and supports liver function in deeper homotoxicoses. Contains Pancreas suis for mental notes of fear of being injured or attacked or of being in narrow places. It is also used for irritability from trifles or on waking (Reckeweg 2002). It may support healing in dermatosis and neurogenic dermatitis, wherein patients suffer irritation, negative emotional responses, and antagonism resultant from altered skin sensations.

Hepeel: Provides support of liver function and detoxification. Contains the homeopathic potency of Veratrum album D5 (psychotic behavior).

Ignatia homaccord: Used for sadness and depression, leading to anger/aggression and restlessness (Pitcairn 2006).

Lachesis-Injeel: Although this remedy is not available in the United States, it deserves mention for cases of thyrotoxicosis.

Lymphomyosot: Used for lymph drainage and endocrine support.

Nervoheel: Indicated for anxiety.

Neuroheel: Provides nervous support.

Nux vomica homaccord: Prescribed for patients that manifest anger and may bite from nervousness (Heel 2003).

Phosporus homaccord: "The phosphorus-type/personality has slender limbs, silky hair, and thin skin; it is nervous, irritable, and fatigues quickly" (Heel 2003). Overexcitability and fear also can be noted (Heel 2003).

Spascupreel: Owing to the constituent Agaricus, used for excessive excitement or to reduce excitability of the nervous system. Also used in sequelae of drug and medication abuse, confused states, or cerebral seizure disorders (Reckeweg 2002). Contains Chamomilla, which is particularly suited to states of nervous agitation as a tranquillizing remedy. Patients are irritable, bad-tempered, irascible, and spiteful. Chamomilla is, in principle, a nerve remedy, indicated for easy agitation without any preexisting organic problem. Reckeweg (2002) states, "the decision to give Chamomilla is based on the discrepancy between the objective findings and the presenting emotional state of the patient."

Thyroidea compositum: Used for endocrine support and matrix drainage in advanced homotoxicoses.

Tonico-Injeel: Indicated for physical and psychic exhaustion.

Ubichinon compositum: Given for mitochondrial support of energy metabolism.

Valerianaheel: Has a mild tranquilizing effect.

Ypsiloheel: Used for central regulation.

Authors' suggested protocols

Nutrition
Brain nerve and behavior/emotional support formula: 1 tablet for each 25 pounds of body weight BID.

Liver support formula: One-half tablet for every 25 pounds of body weight BID.

Lecithin/phosphatidyl choline: One-fourth teaspoon for every 25 pounds of body weight BID.

Phosphatidyl serine (PS): 20 mg for every 15 pounds of body weight SID.

Blue-green algae: One-fourth teaspoon for every 25 pounds of body weight daily.

Chinese herbal medicine

The authors recommend Relaxol at a dose of 1 capsule per 10 to 20 pounds twice daily to effect.

In addition to the herbs mentioned above, Relaxol also contains lily bulb (Bai he), oyster shell (Mu li), haematite (Dai zhe shi), rehmannia (Sheng di huang), anemarrhena (Zhi mu), and fossil teeth (Long chi). Based on clinical observation, this formula helps to modulate behavior and reduce the aggression.

Warning: Any aggressive behavior must be handled very carefully. No single drug can eliminate the aggression entirely. Behavior modification, training, and safety precautions should be applied.

Homotoxicology (10 drops PO for 50-pound dog; 5 drops PO for small dog or cat)

Begin biological therapy in support of known issues. Do behavior modification/training simultaneously. Recheck cases every 14 to 30 days, depending upon progress.

Select the symptom remedy or remedies that best match the case and then select the Detoxification formula based upon the case's location on the Six-Phase Table of Homotoxicology.

Symptom remedy: As determined by case presentation. Contains Nux homaccord (aggression), Aconitum homaccord (fear aggression or history of generalized fever or red rash), Belladona homaccord (history of red spots on skin, sudden lunging attacks), BHI-Calming (hyperactivity and aggression), and Cerebrum compositum (cases with no clear picture).

Detoxification formula (for Phase 1 and 2): Detox Kit, which consists of Lymphomyosot, Nux homaccord, and Berberis homaccord, mixed together and given BID PO for 30 to 60 days, or Hepeel, Reneel, and Coenzyme compositum tablets given orally twice weekly for 30 days.

Deep detoxification formula (for Phases 3,4,5, and 6): Lymphomyosot, Hepar compositum, Solidago compositum, Thyroidea compositum, Coenzyme compositum, and Ubichinon compositum, mixed together and succussed, then administered PO every 3 days for 30 to 120 days or until recovery wanes.

In advanced or deep homotoxicoses consider Glyoxal compositum, given once.

Product sources

Nutrition

Brain/nerve, behavior/emotional, and liver support formulas: Animal Nutrition Technologies. **Alternatives:** Hepatic Support—Standard Process Veterinary Formulas; Hepato Support—Rx Vitamins for Pets, Hepagen—Thorne Veterinary Products.

Lecithin/phosphatidyl choline: Designs for Health.

Phosphatidyl serine (PS): Integrative Therapeutics.

Blue-green algae: Cell Tech (Simplexity) or BlueGreen Foods, Inc.

Chinese herbal medicine

Formula Relaxol: Natural Solutions, Inc.

Homotoxicology remedies

BHI/Heel Inc.

REFERENCES

Western medicine references

Beata CA. Diagnosis and Treatment of Aggression in Dogs and Cats. In: Recent Advances in Companion Animal Behavior Problems, Houpt KA, ed. Ithaca, NY. International Veterinary Information Service (www.ivis.org), 2001; A0808.1201.

Chapman BL. Feline Aggression: classification, diagnosis, and treatment. *Vet Clin North Am Small Anim Pract* 1991;21:315–328.

Eibl-Eibesfeldt I. Biologie du Comportement. 3rd ed. Paris: Ophrys, 1984, www.ivis.org. Document No. A0808.1201.

Houpt K. Domestic Animal Behavior for Veterinarians and Animal Scientists. 3rd ed. Ames: Iowa State University Press, 1998.

Overall KL. Clinical Behavioral Medicine for Small Animals. St Louis: Mosby, 1997.

Overall KL. Feline aggression. Part III: The role of social status in hierarchical systems. *Feline Pract* 1994;22:16–17.

Pageat P. Pathologie du Comportement du Chien. Point Vétérinaire, Maisons-Alfort, 1996.

Nutrition references

Broadfoot P. 1997. Personal communication.

Bruno J. Edible Microalgae: A Review of the Health Research. Center for Nutritional Psychology, 2001, p 23.

Cenacchi T, Bertoldin T, Farina C, et al. Cognitive decline in the elderly: a double-blind, placebo-controlled multicenter study on efficacy of phosphatidylserine administration. *Aging (Milano)* 1993;5:123–33.

Crook TH, Tinklenberg J, Yesavage J, et al. Effects of phosphatidylserine in age-associated memory impairment. *Neurology* 1991;41:644–9.

Crook T, Petrie W, Wells C, Massari DC. Effects of phosphatidylserine in Alzheimer's disease. *Psychopharmacol Bull*
1992;28:61–6.

Delwaide PJ, Gyselynck-Mambourg AM, Hurlet A, et al. Double-
blind randomized controlled study of phosphatidylserine in
senile demented patients. *Acta Neurol Scand* 1986;73:
136–40.

Engel RR, Satzger W, Gunther W, et al. Double-blind cross-over
study of phosphatidylserine vs. placebo in patients with early
dementia of the Alzheimer type. *Eur Neuropsychopharmacol*
1992;2:149–55.

Fünfgeld EW, Baggen M, Nedwidek P, et al. Double-blind study
with phosphatidylserine (PS) in Parkinsonian patients with
senile dementia of Alzheimer's type (SDAT). *Prog Clin Biol
Res* 1989;317:1235–46.

Goldstein R, et al. The BNA Handbook: A Working Manual for
Veterinarians, Animal Nutrition Technologies, Westport, CT.
2000.

Hanin I, Ansell GB. Lecithin: Technological, Biological and
Therapeutic Aspects. 1987. Plenum Press, NY, 180, 181.

Horrocks LA, et al. Phosphatidyl Research and the Nervous
System, 1986, Berlin: Springer Verlach.

Chinese herbal medicine references

Chang Yong Zhong Yao Xian Dai Yan Jiu Yu Lin Chuan
(Recent Study and Clinical Application of Common Traditional Chinese Medicine) 1995; 489:491.

Chen DY, et al. *Journal of Nanjing TCM University*.
1999;15(4):240.

Hao HQ, et al. Curdione's regulatory effect on cats' sleeping
rhythmic electric activity. *Journal of Chinese Materia Medica*.
1994;25(8):423–424.

Ou Yang Guang Ying. Trace elements of 11 tonifying herbs from
the Dunhuang region. *Journal of Gansu College of TCM*.
1990;7(4):24–25.

Wang Niu Wu. *Hunan Journal of TCM and Pharmacy*.
1998;4(5):26–27.

Zhong Yao Tong Bao (*Journal of Chinese Herbology*), 1985;
10(6): 43.

Zhong Yao Xue (*Chinese Herbology*), 1998; 676:677.

Zhong Yao Xue (Chinese Herbology), 1998, 722:725.

Zhong Yao Yao Li Yu Ying Yong (*Pharmacology and Applications of Chinese Herbs*), 1983;888.

Zhong Yao Yao Li Yu Ying Yong (*Pharmacology and Applications of Chinese Herbs*), 1983; 477.

Homotoxicology references

Beata C. 2006a. Ethological and Neurophysiological Basis
of Behavioral Disorders, in proceedings of The North
American Veterinary Conference, Vol 20, Orlando, FL, p
127–8.

Beata C. 2006b. Risk Assessment in Aggressive Dogs, in proceedings of The North American Veterinary Conference, Vol
20, Orlando, FL, pp 137–8.

Beaver B. Canine behaviors associated with hypothyroidism.
J Am Amim Hosp Assoc, 2003;39(5) p 431–4.

Day C. The Homoeopathic Treatment of Small Animals: Principles and Practice. 1990. CW Daniel Company, LTD:Saffron
Walden, Essex, p 127.

Heel. BHI Homeopathic Therapy: Professional Reference. 2002.
Albuquerque, NM: Heel Inc. p 41.

Heel. Veterinary Guide, 3rd English edition. Baden-Baden,
Germany: Biologische Heilmettel Heel GmbH. 2003. p 23,
152.

Kent J. Repertory of the Homoeopathic Materia Medica and a
Word Index. 1921. Paharganj, New Delhi: B. Jain, LTD:,
p vii.

Maciocia G. The Foundations of Chinese Medicine: A comprehensive text for acupuncturists and herbalists. 1989. London:
Churchill Livingstone. p 216.

Palmquist R. Personal discussion regarding aggression and
regressive vicariation observed in behavioral cases. 2003.
Unpublished.

Palmquist R. Homotoxicology: Clinical Case Management, in
proceedings of The North American Veterinary Conference,
2006. Vol 20, Orlando, FL, p 69 (See also taped lecture contents which are more complete).

Palmquist R, Demers J. Personal discussion regarding regressive
vicariations occurring in routine detoxification cases and one
case of seizures in a boxer. 2004. Unpublished.

Pitcairn R. Vegas: The Cat with Homesickness. Advanced
Homeopathy Course, Saguaro. 2006. Eugene, OR.

Reckeweg H. Biotherapeutic Index: Ordinatio Antihomotoxica
et Materia Medica, 5th ed. 2000. Baden-Baden, Germany:
Biologische Heilmittel Heel GMBH, p 343.

Reckeweg H. Homeopathia Antihomotoxica Materia Medica,
4th edition. 2002. Aurelia-Verlag, Baden-Baden, Germany,
p 121, 127, 134–35, 223–34, 287, 350–51, 477.

Roach B. Homotoxicology: Feline Behavior Case, published to
private member Internet list, Complementary Alternative Veterinary Medicine NET, Jan Bergeron, list owner. 2006.
January 30.

Wright J, Wright M. Personal communication from practitioners
well known for successful use of Bach flowers. 2006.

COMPULSIVE DISORDERS

Definition and cause

Compulsive disorders are not a specific diagnosis, and recommending therapy based upon diffuse, descriptive diagnoses often serves to label a patient, but not lead to successful understanding or management of that patient's condition. Generally speaking, it is advisable for professionals to avoid such descriptive diagnoses, especially when recommending therapy.

Compulsive disorders are frequently triggered by stressful conditions such as separation or change of environment, routine, or companionship. Once established, the disorders can become habitual and be present even without a trigger. The end result is a habitual behavior that, in dogs, often takes the form of self trauma such as flank sucking, acral lick granuloma, circling, or nail biting. In cats it takes the form of excessive licking and pulling out hair (Bradshaw 1997, Landsberg 2003).

While the underlying cause is debatable, there is uncertainty as to whether there is a similar underlying neurological disorder or whether the trigger influences the type and location of the compulsive behavior (Landsberg 2003, Luescher 1998).

In all instances of suspected compulsive disorders, it is essential to first rule out any underlying physical or medical causes. A complete physical examination, including blood work and urinalysis, is essential for proper diagnosis.

Medical therapy rationale, drug(s) of choice, and nutritional recommendations

All therapies should be preceded by identifying and eliminating the underlying cause. Medical therapy with tricyclic antidepressants such as Clomipramine have proven successful. Selective serotonin reuptake inhibitors (SSRI) such as Fluoxetine have been shown to be effective with fewer side effects (Overall 1996, Wynchank 1998). In all compulsive disorders, combining medical therapy with behavioral modification techniques and environmental modification offers the best results for controlling the condition.

Anticipated prognosis

In many instances it is not possible to totally eliminate the compulsive behavior; however, good success can be achieved in reducing the frequency as well as the intensity of the episodes.

Integrative veterinary therapies

Integrative therapies should be considered after the diagnosis has been made and complicating conditions such as chronic pain have been confirmed or ruled out. The medical approach of drug and behavior modification techniques do not consider physiological, biochemical, nutritional, and autoimmune reactions such as those from environmental chemical toxins as well as adverse reactions to medications and vaccinations. The inclusion of integrative therapies, nutrition, nutraceuticals, medicinal herbs and homotoxicology remedies, along with drugs and behavior modification therapies or as a freestanding protocol, can improve day-to-day quality of life as well as help to control the compulsive behavior.

Nutrition
General considerations/rationale

The nutritional approach to compulsive disorders consists of nutrient support of the brain and nervous system; enhancement of the gentle detoxification of environmental chemicals, toxins, medication, and vaccinations; and the addition of behavior-modifying or -enhancing natural remedies such as flower essences.

Appropriate nutrients
Nutritional/gland therapies: Glandular brain and pineal supply intrinsic nutrients and can help improve circulation, reduce inflammation, and improve function of the brain and central nervous system (Goldstein 2000) (see Chapter 2, Gland Therapies, for additional information).

Phospholipids found in glandular brain are a source of unsaturated omega-3 fatty acids, which are now thought to play a vital role in the development and maintenance of the central nervous system. High concentrations of phosphatidyl choline and serine are found in brain tissue. Horrocks (1986) reported on the potential clinical use of these nutrients in chronic neurological conditions.

Lecithin/phosphatidyl choline: Phosphatidyl choline is a phospholipid that is integral to cellular membranes particularly of nerve and brain cells. It helps to move fats into the cells and is involved in acetylcholine uptake, neurotransmission, and cellular integrity. As part of the cell membranes, lecithin is an essential nutrient required by cells for general health and wellness (Hanin 1987).

Phosphatidyl serine (PS): Phosphatidyl serine is a phospholipid that is essential for cellular membranes, particularly of brain cells. It has been studied in people with altered mental functioning and degeneration with positive results (Crook 1991, Cenacchi 1993). In people with Alzheimer's disease, the addition of PS to the program provided a mild to significant clinical improvement (Delewaide 1986, Engel 1992, Funfgeld 1989).

Essential fatty acids: Research confirms the benefits of essential fatty acids with regards to their calming effect on the central nervous system (Erasmus 1993).

Chinese herbal medicine
General considerations/rationale
Compulsive disorders are thought to arise from Yin deficiency in the Heart and Qi stagnation in the Liver according to TCM theory. According to the Western interpretation, the Heart houses the Shen, or mind. When there are not enough fluids (Yin) to nourish the Heart, the Shen may be disturbed. This leads to a propensity for the affected individual to have psychological disturbances. The Liver is responsible for overseeing the smooth flow of the Qi. Energy does not flow efficiently when Liver Qi is stagnant. The individual feels constrained and irritable, and she may turn to repetitive actions to try to calm herself. It is necessary to relax the mind to treat these compulsive activities.

Appropriate chinese herbs

Albizzia flower (He huan hua): Depresses the central nervous system (Zhong Yao Xue 1998).

Bupleurum (Chai hu): Contains saikosaponins, which have sedative effects (Zhong Yao Yao Li Yu Ying Yong 1983).

Curcurma root (Yu jin): Contains curdione, which is a sedative in cats (Hao 1994).

Fossil teeth (Long chi): Used for psychological disturbances. Seventy-nine schizophrenic patients were treated with a supplement containing fossilized animal bones, Mu li, Zhi gan cao, Da zao, Xiao mai ± other herbs as determined by the individual doctor. Seventy-eight percent responded well (Zhe Jiang Zhong Yi Yao Za Zhi 1982).

Grass-leaf sweet-flag root (Shi chang pu): Has tranquilizing effects (Zhong Yao Xue 1998).

Polygala root (Yuan zhi): Causes sedation. Its high level of bromine has a tranquilizing effect (Ou 1990).

Polygonum stem (Ye jiao teng): Has demonstrated sedative effects in mice. Experimentally, it decreased the amount of pentobarbital needed to sedate mice (Chen 1999).

White peony (Bai Shao): Has sedative effects in mice and increases sedation time when combined with phenobarbitol (Zhong Yao Tong Bao 1985).

Zizyphus (Suan zao ren): Has been shown to have sedative effects in dogs, cats, rats, rabbits, and guinea pigs. The total flavone portion was proven to inhibit the autonomous activities of mice. Studies have indicated that jujuboside is most likely to be the component responsible for the sedative effects. When combined with barbiturates, zizyphus can increase sedation time in mice. It has been shown to counteract the excitatory effects of caffeine (Zhao 1995, Guo 1998, Chang Yong Zhong Yao Xian Dai Yan Jiu Yu Lin Chuan 1995).

Homotoxicology
General considerations/rationale

No homeopathic or homotoxicology remedies have been specifically studied for use in these conditions in animals. When approaching such cases, the author recommends attempting to identify more precise pathology and select the treatment based upon those findings. In a general sense, the Six-Phase Table of Homotoxicology can be used to guide remedy selection. These disorders fall in nearly any phase, so it is necessary to look carefully for clues in determining the phase of the homotoxicoses. In many cases, these broad general complaints may direct a trained homoeopathic veterinarian to select a specific classical homeopathic remedy, but these are still used on a more or less trial basis and broad clinical protocols cannot be properly formulated at this time.

Every compulsive disorder case should be carefully examined for pain. Generalized, regional, or focal pain may cause irrational or repetitive behavior. Trigger point therapy can involve localizing specific painful points and injecting them with specific antihomotoxic medicines such as Traumeel or Spascupreel (See remarks for *Galium-Heel* below).

Appropriate homotoxicology formulas

Because antihomotoxic medicines are generally nontoxic and free of harmful side effects, it may be appropriate to attempt treatment of these cases using homotoxicology theory and other biological therapies. Clients should be so informed prior to ever beginning therapy. All patients presented for such issues should have a thorough medical and behavioral history (including any known trauma or abuse), full physical and detailed neurological examination, CBC, chemistry, and thyroid determinations, as well as urinalysis and urine culture. Radiographs and other forms of imaging may be needed. Consultation with medical and behavioral specialists may be indicated.

The clinician should be especially aware of the contribution of dietary and other allergies to these cases. Every attempt should be made to determine exposure to potential toxins, both environmental and medical. Adverse reactions to many medical agents can cause neurological and mental signs and cessation of nonessential medications may assist in some cases. Detailed discussion of these remedies is beyond the scope of this text, but several commonly considered remedies are listed below:

Belladona homaccord: Consider if seizures are present in cases associated with focal inflammatory reactions and sudden aggression.

Berberis homaccord: Supports and drains urogenital tissues and supports the adrenal gland.

BHI-Headache II: Indicated for throbbing headache, pain aggravated by noise and light, and restlessness.

Engystol N: Useful in cases of viral impregnation damage, particularly in cases associated with neurological damage from canine distemper virus.

Galium-Heel: Commonly prescribed due to the mental and physical symptom notes provided by Phosphorus, which consist of inflammation of the respiratory, digestive, urinary, and reproductive organs; severe infectious diseases; disorders in convalescence; conditions of exhaustion and rheumatism; spinal complaints, neuralgia; headaches; paralysis; hypersensitivity of the sensory organs; abnormal behavior; emotional discord; or upset (Reckeweg 2002). It is important to consider that many stereotypical behaviors may have roots in discomfort and pain, and since all painful conditions represent Impregnation disorders, *Galium-Heel* is frequently needed in cases involving pain as a phase remedy.

Hepar compositum: Useful in establishing deep drainage, detoxification, and support of hepatic tissues.

Hormeel: Used for hyperactivity, nervous disorders.

Ignatia homaccord: Used for depression, anxiety, hysteria, nervous excitability.

Neuro-Injeel: Contains Valeriana, as well as Ignatia, and both of these homeopathic dilutions are recommended for nervous disorders; also indicated for emotional discord or upset and spasmodic conditions experienced at hollow organs and muscles. Mental notes are great anxiety on waking and are worse after midnight; indicated by business, irritability, restlessness, sensitivity to noise, and possessed of repetitive thoughts (Reckeweg 2002). Ignatia is also found in *Cerebrum compositum* and *Nervoheel*.

Nervoheel: Indicated for depression, restless hands and feet, neuralgia.

Cerebrum compositum: Supports cerebral tissue and detoxification; improves mentation. Embryo suis is a key component of this combination with the mental picture attributed as follows: active and busy, confusion on waking, patient may be discontented and/or demonstrate symptoms showing that the case is better from diversions. Changeable mood, restlessness improve with the condition of the patient. Human patients have thoughts that are persistent, or that are clear but with more emotion (Reckeweg 2002). Also contains Medorrhinum, which has effects on mucosal inflammations of the urinary and reproductive organs, the respiratory passages, and the gastrointestinal tract; rheumatism; abnormal behavior; and premature aging (Reckeweg 2002).

Psorinoheel: Deep remedy for use in Excretion and Impregnation phase disorders; consider if seizures present.

Spascupreel: Contains Agaricus (*Amanita muscaria*). Indicated for patients demonstrating sensitivity to cold air, motor restlessness, chorea, tics, states of agitation, epileptiform attacks, itching, crawling sensations, burning pains, and sensations of numbness (as if frozen). The predominant characteristic is a hyperesthesia of the whole body, with the slightest pressure causing pain. There is general painfulness of all of the limbs, especially the lower extremities; pain is marked on sitting or standing, and gradually subsides on walking. This is accompanied by a feeling of coldness with paresthesia (numbness and crawling sensation) and sensitivity to cold air. There is a general restlessness of the muscles with a compulsion to move in unusual ways (Reckeweg 2002).

Valerianaheel: Used for restlessness and neurasthenia. This remedy takes its name from the herb Valeriana. Its main homeopathic indications are consequences of excitement, insomnia, waking with fear and gagging, and restlessness with compulsive motion (pacing, etc.) (Reckeweg 2002).

Veratrum homaccord: Indicated for gastroenteritis, colitis, diarrhea, paper shredding, collapse, or psychosis.

Ypsiloheel: Improves central nervous system regulation.

BHI-Calming: Used for twitching muscles, headache, mania, and compulsive twitching.

Authors' suggested protocols

Nutrition

Brain nerve and behavior support formulas: 1 tablet for every 25 pounds of body weight BID.

Lecithin/phosphatidyl choline: One-fourth teaspoon for every 25 pounds of body weight BID.

Phosphatidyl serine (PS): 20 mg for every 15 pounds of body weight SID.

Oil of evening primrose: 1 capsule for every 25 pounds of body weight SID.

Chinese herbal medicine

Relaxol: 1 capsule per 10 to 20 pounds twice daily to effect. It may be advisable to consult with an animal behaviorist for complementary therapy. In addition to the herbs mentioned above, Relaxol contains anemarrhena (Zhi mu), haematite (Dai zhe shi), lily (Bai he), oyster shell (Mu li), and rehmannia (Sheng di huang). These additional herbs help increase the efficacy of the formula. They have synergistic actions with the herbs mentioned above.

Homotoxicology (Dose: 10 drops PO for 50-pound dog; 5 drops PO for cat or small dog)

Select the symptom remedy or remedies that best match the case and then select the detoxification formula which is applicable based upon the case's location on the Six-Phase Table of Homotoxicology.

Symptom formula: Select individual formulas based upon the symptoms manifested by the patient from the Appropriate Homotoxicology Formulas (above) or according to further research by the clinician. Cerebrum compositum twice weekly is a safe starting place. Hormeel, Nervoheel, and BHI-Calming are also common first remedies.

Detoxification formula (for cases in phases 1, 2, 3): Lymphomyosot, Berberis homaccord, and Nux vomica homaccord mixed together and given BID for 30 to 60 days, OR Hepeel plus Reneel BID PO. In cases where environmental toxicity may play a part, also give *BHI-Body Pure* BID.

Deep detoxification formula (for cases manifesting homotoxicoses in phases 3, 4, 5, 6): Galium-Heel, Lymphomyosot, Hepar compositum, Solidago compositum, Thryoidea compositum, Coenzyme compositum, and Ubichinon compositum mixed together and given PO every 3 days for 120 days or longer as needed.

In Degeneration or Dedifferentiation phase disorders consider Glyoxal compositum, given once and not repeated until recovery wanes.

Product sources

Nutrition

Brain and behavior support formulas: Animal Nutrition Technologies. **Alternatives:** Composure—Vetri Science Laboratories
Lecithin/phosphatidyl choline—Designs for Health
Phosphatidyl serine (PS)—Integrative Therapeutics
Oil of evening primrose—Jarrow Formulas.

Chinese herbal medicine

Relaxol: Natural Solutions, Inc.

Homotoxicology remedies

BHI/Heel Corporation: Bach flower Remedies—Ellon Bach; Anaflora Flower Essences—Earth Animal, Inc.

REFERENCES

Western medicine references

Bradshaw JWS, Neville PF, Sawyer D. Factors affecting pica in the domestic cat. *J App An Behav Sci*, 1997; 52, 373–379.

Dodman NH, Knowles KE, Shuster L, et al. Behavioral changes associated with complex partial seizures in Bull Terriers. *J Am Vet Med Assoc*, 1996;208, 688–691.

Goldberger E, Rapaport JL. Canine acral lick dermatitis: response to the antiobsessional drug clomipramine. *JAAHA*, 1990;27, 179–182.

Landsberg G. Handbook of Behavior Problems of the Dog and Cat. 2003. WB Saunders Co. Ltd.

Luescher UA. Compulsive behaviour in dogs. *Veterinary International*, 1998;10 (2), 7–12.

Overall KL. Drugs, Pets and Prozac. *Can Pract*, 1996; 21 (5), 20–24.

Paterson S. A placebo-controlled study to investigate clomipramine in the treatment of canine acral lick granuloma. Third World Congress of Veterinary Dermatology Proceedings, 1996, Edinburgh, Scotland, UK, September.

Wynchank D, Berk M. Fluoxetine treatment of acral lick dermatitis in dogs: a placebo-controlled randomized double blind trial. *Depress Anxiety* 1998; 8 (1): 21–3.

Nutrition references

Erasmus U. Fats That Heal, Fats That Kill. Alive Books; revised and updated edition (January 1, 1993). The Complete Lecture, www.udoerasmus.com.

Broadfoot P. 1997. Personal communication.

Bruno J. Edible Microalgae: A Review of the Health Research. Center for Nutritional Psychology, 2001. p 23.

Cenacchi T, Bertoldin T, Farina C, et al. Cognitive decline in the elderly: a double-blind, placebo-controlled multicenter study on efficacy of phosphatidylserine administration. *Aging (Milano)* 1993;5:123–33.

Crook TH, Tinklenberg J, Yesavage J, et al. Effects of phosphatidylserine in age-associated memory impairment. *Neurology* 1991;41:644–9.

Crook T, Petrie W, Wells C, Massari DC. Effects of phosphatidylserine in Alzheimer's disease. *Psychopharmacol Bull* 1992;28:61–6.

Delwaide PJ, Gyselynck-Mambourg AM, Hurlet A, et al. Double-blind randomized controlled study of phosphatidylserine in senile demented patients. *Acta Neurol Scand* 1986;73:136–40.

Engel RR, Satzger W, Gunther W, et al. Double-blind cross-over study of phosphatidylserine vs. placebo in patients with early dementia of the Alzheimer type. *Eur Neuropsychopharmacol* 1992;2:149–55.

Fünfgeld EW, Baggen M, Nedwidek P, et al. Double-blind study with phosphatidylserine (PS) in Parkinsonian patients with senile dementia of Alzheimer's type (SDAT). *Prog Clin Biol Res* 1989;317:1235–46.

Goldstein R., et al. The BNA Handbook: A Working Manual for Veterinarians, Westport, CT: Animal Nutrition Technologies. 2000.

Hanin I, Ansell GB. Lecithin: Technological, Biological, and Therapeutic Aspects 1987. NY: Plenum Press, 180, 181.

Horrocks LA., et al. Phosphatidyl Research and the Nervous System, Berlin: Springer Verlach, 1986.

Chinese herbal medicine references

Chang Yong Zhong Yao Xian Dai Yan Jiu Yu Lin Chuan (Recent Study and Clinical Application of Common Traditional Chinese Medicine), 1995;489:491.

Chen DY, et al. *Journal of Nanjing TCM University*. 1999;15(4):240

Guo SM, et al. The central inhibitory effect of Suan Zao Ren total flavone. *Journal of Traditional Chinese Medicine Material*. 1998;21(11):578–579.

Hao HQ, et al. Curdione's regulatory effect on cats' sleeping rhythmic electric activity. *Journal of Chinese Materia Medica*. 1994;25(8):423–424.

Ou Yang Guang Ying. Trace elements of 11 tonifying herbs from the Dunhuang region. *Journal of Gansu College of TCM*. 1990;7(4):24–25.

Zhao QX, et al. The central inhibitory effect of Suan Zao Ren. *Journal of Xi-An Medical University*. 1995;16(4):432–434.

Zhe Jiang Zhong Yi Yao Za Zhi Zhejiang. *Journal of Chinese Medicine*. 1982; 6:273.

Zhong Yao Tong Bao. *Journal of Chinese Herbology*. 1985; 10(6):43.

Zhong Yao Xue. *Chinese Herbology*. 1998; 676:677.

Zhong Yao Xue. *Chinese Herbology*. 1998, 722: 725.

Zhong Yao Yao Li Yu Ying Yong. *Pharmacology and Applications of Chinese Herbs*. 1983;888.

Homotoxicology references

Heel. BHI Homeopathic Therapy: Professional Reference. 2002. Albuquerque, NM: Heel Inc.

Reckeweg H. *Biotherapeutic Index: Ordinatio Antihomotoxica et Materia Medica*, 5th ed. 2000. Baden-Baden, Germany: Biologische Heilmittel Heel GMBH.

Reckeweg H. *Homeopathia Antihomotoxica Materia Medica*,
4th ed. 2002.Aurelia-Verlag, Baden-Baden, Germany, pp 127,
287, 318, 409, 490, 589.

INAPPROPRIATE URINATION

Definition and cause

Inappropriate urination is defined as urinating outside the
litter box or in particular and specific locations in the
house. It is often a behavioral trait related to normal feline
marking behavior; abnormal, habitual, or compulsive
behavior; or a physical condition. This condition is more
common in cats than dogs and in males than females.

All patients presented for such issues should have a
thorough medical and behavioral history (concentrating
on diet, water intake, environmental stressors, and litter
box medium, location, and cleanliness), physical/neuro-
logical examination, urinalysis, and urine culture/sensitiv-
ity performed. In many cases, further diagnostic evaluation
is necessary and may include urinalysis, urine culture and
sensitivity, CBC, serum chemistry and thyroid/endocrine
determinations, FeLV/FIV virus status, and radiographs
and ultrasound imaging. Blood pressure determination
may reveal hypertension, which can be associated with
behavioral problems. Consultation with medical and
behavioral specialists may be indicated and many of these
patients are greatly assisted with pheromone therapy and
proper litter box handling.

Medical therapy rationale, drug(s) of choice, and nutritional recommendations

The treatment should be based on the proper diagnosis
of any causative medical condition. Most veterinarians
recommend environmental and behavioral modification
techniques before resorting to medications. Techniques
include frequent cleaning of the litter box, strategically
locating litter boxes in heavily soiled areas, and separating
feeding and litter locations. Medication is usually recommended as the last resort.

Medications such as benzodiazepines (Alprazolam) can
be used but can be associated with serious complications
such as liver failure. Other drugs such as Buspirone and
amitriptyline have also been used with varying degrees of
success. Pheromone therapy such as Feliway (Farnum Pet
Products, Phoenix, Ariz.) have been reported to halt the
problem (Cooper 1997; Ekstein 1996; Houpt 1998, 2004;
Overall 1994, 1997, 1998).

Anticipated prognosis

While not a serious condition, this is a very common
condition that often leads to frustration and helplessness

and can result in the decision to euthanize. For this reason
it is important to establish and eliminate any underlying
causes early, and quickly implement behavior and environmental modification techniques that improve the
chances of successful control of the condition (Houpt
2004, Halip 1992, Borchelt 1986).

Integrative veterinary therapies

While the medical approach focuses on the environmental
and behavioral aspects, and the medical route as a last
resort, often, little is done to internally correct the physical
or emotional imbalances that underlie the condition. A
more global view of the condition illustrates the surface
conditions such as the odor of the litter, the physical place-
ment of the litter box, the elimination of boredom, etc. as
the trigger to the behavior. These factors are stresses or
stressors that, when triggered, bring on the condition.

Integrative therapies add the dimension of nourishing,
balancing, and improving the nervous, mental, and emotional stability of the animal. This helps the animal to
become less reactive to stressors and therefore less likely
to initiate episodes of inappropriate urination.

In addition to nutritional and herbal therapies, the
authors advise multiple clean litter boxes, both with and
without covers, to allow cats to satisfy their preference.
Offer the cat both clay and sand litters to avoid substrate
avoidance. In some cases it may be advisable to avoid
perfumed substrates.

Nutrition
General considerations/rationale

The nutritional approach to inappropriate urination
consists of nutrient support of the brain and nervous
system; enhancement of the detoxification of environmental chemicals, toxins, medication and prior vaccinations;
and the addition of behavior-modifying or -enhancing
natural remedies such as flower essences (see Separation
Anxiety, below).

Appropriate nutrients

Nutritional/gland therapies: Glandular brain and pineal
supply intrinsic nutrients and can help improve emotional
status and brain function (see Chapter 2, Gland Therapies). Phospholipids found in glandular brain are a source
of unsaturated omega-3 fatty acids, which are now
thought to play a vital role in the development and maintenance of the central nervous system. High concentrations of phosphatidyl choline and serine are found in
brain tissue. Horrocks (1986) reported on the potential
clinical use of these nutrients in chronic neurological
conditions.

Phosphatidyl serine (PS): Phosphatidyl serine is a phospholipid, an essential ingredient in cellular membranes

and particularly of brain cells. It has been studied in people with altered mental functioning and degeneration with positive results (Crook 1991, Cenacchi 1993). In people with Alzheimer's disease the addition of PS to the program showed a mild to significant clinical improvement (Delewaide 1986, Engel 1992, Funfgeld 1989).

Essential fatty acids: Blue-green algae have been observed to create a generalized feeling of well-being in humans taking the product, and may prove helpful in veterinary patients. Its effects are usually observed to be slower in onset with the resultant benefits taking 3 to 4 weeks to appear. This may be due in part to their natural antihistaminic compounds or their levels of omega-3 fatty acids (Bruno 2001).

Many recent studies have confirmed the beneficial results from these critical fatty acids. Aphanizomenon flos aquae, a blue-green algae, has been shown in clinical settings to have positive effects on brain function. In addition to the omega-3 fatty acids, it contains a full spectrum of essential amino acids, a broad-based mineral content, a rapidly assimilable glyolipoprotein cell wall, and a wide variety of vitamins. It has mild chelating properties so it is valuable in heavy metal toxicoses such as Thimerosol reactions. It is an asset as a micronutrient resource and figures prominently in many treatment programs (Broadfoot 1997).

Chinese herbal medicine
General considerations/rationale

According to TCM theory, inappropriate urination is due to Yin and Blood deficiency in the Heart with Qi stagnation in the Liver. According to the Western interpretation, inappropriate urination is defined in TCM terms as a disturbance in the mind. The Shen, or Mind, is housed in the Heart. Blood and Yin (fluids) are nourishing. The mind is not nourished when there is a Blood and or Yin deficiency in the Heart; therefore, the mind does not function normally. The Liver uses its energy or Qi to ensure the smooth flow of energy and emotions in the body. When the Liver Qi becomes stagnant, the animal becomes irritable, stressed, and nervous. In the case of inappropriate urination, the animal manifests this stress by eliminating in an undesirable location(s). Therefore, treatment must be directed at calming the patients.

Appropriate chinese herbs

Albizzia flower (He huan hua): Has been shown to cause sedation in mice (Zhong Yao Xue 1998).

Grass-leaf sweet-flag root (Shi chang pu): Has demonstrated sedative effects (Zhong Yao Xue 1998).

Polygala root (Yuan zhi): Contains a high level of bromine, which has a tranquilizing effect (Ou 1990). It has been shown to be tranquilizing in mice (Zhong Yao Yao Li Yu Ying Yong 1983).

Polygonum stem (Ye jiao teng): Has tranquilizing effects in mice (Chen 1999).

White peony (Bai shao): Has sedative effects in mice and has a synergistic effect with phenobarbitol in prolonging sleep time. It also protects against cardiazol-induced seizures (Zhong Yao Tong Bao 1985).

Zizyphus (Suan zao ren): Has sedative and hypnotic effects in mice, dogs, cats, rabbits, rats, and guinea pigs. This effect has been attributed to the jujuboside component (Chang Yong Zhong Yao Xian Dai Yan Jiu Yu Lin Chuan 1995). The flavone component combined with pentobarbital sedates the central nervous system and can counteract benzedrine-induced central excitation (Zhao 1995, Guo 1998).

Homotoxicology
General considerations/rationale

When approaching such cases, the author recommends attempting to identify more precise pathology and then recommending treatment based upon those findings. In a general sense we may use the Six-Phase Table of Homotoxicology to guide remedy selection. These disorders fall in nearly any phase, so it is necessary to look carefully for clues in determining the phase of the homotoxicoses.

Most veterinary behavioral specialists reserve the use of drugs in these cases of last resort. Psychoactive drugs are advocated by some authors, but bearing in mind the damage and side effects that these medications can cause in humans, it is recommended that all other options be eliminated before prescribing potentially damaging drugs (Palmquist 2003, Prozactruth.com).

The authors have many cases referred to them in which clients report negative side effects of commonly prescribed psychiatric drugs. While the veterinary literature is lacking in understanding these side effects, it is not unlikely that veterinary patients suffer similar mental side effects, which they are unable to communicate to their owners. Many of these owners have left their prior veterinarian after receiving psychiatric prescriptions and observing lethargy or generalized poor vitality after administering the drugs to their pets. Biological therapy provides another option.

Treating the correct cause, selecting proper symptom remedies, and conducting proper detoxification may prove helpful in cases of inappropriate urination. In some cases, these broad general complaints may direct a trained homoeopathic veterinarian to select a specific classical homeopathic remedy, but these are still more or less used on a trial-and-error basis. Broad clinical protocols cannot be properly formulated at this time.

Appropriate homotoxicology formulas

Because antihomotoxic medicines are generally nontoxic and free of harmful side effects, it may be appropriate to attempt treatment of these cases using homotoxicology theory and other biological therapies. Clients should be so informed prior to ever beginning therapy. Use of homotoxicology remedies without proper diagnosis and dietary therapy is discouraged. Some useful remedies appear below.

Berberis homaccord: Used for support and drainage of urogenital tissues and adrenal gland. Some characteristic indications of Berberis indications are irritations and inflammations of the urinary tract; radiating renal pains, especially pain radiating down the ureters; and tenesmus (physical sensations frequently found in cases suffering from renal colic and urinary gravel), even extending down the urethra and into the testicles. Berberis is one of the main remedies for renal calculi, pyelitis, and cystitis (Reckeweg 2002). The constituent of Berberis is also found in the following antihomotoxic medicines: *Reneel, Solidago compositum,* and *Populus compositum.*

BHI-Calming—(behavioral): Indicated for twitching muscles, headache, mania, and compulsive twitching.

Cantharis compositum: Used for cases with burning urination, stranguria, and hematuria. The formula's primary constituent is Cantharis (Spanish Fly), which principally affects the mucosa of the genito-urinary organs, with indications for violent inflammations with states of irritation and hemorrhagic inflammations. The urinary symptoms are frequently accompanied by cramping and spastic contraction, and are linked with continuous violent urging to urinate. The urine is only passed in drops and violent burning pains persist afterwards, extending possibly as far as the sacrum (Reckeweg 2002). This remedy is contained in the following formulas: *Populus compositum, Reneel,* and *Solidago compositum.*

BHI-Bladder: Used for cystitis complaints.

BHI-Prostate: Used for cases manifesting FUS blockage (once relief of obstruction has occurred), straining, burning, and difficult urination.

Echinacea compositum: Used in cases of bacterial and inflammatory cystitis, especially in Inflammation and Impregnation phases.

Galium-Heel: Used for cellular detoxification and renal tubular support. Specific renal system support comes from several components. Clematis helps with inflammation of the urinary bladder, urethra, testicles, prostate, and epididymis; urethral strictures and pain in the urethra on external pressure; spasmodic narrowing and contraction of the urethra with purulent discharge (urethritis); and tenesmus and pain on urinating, with intermittent stream and involuntary dribbling afterwards. Clematis also helps the mental status parameters, including great irritability, choleric temperament, and the complaints often triggered by anger or vexation. The chief component, Galium aparine, acts especially on the urinary system and is said to be able to dissolve renal calculi. It is also useful in edema, dysuria, and cystitis. Juniperus communis, whose main indications include glomerulonephritis, acts as a diuretic that targets elimination dysfunctions of the urinary tract collection system (Reckeweg 2002). The remedy also contains Phosphorus for inflammations of urinary and reproductive organs; severe infectious diseases; and disorders in convalescence and conditions of exhaustion along with abnormal behavior, emotional discord, or upset (Reckeweg 2002).

Hormeel (behavioral)*:* Used for hyperactivity and nervous disorders by way of its homeopathic constituent Sepia, which is used for the following symptoms: sensation of bearing-down and fullness in the urinary organs; pressure on the bladder and frequent passing of urine with flatulence in the lower abdomen; inflammation of the urinary organs; and the urine contains a sediment like clay and may also be very offensive. Sepia also helps with disorders in voiding from the urinary bladder. In enuresis, the incontinence usually takes place during the first stages of sleep. Mental factors used in prescribing this for humans include exhaustion, disorders of an emotional or otherwise psychological nature, and depressive emotional discord or upset (Reckeweg 2002).

Mucosa compositum: Used in the recovery phase of cystitis or pyelonephritis. Contains Colibacillinumin, which may be given for urinary tenesmus and dark-colored, offensive urine; salpingitis; cystitis; renal calculi; and cholangitis; and in depressive psychoses. It has a strong behavioral component. It is especially indicated after antibiotics and in retoxic damage caused by antibiotics (Reckeweg 2002).

Plantago homaccord: Used in cases demonstrating cystalgia and urinary incontinence. Note that this combination is not currently available in the United States, but it is extremely useful and it is hoped that it will be reinstated as part of Heel's product line.

Populus compositum: Contains Kreosotum, which is useful in cases demonstrating incontinence at night as a prevailing symptom; also for profuse pale urine and violent urge to urinate. *Populus compositum* also contains Mercurius sublimatus corrosivus for affections of the mucosa, acute glomerulonephritis with albuminuria, haematuria, and tenesmus. Mental notes useful to this remedy include shivering, trembling of the limbs, fear, restlessness, unquenchable thirst, brain symptoms. *Populus compositum* is also found in *Solidago compositum* (Reckeweg 2002). Other remedies in this combination include: Equisetum, Solidago, Berberis, and a number of other well-indicated components.

Reneel: Used for kidney support and detoxification. This remedy contains *Causticum,* which is known for its usefulness for disorders of the urinary tract, spasmodic contractions, paralysis, itching of the urethral orifice, tenesmus of urine, raw pain in the bladder, enuresis day or night, and stress incontinence of urine (Reckeweg 2002). In addition, it has the mental notes dictating use in cases manifesting emotional discord or upset, and thus may be valuable in stressed animals.

Solidago compositum: This is a formula for deep drainage and support of urogenital tissues in Deposition, Impregnation, Degeneration, and Dedifferentiation phase cases. Contains Colibacillinum (See Mucosa compositum, above) and Equisetum arvense, with the main indications being use for cystitis; pyelitis with copious discharge of mucus in the urine; dull, raw pain in the bladder; nephrolithiasis; gravel in the urine; and nocturnal enuresis associated with irritation of the bladder. All varieties of Equisetum act primarily on the connective tissue and the urinary tract, with signs of renal pain extending as far as the bladder and urethra. The urge to urinate with violent pains after urination, and passage of urine drop by drop are typical symptoms; there are also violent burning and cutting pains on urination (Reckeweg 2002).

Ubichinon compositum: Provides mitochondrial support and improved cellular energy mechanics in deep phase disorders. Bianchi (1995) recommends this agent for renal damage following vaccinations.

Spascupreel: Used for cases that suffer spasms and painful constriction. *Spascupreel* has an affinity for smooth muscle. The Gelsemium component is particularly indicated in states of paralysis, and in weakness of the bladder and urinary incontinence (Reckeweg 2002).

Authors' suggested protocols

Nutrition
Brain nerve formula: 1 tablet for every 25 pounds of body weight BID.

Behavioral/emotional/stress formula: 1 tablet for every 25 pounds of body weight BID.

Phosphatidyl serine (PS): 20 mg for every 15 pounds of body weight SID.

Blue-green algae: One-fourth teaspoon for every 25 pounds of body weight daily.

Chinese herbal medicine
For psychogenic inappropriate urination the authors recommend Relaxol at a dose of 1 capsule for every 10 to 20 pounds twice a day as needed. In addition to the herbs listed above, Relaxol also contains anemarrhena (Zhi mu), bupleurum (Chai hu), curcuma root (Yu jin), fossil teeth (Long chi), haematite (Dai zhe shi), lily (Bai he), oyster shell (Mu li), and rehmannia (Sheng di huang). These additional herbs improve the efficacy of the formula.

Homotoxicology (dose: 10 drops PO for 50-pound dog; 5 drops PO for cat or small dog)
Select the symptom remedy or remedies that best match the case and then select the detoxification formula which is applicable based upon the case's location on the Six-Phase Table of Homotoxicology.

Symptom formula: Select individual formulas based upon the symptoms manifested by the patient from the Appropriate Homotoxicology Formulas section or according to further research by the clinician. For cystitis, consider Berberis homaccord, possibly combined with BHI-Bladder BID to TID PO. For behavioral issues, consider Valerianaheel and possibly Hormeel or BHI-Calming BID PO.

Detoxification formula (for cases in phases 1, 2, 3): Lymphomyosot, Berberis homaccord, and Nux vomica homaccord mixed together and given BID PO for 30 to 60 days, or Hepeel plus Reneel BID PO. In cases where environmental toxicity may play a part, also give BHI Body Pure BID.

Deep detoxification (for cases in phases 3, 4, 5, 6): Galium-Heel, Lymphomyosot, Hepar compositum, Solidago compositum, Thryoidea compositum, Coenzyme compositum, and Ubichinon compositum mixed together and given PO every 3 days for 120 days or longer as needed.

In Degeneration or Dedifferentiation phase disorders, consider Glyoxal compositum given once and not repeated until recovery wanes.

Product sources

Nutrition
Brain/nerve and behavioral/emotional/stress formulas: Animal Nutrition Technologies. **Alternatives:** Composure—Vetri Science Laboratories
Phosphatidyl serine (PS)—Integrative Therapeutics
Blue-green algae—Simplexity.

Chinese herbal medicine
Relaxol: Natural Solutions, Inc.

Homotoxicology remedies
BHI Heel, Inc.

REFERENCES

Western medicine references
Cooper LL. Feline inappropriate elimination. *Vet Clin North Am Small Anim Pract.* 1997;27:569–600.
Borchelt PL, Voith VL. Elimination behavior problems in cats. *Compend Contin Educ Pract Vet.* 1986;8:3–12.
Eckstein RA, Hart BL. Pharmacologic approaches to urine marking in cats. In: Dodman NH, Shuster L, eds. Psychophar-

macology of animal behavior disorders. Maiden, Mass: Blackwell Science, 1998;264–278.

Halip JW, Luescher UA, McKeown DB. Inappropriate elimination in cats, part I. *Feline Pract*. 1992;20(3):17–21.

Halip JW, Luescher UA, McKeown DB. Inappropriate elimination in cats, part II. *Feline Pract*. 1992;20(4):25–29.

Houpt KA, Honig SU, Reisner IR. Breaking the Human-Companion Animal Bond. *JAVMA* 208.10 (15 May 1996): 1653–1659.

Houpt KA. *JAVMA*, Vol 224, No. 10, May 15, 2004.

Overall KL. Clinical behavioral medicine for small animals. St Louis: Mosby Year Book Inc, 1997;160–194.

Overall KL. Treating feline elimination disorders. *Vet Med*. 1998;93:367–382.

Overall KL. Animal behavior case of the month. Urine spraying by a cat in a multi-cat household. *J Am Vet Med Assoc* 1994; 205:694–696.

Olm DD, Houpt KA. Feline house-soiling problems. *Appl Anim Behav Sci* 1988;20:335–345.

Integrative veterinary medicine/nutrition references

Broadfoot P. 1997. Personal communication.

Bruno J. Edible Microalgae: A Review of the Health Research. Center for Nutritional Psychology, 2001. p 23.

Cenacchi T, Bertoldin T, Farina C, et al. Cognitive decline in the elderly: a double-blind, placebo-controlled multicenter study on efficacy of phosphatidylserine administration. *Aging (Milano)* 1993;5:123–33.

Crook TH, Tinklenberg J, Yesavage J, et al. Effects of phosphatidylserine in age-associated memory impairment. *Neurology* 1991;41:644–9.

Delwaide PJ, Gyselynck-Mambourg AM, Hurlet A, et al. Double-blind randomized controlled study of phosphatidylserine in senile demented patients. *Acta Neurol Scand* 1986;73:136–40.

Engel RR, Satzger W, Gunther W, et al. Double-blind cross-over study of phosphatidylserine vs. placebo in patients with early dementia of the Alzheimer type. *Eur Neuropsychopharmacol* 1992;2:149–55.

Fünfgeld EW, Baggen M, Nedwidek P, et al. Double-blind study with phosphatidylserine (PS) in Parkinsonian patients with senile dementia of Alzheimer's type (SDAT). *Prog Clin Biol Res* 1989;317:1235–46.

Horrocks LA, et al. Phosphatidyl Research and the Nervous System, Berlin: Springer Verlach, 1986.

Chinese herbal medicine references

Chang Yong Zhong Yao Xian Dai Yan Jiu Yu Lin Chuan (Recent Study and Clinical Application of Common Traditional Chinese Medicine) 1995; 489: 491.

Chen DY, et al. *Journal of Nanjing TCM University*. 1999;15(4):240.

Guo SM, et al. The central inhibitory effect of Suan Zao Ren total flavone. *Journal of Traditional Chinese Medicine Material*. 1998;21(11):578–579.

Ou Yang Guang Ying. Trace elements of 11 tonifying herbs from the Dunhuang region. *Journal of Gansu College of TCM*. 1990;7(4):24–25.

Zhao QX, et al. The central inhibitory effect of Suan Zao Ren. *Journal of Xi-An Medical University*. 1995;16(4): 432–434.

Zhong Yao Tong Bao (*Journal of Chinese Herbology*), 1985; 10(6): 43.

Zhong Yao Xue (*Chinese Herbology*), 1998; 676: 677.

Zhong Yao Xue (*Chinese Herbology*), 1998, 722:725.

Zhong Yao Yao Li Yu Ying Yong (*Pharmacology and Applications of Chinese Herbs*), 1983; 477.

Homotoxicology references

Bianchi I. Homeopathic Homotoxicological Repertory. Baden-Baden, Germany: Aurelia-Verlag, 1995.pp 257–268.

Palmquist P. Psychiatric Drugs Impact Veterinary Medicine. Safe Harbor. 2003. http://www.alternativementalhealth.com/articles/vets.htm.

Prozac Drug Truth. The truth about prozac and antidepressants. http://www.prozactruth.com/.

Heel. BHI Homeopathic Therapy: Professional Reference. 2002. Albuquerque, NM: Heel Inc.

Reckeweg H. Biotherapeutic Index: Ordinatio Antihomotoxica et Materia Medica, 5th ed. 2000. Baden-Baden, Germany: Biologische Heilmittel Heel GMBH.

Reckeweg H. Homeopathia Antihomotoxica Materia Medica, 4th ed. Baden-Baden, Germany: Aurelia-Verlag, 2002. pp 165–66, 180–2, 205, 217–220, 243, 290, 314, 316, 337, 379, 390, 420, 463, 490, 529, 531–33.

ACRAL LICK DERMATITIS (ALD OR LICK GRANULOMA)

Definition and cause

Acral lick dermatitis develops secondary to chronic licking. It leads to secondary inflammation and often a non-healing, ulcerated wound, and is most common in larger breeds such as Golden Retrievers, German Shepherds, Labrador Retrievers, and Great Danes. The causes besides allergies, infection, infestation, foreign bodies, etc. are generally linked to emotional or habitual stresses such as boredom, separation anxiety, loss or depression, and appropriately called canine nuerodermatitis. It also has been reported in cats (Paterson 1998; Scott 2000; Virga 2003, 2005).

Medical therapy rationale, drug(s) of choice, and nutritional recommendations

Recommended treatments are most often restrictive collars or bandages coupled with systemic and topical cortisone or bitter/herbal cremes, surgical excision, and antidepressant types of drugs. Many of these approaches are temporary unless the underlying behavior issues are identified and addressed. Success comes from a multi-faceted approach that includes identifying the underlying cause (Dodman 1988, Eckstein 1996, Rappaport 1992, Hewson 1998, Reichling 2004).

Anticipated prognosis

The success of treatment and the prognosis is directly related to the individual animal, identifying the underlying cause, preventing self-mutilation, and correcting the habitual behavior. Improved prognosis will occur if the client increases exercise, seeks professional behavior training, and reduces or eliminates the underlying stress anxiety (Dodman 1988).

Integrative veterinary therapies

Integrative therapies follow the holistic approach and address symptoms and underlying causes such as pruritus, infection, habitual behavior, anxiety, and self-trauma, which propagate the condition. The expanded treatment approach relies upon natural remedies which address the animal's emotional status, reduce cellular inflammation, and improve the animal's ability to heal, all of which are essential for permanent healing.

Nutrition
General considerations/rationale

The nutritional approach to habitual disorders such as acral lick dermatitis should focus upon the nutrient support of the brain and nervous system, reduction of cellular inflammation, enhancement of metabolic elimination via the skin, and addition of behavior-modifying or -enhancing natural remedies such as flower essences (see Separation Anxiety).

Appropriate nutrients
Nutritional/gland therapies: Glandular adrenal, brain and pineal along with intrinsic nutrients can help reduce inflammation, improve metabolic elimination, and improve nervous and emotional function (see Chapter 2, Gland Therapy, for more information).

Fatty acids: Recent studies have shown that adding essential fatty acids (omega-3 and -6) have proven beneficial for the health of the skin and coat. For allergic reactions, fatty acids that contain high amounts of DHA, EPA, and GLA helped reduce the inflammation and pruritus. These fatty acids, when used in conjunction with medications such as cortisone, can reduce the required amounts of those medications (Ackerman 1997, Campbell 1992, Degroot 1998, Mooney 1998).

Lecithin/phosphatidyl choline: Phosphatidyl choline is a phospholipid that is integral to cellular membrane, particularly that of nerve and brain cells. It helps to move fats into the cells, and is involved in acetylcholine uptake, neurotransmission, and cellular integrity. As part of the cell membranes, lecithin is an essential nutrient that is required by the nerves and all of the body's cells for general health and wellness (Hanin 1987).

Phosphatidyl serine (PS): Phosphatidyl serine is a phospholipid and an essential ingredient in cellular membranes, and particularly those of brain cells. It has been studied in people with altered mental functioning and degeneration with positive results (Crook 1991, Cenacchi 1993). In people with Alzheimer's, disease the addition of PS showed a mild to significant clinical improvement (Delewaide 1986, Engel 1992, Funfgeld 1989).

Chinese herbal medicine/acupuncture
General considerations/rationale
According to traditional Chinese medicine theory, acral lick granulomas are a result of Wind and Phlegm in the Liver.

The authors' interpretation is that in traditional Chinese medicine, acral lick dermatitis is a disturbance of the Shen. In Western medicine this means an emotional disturbance. The Liver is charged with assuring the smooth flow of energy (Qi) throughout the body. When the smooth flow is disrupted, the patient feels tense and irritable. Phlegm is, in this case, a symbolic sticky substance that interferes with the Liver's function. It does not exist in a solid form in the Liver, i.e., you will not find pockets of mucus in the liver of dogs with acral lick granulomas. It is more a metaphorical description of what is occurring in the organ. This internal Phlegm is mirrored by the discharge on the skin, which can be clear or, if there is a secondary bacterial infection, yellow or white. The itching sensation felt by the patient is ascribed to wind.

In the case of acral lick granulomas the emotional disturbance is manifested as compulsive licking of the skin. The skin then secondarily becomes damaged and inflamed. The Chinese herbal medicine approach is thus directed at decreasing the inflammation of the skin to eliminate the physical impetus for licking, and calming the mind to address the psychological basis of the licking behavior. Any inciting cause or secondary bacterial infection must also be addressed.

Acupuncture has been used in a variety of dermatological conditions with varying results (Khoe 1976). It may help reduce itching, possibly by decreasing histamine release (Belgreade 1984, Lundeberg 1988). A study at the Glasgow University Veterinary School found that acupuncture can be quite successful in treating acral lick dermatitis (Scott 2001).

Appropriate chinese herbs
Albizia (He huan hua): Has sedative effects. Experiments showed that administration of albizia reduced the activity of mice (Zhong Yao Xue 1998).

Anemarrhena root (Zhi mu): Can increase plasma corticosterone levels and has anti-inflammatory effects in animals with intact adrenal glands. It also decreases adrenocortical hormone, indicating that it stimulates the release of corticosteroids from adrenal glands (Chen Wan Sheng 1999). It also has antibacterial efficacy against Staphylococcus aureus, alpha and beta hemolytic streptococci, E. coli, and Pseudomonas (Yao Xue Qing Bao Tong Xun 1987).

Bupleurum root (Chai hu): Decreases the effect of serotonin and histamine on the permeability of capillaries, thereby decreasing inflammation (Zhong Yao Yao Li Yu Ying Yong 1983).

Grass-leaf sweet-flag root (Shi chang pu): Contains alpha-asarone, which sedates the central nervous system (Yao Xue Tong Bao 1982).

Lily bulb (Bai he): Has been used topically on sores with good results (Hong Cheng Yao Yan Jiu 1985).

Peony root (Bai shao): Has anti-inflammatory effects (Zhong Yao Zhi 1993).

Polygala root (Yuan zhi): Was shown to have sedative effects in mice (Zhong Yao Yao Li Yu Ying Yong 1983). The sedative effect has been proposed to be due to the high level of bromine that the root contains (Ou Yang Guang Ying 1990). It has further application for use in acral lick granulomas for its antibacterial effects. It has been shown to be effective against Staphylococcus aureus, a common cause of dermatitis (Peng Wen Duo 1998).

Polygonum multiforme vine (Ye jiao teng): Has a sedative effect when given to mice at the dosage of 20 g/kg (Chen Dao Yuan 1999).

Rehmannia (Sheng di huang): Reduces swelling and inflammation (Zhong Yao Yao Li Yu Ying Yong 1983).

Sour jujube (Suan da zao): Has significant sedative effects, apparently due to the flavone component (Zhao Qiu Xian 1995, Guo Sheng Ming 1998).

Turmeric (Yu jin): Contains curdione, which seems to have sedative effects (Hao Hong Qian 1994). Furthermore, it contains volatile oils with antibacterial efficacy (Cao Yu 1998).

Homotoxicology
General considerations/rationale
Acral lick dermatitis generally represents Inflammation Phase homotoxicoses. It may appear in Impregnation Phase disorders as well, and is more difficult to treat successfully owing to the permanent alternation in tissue structure and function. Dedifferentiation Phase disorders may yield an important phenomenon known as Alternative Phase, which represents a homotoxicosis in which severe cellular alterations occur in either preneoplastic or neoplastic circumstances. The body may attempt to eliminate material through inflammatory and excretion pathways involving localized areas of the skin during these occurrences. These lesions resemble smaller or larger areas of cutaneous ulceration and they are frequently found on acupuncture meridians or at specific acupuncture points. Alternate phase disorders should be addressed as Dedifferentiation Phase conditions and the surface lesions should not be interfered with because this may cause rapid progressive vicariation in the patient.

Appropriate homotoxicology formulas
Due to the wide variety of homotoxicoses which can be associated in these lesions, the following list contains items that are directly applicable. Further remedies may be required in total case management as vicariation occurs. The clinician must examine the case's presenting symptoms, select appropriate remedies that are equivalent in their provings, and then administer them to the patient. The resulting response by the patient dictates subsequent case programming needs. Further research into materia medicas may be needed.

Berberis homaccord: Provides urinary and hepatic detoxification and adrenal support.

BHI-Allergy: Its components, including Sulphuricum acidum, are indicated for neurodermatitis, and can be used as a cellular regeneration agent (Reckeweg 2002). This complex formula has many remedies that are geared toward itching, burning skin lesions. One such ingredient, Graphites, is used for various skin diseases such as dermatitis with crusty eruptions and discharge of a sticky, honey-like fluid that hardens into scabs and is often found in the folds and creases of the skin. Graphites is also used for itching that is aggravated by warmth.

The ingredient Formicum acidum can change the course of rheumatism and treats neuralgias and allergies in all cellular phases. Thuja is useful for skin diseases within the context of Deposition or Reaction phases and those developing out of Impregnation phases. Thuja is especially useful in treating warts, condylomata, papilloma, mucosal polyps, adenoid growths, epithelial proliferations in the glands, Meibomian cysts, ranula in the sublingual gland and Bartholin cysts, and scabby skin eruptions such as impetigo. It is also used in neuralgias that are limited to small, circumscribed locations and fixed ideas or incipient psychoses, because there are often emotional components to these cases.

Histaminum helps with eczema and other skin diseases, neurodermitis, pemphigus, pyoderma, boils, and carbuncles. It is recommended after contusions, fractures, tissue destruction, and emotional traumas (Reckeweg 2002), so an undiagnosed previous injury might well respond to this remedy. Histaminum is also an ingredient common to *Causticum compositum*, *Hepar compositum*, and *Ubichinon compositum*. It is frequently indicated as an intermediate remedy in all cellular phases, possibly in combination with the intermediary acids of the citric acid cycle and other intermediary catalysts.

Causticum compositum: Treats lesions resembling burns or radiation injury. The component Arsenicum is noted for burning sensations, when there is burning of the skin and itching with burning after scratching, and when skin eruptions and other symptoms are mostly of a stubborn nature, or may even border on the Degeneration Phase or begin to look malignant (Reckeweg 2002).

Coenzyme compositum: This agent is used for metabolic support. It contains several useful remedies, including alpha-Ketoglutaricum acidum and dl-Malicum acidum (malic acid), as an active factor in the citric acid cycle and in redox systems. These are used for all kinds of Impregnation Phases, such as pruritus, skin diseases, psoriasis, pre-cancerous states and neoplasm phases (especially in the early stages). They improve cell respiration, promote cutaneous cell functions, and stimulate regeneration (Reckeweg 2002). Both of these remedies are also found in the combination *Hepar compositum*, below.

Cutis compositum: Used for repair and detoxification of skin. It has Cutis suis, which is indicated in allergic reactions, dermatoses, eczema, pemphigus, fissures, psoriasis, and dermatomycoses. Used after burns (including X-ray burns) and to treat neurodermatitis (Reckeweg 2002). This formula also has many other remedies that are discussed in this section, including Hepar suis, alpha-ketoglutaricum, and a host of other skin therapeutics.

Echinacea compositum: A natural "antibiotic" in Impregnation, Degeneration, Dedifferentiation phase disorders.

Engystol N: Supports skin in allergic disorders.

Galium-Heel: A cellular detoxification agent that is useful for both drainage and repair, especially in geriatric and allergic patients.

Glyoxal compositum: Activates enzymes in deep homotoxicoses.

Hepar compositum: Used for liver detoxification in deeper disorders. The following statement from Reckeweg (2002) details the factors useful in deciding on its use: "On the skin, there is a tendency to fester, (skin slow to heal), the wounds being mostly flat with a pulsating sensation. The edges are sensitive to touch and often surrounded by pimples. The discharges are generally thick and purulent, with a characteristic odor of old cheese" (Reckeweg 2002). This remedy also contains malic acid, alpha-ketoglutaricum (see *Coenzyme compositum*), Histaminum (see BHI-Allergy), and sulphur (see *Psorinoheel*.)

Lymphomyosot: Provides lymph drainage.

Nux vomica homaccord: Used in cases that need hepatic and gastrointestinal detoxification and drainage.

Psorinoheel: Contains Psorinum, from which it gains its name. Used for emotional lability, depression, catatonia, and intransigent neuralgias. Also used for chronic eczema, impetigo and all kinds of skin eruptions, asthma alternating with eczema, psoriasis, boils, acne, seborrhea, etc. Pruritus in Psorinum cases is relieved by scratching until the patient bleeds. Psorinoheel also contains homeopathic Sulphur, which is indicated for itching, in skin

diseases or on its own, often followed by burning (those symptom notes are also common to Phosphorus and Arsenicum album). Other signs that may direct the clinician to Psorinoheel are chronic skin diseases, lichen planus, acne vulgaris, pruritic eczema and suppurative skin diseases, urticaria neurodermitis, dermatoses with much itching (especially at night), behavioral disorders, emotional discord, or upset (Reckeweg 2002). This remedy also contains Thuja (see *BHI-Allergy*) and Bufo, which is homeopathically indicated for certain cases involving itching and burning skin.

Solidago compositum: Used for urogenital detoxification in deeper disorders.

Traumeel S: Used topically or systemically. *Traumeel* may also be injected in small amounts around the lesion. This is known as "circle the dragon" in Traditional Chinese Medicine.

Thyroidea compositum: A powerful matrix drainage and hormonal support antihomotoxic drug used commonly in deeper disorders.

Ubichinon compositum: Used for metabolism support.

Authors' suggested protocols

Nutrition

Skin and behavioral/emotional/stress support formulas: 1 tablet for every 25 pounds of body weight BID.

Lecithin/phosphatidyl choline: One-fourth teaspoon for every 25 pounds of body weight BID.

Phosphatidyl serine (PS): 20 mg for every 15 pounds of body weight SID.

Oil of evening primrose: 1 capsule for every 25 pounds of body weight SID.

Chinese herbal medicine

Relaxol: 1 capsule for every 10 to 20 pounds of body weight BID (to effect). About 50% of dogs respond well. The Relaxol formulation by Natural Solutions, Inc. also contains hematite (Dai zhe shi), dragon's tooth (Long chi), and oyster shell (Mu li), which help to balance the formula and increase the efficacy of the herbs mentioned above.

Acupuncture: The authors are not aware of any well-controlled studies regarding the use of acupuncture for acral lick granulomas. They recommend the following points based upon TCM theory and clinical experience: GV20, LI11, PC6, ST36, SP6, Baihui, GB30, BL15, and BL18.

Homotoxicology

Initial therapy: Traumeel, given orally, topically, and by injection surrounding the lesion. This is called the "circle the dragon" technique in acupuncture.

Detoxification remedy (phase 1 and 2): Hepeel and Coenzyme compositum tablets given orally twice weekly for 30 days, or Detox Kit Lymphomyosot, Nux homaccord, and Berberis homaccord BID PO for 30 to 60 days.

Deep detoxification remedy (phases 3, 4, 5, 6): Galium-Heel, Lymphomyosot, Hepar compositum, Solidago compositum, Thyroidea compositum, Coenzyme compositum, and Ubichinon compositum, given every 3 days for 30 to 120 days or until recovery wanes. In advanced or deep homotoxicoses consider Glyoxal compositum, given once.

Product sources

Nutrition
Skin support formula and behavioral/emotional/stress support formula: Animal Nutrition Technologies. **Alternatives:** Composure—Vetri Science Laboratories; Derma Strength—Vetri Science Laboratories; Canine Dermal Support—Standard Process Veterinary Formulas.

Lecithin/phosphatidyl choline: Designs for Health.

Phosphatidyl serine (PS): Integrative Therapeutics; oil of evening primrose—Jarrow Formulas.

Chinese herbal medicine
Relaxol: Natural Solutions, Inc. **Alternative:** Shen calmer—Jing Tang Herbals, at 0.5 g for every 10 pounds, daily.

Homotoxicology remedies
BHI/Heel Corporation

REFERENCES

Western medicine references
Dodman NH, Shuster L, White SD, Court MH, Parker D, Dixon R. Use of narcotic antagonists to modify stereotypic self-licking, self-chewing, and scratching behavior in dogs. *J Am Vet Med Assoc.* 1988; Oct 1;193(7):815–9.

Eckstein RA, Hart BL. Treatment of canine acral lick dermatitis by behavior modification using electronic stimulation. *J Am Anim Hosp Assoc.* 1996 May-Jun;32(3): 225–30.

Hewson CJ, Luescher UA, Parent JM, Conlon PD, Ball RO. Efficacy of clomipramine in the treatment of canine compulsive disorder. *J Am Vet Med Assoc.* 1998 Dec 15; 213(12):1760–6.

Paterson S. Skin Diseases of the Dog. London: Blackwell Science Ltd. 1998;239–241.

Rappaport JL, Ryland DH, Kriete M. Drug treatment of canine acral lick. An animal model of obsessive-compulsive disorder. *Arch Gen Psychiatry.* 1992 Jul;49(7):517–21.

Reichling J, Fitzi J, Hellmann K, Wegener T, Bucher S, Saller R. Topical tea tree oil effective in canine localised pruritic dermatitis—a multi-centre randomised double-blind controlled clinical trial in the veterinary practice. *Dtsch Tierarztl Wochenschr.* 2004 Oct;111(10): 408–14.

Scott DW, et al. Psychogenic Skin Diseases. In Muller and Kirk's Small Animal Dermatology, 6th ed. Philadelphia: WB Saunders Co. 2000;1058–1064.

Virga V. Self-directed behaviors in dogs and cats. *Vet Med* 2005;100:212–222.

Virga V. Behavioral dermatology. *Vet Clin N A: Small Anim Pract.* 2003;33:231–251.

IVM/nutrition references
Ackerman L. Selecting fatty acid supplements for use in small animal dermatology. Supplement to the Compendium on Continuing Education for the Practicing Veterinarian. 1997;19(3):93–96.

Campbell KL. Therapeutic indications for dietary lipids. In Kirk, RW (ed): Current Veterinary Therapy XI. Philadelphia: WB Saunders Co. PA. 1992;36–39.

Crook TH, Tinklenberg J, Yesavage J, et al. Effects of phosphatidylserine in age-associated memory impairment. *Neurology* 1991;41:644–9.

DeGroot JE. Veterinary medical uses and sources of omega-3 fatty acids. *Veterinary Forum.* 1998; May:42–48.

Delwaide PJ, Gyselynck-Mambourg AM, Hurlet A, et al. Double-blind randomized controlled study of phosphatidylserine in senile demented patients. *Acta Neurol Scand* 1986;73: 136–40.

Engel RR, Satzger W, Gunther W, et al. Double-blind cross-over study of phosphatidylserine vs. placebo in patients with early dementia of the Alzheimer type. *Eur Neuropsychopharmacol* 1992;2:149–55.

Fünfgeld EW, Baggen M, Nedwidek P, et al. Double-blind study with phosphatidylserine (PS) in Parkinsonian patients with senile dementia of Alzheimer's type (SDAT). *Prog Clin Biol Res* 1989;317:1235–46.

Hanin I, Ansell GB. Lecithin : Technological, Biological, and Therapeutic Aspects. NY: Plenum Press. 1987. 180, 181.

Mooney MA, Vaughn DM, Reinhart GA, et al. Evaluation of the effects of omega-3 fatty acid-containing diets on the inflammatory stage of wound healing in dogs. *American Journal of Veterinary Research.* 1998;59:859–863.

Chinese herbal medicine references
Belgreade MJ et al. Effect of acupuncture on experimentally-induced itch (abstract). *Am J Acupuncture* 12:276, 1984.

Cao Yu, et al. The anti-fungal effect of volatile oils of herbs of the curcuma genus, the ginger family. *Journal of Guiyang College of Medicine.* 1998;13(2):157–159.

Chen DY, et al. *Journal of Nanjing TCM University.* 1999;15(4):240.

Chen WS, et al. *Journal of Second Military Medical College.* 1999;20(10):758–760.

Guo SM, et al. The central inhibitory effect of Suan Zao Ren total flavone. *Journal of Traditional Chinese Medicine Material.* 1998;21(11):578–579.

Hao HQ, et al. Curdione's regulatory effect on cats' sleeping rhythmic electric activity. *Journal of Chinese Materia Medica.* 1994;25(8):423–424.

Hong Cheng Yao Yan Jiu (*Research of Chinese Patent Medicine*), 1985;1:45.

Khoe WH. Dermatological conditions successfully treated with acupuncture. *Am J Acupunct* 1976;4(4):362–4.

Lundeberg T et al: Effect of acupuncture on experimentally induced itch (abstract). *Am J Acupuncture* 16:275, 1988.

Ou Yang Guang Ying. Trace elements of 11 tonifying herbs from the Dunhuang region. *Journal of Gansu College of TCM.* 1990;7(4):24–25.

Peng WD, et al. Polygalin's expectorant and anti-tussive effects. *Journal of Pharmacy.* 1998;33(8):491.

Scott S: Developments in Veterinary Acupuncture. *Acupunct Med.* 2001;19(1):27–31.

Yao Xue Qing Bao Tong Xun (*Journal of Herbal Information*), 1987; 5(4):62.

Yao Xue Tong Bao (Report of Herbology), 1982;9:50.

Zhao QX, et al. The central inhibitory effect of Suan Zao Ren. *Journal of Xi-An Medical University.* 1995;16(4):432–434.

Zhong Yao Xue (*Chinese Herbology*), 1998; 676:677.

Zhong Yao Yao Li Yu Ying Yong (*Pharmacology and Applications of Chinese Herbs*), 1983:400.

Zhong Yao Yao Li Yu Ying Yong (*Pharmacology and Applications of Chinese Herbs*), 1983;477.

Zhong Yao Yao Li Yu Ying Yong (*Pharmacology and Applications of Chinese Herbs*), 1983; 888.

Zhong Yao Zhi (*Chinese Herbology Journal*), 1993;183.

Homotoxicology reference

Reckeweg H. 2002. Homeopathia Antihomotoxica Materia Medica, 4th ed. Baden-Baden, Germany: Aurelia-Verlag, 82, 150, 269, 304, 330, 340, 344, 373, 402, 502–3, 560, 575.

SEPARATION ANXIETY

Definition and cause

Dogs and cats have become close members of many families, and as such, when separated from family members to whom they have bonded, they can experience anxiety leading to behavior problems. Behavior abnormalities such as destruction of home furnishing, urination and defecation in the home, vocalization, incessant barking and howling, and depression often result from the distress of being separated.

Before the diagnosis of separation anxiety is made, other causes such as medical or physical problems, inability to reach the litter box, and inadequate training must first be ruled out (Borchelt 1982, Lund 1999, Schwartz 2003).

Medical therapy rationale, drug(s) of choice, and nutritional recommendations

Client compliance is an important part of proper therapy; this includes behavior modification, desensitization, counter-conditioning, habituation, and medications. Drugs should not be the first choice; they should only be prescribed after a well-thought-out behavior modification program has been tried. If the behavior modification program does not completely control of problem, then the use of medication can be considered. The drug of choice is Clomicalm®, which is approved for the treatment of separation anxiety, but side effects of diarrhea can prove problematic (Horwitz 2000, Takeuchi, 2000).

Anticipated prognosis

As with other compulsive disorders, client compliance and adherence to the behavior modification program are essential for control of the condition. In addition, the formulation of a good behavior modification protocol that helps to desensitize the animal is as important as compliance (Lem 2002, Takeuchi 2000).

Integrative veterinary therapies

Separation anxiety is not a specific diagnosis. Recommending therapy based upon diffuse, descriptive diagnoses often serves to label a patient, but may not result in the successful understanding or management of that patient's condition. Generally speaking, it is advisable for professionals to avoid such descriptive diagnoses, especially when recommending therapy.

Excessive anxiety can lead to vocalization, hyperactivity, destructive behavior, and client dissatisfaction. Such activities can originate from natural, survival-oriented behavior in canines, and therefore do not necessarily represent pathological conditions. Puppies left alone or separated from the pack become vulnerable to predation, and it is natural for them to seek pack members for protection. Shredding clothing, especially shoes and undergarments, may actually be the puppy's attempt to get closer to the owner for protection. Most puppies may only need non-drug behavior modification; pheromone aeorsolizers also may be very helpful.

Puppies may have other issues that lead to excessive anxiety behaviors. In some instances there are factors affecting the normal development of the nervous system. Damage in utero, poor nutrition, adverse reactions to food, food allergy, poor environment, excessive stress, improper handling of the puppy in its new environment, and premature removal from the dam may negatively affect the puppy's development and lead to behavioral problems. Genetic factors may play a role. Furthermore, there may be a reaction to vaccination (See Chapter 35, Vaccinations, for more information)

Careful evaluation may be needed to properly approach these cases, and difficult cases should be referred to a behavioral specialist prior to more desperate actions (Mege 2006).

A veterinarian addressing separation anxiety should take a careful medical and behavioral history in addition to conducting a complete physical examination and should attempt to determine any aggravating causes for the anxious behavior (Beata 2006). A therapeutic plan can be initiated once these factors are identified. The addition of therapeutic nutrition, medicinal herbs, and homeopathic remedies can help balance the animals' emotions and make them less reactive to stresses.

Nutrition
General considerations/rationale
The nutritional approach to separation anxiety consists of nutrient support of the brain and nervous system; the gentle detoxification of environmental chemicals, toxins, medication, and vaccinations; and the addition of behavior-modifying or -enhancing natural remedies such as flower essences.

Appropriate nutrients
Nutrition/gland therapies: Glandular brain and pineal supply intrinsic nutrients and can help nourish brain and nerve cells, improve circulation, and reduce inflammation in the central nervous system (see Chapter 2, Gland Therapy, for more information).

Phospholipids in glandular brain are a source of unsaturated omega-3 fatty acids, which are thought to play a vital role in the development and maintenance of the central nervous system. High concentrations of phosphatidyl choline and serine are found in brain tissue. Horrocks (1986) reported on the potential clinical use of these nutrients in chronic neurological conditions.

Phosphatidyl serine (PS): Phosphatidyl serine is a phospholipid that is essential for cellular membranes, particularly those of brain cells. PS has been studied in people with altered mental functioning and degeneration with positive results (Crook 1991, Cenacchi 1993). In people with Alzheimer's disease the addition of PS showed a mild to significant clinical improvement (Delewaide 1986, Engel 1992, Funfgeld 1989).

Blue-green algae: Blue-green algae have been observed to create a generalized feeling of well-being in humans and may prove helpful in veterinary patients. Blue-green algae's effects and benefits are slower in onset, generally taking 3 to 4 weeks to appear. This may be due in part to their content of natural antihistaminic compounds or their levels of omega-3 fatty acids (Bruno 2001).

Many studies in recent years have confirmed the beneficial results from these critical fatty acids. Aphanizomenon flos aquae, a blue-green algae, has been shown in clinical settings to have positive effects on brain function. In addition to the omega-3 fatty acids, it has a full spectrum of essential amino acids, a broad-based mineral content, a rapidly assimilable glyolipoprotein cell wall, and a wide variety of vitamins. It has mild chelating properties and thus, can be valuable in heavy metal toxicoses such as Thimerosol reactions. It is a tremendous asset as a micronutrient resource and figures prominently in many treatment programs (Broadfoot 1997).

Chinese herbal medicine
General considerations/rationale
Separation anxiety is considered to be a combination of Yin deficiency in the Heart and Qi stagnation in the Liver. In the Western interpretation, The Shen or mind is housed in the Heart in TCM terms. Yin can be thought of as nourishment or fluids. When there is a Yin deficiency of the Heart, the mind is not nourished. This leads to anxiety. The Liver is responsible for the smooth flow of emotions. When the Liver Qi is stagnant, the animal feels constrained, frustrated, and irritable. Treatment is aimed at calming the patient.

Appropriate chinese herbs
Albizzia flower (He huan hua): Has been shown to have sedative effects in mice (Zhong Yao Xue 1998).

Bupleurum (Chai hu): Contains saikosaponins, which have sedative effects (Zhong Yao Yao Li Yu Ying Yong 1983).

Curcuma (Yu jin): Contains curdione, which depresses the central nervous system (Hao 1994).

Gardenia (Zhi zi): Sedates the central nervous system. It decreases spontaneous activity in mice (Jiang 1976).

Grass-leaf sweet-flag root (Shi chang pu): Has demonstrated sedative effects (Zhong Yao Xue 1998).

Peony (Bai shao): Has sedative effects and prolongs sleeping time when administered along with phenobarbitol in mice (Zhong Yao Tong Bao 1985).

Polygala root (Yuan zhi): Contains a high level of bromine, which causes sedation (Ou 1990).

Polygonum (Ye jiao teng): Causes sedation. When given to mice it causes a significant decrease in the amount of pentobarbital needed to induce anesthesia (Chen Dao Yuan 1999).

Poria (Fu ling): Has a calming effect. It has been shown to be capable of counteracting the excitatory effects of caffeine in mice (Hu 1957).

Zizyphus (Suan zao ren): Has demonstrated sedative effects in dogs, cats, rats, rabbits, and guinea pigs. It also counteracts the excitatory effects of caffeine and benzedrine. One of the components of zizyphus, jujuboside, is the most likely candidate for the sedative effects (Chang Yong Zhong Yao Xian Dai Yan Jiu Yu Lin Chuan 1995, Zhao Qiu Xian 1995, Guo 1998).

Practitioners have used acupuncture successfully to treat many psychological conditions, among them separation anxiety (Xie 2006).

Homotoxicology
General considerations/rationale

No homotoxicology remedies have been specifically studied for use in separation anxiety in animals, but anxiety as a generality is often addressed homeopathically and a theoretical discussion of these principles follows.

Anxiety can originate from neurodermal impregnation homotoxicoses. In these conditions, the binding of homotoxins to the matrix damages the patient's nervous system. Such binding negatively affects the proper functioning of these elements. Viral particles, toxins (heavy metals), and a host of other possibilities exist. Dyes and food additives may contribute as well. Food allergy is an example of a common Impregnation Phase homotoxicosis seen in clinical practice (Reckeweg 2000). Anxious behavior can temporarily appear and fade away during regressive vicariation and is associated with improved patient condition. During these periods the patient may benefit from improved levels of neurosupportive nutrients (see nutrition discussion).

Antihomotoxic medicines may help establish calm, relieve organ stress, and reduce homotoxin levels. In some cases they provide a psychological benefit to the animal's owner because they provide the owner with something to do while training methods, pheromones, and other treatment plan steps have time to function effectively.

If properly managed, most of these cases do not require psychopharmaceutical agents, which may be associated with progressive vicariation and unpleasant side effects such as diarrhea. In limited cases, especially when there is bona fide, organic nerve damage, the use of such agents may be considered, but it should be recognized that such treatment may be associated with functional nerve damage, a highly undesirable side effect (Gur 1998a, 1998b).

L-theanine, an amino acid in green tea, may also assist some cases. Although it is nonsedating, L-theanine tends to create a calmer mental outlook. The authors have used this agent with limited success in clients looking for natural, nonpharmaceutical solutions to puppy anxiety (Mitchell 2003, Palmquist 2005).

Classical homeopathy may yield surprising responses in some cases of anxiety, and should be considered (Day 1990). This subject is beyond the scope of this text, but it is important to note that anxiety can be a manifestation of many different emotional states (anxiety, fear, anger, frustration, resentment, and antagonism, to name a few), and each of these requires separate consideration in developing a classical homeopathic approach (Kent 1921). Seeking a trained homeopathic practitioner with experience in behavioral cases is advised in such situations (Schoen 1998).

Bach flower essences also have anecdotal use in anxiety. They are used primarily when there are disturbances of a mental, emotional, or behavioral nature. Dr. Bach's original 38 English flower remedies included the popular combination known as *Rescue Remedy*. It consists of 5 flower essences: cherry plum, clematis, impatiens, rock rose, and star of Bethlehem. *Rescue Remedy* is used in situations of high stress and anxiety. It is important to note that it does not have conventional tranquilizing properties, but simply a calming effect that reduces or relieves the sense of stress and anxiety.

Many practitioners use *Rescue Remedy* to settle fractious dogs and cats, and its use is much appreciated by patients, clients, and technicians alike. Each individual flower essence has a particular area of mental, emotional, or behavioral use. For example, Aspen purportedly helps in situations of apprehension or fear, but not of a known entity, more the fear of an unknown. Mimulus, on the other hand, is believed to help with fears of known things. Holly is commonly used in the strong and aggressive emotions of outright anger and jealousy (Wright 2006). Because these agents are safe and nontoxic, therapeutic trial use can prove very helpful, especially in milder cases. Callahan (1997) reports that Recovery Formula helps animals in a state of emotional stress as well as addictive patterns.

Appropriate homotoxicology formulas

Antihomotoxic formulas to consider as starting points include:

Aconitum homaccord: Animals that benefit from this often have fearful cases; nervous conditions; irritation with great agitation; sharp, stabbing pains; paralysis; restlessness; fear of death; and consequences of fright, which may be made much worse by the slightest contact. Patients responding to this remedy may have violent, acute complaints; red skin; and fever.

Apis homaccord: Used for certain nervous disorders, vaccination reactions, urticaria, or angioedema (in combination with *Lymphomyosot*) (Broadfoot 2006).

Atropinum compositum: Used for its Argentum nictricum component, which is indicated in some cases of anxiety, abdominal complaints, diarrhea, and spasm.

BHI-Calming: Indicated for anxiety, but used in humans in cases of swearing mad and mania (Heel 2003).

Cerebrum compositum: Provides support of cerebral tissues and blood flow. This combination contains Hyoscyamus for states of excitement with great restlessness, mobility, vehemence, jealousy, raving, and attacks of fury. At the other end of the scale there may also be depression to the point of melancholia and dull apathy (as in chronic poisoning). The eyes may have a glazed stare and an unusual sheen (Reckeweg 2002). This description may partially fit those animals with "rage" syndromes.

This combination also contains Anacardium, which is indicated for retoxic impregnations after suppressed skin eruptions. It is particularly indicated for cerebral and emotional symptoms with irritability, timidity, and fearfulness of misfortune and danger; along with mental exhaustion; emotional discord or upset; and delusions. Human patients may feel as if they have two wills, each driving them to do opposing things, as is found in schizophrenia (Reckeweg 2002).

Also contained in this formula is Embryo suis, with notes for use in cases demonstrating anxiety on waking, an aversion to or desire for company, and fear that something bad will happen. These cases often are irascible and irresolute. Irritability with a changeable mood may also be seen. Some cases may demonstrate sensitivity to music and noise, while others may be sensitive to touch and have their signs aggravated by physical contact (Reckeweg 2002).

Diarrheel S: Given for diarrhea with neurosis (contains Argenticum nitricum) (Heel 2003).

Gelsemium homaccord: Used for headaches and anxiety (usually in older pets), possibly in reactions to vaccines in which headache or neurogenic swelling occurs.

Hepar compositum: This combination drains and supports liver function in deeper homotoxicoses. Contains Pancreas suis with mental notes for use such as fear of being injured or attacked or of narrow places. Assists with irritability from trifles or on waking (Reckeweg 2002). *Hepar compositum* may support healing in dermatosis and neurogenic dermatitis, which can cause irritation, negative emotional responses, and antagonism resultant from altered skin sensations. It also contains arsenicum, which is associated with nervousness and anxiety (Day 1990).

Ignatia homaccord: More typically used for depression, but cases of aggression originating from sadness exist (Pitcairn 2006). It is logical to consider this agent in some cases of anxiety.

Nervoheel: Used for anxiety.

Phosphor homaccord: Assists with melancholy.

Valerianaheel: Provides mild, gentle sedation through homeopathic and herbal dilutions.

Veratrum homaccord: Used in cases showing some or all of the following: paper shredding, psychotic behavior, collapse, vomiting, and diarrhea.

Authors' suggested protocols

Nutrition

Brain nerve support and behavior support formulas: 1 tablet for every 25 pounds of body weight BID.

Phosphatidyl serine (PS): 20 mg for every 15 pounds of body weight SID.

Blue-green algae: One-fourth teaspoon for every 25 pounds of body weight daily.

Chinese herbal medicine

The authors recommend Relaxol at a dose of 1 capsule for every 10 to 20 pounds twice daily to effect. It is important to combine medical therapy with behavioral therapy for optimal results. Relaxol contains albizia flower (He huan hua), anemarrhena (Zhi mu), bupleurum (Chai hu), curcuma root (Yu jin), fossil teeth (Long chi), grass-leafed sweet-flag root (Shi chang pu), haematite (Dai zhe shi), lily (bai he), oyster shell (Mu li), peony (Bai shao), polygala root (Yuan zhi), polygonum (Ye jiao teng), rehmannia (Sheng di huang), and ziziphus (Suan zao ren).

An alternative therapy is jia wei xiao yao wan, a patent formula. It contains angelica (Dang gui), atractylodes (Chao bai zhu), bupleurum (Chai hu), gardenia (Zhi zi), licorice (Gan cao), moutan (Mu dan pi), peony (Bai shao), and poria (Fu ling). This formula was used in 42 human subjects who reported anxiety. Seventy-four percent experienced significant reduction in anxiety while another 21% received some relief (Xu 1996).

These supplements contain some herbs not mentioned above. The extra herbs serve to increase the efficacy of the formula.

The authors use the following acupuncture points: GV15, GV20, GB20, SP6, and PC6.

Homotoxicology (Dose: 10 drops PO for 50-pound dog; 5 drops PO for small dog or cat)

Symptom formula: Select individual formulas based upon the symptoms manifested by the patient from the Appropriate Homotoxicology Formulas section or according to further research by the clinician. In cases in which no clear picture is evident, begin with Cerebrum compositum at 1 tablet EOD. If no improvement after 2 weeks, adjust the prescription accordingly (Nervo-Heel, BHI-Calming, Ignatia homaccord, Valerianaheel, etc.).

Detoxification formula: Hepeel or *Coenzyme compositum* tablets every day, both given PO in the evening.

Note: The addition of flower essences such as *Rescue Remedy* or *Recovery* may be beneficial.

Product sources

Nutrition

Brain nerve and behavioral/emotional/stress formulas: Animal Nutrition technologies. **Alternative:** Composure—Vetri Science Laboratories.

Phosphatidyl serine (PS): Integrative Therapeutics.
Blue-green algae: Simplexity.

Chinese herbal medicine
Relaxol: Natural Solutions, Inc.
Jia wei xiao yao wan: Mayway Corporation.

Homotoxicology remedies
BHI/Heel Corporation
Bach flower remedies: Ellon Bach.
Anaflora flower essences: Earth Animal, Inc.

REFERENCES

Western medicine references
Borchelt PL, Voith VL. Diagnosis and treatment of separation-related behavior problems in dogs. *Vet Clin North Am Small Anim Pract.* 1982; Nov;12(4):625–35.

Flannigan G, Dodman NH. Risk factors and behaviors associated with separation anxiety in dogs, *J Am Vet Med Assoc.* 2001; Aug 15;219(4):460–6.

Horwitz DF. Diagnosis and treatment of canine separation anxiety and the use of clomipramine hydrochloride (clomicalm). *J Am Anim Hosp Assoc.* 2000; Mar-Apr;36(2): 107–9.

Lem M. Behavior modification and pharmacotherapy for separation anxiety in a 2-year-old pointer cross. *Can Vet J.* 2002; Mar;43(3):220–2.

Lund JD, Jorgensen MC. Behaviour patterns and time course of activity in dogs with separation problems. *Applied Animal Behaviour Science.* 1999; Apr 63(3):219–236.

Schwartz S. Separation anxiety syndrome in dogs and cats. *J Am Vet Med Assoc.* 2003; Jun 1;222(11):1526–32.

Takeuchi Y, Houpt KA, Scarlett JM. Evaluation of treatments for separation anxiety in dogs. *J Am Vet Med Assoc.* 2000; Aug 1;217(3):342–5.

Nutrition references
Bruno J. Edible Microalgae: A Review of the Health Research. 2001. Center for Nutritional Psychology, p 23.

Cenacchi T, Bertoldin T, Farina C, et al. Cognitive decline in the elderly: a double-blind, placebo-controlled multicenter study on efficacy of phosphatidylserine administration. *Aging (Milano)* 1993;5:123–33.

Crook TH, Tinklenberg J, Yesavage J, et al. Effects of phosphatidylserine in age-associated memory impairment. *Neurology* 1991;41:644–9.

Delwaide PJ, Gyselynck-Mambourg AM, Hurlet A, et al. Double-blind randomized controlled study of phosphatidylserine in senile demented patients. *Acta Neurol Scand* 1986;73:136–40.

Engel RR, Satzger W, Gunther W, et al. Double-blind cross-over study of phosphatidylserine vs. placebo in patients with early dementia of the Alzheimer type. *Eur Neuropsychopharmacol* 1992;2:149–55.

Fünfgeld EW, Baggen M, Nedwidek P, et al. Double-blind study with phosphatidylserine (PS) in Parkinsonian patients with senile dementia of Alzheimer's type (SDAT). *Prog Clin Biol Res* 1989;317:1235–46.

Horrocks LA, et al. Phosphatidyl Research and the Nervous System, Berlin: Springer Verlach, 1986.

Chinese herbal medicine references
Chang Yong Zhong Yao Xian Dai Yan Jiu Yu Lin Chuan (Recent study and Clinical Application of Common Traditional Chinese Medicine), 1995;489:491.

Chen DY, et al. *Journal of Nanjing TCM University.* 1999;15(4):240.

Guo SM, et al. The central inhibitory effect of Suan Zao Ren total flavone. *Journal of Traditional Chinese Medicine Material.* 1998;21(11):578–579.

Hao HQ, et al. Curdione's regulatory effect on cats' sleeping rhythmic electric activity. *Journal of Chinese Materia Medica.* 1994;25(8):423–424.

Hu CJ. *Journal of Wuhan Medical College,* 1957;(1):125.

Jiang Su Yi Yao (*Jiangsu Journal of Medicine and Herbology*), 1976;(1):28.

Ou Yang Guang Ying. Trace elements of 11 tonifying herbs from the Dunhuang region. *Journal of Gansu College of TCM.* 1990;7(4):24–25.

Xie, H, Ortiz-Umpierre, C. What acupuncture can and cannot treat. *Journal of the American Animal Hospital Association* 42;244–248 (2006).

Xu YX. *Journal of Integrated Medicine of First Aid Clinical Application.* 1996;3(5):205–206.

Zhao QX, et al. The central inhibitory effect of Suan Zao Ren. *Journal of Xi-An Medical University.* 1995;16(4): 432–434.

Zhong Yao Tong Bao (*Journal of Chinese Herbology*), 1985; 10(6):43.

Zhong Yao Xue (*Chinese Herbology*), 1998; 676:677.

Zhong Yao Xue (*Chinese Herbology*), 1998, 722:725.

Zhong Yao Yao Li Yu Ying Yong (*Pharmacology and Applications of Chinese Herbs*), 1983;888.

Homotoxicology references
Beata C. Ethological and Neurophysiological Basis of Behavioral Disorders. In: Proceedings of The North American Veterinary Conference, 2006; Vol 20, Orlando, FL, pp 127–8.

Broadfoot P. 1997. Personal communication.

Broadfoot P. Puppyactrics: Handling the Vaccination Reaction. *J Biomedical Ther,* 2006; Winter, pp 14–5.

Callahan S. Anaflora Flower Essences, 1997. Mt. Shasta, CA: Sacred Spirit Publishing.,

Day C. The Homoeopathic Treatment of Small Animals: Principles and Practice. Saffron Walden, Essex: CW Daniel Company, LTD. 1990. p 110.

Gur R, Maany V, Mozley P, Swanson C, Bilker W. Subcortical MRI volumes in neuroleptic-naive and treated patients with schizophrenia. *Am J Psychiatry,* 1998a. 155 (12), pp 1711–1717.

Gur R, Cowell P, Turetsky B, Gallacher F, Cannon T, Bilker W. A follow-up magnetic resonance imaging study of schizophrenia. *Arch Gen Psych,* 1998b. 55: pp 145–v152.

Heel. Veterinary Guide, 3rd English edition. Biologische Baden-Baden, Germany: Heilmettel Heel GmbH. 2003. pp 82–84.

Kent J. Repertory of the Homeopathic Materia Medica and a Word Index. Paharganj, New Delhi: B. Jain, LTD. 1921. p vii.

Mege C. Behavioral Disorders in Growing Dogs and Cats. North American Veterinary Conference, Vol 20, Orlando, Florida, 2006. pp 149–50.

Mitchell T. Life Extension Animals Case Studies: The Anxious Basset Hound. *Life Extension Magazine*. 2003. May issue online at www.lef.org.

Palmquist R. Use of Vetri-Science's Composure Liquid in Canine Anxiety. 2005. Unpublished case data.

Pitcairn R. Vegas: The Cat with Homesickness. Advanced Homeopathy Course, Saguaro. 2006. Eugene, OR.

Reckeweg H. Biotherapeutic Index: Ordinatio Antihomotoxica et Materia Medica, 5th ed. Baden-Baden, Germany: Biologische Heilmittel Heel GMBH, 2000. p 83.

Reckeweg H. Homeopathia Antihomotoxica Materia Medica, 4th ed. Baden-Baden, Germany: Aurelia-Verlag, 2002. pp. 134–5, 287, 350–1, 477.

Schoen A, Wynn S. Complementary and Alternative Veterinary Medicine: Principles and Practice. St Louis: Mosby. 1998. pp 494–5, 501, 503.

Wright J, Wright M. 2006. Personal communication from practitioners well known for successful use of Bach flowers.

STORM, NOISE (FIREWORKS), AND OTHER PHOBIAS

Definition and cause

Phobia is not simply a fear of something. By definition it is an extreme fear, one far worse than rationally explained. Storm phobia is a descriptive term and not a specific diagnosis, and as such, cannot be used as a diagnostic criterion in conventional medicine. Abnormal, unwarranted, or excessive fear can occur in many different organic states and can be a sign of abnormality or malfunction of the nervous system. Storm phobia may be associated with other fears or abnormal behaviors in dogs (McCobb 2001). A medical work-up is indicated in these cases as with any other neurological condition.

Medical therapy rationale, drug(s) of choice, and nutritional recommendations

The medical approach to storm phobias focuses on tranquilization, sedation, or anti-anxiety medications. Medications such as Diazepam and Acepromazine are more commonly used by veterinarians. Anti-anxiety and panicolytic drugs such as Alprazolam (Xanax), Amitriptyline (Elavil), Buspirone (Buspar), and Clomipramine (Clomicalm) are gaining popularity.

While these drugs do not address specific causes of the problem, they generally are helpful in preventing injury to a pet that would otherwise be too afraid and reactive to properly control its own behavior. These drugs may have long-term harmful effects not yet understood in vet-erinary medicine; so caution should be exercised in the use of psychoactive drugs in animal patients until further, more thorough research is completed (Gur 1998). Even the experts say that using drugs such as Acepromazine, a dissociative anesthetic, really does not help or address the issue and may make the associated fear worse (Overall 1997).

In addition to medication, veterinary behaviorists recommend behavior modification techniques, desensitization to the noise, proper nutrition, noise-blocking techniques, and counter-conditioning methods, all of which improve the effectiveness of the drugs and success rates (Nash).

Anticipated prognosis

The prognosis is good when conventional medication and other techniques such as behavior modification and desensitization are used; however, client compliance is essential for long-term control.

Integrative veterinary therapies

When dealing with these phobias, it is accepted that medical therapies do not address the underlying cause and their values lie more in the prevention of injury to the animal. Furthermore, there may be harmful side effects that are not known at this point, which could actually worsen the situation. Therefore, precautions must be taken and alternatives should be explored.

Flower remedies may be helpful and some people have also reported anecdotal success with essential oils (Essential Science 2002, Wright 2006). Some of the authors have recommended *Rescue Remedy*, Mimulus (for fear of known things), and rock rose (for terror and panic) with some success. Anaflora's Tranquility also has shown success anecdotally (Callahan 1997).

L-theanine, an amino acid from green tea extracts, may be helpful in this condition, but there are no controlled studies on its use. Peppermint oil has been recommended by several holistic veterinarians and is worth trying (Silver 2004). The authors have not been able to duplicate success using this oil, but exploration of this field may yield useful information in the future. Bluegreen algae may be helpful over longer periods of time owing to its rich mineral and omega-3 fatty acid content (Broadfoot 2003).

A behavioral specialist may provide successful training and destimulation or counter-conditioning drills. The first step is usually environmental controls. Providing a safe space or hiding area may reduce the behavior in many cases (Haug 2006). Caution should always be taken when dealing with phobic pets to avoid unnecessarily stressful or restimulative situations.

A few novel techniques deserve mention. T-Touch™ technique is a method of calming fearful dogs and cats that has been used by thousands of animal owners and professionals with good success (Tellington-Jones 1999). Another novel approach to anxiety and fear is "body wrapping." This may calm some pets by placing pressure on peripheral nerve receptors, and it provides yet another drug-free method of addressing the issue (Farber 2002). Sadly, in some cases there may be no other option but short-term use of a pharmaceutical agent.

Nutrition
General considerations/rationale
If the cause has been identified and medication and behavior modification techniques are being used, nutritional support that focuses upon the brain and the emotions can often improve the animal's general attitude and well-being.

Appropriate nutrients
Nutritional/gland therapies: Glandular brain and pineal supply intrinsic nutrients and can help improve function and reduce inflammation in the brain and central nervous system (see Chapter 2, Gland Therapy).

Phospholipids found in glandular brain are a source of unsaturated omega-3 fatty acids, which are now thought to play a vital role in the development and maintenance of the central nervous system. High concentrations of phosphatidyl choline and serine are found in brain tissue. Horrocks (1986) reported on the potential clinical use of these nutrients in chronic neurological conditions.

Lecithin/phosphatidyl choline and innositol: Lecithin is an essential nutrient required by cells for general health and wellness (Hanin 1987). Innositol, which often is found in combination with lecithin, has been shown to help people with panic attacks. In a double-blind study it has been shown to be effective in relieving symptoms of obsessive-compulsive disorders (Benjamin 1995, Fux 1996)

Phosphatidyl serine (PS): Phosphatidyl serine is a phospholipid that is essential in cellular membranes, particularly those of brain cells. It has been studied in people with altered mental functioning with positive results (Crook 1991, Cenacchi 1993).

Essential fatty acids: Research confirms the benefits of essential fatty acids regarding their calming effect on the central nervous system (Erasmus 1993).

Chinese herbal medicine
General considerations/rationale
According to traditional Chinese Medicine, storm phobias are Heart Yin and Blood deficiency and Liver Qi stagnation. In the Western interpretation, the Liver is charged with ensuring the smooth flow of energy within the body. Anything that interferes with this function can cause constraint, according to Traditional Chinese Medicine. This may be an emotional disorder. Often, people who feel constrained are irritable. Therefore, it is easy to see how the ancient Chinese felt that Liver Qi stagnation caused irritability. The Heart is the seat of the Mind or Shen. When the Heart is not nourished properly due to Yin and Blood deficiency, the patient feels fearful. Treatment is aimed at calming the patient.

In December 1979 the World Health Organization recognized psychological conditions as being responsive to acupuncture therapy. Storm phobias and other phobic conditions fall into this category. Wang and Kain used aural acupuncture in 55 patients to decrease anxiety with good results, based upon the State-Trait Anxiety Inventory scale, which measures tension (Wang 2001). In another study 18 people with insomnia and anxiety above 50 on the Zung Anxiety Self Rating scale were treated with acupuncture with excellent results (Spence 2004).

Appropriate chinese herbs
Albizzia flower (He huan hua): Has sedative effects (Zhong Yao Xue 1998).

Bupleurum (Chai hu): Contains saikosaponins, which have sedative effects (Zhong Yao Yao Li Yu Ying Yong 1983).

Curcuma root (Yu jin): Contains curdione, a compound that sedates the central nervous system. Experiments on cats showed that it inhibits the central nervous system, which affects sleep patterns (Hao 1994).

Grass-leaf sweet-flag root (Shi chang pu): A central nervous system suppressant (Zhong Yao Xue 1998). Grass-leaf sweet-flag root was used along with Shu di huang, Shan zhu yu, Fu ling, Tai zi shen, Suan zao ren, Hu po, Dang gui, Gou qi zi, Wu wei zi, and Zhi gan cao in 48 people with anxiety disorders. Seventy-five percent showed significant improvement and 22% had some improvement (Wang 1998).

Polygala root (Yuan zhi): Causes sedation (Zhong Yao Yao Li Yu Ying Yong 1983). It contains a high level of bromine, which has a tranquilizing effect (Ou 1990).

Polygonum (Ye jiao teng): A tranquilizer. Experiments in mice showed that it could decrease the amount of pentobarbital needed to sedate the animals (Chen 1999).

White peony (Bai shao): Causes sedation, as has been shown experimentally in mice (Zhong Yao Tong Bao 1985).

Zizyphus (Suan zao ren): Has demonstrated sedative effects in various animals (Chang Yong Zhong Yao Xian Dai Yan Jiu Yu Lin Chuan 1995).

Homotoxicology
General considerations/rationale

Classical homeopathy has recognized general mental complaints as important diagnostic criteria since its inception more than 200 years ago. Classical homeopathy contains many remedies associated with fear (Pitcairn 2006). Kent's classic text lists six and one-half pages of remedies that are useful in cases of fear (Kent 1999). Physical diseases may manifest as a restlessness or fear if pain or other abnormal sensations occur as a result. Homeopathic remedies that are considered in physical symptoms due to changes of weather might be considered in light of medical findings. Quinhydrone can be used in sensitivity to weather but should be given in frequent doses. This remedy is complemented by Sulphur and by all homeopathic remedies that have aggravation from wet weather, such as Kalmia, Dulcamara, Rhus tox, Rhododendron, Medorrhinum, Bryonia, and others (Reckeweg 2002).

Homotoxicologists have noted similar findings, and case reports regarding treatment of fear and fear aggression are beginning to appear (Palmquist 2006, Roach 2006). No controlled studies exist for antihomotoxic drugs in these cases, but because homotoxicology formulas and classical homeopathic remedies are nontoxic, it seems prudent to consider them in therapeutic plans for patients in this category. Such therapy is by trial and error at this time, and clients should be informed of the experimental nature of such treatments.

Appropriate homotoxicology formulas

Useful formulas (also see protocols for Separation Anxiety, Compulsive Disorders, and Aggression):

Aconitum homaccord: Used for intense fear.

BHI-Calming: A calming remedy that works more gently than others on this list.

Gelsemium homaccord: Animals likely have baroceptors, which may be hypersensitive in some storm phobia cases. The main constituent in the remedy is a neuractive herb that is diluted homeopathically and used for cases showing sensitivity to falling barometric pressure, fear of thunder, and/or fear of falling. Consider this remedy in cases in which fear begins long before thunder starts (falling barometric pressure).

Cerebrum compositum: Contains Gelsemium (see the listing in this remedy set). It is used for cerebral insufficiency, detoxification, and support. It also contains Thuja. The Impregnation phases that are characteristic of Thuja-responsive cases are found in the typical mood that is observed, which tends toward frequent angry outbursts, despondency and melancholy, discontent, anxiety, restlessness, and peevishness. These may be the consequences of bacterial and animal poisoning, vaccinations, snakebites, etc., and the symptoms are worse in cold and wet weather (Reckeweg 2002).

Mucosa compositum: Used for nervous diarrhea owing to the signs of poisoning demonstrated with Lachesis.

Nux vomica homaccord: Used with the ingredient Bryonia (for fear of thunderstorm), and also in cases with joint or respiratory complaints or nausea/vomiting.

Phosphor homaccord: This is a major remedy for cases showing fear of loud sounds and thunderstorms, thin animals, nervous debility, and neurosis (Boericke 1927, Heel 2003). Phosphorus is the principal remedy selected for use in this formula for patients with the following general symptom picture: emotionally there is a general excitability and irritability, timidity and fearfulness at twilight, and above all during thunderstorms; the patient fears being alone, and is hypersensitive to light, noises, and music, as with Nux vomica (Reckeweg 2002).

Rhododendron homaccord: Used for fear of thunderstorms, joint pain, and problems that originate following vaccinations (Day 1990).

Spigelon: Used with the ingredient Bryonia (used for fear of thunderstorm), and also in cases with joint or respiratory complaints. *Spigelon* is characteristically known for its assistance in migraine headaches in humans.

Valerianaheel: Has a mild calming effect.

Ypsiloheel: Leads to improved central mediation; contains *Lachesis* (Kent 1921).

Authors' suggested protocols

Nutrition

Brain nerve support and behavior support formulas: 1 tablet for every 25 pounds of body weight BID.

Lecithin/phosphatidyl choline: One-fourth teaspoon for every 25 pounds of body weight BID.

Inositol: 100 mg for every 25 pounds of body weight SID/BID.

Phosphatidyl serine (PS): 20 mg for every 15 pounds of body weight SID.

Omega-3,-6,-9: 1 capsule for every 25 pounds of body weight with food.

Chinese herbal medicine

Relaxol: 1 capsule for every 10 to 20 pounds of body weight, twice daily to effect. This therapy must be continued every day. It will not be effective if the supplement is only given before or during the storm.

In addition to the herbs mentioned above, Relaxol also contains anemarrhena (Zhi mu), haematite (Dai zhe shi), lily (Bai he), oyster shell (Mu li), and rehmannia (Sheng di huang). These additional herbs increase the efficacy of the formula by supporting the actions of the other herbs.

The authors use the following acupuncture points in phobic patients: PC6, GV15, SP6, and GB20.

Homotoxicology (Dose: 1 tablet or 10 drops for 50-pound dog; 1 tablet or 5 drops for small dog or cat)

Phosphor homaccord or Cerebrum compositum: Use as a starting prescription, or as indicated by other symptoms.

Product sources

Nutrition

Brain and behavioral/emotional support formulas: Animal Nutrition Technologies. **Alternative:** Composure—Vetri Science Laboratories.

Lecithin/phosphatidyl choline: Designs for Health.
Inositol: Progressive Labs.
Phosphatidyl serine (PS): Integrative Therapeutics.
Omega-3,-6,-9: Vetri Science. **Alternative:** Oil of evening primrose: Jarrow.

Chinese herbal medicine

Relaxol—Natural Solutions, Inc.

Homotoxicology remedies

BHI/Heel Corporation
Bach Flower Remedies: Ellon Bach.
Anaflora Flower Essences: Earth Animal, Inc.

REFERENCES

Western medicine references

Gur R, Cowell P, Turetsky B, Gallacher F, Cannon T, Bilker W. A follow-up magnetic resonance imaging study of schizophrenia. *Arch Gen Psych*, 1998; 55: 145–152.

Horwitz DF. Prognosis of behavior problems. Presented at the Atlantic Coast Veterinary Conference, October, 2001. Atlantic City, NJ.

McCobb E, Brown E, Damiani K, Dodman N. Thunderstorm phobia in dogs: an Internet survey of 69 cases. *J Am Anim Hosp Assoc.* 2001;37(4): pp 319–24.

Nash H. Fear of Thunderstorms and Noise Phobias, Veterinary Services Department, Drs. Foster and Smith, Inc.

Overall KL. Clinical Behavioral Medicine for Small Animals. 1997. St. Louis, MO; Mosby Year Book Inc.

Overall KL, Dunham AE, Frank D. Frequency of nonspecific clinical signs in dogs with separation anxiety, thunderstorm phobia, and noise phobia, alone or in combination. *Journal of the American Veterinary Medical Association.* 2001; August 15;219(4):467–73.

Integrative veterinary medicine references

Broadfoot P. 2003. Personal communication on clinical management of CNS cases.

Callahan S. Anaflora Flower Essences. 1997. Mt. Shasta, CA: Sacred Spirit Publishing.

Essential Science. Essential Oils Desk Reference, 2nd ed. Essential Science Publishing, 2002. pp 33–81.

Farber S. Sports Medicine for Dogs: Part 2, Introduction to Treatment: The Anxiety Wrap™, Golden Retriever News Column: Integrative Care for Golden Retrievers, 2002. http://www.anxietywrap.com/golden_retriever_news_column.htm.

Farber S. Sports Medicine for Dogs: Part 2, Introduction to Treatment: The Anxiety Wrap™, Golden Retriever News Column: Integrative Care for Golden Retrievers 2002. http://www.anxietywrap.com/golden_retriever_news_column.htm.

Haug L. Thunderstorm Fear and Phobia. Texas A&M University 2006. http://www.bcrescuetexas.org/Training/THUNDER-STORM%20PHOBIA.doc.

Silver R. 2004. Personal communication.

Tellington-Jones L. 1999. Getting in Touch With Your Dog, A Gentle Approach to Influencing Behavior, Health, and Performance. North Pomfret, VT: Trafalgar Square Publishing, pp 82–85.

Wright J, Wright M. 2006. Personal communication from practitioners well known for successful use of Bach flowers.

Nutrition references

Benjamin J, Levine J, Fux M, et al. Double-blind, placebo-controlled, crossover trial of inositol treatment for panic disorder. *Am J Psychiatry* 1995;152:1084–6.

Cenacchi T, Bertoldin T, Farina C, et al. Cognitive decline in the elderly: a double-blind, placebo-controlled multicenter study on efficacy of phosphatidylserine administration. *Aging (Milano)* 1993;5:123–33.

Crook TH, Tinklenberg J, Yesavage J, et al. Effects of phosphatidylserine in age-associated memory impairment. *Neurology* 1991;41:644–9.

Erasmus U. Fats That Heal, Fats That Kill. Alive Books; revised and updated edition. January 1, 1993. The Complete Lecture, www.udoerasmus.com.

Fux M, Levine J, Aviv A, Belmaker RH. Inositol treatment of obsessive-compulsive disorder. *Am J Psychiatry* 1996;153:1219–21.

Horrocks LA, et al. Phosphatidyl Research and the Nervous System, Berlin: Springer Verlach, 1986.

Chinese herbal medicine references

Chang Yong Zhong Yao Xian Dai Yan Jiu Yu Lin Chuan (Recent Study and Clinical Application of Common Traditional Chinese Medicine), 1995; 489:491.

Chen DY, et al. *Journal of Nanjing TCM University.* 1999;15(4):240.

Hao HQ, et al. Curdione's regulatory effect on cats' sleeping rhythmic electric activity. *Journal of Chinese Materia Medica.* 1994;25(8):423–424.

Ou Yang Guang Ying. Trace elements of 11 tonifying herbs from the Dunhuang region. *Journal of Gansu College of TCM.* 1990;7(4):24–25.

Spence D, Warren MA, Kayumov L, Chen A, Lowe A, Jain U, Katzman MA, Shen J, Perelman B, Shapiro CM. Acupuncture increases nocturnal melatonin secretion and reduces insomnia and anxiety: a preliminary report. *J Neuropsychitry Clin Neurosci*. February 2004; 16:19–28.

Wang NW. *Hunan Journal of TCM and Pharmacy*. 1998;4(5):26–27.

Wang SM, Kain ZN. Auricular acupuncture: a potential treatment of anxiety. *Anesthesia and Analgesia* February 2001;92(2):548–553.

Zhong Yao Tong Bao (*Journal of Chinese Herbology*), 1985; 10(6): 43.

Zhong Yao Xue (*Chinese Herbology*), 1998; 676:677.

Zhong Yao Xue (*Chinese Herbology*), 1998, 722:725.

Zhong Yao Yao Li Yu Ying Yong (*Pharmacology and Applications of Chinese Herbs*), 1983;888.

Zhong Yao Yao Li Yu Ying Yong (*Pharmacology and Applications of Chinese Herbs*), 1983; 477.

Homotoxicology references

Boericke W. Materia Medica with Repertory, 9th ed. Santa Rosa, CA: Boericke and Tafel, Inc. 1927. pp 407–10.

Day C. The Homeopathic Treatment of Small Animals: Principles and Practice. Saffron Walden, Essex: CW Daniel Company, LTD, 1990. p 128.

Essential Science. Essential Oils Desk Reference, 2nd ed. Essential Science Publishing, 2002. pp 33–81.

Gur R, Cowell P, Turetsky B, Gallacher F, Cannon T, Bilker W., A follow-up magnetic resonance imaging study of schizophrenia. *Arch Gen Psych*, 1998, 55: 145–152.

Haug L. Thunderstorm Fear and Phobia. Texas A&M University, 2006. http://www.bcrescuetexas.org/Training/THUNDERSTORM%20PHOBIA.doc.

Heel. Veterinary Guide, 3rd ed. Baden-Baden, Germany: Biologische Heilmettel Heel GmbH, 2003. p 104.

Kent J. Repertory of the Homeopathic Materia Medica and a Word Index. Paharganj, New Delhi: B. Jain, LTD, 1921. p 47.

McCobb E, Brown E, Damiani K, Dodman N. Thunderstorm phobia in dogs: an Internet survey of 69 cases. *J Am Anim Hosp Assoc*. 2001, 37(4): pp 319–24.

Palmquist R. Homotoxicology: Clinical Case Management. In: Proceedings of The North American Veterinary Conference, Vol 20, Orlando, FL, 2006. p 69 (See also taped lecture contents, which are more complete).

Pitcairn R. Vegas: The Cat with Homesickness. Advanced Homeopathy Course, Saguaro, 2006. Eugene, OR.

Reckeweg H. Homeopathia Antihomotoxica Materia Medica, 4th ed. Baden-Baden, Germany: Aurelia-Verlag, 2002. pp 231, 490, 573–4.

Roach B. Homotoxicology: Feline Behavior Case, published to private member internet list, Complementary Alternative Veterinary Medicine NET, Jan Bergeron, list owner. 2006. January 30.

Tellington-Jones L. Getting in Touch With Your Dog, A Gentle Approach to Influencing Behavior, Health, and Performance. North Pomfret, VT: Trafalgar Square Publishing, 1999. pp 82–85.

Wright J, Wright M. 2006. Personal communication from practitioners well known for successful use of Bach flowers.

Chapter Nine

Diseases of the Cardiovascular System

CARDIAC ARRHYTHMIAS

Definition and cause

Cardiac arrhythmias can occur for many reasons (Keating 2001, Bhatt 2005). Hypoxia, trauma, biochemical insult resulting in tissue injury, metabolic disturbances, genetic alteration, reactions to medications, hyperthermia, neuroendocrine imbalances, nutritional deficiencies, and neoplasia are only a few of the possible causes. Disturbances of cellular function lead to improper cellular responses, which can subsequently lead to rhythm disturbances (Bhatt 2005).

Medical therapy rationale, drug(s) of choice, and nutritional recommendations

Many cardiac arrhythmia patients require cardiac medications once a proper diagnosis has been reached (Vaughan-Williams 1970). These should be used as necessary to stabilize, preserve, and prolong life. In other cases, it is possible that the condition will resolve once the primary causative factors have been handled. Periodic monitoring of physical health, laboratory data, and cardiac testing such as electrocardiographic, echocardiographic, and radiographic imaging are helpful in following the progress and adjusting the treatment programs.

Anticipated prognosis

The prognosis depends upon the underlying cause. The arrhythmias usually are resolved if the cause is corrected.

Integrative veterinary therapies

An integrative approach to cardiac arrhythmias should be prescribed only after a definitive diagnosis and the underlying cause have been determined. This integrative approach focuses upon both the underlying cause and the physiological cellular changes that have occurred in both nerve and cardiac cells that result in the arrhythmia. Nutrients, nutraceuticals, medicinal herbs, and combination homeopathics can reduce cellular inflammation, improve mineral and nutrient passage through membranes, protect cells, and work alone or in combination with medication, when indicated, to improve the animal's clinical condition.

Nutrition
General considerations/rationale

After the cause of the arrhythmia has been established and addressed, nutritional support can be recommended to address both the cause and the arrhythmia. Nutrients that are required for the proper functioning and nourishment of cardiac and nerve cells, as well as antioxidants to reduce free-radical-induced inflammation, often help to stabilize the condition.

Appropriate nutrients

Nutritional/gland therapy: Glandular heart and nutrients such as magnesium, potassium, carnitine, taurine, and antioxidants can help neutralize immune cellular inflammation and eventual cellular degeneration and organ (see Gland Therapy, Chapter 2).

Coenzyme Q10: Much of the clinical research on CoQ10 has been in human heart disease. Research has shown that it is beneficial in cardiovascular disease and in controlling cardiac arrhythmias (Gaby 1996).

Taurine: Deficiencies of taurine have been clinically linked to cardiac disease in animals (Fox 1992, Novotny 1994).

L-carnitine: L-carnitine is proven to improve cardiac function. Research has shown that the cardiac reserves of carnitine are depleted when oxygen levels in the body are reduced. Orlando (1986) showed a benefit to heart patients with L-carnitine supplementation and McEntee (1995) reported on low levels of L-carnitine in a dog with cardiomyopathy. The dog showed clinical improvement after L-carnitine therapy at 50 mg/kg/TID.

Vitamin E: Vitamin E is involved in the proper functioning of the heart muscle; it particularly improves cardiac output and circulation (Traber 2001).

Magnesium: Bashir (1993) showed that people taking magnesium supplementation had a reduction of more than 30% in arrhythmias. In a large population study, Tsuji (1994) associated low serum levels of magnesium with an increased rate of arrhythmias. Tzivoni (1990), in a peer-reviewed study, showed that magnesium may definitively reduce drug-induced arrhythmias.

Fish oil: In a double-blind trial, people with ventricular premature complexes had a reduction of 70% in abnormal heartbeats when fish oil was added to their diets (Sellmayer 1995).

Potassium: Lumme (1989) showed that the addition of potassium to the diet also significantly reduced arrhythmias.

Chinese herbal medicine
General considerations/rationale
In Traditional Chinese Medicine terms, cardiac arrhythmias are caused by Qi deficiency and Blood and Qi stagnation affecting the Heart. Under the Western interpretation, Qi deficiency can be translated into weakness or fatigue. Qi stagnation in the Heart may lead to irregular beating. The Heart may not beat while the Qi is blocked, but may then beat faster as the Qi breaks through. An arrhythmia results. Blood stagnation prevents normal blood flow, which leads to chest pain. Treatment is aimed at restoring blood flow by strengthening the heart contraction, increasing cardiac output, and normalizing the cardiac rhythm.

Appropriate Chinese herbs
Aconite (Fu zi): Can cause positive inotropic and chronotropic effects (Yao Xue Xue Bao 1983).

Astragalus (Huang qi): In a study of 14 human patients with heart failure, astragalus led to increases in cardiac output, cardiac index, stroke output, and stroke index. Experiments on animals show that astragalus can increase coronary blood flow and decrease coronary circulation resistance (Modern TCM Pharmacology 1997, Xu 1999, Luo 1999).

Carthamus (Hong hua): Has positive inotropic effects at low doses (Zhong Cheng Yao Yan Jiu 1983).

Cinnamon twig (Gui zhi): Has cardiotonic effects and vasodilatory properties (Zhong Yao Xue 1998).

Cnidium (Chuan xiong): Contains chuanxiongzine, which can inhibit the thoracic aorta's contraction when it is induced experimentally by noradrenalin, potassium chloride, or calcium chloride. It was shown to dilate pulmonary vessels in rats (Zou 1984, Chen 1990, Wang 1990). Additionally, it improved coronary blood flow in experiments using isolated rat and hamster hearts (Gao 1987).

Codonopsis (Dang shen): Has been shown to increase cardiac output and improve blood perfusion in cats (Zhong Yao Xue 1998).

Licorice (Gan cao): Used with good results in 23 humans with arrhythmia (Bei Jing Zhong Yi Xue Yuan Xue Bao 1983). Licorice can decrease myocardial oxygen consumption and improve the general condition of blood vessels (Xu 1997).

Notoginseng (San qi): Improves arrhythmia due to decreased cardiac output (Zhong Yao Xue 1998).

Ophiopogon (Mai men dong): Treats drug-induced arrhythmia in rats (Zhong Cao Yao 1982).

Peach kernel (Tao ren): Has been shown experimentally to be able to increase the blood flow in dogs' femoral arteries and rabbits' auricular arteries by reducing vascular resistance (Liu 1989).

Peony (Chi shao): Increases resistance to hypoxia in animals (Zhong Cheng Yao Yan Jiu 1980).

Rehmannia (Sheng di huang): Has demonstrated cardiotonic effects (Zhong Yao Xue 1998).

Salvia (Dan shen): Increases perfusion of coronary arteries, thereby decreasing damage from cardiac ischemia (Gou Wai Yi Xue Zhong Yi Zhong Yao Fen Ce 1991).

White peony (Bai shao): Dilates peripheral blood vessels, thereby decreasing vascular resistance (Zhong Guo Yao Li Xue Tong Bao 1986).

Zizyphus (Suan zao ren): Has been shown to decrease experimentally induced arrhythmias (Zhong Guo Shou Yi Za Zha 1988).

Homotoxicology
General considerations/rationale
Most commonly encountered clinical veterinary cardiac arrhythmias represent Impregnation, Degeneration, or Dedifferentiation phase disorders. Clinicians should conduct full medical evaluations so they possess the most accurate information concerning the patient's condition. Diagnostic data is critical to properly treating these pets. Some arrhythmia patients can taper medications and continue on only their antihomotoxic support, while others require continued allopathic support.

Clinicians should not hesitate to mix antihomotoxic medications and pharmaceutical cardiac agents in a patient's treatment program. When prescribing cardiac glycosides, it may be observed that much lower doses are sufficient due to the synergistic effects of antihomotoxic drugs. Monitoring levels is advised in all patients that receive digitalis type drugs. In the author's practice, digoxin is rarely required to handle most cardiac patients.

Homotoxicology readily integrates with many different fields of healing, and Demers and Ben-Yakir have presented data regarding integration of homotoxicology with Traditional Chinese Medicine (Demers, 2005, Ben-Yakir, 2005ab). Factually, many patients that receive integrative treatment protocols feel better and require less medication. Cardiac healing and repair can occur as a result of homotoxicology treatment and have been reported (Palmquist 2005, 2006). Homotoxicology and other biological therapies are increasing in popularity, providing an exciting set of alternatives for handling cardiac issues in veterinary practice. Future research should prove interesting.

Appropriate homotoxicology formulas

Because arrhythmias can result from many different causes, this list primarily concerns those conditions that relate directly to the heart (see other protocols as indicated by the specific case):

Aconitum homaccord: Used for anxiety, fear, fever, generalized erythema, and Inflammation phase homotoxicoses. Active ingredient is Aconitine and causes death by respiratory paralysis and ventricular fibrillation (Dorland 2006).

Aesculus compositum: Used for peripheral vascular repair.

Angio-Injeel (AngioHeel): Currently not available in the United States. Used for angina, arterial hypertension, left-sided cranial pains, cardiac circulatory issues, anxiety, palpitations in the neck (these sometimes occur and lead to feline patients vocalizing in distress), and in allergic or sensitive patients. Glonoin (Nitroglycerin), an ingredient in this remedy, may assist in managements of these cats. Glonoin is also contained in *Cactus compositum*, *Cardiacum-Heel*, *Cor compositum*, *Glonoin homaccord*, *Strophanthus compositum*, and *Ypsiloheel* (Reckeweg 2000).

Aurumheel: Used for hypotension, hypertension, and cardiac arrhythmias. The ingredient Convallarea majalis (lily of the valley) is known to assist in myocardial weakness and is used as a Western herb to increase cardiac performance and strength. It also treats hypertrophy and decompensation. It is part of the recommended human protocol for atrial fibrillation (Reckeweg 2000, Broadfoot 2005). The main indications are: weakness of myocardium, endocarditis, nervous palpitation, and athlete's heart (hypertrophy). The patient's history may include dyspnea with a feeling of faintness and palpitations, along with air hunger on the slightest movement, fluttering in the heart on exertion, then flushing of the face, and a sensation as if the heart were about to stop beating, then it would suddenly beat strongly again, and be accompanied by a feeling of faintness. Arrhythmia and cardiac insufficiency are the defining symptoms (Reckeweg 2002).

Cactus compositum: Indicated for angina and weakness in coronary blood flow/supply. Kalium carbonicum supports cardiac arrhythmias; Glonoin (Nitroglycerin) is indicated for anginal pain and palpitations involving the neck. Also contains Crataegus, as in *Cralonin* (below) (Reckeweg 2000, Broadfoot 2005).

Carbo compositum: Currently not currently available in the United States. Used in hypertensive patients and for cardiocirculatory disturbances.

Cardiacumheel: Indicated for cardiac pain, angina, pain radiating up the neck, arrhythmia, intercostal pain (Ranunculus), cardiac pain with *China homaccord*, exhaustion, and weakness with lowered ability to function. It is useful after loss of body fluids (China), and to treat the origins of pain in vertebral area.

Coenzyme compositum: Used to repair enzyme systems associated with metabolism. It is useful in all cellular phases. Its spectrum includes Natrum pyruvicum; in its sphere of use, Natrum pyruvicum has certain similarities to the indications for Sulphur in that pyruvic acid is situated at a focal point in the citric acid cycle, and Sulphur-like symptoms occur when there is an accumulation of pyruvates, e.g. in iatrogenic damage. Thus, Natrum pyruvicum can be combined with *Engystol*, Sulphur, and possibly Hepar Sulph., and all sarcodes and numerous nosodes. It is especially indicated in cellular phases of all kinds, and in chronic conditions, including Impregnation Phases such as asthma, angina pectoris, pruritus, skin diseases, and psoriasis. It is also indicated in other Degeneration Phases, e.g. organic nervous diseases, and in precancerous states and neoplasm phases.

The regressive vicariations that follow should be tackled with suitable single remedies. The homotoxins that require Natrum pyruvicum are not characterized so much by disorders of the direct energy extraction and use as they are by respiratory disorders, but rather they concern an integral part of the energy extraction which precedes the introduction of the decomposing carbohydrates into the citric acid cycle (Reckeweg 2002). A recent study from the *Annals of Thoracic Surgery* showed that administration of pyruvate upon reperfusion after cardioplegic arrest mitigated oxidative stress, protected mitochondrial enzymes, and increased the myocardial energy state, which supports Reckeweg's therapeutic application of pyruvates, particularly after cardioplegic arrest (Knott 2006).

Cor compositum: Initiates repair and provides detoxification and drainage of the cardiac tissues. Its indications include hypertension, cardiac circulatory disorders, post-infectious and post-toxic cardiac disease, myocarditis, preinsufficiency, dyspnea, and anxiety associated with cardiac weakness, dyspnea, arrhythmia, and collapse (Reckeweg 2000). *Cor compositum* works similarly to carnitine. Due to its ingredient Cor suis (heart), it may theoretically contribute to cellular repair.

Cor compositum contains Kali carbonicum, which is also contained in *Cactus compositum, cardiacum,* and *Cralonin.* This remedy targets heart symptoms. It can treat some perpetual arrhythmias, possibly interspersed with paroxysmal tachycardia, as well as defects of the valves that are associated with myocardial weakness pains in the heart. The Kali salts have a general prophylactic action in respect to heart attack. Problems arise most frequently around 3 a.m. in patients responsive to this agent.

Another strong contributor to this far-reaching remedy is DL-malicum acidum (malic acid), which is also found in *Coenzyme compositum.* It is an active factor in the citric acid cycle and in redox systems, and is useful in Impregnation Phases including asthma and angina pectoris, and neoplasm phases (especially in the early stages) to improve cell respiration. It has a diuretic action and should be given in conjunction with fumaric acid, which is also found in *Cor compositum* and *Coenzyme compositum,* because they aid in general detoxification and oxygenation of glandular and muscular tissues. Malic acid is also used to treat angina pectoris, myocardial weakness with dyspnea, tachycardia from metabolic and post-infective weakness of the myocardium, circulatory collapse, and bradycardia in athletes. Cold hands and feet and cyanosis of the skin are all typical symptoms (Reckeweg 2002).

Cralonin: Supports cardiac strength in geriatric conditions and positive ionotrope through action of Crataegus (Hawthorne, also known as Whitethorn). *Cralonin* is useful in nearly all cardiac complaints, hypertension, fatigue, and anemia, and as emergency injection in acute cases (Reckeweg 2000, Schroder 2003, Broadfoot 2005). Crataegus' action is not confined to the circulation, but extends to other systems. Therefore, in addition to cardiac function, there is a general toning action on the circulation, and a regulating effect on the blood pressure. As a result, it also relieves tension in the peripheral circulation, as blood pressure is controlled both centrally and peripherally. Thus, it affects arrhythmia, angina pectoris, and dysarteriotomy.

The indications are as follows: weakness of the heart muscle, including that of a toxic nature (infectious toxic weakness of the heart muscle), myocarditis, cardiomyopathy, senile heart syndromes, athlete's heart, fatty degeneration of the heart, hypertension, general arteriosclerosis, and myocardial ischemia and disturbances of coronary circulation with angina pectoris. It is useful after infectious diseases such as influenza and pneumonia and after fever (Reckeweg 2002). Crataegus is also found in *Angio-Heel, Aurumheel, Cactus compositum, Cor compositum, Cralonin, Glonoin homaccord,* and *Melilotus homaccord.*

Engystol: May be valuable in cases that could have a viral onset with subsequent alteration of cardiac conductivity (e.g., rheumatic fever in humans).

Glonoin (**nitroglycerin**): An agent that bridges homeopathic and allopathic practice (Schuppel 1997). The name *Glonoin* is based on the three components: Gl = glycerol, O = oxygen, and N = nitrogen. It can be helpful in cases of chest pain, tachycardia, arrhythmias associated with hyperthyroidism in cats (Lycopus), and nocturnal howling in elderly cats (perhaps through action on palpitations reaching up the neck) (Reckeweg 2000, Palmquist 2005).

Melilotus homaccord: Contains cardiac glycosides, which makes it useful in tachycardia (*Strophanthus*), angiospasms, arrhythmia (*Arsenicum album*), periendocarditis, collapse, asthma, and emphysema (*Carbo vegetalis*) (O'Hanlon 1952, Norn 2004). It can be used as an antistress remedy in acute failure and vasodilates. Strophanthus is a primary component, with indications for cardiac decompensation, palpitations, tachycardia, cardiac insufficiency, and anticipatory anxiety (Reckeweg 2002). This formula also contains Crataegus, which is used primarily for hypertensive states with arrhythmias.

Rauwolfia compositum: Takes its name from Rauwolfia serpentina, long recognized as a very efficient regulator of blood pressure. It also contains, among other components, Melilotus, which has a characteristic action on the kidneys and to some extent opens the glomeruli for a more generous flow of blood. It has not yet been experimentally clarified whether the decrease in blood flow might be due to spastic contractions of the arterioles. After Melilotus has been given the congestion usually improves, so that Melilotus can also be helpful in chronic kidney conditions, e.g., renal hypertension (Reckeweg 2002). This remedy also contains Ren suis and Hepar suis to help drain the organ systems. Viscum album is the anti-arrhythmic component, which is useful for Impregnation phases and is indicated for hypotension and hypertension, sensations of vertigo, coronary stenosis, arrhythmia, and articular diseases of attrition (Reckeweg 2002).

Ubichinon compositum: This remedy is deeper reaching than *Coenzyme compositum* in supporting metabolism and mitochondrial functions in Degeneration and Dedifferentiation phase homotoxicoses. Seventy-nine percent of patients who were suffering from chronic disorders with metabolic problems and were treated with *Coenzyme compositum* showed improvement.

Authors' suggested protocols

Nutrition

Cardiac support formula: 1 tablet for every 25 pounds of body weight.

Coenzyme Q10: 15 mg for every 10 pounds of body SID.

Eskimo fish oil: One-half to 1 teaspoon per meal for cats. One teaspoon for every 35 pounds of body weight for dogs.

Vitamin E: 50 IU for every 20 pounds of body weight SID.

Chinese herbal medicine

H110 Arrhythmia: Recommended at a dose of 1 capsule per 10 to 20 pounds of body weight twice daily. In addition to the herbs mentioned above, H110 Arrhythmia also contains amber (Hu po), cnidium (Chuan xiong), fossil bones (Long gu), oyster shell (Mu li), and schisandra (Wu wei zi).

Homotoxicology (Dose: 10 drops for 50-pound dog; 5 drops for cat or small dog)

Symptom remedy (general arrhythmia): Cralonin, Cardiacum-Heel, Aesculus compositum, and Aurumheel mixed together and given TID PO. Cor compositum given by injection or orally acutely and then repeated twice weekly as needed. For ventricular fibrillation, consider adding Aconitum homaccord (give at close intervals until effect is noted, then taper dose) in addition to drugs. *Crataegus* remedies given I.V. are the best choice for fibrillation. Cor compositum serves as a rescue medication in these cases (Broadfoot 2005).

For those that are possibly hypertensive, the remedy Melilotus, with *Crataegus*, Melilotus homaccord, and Strophanthus, may be a valuable therapeutic tool, in conjunction with Coenzyme compositum for the mitochondrial support in a crisis. For impending circulatory collapse, a remedy which is unfortunately unavailable at this time is Strophanthus compositum. That remedy contained *Carbo* and *Veratrum*, the homeopathic equivalent for shock, along with *Strophanthus, Cactus, Glonoinum, Aconitum, Latrodectus,* and *Aethusa.*

Symptom remedy (atrial fibrillation): Aurumheel and Chelidonium, with alternating remedies of Cardiacumheel (for anxiety, pressure, or stabbing chest pains), Hepeel, and Cralonin (Reckeweg 2000).

Symptom remedy (paroxysmal tachycardia): Cardiacumheel, Belladonna homaccord, Aurumheel, Gastricumheel, and Psorinoheel. Give Glonoin if pulsating neck pains or in hyperthyoidism/thryotoxicosis (Reckeweg 2000).

Detoxification remedy: Uses as indicated by other conditions and phases of homotoxicoses present. Most patients should receive Galium-Heel in combination with other remedies. Coenzyme compositum, Ubichinon compositum are indicated in most cases, as well.

Product sources

Nutrition
Cardiac support formulas: Animal Nutrition Technologies. **Alternatives:** Formula CV—Rx Vitamins for Pets; Cardiac Support formula—Standard Process Veterinary Formulas; Cardio-Strength—Vetri Science Laboratories; Bio-Cardio—Thorne Veterinary Products.

Coenzyme Q10: Vetri Science; Rx Vitamins for Pets; Integrative Therapeutics; Thorne Veterinary Products.

Eskimo fish oil: Tyler Encapsulations.

Chinese herbal medicine
Formula H110 Arrhythmia: Natural Solutions, Inc.

Homotoxicology remedies
BHI/Heel, Inc.

REFERENCES

Western medicine references
Bhatt L, Nandakumar K, Bodhankar S. Experimental animal models to induce cardiac arrhythmias. *Indian J Pharmacol*, 2005. 37: pp 348–357.

Keating M, Sanguinetti M. Molecular and cellular mechanisms of cardiac arrhythmias. *Cell*, 2001. 104: pp 569–80.

Vaughan-Williams E. Classification of antiarrhythmic drugs. In: sandöe E, Flensted-Jensen E, Olesen KH, editors. Symposium on cardiac arrhythmias. 1970. Elsinore, Denmark: AB Astra, Sfdertdlje, Sweden.

IVM/nutrition references
Bashir Y, Sneddon JF, Staunton A, et al. Effects of long-term oral magnesium chloride replacement in congestive heart failure secondary to coronary artery disease. *Am J Cardiol* 1993;72:1156–62.

Fox PR, Sturman JA, Myocardial taurine concentrations in cats with cardiac disease and in healthy cats fed taurine-modified diets, *Am J Vet Res*; 1992. Feb;53(2):237–41.

Gaby AR. The role of coenzyme Q10 in clinical medicine: part II. Cardiovascular disease, hypertension, diabetes mellitus and infertility. *Altern Med Rev* 1996;1:168–75

Lumme JA, Jounela AJ. The effect of potassium and potassium plus magnesium supplementation on ventricular extrasystoles in mild hypertensives treated with hydrochlorothiazide. *Int J Cardiol* 1989;25:93–8.

McEntee K, et al. Clinical Electrocardiographic and Echocardiographic Improvement after L-Carnitine Supplementation in a Cardiomyopathic Labrador. *Canine Pract.* 20: 12, 1995.

Novotny MJ, Hogan PM, Flannigan G., Echocardiographic evidence for myocardial failure induced by taurine deficiency in domestic cats, *Can J Vet Res* 1994 Jan;58(1): 6–12.

Orlando G, Rusconi C. Oral L-Carnitine in the Treatment of Chronic Cardiac Ischemia in Elderly Patients. *Clin. Trials J.*, 1986; 23:238–244.

Sellmayer A, Witzgall H, Lorenz RL, Weber PC. Effects of dietary fish oil on ventricular premature complexes. *Am J Cardiol* 1995;76:974–7.

Traber MG. Vitamin E. In: Shils M, Olson JA, Shike M, Ross AC, eds. Nutrition in Health and Disease. 9th ed. Baltimore: Williams and Wilkins; 1999:347–362.

Tsuji H, Venditti FJ, Evans JC, et al. The associations of levels of serum potassium and magnesium with ventricular premature complexes (the Framingham Heart Study). *Am J Cardiol* 1994;74:232–5.

Tzivoni D, Keren A. Suppression of ventricular arrhythmias by magnesium. *Am J Cardiol* 1990;65:1397–9 [review].

Chinese herbal medicine references

Bei Jing Zhong Yi Xue Yuan Xue Bao (*Journal of Beijing University School of Medicine*), 1983;2:24.

Chen BH, et al. *China Journal of Tuberculosis and Respiration.* 1990;13(5):268.

Gou Wai Yi Xue Zhong Yi Zhong Yao Fen Ce (*Monograph of Chinese Herbology from Foreign Medicine*), 1991; 13 (3):41.

Gao ZP, et al. *China Pharmacology Bulletin.* 1987;3(6): 363.

Liu CH, et al. The pharmacology of Tao Ren. *Journal of Pharmacology and Clinical Application of TCM.* 1989;(2): 46–47.

Luo XP, et al. *China Journal of Pathology and Physiology.* 1999; 15(7):639–643.

Modern TCM Pharmacology. 1997. Tianjin: Science and Technology Press.

Wang DX, et al. Medical Research Update. 1990;19(6):20.

Xu L, et al. *Journal of Research in Chinese Medicine.* 1997;10(2):31–32.

Xu SA, et al. *China Journal of Pharmacy.* 1999;34(10)663–665.

Yao Xue Xue Bao (*Journal of Herbology*), 1983; 18(5):394.

Zhong Cao Yao (*Chinese Herbal Medicine*), 1982; 3(9); 27–32.

Zhong Cheng Yao Yan Jiu (*Research of Chinese Patent Medicine*), 1980;1:32.

Zhong Cheng Yao Yan Jiu (*Research of Chinese Patent Medicine*), 1983;12:31.

Zhong Guo Shou Yi Za Zha (*Chinese Journal of Husbandry*), 1988; 14 (6):44.

Zhong Guo Yao Li Xue Tong Bao (*Journal of Chinese Herbal Pharmacology*), 1986; 2(5):26.

Zhong Yao Xue (*Chinese Herbology*), 1998;65:67.

Zhong Yao Xue (*Chinese Herbology*), 1998; 156:158.

Zhong Yao Xue (*Chinese Herbology*), 1998; 507:512.

Zhong Yao Xue (*Chinese Herbology*), 1998;739:741.

Zou AP, et al. *Journal of Wuhan Medical College.* 1984;13(4):282.

Homotoxicology references

Ben-Yakir S. Homotoxicology: Homeosiniatry, the Bridge Between Acupuncture and Homeopathy. In: Proceedings 142nd AVMA Annual Convention and 28th World Veterinary Congress, Minneapolis, MN, USA, 2005a. July 16–20.

Ben-Yakir S. Veterinary Homeosiniatry. In: Proceedings of the 31st Annual International Congress of Veterinary Acupuncture, International Veterinary Acupuncture Society (IVAS), 2005b. Sept 21–24, USA, pp 129–135.

Broadfoot P. Heart Happy Homotoxicology. In: Proceedings of AHVMA/Heel Annual Homotoxicology Seminar, 2005. May 27–29, Denver, CO, pp 75–7, 80–1, 86, 90.

Broadfoot P. Puppyatrics—Handling the vaccination reaction. *J Biomed Ther*, 2006. Winter, pp 14–5.

Demers J. Cardiovascular Disease: Homotoxicology and TCM. In: Proceedings of AHVMA/Heel Homotoxicology Seminar, 2005. Denver, CO, May 27–28, pp 98–103.

Dorland's Illustrated Medical Dictionary, 25th edition. WB Saunders, Philadelphia. 1974.

Knott EM, Sun J, Lei Y, Ryou MG, Olivencia-Yurvati AH, Mallet RT. Pyruvate mitigates oxidative stress during reperfusion of cardioplegia-arrested myocardium. *Ann. Thorac.Surg.* 2006; Mar.81 (3) 928–934.

Melcart D, Linde K, Worku F, Sarkady L, Holzmann M, Jurcic K, Wagner H. Results of five randomized studies on the immunomodulatory activity of preparations of Echinacea, *J Altern Complement Med*, 1995. Summer;1(2): pp 145–60.

Norn S, Kruse P. Cardia glycosides: From ancient history through Withering's foxglove to endogenous cardiac glycosides, translated from Danish. *Dan Medicinhist Arbog*, 2004;pp 119–32.

O'Hanlon A. A short proving of Strophanthus sarmentosus, *Br Homeopath J*, 1952. Jan;42(1): pp 13–5.

Palmquist R. Case report. In: Proceedings of AHVMA/Heel Homotoxicology Seminar, Denver, O, 2005. May 27–29, pp 106–8.

Palmquist R. 2005. Unpublished case report.

Palmquist R. Use of homotoxicology and biological therapy in treatment of feline hypertrophic cardiomyopathy: A clinical case report, *JAHVMA*, 2006.

Pedalino C, Perazzo F, Carvalho J, Martinho K, Massoco C, Bonamin L. Effect of Atropa belladonna and Echinacea angustifolia in homeopathic dilution on experimental peritonitis, *Homeopathy*, 2004. Oct;93(4): pp 193–8.

Reckeweg H. *Biotherapeutic Index: Ordinatio Antihomotoxica et Materia Medica*, 5th ed. 2000. Baden-Baden, Germany: Biologische Heilmittel Heel GMBH, pp 95–6, 264, 258, 298–90, 302, 311, 319–20, 320–21, 342, 533.

Reckeweg H. *Homeopathia Antihomotoxica Materia Medica*, 4th edition. 2002. Baden-Baden, Germany: Aurelia-Verlag, pp 148–9, 256–7, 260–1, 367, 402, 450, 551, 598–99.

Schroder D, Weiser M, Klein P. Efficacy of a homeopathic Crataegus preparation compared with usual therapy for mild (NYHA II) cardiac insufficiency: results of an observational cohort study. *Eur J Heart Fail*, 2003. Jun;5(3):319–26.

Schuppel R. Significance of cognitive processes in drug research in the 19th century-emplified by nitroglycerin, translation from German, *Gesnerus*, 1997.54(1–2): pp 59–73.

Van Wassenhoven M. Towards evidence-based repertory: Clinical evaluation of Veratrum album, *Homeopathy*, 2004. Apr;93(2): pp 71–7.

CARDIOMYOPATHIES, CONGENITAL HEART DISEASES, CARDIAC ARRHYTHMIAS, CONGESTIVE HEART FAILURE

Definition and cause

Because of the similarity in the approach of integrative therapies, heart disease (congenital, congestive and cardiomyopathy) is described together in this section.

Cardiomyopathy: Several forms of myocardial disease exist, including "idiopathic dilated cardiomyopathy (DCM), arrhythmogenic cardiomyopathy (ACM) (Boxer, English Bulldog, and Doberman Pinscher), lone atrial fibrillation (AF)(Wolfhound), or ventricular ectopia (Doberman Pinscher) without obvious echocardiographic evidence of myocardial failure" (Bonagura 2001). It is currently felt that most cases of cardiomyopathy have multiple causal factors, including genetics, diet, body type, breed, and sex. DCM and ACM are most common in dogs, while hypertrophic cardiomyopathy (HCM) is most common in cats and is more commonly seen in dogs of the Boston Terrier breed (Bonagura 2001, Pion 1987). Sudden death can occur in both species without prior symptomology being noted by veterinarian or client.

A full medical evaluation is indicated for the clinician to assess the patient's condition. Feline patients with an arrhythmia or murmur noted on routine physical examination should have a cardiac work-up, because many of these cats are asymptomatic cardiac cases. Diagnostic data is critical to properly treating these pets. Tumor (hemangiosarcoma), electrolyte imbalances, post trauma or postoperative ventricular arrhythmia, medication reactions, and thyroid imbalances may all contribute to the disease process. Once a proper diagnosis is reached, many of these patients require cardiac medications. These should be used as necessary to stabilize the patient and preserve and prolong life (DeFrancesco 2003, Pion 1987).

Congenital heart disease: Surgery can be attempted for congenital defects and consultation with a surgeon and cardiologist is recommended early in the course of therapy. Dilated cardiomyopathy in dogs is one of the more common congenital heart diseases. It is most often idiopathic, but there are indications that there may be underlying causes such as familial protein abnormalities or nutritional deficiencies of taurine and/or L-carnitine (Miller 2003, Sissan 1999). Certainly any pediatric patient should be examined fully and this examination should include auscultation and determination of pulse quality. Abnormalities in these areas should prompt advice to proceed with a cardiac work-up including radiography, echocardiography, and possibly electrocardiography. The clinician should search further for other congenital abnormalities in such patients.

Congestive heart disease: Valvular lesions in animals commonly result in heart failure. This can be so-called "endocardiosis," an alteration of the valve leaflet caused by changes in the matrix or by interference with valvular function by a vegetative lesion consisting of infection or tumor. Rupture of the chordae tendonae can lead to rapid congestive heart failure and sudden death. Other causes are secondary to dilated cardiomyopathy, chemotherapy such as doxorubicin, or hyperthyroidism (Smith 2003).

Autoaggressive disease can damage valve function as well, as can deterioration of the heart's lining in endocarditis. Feline congestive heart failure is usually the result of cardiomyopathy, but other valve defects and congenital defects can also occur in cats, too (see congenital heart disease protocols).

Periodic monitoring of laboratory data and blood pressure, as well as physical examination and cardiac testing such as electrocardiographic, echocardiographic, and radiographic imaging are helpful in following the progress and adjusting treatment programs for best effect. Careful attention to other body systems is warranted because congestive heart failure affects multiple organ systems. Screening kidney values is important, especially for those patients treated with cardiac pharmaceuticals, such as enalapril and diuretics, which may cause exacerbation of renal function. Altered renal function may require adjustment of drug dosages as well, as in the case of digoxan. Concurrent dental disease can be aggravating or causative in valvular disease, and proper dental care is an important part in the prevention and management of cardiac disease in veterinary patients.

Medical therapy rationale, drug(s) of choice, and nutritional recommendations

Medical therapy is dictated by the condition and complicating factors such as hypoxemia, pleural effusion, ascites, pulmonary edema, arrhythmia, elevated blood pressure, etc. Medically matched drugs such as adrenergic blockers, beta-blockers, anti-arrhythmics, calcium channel blockers, ACE inhibitors, and diuretics are recommended. The use of nutritional supplementation such as taurine, carnitine, and Coenzyme Q10 remains controversial. Cats and American Cocker Spaniels, however, respond quite well to taurine supplementation (See Nutrition, below). All cats with heart disease should be placed on taurine supplementation (DeFrancesco 2003, Miller 2003).

Anticipated prognosis

The prognosis for dogs and cats varies considerably with the underlying cause and the clinical status of the disease.

Cats with hypertrophic cardiomyopathy can do well for years, even after medication is withdrawn. Dogs with dilated cardiomyopathy is listed in the literature as always fatal within 6 months to 2 years after diagnosis (Kienle 2003, Miller 2003).

Integrative veterinary therapies

While the veterinary literature contains many references relating to cardiovascular pathology and diagnostic techniques, there is little focus on alternative therapies, except taurine supplemental therapy in cats. The lack of acceptable evidenced-based studies has been the deterrent.

The heart, a muscle that is continually contracting with no periods of rest, has very specific metabolic needs. Proper function relies upon a steady supply of nutrients to fuel cardiac cells as well as good perfusion for metabolic waste removal. The heart requires glandular and hormonal support to maintain proper function, because blood supply to the body's vital organs and tissues is critical for life. No other organ exemplifies the importance of reducing inflammation and enhancing elimination than the heart. Free radical production has been clinically proven to set the stage for degeneration of heart tissue, be it the heart muscle, the valves, or the conduction system itself (Facino 1994).

An integrative approach to cardiac disease considers not only the medical control of the symptoms associated with compromised cardiac function, but also the underlying causes in the heart itself, i.e., nutritional requirements; inflammatory or degenerative processes in the heart muscle, nerves, and conduction system; or valvular efficiency and integrity. The use of nutrients, nutraceuticals, medicinal herbs, and combination homeopathics that have anti-inflammatory and tissue protective effects on cells can often aid in the control of the clinical signs, reduce dependency on medication, and improve the day-to-day quality of life.

Many patients with congestive heart failure require cardiac medications for stabilization, and to preserve and prolong life. Some animals with CHF and cardiomyopathy may be able to be weaned off medications and be maintained on protocols of nutritional supplementation, Chinese herbal medicine, and/or homotoxicology support, while others may require continued ongoing medical support. When the cardiac condition is caused by other factors (i.e., endocarditis secondary to periapical dental abscessation), it is possible that the condition will resolve upon handling of the primary causative factors, but in most cases of valvular disease, the alterations are not reversible.

Periodic monitoring of laboratory data, and physical examination and cardiac testing such as electrocardiographic, echocardiographic, and radiographic imaging is helpful in following progress and adjusting treatment programs. (See Homotoxicology References for Ben-Yakir 2005; Broadfoot 2005; Demers 2005; Knott 2006; Norn 2004; Palmquist 2005, 2006; Reckeweg 2000, 2002; Schroder 2003; Van Wassenhoven 2004.)

Nutrition
General considerations/rationale
Nutritional support required for the proper functioning and nourishment of cardiac cells, and antioxidants to reduce free-radical-induced inflammation and help in cellular regeneration can help to stabilize the heart condition after the cause of the heart disease has been established and addressed.

Note: Because heart disease can be severe and involve organ failure, it is recommended that blood be analyzed both medically and physiologically to determine related organ involvement and disease. This allows for a more specific gland and nutritional support protocol (see Nutritional Blood Testing, Chapter 2).

Appropriate nutrients
The heart requires a continuous supply of bioavailable proteins and amino acids, essential fatty acids, and essential minerals.

Nutritional/glandular therapy: Glandular heart and other important nutrients such as L-carnitine and Coenzyme Q10 help to nourish heart cells, reduce free-radical-induced inflammation, and neutralize a cellular immune attack. It is this process at the cellular level that is one of the initiating causes of inflammation, leading to cellular weakness and breakdown, antibody production, and finally an auto-immune attack on heart cells. Gland therapy can help spare the heart, reduce inflammation, and help prevent eventual organ degeneration (see Chapter 2, Gland Therapy, for more details).

Essential fatty acids: In people with heart disease, fish oil been shown to be beneficial in slowing the progression of arteriosclerosis and improving disease symptoms (Leaf 1988, von Schacky 1999). In studies on animals, seabuckthorne oil has been shown to improve cardiac function, contractility, and oxygen utilization (Wu 1994, 1997).

Taurine: Low levels of taurine have been clinically proven to cause cardiomyopathy. Ryan (1989), Simpson (1993), Pion (1992), and Wysong (1989) found a direct link between low levels of taurine in the body and cardiac disease (Fox 1992, Novotny 1994).

L-carnitine: L-carnitine has proven effective in improving the functioning of the heart by allowing heart muscle to use lower levels of oxygen more efficiently. Cherchi (1985) and Orlando (1986) showed a benefit to heart patients with L-carnitine supplementation and McEntee (1995) reported on low levels of L-carnitine in a dog with cardiomyopathy and clinical improvement after L-carnitine therapy at 50 mg/kg/TID.

Studies on heart disease have shown that the addition of L-carnitine to the diet can reduce heart damage in animals (Lopaschuk 2000). In a study of human patients with heart disease Davini (1992) found that the introduction of L-carnitine after the diagnosis of heart disease resulted in a significant improvement over standard drug therapy: the mortality rate in the L-carnitine-supplemented group was 1.2% as compared to 12.5% in the group that did not recieve supplements (Davini 1993).

Potassium: Potassium plays an important role in the transmission of electrical impulses in the heart and the regulation and lowering of blood pressure in people. (Whelton 1997). It is also important in maintaining a regular heart rhythm.

Magnesium: Magnesium has been extensively researched with regards to pathogenesis and treatment and its beneficial effects in the treatment of cardiovascular disease in people (Altura 1985; Seelig 1980, 1989; Sjogren 1989). Because of its inverse relationship with calcium, magnesium can act as a calcium channel blocker and help reduce blood pressure(Kawano 1998).

CoEnzyme Q10 (CoQ10 or ubiquinone): CoEnzyme Q10 is a strong antioxidant that helps reduce the associated inflammation that precedes many chronic diseases. CoQ10 has indications in the prevention and treatment of common diseases such as gingivitis and periodontal disease, heart disease, arthritis, diabetes, and many types of cancer (Gaby 1998, Shigeta 1966).

Clinical research in people has shown that CoQ10 is beneficial in controlling cardiac arrhythmias, congestive heart disease, and cardiomyopathy (Gaby 1996, Giugliano 2000, Greenberg 1990, Folkers 1985, Harker-Murray 2000, Hofman-Bang 1995, Kim 1997, Khatta 2000, Mortensen 1985, Morisco 1993, Permanetter 1992, Soja 1997). Results of these clinical studies showed an improvement in the related symptoms of the heart diseases, such as reducing dyspnea and edema, improving blood pressure, and helping to normalize heart rate. Harker-Murray (2000) showed that in dogs, while a CoQ10 deficiency does not appear to be present in dogs with heart disease, supplementation does appear to lessen the resultant hypertrophic response.

Vitamin E: Besides its antioxidant functions, vitamin E is involved in the proper functioning of the heart muscle, particularly in improving cardiac output and circulation and helping to reduce platelet aggregation. Vitamin E works by helping vessels to dilate and reduce the agglutination of blood platelets (Traber 1999, 2001).

Chinese herbal medicine
General considerations/rationale
Cardiomyopathy: Cardiomyopathy is a combination of Qi and Yang deficiency in the Heart with accompanying Blood stagnation. According to the author's interpretation, Qi and Yang are energy. When there is a deficiency in the Heart, it becomes too weak to move the Blood. One result is the stagnation of Blood, which leads to pain—in this case, angina. Another consequence of the Heart deficiency is the inability of the Blood to nourish the body because the Heart cannot ensure proper circulation. This leads to the clinical signs of exercise intolerance and weakness.

Congenital heart disease: In the case of congenital heart disease there may also be an Essence deficiency. According to the author's interpretation, Essence is the genetic potential an individual is born with. Therefore, it stands to reason that a congenital problem is attributed to a deficiency of Essence.

Congestive heart disease: This is basically the decompensated form of cardiac disease. At this point, the Lung is not being nourished, which leads to dyspnea because the Lung is responsible for water distribution. If the Lung is deficient, it may allow the buildup of "water" or, in Western terms, pulmonary edema and pleural effusion or ascites. Concurrently, the Liver is not being nourished, causing elevated hepatic enzymes, and stagnation of Blood in the Liver may lead to the hepatomegaly that is often seen in affected patients.

Treatment involves strengthening the heart muscle, decreasing peripheral vascular resistance, and treating sequellae such as pleural effusion and hepatomegaly.

Appropriate Chinese herbs
Alisma (Ze xie): Has a diuretic effect in humans (Shi 1962). It decreases blood pressure (Zhong Yao Yao Li Yu Ying Yong 1983). In one experiment on rabbits, it increased blood flow in the coronary arteries (Yamahara 1991).

Astragalus (Huang qi): Has been shown to decrease hypertension and improve cardiac output. It increases coronary circulation (Xu 1999, Luo 1999). It also has been shown to have diuretic effects in people (Modern TCM Pharmacology 1997).

Atractyoldes (Bai zhu): Has diuretic properties (Zhong Hua Yi Xue Za Zhi 1961). It may help decrease pulmonary edema.

Carthamus (Hong hua): Can have a positive inotropic effect if given in small doses. Larger doses have a negative effect (Zhong Cheng Yao Yan Jiu 1983).

Cnidium (Chuan xiong): Causes vasodilation and decreases blood pressure. It also increases blood flow to the coronary arteries (Zhong Yao Yao Li Yu Ying Yong 1989).

Codonopsis (Dang shen): Decreases blood pressure, thereby improving cardiac output (Zhong Yao Xue 1998).

Cultivated cordyceps (Dong cong xia cao): Decreases heart rate, blood pressure, and myocardial oxygen requirements (Zhong Cao Yao 1986). In one study it controlled arrhythmia in 37 of 57 patients (Zhong Cao Yao 1983).

Lepidium (Ting li zi): Increases the strength of cardiac contraction while slowing the heart rate (Wu Han Yi Xue Yuan Xue Bao 1963). It also has diuretic effects (Zhong Yao Zhi 1984).

Poria (Fu ling): Has diuretic effects (Lu 1987). It may help decrease pulmonary edema.

Red peony (Chi shao): Decreases blood pressure and dilates coronary arteries. It also increases the patients' resistance to hypoxia (Zhong Cheng Yao Yan Jiu 1980).

Salvia (Dan shen): Decreases heart rate and blood pressure (Guo Wai Yi Xue Zhong Yi Zhong Yao Fen Ce 1991). In rabbits it was shown experimentally to decrease EKG abnormalities and the severity of myocardial necrosis after myocardial infarction (Wei 1999).

Scrophularia (Xuan shen): Slows tachycardia and lowers blood pressure. It also improves the patients' ability to tolerate hypoxia (Zhang 1959, Gong 1981).

Acupuncture

Acupuncture may improve cardiac function (Ballegaard 1998). Acupuncture at PC6 has been shown by serial equilibrium radionuclide angiography to improve cardiac function (Ho 1999). In one trial 15 people with left-sided heart failure were treated by acupuncture at PC6 and Lu 7. Tachycardia decreased in all of the participants (Hu 1997).

Homotoxicology
General considerations/rationale

Cardiomyopathy: Most cases of cardiomyopathy represent primary disorders of the myocardium; thus, they fall in the category of Degeneration Phase disorders. Clinicians should not hesitate to mix antihomotoxic medications and pharmaceutical cardiac agents in a patient's treatment program. When prescribing cardiac glycosides, it may be observed that much lower doses are sufficient due to the synergistic effects of antihomotoxic drugs. Monitoring levels is advised in all patients receiving digitalis-type drugs. In the authors' practice, digoxin is rarely required to handle most cardiac patients.

Homotoxicology readily integrates with many different fields of healing and Demers and Ben-Yakir have presented data regarding integration of homotoxicology with Traditional Chinese Medicine (Demers 2005, Ben-Yakir 2005ab). Factually, many patients receiving integrative treatment protocols feel better and require less medication. Cardiac healing and repair can occur as a result of homotoxicology treatment and has been reported (Palmquist 2005, 2006). Since the effectiveness of early intervention is controversial in asymptomatic cardiomyopathy cases, homotoxicology and other biological thera-

pies may provide an exciting set of alternatives for consideration of handling cardiac issues in veterinary practice. Future research should prove helpful in determining more precise treatment protocols in integrative veterinary medicine.

Congenital heart disease: Congenital heart diseases represent Degeneration Phase homotoxicoses. Homotoxicology theory can be applied in early cases to attempt to alter the tissue state, but the authors are unaware of any studies showing reversal of congenital cardiac defects resulting from antihomotoxic medications.

The possibility for activation of stem cell elements and resumption of autoregulation in developmental disorders has been raised, but such therapy would need to be done early in the course of disease. A trial of stem-cell activating remedies such as Discus compositum, Zeel, Tonsilla compositum, Cor compositum, and Placenta compositum might be useful for determining future areas of investigation, but for now the clinician can concentrate on handling cardiac insufficiency as it arises in these cases. Psorinoheel may also have some effects on genetic defects owing to its effects on constitutional disorders. Another interesting area for exploration is the use of Traumeel in patent ductus arteriosis. Because aspirin may be used to close the ductus arteriosis in cases with early diagnosis, Traumeel may have an application due to its nonsteroidal anti-inflammatory nature. There is currently no data regarding this theory, however.

Congestive heart disease: Congestive heart failure can occur for many reasons. Most commonly encountered clinical veterinary cases represent Impregnation, Degeneration or Dedifferentiation phase disorders, and a full medical evaluation is needed to diagnose the patient's condition. Diagnostic data is critical to properly treating these pets.

Appropriate homotoxicology formulas

Antihomotoxic formulas with actions in cardiovascular disease include:

Aconitum homaccord: Indicated for anxiety, fear, fever, generalized erythema, and Inflammation Phase homotoxicoses. The active ingredient is Aconitine, which causes death by respiratory paralysis and ventricular fibrillation (Dorland 2006).

Aesculus compositum: Used for peripheral vascular repair.

Angio-Injeel (AngioHeel): Treats angina, arterial hypertension, left-sided cranial pains, cardiac circulatory issues, anxiety, and palpitations in the neck (these sometimes occur and lead to feline patients vocalizing in distress). It is also used in allergic or sensitive patients. The Glonoinum (nitroglycerin) in this remedy may assist in management of these cats, and is also contained in *Cactus compositum, Cardiacum-Heel, Cor compositum, Glonoin homaccord, Strophanthus compositum*, and *Ypsiloheel* (Reckeweg 2000).

Apis homaccord: This remedy has a wide variety of uses due to the action of Apis (Bee venom). It is a powerful agent in mobilizing edema (angioedema, pulmonary edema, cerebral edema, positional swelling), and this effect is accentuated in combination with lymph-moving remedies such as Lymphomyosot (Broadfoot 2006). Patients that are allergic to bee stings should use this remedy with extreme caution.

Arnica-Heel: The ingredient Solanum dulcamara (Bittersweet) helps to reduce subacute and chronic inflammatory conditions, especially those that worsen in wet weather.

Aurumheel: Used for hypotension, hypertension, hypertrophy, decompensation, and cardiac arrhythmias. The ingredient Convallarea majalis (Lily of the Valley) is known to assist in myocardial weakness and is used as a Western herb to increase cardiac performance and strength. It is part of the recommended human protocol for atrial fibrillation (Reckeweg 2000, Broadfoot 2005). The main indications are weakness of myocardium, endocarditis, nervous palpitation, and athlete's heart (hypertrophy). The patient's history may include dyspnea with a feeling of faintness and palpitations, along with air hunger on the slightest movement, fluttering in the heart on exertion, then flushing of the face, and a sensation as if the heart were about to stop beating. Then it would suddenly beat strongly again, with a feeling of faintness. Arrhythmia and cardiac insufficiency are the defining symptoms (Reckeweg 2002).

Belladonna homaccord: The ingredient Echinacea angustifolia helps treat localized inflammatory reactions and septic processes (Melchart 1995, Pedalino 2004).

Berberis homaccord: Used for hepatic, urogenital, and adrenal gland support and drainage and to treat painful urination.

Cactus compositum: Used for angina and weakness in coronary blood flow/supply. Kalium carbonicum supports cardiac arrhythmias.

Carbo compositum: Used in hypertensive patients for cardiocirculatory disturbances.

Cardiacumheel: Treats cardiac pain, angina, pain radiating up the neck, arrhythmia, intercostal pain (Ranunculus). Also treats cardiac pain, exhaustion, and weakness with loss of ability to function (China). Useful after major loss of body fluids (China), and pain originating in the vertebral area.

Chelidonium homaccord: Provides drainage of the gall bladder, support of biliary tree, and assistance for arrhythmia patients through support of liver function. Bile acids contribute to the correction of cardio rhythms. This complex remedy is indicated for arrhythmia cordis (Reckeweg 2000).

Coenzyme compositum: Helps repair enzyme systems associated with metabolism and is useful in all cellular phases. It contains Natrum pyruvicum. A recent study showed that administration of pyruvate upon reperfusion after cardioplegic arrest mitigated oxidative stress, protected mitochondrial enzymes, and increased the myocardial energy state, which supported Reckeweg's theoretical, therapeutic application of pyruvates, particularly after cardioplegic arrest (Knott, Sun, et al. 2006).

Cor compositum: Initiates repair, detoxification, and drainage of the cardiac tissues. It has indications for hypertension; cardiac circulatory disorders; post-infectious and post-toxic cardiac disease; myocarditis; preinsufficiency dyspnea; and anxiety associated with cardiac weakness and dyspnea, arrhythmia, and collapse (Reckeweg 2000). The ingredient Cor suis (Heart) may contribute to cellular repair. It works similarly to carnitine.

Cralonin: Supports cardiac strength in geriatric conditions and positive ionotrope through action of Crataegus (Hawthorne, also known as Whitethorn). *Cralonin* is useful in nearly all cardiac complaints, hypertension, fatigue, and anemia, and as emergency injection in acute cases (Reckeweg 2000, Schroder 2003, Broadfoot 2005). Crataegus' action is not confined to the circulation, but extends to other systems. Therefore, in addition to cardiac function, there is a general toning action on the circulation, and a regulating effect on the blood pressure. As a result, it also relieves tension in the peripheral circulation, as blood pressure in controlled both centrally and peripherally. Thus, it affects arrhythmia, angina pectoris, and dysarteriotomy.

The indications are as follows: weakness of the heart muscle, including that of a toxic nature (infectious toxic weakness of the heart muscle), myocarditis, cardiomyopathy, senile heart syndromes, athlete's heart, fatty degeneration of the heart, hypertension, general arteriosclerosis, and myocardial ischemia and disturbances of coronary circulation with angina pectoris. It is useful after infectious diseases such as influenza and pneumonia and after fever(Reckeweg 2002). Crataegus is also found in *Angio-Heel, Aurumheel, Cactus compositum, Cor compositum, Cralonin, Glonoin homaccord*, and *Melilotus homaccord*.

Echinacea compositum: Simulates immune response in febrile and bacterial diseases.

Engystol N: May be valuable in cases that could have a viral onset with subsequent alteration of cardiac conductivity.

Glonoin (**nitroglycerin**): Indicated for anginal pain and palpitations involving the neck. Also contains Crataegus, as in *Cralonin*, above (Reckeweg 2000, Broadfoot 2005). *Glonoin* is an agent that bridges homeopathic and allopathic practice (Schuppel 1997). It can be helpful in tachycardia, arrhythmias associated with hyperthyroidism in cats (Lycopus), and cases of nocturnal howling in elderly cats (perhaps through action on palpitations reaching up the neck) (Reckeweg 2000, Palmquist 2005).

Glonoin's main characteristic symptoms are palpitations extending to the neck, which can be seen in the pulsating carotid arteries, and a tendency to sudden violent irregularities in the circulation, with a sensation of fullness in the precordium and strong pulsations throughout the body, as if the chest would burst. It is linked with pains radiating out into the arms and throat (Reckeweg 2002).

Glyoxal compositum: Used for decoupling polymerized homotoxins and blocked enzymes in deep homotoxicoses. Such activity exposes blocked membrane receptors and transport proteins for reactivation. It may help clear impregnated viral stages.

Hepar compositum: Indicated for liver support and drainage in more chronic diseases.

Lymphomyosot: Provides lymph drainage and detoxification in Excretion, Deposition, Degeneration, and Dedifferentiation phase disorders. It also supports thyroid function. Combined with *Apis homaccord*, it can be helpful in edema management. Consider trying this combination in pericardial fluid accumulations in combination with conventional therapy.

Melilotus homaccord: Contains cardiac glycosides, which are useful in tachycardia (Strophanthus), angiospasms, arrhythmia (Arsenicum album), periendocarditis, collapse, asthma, and emphysema (Carbo vegetalis) (O'Hanlon 1952, Norn 2004). Helps with antistress and vasodilation in acute failure. Strophanthus is a primary component, with the following indications: cardiac decompensation, palpitations, tachycardia, cardiac insufficiency, anticipatory anxiety (Reckeweg 2002). This remedy also contains Crataegus, which is used primarily for hypertensive states with arrhythmias.

Mucosa compositum: Provides repair and drainage of mucosal elements throughout the body. It contains E. coli nosode for use in mucosal infections. Due to the energetic organ connection of the heart and small intestine, this remedy is frequently used in regimens directed at Degeneration Phase cardiac disorders.

Nux vomica homaccord: Provides drainage and support of the gastrointestinal system. It is also used in angry pets and people.

Pectus-Heel: Treats anxiety, precardialgia, spasm, stress, emotional issues. This agent has sympathicotonic (similar to beta-blockers) characteristics. Can also be used in cases manifesting sudden angina (Broadfoot 2005).

Psorinoheel: Used in Excretion and Dedifferentiation phase disorders, constitutional cardiac issues, anginal disorders in humans (the pertinent ingredient is Oleander), bacterial issues through Bacillinum, skin disorders, seborrhea, headaches, post-vaccinal issues, and convulsions.

Pulsatilla compositum: Treats regulation rigidity cases in which there is no response to *Traumeel* S, migrating disorders, and therapeutic damage from corticoid hormones or drugs. It is helpful in many chronic diseases, and in cellular activation. It may initiate desirable regressive vicariation syndromes in which use of *Traumeel* S is desirable.

Rauwolfia compositum: Takes its name from Rauwolfia serpentina, long recognized as a very efficient regulator of blood pressure. It also contains Melilotus, which has a characteristic action on the kidneys and to some extent opens the glomeruli for a more generous flow of blood. The components Ren suis and Hepar suis provide additional regulating functions of the drainage organ systems. The arrhythmic component is primarily covered by the addition of Viscum album, which is useful for Impregnation phases and is indicated for hypotension and hypertension, sensations of vertigo, coronary stenosis, arrhythmia, and articular diseases of attrition (Reckeweg 2002).

Traumeel S: A nonsteroidal anti-inflammatory agent that activates sulfide-containing enzymes in all phases. Can be alternated with *Arnica Heel* in inflammatory cardiac conditions. Arnica constitution is usually muscular, athletic and plethoric and tends to hypertension. It treats the consequences of overexertion, e.g. muscular ache and sportsman's heart. Indications include injuries of every kind, such as hemorrhages, those to the soft tissues, concussion, dislocations, contusions, fractures, subluxations, and others (Reckeweg 2002). Arnica is found in *Traumeel, Arnica Heel, Aesculus compositum, Aurumheel, Carbo compositum, Cor compositum, Rauwolfia compositum, Secale compositum*, and *Spigelia compositum*, all of which are circulatory remedies.

Ubichinon compositum: This remedy is deeper reaching than *Coenzyme compositum*, and supports metabolism and mitochondrial functions in Degeneration and Dedifferentiation phase homotoxicoses. Seventy-nine percent of patients suffering from chronic disorders with metabolic problems who were treated with *Coenzyme compositum* and *Ubichinon compositum* showed improvement.

Authors' suggested protocols

Nutrition

Cardiac support formula (contains Heart, K, Mg, Carnitine, Taurine): 1 tablet for every 25 pounds of body weight BID.

Coenzyme Q10: 15 mg for every 10 pounds of body weight daily.

Additional vitamin E: 50 IU for every 25 pounds of body weight.

Eskimo fish oil: One-half to 1 teaspoon per meal for cats. 1 teaspoon for every 35 pounds of body weight for dogs.

Beyond essential fats: One-half teaspoon for every 35 pounds of body weight with food.

Chinese herbal medicine

H64 HeartAssist: This formula, which is used by the authors, may be used with vasodilators and diuretics if needed. Do not combine it with digitalis. Give 1 capsule for every 10 to 20 pounds twice daily. In addition to the herbs discussed above, HeartAssist also includes aquilaria (Chen xiang), fossil bones (Long gu), leech (Shui zhi), oyster shell (Mu li), and tortoise shell (Bie jia). These herbs increase the efficacy of the formula.

Acupuncture points to consider include BL14, BL15, PC6, ST36, and PC5 (Handbook of TCM Practitioners 1987).

Homotoxicology

Cardiomyopathy (Dose: 10 drops for 50-pound dog; 5 drops for cat or small dog): Because cardiomyopathy represents deep homotoxicoses, consider autosanguis therapy where allowed by law. The following represent starting formulas, which should be adjusted according to patient response as the case progresses:

Symptom formula for canine DCM: (The goal is to manage cardiac function and address congestive heart failure and rhythm disturbances as indicated as with conventional pharmacologic interventions such as digoxin, benazepril, enalapril, spironolactone and or furosemide as indicated; treat arrhythmias if present and significant with agents such ascarvedilol, propanolol, metoprolol, mexiletine, sotalol, etc.) Cralonin, Aurumheel, Cactus homaccord, Cardiacumheel or China Homaccord, mixed together and given orally BID.

Lymphomyosot and Apis homaccord in cases with pulmonary edema. Orally QID to TID initially and then reduce to BID when stable.

Psorinoheel may be helpful in constitutional (genetic) cases.

Traumeel may be helpful in early cases.

Symptom formula for canine ACM (tachycardia): (The major goal is to slow heart rate with beta-blocking drugs such as atenalol or metoprolol.) Cardiacumheel, Cralonin, Aurumheel as a mixture used BID PO.

Cardiacumheel can be given every 5 to 10 minutes in acute cases to gain control of the situation.

Give Pectus-Heel if heart rate stays high; consider BID PO.

Symptom formula for atrial fibrillation: Aurumheel, Chelidonium homaccord, given orally BID.

Cralonin can be used, alternating with Cardiacumheel and Hepeel intermittently.

Symptom formula for HCM (feline or canine): (The major conventional goal is to slow the heart rate with beta blockers such as atenolol.) Cralonin, Aurumheel, and China homaccord, combined and taken orally BID.

Engystol N can be given intermittently if there is viral disease or allergy in the history.

Deep detoxification formula: Galium-Heel, Lymphomyosot, Hepar compositum, Solidago compositum, Thyroidea compositum, Coenzyme compositum, Ubichinon compositum, and Cor compositum, mixed together and taken twice weekly PO. If frequent infections or other indications of lowered immune response, substitute Tonsilla compositum for Thyroidea compositum for 30 to 60 days.

Congenital heart disease: (Dose: 10 drops for 50-pound dog; 5 drops for cat or small dog)

Specific treatment of congenital cardiac cases is not indicated based upon clinical experience. However, Cor compositum, Tonsilla compositum, Traumeel, Discus compositum, and Placenta compositum may be tried early on in pediatric cases to attempt to activate stem cells, along with the catalysts, particularly Ubichinon comp. The client should be informed that this is experimental treatment, which may have no effect whatsoever. Any positive results from such treatment should be submitted for publication. Cralonin, Aesculus comp and other cardiac formulas may be used as needed to manage other cardiac insufficiency signs (See Congestive Heart Failure).

Congestive heart failure (Dose: 10 drops for 50-pound dog; 5 drops for cat or small dog):

Symptom remedy: Cardiacumheel, Aurumheel, used BID PO in all cases. In mild cases, Cactus compositum and China homaccord are commonly needed additions to this basic protocol.

Cralonin alone may be adequate to improve cardiac blood flow in early or mild cases. Use BID PO.

Apis homaccord and Lymphomyosot can be given QID to TID for pulmonary edema initially and reduced to BID as condition improves.

Cor compositum may be given as an injection therapy 2 to 3 times weekly, along with Coenzyme comp, possibly alternating with Ubichinon comp. These adjunctive therapies can be very helpful in heartworm cases with cardiac damage.

Detoxification: Lymphomyosot, Galium-Heel, Hepar compositum, Solidago compositum, Thyroidea compositum, Coenzyme compositum, Ubichinon compositum combined and given twice weekly PO.

Hepeel twice daily.

Product sources

Nutrition

Cardiac support formula: Animal Nutrition Technologies. **Alternatives:** Cardio Strength—Vetri Science; Canine cardiac support—Standard Process Veterinary Formulas; Formula CV—RxVitamins; Bio Cardio—Thorne Veterinary Products.

  Coenzyme Q10: Vetri Science; Rx Vitamins for Pets; Integrative Therapeutics; Thorne Veterinary Products.
Eskimo fish oil: Tyler Encapsulations.
Beyond essential fats: Natural Health Products.

Chinese herbal medicine

Formula H64 HeartAssist: Natural Solutions, Inc.

Homotoxicology

BHI/Heel Inc.

REFERENCES

Western medicine references

Bonagura J. Canine Cardiomyopathy. In: Proceedings of World Small Animal Veterinary Association Congress, World Small Animal Veterinary Association, Vancouver, Canada, 2001. http://vin.com/VINDBPub/SearchPB/Proceedings/PR05000/Pr00034.htm.

DeFrancesco, TC. Cardiomyopathy Dilated Cats, In: Tilley L, Smith F, The 5-Minute Veterinary Consult: Canine and Feline, 2003. Blackwell Publishing.

Keene BW, Bonagura JD. Therapy of heart failure. In: Bonagura JD, ed. Current Veterinary Therapy XII. Philadelphia: WB Saunders, 1995.

Kienle, RD. Cardiomyopathy, Hypertrophic—Dogs, In: Tilley L, Smith F, The 5-Minute Veterinary Consult: Canine and Feline, 2003. Blackwell Publishing.

Miller, MW. Cardiomyopathy, Dilated—Dogs, In: Tilley L, Smith F, The 5-Minute Veterinary Consult: Canine and Feline, 2003. Blackwell Publishing.

Miller, MW. Cardiomyopathy, Hypertrophic—Cats, In: Tilley L, Smith F, The 5-Minute Veterinary Consult: Canine and Feline, 2003. Blackwell Publishing.

Smith FWK, Keene BW. Congestive Heart Failure, Left-Sided, In: Tilley L, Smith F, The 5-Minute Veterinary Consult: Canine and Feline, 2003. Blackwell Publishing.

Smith FWK, Keene BW. Congestive Heart Failure, Right-Sided, In: Tilley L, Smith F, The 5-Minute Veterinary Consult: Canine and Feline, 2003. Blackwell Publishing.

Sisson DD, Thomas WP. Myocardial Diseases, In: Fox PR, Sisson DD, Moise NS, eds. Canine and Feline Cardiology 2nd ed. 1999. Philadelphia: WB Saunders.

IVM and nutrition references

Altura BM, Altura BT. New perspectives on the role of magnesium in the pathophysiology of the cardiovascular system. *Magnesium* 4, 1985; 226–244.

Budwig J. Flax oil as a true aid against arthritis, heart infarction, cancer and other diseases. 1992. Vancouver: Apple Publ.

Capron L. Marine Oils and Prevention of Cardiovascular Disease. *Revue Practicien.*, 1993; 43: 164.

Cherchi A, et al. Effects of L-Carnitine on exercise tolerance in chronic stable angina: A multi-center, double blind, randomized, placebo controlled, cross-over study. *Int. J. of Clin. Pharm. Ther Toxicol* 1985;23:569–72.

Davini P, Bigalli A, Lamanna F, Boem A. Controlled study on L-carnitine therapeutic efficacy in post-infarction. *Drugs Exp Clin Res.* 1992;18(8):355–365.

Folkers K, et al. Biochemical Rationale and Mitochondrial Tissue Data on the Effective Therapy of Cardiomyopathy with Coenzyme Q10, *Proc. Nat'l. Acad. Sci.* 1985;82: 901.

Folkers K, Yamancria Y. Biomedical and Clinical Aspect of Coenzyme Q10, 5th ed., 1986. NY: Elsevier.

Fox PR, Sturman JA. Myocardial taurine concentrations in cats with cardiac disease and in healthy cats fed taurine-modified diets, *Am J Vet Res* 1992; Feb;53(2):237–41.

Gaby AR. Coenzyme Q10. In: A Textbook of Natural Medicine, Pizzorno JE, Murray MT, eds. Seattle: Bastyr University Press, 1998, V:CoQ10-1–8.

Gaby AR. The role of coenzyme Q10 in clinical medicine: part II. Cardiovascular disease, hypertension, diabetes mellitus and infertility. *Altern Med Rev* 1996;1:168–75.

Giugliano D. Dietary antioxidants for cardiovascular prevention. *Nutr Metab Cardiovasc Dis.* 2000 Feb;10(1):38–44.

Greenberg S, Frishman WH. Co-enzyme Q10: a new drug for cardiovascular disease. *J Clin Pharmacol.* 1990; Jul;30(7): 596–608.

Harker-Murray AK, Tajik AJ, Ishikura F, Meyer D, Burnett JC, Redfield MM. The role of coenzyme Q10 in the pathophysiology and therapy of experimental congestive heart failure in the dog. *J Card Fail.* 2000 Sep;6(3):233–42.

Herman HA, et al. The Influence of Dietary Omega-6: Omega-3 Ratio in Lameness in Dogs with Osteoarthrosis of the Elbow Joint, Recent Advances in Canine and Feline Nutrition Volume II, 1998. Iams Proceedings p 325.

Hofman-Bang C, Rehnqvist N, Swedberg K, Wiklund I, Astrom H. Coenzyme Q10 as an adjunctive in the treatment of chronic congestive heart failure. The Q10 Study Group. *J Card Fail.* 1995; Mar;1(2):101–7.

Kawano Y, Matsuoka H, Takishita S, Omae T. Effects of magnesium supplementation in hypertensive patients. Hypertension 1998;32:260–5.

Khatta M, Alexander BS, Krichten CM, Fisher ML, Freudenberger R, Robinson SW, Gottlieb SS. The effect of coenzyme Q10 in patients with congestive heart failure. *Ann Intern Med.* 2000 Apr 18;132(8):636–40.

Kim Y, Sawada Y, Fujiwara G, Chiba H, Nishimura T. Therapeutic effect of co-enzyme Q10 on idiopathic dilated cardiomyopathy: assessment by iodine-123 labelled 15-(p-iodophenyl)-3(R,S)-methylpentadecanoic acid myocardial single-photon emission tomography. *Eur J Nucl Med.* 1997; Jun;24(6):629–34.

Leaf A, Weber PC. Cardiovascular effects of n-3 fatty acids. *N Engl J Med* 1988;318:549–57.

Lopaschuk G. Regulation of carbohydrate metabolism in ischemia and reperfusion. *Am Heart J.* 2000;139(2 Pt 3): S115–119.

McEntee, K et al. Clinical Electrocardiographic and Echocardiographic Improvement after L-Carnitine Supplementation in a Cardiomyopathic Labrador. *Canine Pract.* 1995;20: 12.

Monson W. Taurine's Role in the Health of Cats. *Vet. Med.,* 1989; 84(10): 1013–105 Oct.

Morisco C, Trimarco B, Condorelli M. Effect of coenzyme Q10 in patients with congestive heart failure: a long-term multicenter randomized study. *Clin Investig* 1993;71:S134–6.

Morris JG, Rogers QR, Pacioretty LM. Taurine: An Essential Nutrient for Cats, 1989. *J. Sm. Anim. Practice,*

Mortensen SA, Vadhanavikit S, Baandrup U, Folkers K. Long-term coenzyme Q10 therapy: a major advance in the management of resistant myocardial failure. *Drug Exptl Clin Res* 1985;11:581–93.

Novotny MJ, Hogan PM, Flannigan G. Echocardiographic evidence for myocardial failure induced by taurine deficiency in domestic cats, *Can J Vet Res* 1994; Jan;58(1):6–12.

Orlando G, Rusconi C. Oral L-Carnitine in the Treatment of Chronic Cardiac Ischemia in Elderly Patients. *Clin. Trials J.,* 1986; 23:238–244.

Permanetter B, Rossy W, Klein G, et al. Ubiquinone (coenzyme Q10) in the long-term treatment of idiopathic dilated cardiomyopathy. *Eur Heart J* 1992;13:1528–33.

Pion PD, Kittleson MD, Skiles ML, Morris JG. Dilated cardiomyopathy associated with taurine deficiencies in the domestic cat: relationship of diet and myocardial taurine content. *Advances in Experimental Medicine and Biology* 1992; 315:63–73.

Pion PD, Kittleson MD, Thomas WP, Skiles ML, Rogers QR. Clinical findings in cats with dilated cardiomyopathy and relationship of findings to taurine deficiency. *J Am Vet Med Assoc.* 1992; Jul 15;201(2):267–74.

Pion PD, Kittleson MD, Thomas WP, Delellis LA, Rogers QR. Response of cats with dilated cardiomyopathy to taurine supplementation, *J Am Vet Med Assoc* 1992; Jul 15;201(2):275–84.

Reinhart GA. A Controlled Dietary Omega-6:Omega-3 Ratio Reduces Pruritus in Non-Food Allergic Atopic Dogs, Recent Advances in Canine and Feline Nutritional Research: Iams Proceedings, 1996. p 277.

Ryan JA. Taurine Deficiency in Cats. *Comp. Anim. Pract.,* Apr/May 1989. 19(4 and 5): 28–31.

Seelig MS. Magnesium Deficiency in the Pathogenesis of Disease: Early Roots of Cardiovascular Skeletal, and Renal Abnormalities. New York: Plenum Medical Book Company 1980, 1–24,141–266.

Seelig M. Cardiovascular consequences of magnesium deficiency and loss: Pathogenesis, prevalence and manifestations—magnesium and chloride loss in refractory potassium repletion. *Am J Cardiol* 1989;63, 4G–21G.

Simpson J, Anderson R, Markwell P. Clinical Nutrition of the Dog and Cat. 1993. London: Blackwell Scientific.

Simpson JW, et al. Clinical Nutrition of the Dog and Cat. 1993. Santa Barbara: Veterinary Practice Publ. Co.

Shigeta Y, Izumi K, Abe H. Effect of coenzyme Q7 treatment on blood sugar and ketone bodies of diabetics. *J Vitaminol* 1966;12:293–8.

Sjogren A, Edvinsson L, Fallgren B. Magnesium deficiency in coronary artery disease and cardiac arrhythmias. *J Int Med* 1989;226, 213–222.

Soja AM, Mortensen SA. Treatment of chronic cardiac insufficiency with coenzyme Q10, results of meta-analysis in controlled clinical trials. *Ugeskr Laeger* 1997;159: 7302–8.

Traber MG. Does vitamin E decrease heart attack risk? Summary and implications with respect to dietary recommendations. *J Nutr.* 2001;131(2):395S–397S.

Traber MG. Vitamin E. In: Shils M, Olson JA, Shike M, Ross AC, eds. Nutrition in Health and Disease. 9th ed. Baltimore: Williams and Wilkins; 1999:347–362.

von Schacky C, Angerer P, Kothny W, et al. The effect of dietary omega-3 fatty acids on coronary atherosclerosis. A randomized, double-blind, placebo-controlled trial. *Ann Intern Med* 1999;130:554–62.

Whelton PK, He J, Cutler JA, et al. Effects of oral potassium on blood pressure: meta-analysis of randomized controlled clinical trials. *JAMA* 1997;277:1624–32.

Wu Y, Wang Y, Wang B, Lei H, Yang Y. Effects of total flavones of fructus Hippophae (TFH) on cardiac function and hemodynamics of anesthetized open-chest dogs with acute heart failure. Chung Kuo Chung Yao Tsa Chih. 1997 Jul;22(7):429–31, 448.

Wu J, Yu XJ, Ma X, Li XG, Liu D. Electrophysiologic effects of total flavones of Hippophae rhamnoides L on guinea pig papillary muscles and cultured rat myocardial cells. Chung Kuo Yao Li Hsueh Pao. 1994 Jul;15(4):341–3.

Wysong R. Taurine and Arterial Thromboembolism in Cats. *JAVMA,* 1989; 195(11): 1463–1464, Dec. 1.

Chinese herbal medicine/acupuncture references

Ballegaard S. Acupuncture and the cardiovascular system: a scientific challenge. *Acupuncture-Medicine,* 1998, 16(1):2–9.

CHM Handbook of TCM Practitioners, Oct 1987. Hunan College of TCM. Shanghai Science and Technology Press.

Gong WG, et al. *Zhejiang Journal of Medicine.* 1981;3(1):11.

Guo Wai Yi Xue Zhong Yi Zhong Yao Fen Ce (*Monograph of Chinese Herbology from Foreign Medicine*), 1991; 13(3):41.

Ho FM et al. Effect of acupuncture at nei-kuan on left ventricular function in patients with coronary artery disease. *American Journal of Chinese Medicine,* 1999,27(2):149–156.

Hu YW. *Hunan TCM News.* 1997;3(2–3):102.

Lu D, et al. *Journal of China Medical Academy.* 1987; 9(6):433.

Luo XP, et al. *China Journal of Pathology and Physiology.* 1999; 15(7):639–643.

Modern TCM Pharmacology. 1997. Tianjin: Science and Technology Press.

Shi JL, et al. *Haerbin Journal of Traditional Chinese Medicine.* 1962;(1):60–61.

Wei X, et al. Dan Shen's effects on experimental cardiac ischemia in rabbits. *Journal of Hengyang Medical College.* 1999;27(4): 383–385.

Wu Han Yi Xue Yuan Xue Bao (*Journal of Wuhan University School of Medicine*), 1963; (20):9.

Xu SA, et al. *China Journal of Pharmacy*. 1999;34(10)663–665.

Yamahara J. *Journal of Foreign Medicine*. 1991;6(2):86.

Zhang Bao Heng. *Journal of Beijing Medical College*. 1959;(1):59.

Zhong Cao Yao (*Chinese Herbal Medicine*), 1983; 14(5):32.

Zhong Cao Yao (*Chinese Herbal Medicine*), 1986; 17(5): 17.

Zhong Cheng Yao Yan Jiu (*Research of Chinese Patent Medicine*), 1980;1:32.

Zhong Cheng Yao Yan Jiu (*Research of Chinese Patent Medicine*), 1983; 12:31.

Zhong Hua Yi Xue Za Zhi (*Chinese Journal of Medicine*), 1961; 47(1):7.

Zhong Yao Xue (*Chinese Herbology*), 1998; 739: 741.

Zhong Yao Yao Li Yu Ying Yong (*Pharmacology and Applications of Chinese Herbs*), 1983: 718.

Zhong Yao Yao Li Yu Ying Yong (*Pharmacology and Applications of Chinese Herbs*), 1989; (2):40.

Zhong Yao Zhi (*Chinese Herbology Journal*), 1984; 625.

Homotoxicology references

Ben-Yakir S. Homotoxicology: Homeosiniatry, the Bridge Between Acupuncture and Homeopathy. In: Proceedings 142nd AVMA Annual Convention and 28th World Veterinary Congress, 2005a. Minneapolis, MN, USA, July 16–20.

Ben-Yakir S. Veterinary Homeosiniatry. In: Proceedings of the 31st Annual International Congress of Veterinary Acupuncture, International Veterinary Acupuncture Society (IVAS), 2005b. Sept 21–24, USA, pp 129–135.

Broadfoot P. Heart Happy Homotoxicology. In: Proceedings of AHVMA/Heel Annual Homotoxicology Seminar, 2005. May 27–29, Denver, CO, pp 75–7, 80–1, 86, 90.

Broadfoot P. Puppyatrics—Handling the vaccination reaction. *J Biomed Ther*, 2006. Winter, pp 14–5.

Demers J. Cardiovascular Disease: Homotoxicology and TCM, in proceedings of AHVMA/Heel Homotoxicology Seminar, Denver, CO, 2005. May 27–28, pp 98–103.

Knott E, Sun J, Lei Y, Ryou M, Olivencia-Yurvati A, Mallet R. Pyruvate mitigates oxidative stress during reperfusion of cardioplegia-arrested myocardium. *Ann Thorac Surg*. 2006. Mar;81(3):928–34.

Norn S, Kruse P. Cardia glycosides: From ancient history through Withering's foxglove to endogenous cardiac glycosides, translated from Danish, *Dan Medicinhist Arbog*, 2004. pp 119–32.

Palmquist R. Case report. In: Proceedings of AHVMA/Heel Homotoxicology Seminar, Denver, CO, 2005. May 27–29, pp 106–8.

Palmquist R. 2005. Unpublished case report.

Palmquist R. Use of homotoxicology and biological therapy in treatment of feline hypertrophic cardiomyopathy: A clinical case report, *JAHVMA*, 2006, accepted for publication Spring 2006.

Reckeweg H. Biotherapeutic Index: Ordinatio Antihomotoxica et Materia Medica, 5th ed. 2000. Baden-Baden, Germany: Biologische Heilmittel Heel GMBH, p 95–6, 264, 258, 298–90, 302, 319–20, 320–21, 342, 533.

Reckeweg H. Homeopathia Antihomotoxica Materia Medica, 4th ed. 2002. Baden-Baden, Germany: Aurelia-Verlag, pp 148–9, 256–7, 260–1, 325–7, 367,402, 450, 551, 598–99

Schroder D, Weiser M, Klein P. Efficacy of a homeopathic *Crataegus* preparation compared with usual therapy for mild (NYHA II) cardiac insufficiency: results of an observational cohort study *Eur J Heart Fail*, 2003. Jun;5(3):319–26.

Van Wassenhoven M. Towards evidence-based repertory: Clinical evaluation of Veratrum album, *Homeopathy*, 2004. Apr;93(2): pp 71–7.

HEARTWORM DISEASE

Definition and cause

Caused by *Dirofilaria immitis* which obstruct blood flow, causing secondary heart and pulmonary issues such as thrombosis and hypertension and signs such as coughing, rapid breathing, dyspnea, loss of energy, lethargy, and weight loss. Generally more adult worms occur in dogs then in cats (Calvert 1994, Clay 2003, Dillon 2000, Miller 2003, Soulsby 1982).

Medical therapy rationale, drug(s) of choice, and nutritional recommendations

The treatment of choice is the adulticide Immiticide for dogs and Thiacetarsamide sodium (Caparsolate®) for cats. In most cases, adulticide medication is not recommended for asymptomatic cats. Symptomatic treatment with anti-inflammatories such as corticosteroids and diuretics is often recommended (Blagburn 2003, Clay 2003, Dillon 2000, Lok 1997, Miller 2003).

Anticipated prognosis

Treated dogs and asymptomatic cats usually have a good prognosis. Symptomatic cats and severely infested dogs have a more guarded prognosis (Calvert 1994, Clay 2003, Dillon 2000).

Integrative veterinary therapies

Medical therapies for heartworm disease treatment and control are safe and effective. Therefore, integrative approaches take into consideration the immune system, secondary inflammation, and cellular protection of the involved organs, from not only the parasite but also from the required medications. Not all animals bitten by infested mosquitoes develop the disease; and therefore, there is an immune component that should be addressed on the prevention side of the equation. The use of nutrients, nutraceuticals, medicinal herbs, and combination homeopathics that have anti-inflammatory, tissue-sparing, and immune-enhancing effects should be used in conjunction with conventional prevention and treatment protocols

Nutrition
General considerations/rationale
The nutritional approach to heartworm disease adds nutrients, antioxidants, and gland support for the heart and organs of the immune system, and for the reduction of inflammation.

Appropriate nutrients
Nutritional/gland therapy: Glandular heart, lung, adrenal, thymus, and spleen supply intrinsic nutrients that improve organ function and reduce cellular inflammation. This helps to spare these organs from cascading inflammation and eventual degeneration (see Gland Therapy, Chapter 2, for a more detailed explanation).

Essential fatty acids: Fish and flaxseed oil have been shown to slow the progression of arteriosclerosis and improve disease symptoms in people with heart disease(Budwig 1992, Capron 1993, Leaf 1988, von Schacky 1999). In studies on animals, seabuckthorne oil has been shown to improve cardiac function and contractility and oxygen utilization (Wu 1994, 1997).

Coenzyme Q10 (CoQ10 or ubiquinone): Clinical research in people has shown that CoQ10 is beneficial in controlling cardiac disease. Results of clinical studies showed an improvement in the related symptoms of the heart diseases, such as a reduction in dyspnea and edema and well as improvements in blood pressure and helping to normalize heart rate (Gaby 1996, Giugliano 2000).

L-carnitine: L-carnitine has proven effective in improving the functioning of the heart. Heart muscle relies on fatty acids for energy, and L-carnitine is required for the transport of these fatty acids. Research has shown that when oxygen levels in the body are reduced, the cardiac reserves of carnitine are depleted. When L-carnitine is supplemented in the diet, it allows the heart muscle to use lower levels of oxygen more efficiently. Cherchi (1985) and Orlando (1986) showed a benefit to heart patients with L-carnitine supplementation. In studies in heart disease the addition of carnitine to the diet in these patients has been found to reduce heart damage in animals (Lopaschuk 2000).

Taurine: Low levels of taurine have been clinically proven to cause cardiomyopathy, and dietary supplementation with taurine led to clinical improvement (Ryan 1989, Simpson 1993, Pion 1992, Wysong 1989). Fox (1992) and Novotny (1994) found a direct link between low levels of taurine in the body and cardiac disease.

Potassium: Potassium plays an important role in the transmission of electrical impulses in the heart and the regulation and the lowering of blood pressure in people (Whelton 1997). It is also important in maintaining a regular heart rhythm.

Magnesium: Magnesium has been extensively researched with regards to the pathogenesis and its beneficial effects in the treatment of cardiovascular disease in people (Altura 1985; Seelig 1980, 1989; Sjogren 1989). Because of its inverse relationship with calcium, magnesium can act as a calcium channel blocker and help in the reduction of blood pressure (Kawano 1998).

Chinese herbal medicine/acupuncture
General considerations/rationale
Both schools of medicine recognize parasites as the cause, and both recommend eradicating the parasites. It is also necessary to control the inflammatory reaction to the dying parasites.

Appropriate Chinese herbs
Areca seed (Bing lang): Has been used to eliminate hookworms, roundworms, and tapeworms (Jiang Su Zhong Yi Za Zhi 1960, Zhong Hua Yi Xue Za Zhi,, 1957, Zhe Jiang Yi Ke Da Xue Xue Bao 1980). It may also be useful against other parasites.

Atractylodes root (Bai zhu): Can increase the phagocytic function of macrophages (Tang 1998). This may help the body eliminate dead worms.

Bupleurum (Chai hu): Has anti-inflammatory effects. It was shown to decrease dimethyl benzene-induced ear swelling in mice (Liu 1998), which may help control the inflammatory response to the dying worms.

Garlic (Da suan): Prevents the eggs of some parasites from hatching (Bastidas 1969). It is possible that it may have efficacy against parasites such as Dirofilaria immitus.

Slough of snake (She tui): Has an anti-inflammatory effect (Guo Wai Yi Xue Zhong Yao Fen Ce 1981), which may help prevent adverse reactions to the dead parasites.

Walnut (Hu tao ren): Has anti-inflammatory properties (Zhong Yao Tong Bao 1986).

Wormwood (Yin chen hao): Has anti-inflammatory effects. It inhibits carrageenin-induced foot swelling in rats (Wan 1987, Shan 1982).

Homotoxicology
General considerations/rationale
Heartworm disease is a Deposition Phase disorder. There are no published protocols for heartworm disease using homotoxicology formulas. Furthermore, bearing in mind the safe and efficacious nature of conventional heartworm control and treatment, one would be hard pressed to vary from established protocols. Antihomotoxic medications can be used in the handling of many of the complications

originating from heartworm infestation and treatment, however.

Appropriate homotoxicology formulas

A wide variety of situations may benefit from use of homotoxicology formulas in heartworm disease. The remedies below have particularly common applications:

Aesculus compositum: Used for circulatory disorders, post infarction.

Apis homaccord: Used to treat acute swelling and edema or hypersensitivy reactions, especially when combined with Lymphomyosot.

BHI-Circulation: Used for angina, arrhythmia, tachycardia (Heel 2002).

BHI-Recovery: Used for post-embolic events.

Carbo compositum: An antihomotoxic regulation following embolic crisis.

Cactus homaccord: Indicated for coronary circulatory disorders.

Berberis homaccord: Provides adrenal support and detoxification of the urinary tract and liver.

Cardiacumheel: Provides cardiac support.

China homaccord: Used for exhaustion and collapse.

Circulo-Injeel: Used for circulation disorders.

Cralonin: Provides support of heart function.

Cor compositum: Provides heart and circulatory support.

Galium-Heel: Used for allergies and glomerulonephritis. It is a cellular detoxification and drainage agent and a phase remedy for Deposition Phase diseases.

Hepar compositum: Provides detoxification and support of liver function, and repair after iatrogenic injury.

Lymphmyosot: Used to reduce swelling, and for lymph drainage, and for edema when combined with *Apis homaccord*.

Nux homaccord: Provides gastrointestinal and hepatic detoxification.

Placenta compositum: Used for vascular repair, particularly of peripheral circulation. It is a phase remedy for Deposition Phase diseases.

Solidago compositum: Provides drainage and support of urinary tissues, and treats glomerulonephritis (Heel 2003). It is a phase remedy for Deposition Phase diseases.

Traumeel S: Used for inflammation and modulation of inflammation. This is a natural nonsteroidal anti-inflammatory medication. To prevent clots and embolic issues, conventional agents such as aspirin may be superior, but *Traumeel* has the potential to stabilize a wide variety of conditions. Further research is indicated. It also may decrease pain and speed healing associated with the parasite and with deep intramuscular injection of heartworm adulticide.

Authors' suggested protocols

Nutrition

Heart and bronchus/lung support formulas: 1 tablet for every 25 pounds of body weight BID.

Immune support formula: One-half tablet for every 25 pounds of body weight BID.

Coenzyme Q 10: 25 mg for every 10 pounds of body weight daily.

Eskimo fish oil: One-half to 1 teaspoon per meal for cats. 1 teaspoon for every 35 pounds of body weight for dogs.

Beyond essential fats: One-half teaspoon for every 35 pounds of body weight with food (maximum 100 pounds).

Additional vitamin E: 50 IU for every 25 pounds of body weight.

Chinese herbal medicine

Recommended formula: Garden Balsam seeds (Tou gu cao) 30%, atractylodes root (Bai zhu)16%, scorpion (Quan xie) 5%, slough of snake (She tui) 16%, bupleurum (Chai hu) 30%, and centipede (Wu gong) 3%. For the average 60-pound dog, the dose is 2 g of 1:5 ratio of extracted powder daily (Yang 1996). The author recommends adding areca seed (Bing lang), areca husks (Da fu pi), garlic (Da suan), walnut (Hu tao ren), and wormwood (Yin chen hao) to increase efficacy and decrease the inflammatory reaction to the dying parasite.

Homotoxicology

(See Congestive Heart Disease, Arrhythmia, Hepatitis, Vomiting, etc.) Treat conventionally and handle conditions as they arise. For most cases consider:

Traumeel S: Give orally BID on the day of adulticide injection and for 3 days afterward.

Coenzyme compositum: Give daily.

Hepar compositum and Solidago compositum: 1 tablet every 3 days for detoxification and support for 30 days following treatment.

Galium-Heel: Give daily for 30 days after treatment, especially in patients that are more ill.

Cactus compositum, Cralonin, Aurumheel: Mix together and give orally BID to TID if symptoms of cardiac distress are present.

Product sources

Nutrition

Heart, bronchus/lung, and immune support formulas: Animal Nutrition Technologies. **Alternatives:** Formula CV—Rx Vitamins for Pets; Cardiac Support formula—Standard Process Veterinary Formulas; Cardio-Strength—

Vetri Science Laboratories; Bio-Cardio—Thorne Veterinary Products.

Coenzyme Q10: Vetri Science, Rx Vitamins for Pets, Integrative Therapeutics, Thorne Veterinary Products.

Eskimo fish oil: Tyler Encapsulations.

Beyond essential fats: Natural Health Products.

Chinese herbal medicine

The powder can be made by the practitioner or ordered from Mayway Company.

Homotoxicology

BHI/Heel Corporation

REFERENCES

Western medicine references

Blagburn BL. Important heartworm basics for the practicing veterinarian. *DVM Best Practice.* 2003;March:12–15.

Calvert CA. Heartworm Disease. In Birchard SJ, Sherding RG, eds. Saunders Manual of Small Animal Practice. Philadelphia, PA: WB Saunders Co.; 1994;487–493.

Clay A, Calvert CA, Rawlings CA. Heartworm Disease—Dogs, In: Tilley L, Smith F, 2003. The 5-Minute Veterinary Consult: Canine and Feline, Blackwell Publishing.

Dillon R. Dirofilariosis in dogs and cats. In: Ettinger SJ, Feldman EC, eds. Textbook of canine and feline veterinary internal medicine. 2000. Philadelphia: Saunders.

Lok JB, Knight DH. A review of the treatment options for heartworm infections. *Supplement to Veterinary Medicine.* June 1997:15–25.

Miller MW. Heartworm Disease—Cats, In: Tilley L, Smith F, The 5-Minute Veterinary Consult: Canine and Feline, 2003. Blackwell Publishing.

Soulsby EJL. Helminths, arthropods and protozoa of domesticated animals. Philadelphia: Lea and Febiger. 1982;307–312.

IVM/nutrition references

Altura BM, Altura BT. New perspectives on the role of magnesium in the pathophysiology of the cardiovascular system. *Magnesium.* 1985;4, 226–244.

Budwig J. Flax Oil as a true aid against arthritis, heart infarction, cancer and other diseases. 1992. Vancouver: Apple Publ.

Capron L. Marine Oils and Prevention of Cardiovascular Disease, *Revue Practicien.,* 1993; 43: 164.

Cherchi A, et al. Effects of L-Carnitine on Exercise Tolerance in Chronic Stable Angina: A Multicenter, Double-blind, Randomized, Placebo-controlled, Crossover Study. *Int'l. J. of Clin. Pharm. Ther Toxico* 1985;23: 569–72.

Fox PR, Sturman JA. Myocardial taurine concentrations in cats with cardiac disease and in healthy cats fed taurine-modified diets, *Am J Vet Res* 1992 Feb;53(2):237–41.

Gaby AR. Coenzyme Q10. In: A Textbook of Natural Medicine; Pizzorno JE, Murray MT, eds. Seattle: Bastyr University Press, 1998, V:CoQ10-1–8.

Giugliano D. Dietary antioxidants for cardiovascular prevention. *Nutr Metab Cardiovasc Dis.* 2000 Feb;10(1):38–44.

Kawano Y, Matsuoka H, Takishita S, Omae T. Effects of magnesium supplementation in hypertensive patients. *Hypertension* 1998;32:260–5.

Lopaschuk G. Regulation of carbohydrate metabolism in ischemia and reperfusion. *Am Heart J.* 2000;139(2 Pt 3): S115–119.

Orlando G, Rusconi C. Oral L-Carnitine in the Treatment of Chronic Cardiac Ischemia in Elderly Patients. *Clin. Trials J.,* 1986; 23:238–244.

Novotny MJ, Hogan PM, Flannigan G. Echocardiographic evidence for myocardial failure induced by taurine deficiency in domestic cats, *Can J Vet Res* 1994; Jan;58(1):6–12.

Pion PD, Kittleson MD, Skiles ML, Morris JG. Dilated Cardiomyopathy Associated with Taurine Deficiencies in the Domestic Cat: Relationship of Diet and Myocardial Taurine Content. *Advances in Experimental Medicine and Biology,* 1992; 315:63–73.

Pion PD, Kittleson MD, Thomas WP, Skiles ML, Rogers QR. Clinical findings in cats with dilated cardiomyopathy and relationship of findings to taurine deficiency. *J Am Vet Med Assoc,* 1992; Jul 15;201(2):267–74.

Pion PD, Kittleson MD, Thomas WP, Delellis LA, Rogers QR. Response of cats with dilated cardiomyopathy to taurine supplementation, *J Am Vet Med Assoc* 1992; Jul 15;201(2): 275–84.

Ryan JA. Taurine Deficiency in Cats. *Comp. Anim. Pract.,* 198919(4 and 5): 28–31, Apr/May.

Seelig MS. Magnesium Deficiency in the Pathogenesis of Disease: Early Roots of Cardiovascular, Skeletal, and Renal Abnormalities. New York: Plenum Medical Book Company, 1980,1–24,141–266.

Seelig M. Cardiovascular consequences of magnesium deficiency and loss: Pathogenesis, prevalence and manifestations—magnesium and chloride loss in refractory potassium repletion. *Am J Cardiol* 1989;63, 4G–21G.

Simpson J, Anderson R, Markwell P, Clinical Nutrition of the Dog and Cat. 1993. London: Blackwell Scientific.

Simpson JW, et al. Clinical Nutrition of the Dog and Cat. 1993. Santa Barbara: Veterinary Practice Publ. Co.

Sjogren A, Edvinsson L, Fallgren B. Magnesium deficiency in coronary artery disease and cardiac arrhythmias. *J Int Med* 1989;226, 213–222.

Whelton PK, He J, Cutler JA, et al. Effects of oral potassium on blood pressure: meta-analysis of randomized controlled clinical trials. *JAMA* 1997;277:1624–32.

Wu Y, Wang Y, Wang B, Lei H, Yang Y. Effects of total flavones of fructus Hippophae (TFH) on cardiac function and hemodynamics of anesthetized open-chest dogs with acute heart failure. Chung Kuo Chung Yao Tsa Chih. 1997 Jul;22(7):429–31, 448.

Wu J, Yu XJ, Ma X, Li XG, Liu D. Electrophysiologic effects of total flavones of Hippophae rhamnoides L on guinea pig papillary muscles and cultured rat myocardial cells. Chung Kuo Yao Li Hsueh Pao. 1994 Jul;15(4):341–3.

Wysong R. Taurine and Arterial Thromboembolism in Cats. *JAVMA*, Dec. 1, 1989;195(11): 1463–1464.

Chinese herbal medicine/acupuncture references
Bastidas GJ. Effect of ingested garlic on Necator americanus and Ancylostoma caninum. *Am. J. Trop. Med. Hyg.*, 1969;18(6): 920–923.
Guo Wai Yi Xue Zhong Yao Fen Ce (*Monograph of Chinese Herbology from Foreign Medicine*), 1981.
Jiang Su Zhong Yi Za Zhi (*Jiangsu Journal of Chinese Medicine*), 1960;(5):30.
Liu W, et al. *Henan Journal of TCM Pharmacy*. 1998;13(4):10–12.
Shan YT E, et al. *Journal of Pharmacy*. Japan. 1982;102(3): 285.
Tang XH. *Journal of Research in Traditional Chinese Medicine*. 1998;11(2):7–9.
Wan YD. The antipyretic effects of capillarin. *Pharmacy Bulletin*. 1987;(10):590–593.
Yang SS. Chinese Modern Famous Doctors Formulas Collection, Hubei Science and Technology Press, Feb 1996, p. 121.
Zhe Jiang Yi Ke Da Xue Xue Bao (*Journal of Zhejiang Province School of Medicine*),1980;9(1):1.
Zhong Hua Yi Xue Za Zhi (*Chinese Journal of Medicine*), 1957;43(5):371.
Zhong Yao Tong Bao (*Journal of Chinese Herbology*), 1986; 11(11): 37.

Homotoxicology references
Heel. BHI Homeopathic Therapy: Professional Reference. 2002. Albuquerque, NM: Heel Inc., p 67.
Heel. Veterinary Guide, 3rd English edition. 2003. Baden-Baden, Germany: Biologische Heilmettel Heel GmbH, p 108.

HYPERTENSION

Definition and cause

Hypertension is defined as continual elevation in arterial blood pressure. Often, hypertension is secondary to other diseases such as renal disease, hyperthyroidism, and hyperadrenocorticism (Cowgill 1983; Henik 1997; Hypertension Consensus Panel 2002; Snyder 1991, 2003).

Hypertension is an important diagnosis, and small-animal clinicians should regularly screen their geriatric population for this condition. Renal disease is the most commonly found condition associated with hypertension in animals, especially in cats, and any patient with renal disease should be carefully monitored for the appearance of hypertension (Littman 1994, Mishina 1998). Patients presenting for various other complaints such as hyperthyroidism, acute or chronic loss of vision, detached retina, retinal hemorrhage, cerebrovascular embolic or hemorrhagic disease, altered behavior, vocalization, diabetes mellitus, hyperlipidemia, and obesity should also be screened (Acierno 2005, Kobayashi 1990, Littman 1994, Snyder 2003).

Medical therapy rationale, drug(s) of choice, and nutritional recommendations

The preferred drugs of choice are calcium channel blockers and/or ACE inhibitors. Dietary adjustments include feeding of low-sodium foods (Acierno 2005, Cowgill 1983, Snyder 2003).

Anticipated prognosis

The prognosis depends upon the underlying cause and is often controlled well with medication. Client compliance is essential (Acierno 2005, Snyder 2003).

Integrative veterinary therapies

Determining the underlying cause is important when selecting alternative therapies. Adequate water intake, proper diet (sodium restricted), and appropriately chosen pharmaceutical agents should be used to control blood pressure because this is a potentially life-threatening condition. The clinician should integrate nutritional, herbal, and biological therapy, and in some cases may find that less medication is needed to stabilize the blood pressure. In some cases the hypertensive condition will resolve, and can be maintained without pharmaceutical agents. Many patients require lifetime therapy and regular monitoring of their medical condition.

Nutrition
General considerations/rationale
After the causes of the hypertension are established and medical therapy started to control the condition, nutritional and metabolic support of the heart should be started.

Appropriate nutrients
Nutritional/gland therapy: Glandular heart, pituitary, and hypothalamus supply intrinsic nutrients that help to improve organ function and reduce cellular inflammation (see Gland Therapy, Chapter 2, for a more detailed explanation). Because hypertension may have multiple causes and contributing factors, a medical and physiological blood evaluation is recommended to assess glandular health. This helps clinicians to formulate therapeutic nutritional protocols that address the local lesions as well as underlying organ conditions that may be ultimately responsible for elevated blood pressure.

Coenzyme Q10: Supplementation with Coenzyme Q10 leads to a significant reduction in blood pressure in people with hypertension (Folkers 1981, Langsjoen 1994, Digiesi 1994).

Essential fatty acids: Morris (1993) found that people who supplemented their diet with fish oil that is rich in the essential fatty acids EPA and DHA significantly lowered their blood pressure.

Arginine: Some amino acids have been shown to affect blood pressure. Abe (1987) demonstrated that animals supplemented with taurine had lower blood pressure. Kohashi (1983) showed similar results on blood pressure in people. Arginine is believed to have a dilating effect on blood vessels and a resultant decrease in blood pressure. In a controlled trial, Pezza (1998) showed that people who were not responding to medical therapies did respond positively with reduced blood pressure when arginine was added to the diet.

Vitamin E: A double-blind study showed that 200 IU of vitamin E per day was significantly more effective than a placebo in reducing both diastolic and systolic blood pressure (Boshtam 2002).

Note: Hypertension is often secondary to other organ conditions. It is recommended that blood be analyzed both medically and physiologically to determine associated organ involvement and disease. This will allow for a more specific gland and nutritional support protocol (see Chapter 2, Nutritional Blood Testing, for more information).

Chinese herbal medicine/acupuncture
General considerations/rationale

Hypertension may be due to stress, improper diet, lifestyle, Yang excess or Yin deficiency leading to Yin-Yang disharmony, fire rising up from the Liver, or Phlegm accumulation. The authors note that stress, improper diet, and lifestyle are discussed in Western medical journals as causes of hypertension. Yin-Yang disharmony is a relative excess of either Yin or Yang. As Yang is heat, motion, activity, energy when Yang is in excess, the Blood may move faster and pressure may be higher. The Liver is charged with maintaining a harmonious flow of Qi. When the Liver heat flares up, this smooth flow is disrupted. Just as a fire heats up air and causes rapid and irregular gusts of wind, Liver fire flaring up can cause rapid and reckless flow of Qi and Blood, or hypertension. Phlegm (cholesterol plaques) may accumulate in blood vessels, leading to strokes and heart attacks, although this is more common in humans and possibly birds than most animals. Treatment involves lowering blood pressure, treating both potential causes, and preventing sequellae of the disorder.

Appropriate Chinese herbs

Alisma (Ze xie): Has a mild antihypertensive effect (Zhong Yao Yao Li Yu Ying Yong 1983).

Angelica root (Dang gui): Causes vasodilation (You 1981), which helps decrease the blood pressure.

Chinese yam (Shan yao): Has been shown to lower the blood pressure in mice (Zhang 1997).

Cinnamon bark (Rou gui): Causes peripheral vasodilation and a reduction in blood pressure and heart rate (Zhong Yao Tong Bao 1981).

Cornus (Shan zhu yu): Has diuretic actions (Zhang Yong Zhong Yao Cheng Fen Yu Yao Li Shou Ce 1994). Diuretics are commonly prescribed to lower blood pressure in Western medicine.

Eucommia bark (Du Zhong): Can lower blood pressure. In humans, the erythrocyte zinc:copper ratio of hypertensive patients is higher than that of healthy people. This herb decreases both the zinc:copper ratio and blood pressure (Wang 1997). It has also been shown to decrease the blood pressure of anesthetized dogs (Fan 1979).

Gentian root (Long dan cao): Has a diuretic effect (Zhong Yao Yao Li Yu Ying Yong 1983).

Licorice (Zhi gan cao): Decreases myocardial oxygen consumption and helps to prevent arrhythmias. It also helps protect blood vessels (Jiang Su Zhong Yi Za Zhi 1987, Xu 1997).

Rehmannia(cooked) (Shu di huang): Reduces blood pressure (Chang Yong Zhong Yao Cheng Fen Yu Yao Li Shou Ce 1994). It also lowers the concentration of serum T3 while simultaneously increasing serum T4 (Qu 1998, Zhang 1999, Hou 1992). Because T3 is about 4 times as active as T4, the overall effect is to counteract hyperthyroidism, which is a common cause of hypertension in animals.

Wolfberry (Gou qi zi): Lowers blood pressure (Zhong Yao Zhi 1984).

Acupuncture

Acupuncture has been used to treat hypertension (Dan 1998). It has been theorized that acupuncture works by regulating serum nitrogen monoxide (Cai 1998).

Homotoxicology
General considerations/rationale

Hypertension is considered to be an Impregnation or Degeneration phase disorder. High systolic blood pressure resulting from a functional thyroid tumor is an example of a Dedifferentiation Phase condition. When this is confusing, further examination of the patient and an inventory of other historical and diagnostic findings will lead the practitioner toward the correct therapy.

Appropriate homotoxicology formulas (Dose: 10 drops PO for 50-pound dog; 5 drops PO for small dog or cat)

Angio-Injeel: Alternated with *Circulo-Injeel* in some cases.

Berberis homaccord: Used for detoxification of the urinary system, in cases with pigmented axillary regions. The ingredient Berberis is contained in *Reneel* and *Solidago compositum* as well.

Circulo-Injeel: Alternated with *Angio-Injeel* in difficult cases.

Coenzyme compositum: Provides energy metabolism support.

Cralonin: Provides support of cardiac muscle.

Engystol N: Used for constitutional hypertension (not common in animals).

Galium-Heel: Provides cellular drainage and support, especially of kidney and renal tubular pathologies. Has been used in 2 cases of congenital polycystic kidney disease of Persian cats; improved and prolonged the quality of life (Palmquist 2006).

Glonoin homaccord: Used for palpitations and in hyperthyroidism.

Hepar compositum: Provides liver drainage and support, and is part of the Deep Detoxification Formula.

Hepeel: Provides liver detoxification and repair. It can be altered with *Hepar compositum* or used singly. It is part of the Deep Detoxification Formula.

Melilotus: Used for congestive headache, which is better following nosebleed; consider in cases of retinal hemorrhage or detachment with hypertension.

Rauwolfia compositum: The primary agent in hypertension (Rauwolfia serpentina-Indian snakeroot), this rapidly lowers blood pressure when injected (use with caution by prescription only). Use caution in individuals sensitive to compounds that contain iodine (Reckeweg 2000).

Reneel: Provides kidney detoxification and support.

Solidago compositum: This is an important phase remedy in Deposition Phase cases and in the Deep Detoxification Formula. It detoxifies and assists in the repair of renal and other urogenital tissues.

Traumeel S: Used in constitutional hypertension (not common in animals).

Ubichion compositum: Used for mitochondrial energy production and autoimmune issues.

Authors' suggested protocols

Nutrition
Cardial (contains taurine and carnitine) and pituitary/hypothalamus/pineal support formulas: 1 tablet for every 25 pounds of body weight BID.

Coenzyme Q10: 15 mg for every 10 pounds of body weight daily.

Beyond essential fats: One-half teaspoon for every 35 pounds of body weight, with food.

Eskimo fish oil: One-half to 1 teaspoon per meal for cats. 1 teaspoon for every 35 pounds of body weight for dogs.

Arginine: 50 mg per 10 pounds of body weight daily.

Additional taurine: 100 mg per 10 pounds of body weight daily.

Vitamin E: Additional vitamin E—50 IU for every 25 pounds of body weight.

Chinese herbal medicine
Severely elevated blood pressure should be managed with Western medications in addition to herbs. The patient may be weaned off Western medications once the blood pressure is out of critical ranges.

Acute and young patients can be treated with Long Dan Xie Gan Tang, which contains alisma (Ze xie), angelica root (Dang gui), bupleurum (Chai hu), gentian root (Long dan cao), licorice (Gan cao), and plantago seed (Che qian zi).

In chronic hypertension or in older patients, the patent formula You Gui Yin is appropriate. It contains aconite (Fu zi), Chinese yam (Shan yao), cinnamon bark (Rou gui), cornus (Shan zhu yu), eucommia bark (Du Zhong), licorice (Zhi gan cao), rehmannia(cooked) (Shu di huang), and wolfberry (Gou qi zi). The aconite helps prevent the side effect of hypotension.

These formulas are dosed as per the manufacturer's recommendations.

Acupuncture points that are recommended include GB20, LI11, ST36, LI3, PC6, GB34, SP6, and Baihui (Handbook of TCM Practitioner 1987).

Homotoxicology (Dose: 10 drops for 50-pound dog; 5 drops for small dog or cat)
Determine the cause of hypertension and address that primary condition. Use pharmaceutical agents as needed to safely decrease and control the hypertension.

Symptom remedy: Rauwolfia compositum by injection or tablet, given 1 to 3 times weekly. In acute cases, this may be given daily, but blood pressure and patient condition should be monitored to avoid rapid decline in blood pressure and weakness associated with too rapid a drop in systolic pressure. IV administration is associated with hypersensitivity reactions in rare patients and is not recommended routinely. Patients sensitive to iodine should receive this agent with caution.

Deep detoxification formula: Galium-Heel, Lymphomyosot, Hepar compositum, Thyroidea compositum, Solidago compositum, Coenzyme compositum, and Ubichinon compositum given every 2 to 3 days for 120 days or longer as indicated by case responses.

Product sources

Nutrition

Cardiac and pituitary/hypothalamus/pineal support formulas: Animal Nutrition Technologies. **Alternatives:** Formula CV—Rx Vitamins for Pets; Cardiac Support formula—Standard Process Veterinary Formulas; Cardio-Strength—Vetri Science Laboratories; Bio-Cardio—Thorne Veterinary Products.

CoEnzyme Q10: Vetri Science, Rx Vitamins for Pets, Integrative Therapeutics, Thorne Veterinary Products.

Eskimo fish oil: Tyler Encapsulations.

Beyond essential fats: Natural Health Products.

Vitamin E, arginine: Over the counter.

Chinese herbal medicine

Long Dan Xie Gan Tang: Mayway Company.
You gui yin: Blue Poppy Enterprises.

Homotoxicology
BHI/Heel Corporation

REFERENCES

Western medicine references

Acierno M, Labato M. Hypertension in renal disease: diagnosis and treatment. *Clin Tech Small Anim Pract.* 2005 Feb;20(1): pp 23–30.

Cowgill LG, Kallet AJ. Recognition and management of hypertension in the dog. In: Kirk RW, Bonagura JD, eds. Current Veterinary Therapy VIII: Small Animal Practice. Philadelphia: WB Saunders Company; 1983;1025–1028.

Henik RA. Systemic hypertension and its management. *Vet Clin NA, Sm Anim Prac* 1997;27:1355–1372.

Hypertension Consensus Panel, American College of Veterinary Internal Medicine. Current recommendations for diagnosis and management of hypertension in cats and dogs (report). 2002. Dallas, TX, 20th Annual Veterinary Medical Forum.

Kobayashi DL, Peterson ME, Graves TK, et al. Hypertension in cats with chronic renal failure or hyperthyroidism. *J Vet Int Med* 1990;4:58–62.

Littman MP. Spontaneous systemic hypertension in 24 cats. *J Vet Int Med* 1994;8:79–86.

Mishina M, Watanabe T, Fujii K, et al. Non-invasive blood pressure measurements in cats: Clinical significance of hypertension associated with renal failure. *J Vet Med Sci* 1998;60:805–808.

Snyder PS. Canine hypertensive disease. *Compend Cont Ed Pract Vet* 1991;13:1785–1793.

Snyder PS, Thornhill JA. Hypertension, Systemic, In: Tilley L, Smith F, The 5-Minute Veterinary Consult: Canine and Feline, 2003. Blackwell Publishing.

IVM/nutrition references

Abe M, Shibata K, Matsuda T, Furukawa T. Inhibition of hypertension and salt intake by oral taurine treatment in hypertensive rats. *Hypertension* 1987;10:383–9.

Boshtam M, Rafiei M, Sadeghi K, Sarraf-Zadegan N. Vitamin E can reduce blood pressure in mild hypertensives. *Int J Vitam Nutr Res* 2002;72:309–14.

Folkers K, Drzewoski J, Richardson PC, et al. Bioenergetics in clinical medicine. XVI. Reduction of hypertension in patients by therapy with coenzyme Q10. *Res Commun Chem Pathol Pharmacol* 1981;31:129–40.

Langsjoen P, Langsjoen P, Willis R, Folkers K. Treatment of essential hypertension with coenzyme Q10. *Mol Aspects Med* 1994;15 Suppl:s265–72.

Digiesi V, Cantini F, Oradei A, et al. Coenzyme Q10 in essential hypertension. *Molec Aspects Med* 1994;15 Suppl:s257–63.

Kohashi N, Katori R. Decrease of urinary taurine in essential hypertension. *Jpn Heart J* 1983;24:91–102.

Morris MC, Sacks F, Rosner B. Does fish oil lower blood pressure? A meta-analysis of controlled trials. *Circulation* 1993;88:523–33.

Pezza V, Bernardini F, Pezza E, et al. Study of supplemental oral l-arginine in hypertensives treated with enalapril + hydrochlorothiazide. *Am J Hypertens* 1998;11:1267–70 [letter].

Chinese herbal medicine references

Cai QC, et al. The regulatory effects of acupuncture on blood pressure and serum nitrogen monoxide levels in patients with hypertension. *Chinese Acupuncture and Moxibustion*, 1998, 18(1):9–11 (in Chinese).

Chang Yong Zhong Yao Cheng Fen Yu Yao Li Shou Ce (A Handbook of the Composition and Pharmacology of Common Chinese Drugs), 1994; 792–793.

Dan Y. Assessment of acupuncture treatment of hypertension by ambulatory blood pressure monitoring. *Chinese Journal of Integrated Traditional and Western Medicine*, 1998, 18(1):26–27 (in Chinese).

Fan Wei Heng. *Pharmacy Bulletin.* 1979;14(9):404.

Handbook of TCM Practitioner, Hunan College of TCM, Shanghai Science and Technology Press, Oct 1987, p 291–293.

Hou SL, et al. *China Journal of Materia Medica.* 1992;17(5):301.

Jiang Su Zhong Yi Za Zhi (*Jiangsu Journal of Chinese Medicine*), 1987; 8(10): 688.

Qu FY, et al. *Heilongjiang Journal of TCM.* 1998;21(5):6.

Wang CL, et al. *Journal of Trace Elements and Health Research.* 1997;14(4):33–34.

Xu L, et al. *Journal of Research in Chinese Medicine.* 1997;10(2):31–32.

You GX, et al. 52 cases of migraine treated with Dang Gui Si Ni Tang. *China Journal of Medicine* 1981;(1):57.

Zhang H, et al. *Journal of Shizhen Medicinal Material Research.* 1997;8(1):71–72.

Zhang PX, et al. *China Journal of Gerontology.* 1999;19(3):174–175.

Zhang Yong Zhong Yao Cheng Fen Yu Yao Li Shou Ce (A Handbook of the Composition and Pharmacology of Common Chinese Drugs), 1994; 368:376.

Zhong Yao Tong Bao *Journal of Chinese Herbology*, 1981; 6(5): 32.

Zhong Yao Yao Li Yu Ying Yong (*Pharmacology and Applications of Chinese Herbs*), 1983; 295.

Zhong Yao Yao Li Yu Ying Yong (*Pharmacology and Applications of Chinese Herbs*), 1983:718.

Zhong Yao Zhi (*Chinese Herbology Journal*), 1984:484.

Homotoxicology references

Palmquist R. Experimental Application of Galium-Heel: Two cases of PKD in cats with one surviving over 16 years. 2006. Unpublished case file.

Reckeweg H. Biotherapeutic Index: Ordinatio Antihomotoxica et Materia Medica, 5th ed. 2000. Baden-Baden, Germany: Biologische Heilmittel Heel GMBH, p 394–5.

PERICARDIAL EFFUSION

Note: When secondary to neoplasia, see Section 5, Heart Base Tumor.

Definition and cause

Pericardial effusion is defined as excessive fluid in the pericardial sac and often cardiac tamponade. Common causes are idiopathic infections such as FIP or bacterial pericarditis, congestive heart failure, and neoplasia (Miller 1995, Smith 1999, Rush 2003).

Medical therapy rationale, drug(s) of choice, and nutritional recommendations

Pericardiocentesis and pericardectomy are often the recommended choice because of the serious nature of the tamponade. Medical management is generally recommended to help control the fluid build-up (Miller 1995, Smith 1999, Rush 2003).

Anticipated prognosis

The prognosis is fair to good with pericardiocentesis and pericardectomy. Neoplasia carries a more guarded prognosis. (Rush 2003).

Integrative veterinary therapies

An integrative approach to pericardial effusion is to use therapeutic nutrition and herbal and biological therapies in support of surgery and medical control of the condition. Once the effusion is controlled, integrative therapies can help maintain control and minimize the necessity for ongoing pericardiocentesis and the chronic use of medication.

Nutrition
General considerations/rationale

After the causes of the pericardial effusion are established and medical or surgical therapy has been selected to control the condition, nutritional support focuses on metabolic support of the heart. Support is also directed toward reducing associated inflammation, especially when the cause is unknown or is determined to be pericarditis.

Appropriate nutrients

Nutritional/gland therapy: Glandular heart and lung supply intrinsic nutrients that improve organ function and reduce cellular inflammation (see Gland Therapy, Chapter 2, for a more detailed explanation).

Coenzyme Q10 (CoQ10 or ubiquinone): Clinical research in people has shown that CoQ10 is beneficial in controlling cardiac disease. Results of clinical studies showed an improvement in the related symptoms of the heart diseases such as a reduction in dyspnea and edema and well as improvements in blood pressure and helping to normalize heart rate (Gaby 1996, Giugliano 2000).

Essential fatty acids: Fish and flaxseed oil have been shown to slow the progression of arteriosclerosis and improve disease symptoms in people with heart disease(Budwig 1992, Capron 1993). In studies on animals, seabuckthorne oil has been shown to improve cardiac function and contractility and oxygen utilization (Wu 1994, 1997).

Vitamin E: Besides its antioxidant functions, vitamin E is involved in the proper functioning of the heart muscle, particularly improving cardiac output and circulation and helping to reduce platelet aggregation (Traber 2001).

Chinese herbal medicine/acupuncture
General considerations/rationale

According to TCM theory, pericardial effusion is due to Qi and Yin deficiency with Phlegm and fluid accumulation in the upper burner. There may be internal Heat, Qi, and Blood stagnation and/or Toxin accumulation. In the author's interpretation, the upper burner contains the Heart, Pericardium, and Lungs. In this case the Fluid accumulates in the pericardial space. This fluid is termed Phlegm because the Qi deficiency makes the patient too weak to transform fluids. In addition, the Yin is deficient so the body fluids become thick, leading to Phlegm. Heat (inflammation) or Toxin accumulation (bacterial infection, for example) further dries fluids and may cause the patient to develop stagnation of Qi and Blood. Stagnation can lead to pain and/or an irregular heartbeat. The Qi deficiency can also cause weakness and exercise intolerance.

Appropriate Chinese herbs

For pericardial effusion:

Angelica root (Dang gui): Was 83% effective in a study of 100 patients in controlling cardiac arrhythmias (Zhong Yi Za Zhi 1981). It may help stabilize cardiac function in cases of pericardial effusion.

Astragalus (Huang qi): Can increase cardiac output and coronary blood flow (Xu 1999, Luo 1999). This may help preserve cardiac function.

Codonopsis (Dang shen): Increases cardiac output and blood perfusion (Zhong Yao Xue 1998).

Ophiopogon (Mai men dong): Can control drug-induced arrhythmias (Zhong Cao Yao 1982). It also has positive inotropic effects (Hua Xi Yao Xue Za Zhi 1991) and some antibacterial effects (Zhong Yao Xue 1998). This may help in the rare case of bacterial causes of pericardial effusion.

Platycodon root (Jie geng): Has anti-inflammatory effects. It increases the secretion of corticosterone in rats (Li 1984, Zhang 1984), which may be beneficial in cases of immune-mediated pericardial effusion.

Scutellaria (Huang qin): May be beneficial for several reasons. It contains baicalin and baicalein, which have been shown to be anti-inflammatory (Kubo 1984). This may help in inflammatory or immune-mediated pericardial effusion. Baicalein has also been shown to have the ability to inhibit cancer cells (Zi 2005). It may help with heart-based neoplasia. In addition, baicalin has antibiotic properties (Liu 2000). One interesting effect of Scutellaria is that it increases the ability of animals to withstand hypoxia (Liu Xiao Juan 1999). This is extremely useful because pericardial effusion decreases cardiac function and impairs blood flow.

Talc (Hua shi): Has antibacterial efficacy (Microorganism Group 1959). It may help in cases of bacterial infections.

Trichosanthes root (Tian hua feng): Has anti-neoplastic effects (Xu Zhen Wu 1997, Bi 1998) and may be useful in neoplastic etiologies. It has shown antiviral effects against the AIDS virus in humans (Modern TCM Pharmacology. 1997). It may be useful for pericardial effusions of viral etiology if it has efficacy against other viruses.

White peony (Bai shao): Contains paeoniflorin, which has anti-inflammatory actions (Zhong Yao Zhi 1993). It may help in inflammatory or immune-mediated pericardial effusion.

H60 Anticancer/generic:

Antler powder (Lu jiao shuang): May have some efficacy as an adjuvant cancer therapy (Du 1981).

Astragalus (Huang qi): Enhances the immunity of mice with solid tumors (Ying 1999). It also has direct anticancer effects on some tumors (Liu Hui 1999, Shi 1999).

Barbat skullcap (Ban zhi lian): May inhibit tumor growth (Ren Min Wei Sheng Chu Ban She 1988).

Centipede (Wu gong): Has demonstrated anticancer effects in vitro (Chang Yong Zhong Yao Cheng Fen Yu Yao Li Shou Ce 1994).

Coix (Yi yi ren): Can inhibit the growth of tumor cells and enhance natural killer cell function (Lu 1999).

Cornus (Shan zhu yu): Has positive inotropic effects (Hu 1988).

Ginseng (Ren shen): Has positive inotropic effects (CA 1992).

Honeysuckle (Jin yin hua): Has demonstrated anti-inflammatory effects (Shan Xi Yi Kan 1960). It may help decrease inflammation of the pericardium.

Hornet nest (Lu feng fang): Can inhibit tumor growth, possibly by enhancing macrophage activity (Li 1999).

Licorice (Gan cao): Can improve the heart function and decrease myocardial oxygen consumption (Xu Ling 1997). It prevented aconitine-induced arrhythmia (Hu 1996). It may also help with arrhythmias secondary to pericardial effusion.

Poria (Fu ling): Contains pachyman. This can be used to inhibit cancers (Chen 1986).

Reishi mushroom (Ling zhi): Seems to be effective for preventing and treating cancer. A polysaccharide extract called ganopoly has been shown to have anti-oxidant and radical scavenging effects. It also increases the function of T cells, macrophages, and natural killer cells. There is some evidence of direct cytotoxicity and it may induce apoptosis. It may also have anti-angiogenic capabilities (Gao 2004).

Salvia (Dan shen): Inhibits the growth of cancer cells (Li Xu Fen 1999).

Scorpion (Quan xie): Has been used to treat sarcoma in mice (Jiang Su Yi Yao 1990). It may have efficacy against other tumors.

Homotoxicology
General considerations/rationale

The pericardium originates from mesothelial elements that have development in common with the kidney, reproductive system, heart, and other serous membranes. Pericarditis represents an Inflammation Phase disorder. Pericardial fluid accumulations can also occur in Deposition, Impregnation, Degeneration, and Dedifferentiation phase homotoxicoses. The primary pathology directs the clinician in determining the correct phase for designing the most effective treatment plans. Medical and surgical methods can be used, depending upon the animal's diagnosis. Prognosis is guarded to grave. In many cases, it is appropriate to deliver emergency care and refer these patients to the proper internist and/or surgeon for support and therapy. Emergency treatment can include the protocol listed below in addition to proper conventional medical and surgical care.

Clinicians should be aware that several commonly used medications can be associated with hemothorax, pleural/pericardial effusion or thickening, ascites, and drug-induced lupus syndrome. The list of these medications is long and contains commonly used medications such as angiotensin converter enzyme inhibitors, beta-blockers, chlorpromazine, hydralazine, minocycline, procainamide, propranolol, sulfamides-sulfonamides, sulfasalazine, and tetracycline (Foucher, Camus 2006). Smallpox vaccination has been associated with pericarditis in humans; clinicians should be aware of the historical importance of prior vaccination in certain cases of pericarditis and pericardial effusion (CDC 2003).

Appropriate homotoxicology formulas (Dose: for 50-pound dog; 5 drops PO for small dog or cat)

See cardiac protocols.

Aesculus compositum: Provides vessel support. Acidum benzoicum is indicated in autoimmune disorders (Wemmer 1996).

Angio-Injeel: Contains Acidum formicicum, which is indicated in autoimmune vasculitis (Wemmer 1996).

Apis homaccord: Mobilizes fluid from body spaces, especially when combined with Lymphomyosot. Is used to treat pulmonary edema.

Arnica-Heel: Used for generalized or localized inflammation reactions (Reckeweg 2000). Mercurialis perennis is indicated in endocarditis and pericarditis (Reckeweg 2002).

Aurumheel: Has anti-arrhythmic qualities.

Bryaconeel: Used in conditions involving serous membrane inflammation and coughs worsened by chill. Rheumatism is associated in many cases. Connections between polyarthritis and inflammation of serous membranes in pericarditis exist and have been known for more than 100 years (Mihoc 1986).

Cactus compositum: Treats coronary circulatory disorders.

Cardiacum-Heel: Supports cardiac functions.

Coenzyme compositum: Provides metabolism support of citric acid cycle cytosol components.

Cor compositum: Provides cardiac support. See *Spigelon* for details regarding Spigelia anthelmia. The component of Cactus benefits autoimmune cases (also present in *Cactus compositum*, *Cardiacum-Heel*, and *Strophanthus compositum*). (Wemmer 1996)

Cralonin: Cardiac support. See Spigelon, below, for details regarding Spigelia anthelmia.

Echinacea compositum: Used for bacteria endocarditis and infections or sepsis.

Engystol: Supportive in viral conditions.

Galium-Heel: Provides powerful immune support and cellular drainage formula.

Glyoxal compositum: Used for decoupling and enzyme activation.

Hepar compositum: Provides liver drainage and support.

Lymphomyosot: Provides lymph drainage and detoxification, and is used to mobilize edema when combined with *Apis compositum*.

Molybdan compositum: Provides trace mineral metabolism support and supplementation.

Mucosa compositum: Supports excretory mucosal surfaces. In Traditional Chinese Medicine, the Heart and Small Intestine are paired, and the Pericardium and Triple Heater are paired. Support of the energy metabolism and gastro-intestinal excretion pathways are advantageous.

Pectus-Heel: Contains Spigelia anthelmia (see *Spigelon*), Arnica montana (see *Anica-Heel*), and Aconitum napellus for stabbing pains, fever, and cardiac disorders. (Reckeweg 2000).

Placenta compositum: Provides support for vessels and activation of stem cell elements.

Psorinoheel: Used in Excretory and Impregnation phase disorders.

Ranunculus homaccord: A minor remedy for pericardial effusion that is more directed at pleuritis and pain associated with chest wall pathology through Ranunculus bulbosus. Also used if there is sciatica. Use with caution in combination with other remedies because Ranunculus is believed to antidote Bryonia, Camphor, and Rhus (Boericke 1927).

Solidago compositum: Provides urogenital support and detoxification. Contains Coxsackie virus B1-B5, which in human medicine is associated with myocarditis and infectious pericarditis. Because kidney tissue arises from mesothelial elements, support of renal tissue may prove to be helpful in such cases.

Spigelon: Contains Spigelia anthelmia, which is indicated in cases manifesting precordial pain, pericariditis (with sharp pains and dyspnea), sore left side, neuralgia, and a preference to lie on the left side (Boericke 1927). Functions by targeting tissues in the pericardium, endocardium, trigeminal nerve, and central nervous system (Hamalcik 1990). Spigelia anthelmia is also present in *Angio-Heel, Cactus compositum, Cardiacum-Heel, Cor compositum, Cralonin, Oculoheel, Pectus-Heel, Strophanthus compositum, BHI-Heart,* and *BHI-Neuralgia* (Reckeweg 2000).

Thyroidea compositum: Provides endocrine support and matrix drainage in precancerous cases. There is a possible connection to the Triple Heater Meridian in Traditional Chinese Medicine.

Tonsilla compositum: Used in deeply immunosuppressed individuals and to support the spleen, which in Traditional Chinese Medicine is thought to control the blood vessels and hold in fluids. Also used in Impregnation and Dedifferentiation phase disorders.

Traumeel S: Used in traumatic incidents as a nonsteroidal anti-inflammatory agent, in infections, and in chronic conditions to activate blocked enzymes (Mihoc 1986).

Ubichinon compositum: Provides mitochondrial support and conditioning.

Authors' suggested protocols

Nutrition

Heart and bronchus/lung support formulas: 1 tablet for every 25 pounds of body weight BID.

Coenzyme Q10: 15 mg for every 10 pounds of body weight daily.

Beyond essential fats: One-half teaspoon with food for every 35 pounds of body weight (maximum, 100 pounds).

Vitamin E: 50 IU for every 20 pounds of body weight SID.

Chinese herbal medicine/acupuncture

If the pericardial effusion is secondary to cardiac disease or pericarditis, the authors use H38 Pleural effusion/cardiac at a dose of 1 capsule for every 10 to 20 pounds twice daily.

H38 Pleural effusion/cardiac contains angelica root (Dang gui), astragalus (Huang qi), codonopsis (Dang shen), dianthus (Qu mai), fritillaria (Bei mu), lily bulb (Bai he), ophiopogon (Mai men dong), pharbitis (Qian niu zi), platycodon root (Jie geng), scutellaria (Huang qin), talc (Hua shi), trichosanthes root (Tian hua feng), and white peony (Bai shao).

If the effusion is secondary to a heart-based tumor or is idiopathic, the authors use a combination of the H38 Pleural effusion/cardiac and H60 Anticancer at a dose of 1 capsule of each formula per 10 to 20 pounds twice daily.

H60 Anticancer contains antler powder (Lu jiao shuang), arisaema (Dan nan xing), astragalus (Huang qi), barbat skullcap (Ban zhi lian), centipede (Wu gong), coix (Yi yi ren), cornus (Shan zhu yu), dandelion (Pu gong ying), dioscoria (Shan yao), ginseng (Ren shen), honeysuckle (Jin yin hua), hornet nest (Lu feng fang), licorice (Gan cao), mugwort (Liu ji nu), poria (Fu ling), rehmannia (Shu di huang), reishi mushroom (Ling zhi), salvia (Dan shen), scorpion (Quan xie), and tortoise shell (Bie jia).

The herbs not discussed above are added to the respective formulas to increase efficacy.

Homotoxicology (Dose: 10 drops PO for 50-pound dog; 5 drops PO for small dog or cat dose)

Emergency treatment including drainage and other drugs should be instituted while fluid analysis, cytology, culture, and other imaging is in progress. Autosanguis may prove helpful in advanced cases.

Symptom remedy (all cases): Apis homaccord, Lymphomyosot, Cactus compositum, Cralonin give every 15 to 30 minutes until response is noted, and then 2 to 6 times daily.

Symptom remedy (additional in infectious cases): Consider Engystol N (viral or allergic) BID, Echinacea compositum or Tonsilla compositum (bacterial) once daily by injection or PO BID by tablet.

Symptom remedy (traumatic cases): Traumeel S IV, IM, SQ, or PO.

Symptom remedy (hemorrhagic cases): Cinnamomum compositum plus Traumeel S by injection.

Symptom remedy (neoplasia cases): Tonsilla compositum and Viscum compositum by injection (plus above symptom remedies as indicated) (See Cancer, Section 5).

Deep detoxification formula: Galium-Heel, Lymphomyosot, Hepar compositum, Thyroidea compositum, Solidago compositum, Coenzyme compositum, and Ubichinon compositum given every 2 to 3 days for 120 days or longer as indicated by case responses.

Product sources

Nutrition

Cardiac and bronchus/lung support formulas: Animal Nutrition Technologies. **Alternatives:** Cardio Strength—Vetri Science; Canine Cardiac Support—Standard Process Veterinary Formulas; Formula CV—RxVitamins; Bio Cardio; Thorne Veterinary Products.

Coenzyme Q10: Vetri Science; Rx Vitamins for Pets; Integrative Therapeutics; Thorne Veterinary Products.

Beyond essential fats: Natural Health Products. **Alternatives:** Oil of Evening Primrose, Hemp Oil, Flax Oil, Fish Oil.

Chinese herbal medicine

Formula H38 and H60: Natural Solutions, Inc.

Homotoxicology

BHI/Heel Corporation

REFERENCES

Western medicine references

Miller MW, Sisson DD. Pericardial disorders. In: Ettinger SJ, Feldman EC, eds. Textbook of veterinary internal medicine. 4th ed. Philadelphia: Saunders, 1995:1032–1045.

Smith FWK Jr, Rush JE. Diagnosis and treatment of pericardial effusion. In: Bonagura JD, ed. Kirk's current veterinary therapy XIII. Philadelphia: Saunders, 1999:772–777.

Rush JE. Pericardial Effusion. In: Tilley L, Smith F, The 5-Minute Veterinary Consult: Canine and Feline, 2003.Blackwell Publishing.

IVM/nutrition references

Budwig J. Flax oil as a true aid against arthritis, heart infarction, cancer and other diseases. 1992. Vancouver: Apple Publ.

Capron L. Marine Oils and Prevention of Cardiovascular Disease, *Revue Practicien.*, 1993,43: 164.

Gaby AR. Coenzyme Q10. In: *A Textbook of Natural Medicine. In:* Pizzorno JE, Murray MT, eds. Seattle: Bastyr University Press, 1998, V:CoQ10-1–8.

Giugliano D. Dietary antioxidants for cardiovascular prevention. *Nutr Metab Cardiovasc Dis.* 2000 Feb;10(1):38–44.

Traber MG. Does vitamin E decrease heart attack risk? Summary and implications with respect to dietary recommendations. *J Nutr.* 2001;131(2):395S–397S.

Wu Y, Wang Y, Wang B, Lei H, Yang Y. Effects of total flavones of fructus Hippophae (TFH) on cardiac function and hemodynamics of anesthetized open-chest dogs with acute heart failure. *Chung Kuo Chung Yao Tsa Chih.* 1997; Jul;22(7):429–31, 448.

Wu J, Yu XJ, Ma X, Li XG, Liu D. Electrophysiologic effects of total flavones of Hippophae rhamnoides L on guinea pig papillary muscles and cultured rat myocardial cells. *Chung Kuo Yao Li Hsueh Pao.* 1994; Jul;15(4):341–3.

Chinese herbal medicine/acupuncture references

Bi LQ, et al. *China Journal of Integrated Medicine.* 1998;18(1):35–37.

CA, 1992; 116: 34223d.

Chang Yong Zhong Yao Cheng Fen Yu Yao Li Shou Ce (A Handbook of the Composition and Pharmacology of Common Chinese Drugs), 1994; 1725:1728.

Chen CX. *Journal of Chinese Materia Medica.* 1986;16(4):40.

Du YT. Lu Jiao Jiao injection's effect on the phagocytosis of macrophagocytes in patients of mammary cancer. *Journal of Traditional Chinese Medicine.* 1981;(3):36.

Gao YH and Zhou SF. Chemopreventive and Tumoricidal Properties of Ling Zhi Mushroom *Ganoderma lucidum* (W.Curt.: Fr.) Lloyd (Aphyllophoromycetideae). Part II. Mechanism Considerations (Review). *International Journal of Medicinal Mushrooms* 2004; vol 6 issue 3.

Hu SY, et al. *Journal of Nanjing University of TCM.* 1996;12(5):23–24.

Hu XY, et al. *Journal of Nanjing College of TCM.* 1988;(3):28–29.

Hua Xi Yao Xue Za Zhi (*Huaxi Herbal Journal*), 1991; 6(1):13.

Jiang Su Yi Yao (*Jiang Su Journal of Medicine and Herbology*), 1990;16 (9):513.

Kubo M, Matsuda H, Tanaka M, Kimura Y, Okuda H, Higashino M, Tani T, Namba K, Arichi S. Studies on Scutellariae radix. VII. Anti-arthritic and anti-inflammatory actions of methanolic extract and flavonoid components from Scutellariae radix. *Chem Pharm Bull*, 1984; 32(7):2724–9.

Li L, et al. *Journal of Beijing Medical University.* 1999;22(3):38–40.

Li XF, et al. In vitro anti-tumor effects of Dan Shen and Dan Shen compound injection. *Zhejiang Journal of Integrated Medicine.* 1999;9(5):291–292.

Li YF (translator). Foreign Medicine, vol. of TCM. 1984; 6(1):15–18.

Liu H. *Journal of Stomatology.* 1999;19(2):60–61.

Liu IX, Durham DG, Richards RM. Baicalin synergy with beta-lactam antibiotics against methicillin-resistant Staphylococcus aureus and other beta-lactam-resistant strains of S. aureus. *J Pharm Pharmacol.* 2000; Mar;52(3):361–6.

Liu XJ, et al. *Journal of Jingzhou Medical College.* 1999;20(3):16–18.

Lu Y, et al. Yi Yi Ren oil's anti-tumor effects. *Journal of Pharmacology and Clinical Application of TCM.* 1999;15(6):21–23.

Luo XP, et al. *China Journal of Pathology and Physiology.* 1999;15(7):639–643.

Microorganism Group, Shandong Medical College. Experiments on 110 Chinese medicinal materials' bacteriostatic effect. *Journal of Shandong Medical College.* 1959;(8):42.

Modern TCM Pharmacology. 1997. Tianjin: Science and Technology Press.

Ren Min Wei Sheng Chu Ban She (*Journal of People's Public Health*), 1988;302.

Shan Xi Yi Kan (*Shanxi Journal of Medicine*), 1960; (10):32.

Shi Ren Bing. *Journal of Beijing University of TCM.* 1999;22(2):63–64.

Xu L, et al. *Journal of Research in Chinese Medicine.* 1997;10(2):31–32.

Xu SA, et al. *China Journal of Pharmacy.* 1999;34(10)663–66.

Xu ZW, et al. *Zhejiang Journal of Oncology.* 1997;3(2):110–111.

Ying ZZ, et al. *Journal of Shizhen Medicine.* 1999;10(10):732–733.

Zhang SC, et al. *Journal of Chinese Patent Medicine Research.* 1984;(2):37.

Zhong Cao Yao (*Chinese Herbal Medicine*), 1982; 13(9);27–3.

Zhong Yao Xue (*Chinese Herbology*), 1998; 739:741.

Zhong Yao Xue (*Chinese Herbology*), 1998; 845:848.

Zhong Yao Zhi (*Chinese Herbology Journal*), 1993:183.

Zhong Yi Za Zhi (*Journal of Chinese Medicine*), 1981;7:54.

Zi M, Ken-ichiro Otsuyama, Shangqin Liu, Saeid Abroun, Hideaki Ishikawa, Naohiro Tsuyama, Masanori Obata, Fu-Jun Li, Xu Zheng, Yasuko Maki, Koji Miyamoto, and Michio M. Kawano. Baicalein, a component of *Scutellaria* radix from Huang-Lian-Jie-Du-Tang (HLJDT), leads to suppression of proliferation and induction of apoptosis in human myeloma cells. *Blood.* 2005; 105:3312–3318.

Homotoxicology references

Boericke W. Materia Medica with Repertory, 9th ed. 1927. Santa Rosa, CA: Boericke and Tafel, pp 438, 482.

CDC. Cardiac adverse events following smallpox vaccination—United States, 2003, *Morbid Mortal Wkly Rep*, 2003. March 28;52:248–50.

Foucher P, Camus P. Drug-Induced Lung Diseases. Department of Pulmonary Diseases and Intensive Care Unit. University Hospital. Dijon, France. http://www.pneumotox.com/indexf.php?fich=clin0andlg=en.

Hamalcik P. The biological therapy of cardiac, circulatory, and vascular disorders. *Biol Ther*. 1990; 10(21992): pp 244–6.

Mihoc M. Treatment of Inflammatory Rheumatic Diseases with Traumeel. *Biol Ther*. 1986. 4(3/4): pp 53–6.

Reckeweg H. Biotherapeutic Index: Ordinatio Antihomotoxica et Materia Medica, 5th ed. 2000. Baden-Baden, Germany: Biologische Heilmittel Heel GMBH, pp 293, 382, 537.

Reckeweg H. Homeopathia Antihomotoxica Materia Medica, 4th ed. 2002. Baden-Baden, Germany: Aurelia-Verlag, p 414.

Wemmer U. Systemic lupus erythematosus: the clinical picture. *Biol Medizin*. 1996. December: pp 256–258.

Chapter Ten

Diseases of the Dermatological System

ALLERGIC DERMATITIS, ATOPY, AND FLEA BITE DERMATITIS

Definition and cause

The basic underlying cause for allergic dermatitis in dogs and cats is an exaggerated immune response to allergens such as pollen, dander, molds, dust mites and other environmental allergens and chemicals. The basic exaggerated immune response is believed to involve T- and B-lymphocytes, the production of IgE, and the stimulation of mast cells and eosinophils, causing the local, cutaneous reaction (Hnilica 1997, 1998; Ihrke 1995; Plant 2003; Reedy 1997; Scott 1995).

The result is that sensitized animals react in receptor sites in the skin, leading to pruritus and secondary issues. There is also an inherited component; many popular breeds such as Golden Retrievers, Irish Setters, and Old English Sheepdogs are more prone to the condition (Reedy 1997, Scott 1995).

Medical therapy rationale, drug(s) of choice, and nutritional recommendations

The central focus of standard therapy is to identify and eliminate the causative agent in combination with antihistamines and oral and topical immune-suppressing drugs such as corticosteroids and cyclosporine. In addition, allergen desensitizing (immunotherapy) injections are favored by some dermatologists. Dietary recommendations include hypoallergenic diets in combination with omega-3-rich sources of fatty acids (Ihrke 1995, Paterson 1995, Plant 2003, Reedy 1997, Saevik 2004, Scott 1995).

Anticipated prognosis

Most animals with allergic dermatitis respond well to topical and oral therapy in combination with avoidance of exposure to allergens. Allergic dermatitis is a progressive condition and most often requires ongoing medical therapy to control the allergic response (Reedy 1997).

Integrative veterinary therapies

Pollutants, preservatives, food additives, and a host of compounds can lead to tissue injury and activate the immune response. The mucosa is the primary barrier and location of many immune elements, and anything that injures the mucosal integrity can lead to immune dysfunction.

Once allergens gain access to these tissues, they can be removed and processed by macrophages in a wide variety of locations (especially the gut, liver, spleen, and lung). In cases in which the damage is rapidly repaired, there is a reduced likelihood of chronic allergies developing, but if a chronic defect in mucosal integrity occurs, then allergies can develop more easily. Genetic predisposition is a factor in this situation.

The liver is responsible for processing much of the material that originates from mucosal borders. The hepatic macrophage system of Kupfer cells is very efficient in removing and processing antigens. The liver can metabolize, conjugate, and excrete many homotoxins, and support of liver function and excretion is a critical portion of any allergic therapy.

Macrophages present the antigen components to lymphocytes and these dictate the development of immune response through the action of T-lymphocytes (TH-0, TH-1, and TH-2 cells). Alteration of the T-helper cell can determine the type of immune response by the organism. Homotoxins that are not removed by first passage through the liver can also be excreted by the kidney, skin, and lung. Homotoxins that have been eliminated by the liver but reabsorbed through the enterohepatic circulation also enter the system at this level.

Support of mucosal tissues is critical, and therefore one of the first areas requiring attention in allergic patients is the intestinal tract. The patient should be fed an easily digested ration which ideally lacks excessive amounts of allergens. This allows for improved intestinal function and reduces homotoxins presented to the liver. It also allows for improved mucosal integrity. In managing airborne allergens, it is advisable to reduce the level of homotoxins such as pollens, scented products and incenses, and toxic agents such as ozone and pollutants, which might damage mucosal integrity.

Adequate water consumption is also important in maintaining proper immune function and repairing damaged tissue. Probiotics may greatly assist in protecting the mucosal border and local immune system and are useful in most immune imbalance cases. Antioxidant agents such as vitamins and minerals, as well as other nutraceuticals, herbals, and whole foods, provide needed protection from oxidative damage and assist in repairing tissues.

Support of liver function assists greatly in handling allergic cases and in many clinical situations support of the enterohepatic system is the first action in preparing a case.

Providing attention to the renal system further assists detoxification, and is especially necessary in cases that are undergoing regressive vicariation from the Impregnation Phase to the Deposition and Inflammation phases. Providing adequate levels of fatty acids, especially omega-3 fatty acids, assists in repairing cell membranes and in decreasing levels of tissue inflammation.

Unnecessary or redundant vaccinations should be avoided in all patients, but this is particularly true in allergic pets. Risk for vaccination reaction is higher in atopic pets. In 1983, a study showed that allergies (such as atopic dermatitis) develop in dogs when vaccinated for distemper, hepatitis, and leptospirosis just prior to, but not after, exposure to pollen extracts. Dogs predisposed to atopy produce excess amounts of IgE antibodies in response to antigens, resulting in chronically irritating skin inflammations. Other organs may exhibit signs of hypersensitivity causing, for example, conjunctivitis or rhinitis, as exhibited in further studies by this group (Frick 1983). A recent study demonstrated no increase in the rate of atopy in children receiving vaccinations (Adler 2005). Good medical practice dictates caution in the use of any agent in patients that are known to be prone to allergic reactions (see Vaccinations, Chapter 35).

Note: See Homotoxicology for the "4 Rs" approach to an allergic patient.

Nutrition
General considerations/rationale
While the target tissue is often the skin or intestinal tract, allergies are metabolically a systemic disease. They often involve multiple organs, particularly the liver, which shares the same detoxification enzyme systems (Ahmad 2004). In addition, the elimination of toxins, allergens, and metabolic wastes often burdens the organs of detoxification, namely the bowel, kidney, lung, and skin. The use of immune-suppressing drugs such as cortisone, while often necessary because of self-trauma, actually exacer-bate the condition by slowing elimination and covering up the inflammation. Because allergies are metabolically a multi-organ disease, a physiological evaluation of the blood is recommended to more closely address nutritional deficiencies and required gland support (see Chapter 2, Nutritional Blood Testing, for additional information).

Appropriate nutrients
Nutritional/gland therapy: Glandular intestines, kidney, adrenal, thymus, liver, and pituitary supply intrinsic nutrients that improve organ function, reduce cellular inflammation, and promote and enhance detoxification (see Gland Therapy, Chapter 2, for a more detailed explanation).

Probiotics: Administration of the proper combination of probiotics has been reported to have a positive impact on the intestines and the digestive process (Goldin 1984, Perdigon (1987). Probiotics have been shown to improve and enhance the digestive process by secreting their own source of enzymes (McDonough 1987).

Sterols: Plant-derived sterols such as betasitosterol show anti-inflammatory properties, which appear to be similar to corticosteriods (Gupta 1980). A cortisone-like effect without the associated immune-suppressing effects is beneficial in all allergic reactions. Bouic (1996) reports on the immune-enhancing and balancing effect of plant sterols, which are also beneficial to animals with allergic reactions or responses.

Evening primrose oil (EPO): Evening primrose oil has been proven to have both anti-inflammatory and anti-pruritic effects. As part of a balanced nutritional program, EPO can exert a positive effect on animals with skin disease. Studies suggest that EPO is beneficial in people with atopic dermatitis and eczema (Hederos 1996, Humphreys 1994, Morse 1989).

Quercetin: Quercetin is a flavonoid and has potent antioxidant properties (see Chapter 2, Phytonutrients). Quercetin also functions similar to an antihistamine in that it can inhibit cells from releasing histamines (Middleton 1986, Ogasawara 1985). This antihistamine attribute helps treat allergic conditions such as asthma, dermatitis, and eczema.

Chinese herbal medicine
General considerations/rationale
Practitioners of Traditional Chinese Medicine consider allergic dermatitis to be a combination of Wind, Heat, and Damp. Allergy generally is considered to be an immune disorder. Heat refers to the inflammation, which tends to be red and may be warm to the touch. Dampness describes the greasy nature of some allergic dermatitis patients. It can also apply to skin with serous discharge, i.e., "weepy" sores or purulent debris in pustules. Wind translates into itching, in modern terms.

Appropriate Chinese herbs and acupuncture

Angelica (Bai zhi): Has been shown to have anti-inflammatory and antipruritic effects in mice. (Zhong Guo Zhong Yao Za Zhi 1991).

Atractylodes (Cang zhu): Has activity against Staphylococcus aureus and dermatophytes (Zhong Yao Xue 1998).

Bupleurum (Chai hu): Decreases the effect of histamine release (Zhong Yao Yao Li Yu Ying Yong 1983) and has antibiotic effects against streptococci (Zhong Yao Xue 1998).

Cicada slough (Chan tui): Has been used successfully in humans to treat chronic urticaria (Pi fu Bing Fang Zhi Yan Jiu Tong Xun 1972).

Licorice (Gan cao): Inhibits the growth of Staphylococcus aureus (Zhong Yao Zhi, 1993). It contains glycyrrhizine and glycyrrhentinic acid, which have corticosteroid activity (Zhong Cao Yao 1991).

Lonicera flower (Jin yin hua): Has antibiotic effects against Staphylococcus aureus, E. coli, and Pseudomonas aeruginosa (Xin Yi Xue 1975) and is anti-inflammatory (Shan Xi Yi Kan 1960).

Mint (Bo he): Relieves itching (Zhong Cao Yao Xue 1980) and has anti-inflammatory effects (Zhong Yao Xue 1998).

Moutan (Mu dan pi): Demonstrates anti-inflammatory actions via inhibition of prostaglandin synthesis and decreases vascular permeability (Sheng Yao Xue Za Zhi 1979, Zhong Guo Yao Ke Da Xue Xue Bao 1990). It inhibits the growth of Staphylococcus aureus, streptococci, and dermatophytes (Zhong Yao Cai 1991).

Platycodon (Jie geng): Decreases allergic reactions (Zhong Yao Yao Li Yu Ying Yong 1983).

Poria (Fu ling): Has inhibitory effects on Staphylococcus aureus (Zhong Yao Cai, 1985).

Rehmannia (Sheng di huang): Has shown anti-inflammatory activity in mice (Zhong Yao Yao Li Yu Ying Yong 1983).

Siegesbeckia (Xi xian cao): Inhibits the growth of Staphylococcus aureus (Phytochemistry, 1979).

White peony (Bai shao): Contains paeoniflorin, which is a strong anti-inflammatory (Zhong Yao Zhi 1993). It also has antibiotic effects against Staphylococcus aureus, some streptococci, E. coli, Pseudomonas aeruginosa and some dermatophytes. (Xin Zhong Yi 1989).

Acupuncture has been used to treat skin allergies (Lundesberg 1988). By stimulating specific acupuncture points, it is possible to stimulate the pet's immune system and reduce the itching and inflammation associated with allergic dermatitis.

The authors have used GV14, SP9, and SP10 to control inflammation (Clear Heat in TCM terms). LI11 can be used to stop itching and HT7 can be used to calm the animal so it does not lick or scratch and irritate the skin further.

Local points can be used. These include LI4 for the front legs, GB34 for the back legs, and GB20 for the neck (Schoen 1994).

Homotoxicology
General considerations/rationale

The basic biophysiology of allergies is well described. Allergic reactions represent Impregnation Phase homotoxicoses as IgE binds to mast cells and alters the response of the connective tissue to allergens. Numerous homotoxins are released as part of the allergic response; histamine is a major homotoxin that requires detoxification and elimination. Excessive amounts of histamine lead to tissue injury and progressive vicariation.

Understanding the elimination pathways for homotoxins is critical to properly handling allergic cases. Biological therapy for allergies involves decreasing the levels of homotoxins, improving detoxification pathways, increasing elimination of homotoxins, and supporting repair of injured tissues and organs.

4 Rs: This system for approaching allergic cases consists of:

Remove: Remove toxic materials, antigenic substances, pathogens, disease-causing stressors, and other factors that favor pathology. This allows for a cessation or reduction in tissue injury, and calming of the overtaxed immune response. Healing occurs best in a safe environment at a microscopic and macroscopic level. Avoidance of unnecessary vaccinations and unnecessary symptom-suppressive medicants, and use of limited-antigen and more natural diets, air filters, hygiene, endoparasite control, ectoparasite control, as well as an altered environment, are all examples of this step. In some cases, all that is needed for recovery is removal of the antigenic stimulation (flea allergy, mild pollen or food allergy). This is an important first step in handling all allergy patients. Detoxification therapy is useful in this step and it has been frequently observed that allergic pets do better clinically if they are given routine detoxification therapy at regular intervals (at least twice yearly). In mild cases, the easiest form of detoxification is the Detox Kit. In deeper homotoxicoses, the deep detoxification formula is recommended (see below).

Repopulate/Revive: Provide adequate probiotic bacteria to repopulate a proper intestinal and mucosal flora, and revive function of chief excretory organs such as the liver and intestine. Probiotic bacteria also provide a means of reactivating damaged enzyme systems from earlier disease elements such as bacterial or fungal toxins and pharmaceutical agents such as cortisone, NSAIDs, and antibiotics.

Rebalance/Repair: Assist the natural bio-oscillation of inflammation and pH fluctuations, eliminate diseased tissue elements, clear the matrix of debris, promote collagen repair and replacement and provide improved circulation of hemic-lymphatic components, and provide adequate raw materials for enzyme production and tissue repair.

Reorganize: Cycles of repair continually improve the status of the diseased tissue and its relationship to the body as a whole. Hering's Law of Cure manifests at this level as we see the body repair from inside to outside, from most important organ to least important organ, from the head down and in reverse order of present pathologic history. This is a useful tool for the clinician in determining whether a patient is undergoing regressive vicariation (in which case the clinician would simply continue therapy), or undergoing less desirable progressive vicariation (in which case the clinician would need to intervene and address the patient's worsening condition).

In patients that are already on symptom-suppressing drugs such as corticosteroids, antihistamines, antibiotics, or cyclosporin, it is advisable to begin therapy gently and not to stop these medications initially. After the system has been sufficiently strengthened, the dosages can be gradually reduced until many patients no longer require as much medication to manage their cases. In some instances they may no longer need symptom-suppressing medications to maintain a healthy lifestyle. Not all allergic patients can be cured, but it is a worthwhile goal to simply improve their quality of life and when possible reduce their dependency on pharmaceutical agents.

Allergic patients can be greatly assisted by proper use of biological therapies and many make surprising recoveries if they are allowed to go through regressive vicariation and are not subjected to further suppression of their body's natural healing responses. Homeopathy has been used for many years to treat allergies in human and veterinary patients (Witt 2005). Clinicians should advise clients that this process might take from 1 to 3 years, and ascertain if the clients are dedicated to the process before embarking on such a program. It may be more expedient for some clients to simply suppress symptoms, but for those who desire maximizing the health of their pet, it is very rewarding and challenging work. Biological therapy options should be discussed with clients as part of the informed consent procedure as an option to administering potentially damaging pharmaceutical agents.

Appropriate homotoxicology formulas

A large number of antihomotoxic formulas may be needed to manage a case of allergic skin disease. Autosanguis therapy can be particularly useful. (Also see sections on Otitis externa and Otitis media, Chapter 12; vomiting and diarrhea, Chapter 11; coughing, Chapter 14; and seborrhea, throughout this chapter). Careful attention to phase and phase shifting is needed to guide remedy selection. A list of commonly used agents follows:

Aesculus homaccord: Promotes improved circulation and lymph drainage.

Apis homaccord: Used for urticarial reactions (especially when combined with Lymphomyosot)(Broadfoot 2005). Also used for pruritic dermatitis, pustular dermatitis, and bullous eczema (Reckeweg 2000).

Belladonna homaccord: Treats intensely red lesions, furunculosis, boils; the skin is dry, red, and hot; patients resent being touched. The ears may itch intensely, to the point that the pet drills things into the ears or rubs excessively. There is excessive head shaking.

Berberis homaccord: Part of Heel's *Detox Kit* used for adrenal support and detoxification of the renal system and liver, in cases with pigmentation of the axillary area.

BHI-Allergy: Used for skin rashes and hives, and respiratory and ocular allergy symptoms (Heel 2002). In the authors' experience, this remedy is usually not sufficient to use as a single agent, except in mild, acute cases, and works best when combined with other remedies in management of allergy symptoms. Contains Sulphur 12X, which is useful in a wide variety of skin conditions and chronic illnesses.

BHI-Inflammation: Used for pyoderma, itching, inflammation, and atopy (especially when there is a tendency toward pyoderma with multiple small lesions). Can be used like an antihistamine in these cases, before other drugs are tried. Response can be seen within 1 week. Provides long-term control of itching in some patients as a simple nontoxic strategy (Palmquist 2003).

BHI-Skin: Used for "eczema, blisters and cold sores, rashes and hives" (Heel 2002).

Coenzyme compositum: Provides metabolic support (Reinhart 2005).

Cutis compositum: A wide-reaching formula that stimulates nonspecific defenses in a variety of cutaneous conditions. Can be used in any phase homotoxicosis; opens skin to drainage and repair. Supports regeneration and repair of organs involved in skin health. Contains Cutis suis, Hepar suis, Splen suis, Placenta suis, Glandula suprarenalis suis, and Funiculus ubilicalis suis. Also contains Sulfur to repair blocked enzyme systems and Cortisonum aceticum to repair damage from prior corticosteroid exposure. The ingredient Aesculus hipposcastanum supports circulation and drainage (Reckeweg 2000).

Detox Kit: A combination of *Lymphomyosot* for lymph drainage, *Nux vomica homaccord* to support the gastrohepatic system, and *Berberis homaccord* for adrenal, renal, and hepatic support that is used as a method of general detoxification.

Echinacea compositum: Used to control bacteria infections and for immune normalization.

Engystol N: Supports immunity. Through Sulphur, acts as a catalyst in chronic diseases (Reihnart 2005). Useful in viral infections and allergic disorders.

Galium-Heel: This remedy is indicated in most allergic cases. It is a phase remedy for Deposition to Dedifferentiation phases. It has diuretic effects due to Galium aparine, Sempervivum tectorum, Ononis spinosa, Juniperus communis, Betula alba, Saponaria officinali, and Acidum nitricum, and detoxifying effects due to Galium mullugo. It supports parenchyma (lung, liver, kidney, and heart) through Phosphorus. *Galium-Heel* is used for edema and to create drainage through connective tissue. It also is used for itching (Apis mellifica), infectious Inflammatory phases (Pyrogenium-Nosode), and eczema and dermatosis (Urtica urens) (Reckeweg 2000). Finally, it is also a cellular drainage and repair agent.

Graphites homaccord: Used in obese patients with alopecia, oozing purple-colored lesions, and erosions that develop into suppurative sores (Macloed 1983).

Hepar compositum: Provides drainage and repair of the liver, support of metabolism, and reversal of prior corticosteroid therapeutic damage. It is critical as a first line of defense in skin repair, because it bears the brunt of detoxification.

Hepeel: Provides liver detoxification.

Histamin-Injeel: A homeopathically prepared histamine that assists in reversal of damages from histamine excess in allergic patients. When combined with *BHI-Allergy* vials it may produce a more potent Histaminum homaccord.

Lymphomyosot: Provides lymph drainage and support, as well as support of the thyroid function.

Mucosa compositum: Supports mucous membranes throughout the body. Used intermittently during repair stages.

Nux vomica homaccord: Provides detoxification of the liver and gastrointestinal tract; is part of the Detox Kit.

Psorinoheel: An exudation and cellular phase remedy that is used for itching, precancerous conditions, chronic skin conditions, acne, seborrhea, eczema, and pruritus.

Pusatilla compositum: Reverses the effects of prior cortisone therapy and regulates rigidity cases to move them toward inflammation and regressive vicariation.

Reneel: Provides kidney and urinary tract detoxification.

Schwef-Heel: Contains a homaccord of Sulphur, which is widely used in homeopathic practice (Becker-Witt 2004). It is used for dermatosis with eczema, pyoderma, and red skin (Reckeweg 2000). It has great affinity for skin and adnexal tissues, and is known for working from the inside out on dirty and filthy animals prone to skin infections (Boericke 1927). Helps with redness and itching made worse by heat and red body orifices, and often is useful in concomitant use with other remedies in opening cases (Macleod 1983).

Solidago compositum: Provides renal support and is a phase remedy for Deposition Phase disorders.

Sulfur Heel: Used for eczema, pruritus, neuralgia with sensitivity to cold air (Daphne mezereum), urticaria with burning and itching skin (Arsenicum album), and irritating eczema (wood tar). It is also useful in scabies dermatitis (Reckeweg 2000).

Thyroidea compositum: Provides endocrine support and deep matrix cleansing. It is a phase remedy in Impregnation Phase disorders.

Traumeel S: Provides nonsteroidal anti-inflammatory action, activates and regulates normal inflammatory responses, and unblocks enzyme systems.

Ubichinon compositum: Provides metabolic support.

Authors' suggested protocols

Nutrition

Skin and immune support formulas: 1 tablet for every 25 pounds of body weight BID.

Intestinal and/or liver support formulas: One-half tablet for every 25 pounds of body weight BID. When required, kidney and pituitary support can be added.

Probiotic MPF: One-half capsule for every 25 pounds of body weight with food.

Oil of evening primrose: 1 capsule for every 25 pounds of body weight SID.

Betathyme: 1 capsule for every 35 pounds of body weight BID. (maximum 2 capsules BID)

Quercetin: 50 mg for every 10 pounds of body weight daily.

Chinese herbal medicine/acupuncture

The authors advise a combination of two herbal preparations: ImmunoDerm and Dermguard. In addition to the herbs discussed above, these preparations contains scutellaria (Huang Qin), fleece flower root (He shou wu), siler (Fang feng), tokoro (Bi xie), schizonepeta (Jing jie), dandelion (Pu gong ying), oldenlandia (Bai hua she cao), kochia (Di fu zi), xanthium fruit (Cang Er zi), bitter orange (Zhi ke), angelica radix (Dang gui), buffalo horn shavings (Sui Niu jiao), earthworm (Di long), silkworm (Jiang can), and cnidium (Chuan xiong). The combination of these 2 formulas has anti-inflammatory, antipruritic, and antibacterial effects.

Homotoxicology (Dose: 10 drops PO for 50-pound dog; 5 drops PO small dog or cat)

An autosanguis with Traumeel S, Engystol N, Hepar compositum, and Cutis compositum is quite useful in many allergy cases. Open the case as follows for 3–6 months, and use other antihomotoxic medications as listed above depending upon the patient's specific symptom picture:

Traumeel S: Give orally once on Monday and Thursday.

Engystol N: Give orally once on Monday and Thursday.

Hepeel and Coenzyme compositum or BHI-Enzyme: Give each evening for 30 days.

Detox Kit (Lymphomyosot, Nuv vomica homaccord, Berberis homaccord): Give orally twice daily.

Galium-Heel: Give orally twice daily.

In the case of chronic or deep homotoxicoses, use:

Deep detoxification formula: Galium-Heel, Lymphomyosot, Hepar compositum, Thyroidea compositum, Solidago compositum, Coenzyme compositum, Ubichinon compositum, given orally twice weekly for 60 to 120 days and then alternated with Detox Kit above.

In the event of severe pruritus, give:

BHI-Allergy plus Histamin-Injeel, Cutis compositum, and Psorinoheel: Give as an injection; often gives sufficient relief so that biological therapy can continue. This can be repeated twice weekly as needed.

Product sources

Nutrition

Skin, immune, intestinal, kidney, liver, and pituitary support formulas: Animal Nutrition Technologies. **Alternatives:** Enteric Support—Standard Process Veterinary Formulas; NutriGest—Rx Vitamins for Pets; Derma Strength—Vetri Science Laboratories; Canine Dermal Support—Standard Process Veterinary Formulas.

Hepatic support: Standard Process Veterinary Formulas; Hepato Support—Rx Vitamins for Pets; Hepagen—Thorne Veterinary Products; Immune System Support Standard Process Veterinary Formulas; Immuno Support—Rx Vitamins for Pets; Immugen—Thorne Veterinary Products.

Probiotic MPF: Progressive Labs; Rx Biotic Rx Vitamins for Pets.

Oil of evening primrose: Jarrow Formulas.

Betathyme: Best for Your Pet—Alternative: Moducare Thorne Veterinary Products.

Quercetin: Source Naturals; Quercitone—Thorne Veterinary Products.

Chinese herbal medicine
ImmunoDerm and Derm Guard: Natural Solutions, Inc.

Homotoxicology
BHI/Heel Inc.

REFERENCES

Western medicine references
Hnilica KA, Angarano DW. Advances in Immunology: Role of T-helper Lymphocyte Subsets. *Compendium of Continuing Education for the Practicing Veterinarian.* 19:1;87–93, 1997.

Hnilica KA. Advances in allergy diagnosis and treatment. *The Compendium.* 1998. 20: 258–259.

Ihrke PJ. Pruritis. In: Ettinger EJ, Feldman EC, eds. Textbook of Veterinary Internal Medicine, 1995. Toronto: WB Saunders Co. pp. 214–219.

Lundesberg T, et al. Effect of acupuncture on experimentally induced itch (Abstract). *Am J Acupuncture* 1988; 16:275.

Plant J, Reedy L. In: Tilley L, Smith F, The 5-Minute Veterinary Consult: Canine and Feline, 2003. Blackwell Publishing.

Reedy LM, Miller WH, Willemse T. Allergic skin diseases of dogs and cats. 2nd ed. 1997: Philadelphia: Saunders.

Schoen A. Veterinary Acupuncture: Ancient Art to Modern Medicine. 1994. California: American Vet Pub, Inc., p. 252

Scott DW, Miller WH, Griffin CE. Immunologic Skin Diseases. *In:* Muller and Kirk's Small Animal Dermatology Toronto: WB Saunders Co., 1995. p. 500–518.

IVM/nutrition references
Adler UC. The influence of childhood infections and vaccination on the development of atopy: a systematic review of the direct epidemiological evidence. *Homeopathy,* 2005. Jul;94(3): pp 182–95.

Ahmad N, Mukhtar H. Cytochrome P450: A Target for Drug Dermatology. 2004. 123, 417–425.

Bouic PJD, et al. Beta-sitosterol and beta-sitosterol glucoside stimulate human peripheral blood lymphocyte proliferation: Implications for their use as an immunomodulatory vitamin combination. *International Journal of Immunopharmacology* 1996;18:693–700.

Frick OL, Brooks DL. Immunoglobulin E antibodies to pollens augmented in dogs by virus vaccines. *Am J Vet Res.* 1983;44:440–445.

Golden BR, Gorbach SL. The Effect of Milk and Lactobacillus Feeding on Human Intestinal Bacteria Activity. *Am. J. of Clin. Nutr.,* 1984; 39: 756–61.

Gupta MB, Nath R, Srivastava N, et al. Anti-inflammatory and antipyretic activities of β-sitosterol. *Planta Medica* 1980;39:157–163.

Hederos CA, Berg A. Epogam evening primrose oil treatment in atopic dermatitis and asthma. *Arch Dis Child* 1996; 75(6):494–497.

Humphreys F, Symons J, Brown H, et al. The effects of gamolenic acid on adult atopic eczema and premenstrual exacerbation of eczema. *Eur J Dermatol* 1994;4(598):603.

McDonough FE, Hitchins AD, Wong NP, et al. Modification of sweet acidophilus milk to improve utilization by lactose-intolerant persons. *Am J Clin Nutr* 1987;45:570–4.

Morse PF, Horrobin DF, Manku MS, et al. Meta-analysis of placebo-controlled studies of the efficacy of Epogam in the treatment of atopic eczema: relationship between plasma essential fatty acid changes and clinical response. *Br J Dermatol* 1989;121(1):75–90.

Middleton E Jr. Effect of flavonoids on basophil histamine release and other secretory systems. *Prog Clin Biol Res.* 1986;213:493–506.

Ogasawara H, Middleton E Jr. Effect of selected flavonoids on histamine release (HR) and hydrogen peroxide (H2O2) generation by human leukocytes [abstract]. *J Allergy Clin Immunol.* 1985;75(suppl):184.

Perdigon GN, de Masius N, Alvarez S, et al. Enhancement of Immune Response in Mice fed with S. Thermophilus and L. Acidophilus, *J. of Dairy Sci.*, 1987; 70: 919–926.

Chinese herbal medicine/acupuncture references

Kim JH, Han KD, Yamasaki K, Tanaka O. Darutoside, a. diterpenoid from Siegesbeckia pubescens and its structure. *Phytochemistry*, 1979; 18(5): 894.

Lundesberg T, et al. Effect of acupuncture on experimentally induced itch (Abstract). 1988 *Am J Acupuncture.*

Pi fu Bing Fang Zhi Yan Jiu Tong Xun *(Research Journal on Prevention and Treatment of Dermatological Disorders)*, 1972; 3: 215.

Shan Xi Yi Kan *(Shanxi Journal of Medicine)*, 1960; (10): 32.

Sheng Yao Xue Za Zhi *(Journal of Raw Herbology)*, 1979; 33(3): 178.

Schoen A. Veterinary Acupuncture: Ancient Art to Modern Medicine. *American Vet Pub, Inc*, California, 1994.

Xin Yi Xue *(New Medicine)*, 1975; 6(3): 155.

Xin Zhong Yi *(New Chinese Medicine)*, 1989; 21(3): 51.

Zhong Cao Yao *(Chinese Herbal Medicine)* 1991; 22 (10): 452.

Zhong Cao Yao Xue *(Study of Chinese Herbal Medicine)*, 1980;932.

Zhong Guo Yao Ke Da Xue Xue Bao *(Journal of University of Chinese Herbology)*, 1990;21 (4):222.

Zhong Guo Zhong Yao Za Zhi *(People's Republic of China Journal of Chinese Herbology)*, 1991; 16(9): 560.

Zhong Yao Cai *(Study of Chinese Herbal Material)*, 1985; (2): 36.

Zhong Yao Cai *(Study of Chinese Herbal Material)*, 1991; 14(2): 41.

Zhong Yao Xue *(Chinese Herbology)*, 1998; 89:91.

Zhong Yao Xue *(Chinese Herbology)*, 1998;103:106.

Zhong Yao Xue *(Chinese Herbology)*, 1998; 318: 320.

Zhong Yao Yao Li Yu Ying Yong *(Pharmacology and Applications of Chinese Herbs)*, 1983: 400.

Zhong Yao Yao Li Yu Ying Yong *(Pharmacology and Applications of Chinese Herbs)*; 1983; 866.

Zhong Yao Yao Li Yu Ying Yong *(Pharmacology and Applications of Chinese Herbs)*, 1983; 888.

Zhong Yao Zhi *(Chinese Herbology Journal)* 1993:183.

Zhong Yao Zhi *(Chinese Herbology Journal)*, 1993; 358.

Homotoxicology references

Boericke W. Materia Medica with Repertory, 9th ed. 1927. Santa Rosa, CA: Boericke and Tafel, pp 597–500.

Becker-Witt C, Ludtke R, Weisshuhn T, Willich S. Diagnoses and treatment in homeopathic medical practice. *Forsch Komplementarmed Klass Naturheilkd*, 2004. Apr;11(2): pp 98–103.

Broadfoot P. Homotox and Skin. 2005. Heel Veterinary Congress, Memphis, TN.

Heel. BHI Homeopathic Therapy: Professional Reference. Albuquerque, NM: Heel Inc. 2002. pp 28–9, 96.

Macleod G. A Veterinary Materia Medica and Clinical Repertory with a Materia Medica of the Nosodes. Safron, Walden: CW Daniel Company, LTD. 1983. p 77–8, 150.

Palmquist R. 2003. Unpublished case series using BHI Inflammation before prescription of antihistamine for control of pruritus in atopic dogs with mild signs.

Paterson S. Additive Benefits of EFAs In Dogs With Atopic Dermatitis After Partial Response to Antihistamine Therapy, *J Small Anim Pract.* 1995; Sep;36(9):389–94.

Reckeweg H. Biotherapeutic Index: Ordinatio Antihomotoxica et Materia Medica, 5th ed. Baden-Baden, Germany: Biologische Heilmittel Heel GMBH, 2000. pp 292–3, 337–8, 399–400, 407–8.

Reinhart E. Liver and Metabolic Diseases. In: Proceedings of 1st Annual Veterinary Congress, Memphis, TN. 2005. Nov 11-13, Heel, pp 22.

Saevik BK, Bergvall K, Holm BR, Saijonmaa-Koulumies LE, Hedhammar A, Larsen S, Kristensen F. A randomized, controlled study to evaluate the steroid sparing effect of essential fatty acid supplementation in the treatment of canine atopic dermatitis. *Veterinary Dermatology* 2004. 15 (3), 137–145.

Witt C, Ludtke R, Baur R, Willich S. Homeopathic medical practice: long-term results of a cohort study with 3981 patients. *BMC Public Health*, 2005. Nov 3(5): pp 115.

ALOPECIA

Definition and cause

Alopecia is one of the most common conditions seen by veterinarians. It is often a result of multiple underlying causes with the secondary ramification of loss of hair. The broad categories of alopecia are (1) genetic predisposition, and (2) acquired, such as inflammatory, infectious (bacterial, fungal), immune-mediated, hormonal imbalances, parasitic, and secondary to other diseases such as hypothyroidism, Cushing's, etc. (Griffin 1993, Helton-Rhodes 1990, McKeever 1998, Paterson 2000, Schmeitzel 1994, Scott 1995, Tilley 2003).

Medical therapy rationale, drug(s) of choice, and nutritional recommendations

Therapy for alopecia relies upon the proper and accurate diagnosis, because the underlying cause dictates the course of therapy. Please refer to other sections in this book for underlying causes and their appropriate therapies.

Anticipated prognosis

Because alopecia is most often secondary to multiple underlying causes, the prognosis varies with the primary cause.

Integrative veterinary therapies

An integrative approach to alopecia starts with a determination of the underlying cause. If the cause can be identified and addressed, the alopecia usually resolves.

The use of nutrients, nutraceuticals, medicinal herbs, and combination homeopathics that help balance gland function, reduce inflammation, and prevent cellular degeneration should be part of the therapeutic approach to alopecia.

Nutrition
General considerations/rationale
When searching for the underlying cause and proper diagnosis, a medical and physiological blood evaluation should be included as part of the clinician's diagnostic protocol. This nutrition-based information gives clinicians the ability to formulate therapeutic nutritional protocols that address the local lesions as well as underlying organ conditions that may be ultimately responsible for the surface condition. For example, identifying early thyroid and pituitary weakness and supporting their function with appropriate nutrients, antioxidants, and gland support can help re-establish a normal coat. (See chapter 2, Nutritional Blood Testing for more information.)

Appropriate nutrients
Nutritional/gland therapy: Glandular hypothalamus, pituitary, and lymph provide intrinsic nutrients that nourish and help neutralize cellular immune inflammation and help improve organ function (see Gland Therapy, Chapter 2, for a more detailed explanation).

Zinc: Zinc is a mineral that particularly benefits metabolism and skin health. Zinc-responsive dermatosis is a common deficiency disease in animals; it is found often in huskies, malamutes, and large-breed puppies (Griffin 1993, Werner 2003).

Essential fatty acids: Research has been conducted on the importance of essential fatty acids in the daily diet, and on the clinical management of various degenerative diseases (Reinhart 1996, Holub 1995, Herman 1998). The importance of the ratio between omega-6 and omega-3 fatty acids has been substantiated. Research on polyunsaturated fatty acids has shown their beneficial and antipruritic affects on skin (Reinhart 1996, Schick 1996).

Chinese herbal medicine
General considerations/rationale
According to TCM theory, alopecia is a result of Yin and Blood deficiency in the Liver and Kidney, accompanied by blockage of the meridians. The Liver and Kidney control the Blood. The fur is the end of the Blood, according to TCM. Without Blood and fluids (Yin), there is no fluid to nourish the skin. Similarly, if the meridians are blocked, nourishment cannot get to the skin to allow the fur to grow. Without nourishment, the follicles become inactive.

The etiology of the Yin and Blood deficiency must be corrected to heal the patient. In Western practice this means that not only is the hair loss treated, but the cause of the alopecia must also be addressed. To modern practitioners, this means any immune dysfunction, pathogen infection, or hormonal imbalance must be corrected.

Appropriate Chinese herbs
Actractylodes (Cang zhu): Has anti-inflammatory effects. Experimentally, it has been shown to ameliorate swelling caused by treatment with xylene, carrageenin, and acetic acid (Zhang 1998). It also inhibits Staphylococcus aureus and some dermatophytes (Zhong Yao Xue 1998).

Angelica (Bai zhi): Has demonstrated anti-inflammatory properties in mice (Zhong Guo Zhong Yao Za Zhi 1991), which suggests efficacy in any inflammatory type of alopecia.

Angelica root (Dang gui): Was used in 40 patients with alopecia areata, an immune-mediated skin disease in which the follicles are attacked, leading to baldness or hair loss on the entire body. In this trial, all 40 patients had improvement in their symptoms (Shan Xi Zhong Yi 1987).

Buffalo horn shavings (Shui niu jiao): Has anti-inflammatory effects. It has been shown to decrease experimentally induced edema in the ears and feet of mice (Mao 1997). It may help promote cellular immunity. It increases the leukocyte count (Wu 1985), which may help in cases of infectious alopecia.

Bupleurum (Chai hu): Stimulates both humoral and cellular immunity in mice (Shang Hai Yi Ke Da Xue Xue Bao 1986), which may help in cases of alopecia of infectious etiology. In addition it has been shown to inhibit various bacteria (Zhong Yao Xue 1988). Bupleurum has anti-inflammatory effects, as was demonstrated in a mouse model using dimethyl-benzene-induced ear swelling (Liu 1998).

Cnidium (Chuan xiong): Stimulates the cellular immunity. It increases phagocytic function of macrophages (Lang 1991, Zhao 1993, Cheng 1993). It also stimulates the humoral immune system. It can also promote the formation of sheep red blood cells (SRBC) antibody in mice (Lang 1991).

Dandelion (Pu gong ying): Has demonstrated antibacterial efficacy against many bacteria, including Staph aureus and beta-hemolytic streptococci (Zhong Yi Yao Xue Bao 1991).

Earthworm (Di long): Has immunostimulant properties. It improves macrophage function (Zhang Feng Chun 1998). It also promotes wound healing. Earthworm was shown to enhance the production of fibroblasts and capillaries in experimentally induced wounds in rabbits. It also increased the healing rate of the skin (Zhang 1999).

Fleece flower root (He shou wu): Increases thyroid hormone secretion (Zhong Yao Yao Li Yu Lin Chuang 1989). This may be beneficial in cases of hypothyroid-induced alopecia. Furthermore, it has been shown to inhibit a variety of bacteria including Staphylococcus aureus (Zhen 1986). It may prove efficacious in cases of bacterial pyoderma.

Honeysuckle (Jin yin hua): Has demonstrated antibacterial properties. This is due in large part to the action of chlorogenic acid and isochlorogenic acid. Among the bacteria these compounds inhibit are Staphylococcus aureus, beta-hemolytic streptococci, and E coli (Xin Yi Xue 1975, Jiang 1960).

Kochia (Di fu pi): Has been shown to inhibit some dermatophytes (Yun Nan Zhong Yao Zhi 1990).

Licorice (Gan cao): Has demonstrated a complex effect on the immune system. It has shown the ability to both stimulate and inhibit the phagocytic activity of macrophages (Zhong Yao Xue 1998). It also contains glycyrrhizin and glycyrrhetinic acid, which have approximately 10% of the corticosteroid activity of cortisone and decrease the permeability of blood vessels and interfere with histamine action (Zhong Cao Yao 1991). These actions suggest that licorice may be useful in allergic, immune-mediated, and infectious alopecia. In addition it has antibiotic effects on different bacteria including Staphylococcus aureus (Zhong Yao Zhi 1993).

Mint (Bo he): Has demonstrated anti-inflammatory properties (Zhong Yao Xue 19981). This may make it useful in inflammation-mediated alopecic condition.

Mouton (Mu dan pi): Reduces inflammation. In mice it was shown to decrease dimethylbenzene-induced inflammation in the ear (Wu 1990). It also may treat bacterial dermatitis. It has a direct inhibitory effect on multiple strains of bacteria including Staphylococcus aureus and beta-hemolytic streptococci (Zhong Yao Cai 1991). It has been shown to enhance phagocytosis of peripheral neutrophils on Staphylococcus aureus (Li 1994).

Platycodon (Jie geng): Prevents allergic reactions and decreases capillary permeability (Zhong Yao Yao Li Yu Ying Yong 1983). It has been shown to promote the secretion of corticosterone in rats (Li 1984, Zhang 1984, Zhou 1979), which suggests that it is indicated in cases of allergic pyoderma.

Poria (Fu ling): Inhibits Staphylococcus aureus, among other bacteria (Nanjing College of Pharmacy 1976).

Rehmannia (Sheng di huang): Increases the level of estradiol in females and testosterone in male rats (Chen 1993). This may be applicable in cases of hormone-responsive alopecia. It also has anti-inflammatory properties. It reduces swelling and inflammation (Zhong Yao Yao Li Yu Ying Yong 1983).

Schizonepeta (Jing jie): Decreases the signs in cases of pruritic rashes and itching (Zhong Yi Za Zhi 12:18).

Scutellaria (Huang qin): Contains biacalin, which has antibiotic activity against Stapylococcus aureus, b-hemo-

lytic streptococcus, as well as other bacteria and some dermatophytes. Biacilin can have synergistic effects with ampicillin, amoxicillin, methacillin, and cefotaxime. It can help overcome B lactam resistance (Zhong Yao Xue 1988, Liu 2000). Biacalein has an added benefit of suppressing inflammation (Kubo 1984). It has been shown experimentally to decrease swelling induced by dimethylbenzene and formaldehyde (Cao 1999). While decreasing inflammation, it also enhances cellular immunity. It enhances production of IL2, which stimulates the cellular immune system (Pan Ju Fen 1991).

Siegesbeckia (Xi xian cao): Possesses anti-inflammatory properties. It has been shown to decrease swelling in rats. (Zhong Yao Yao Li Yu Ying Yong 1983). It decreases both humoral and cellular immunity in mice (Zhong Guo Zhong Yao Za Zhi 1989), which suggests that it may be of use in immune-mediated cases of alopecia. Furthermore, it has antibiotic actions and may be of benefit in bacterial etiologies (Kim 1979).

Siler (Fang feng): Has been shown to inhibit various bacteria, including Staphylococcus aureus (Zhong Yao Tong Bao 1988).

Silkworm (Jiang can): Has antibiotic effects. It has been shown to affect Staphylococcus aureus and other bacteria (Zhong Yao Xue 1998).

White peony (Bai shao): Has antibiotic properties against a variety of bacterian including both Staphylococcus aureus and beta-hemolytic streptococci. It also inhibits some dermatophytes (Xin Zhong Yi 1989). It contains Paeoniflorin, which is a strong anti-inflammatory (Zhong Yao Zhi 1993). These capabilities may make it useful for bacterial, fungal, allergic, and immune-mediated alopecia.

Xanthium (Cang er zi): Decreases histamine-mediated increases in capillary permeability (Huang 1996). This indicates that it may be of use in allergy-mediated alopecic conditions.

Homotoxicology
General considerations/rationale
Alopecia can occur as a consequence of Inflammation, Deposition, Impregnation, Degeneration, or Dedifferentiation phase disorders. Proper diagnosis is needed to select therapy. In Inflammation Phase disorders, simply treating the primary cause usually results in regrowth of hair. In deeper homotoxicoses, hair growth may be delayed or may not occur.

Appropriate homotoxicology formulas
(Also see other protocols such as Cushing's, hypothyroidism, pancreatic insufficiency, etc).

Cutis compositum: Stimulates healing and detoxification of the skin.

Aesculus homaccord: Supports vascular repair.

BHI-Hair and -Skin: Used for alopecia, dandruff, acne, poor toenails, dry hair coat, postvaccinal hair loss, and hair loss after severely debilitating disease (Heel 2002).

BHI-Skin: Treats eczema, rashes and redness, blisters, and cold sores.

Cerebrum compositum: Supports cerebral tissues.

Coenzyme compositum: Provides metabolic support.

Galium-Heel: Used for cellular and matrix drainage and detoxification, and after vaccination reactions.

Hepar compositum: Supports hepatic tissue.

Lymphomyosot: Provides lymph drainage and support.

Ovarium compositum: Treats endocrine alopecia in females.

Placenta compositum: Used to improve vascularization of extremities.

Psorinoheel: Phase remedy in Excretion and Impregnation phase disorders, intense pruritus of elbows and legs, warts, and excretion of malodorous material.

Pulsatilla compositum: Used for type two regulation rigidity.

Selenium homaccord: Used in conjunction with *Psorinoheel*.

Solidago compositum: Provides support of renal tissues.

Sulfur Heel: Provides general support of mesenchymal structures.

Testis compositum: Supports endocrine alopecias in males.

Thuja homaccord: Used in post vaccinal alopecia.

Thyroidea compositum: Provides endocrine support and deep detoxification and matrix drainage.

Tonsilla compositum: Supports endocrine and central controls.

Traumeel S: Used for type one regulation rigidity and after inflammatory skin issues such as allergies or vaccination reactions.

Ubichinon compositum: Provides metabolic support.

Ypsiloheel: Used for central regulation.

Authors' suggested protocols

Nutrition

Pituitary/hypothalamus/pineal and skin support formula: 1 tablet for every 25 pounds of body weight BID. When indicated, lymph and thyroid support formulas may be added.

Zinc: 15 mg for every 25 pounds of body weight SID.

Eskimo fish oil: One-half to 1 teaspoon per meal for cats. 1 teaspoon for every 35 pounds of body weight for dogs.

Omega-3,-6,-9: 1 capsule for every 25 pounds of body weight with food.

Chinese herbal medicine

The authors recommend a full diagnostic work-up to determine the cause of alopecia because it is a symptom, not a diagnosis. For most causes of alopecia the authors recommend a combination of DermGuard and Immuno-Derm at a dose of 1 capsule of each herbal supplement per 10 to 20 pounds twice daily.

DermGuard contains angelica (Bai zhi), angelica root (Dang gui), aurantium fruit (Zhi qiao), bupleurum (Chai hu), cicada (Chan tui), cnidium (Chuan xiong), honeysuckle (Jin yin hua), licorice (Gan cao), mint (Bo he), moutan (Mu dan pi), platycodon (Jie geng), poria (Fu ling), schizonepeta (Jing jie), scutellaria (Huang qin), siegesbeckia (Xi xian cao), siler (Fang feng), silkworm (Jiang can), and xanthium fruit (Cang er zi).

ImmunoDerm contains atractylodes (Cang zhu), angelica root (Dang gui), buffalo horn shavings (Shui niu jiao), bupleurum (Chai hu), dandelion (Pu gong ying), earthworm (Di long), fleece flower root (He shou wu), honeysuckle (Jin yin hua), kochia (Di fu zi), licorice (Gan cao), moutan (Mu dan pi), oldenlandia (Bai hua she cao), poria (Fu ling), rehmannia—raw (Sheng di huang), scutellaria (Huang qin), siegesbeckia (Xi xian cao), tokoro (Bi xie), white peony (Bai shao), and xanthium fruit (Cang er zi).

Homotoxicology (Dose: 10 drops PO for 50-pound dog; 5 drops PO small dog or cat)

Symptom formula: Psorinoheel, Selenium homaccord, Galium-Heel, BHI-Hair and Skin, and Sulfur-Heel mixed together and given BID PO. In acute cases, Traumeel or BHI-Hair and Skin as single agents may suffice.

Deep detoxification formula: Thyroidea compositum, Solidago compositum, and Hepar compositum given every three days. Cutis compositum given every seven days.

Product sources

Nutrition

Pituitary/hypothalamus/pineal, skin, lymph and thyroid support formulas: Animal Nutrition Technologies. **Alternatives**: Derma Strength—Vetri Science Laboratories; Canine Dermal and Thyroid Support—Standard Process Veterinary Formulas.

Omega-3,-6,-9: Vetri Science. **Alternatives**: Eskimo fish oil—Tyler Encapsulations; flax oil—Barlean's Organic Oils; hemp oil—Nature's Perfect Oil; Ultra EFA—Rx Vitamins for Pets.

Chinese herbal medicine

Derm Guard and ImmunoDerm: Natural Solutions, Inc.

Homotoxicology

BHI/Heel Corporation

REFERENCES

Western medicine references

Griffin C, Kwochka K, Macdonald J. Current Veterinary Dermatology. 1993. Linn, MO: Mosby Publications.

Helton-Rhodes KA. Cutaneous manifestations of canine and feline endocrinopathies. In: Nichols R, ed. *Probl Vet Med* 1990;12:617–627.

McKeever PJ, Harvey RG. Skin Diseases of the Dog and Cat. 1998. Ames, IA: Iowa State University Press.

Paterson S. Skin Diseases of the Cat. 2000. London: Blackwell Science Ltd.

Schmeitzel LP. Growth hormone responsive alopecia and sex hormone associated dermatoses. In: Birchard SJ, Sherding RG, eds. Saunders manual of small animal practice, Philadelphia: Saunders, 1994:326–330.

Scott DW, Griffin CE, Miller BH. Acquired alopecia. In: Muller and Kirk's small animal dermatology. 5th ed. Philadelphia: Saunders, 1995:720–735.

Scott DW, Griffin CE, Miller BH. Keratinization defects. In: Muller and Kirk's small animal dermatology. 5th ed. Philadelphia: Saunders, 1995:736–805.

Tilley L, Smith F. The 5-Minute Veterinary Consult: Canine and Feline, Blackwell Publishing, 2003.

IVM/nutrition references

Griffin CE, Kwochka KW, Macdonald JM. Current veterinary dermatology: the science and art of therapy. 1993. St. Louis: Mosby.

Werner AH. Dermatosis, Exfoliative, In: Tilley L, Smith F. The 5-Minute Veterinary Consult: Canine and Feline, 2003. Blackwell Publishing.

Herman HA, et al. The Influence of Dietary Omega-6:Omega-3 Ratio in Lameness in Dogs with Osteoarthrosis of the Elbow Joint. Recent Advances in Canine and Feline Nutrition, 1998, Volume II, Iams Proceedings p 325.

Holub B. The Role of Omega-3 Fatty Acids in Health and Disease. 1995.Proceeding of the 13th Annual American College of Veterinary Medicine.

Reinhart GA. A Controlled Dietary Omega-6:Omega-3 Ratio Reduces Pruritus in Nonfood Allergic Atopic Dogs. Recent Advances in Canine and Feline Nutritional Research: Iams Proceedings, 1996. p 277.

Schick MP, Schick R. Reinhart G. The Role of Polyunsaturated Fatty Acids in the Canine Epidermis, Recent Advances in Canine and Feline Nutritional Research: Iams Proceedings, 1996. p 267.

Chinese herbal medicine/acupuncture references

Cao ZS, et al. *Strait Journal of Pharmacology.* 1999;11(3): 53–54.

Chen J, Zang Y, Wu Q. Effect of jingui shenqi pills on sex hormone in aged rats, *China Journal of Chinese Materia Medica* 1993;18(10) 619.

Cheng JX, et al. *Journal of Practical Integrated Medicine.* 1993;6(5):261.

Huang SY, et al. *Journal of TCM Pharmacology and Clinical Application.* 1996;12(3):28–29.

Jiang Xi Xin Yi Yao *(Jiangxi New Medicine and Herbology),* 1960 (1):34.

Kim JH, Han KD, Yamasaki K, Tanaka O. *Phytochemistry,* 1979; 18(5):894.

Kubo M, Matsuda H, Tanaka M, Kimura Y, Okuda H, Higashino M, Tani T, Namba K, Arichi S. Studies on Scutellariae radix. VII. Anti-arthritic and anti-inflammatory actions of methanolic extract and flavonoid components from Scutellariae radix. *Chem Pharm Bull,* 1984; 32(7):2724–9.

Lang XC, et al. *Journal of Hebei Medical College.* 1991;12(3): 140.

Li FC, et al. *China Journal of Integrated Medicine.* 1994;14(1): 37–38.

Li YF (translator). *Foreign Medicine, vol. of TCM.* 1984;6(1): 15–18.

Liu IX, Durham DG, Richards RM. Baicalin synergy with beta-lactam antibiotics against methicillin-resistant Staphylococcus aureus and other beta-lactam-resistant strains of S. aureus. *J Pharm Pharmacol.* 2000; Mar;52(3):361–6.

Liu W, et al. *Henan Journal of TCM Pharmacy.* 1998;13(4): 10–12.

Mao XJ, et al. Experimental research on mixture of Cao Wu and Shui Niu Jiao. *Journal of Yunnan College of TCM.* 1997; 19(7):33–34.

Nanjing College of Pharmacy. Materia Medica, vol. 2. Jiangsu: People's Press; 1976.

Pan JF, et al. *Tianjin Journal of Medicine.* 1991;19(8): 468–470.

Shan Xi Zhong Yi *(Shanxi Chinese Medicine),* 1987;9:419.

Shang Hai Yi Ke Da Xue Xue Bao *(Journal of Shanghai University of Medicine),* 1986; 13(1): 20.

Wu GZ, et al. *Journal of University of Pharmacology of China.* 1990;21(4).

Wu XY, et al. Brief discussion on Shui Niu Jiao. *Journal of Traditional Chinese Medicine Material.* 1985;(5):41,38.

Xin Yi Xue *(New Medicine),* 1975; 6(3): 155.

Xin Zhong Yi *(New Chinese Medicine),* 1989; 21(3):51.

Yun Nan Zhong Yao Zhi *(Yunnan Journal of Chinese Herbal Medicine),* 1990;244.

Zhang FC, et al. Di Long's enhancing effect on macrophages' immune activity. *China Journal of Pharmacy.* 1998;33(9): 532–535.

Zhang FC, et al. Research into Di Long's mechanism in its recovery effects on rabbit back injury. *China Journal of Pharmacy.* 1999;34(2):93–96.

Zhang MF, et al. *Journal of Pharmacology and Clinical Application of TCM.* 1998;14(6):12–16.

Zhang SC, et al. *Journal of Chinese Patent Medicine Research.* 1984;(2):37.

Zhao ZB, et al. *Sichuan Journal of Traditional Chinese Medicine.* 1993;11(11):13.

Zhen HC, et al. *Chinese Medicine Bulletin.* 1986;(3):53.

Zhong Cao Yao *(Chinese Herbal Medicine),* 1991;22 (10):452.

Zhong Guo Zhong Yao Za Zhi *(People's Republic of China Journal of Chinese Herbology),* 1989; 14(3):44.

Zhong Guo Zhong Yao Za Zhi *(People's Republic of China Journal of Chinese Herbology),* 1991; 16(9):560.

Zhong Yao Cai *(Study of Chinese Herbal Material),* 1991; 14(2):41

Zhong Yao Tong Bao *(Journal of Chinese Herbology)*, 1988:13(6):364.

Zhong Yao Xue *(Chinese Herbology)*, 1988;103:106.

Zhong Yao Xue *(Chinese Herbology)*, 1988; 137:140.

Zhong Yao Xue *(Chinese Herbology)*, 1998; 89:91.

Zhong Yao Xue *(Chinese Herbology)*, 1998; 318:320.

Zhong Yao Xue *(Chinese Herbology)*, 1998; 706:708.

Zhong Yao Xue *(Chinese Herbology)*, 1998; 759:766.

Zhong Yao Yao Li Yu Ying Yong *(Pharmacology and Applications of Chinese Herbs)*, 1983:400.

Zhong Yao Yao Li Yu Ying Yong *(Pharmacology and Applications of Chinese Herbs)*; 1983;866.

Zhong Yao Yao Li Yu Lin Chuang *(Pharmacology and Clinical Applications of Chinese Herbs)*, 1989; 5(1):24.

Zhong Yao Yao Li Yu Ying Yong *(Pharmacology and Applications of Chinese Herbs)*, 1983:1221.

Zhong Yao Zhi *(Chinese Herbology Journal)*, 1993:183.

Zhong Yao Zhi *(Chinese Herbology Journal)*, 1993;358.

Zhong Yi Yao Xue Bao *(Report of Chinese Medicine and Herbology)*, 1991;(1):41.

Zhong Yi Za Zhi *(Journal of Chinese Medicine)*, 12:18.

Zhou WZ, et al. *Pharmacy Bulletin.* 1979;14(5):202–203.

Homotoxicology reference

Heel. *BHI Homeopathic Therapy: Professional Reference.* 2002. Albuquerque, NM: Heel Inc. p 62.

CHRONIC PYODERMA

Definition and cause

Broadly defined as a secondary bacterial infection of the skin, pyoderma is one of the most common diseases seen in dogs. It is less common in cats. In most instances the surface of the skin has been compromised and bacteria infections are initiated. Pyodermas are classified as superficial and deep, and arise secondary to allergies and/or in combination with compromised immune function. The most common canine bacterial skin infection is caused by staphylococci. Some pyodermas can be secondary to other diseases such as hypothyroidism and Cushing's disease. (Carlotti 1996; Codner 2003; Day 1994; Ihrke 1978, 1987, 1996; Kwochka 1993; Miller 1991; Muller 1989).

Medical therapy rationale, drug(s) of choice, and nutritional recommendations

The approach to pyodermas is often topical, local, and systemic. The treatment of choice is the use of medicated shampoos and lotions such as chlorhexidine or benzoyl peroxide in combination with systemic antibiotics. Corticosteroids are not recommended due to the potential exacerbation of the infection. The dietary recommendation is a high-quality, hypoallergenic type of diet. Immunotherapy with bacterins such as Staph Lysate has proven to be successful in superficial pyodermas (Staph-age Lysate©) (Day 1994; Krishnan 1994; Lloyd 1992; Mason 1989, 1990; Morales 1994; Nesbitt 1983; Van Kampen 1997).

Anticipated prognosis

Pyodermas, especially the superficial types, are quite responsive to therapy. However, both superficial and deep pyodermas tend to recur, become chronic, and are often less responsive to medical therapy. This may be due to compromised local and immune system function.

Integrative veterinary therapies

In Western medical terms, the bacterial growth on the skin is the focus of therapy. In IVM therapies, the bacteria is viewed as secondary to the skin's detoxification process. Bacteria are attracted and replicate in areas that favor their growth. Patients that exude material onto their skin in an attempt to detoxify themselves, with faulty digestion, with defective cutaneous function, or that suffer from altered immunity from a wide variety of causes, are all prone to pyoderma. Parasites, food sensitivities, allergies, endocrinopathies, and a host of other causes such as adverse reactions to drugs, vaccinations, herbs, and some supplements may be involved in chronic recurring pyoderma.

Careful historical and physical evaluation is indicated in all cases, and skin scraping is recommended. In more advanced cases, full laboratory evaluation including CBC, serum chemistries, and thyroid testing are always indicated. Other tests such as further endocrine evaluation, urinalysis, culture and sensitivity, and skin biopsy may be needed. Insufficient treatment duration or client noncompliance is also a common reason for recurrent infections of the skin.

Topical therapy is an important part of any treatment plan. Gentle products that remove exudates are desirable. In more serious cases products that flush the pores and remove debris such as benzoyl peroxide are useful. Antibiotic, antifungal, and antibacterial shampoos should be reserved for cases that do not respond to biological therapy to avoid further intoxification of the cutaneous tissues. In cases requiring systemic antibiotics, it is necessary to treat for at least 3 weeks to get full resolution. Probiotics are recommended in cases undergoing antibiotic therapy because antibiotics can damage the intestinal mucosa and lead to alterations in digestive and immune system function.

Nutrition
General considerations/rationale

While medical therapy is focused externally, therapeutic nutrition adds nutrients, antioxidants, and organ support to help reduce inflammation and enhance detoxification and elimination. In addition, the skin, which is the largest and most visible organ, is often a barometer of internal imbalances, inflammation, and disorders. Therefore, it is especially important in chronic recurrent pyodermas to look past the skin and assess all internal organs for early or overt inflammation or disease. It is therefore recommended that clinicians evaluate the blood both medically and physiologically as a method of assessing glandular health. This information gives clinicians the ability to formulate therapeutic nutritional protocols that address the local lesions as well as underlying organ conditions that may be ultimately responsible for the surface condition (see Chapter 2, Nutritional Blood Testing).

Appropriate nutrients

Nutritional/gland therapy: Glandular adrenal, thymus, and lymph provide intrinsic nutrients that nourish and help neutralize cellular immune inflammation and degeneration (see Gland Therapy, Chapter 2, for a more detailed explanation).

Lecithin/phosphatidyl choline: Phosphatidyl choline is a phospholipid that is integral to cellular membranes, particularly those of nerve and brain cells. It helps to move fats into the cells, and it is involved in neurotransmission and acetylcholine, and particularly with cellular integrity. Lecithin, which is part of the cell membranes, is an essential nutrient required by the skin and all of the cells of the body for general health and wellness (Hanin 1987).

Sterols: Plant-derived sterols such as betasitosterol show anti-inflammatory properties which appear to be similar to corticosteriods (Gupta 1980). A cortisone-like effect without the associated immune-suppressing effects is beneficial in immune-mediated conditions. Bouic (1996) reports on the immune-enhancing and balancing effect of plant sterols, which are also beneficial to animals with immune-mediated disease.

Probiotics: Administration of the proper combination of probiotics has been reported to have a positive impact on the intestines and the digestive process (Goldin 1984, Perdigon 1987). Probiotics have been shown to improve and aid the digestive process by secreting their own source of enzymes, which is beneficial for immune-compromised animals (McDonough 1987).

Evening primrose oil (EPO): In diseases of the skin, evening primrose oil has been proven to have both anti-inflammatory and anti-pruritic effects, and is part of a balanced nutritional program that can exert a positive effect on animals with skin disease. Studies suggest that EPO is beneficial in people with atopic dermatitis and eczema (Hederos 1996, Humphreys 1994, Morse 1989).

Chinese herbal medicine/acupuncture
General considerations/rationale

Practitioners of TCM consider pyoderma to be caused by Heat and Toxins in the Lung. In general, skin infections are related to either immune deficiency or immune disorders with secondary bacterial infection. There is also often an allergic factor. The Lung controls the Skin, so Heat in the Lung translates to inflammation on the Skin. Toxins refer to the inflammatory mediators seen in dermatitis.

Appropriate Chinese herbs

Angelica (Bai zhi): Inhibits multiple strains of bacteria (Zhong Yao Yao Li Yu Ying Yong 1983) and is anti-inflammatory (Zhong Guo Zhong Yao Za Zhi 1991).

Angelica root (Dang gui): Stimulates the immune system by increasing the phagocytic activity of macrophages (Zhong Hua Yi Xue Za Zhi 1978). It also inhibits many types of bacteria (Hou 1981).

Atractylodes (Cang zhu): Has activity against Staphylococcus auerus and dermatophytes (Zhong Yao Xue 1998).

Bupleurum (Chai hu): Has antibiotic effects against streptococci (Zhong Yao Xue 1998).

Cnidium (Chuan xiong): Enhances the immune system. It increases the phagocytic ability of macrophages and increases antibody formation (Lang 1991, Zhao 1993, Cheng 1993, Lang 1991).

Dandelion (Pu gong ying): Has antibiotic activity against a variety of bacteria including Staphylococcus aureus, b-hemolytic streptococci, and Pseudomonas aeruginosa (Zhong Yi Yao Xue Bao 1991). In addition, it may possess anti-inflammatory actions (Mascolo 1987).

Earthworm (Di long): Stimulates the immune system. It has been shown to increase the phagocytic activity of macrophages in mice. It may also shorten the inflammation period, promote fibroblast activity, and enhance the healing rate of the epidermis, thereby promoting the resolution of dermatological lesions (Zhang 1998).

Honeysuckle (Jin yin hua): Has antibiotic effects against Staphylococcus aureus, E. coli, and Pseudomonas aeruginosa (Xin Yi Xue 1975), and is anti-inflammatory (Shan Xi Yi Kan 1960).

Kochia (Di fu zi): Inhibits some dermatophytes and fungi (Yun Nan Zhong Yao Zhi 1990).

Licorice (Gan cao): Inhibits the growth of Staphylococcus aureus (Zhong Yao Zhi 1993).

Mint (Bo he): Has anti-inflammatory effects (Zhong Yao Xue 1998).

Moutan (Mu dan pi): Inhibits the growth of Staphylococcus aureus, streptococci, and dermatophytes (Zhong Yao Cai 1991).

Platycodon (Jie geng): Decreases inflammation by increasing the secretion of corticosterone (Li 1984, Zhang 1984, Zhou 1979).

Polygonum (He shou wu): Increases hormonal secretion by the thyroid gland (Zhong Yao Yao Li Yu Lin Chuang 1989). Many animals are hypothyroid and it is necessary to address this imbalance to gain control over the disease process. This herb also enhances immunity. It increases the total white cell count, especially the T-cells. It also increases the phagocytic activity of macrophages (Zhong Yao Yao Li Yu Lin Chuang 1989) and it stimulates the activity of B cells (Zhou 1989).

Poria (Fu ling): Has inhibitory effects on Staphylococcus aureus (Zhong Yao Cai 1985).

Rehmannia (Sheng di huang): Has shown anti-inflammatory activity in mice (Zhong Yao Yao Li Yu Ying Yong 1983).

Schizonepeta (Jing jie): Has been shown to have efficacy against pruritic dermatological conditions (Zhong Yi Za Zhi).

Scutellaria (Huang qin): Contains biacalin, which has antibiotic activity against many bacteria including Stapylococcus aureus and some dermatophytes. This compound not only acts on its own, but also is synergistic with some penicillins and can help overcome B lactam resistance (Zhong Yao Xue 1988, Liu 2000). Biacalin, along with another component of scutellaria, biacalein, have anti-inflammatory effects (Kubo 1984). Patients with chronic pyoderma may benefit from stimulation of the immune system to help the body fight the pathogens. Scutellaria enhances the cellular immunity and increases production of IL2 (Pan 1991).

Siegesbeckia (Xi xian cao): Inhibits the growth of Staphylococcus aureus (Kim 1979).

Siler (Fang feng): Inhibits bacteria, including Staphylococcus aureus (Zhong Yao Tong Bao 1988).

Silkworm larva (Jiang can): Inhibits bacteria, including Stapylococcus aureus, E. coli, and Pseudomonas aeruginosa (Zhong Yao Xue 1998).

Water buffalo horn (Shui niu jiao): Enhances immunity. It increases the total white blood cell count (Mao 1997). A second experiment by Wu Xiao Yi showed that this increase in white blood cell count was accompanied by an increase in antibody production (Wu 1985).

White peony (Bai shao): Contains paeoniflorin, which is a strong anti-inflammatory (Zhong Yao Zhi 1993:183). It also has antibiotic effects against Staphylococcus aureus, some streptococci, E. coli, Pseudomonas aeruginosa, and some dermatophytes (Xin Zhong Yi 1989).

Homotoxicology
General considerations/rationale

Simple pyoderma is an Inflammation Phase disorder. Aggravations caused by homeopathic substances can result in pyoderma. The appearance of pustular lesions may represent phase shift toward Inflammation Phase, which is a desirable step toward healing. The clinician must evaluate other signs to determine the most appropriate action in these regressive vicariation cases.

Chronic cases represent Impregnation or Degeneration phase homotoxicoses. So-called Alternative Phase disorders occur when deep, unseen homotoxicoses (neoplasia or precancerous conditions) shift their attempt to excrete toxic materials to the outside. Inhibiting Alternative Phase conditions can suppress needed excretory actions, internalize homotoxins, and lead to rapid progressive vicariation. Caution should be exercised when confronted with elderly pets presenting with recurring, focal, moist, eczema-type lesions. A careful search for other pathological conditions is advised in all such cases.

Appropriate homotoxicology formulas

Belladonna homaccord: Used for focal carbuncles and boils, and larger and more intensely red lesions.

BHI-Infection: Is similar to Echinacea compositum.

BHI-Inflammation: Small pustules, itchy skin, and possible lameness are signs to consider for this remedy. An older formulation contained Staph and Strep nosodes, but the new formulation no longer contains these ingredients, a change that has a negative impact on this product's efficacy in pyoderma cases. The authors hope that eventually the company will restore the original formula.

BHI-Skin: Used for skin infections, redness, eczema, and blisters.

Cutis compositum: Contains Hepar sulph and Histaminum, both of which indicated in pyodermas (Reckeweg 2002).

Echinacea compositum: Used for bacterial infections as a substitute for antibiotics.

Psorinoheel: an excretion Phase and Impregnation Phase remedy that is useful in a wide number of skin issues.

Schwef-Heel: Contains Sulphur, which is useful for minor pustular lesions, dry skin with red color, and malodorous pets.

Tonsilla compositum: Contains Baryta carbonica, Funiculus umbicalis suis, Geranium, Hepar suis, Mercurius solubilis, and Psorinum nosode, all of which have very strong indications for pustular skin diseases (Reckeweg 2002). This is often used as an initial autosanguis, or blood therapy.

Traumeel S: All pustular inflammations benefit from *Traumeel* due to its anti-inflammatory characteristics.

Authors' suggested protocols

Nutrition

Immune and skin support formulas: 1 tablet for every 25 pounds of body weight BID.

Lymph support formula: One-half tablet for every 25 pounds of body weight BID.

Lecithin/phosphatidyl choline: One-fourth teaspoon for every 25 pounds of body weight BID.

Betathyme: 1 capsule for every 35 pounds of body weight BID. (maximum 2 capsules BID)

Probiotic MPF: One-half capsule for every 25 pounds of body weight with food.

Oil of evening primrose: 1 capsule for every 25 pounds of body weight SID.

Chinese herbal medicine/acupuncture

The authors use a combination of ImmunoDerm and DermGuard, which stimulates and modulates the immune system and has anti-inflammatory effects and antibacterial function. It helps to control itch. The combination is administered at a dose of 1 capsule of each for every 10 to 20 pounds twice a day.

In addition to the herbs discussed above, these preparations contains bitter orange (Zhi ke), cicada slough (Chan tui), oldenlandia (Bai hua she cao), tokoro (Bi xie), and xanthium fruit (Cang er zi).)

Homotoxicology (Dose: 10 drops PO for 50-pound dog; 5 drops PO small dog or cat)

Therapy depends upon the primary causation. (See also allergy, atopy, food allergy, hypothyroidism, Cushing's Disease, etc.). In recurring cases autosanguis therapy is worthy of consideration. It is particularly useful to start with Tonsilla compositum and the catalysts Coenzyme compositum and/or Ubichinon compositum. Consider the following in combination with appropriate topical therapy:

Acute pyoderma: Psorinoheel plus Schwef-Heel plus Traumeel S BID PO. Cutis compositum once weekly. Also use Detox Kit BID PO.

Recurrent pyoderma: Psorinoheel plus Schwef-Heel plus BHI-Inflammation or Echinacea compositum plus Traumeel S BID PO. Cutis compositum every two weeks. Also use Deep Detox Formula (below).

Deep detoxification formula: Galium-Heel plus Lymphomyosot plus Thyroidea compositum plus Hepar compositum plus Solidago compositum plus Coenzyme compositum mixed together and taken orally twice weekly for 60 to 120 days.

Product sources

Nutrition

Immune, skin and lymph support formulas: Animal Nutrition Technologies. **Alternatives**: Immune system and Dermal support—Standard Process; Immuno support—Rx Vitamin for Pets; Derma Strength—Vetri Science; Immugen—Thorne Veterinary Products.

Lecithin/phosphatidyl choline: Designs for Health.

Betathyme: Best for your Pet. **Alternative**: Moducare—Thorne Veterinary Products.

Probiotic MPF: Progressive Labs, Rx Biotic, Rx Vitamins for Pets.

Oil of evening primrose: Jarrow Formulas.

Chinese herbal medicine

Immunoderm and DermGuard: White Crane Herbs; Natural Solutions, Inc.

Homotoxicology

BHI/Heel Corporation

REFERENCES

Western medicine references

Carlotti DN. New Trends in Systemic Antibiotic Therapy of Bacterial Skin Diseases in Dogs. *Supplement of the Compendium on Continuing Education for the Practicing Veterinarian* 1996.18: 40–47.

Codner EC. In: Tilley L, Smith F. The 5-Minute Veterinary Consult: Canine and Feline, Blackwell Publishing, 2003.

Day MJ. An immunopathological study of deep pyoderma in the dog, *Research in Veterinary Sciences* 56: 18–23, 1994.

Ihrke PJ, Schwartzman RM, McGinley KM, et al. Microbiology of Normal and Seborrheic Canine Skin. *American Journal of Veterinary Research*, 39: 1487–1489, 1978.

Ihrke PJ. Bacterial Skin Disease in the Dog—A Guide to Canine Pyoderma. Bayer/Veterinary Learning Systems, 1996.

Ihrke PI, White SD. Contemporary Issues in Small Animal Practice: Dermatology, Vol. 8. Nesbitt GH, ed. 1987. New York: Churchill Livingstone.

Krishnan G, et al. Cytokines produced by Staphage Lysate, 12th European Immunology Meeting. 1994. Abstracts, Barcelona, Spain, p 395.

Kwochka KW. Recurrent pyoderma. In: Griffin CE, Kwochka KW, MacDonald JM, eds. Current Veterinary Dermatology. The Science and Art of Therapy. St Louis: Mosby Year Book, 1993. 3–21,

Lloyd DH. Therapy for canine pyoderma. In Kirk, RW, Bonagura, JD, eds. Current Veterinary Therapy XI. Philadelphia: WB Saunders Company, 1992. 539–544.

Lloyd DH, Garthwaite G. Epidermal structure and surface topography of canine skin. *Research in Veterinary Science* 1982; 33: 99–104.

Mason IS, Lloyd DH. The role of allergy in the development of canine pyoderma. *Journal of Small Animal Practice* 1989; 30: 216–218.

Mason IS, Lloyd DH. Factors influencing the penetration of bacterial antigens through canine skin. In: Von Tscarner C, Halliwell REW, eds. Advances in Veterinary Dermatology, 1990. Vol. 1, 370–374.

Miller WH. Deep pyoderma in two German shepherd dogs associated with a cell-mediated immunodeficiency, *J. An. Anim. Hosp. Assoc.* 1991; 27: 513–17.

Morales CA, Shultz KT, DeBoer DJ. Anti-staphylococcal antibodies in dogs with recurrent staphylococcal pyoderma. *Vet. Immunol Immunopathol*; 1994; 42(2):137–47.

Nesbitt GH. Canine and Feline Dermatology: A Systematic Approach. 1983. Philadelphia: Lea and Febiger.

Muller GH, Kirk RW, Scott DW. Small animal dermatology. 4th ed. 1989. Philadelphia: Saunders.

Scott DW, Miller WH, Griffin CE. Muller and Kirk's Small Animal Dermatology 6th ed. Philadelphia: WB Saunders Company, 2001. p 230–232, 274–335, 647–650.

Van Kampen, KR. Immunotherapy and Cytokines. *Seminars in Veterinary Medicine and Surgery (Small Animal)*, 1997; Vol. 12, No. 3:186–192.

IVM/nutrition references

Bouic PJD, et al. Beta-sitosterol and beta-sitosterol glucoside stimulate human peripheral blood lymphocyte proliferation: Implications for their use as an immunomodulatory vitamin combination. *International Journal of Immunopharmacology* 1996; 18:693–700.

Golden BR, Gorbach SL. The Effect of Milk and Lactobacillus Feeding on Human Intestinal Bacteria Activity. *Am. J. of Clin. Nutr.*, 1984;39: 756–61.

Gupta MB, Nath R, Srivastava N, et al. Anti-inflammatory and antipyretic activities of β-sitosterol. *Planta Medica* 1980;39: 157–163.

Hederos CA, Berg A. Epogam evening primrose oil treatment in atopic dermatitis and asthma. *Arch Dis Child* 1996; 75(6):494–497.

Hanin I, Ansell GB. Lecithin: Technological, Biological, and Therapeutic Aspects, NY: Plenum Press, 1987, 180, 181.

Humphreys F, Symons J, Brown H, et al. The effects of gamolenic acid on adult atopic eczema and premenstrual exacerbation of eczema. *Eur J Dermatol* 1994;4(598):603.

McDonough FE, Hitchins AD, Wong NP, et al. Modification of sweet acidophilus milk to improve utilization by lactose-intolerant persons. Am J Clin Nutr 1987;45:570–4.

Morse PF, Horrobin DF, Manku MS, et al. Meta-analysis of placebo-controlled studies of the efficacy of Epogam in the treatment of atopic eczema: relationship between plasma essential fatty acid changes and clinical response. *Br J Dermatol* 1989;121(1):75–90.

Perdigon GN, de Masius N, Alvarez S, et al. Enhancement of Immune Response in Mice Fed with S. Thermophilus and L. Acidophilus, *J. of Dairy Sci.*, 1987; 70: 919–926.

Chinese herbal medicine/acupuncture references

Cheng JX, et al. *Journal of Practical Integrated Medicine.* 1993;6(5):261.

Hou Xue Hua Yu Yan Jia *(Research on Blood-Activating and Stasis-Eliminating Herbs)*, 1981:335.

Kim JH, Han KD, Yamasaki K, Tanaka O. Darutoside, a. diterpenoid from Siegesbeckia pubescens and its structure. *Phytochemistry*, 1979; 18(5):894.

Kubo M, Matsuda H, Tanaka M, Kimura Y, Okuda H, Higashino M, Tani T, Namba K, Arichi S. Studies on Scutellariae radix. VII. Anti-arthritic and anti-inflammatory actions of methanolic extract and flavonoid components from Scutellariae radix. *Chem Pharm Bull*, 1984; 32(7):2724–9.

Lang XC, et al. *Journal of Hebei Medical College.* 1991; 12(3):140.

Li YF (translator). *Foreign Medicine, vol. of TCM.* 1984;6(1):15–18.

Liu IX, Durham DG, Richards RM. Baicalin synergy with beta-lactam antibiotics against methicillin-resistant Staphylococcus aureus and other beta-lactam-resistant strains of S. aureus. *J Pharm Pharmacol.* 2000 Mar;52(3):361–6.

Mao XJ, et al. Experimental research on mixture of Cao Wu and Shui Niu Jiao. *Journal of Yunnan College of TCM.* 1997;19(7):33–34.

Mascolo N, Autore G, Capasso F, et al. Biological screening of Italian medicinal plants for anti-inflammatory activity. *Phytotherapy Res* 1987;1(1):28–31.

Pan JF, et al. *Tianjin Journal of Medicine.* 1991;19(8): 468–470.

Shan Xi Yi Kan *(Shanxi Journal of Medicine)*, 1960; (10):32.

Wu XY, et al. Brief discussion on Shui Niu Jiao. *Journal of Traditional Chinese Medicine Material.* 1985;(5):41,38.

Xin Yi Xue *(New Medicine)*, 1975; 6(3):155.

Xin Zhong Yi *(New Chinese Medicine)*, 1989; 21(3):51.

Yun Nan Zhong Yao Zhi *(Yunnan Journal of Chinese Herbal Medicine)*, 1990; 244.

Zhang FC, et al. Di Long's enhancing effect on macrophages' immune activity. *China Journal of Pharmacy.* 1998;33(9): 532–535.

Zhang SC, et al. *Journal of Chinese Patent Medicine Research.* 1984;(2):37.

Zhong Guo Zhong Yao Za Zhi *(People's Republic of China Journal of Chinese Herbology)*, 1991;16(9):560.

Zhong Hua Yi Xue Za Zhi *(Chinese Journal of Medicine)*, 1978;17(8):87.

Zhong Yao Cai *(Study of Chinese Herbal Material)*, 1985; (2):36.

Zhong Yao Cai *(Study of Chinese Herbal Material)*, 1991; 14(2):41.

Zhong Yao Tong Bao *(Journal of Chinese Herbology)*, 1988:13(6):364.

Zhong Yao Xue *(Chinese Herbology)*, 1988; 137:140.

Zhong Yao Xue *(Chinese Herbology)*, 1998; 89:91.

Zhong Yao Xue *(Chinese Herbology)*, 1998;103:106.

Zhong Yao Xue *(Chinese Herbology)*, 1998; 318:320.

Zhong Yao Xue *(Chinese Herbology)*, 1998; 706:708.

Zhong Yao Yao Li Yu Ying Yong *(Pharmacology and Applications of Chinese Herbs)*, 1983: 400.

Zhong Yao Yao Li Yu Ying Yong *(Pharmacology and Applications of Chinese Herbs)*, 1983:796.

Zhong Yao Yao Li Yu Lin Chuang *(Pharmacology and Clinical Applications of Chinese Herbs)*, 1989; 5(1):24.

Zhong Yao Zhi *(Chinese Herbology Journal)*, 1993:183.

Zhong Yao Zhi *(Chinese Herbology Journal)*, 1993; 358.

Zhong Yi Yao Xue Bao *(Report of Chinese Medicine and Herbology)*, 1991;(1):41.

Zhong Yi Za Zhi *(Journal of Chinese Medicine)*, 12:18.

Zhou WZ, et al. *Pharmacy Bulletin.* 1979;14(5):202–203.

Zhou ZW, et al. *Journal of TCM Pharmacology and Clinical Application.* 1989;5(1):24.

Zhao ZB, et al. *Sichuan Journal of Traditional Chinese Medicine.* 1993;11(11):13.

Homotoxicology reference

Reckeweg H. Homoeopathia Antihomotoxica Materia Medica, 4th ed. Baden-Baden, Germany: Aurelia-Verlag GMBH, 2002. p 168, 310–13, 317–20, 338–40, 343–4, 418–20, 500–3.

EOSINOPHILIC GRANULOMA

Definition and cause

Feline eosinophilic granuloma is an inflammatory disease that most commonly occurs in cats but can occur in dogs and other species. While the proven cause is not known, it is believed that the underlying cause is related to an allergic reaction (food, insect, environmental) (MacEwen 1987, Song 1994, Werner 2003). Other suspected causes include genetic predisposition, infection, or an auto-immune response. The body's inflammatory response involves infiltration by eosinophils (Gelberg 1985, Scott 2001, Song 1994).

Medical therapy rationale, drug(s) of choice, and nutritional recommendations

Treatment is usually with systemic, interlesional, and/or topical corticosteroids. More resistant or deeper lesions often require immunosuppressant medication such as Cyclophosphamide or immunomodulating therapy such as Levamisole (Scott 2001, Song 1994). Omega-3 and -6 fatty acids have been shown to improve the condition and reduce the reliance on corticosteroids (Scott 2001).

Anticipated prognosis

The prognosis depends upon determining the underlying cause. Allergically incited lesions often respond well so long as the underlying cause of the allergy is controlled. Often, however, control is achieved with ongoing medication, and recurrences are common (Scott 2001, Werner 2003).

Integrative veterinary therapies

Eosinphilic granuloma is chronic inflammation secondary to antigens, which may gain access to the body through a wide variety of portals. Direct injury as in insect bite hypersensitivity is a classical example. As a flea feeds on the host, it releases anticoagulants and other proteins, which are detected by the immune system as it performs its police function at the injury site. In its attempt to prevent further injury, the immune system codes for antibody against these foreign proteins. Immunoglobulins are produced and IgE binds to mast cells in the skin, creating a future hypersensitivity reaction. Chemotactic factors lead to the infiltration of the tissue by eosinophils and the appearance of a lesion. Further contact with the offending antigen can trigger the disease state. (For additional information on the immune system's production of auto-antibodies and cellular immune processes inciting disease, see Chapter 2 for Gland Therapy and Free Radicals.)

Antigen can be presented by other methods as well. Direct contact, inhalation, and ingestion are all possible genesis points for the condition. The gastrointestinal (GI) and integumentary systems are intricately involved with the basic homeostasis of the organism. Lymphocytes and macrophages are active in both the skin and intestinal tract. Dendritic cells in the intestine communicate with lymphocytes and often encode a "tolerance" response on the part of the organism to antigens, which enter through the digestive system. If this system is imbalanced, then hyperactivity and proinflammatory reactions may occur.

Food allergy, adverse reactions to food, injury to the normal functions of digestion and absorption, and bacterial overgrowth, along with ingestion of toxic substances such as food additives, aflatoxins, and preservatives can all permit the presentation of antigen to the immune system, which can result in inflammatory reactions in several areas of the body. Holistic doctors have long recognized the connection of the intestinal system and allergic symptomology, and successful handling of many patients commonly involves honoring this relationship by beginning therapy with attention to bowel health and diet. This syndrome of pathology resulting from altered permeability and digestion is often described as "leaky gut." Conventional medicine also recognizes the importance of food trials, and is beginning to appreciate the relationship of intestinal injury from other factors such as adverse reactions caused by drugs (i.e., corticosteroids and NSAIDs).

Psychoneuroendocrine and immune factors also affect the skin. Stress can cause increased intestinal permeability and a corresponding onset of inflammatory pathologies.

Phylogenetically, there is an association with the excretory system, and in Traditional Chinese Medicine the Skin is governed by functions of the Kidney Zang Fu organ. When confronting eosinphilic granuloma complex issues, the clinician must recall all these factors in the maintenance of homeostasis. As the body attempts to handle homotoxins, it is common to see involvement of skin as both a barrier and an excretory organ. Furthermore, inflammation frequently can be observed in the integument. Eosinophils are frequently involved in cats. (See Homotoxicology, below, in this section.)

The clinical approach to such lesions involves looking for obvious agents such as fleas, gnats, and mosquitoes. Simple steps should be taken to remove them from the patient and time should be provided to see if recovery occurs. Use of proper insecticide can be the difference between a need for large amounts of immunosuppressive drugs and no medication whatsoever. Many patients begin to improve within 2 weeks after application of an effective spot treatment insecticide. Gentle, natural methods of parasite control (borax powder, diatomaceous earth, etc.) can be used and may be helpful, but care should be used with essential oils because these can be very toxic to some individuals, and in particular feline patients. Some pets are chemically sensitive and can be made ill by insecticides. Some of these individuals may genetically lack appropriate detoxification systems.

Elimination diets—limited antigen or hydrolyzed diets—are useful in cases of food allergy or adverse reactions to food or food additives. Success is gained with both approaches and no single diet assures positive results, so several trials are indicated. Home-prepared diets can be used (Strombeck 1999). Some animals worsen when placed on the correct diet as they undergo regressive vicariation to the Excretion Phase, so the development of diarrhea does not necessarily mean that the diet should be changed (See Homotoxicology in this section).

Other conditions such as pancreatitis can result as the body flushes homotoxins from the system. Blood testing for food allergy is notoriously inaccurate and should not be taken too seriously. Such tests may guide the clinician, but often lead to confusion on the part of the client and other doctors. The client should be informed before blood testing is done.

Searching out other toxins in the environment is frequently beyond the ability of a busy clinician, but many antigens and haptens may be involved. Perfumes, tobacco smoke, cleaners (particularly heavily scented products and those that contain pine oil), perfumed laundry detergent, perfumed fabric rinses, dryer clothing treatments, carpet deodorizers, disinfectants, cosmetics, hair sprays, incense, and aroma therapy units may be key causative agents. Chronic exposure to certain environmental toxins (petroleum distillates or tar) should be evaluated in difficult cases. Advise clients to remove all such items.

Contact antigens and inhaled antigens should be considered. Wool in carpets, clothes, or bedding should be removed. Pet beds that contain cedar chips have been associated in the author's practice, as well. Tree saps and contact with outdoor plants may also aggravate these cases.

Reactions to prescription drugs, vaccinations, nutritional supplements, herbal products, or other medicants should be considered. In some cases, there is a suspicion that injury resulting from such agents can sensitize the patient so that eosinophilic disease manifests at a later date. This relationship is hard to demonstrate but has some support in cases where application of homoeopathic dilutions of therapeutic agents lead to rapid recovery.

Nutrition
General considerations/rationale
While medical therapy is focused locally upon the external lesion, the nutritional approach adds nutrients, antioxidants, and gland support for the organs of the immune system and to help control inflammation. Because eosinophilic granuloma can have multiple causes as well as an exaggerated immune response from multiple imbalanced organs, a medical and physiologically blood evaluation is recommended to assess glandular health. This information gives clinicians the ability to formulate therapeutic nutritional protocols that address the local lesions as well as underlying organ conditions that may be ultimately responsible for the surface condition (see Chapter 2, nutritional blood testing, for more detailed information).

Appropriate nutrients
Nutritional/gland therapy: Glandular adrenal, thymus, spleen, and lymph provide intrinsic nutrients that nourish and help balance the immune response, neutralize cellular inflammation, and prevent degeneration (see Gland Therapy, Chapter 2, for a more detailed explanation).

Sterols: Plant-derived sterols such as betasitosterol show anti-inflammatory properties which appear to be similar to corticosteroids (Bouic 1996, Gupta 1980). A cortisone-like effect without the associated immune-suppressing effects is beneficial in immune-mediated conditions.

Quercetin: Quercetin is a flavonoids that has antioxidant properties. It also functions like an antihistamine, and has been shown to inhibit cells from releasing histamines (Middleton 1986, Ogasawara 1985). Therefore, it is beneficial in the treatment of allergic skin conditions.

Essential fatty acids: Much research has been conducted on the importance of essential fatty acids in the daily diet, and on the clinical management of various degenerative diseases (Reinhart 1996, Holub 1995, Herman 1998). Seabuckthorne oil can be used to treat burns and skin irritations (Wu Fuheng 1991). It is a clinically approved in Russia for use in reducing inflammation and protecting against radiation damage (Yance 2005).

Chinese herbal medicine/acupuncture
General considerations/rationale
According to TCM theory, eosinophilic granulomas are due to Wind, Heat, and Toxin invading the body. Lesions come and go and they spread. The term Wind is used to describe this behavior because wind has the properties of waning and gusting—coming and going. Additionally, Wind can blow the lesions from place to place, much as the wind blows leaves over the yard. Heat refers to the inflammation. Toxins are the inflammatory mediators and any secondary bacterial invaders that may contaminate the lesions secondary to the self-trauma from pruritis. An herbal supplement designed for eosinophilic granulomas must stop the pruritis, decrease the inflammation, and address any secondary infections.

In Traditional Chinese Medicine, the Skin and Mouth are under the control of separate organ systems. Therefore, lesions in the Mouth are treated differently than those on the Skin, necessitating different formulas. To the authors' knowledge, no Western studies have been performed to investigate this belief so there is no discussion of this in the section on appropriate herbs.

Appropriate chinese herbs

Angelica (Bai zhi): Has anti-inflammatory properties (Zhong Guo Zhong Yao Za Zhi 1991).

Atractylodes (Cang zhu): Has demonstrated anti-inflammatory effects in the laboratory. It was shown to prevent xylene-induced auricular swelling, carrageenin-induced foot swelling, and acetic-acid-induced increase in abdominal capillary permeability in 1 trial (Zhang 1998).

Bupleurum (Chai hu): Has anti-inflammatory effects (Liu 1998). In addition, it has demonstrated antibiotic activity against several bacteria including B-hemolytic streptococci (Zhong Yao Xue 1988).

Cicada slough (Chan tui): Was used in a trial of 30 human patients with chronic urticaria. In this investigation 23% of the patients had significant improvement while another 50% had moderate improvement (Pi fu Bing Fang Zhi Yan Jiu Tong Xun 1972).

Dandelion (Pu gong ying): Has shown evidence of anti-inflammatory actions (Mascolo 1987).

Earthworm (Di long): Has been shown to increase the rate of wound healing. In rabbits with experimentally induced skin wounds it promoted the growth of fibroblasts, capillaries, and collagen fibers (Zhang 1999).

Forsythia (Lian cao): Has anti-inflammatory and analgesic effects. It can decrease inflammatory exudate and edema (Ma 1982, Rui 1999). In addition, it has demonstrated antibiotic effects against common skin bacteria such as Staphylococcus aureus and hemolytic streptococcus in vitro (Ma 1982).

Honeysuckle (Jin yin hua): Has been shown experimentally to have anti-inflammatory effects in rabbits and mice (Shan Xi Yi Kan 1960).

Licorice (Gan cao): Contains glycyrrhizin and glycyrrhetinic acid, which have anti-inflammatory effects. They prolong the effect of cortisones in the body either by decreasing its metabolism in the liver or by increasing the plasma concentration by decreasing protein binding (Zhong Yao Zhi 1993). They have approximately 10% of the corticosteroid activity of cortisone. They decrease edema by decreasing the permeability of blood vessels and interfering with histamine action (Zhong Cao Yao 1991).

Mouton (Mu dan pi): Has demonstrated anti-inflammatory effects in several studies. The mechanism of action seems to be through the ability to inhibit prostaglandin synthesis and decrease the permeability of blood vessels (Wu 1990, Sheng Yao Xue Za Zhi 1979, Zhong Guo Yao Ke Da Xue Xue Bao 1990). In addition, it may help control secondary bacterial infections (Zhong Yao Cai 1991).

Platycodon (Jie geng): Causes anti-inflammatory effects by increasing the secretion of corticosterone. This effect has been proven in rats (Li 1984, Zhang 1984, Zhou 1979). It suppresses allergic reactions and decreases capillary permeability (Zhong Yao Yao Li Yu Ying Yong 1983).

Polygonum (He shou wu): Enhances adrenocortical function. Experimentally, this herb has been shown to increase the size of mice's adrenal glands (Shen 1982). It also increases hormonal secretion by the adrenal gland. These effects can increase endogenous serum cortisol levels (Zhong Yao Yao Li Yu Lin Chuang 1989).

Prunella (Xia ku cao): Has immunosuppressive activity. When administered by abdominal injection it was shown to significantly raise the level of plasma cortisol (Jiang 1988).

Rehmannia (Sheng di huang): Increase the plasma levels of adrenocortical hormone. This may lead to increased endogenous cortisol levels. It reduces swelling and inflammation (Zhong Yao Xue 1998, Zhong 1983).

Scutellaria (Huang qin): Contains biacalin and biacalein, which suppress inflammation in mice (Kubo M 1984). These can significantly inhibit histamine-induced increase in capillary permeability (Huang 1996). In addition, biacalin has antibiotic activity against Stapylococcus aureus and may have synergistic effects with ampicillin, amoxicillin, methacillin, and cefotaxime. It can help overcome B lactam resistance (Zhong Yao Xue 1988, Liu 2000).

Schizonepeta (Jing jie): Has been shown to help control rashes and itching (Zhong Yi Za Zhi).

Siegesbeckia (Xi xian cao): Has both anti-inflammatory and immunosuppressive effects. It has been shown to decrease swelling in rats (Zhong 1983). It also decreases both humoral and cellular immunity in mice (Zhong 1989).

Siler (Fang feng): Has demonstrated antibiotic efficacy against common skin pathogens such as Staphylococcus aureus (Zhong Yao Tong Bao 1988).

White mustard seed (Bai jie zi): Has anti-inflammatory effects. One of the components, sinapine, seems to be responsible for this effect (Zhang 1996). It also has antifungal and antibacterial effects (Mei 1998).

White peony (Bai shao): Contains paeoniflorin, which is a strong anti-inflammatory (Zhong 1993).

Xanthium (Cang er zi): Decreases inflammatory swelling. It inhibits the effect of histamine on the capillaries, thereby preventing an increase in capillary permeability (Huang 1996).

Zedoaria (E zhu): Was used in 48 people with neurodermatits, a chronic dermatological disorder in which the skin is pruritic. It may thicken the way an eosinophilic granuloma does in animals. In this experiment, 21 of the 48 patients experienced excellent results, and 9 more had moderate improvement in their signs after injections of E zhu and Sal leng into acupuncture points (Pi Fu Bing Fang Zhi Yan Jiu tong Xun 1979).

Homotoxicology
General considerations/rationale
Eosinophilic granuloma marks a chronic inflammation reaction to particular antigens, which may gain access to the body through a wide variety of portals. This represents Impregnation Phase disease as the body responds to homotoxins that have bound to other elements and damaged the body's ability to eliminate the offending substances. The body responds through a chronic inflammatory reaction in the attempt to remove damaged elements and repair these affected tissues.

In the authors' practices, we frequently diagnose veterinary homotoxicoses related to flea collars. The most common signs are depression following application of the collar, but patients may have inappetance, seizures, anxiety, depression, vomiting, diarrhea, and upper respiratory signs, which vanish rapidly after removal of the collar. Careful questioning of humans residing in the home may reveal similar symptoms and especially chronic, recurring pharyngitis, rhinitis, tonsillitis, and headaches in people sleeping with these pets. When this is noted the people involved should be referred to appropriate medical care and the collar removed until accurate diagnosis can occur. Palmquist is especially sensitive to many chemical poison flea collars and develops a headache and sore throat within a few minutes of exposure. Many other people and animals seem to be so affected. Considering that most flea collars are ineffective in flea control, their use should not be promoted in most situations.

As with all Impregnation Phase disorders, eosinophilic granuloma complex may be recurrent and frustrating to treat; however, if the clinician integrates antihomotoxic medicines over long periods of time, a substantial percentage of patients will show improvement and reduced exacerbation in successive seasons, and some patients will exhibit remarkable responses. Because such treatment is without dangerous side effects, clients often opt for biological therapy instead of chronic use of immunosuppressive agents.

Appropriate homotoxicology formulas
Due to the wide variety of possible treatments needed in these patients, the reader is referred to the list of remedies at the end of the gastrointestinal chapter, as well as those in the allergies protocol. Pharmaceuticals may be needed for symptom control and can be safely used while integrating antihomotoxic agents.

Coenzyme compositum: The ingredient Citricum acidum is useful for dental problems and gingivitis. This remedy also is useful for scurvy; blackening of teeth; heavy deposits of dental plaque; painful, and herpetic vesicles around the lips; as well as nausea, painful cramping in the umbilical area, and distension.

Cutis compositum: A wide-reaching formula that stimulates nonspecific defenses in a variety of cutaneous conditions. Can be used in any phase homotoxicosis. Opens skin to drainage and repair. Contains Cutis suis, Hepar suis, Splen suis, Placenta suis, Glandula suprarenalis suis, and Funiculus ubilicalis suis to support regeneration and repair of organs involved in skin health. Contains Sulfur for repair of blocked enzyme systems and Cortisonum aceticum for repair of damage from prior corticosteroid exposure. Aesculus hipposcastanum supports circulation and drainage (Reckeweg 2000).

Echinacea compositum: Used to bacterial infection control and immune normalization. It is a phase remedy for the Inflammation Phase.

Engystol N: Used for viral origin gastroenteritis and allergic dermatitis. It contains Sulphur in a higher potency, which is helpful for many chronic diseases and skin conditions. In some cases this agent by itself causes marked improvement. It combines readily with Cutis compositum and Ubichinon compositum to resolve difficult cases (Palmquist 2005).

Galium-Heel: Indicated in most allergic cases. It is a phase remedy for Deposition to Dedifferentiation phases. Galium aparine, Sempervivum tectorum, Ononis spinosa, Juniperus communis, Betula alba, Saponaria officinali, and Acidum nitricum give it a diuretic effect, and Galium mullugo provides a detoxifying effect. Phosphorus supports parenchyma (lung, liver, kidney, and heart), and Apis mellifica helps with itching. Pyrogenium-Nosode helps with infectious Inflammatory Phases, and Urtica urens treats eczema and dermatosis (Reckeweg 2000). It is also a cellular drainage and repair agent and it is used for edema and to create drainage through connective tissue.

Hepar compositum: Used for detoxification and drainage of hepatic tissues, organ support, and metabolic support. It is useful in most hepatic and gall bladder pathologies. It is also an important part of the deep detoxification formula. Hepar compositum is used to treat duodenitis, pancreatitis, cystic hepatic ducts, cholelithiasis, cholangitis, cholecystitis, vomiting, and diarrhea (Demers 2004, Broadfoot 2004). This combination contains Natrum oxalaceticum (also found in Coenzyme compositum, Ubichinon compositum, and Mucosa compositum) for changes in appetite and stomach distension due to air. Chelidonium has proapototic characteristics (Habermehl 2006).

Hepeel: Provides liver drainage and detoxification. It is used in a wide variety of conditions including cancer of the liver, where *Hepeel* was found to be antiproliferative, hepatoprotective, and an antioxidant when tested in human HepG2 cells (Gebhardt 2003).

Lamioflur: Used for ulcerations of mucocutaneous areas, diseases of the skin, and mucous membranes. Contains Hepar sulphuris for skin ulcerations and pustular eczema; Acidum nitricum for lesions on mucocutaneous junctions; and Kreosotum for eczema of the hands and mucosa margins (Reckeweg 2000).

Lymphomyosot: Used for lymph drainage and endocrine support, and to treat edema.

Mezereum homaccord: Treats herpes, dermatitis, ulcerative eczema, and pruritus (Reckeweg 2000).

Mucosa compositum: Broadly supports repair of mucosal elements. Used in cellular cases and in recovery periods following active disease (Reckeweg 2000). This remedy contains Kali bichromicum, which is indicated for ulcers found on the gums, the tongue, the lips, and even on the gastric mucosa (gastric or duodenal ulcer). The tongue may have a thick, yellow, mucous coating, or, in ulcerative stomatitis or tonsillitis, it may be dry, smooth, shiny, or fissured. *Kali* has been used effectively in acute gastroenteritis associated with vomiting of clear, light-colored fluid or quantities of mucous bile, and in cases with hematemesis, flatulent colics, and dysenteric stools with tenesmus (Reckeweg 2002).

It also contains Hydrastis for mucosal support of oral problems such as stomatitis; mucosal suppuration accompanied by ulceration, inflammations, and colic of the hepatobiliary system and the gastrointestinal tract; and polyp formation (Reckeweg 2002). The Kreosotum component is for chronic gastritis with gastric hemorrhages and vomiting of brown masses. It also has a dental implication in cases with spongy gums and carious teeth and neuralgias proceeding from them, causing a burning toothache with deep caries, black patches, on the teeth and fetid discharges. The single remedy Phosphorus is broadly useful for dyspepsia and for jaw problems in dental disease (Reckeweg 2002). Phosphorus is found in many other remedies including *Echinacea compositum*, *Leptandra homaccord*, and several others. It is rich in suis organ preparations for mucosal support, plus a large variety of remedies with indications in the gastrointestinal sphere.

Also contained in this broad remedy is Argentum nitricum, (also in *Atropinum compositum*, *Diarrheel*, *Duodenoheel*, *Gastricumeel*, *Momordica compositum*, *BHI-Nausea*, and several other combinations). It is for distension in the upper abdomen, gastro-cardiac symptom-complex, amelioration from eructations, and gastric crises (Reckeweg 2002).

Psorinoheel: An exudation and cellular phase remedy. It treats itching, precancerous conditions, chronic skin conditions, acne, seborrhea, eczema, and pruritus.

Pulsatilla compositum: Used for regulation rigidity. If signs suddenly shift to inflammatory regressive vicariation, shift to *Traumeel*. This remedy contains homeopathically diluted Cortisonum for repair of prior therapeutic damage, which may block recovery. it stimulates the mesenchymal tissues strongly toward healing. Patients frequently develop respiratory Excretion Phase discharges of mucus. The ingredient Sulfur is a reagent in allchronic diseases (Reckeweg 2000).

Schwef-Heel: Used for chronic diseases of skin and liver. This remedy should be interposed in most skin and liver cases (Reckeweg 2000). Patients that need this remedy may look dirty and have scruffy skin conditions, red lips, a white tongue with red tip, itching and burning of the rectal area with morning diarrhea, and prolapsed rectum (Boericke 1927). Sulfur is contained in this and several other antihomotoxic formulas including *Coenzyme compositum*, *Echinacea compositum*, *Engystol*, *Ginseng compositum*, *Hepar compositum*, *Molybdan compositum*, *Mucosa compositum*, *Paeonia Heel*, *Proctheel*, *Psorinoheel*, *Sulfur-Heel*, *Thyroidea compositum*, and *Ubichinon compositum* (Reckeweg 2000).

Solidago compositum: Supports the kidney and urinary system. It is part of the deep detoxification formula. The ingredient Berberis is antihistaminic and anticholinergic (Shamsa, Ahmadiani, Khosrokhavar 1999).

Thyroidea compositum: Provides drainage of matrix and support of the endocrine system. It is a phase remedy for Impregnation Phases and it is part of the deep detoxification formula.

Traumeel: A nonsteroidal anti-inflammatory that is useful in all phases. It is helpful for regulation rigidity cases. It activates blocked enzymes in chronic disease states.

Ubichinon compositum: Provides support of energy-producing components.

Authors' suggested protocols

Nutrition

Immune and lymph support formulas: 1 tablet for every 25 pounds of body weight BID.

Skin support formula: One-half tablet for every 25 pounds of body weight BID.

Betathyme: 1 capsule for every 35 pounds of body weight BID. (maximum 2 capsules BID.)

Quercetin: 50 mg for every 10 pounds of body weight SID.

Beyond essential fats: One-half teaspoon for every 35 pounds of body weight with food (maximum, 2 teaspoons).

Chinese herbal medicine/acupuncture

For lesions on the skin, Formulas H52 ImmunoDerm and H67 DermGuard given at a dose of 1 capsule of each for every 10 to 20 pounds twice daily.

For oral lesions formula, H33 Eosinophilic granuloma is used at a dose of 1 capsule for every 10 to 20 pounds twice daily.

The ingredients of each formula follow. They contain herbs not mentioned above, but which increase the efficacy and minimize the side effects of the respective formulas.

H33 Eosinophilic granuloma: Angelica radix (Dang gui), burreed tuber (San leng), cicata (Chan tui), dahurian angelica root (Bai zhi), dittany bark (Bai xian pi), forsythia (lian qiao), fritillaria (Bei mu), kochia (Di fu zi), licorice (Gan cao), oyster shell (Mu li), prunella (Xia ku cao), red peony (Chi shao), siler (Fang feng), white mustard seed (Bai jie zi), and zedoaria (E zhu).

H52 ImmunoDerm: Angelica radix (Dang gui), atractylodes (Cang zhu), buffalo horn shavings (Sui niu jiao), bupleurum (Chai hu), dandelion (Pu gong ying), earthworm ((Di long), fleece flower root (He shou wu), honeysuckle (Jin yin hua), kochia (Di fu zi), licorice (Gan cao), moutan (Mu dan pi), oldenlandia (Bai hua she cao), poria (Fu ling), rehmannia (Sheng di huang), scutellaria (Huang qin), siegesbeckia (Xi xian cao), tokoro (Bi xie), white peony (Bai shao), and xantium fruit (Cang er zi).

H67 DermGuard: Angelica radix (Dang gui), aurantium fruit (Zhi qiao), bupleurum (Chai hu), cicada (Chan tui), cnidium (Chauan xiong), dahurian angelica (Bai zhi), honeysuckle (Jin yin hua), licorice (Gan cao), mint (Bo he), moutan (Mud an pi), platycodon (Jie geng), poria (Fu ling), schizonepeta (Jing jie), scutellaria (Huang qin), siegesbeckia (Xi xian cao), siler (Fang feng), silkworm (Jiang can), and xanthium fruit (Cang er zi).

Homotoxicology (Dose: 10 drops PO for 50-pound dog; 5 drops PO small dog or cat)

Treatment must be individualized, but the following represent good starting therapies, which can be readily adapted based upon clinical response.

Simple oral protocol: Engystol N, Lamioflur, and Traumeel S mixed together and given BID orally. Also deeper detoxification formula consisting of Galium-Heel, Coenzyme compositum, Ubichinon compositum, Solidago compositum, Hepar compositum, and Thyroidea compositum mixed together and given orally every 3 days. In addition, Cutis compositum given twice weekly to every other week. In difficult cases, Pulsatilla compositum may move the case toward regressive vicariation. Control of allergens is critical to success.

Autosanguis and oral combination therapy per Broadfoot (best option): Perform autosanguis therapy as follows:

Stage 1: Traumeel S IV
Stage 2: Tonsilla compositum or Pulsatilla compositum (consider Tonsilla compositum for first run and use Pulsatilla compositum as an alternative if no or poor response)
Stage 3: Engystol N and Galium-Heel combined
Stage 4: Cutis compositum
Stage 5: Coenzyme compositum

For each step above (2 through 5), inject half of this mixture into the patient subcutaneously (in cases involving one large lesion, consider injecting small amounts around the periphery of the lesion, a technique known as "circling the dragon" in Chinese medicine), and add the remaining half to an oral cocktail of the following ingredients: Psorinoheel, Lamioflur (contains *Mezereum*), and Echinacea compositum Forte tablets. Mix together and succuss it 10 times. Give 5 to 7 drops of this resulting final mixture orally BID to TID. Also treat the lesion topically with Euphorbium compositum BID. Broadfoot reports best results are when this is combined with oral blue-green algae and Gluta-DMG.

Product sources

Nutrition

Immune and lymph support formulas: Animal Nutrition Technologies. **Alternative:** Immune system support—Standard Process Veterinary Formulas; Immungen—Thorne Veterinary Products;

Betathyme—Best for Your Pet. **Alternative:** Moducare—Thorne Veterinary Products.

Quercetin: Source Naturals; Quercitone—Thorne Veterinary Products.

Beyond essential fats: Natura Health Products. **Alternatives:** Oil of Evening Primrose—Jarrow Formulas.

Chinese herbal medicine

Derm Guard, Immunoderm, and Eosinophilic granuloma: Natural Solutions Inc.

Homotoxicology remedies

BHI/Heel Corporation

REFERENCES

Western medicine references
Gelberg HB, Lewis RM, Felsburg PJ, Smith CA. Antiepithelial autoantibodies associated with the feline eosinophilic granuloma complex. *Am J Vet Res* 46:263–265, 1985.
MacEwen EG, Hess PW. Evaluation of effect of immunomuodulation on the feline eosinophilic granuloma complex. *J Am Anim Hosp Assoc* 23:519–525,1987.
Scott DW, Miller WH, Griffin CE. Small Animal Dermatology. Philadelphia: WB Saunders, 2001, pp. 1148–1153.

Song MD. Diagnosing and treating feline eosinophilic granuloma complex. *Vet Med* 89:1141–1145, 1994.

Werner AH. In: Tilley L, Smith F. The 5-Minute Veterinary Consult: Canine and Feline, 2003. Blackwell Publishing.

IVM/nutrition references

Bouic PJD, et al. Beta-sitosterol and beta-sitosterol glucoside stimulate human peripheral blood lymphocyte proliferation: Implications for their use as an immunomodulatory vitamin combination. *International Journal of Immunopharmacology* 18:693–700, 1996.

Gupta MB, Nath R, Srivastava N, et al. Anti-inflammatory and antipyretic activities of β-sitosterol. *Planta Medica* 1980;39: 157–163.

Herman HA, et al. The Influence of Dietary Omega-6:Omega-3 Ratio in Lameness in Dogs with Osteoarthrosis of the Elbow Joint Recent Advances in Canine and Feline Nutrition, Volume II, Iams Proceedings 1998. p 325.

Holub B. The Role of Omega-3 Fatty Acids in Health and Disease. 1995. Proceeding of the 13th Annual American College of Veterinary Medicine.

Middleton E Jr. Effect of flavonoids on basophil histamine release and other secretory systems. *Prog Clin Biol Res.* 1986;213:493–506.

Ogasawara H, Middleton E Jr. Effect of selected flavonoids on histamine release (HR) and hydrogen peroxide (H2O2) generation by human leukocytes [abstract]. *J Allergy Clin Immunol.* 1985;75(suppl):184.

Reinhart GA. A Controlled Dietary Omega-6:Omega-3 Ratio Reduces Pruritus in Nonfood Allergic Atopic Dogs, Recent Advances in Canine and Feline Nutritional Research: Iams Proceedings, 1996. p 277.

Strombeck D. Home-Prepared Dog and Cat Diets: The Healthful Alternative. 1999. Ames, Iowa: Iowa State University Press.

Yance D. Reported in Natural Health Products, 2005. Ashland, Oregon.

Chinese herbal medicine/acupuncture references

Huang SY, et al. *Journal of Pharmacology and Clinical Application of TCM.* 1996;12(3):28–29.

Jiang Y, et al. *Gansu Journal of TCM.* 1988;7(4):4–7.

Kubo M, Matsuda H, Tanaka M, Kimura Y, Okuda H, Higashino M, Tani T, Namba K, Arichi S. Studies on Scutellariae radix. VII. Anti-arthritic and anti-inflammatory actions of methanolic extract and flavonoid components from Scutellariae radix. *Chem Pharm Bull*, 1984; 32(7):2724–9.

Li YF (translator). Foreign Medicine, vol. of TCM. 1984;6(1):15–18.

Liu IX, Durham DG, Richards RM. Baicalin synergy with beta-lactam antibiotics against methicillin-resistant Staphylococcus aureus and other beta-lactam-resistant strains of S. aureus. *J Pharm Pharmacol.* 2000 Mar;52(3):361–6.

Liu W, et al. *Henan Journal of TCM Pharmacy.* 1998;13(4): 10–12.

Mascolo N, Autore G, Capasso F, et al. Biological screening of Italian medicinal plants for anti-inflammatory activity. *Phytotherapy Res* 1987;1(1):28–31.

Ma ZY. *Shannxi Journal of Traditional Chinese Medicine and Herbs.* 1982;(4):58.

Mei QX, et al (ed). Modern TCM Pharmacology. China: TCM Press; 1998:10.

Pi Fu Bing Fang Zhi Yan Jiu tong Xun (*Research Journal on Prevention and Treatment of Dermatological Disorders*), 1979;3:152.

Pi fu Bing Fang Zhi Yan Jiu Tong Xun (*Research Journal on Prevention and Treatment of Dermatological Disorders*), 1972; 3:215.

Rui J. *Journal of Chinese Materia Medica.* 1999;30(1):43–45.

Shan Xi Yi Kan (*Shanxi Journal of Medicine*), 1960; (10):32.

Shen DX, et al. *Journal of Chinese Patent Formulas.* 1982;(1):21.

Sheng Yao Xue Za Zhi (*Journal of Raw Herbology*), 1979; 33(3):178.

Wu GZ, et al. *Journal of University of Pharmacology of China.* 1990;21(4).

Zhang FC, et al. Research into Di Long's mechanism in its recovery effects on rabbit back injury. *China Journal of Pharmacy.* 1999;34(2):93–96.

Zhang MF, et al. *Journal of Pharmacology and Clinical Application of TCM.* 1996;12(1):29.

Zhang MF, et al. *Journal of Pharmacology and Clinical Application of TCM.* 1998;14(6):12–16.

Zhang SC, et al. *Journal of Chinese Patent Medicine Research.* 1984;(2):37.

Zhong Cao Yao (*Chinese Herbal Medicine*) 1991;22 (10):452.

Zhong Guo Yao Ke Da Xue Xue Bao (*Journal of University of Chinese Herbology*), 1990;21(4):222.

Zhong Guo Zhong Yao Za Zhi (*People's Republic of China Journal of Chinese Herbology*), 1989; 14(3):44.

Zhong Guo Zhong Yao Za Zhi (*People's Republic of China Journal of Chinese Herbology*), 1991; 16(9):560.

Zhong Yao Cai (*Study of Chinese Herbal Material*), 1991; 14(2):41.

Zhong Yao Tong Bao (*Journal of Chinese Herbology*), 1988:13(6):364.

Zhong Yao Xue (*Chinese Herbology*), 1988;103:106.

Zhong Yao Xue (*Chinese Herbology*), 1988; 137:140.

Zhong Yao Xue (*Chinese Herbology*), 1998;156:158.

Zhong Yao Yao Li Yu Lin Chuang (*Pharmacology and Clinical Applications of Chinese Herbs*), 1989;5(1):24.

Zhong Yao Yao Li Yu Ying Yong (*Pharmacology and Applications of Chinese Herbs*), 1983:400.

Zhong Yao Yao Li Yu Ying Yong (*Pharmacology and Applications of Chinese Herbs*); 1983:866.

Zhong Yao Yao Li Yu Ying Yong (*Pharmacology and Applications of Chinese Herbs*), 1983:1221.

Zhong Yao Zhi (*Chinese Herbology Journal*), 1993:183.

Zhong Yao Zhi (*Chinese Herbology Journal*), 1993;358.

Zhong Yi Za Zhi (*Journal of Chinese Medicine*), 12:18.

Zhou WZ, et al. *Pharmacy Bulletin.* 1979;14(5):202–203.

Homotoxicology references

Broadfoot PJ. Inflammation: Homotoxicology and Healing. In: Proceedings AHVMA/Heel Homotoxicology Seminar. 2004. Denver, CO, p 27.

Demers J. Homotoxicology and Acupuncture. In: Proceedings of the 2004 Homotoxicology Seminar. AHVMA/Heel. 2004. Denver, CO, p 5, 6.

Gebhardt R. Antioxidative, antiproliferative and biochemical effects in HepG2 cells of a homeopathic remedy and its constituent plant tinctures tested separately or in combination. *Arzneimittelforschung.* 2003. 53(12): pp 823–30.

Habermehl D, Kammerer B, Handrick R, Eldh T, Gruber C, Cordes N, Daniel PT, Plasswilm L, Bamberg M, Belka C, Jendrossek V. Proapoptotic activity of Ukrain is based on Chelidonium majus L. alkaloids and mediated via a mitochondrial death pathway. *BMC Cancer.* 2006. Jan 17;6: p 14.

Palmquist R. Health is the Goal: Dermatology Notes; The Case of Judy Blue Eyes—Chronic Ulcerative Dermatopathy in a Cat. In: Proceedings of Heel/AHVMA Homotoxicology Seminar, Denver, CO, 2005. pp 49–51.

Reckeweg H. Biotherapeutic Index: Ordinatio Antihomotoxica et Materia Medica, 5th ed. 2000. Baden-Baden, Germany: Biologische Heilmittel Heel GMBH, pp. 323–4, 337, 357, 392–3.

Shamsa F, Ahmadiani A, Khosrokhavar R. Antihistaminic and anticholinergic activity of barberry fruit (Berberis vulgaris) in the guinea-pig ileum. *J Ethnopharmacol.* 1999. Feb;64(2):pp 161–6.

FUNGAL INFECTIONS

Definition and cause

Dermatophytosis is a cutaneous fungal infection caused by *Mycosporum canis* and other dermatophte fungi. This fungal infection is contagious, and generally the only clinical manifestation is hair loss and a crusted lesion (Dunbar Gram 2003, Scott 1995). Other fungi can cause infections, which can also become systemic and can cause disease in other organs, such as the sinus and the lungs.

Medical therapy rationale, drug(s) of choice, and nutritional recommendations

Systemic treatment with Griseofulvin, Ketoconazole, and Itraconazole are often prescribed. While fairly effective, they have potential side effects such as anemia and white blood cell suppression (with Griseofulvin) and hepatopathy (with Ketoconazole and Itraconazole). Topical cleaning, clipping the hair, and applying topical agents such as lime sulfur is also effective (Dunbar Gram 2003, Moriello 1994, Scott 1995).

Anticipated prognosis

Most infestations are self limiting and the prognosis is good (Dunbar Gram 2003, Scott 1995).

Integrative veterinary therapies

According to the American Academy of Allergy, Asthma and Immunology, sinusitis in humans and fungal infections are on the rise. This indicates that the common treatments, e.g. antifungals, are not getting to the root of the problem, which is not caused by infection, but is actually an immune disorder caused by fungus. Researchers have found that fungal organisms were present in the mucus of 96% of patients who had surgery for chronic sinusitis, and inflammatory cells were clumped around fungi, suggesting an immune disorder caused by fungus.

This is easy to comprehend when we consider that mold spores contain numerous digestive enzymes that directly attack and damage tissue. A healthy immune system should be able to aggressively defend itself against mold spores. Direct damage by fungal spores coupled with environmental toxins is a perfect formula to initiate allergic responses. As this damage progresses we see an excellent example of progressive vicariation, which rapidly can attain the Degeneration Phase and may predispose to Degeneration Phase disease processes (see Homotoxicology, General Considerations, below).

In the veterinary field, we see an array of fungal conditions, not only in the skin but also systemic forms, and as the body attempts to destroy the fungus, the immune system damages the surrounding tissues. The integrative approach to such fungal infestations, either local or systemic, is to reduce exposure to infectious agents, support immune function, and improve and enhance the elimination of toxins from the body.

Nutrition
General considerations/rationale
The nutritional support used to address fungal infection is usually done in combination with medical therapy, although in this approach, topical medication is preferred. The therapeutic nutritional approach is to help reduce inflammation locally and balance and enhance immune function systemically.

Some approaches to fungal infection involve dietary changes, because high-carbohydrate diets may contribute to fungal overgrowth, and supplementing with a high level of omega-3 fatty acids can improve immune function. Several foods rank high on the list for dietary avoidance, including: corn, which is highly contaminated with fumonisin, aflatoxins, and other fungal toxins (Council for Agricultural Science 2003); wheat and wheat products, because wheat is often contaminated with mycotoxins; barley; cottonseed; sugar cane; sorghum; and sugar beets.

Many disease entities have been linked to fungal overgrowth. To learn more about their sources, read *Diseases Caused by Fungi and Their Mycotoxins* by Costantini (1998) (see Product Sources).

Appropriate nutrients
Nutrition/gland therapy: Glandular therapy support of the skin as well as the immune system organs (adrenals,

thymus, and lymph) is indicated (see Chapter 2, Gland Therapy, for additional information).

Quercetin: Quercetin is in the flavonoids family (see Chapter 2, Phytonutrients). It functions like an antihistamine and has antioxidant properties. It has been shown to inhibit cells from releasing histamines (Middleton 1986, Ogasawara 1985), so it is beneficial in the treatment of allergic conditions such as dermatitis, eczema, and asthma.

Phosphatidyl choline: This phospholipid is integral to cellular membranes and is an essential nutrient for healthy skin (Hanin 1987).

Evening primrose oil: EPO has been proven to have both anti-inflammatory and anti-pruritic effects and, as part of a balanced nutritional program, can exert a positive effect on animals with skin disease. Studies suggest that EPO is beneficial in people with atopic dermatitis and eczema (Hederos 1996, Humphreys 1994, Morse 1989).

Chinese herbal medicine/acupuncture
General considerations/rationale
Fungal infections are a result of Wind, Heat, and Damp invading the body. Wind blows the pathogen into the body. Heat and Damp refer to the inflammation and moist skin lesions, respectively. Treatment is aimed at eliminating the pathogen, clearing inflammation, and preventing secondary bacterial infections.

Appropriate Chinese herbs
Anemarrhena rhizome (Zhi mu): Has demonstrated inhibitory effects against some dermatophytes and some bacteria, including Staphylococcus aureus (Yao Xue Qing Bao Tong Xun 1987). This herb can attack the primary pathogen while simultaneously preventing secondary bacterial infections.

Angelica root (Dang gui): An immunostimulant (Zhong Hua Yi Xue Za Zhi 1978) that may help the patient eliminate the infection.

Arctium (Niu bang zi): Inhibits bacteria, including Staphylococcus aureus and beta streptococcus, and various fungi (Group of Internal Medicine 1960, Group of Virology 1973, Cao 1957).

Atractylodes rhizome (Cang zhu): Inhibits Staphylococcus aureus and some dermatophytes (Zhong Yao Xue 1998 318:320). It can decrease xylene-induced ear swelling and carrageenin-induced foot swelling (Zhang 1998). It may decrease the inflammation associated with fungal infections.

Gypsum (Shi gao): Has dual activities of decreasing inflammation and stimulating immunity. It increases the phagocytic activity of macrophages (Zhong Yao Xue 1998). At the same time it decreases inflammation. In 1 trial 126 human patients with various inflammatory disease processes were treated with gypsum. Most showed improvement (Zhong Hua Wai Ke Za Zhi 1960).

Licorice (Gan cao): Can inhibit Staphylococcus aureus (Zhong Yao Zhi 1993).

Rehmannia (Sheng di huang): Reduces swelling and inflammation (Zhong Yao Yao Li Yu Ying Yong 1983).

Schizonepeta stem (Jing jie hui): Decreases acute and chronic inflammation (Zeng 1998, Xie 1983).

Siler (Fang feng): Inhibits Staphylococcus aureus (Zhong Yao Tong Bao 1988).

Sophora root (Shan dao gen): Increases IgM and IgG levels (Guo Wai Yi Xue Zhong Yi Zhong Yao Fen Ce 1989). It also has antibiotic activity (Xian Dai Shi Yong Yao Xue 1988).

Homotoxicology
General considerations/rationale
Fungal infections may occur if an overwhelming amount of infectious fungal agent gains access to the body. Simple dermatophytosis is a Reaction Phase disorder, while chronic, recurrent, or refractory cases indicate more serious systemic involvement.

Immune suppression by a wide variety of causes predisposes to fungal infection as does residing in a contaminated area. Systemic mycoses involve both of these factors. Many fungal infections occur following compromise of the greater defense system and are more common in Deposition, Impregnation, Degeneration, and Dedifferentiation phases. Yeast infections are commonly associated with allergic disorders, wherein homotoxins accumulate and alter the connective tissue's responses.

Homotoxicology agents are viewed as additional therapy in these cases, because antifungal drugs are both important and useful in treating systemic and topical forms. However, the clinician must remember that these drugs are homotoxins and can cause further damage to the body, particularly the liver and kidney. No cases of successful use of antihomotoxic therapy could be found in the veterinary literature at this time, but one case of feline cryptococcal encephalitis was treated successfully using an integrative approach by the author (Palmquist 2005).

Appropriate homotoxicology formulas
The best known of the classical homeopathic remedies for fungal infection/dermatophytosis are: Sepia for brown, scaly patches; Tellurium for prominent, well-defined, reddish sores; Graphites for thick scales or heavy discharge; and Sulphur for excessive itching (Cummings et al. 1984).

BHI-Allergy: A remedy that contains Arnica for itching, burning skin, and a host of other remedies for skin irritations and eruptions. It also contains, most notably, Tellurium metallicum, which is mentioned in classical reportories. Marked skin (*Herpes circinatus*) is another indication for this remedy, as is a very sensitive back, itching of hands and feet, herpetic spots, ringworm (*Tuberc*), ring-shape lesions, offensive odors from affected parts, and circular patches of eczema. Lesions tend to be equally distributed on either side of the body. Also recommended for Pityriasis versicolor and eruptions—herpetic. (Bianchi 1995). *BHI-Allergy* also contains Graphites (see *Graphites homaccord*) and Sulphur (see *Sulphur heel* and *Engystol N*).

BHI-Skin: A good support remedy that includes Rhus Toxicodendron (also in *Aesculus compositum*, *Arnica-Heel*, *Echinacea compositum*, *BHI-Inflammation*, *BHI-Skin*, et. al.) Rhus toxicodendron (poison ivy) contains rhoitannic acid. A component of the sap, urushiol, is a strong skin irritant. It has been recommended for violent itching, and possibly for an eruption like measles all over the body, a vesicular eruption (herpes), a crusty eruption on the head, and eruptions of a vesicular nature, particularly when the eruptions are bluish-grey in color. It is one of the main remedies for Herpes zoster. However, Rhus toxicodendron is also valuable in chronic skin diseases, especially in eczema with vesicle formation. It is also a main remedy for facial and frontal impetigo if there is violent itching. This remedy also contains Graphites (see *Graphites homaccord*) and sulphur (see *Sulphur-Heel* and *Engystol N*).

Coenzyme compositum: Provides metabolic support and repair of damage to mitochondria by therapeutic agents.

Cutis compositum: Provides support and drainage of the skin and associated adnexa (Heel 2003). This remedy is of huge value in skin disorders, as one might expect from the name. It contains Cutis suis, for which the principal indications are: allergic reactions, dermatoses, eczema, seborrhea, dermatomycoses, neurodermatitis, and other chronic problems. It also has Hepar suis (found in *Hepar compositum*, *Syzygium compositum*, *Thyreoidea compositum*, *Tonsilla compositum*, etc.) for chronic eczemas, neurodermatitis, psoriasis, erythemas, dermatomycoses, and eruptions that are papular or in blotches which itch and that appear on the head, face, back, female genitalia, or extremities. It also contains Sulphur (see *Sulphur Heel*) and Graphites (see *Graphites Homaccord*). The ingredient Thuja can also be of value in chronic skin conditions. The oil from the red cedar, from which Thuja is taken, is known as an antifungal agent.

Echinacea compositum: Provides immune support in Reaction and Impregnation phases.

Galium-Heel: Contains *Aurum metallicum*, which has been used successfully in a case of Feline Aspergillosis (Hoare).

Graphites homaccord: Used to treat dry, crusty or weepy patches of pigmented dermatitis. Graphites (also found in *BHI-Allergy*, *BHI-Skin*, *Cutis compositum*, *Placenta compositum*, *Thyroidea compositum*, *Tonsilla compositum*, etc.) shares indications with Carbo vegetabilis and other anti-psorics, particularly Sulphur. There is a tendency toward the formation of cracks, and to various skin diseases, proceeding with crusty eruptions and the discharge of a sticky, honey-like fluid, which hardens into scabs. These are often localized in the folds and creases of the skin. Itching is aggravated by heat. There may be general loss of hair, which is hard and brittle, and alopecia areata, and possibly chronic ear discharge smelling like herring-brine.

Graphites, as a constituent, is also a remedy indicated for eczema capitis, fissures in general, intertrigo and fungal infections of the nails, and psoriasis on fingertips, nipples, corners of the mouth, and between the toes. Another important constituent, *Sepia* (in BHI-Skin and others) is one of the most frequently needed homeopathic remedies, and is mainly used for chronic diseases and dyscrasias (i.e., both cellular and also chronic humoral phases such as chronic eczemas and chronic discharges such as leucorrhoea). Worthy of particular note are the skin symptoms of Sepia, namely soreness and itching, which is frequently transformed into burning as a result of scratching (cf. Sulphur), with localization in the creases of the knees. These patients may show large, suppurating pustules, which repeatedly relapse; brown patches on the face, chest, and abdomen; and vesicles and scabies-like conditions, particularly if Sulphur has not completed the cure. The skin symptoms may express in the form of pustules, eczema, neurodermitis, herpes, yellowish-brown scaly patches, or sloughing of the epidermis in round patches on the hands and fingers, possibly associated with painless ulcers. Chronic dermatophytosis is another condition that may respond to this remedy. (Reckeweg 2002)

Lymphomyosot: Used in lymph draining and in eczema.

Psorinoheel: A phase remedy in Excretion Phase disorders and in chronic, constitutional cases. One of the most useful components is Bacillinum, which is used in eczema and impetigo and is indicated in alopecia. It is useful for Pityriasis versicolor and other skin disorders, as well as general weakness and debilitation. The ingredient Bufo has been used for purulent blisters (pemphigus) on the skin and mucosa, and for paronychia and glandular and dermal inflammations accompanied by a tendency toward suppuration.

Psorinum nosode (also in Tonsilla compositum (was introduced into the homeopathic Materia Medica by Hering in 1833–34, and was the first nosode to be so included. It is said to be useful in chronic and acute eczemas with violent itching, especially at night, that is relieved by scratching until it bleeds. Other skin dyscrasias also respond well to intercurrent doses of Psorinum. According to some popular materia medicas, there is a wide variety of relationships with well-known polychrests, such as: Arsenicum album (complaints and restlessness at night, fear of death, desquamating skin eruptions); Petroleum (dry skin with cracks and oozing eruptions); and Sulphur, which is the most closely related remedy regarding discharges, burning of the skin, eruptions, vicarious conditions, and general chronicity. Thus, it is appropriately used in chronic eczema, impetigo, all kinds of skin eruptions, asthma alternating with eczema, psoriasis, boils, acne, seborrhoea, etc. (Reckeweg 2002). Also contains Sulphur (see *Sulphur-Heel, Engystol N, and Schwef-Heel*).

Schwef-Heel A Sulphur-containing remedy for red, itchy skin. It is used as a catalyst, and is given intermittently in skin conditions. This is a homaccord of Sulphur, which has deeper reaching potencies than other antihomotoxic formulas.

Sulphur-Heel: Named for Sulphur, one of the most important single remedies in homeopathy. This is easily appreciated when one discovers the number of antihomotoxic agents that contain it, such as *Causticum compositum, Cutis compositum, Echinacea compositum, Engystol, Ginseng compositum, Hepar compositum, Mucosa compositum, Psorinoheel, Pulsatilla compositum, Schwef-Heel, Thyreoidea compositum, Tonsilla compositum, BHI-Allergy, BHI-Enzyme, BHI-Skin*, and many others.

Typical of Sulphur indications in Impregnation phases is the affection of the skin, which itches and then burns after being scratched. The body is trying to eliminate intermediate homotoxins, particularly histamine, via the skin, causing a wide variety of discharges, which are excoriating and cause reddening of the orifices and an offensive body odor. Sulphur should be given intercurrently, e.g. as an intravenous injection, in cases that do not respond to well-indicated biotherapeutic or antihomotoxic remedies. This should be done regardless of the system, e.g. chronic heart disease; skin diseases such as lichen planus, acne vulgaris, eczema, neurodermitis, and dermatoses; and liver disease. (Reckeweg 2002).

This combination also contains a variety of remedies that are useful in itchy, eczematous, eruptive skin lesions, such as Caladium, Pix liquida, Mezereum, Arsenicum, and others.

Tonsilla compositum: Provides immune support in Impregnation, Degeneration, and Dedifferentiation phases. It contains Conium (also in *Ginseng compositum, Testis compositum, Thyroidea compositum, Ubichinon compositum*, and others), which is used for glandular swellings and induration, prickling and stinging, and conditions that are stony-hard to the touch (Reckeweg 2002). *Tonsilla compositum* also contains the aforementioned Graphites, Hepar suis, Psorinum, and Sulphur. Funiculus

umbicalis suis is included for regeneration of damaged tissues (Smit 2004).

Traumeel S: Used as a phase remedy and in cases of regulation rigidity.

Authors' suggested protocols

Nutrition
Skin and immune support formulas: 1 tablet for every 25 pounds of body weight BID.

Lymph support formula: One-half tablet for every 25 pounds of body weight BID.

Quercetin: 50 mg for every 10 pounds of body weight SID.

Lecithin/phosphatidyl choline: One-fourth teaspoon for every 25 pounds of body weight BID.

Oil of evening primrose: 1 capsule for every 25 pounds of body weight SID.

Chinese herbal medicine/acupuncture
The patent formula is Xiao Feng San. It contains 3 g each of angelica root (Dang gui), rehmannia (Sheng di huang), siler (Fang feng), cicada (Chan tui), anemarrhena rhizome (Zhi mu), sophora root (Shan dao gen), sesame seeds (Hei zhi ma), schizonepeta stem (Jing jie hui), atractyloides rhizome (Cang zhu), arctium (Niu bang zi), and gypsum (Shi gao), and 1.5 g of licorice (Gan cao) (Handbook of TCM Practitioners 1987). It is dosed according to the supplier's recommendations.

Homotoxicology (Dose: 10 drops PO for 50-pound dog; 5 drops PO small dog or cat)
Graphites homaccord, Psorinoheel, Cutis compositum autosanguis: Give every 2 to 4 weeks, as needed.

Echinacea compositum: Give every 3 days orally.

Hepeel compositum: Give every 3 days.

Coenzyme compositum and Ubichinon compositum: Give on alternate days.

Detox Kit and Galium-Heel: Give daily BID PO for 30 days, possibly with the aforementioned autosanguis mixed in.

Echinacea comp forte, Traumeel plus Mucosa compositum and Chelidonium homaccord (for intestinal mycosis): Injected e.o.d., preferably as an autosanguis. European practitioners have reported good results from this combination (Guray 2003).

Product sources

Nutrition
Skin, immune, and lymph support formulas: Animal Nutrition Technologies. **Alternatives:** Immune System Support—Standard Process Veterinary Formulas; Immuno Support—Rx Vitamins for Pets; Immugen—Thorne

Veterinary Products; Derma Strength—Vetri Science Laboratories; Canine Dermal Support—Standard Process Veterinary Formulas.

Quercetin: Source Naturals; Quercetone—Thorne Veterinary Products.

Lecithin/phosphatidyl choline: Designs for Health.

Oil of evening primrose: Jarrow Formulas.

Chinese herbal medicine
Patent formula: Xiao Feng San—Mayway.

Homotoxicology
BHI/Heel Corporation

REFERENCES

Western medicine references
Dunbar Gram W. Dermatophytosis. In: Tilley L, Smith F. The 5-Minute Veterinary Consult: Canine and Feline, 2003. Blackwell Publishing.

Moriello KA, DeBoer DJ. Dermatophytosis. In: August JR, ed. Consultations in feline internal medicine 2. Philadelphia: Saunders, 1994:219–225.

Scott DW, Miller WH, Griffin CE, eds. Fungal skin diseases. In: Muller and Kirk's small animal dermatology 5th ed. Philadelphia: Saunders, 1995:332–350.

Nutrition references
Middleton E Jr. Effect of flavonoids on basophil histamine release and other secretory systems. *Prog Clin Biol Res.* 1986;213:493–506.

Ogasawara H, Middleton E Jr. Effect of selected flavonoids on histamine release (HR) and hydrogen peroxide (H2O2) generation by human leukocytes [abstract]. *J Allergy Clin Immunol.* 1985;75(suppl):184.

Hanin I, Ansell GB. Lecithin : Technological, Biological, and Therapeutic Aspects, NY: Plenum Press. 1987, 180, 181.

Hederos CA, Berg A. Epogam evening primrose oil treatment in atopic dermatitis and asthma. *Arch Dis Child* 1996; 75(6):494–497.

Humphreys F, Symons J, Brown H, et al. The effects of gamolenic acid on adult atopic eczema and premenstrual exacerbation of eczema. *Eur J Dermatol* 1994;4(598):603.

Morse PF, Horrobin DF, Manku MS, et al. Meta-analysis of placebo-controlled studies of the efficacy of Epogam in the treatment of atopic eczema: relationship between plasma essential fatty acid changes and clinical response. *Br J Dermatol* 1989;121(1):75–90.

Chinese herbal medicine/acupuncture references
Cao RL, et al. *China Journal of Dermatology.* 1957;(4):286.

Guo Wai Yi Xue Zhong Yi Zhong Yao Fen Ce (*Monograph of Chinese Herbology from Foreign Medicine*), 1989; 11(2): 59.

Group of Internal Medicine, Chongqing Medical University Hospital, No. 1. *Journal of Microbiology.* 1960;8(1):52.

Group of Virology. Institute of Pharmacy. Academy of Traditional Chinese Medicine. *Journal of Modern Medicine and Pharmacology.* 1973;(12):38.

Handbook of TCM Practitioners, Hunan College of TCM, Shanghai Science and Technology Press, Oct 1987, p 604–605.

Xian Dai Shi Yong Yao Xue (*Practical Applications of Modern Herbal Medicine*), 1988; 5(1):7.

Xie ZZ. *Sichuan Journal of TCM.* 1983;1(2):56.

Yao Xue Qing Bao Tong Xun (*Journal of Herbal Information*), 1987; 5(4):62.

Zeng N, et al. *Journal of TCM Pharmacology and Clinical Application.* 1998;14(6):24–26.

Zhang MF, et al. *Journal of Pharmacology and Clinical Application of TCM.* 1998;14(6):12–16.

Zhong Hua Wai Ke Za ZHi (*Chinese Journal of External Medicine*), 1960;4:366.

Zhong Hua Yi Xue Za Zhi (*Chinese Journal of Medicine*), 1978;17(8):87.

Zhong Yao Tong Bao (*Journal of Chinese Herbology*), 1988:13(6):364.

Zhong Yao Xue (*Chinese Herbology*), 1998, 115: 119.

Zhong Yao Xue (*Chinese Herbology*), 1998; 318:320.

Zhong Yao Yao Li Yu Ying Yong (*Pharmacology and Applications of Chinese Herbs*), 1983:400.

Zhong Yao Zhi (*Chinese Herbology Journal*), 1993;358.

Homotoxicology references
Bianchi I. Homeopathic, Homotoxicological Repertory Homotoxicological Materia Medica. Baden-Baden, Germany: Aurelia Publishers Ltd. 1995, p 574.

Boericke W. Materia Medica with Repertory, 9th ed. 1927. Santa Rosa, CA: Boericke and Tafel. http://www.homeoint.org/books/boericmm/t/tell.htm.

Council for Agricultural Science and Technology. Mycotoxins: Risks in Plant, Animal and Human Systems. Task Force Report Jan 2003. No. 139. Ames, IA.

Cummings S, Ullman D. Everybody's Guide to Homeopathic Medicine. 1984. Los Angeles: Jeremy P. Tarcher.

Guray J. 2003. Personal communication regarding systemic fungal infections.

Heel. Veterinary Guide, 3rd English edition. Baden-Baden, Germany: Biologische Heilmettel Heel GmbH. 2003. p 34.

Hoare J. Communication on therapy of Feline Aspergillosis.

Mercola J, Droege R. Fungus May be Causing Your Sinus Infections—Here's What Can Help. 2005. Mercola.com.

Palmquist R. A case of feline Cryptococcal encephalitis successfully treated integratively using fluconazole and autosanguis therapy. 2005. Unpublished.

Reckeweg H. Homeopathia Antihomotoxica Materia Medica, 4th Completely Revised Edition. Baden-Baden, Germany: Aurelia-Verlag, 2002. pp. 164, 190–1, 330–1, 338–40, 500–3, 512–14, 532–3, 555–60.

Rubik B. Report on the status of research on homeopathy with recommendations for future research. *Biol Ther*, 1989. 7(2): pp 25–30, 46.

Smit A. General Protocol for Fungal Infections. 2004. Heel.

SEBORRHEIC DERMATITIS

Definition and cause

Seborrheic dermatitis is characterized by excessive dry or oily sebum, commonly caused by a combination of Staph pyoderma and Malassezia dermatitis. It is fairly common in dogs and rare in cats (Mason 2003, Scott 1995).

Medical therapy rationale, drug(s) of choice, and nutritional recommendations

The recommended treatments are topical shampoos such as selenium sulfide in combination with ketaconizole when secondary yeast infections are involved. Antibacterial shampoos may also be indicated based upon the status of the skin and secondary bacterial infection. The potential of hepatopathies with ketaconizole is a precaution that should be discussed.

Anticipated prognosis

Regular antifungal or antibacterial shampoos can be used to control seborrheic dermatitis, although recurrences are common (Mason 2003).

Integrative veterinary therapies

Proper diagnostic evaluation is required to properly diagnose and treat these cases. Obtaining a full medical history and conducting a physical exam, skin scraping, and blood evaluation with thyroid levels are recommended in most cases. Impression smears and cytology may yield yeast overgrowth and secondary bacterial infections as microorganisms congregate around the exudative process in an attempt to ingest and process homotoxins being excreted or stored in affected tissues. Many chronic dermatitis cases undergo regressive vicariation and produce severe oily material (see Homotoxicology, below).

Gently cleansing the oily material away on a regular basis decreases retoxification from rancid, oxidized fatty acids, and reduces nutritional support of pathogens such as yeast and bacteria. Avoid topical agents that suppress the secretion of material (such as coal tar, corticosteroids, and antihistamines) unless their use is absolutely necessary, because these inhibit the body's natural ability to remove fat-soluble homotoxins through the skin and can be absorbed, causing further injury to the cutaneous defenses. Antihistamines are the least harmful of the aforementioned group.

The addition of therapeutic nutrition and biological therapies helps to boost immune function and improve the elimination of toxins via the skin. These improvements often minimize exacerbation and recurrences.

Nutrition
General considerations/rationale

While medical therapy is focused locally upon the skin (inflammation, pruritus, sebum), the nutritional approach adds gland support for the organs of the immune system and nutrients to help decrease local inflammation and enhance toxin elimination, especially via the skin.

Appropriate nutrients

Nutritional/gland therapy: Glandular adrenal and lymph provide intrinsic nutrients for the glands of the immune system and the skin. These nutrients help enhance the elimination of toxins via the skin (see Gland Therapy and the Enhancement of Elimination, Chapter 2).

Lecithin/phosphatidyl choline: Phosphatidyl choline is a phospholipid that is integral to cellular membranes. It helps to move fats into the cells and is important for cellular integrity. Lecithin is an essential nutrient required by the skin and all of the body's cells of the body for general health and wellness (Hanin 1987). Studies with lecithin have shown that it can emulsify fats which are important for the skin's health (Brook 1986, Spilburg 2003).

Evening primrose oil: EPO has been proven to have both anti-inflammatory and anti-pruritic effects and, as part of a balanced nutritional program, can exert a positive effect on animals with skin disease. Studies suggest that EPO is beneficial in people with atopic dermatitis and eczema (Hederos 1996, Humphreys 1994, Morse 1989).

Chinese herbal medicine/acupuncture
General considerations/rationale

Seborrheic dermatitis is due to Heat and Wind invading the Liver and Lungs. This leads to Yin and Blood deficiency. The Lungs control the skin, so Lung pathology can cause dermatitis. The Liver is the organ most likely to suffer from Wind. When the Liver is invaded by Wind, the result is pruritis.

Blood and Yin are fluids. If they are deficient in the Skin it causes dryness because the skin cannot remain healthy when it is not nourished.

Treatment is aimed at reversing the fluid deficiency, or normalizing the skin and soothing the itch. It is also necessary to control secondary infections.

Appropriate Chinese herbs

Angelica (Bai zi): Has anti-inflammatory properties (Zhong Guo Zhong Yao Za Zhi 1991). It may decrease inflammation of the skin.

Atractylodes (Cang zhu): Has activity against Staphylococcus auerus and dermatophytes (Zhong Yao Xue 1998). It may help prevent secondary infections.

Bupleurum (Chai hu): Decreases the effect of histamine release (Zhong Yao Yao Li Yu Ying Yong 1983) and has antibiotic effects against streptococci (Zhong Yao Xue 1998). It may help decrease pruritis and prevent secondary skin infections.

Cicada slough (Chan tui): Has been used successfully in humans to treat chronic urticaria (Pi fu Bing Fang Zhi Yan Jiu Tong Xun 1972), which indicates that it has a beneficial effect on the skin. It may be of use in seborrheic dermatitis to help protect the skin or prevent itching due to secondary bacterial infections.

Honeysuckle (Jin yin hua): Has antibiotic effects against Staphylococcus aureus, E. coli, and Pseudomonas aeruginosa (Xin Yi Xue 1975), and is anti-inflammatory (Shan Xi Yi Kan 1960).

Licorice (Gan cao): Inhibits the growth of Staphylococcus aureus (Zhong Yao Zhi 1993). It contains glycyrrhizine and glycyrrhentinic acid, which have corticosteroid activity (Zhong Cao Yao 1991). This may help prevent secondary infections and decrease pruritis.

Mint (Bo he): Relieves itching (Zhong Cao Yao Xue 1980) and has anti-inflammatory effects (Zhong Yao Xue 1998).

Moutan (Mu dan pi): Demonstrates anti-inflammatory actions via inhibition of prostaglandin synthesis and decreases vascular permeability (Sheng Yao Xue Za Zhi 1979, Zhong Guo Yao Ke Da Xue Xue Bao 1990). It inhibits the growth of Staphylococcus aureus, streptococci, and dermatophytes (Zhong Yao Cai 1991).

Platycodon (Jie geng): Decreases allergic reactions (Zhong Yao Yao Li Yu Ying Yong 1983), and may help with skin inflammation.

Poria (Fu ling): Has inhibitory effects on Staphylococcus aureus (Zhong Yao Cai 1985).

Rehmannia (Sheng di huang): Has shown anti-inflammatory activity in mice (Zhong Yao Yao Li Yu Ying Yong 1983).

Siegesbeckia (Xi xian cao): Inhibits the growth of Staphylococcus aureus (Kim 1979).

White peony (Bai shao): Contains paeoniflorin, which is a strong anti-inflammatory (Zhong Yao Zhi 1993). It also has antibiotic effects against Staphylococcus aureus, some streptococci, E. coli, Pseudomonas aeruginosa, and some dermatophytes (Xin Zhong Yi 1989).

Acupuncture has been used to treat skin allergies (Lundesberg 1988). By stimulating specific acupuncture points, it is possible to stimulate the pet's immune system and reduce the itching and inflammation associated with dermatitis. This may be applicable to the skin inflammation seen in seborrheic dermatitis or help with itching secondary to bacterial invasion of the abnormal skin.

The authors have used GV14, SP9, and SP10 to control inflammation (clear Heat in TCM terms). LI11 can be used to stop any itching and HT7 can be used to calm the animal so it does not lick or scratch and irritate the skin further. Local points can be used; these include LI4 for the front legs, GB34 for the back legs, and GB20 for the neck (Schoen 1994).

Homotoxicology
General considerations/rationale
Seborrhea means "to run oil," and represents Excretion Phase or Inflammation Phase homotoxicoses. Seborrhea often occurs in chronic cases of dermatitis, and this condition can represent genetic or breed-related issues. In those cases, it represents the Degeneration Phase on the Six-Phase Table.

An important sign of healing is represented by an oily secretion, which begins as thick waxy material and slowly becomes progressively more liquid and lighter in viscosity. If the clinician observes such changes, especially when hair regrowth and depigmentation of hyperpigmented areas are noted, the client should be properly advised and therapy should be continued in earnest.

Appropriate homotoxicology formulas
(See also the protocols for Hypothyroidism, Cushing's disease, Addison's disease, allergic dermatitis, and otitis externa.)

Abropernol: Hyperhydrosis, hyperkeratosis, and eczema are all indications. The ingredient Pulsatilla pratensis is classically used for urticarial eczema, which may occur following the ingestion of rich food (diarrhea may be present). This is a useful remedy in many conditions where response to treatment (case change) is not apparently forthcoming. Ocular discharge may be present, as may be heavy, bland ear discharges (Macleod 1983). Calcium fluoratum is useful for stony swelling of glands, calcified ear canals, chronic suppurative otitis media, anal itching, fissures and cracks on the anus and foot pads, and excessive scar tissue (Boericke 1927).

BHI-Hair and -Skin: The ingredient Thuja occidentalis treats dry hair, hair loss, dandruff (due to Selenium), urticarial reactions, eczema located around the mouth and face, and epitherliomas. Petroleum rectifacatum is included for eczema that is worse in the winter and excessive sweating from the axillae and feet (Reckeweg 2000). Acidum nitricum treats jagged warts that bleed easily, foul skin secretions, and poorly healing granulomas (Macleod 1983). The presence of Hamamelis virginiana is useful for traumatic inflammations and venous disturbances. This remedy also treats blistery eruptions and dry skin (Macloed 1983).

BHI-Skin: Used for eczema; rashes and hives; skin eruptions; red rash all over the body; pustules; acute and chronic skin lesions; moist, suppurating lesions; and herpetic ulcers. This is a very useful remedy that contains Berberis vulgaris for itchy blisters, anal eczema, and pigmenting eczema. Berberis is supportive of cutaneous, hepatobiliary, renal, and adrenal systems, and greatly assists in excretion of homotoxins via these routes. Rhus tox is useful for red rashes, itching, and contact hypersensitivity reactions. Arsenicum album is a classic remedy for dry skin, eruptions, and boils/carbuncles. Sulfur is a useful agent in chronic dermatitis because it activates blocked enzyme systems. It is useful in eczema with intense itching and vesicular eruptions, and for patients that frequently have a bad smell. Sepia, Petroleum, and Kreosotum all assist in eczema. Hydrofluoricum acidum is useful for brittle nails. Graphites (see *Graphites homaccord*) is also included (Heel 2002).

Coenzyme compositum: Provides metabolic support and reversal of iatrogenic factors. *Hepeel* and *Coenzyme compositum* may be used in conditions to reduce pruritus (Reinhart 2005).

Cutis compositum: A broad remedy that is indicated in all cutaneous diseases to establish drainage and stimulate healing of the skin. It is a wide-reaching formula that stimulates nonspecific defenses in a variety of cutaneous conditions. *Cutis compositum* can be used in any phase homotoxicosis; it opens skin to drainage and repair. It supports regeneration and repair of organs involved in skin health (Cutis suis, Hepar suis, Splen suis, Placenta suis, Glandula suprarenalis suis, Funiculus ubilicalis suis). It contains Sulfur to repair blocked enzyme systems and Cortisonum aceticum to repair damage from prior corticosteroid exposure. It supports circulation and drainage (Aesculus hipposcastanum) (Reckeweg 2000).

Engystol N: Provides support to the immune system. Sulfur assists in allergic dermatitis and eczema, as well as in viral infections and in cases associated with vaccinosis.

Graphites homaccord: Contains Graphites, which is indicated for loss of hair, oozing cutaneous discharges, and sticky eczema behind the ear pinnae (Macloed 1983). Treats dry, chronic dermatitis and eczema; obese patients; constipation; honey-yellow crusts on dermatitis; dermatitis of the ear's meatus; moist and cold feet with poorly healing wounds; and easily ulcerating skin (Reckeweg 2000). Patients that require Graphites frequently have a tendency to obesity and constipation. Tiny abrasions may be more susceptible to infection and oozing. The patients may have dry ear canals in which otoscopic examination may show white concretions on the tympanum (Boerike 1927). Calcium carbonicum Hahnemanni complements Graphites; this assists in cases showing exudative dermatitis and facial rashes/eczema, poor-healing wounds, petechial eruption, and boils.

Hepar compositum: Used for liver drainage and support during detoxification (see Hepatitis protocols).

Hormeel S: Has a normalizing effect on the endocrine system.

Lymphomyosot: Promotes lymphatic drainage and contains homeopathically diluted thyroid hormone and iodine to activate suppressed thyroid and immune functions.

Psorinoheel: A deep-acting remedy with Psorinum and sulfur that is indicated in constitutional cases as well as the Excretion Phase.

Schwef-Heel: Contains sulfur, which is indicated in seborrhea activates many blocked enzymes systems. Oily skin, red skin, foul odors are all indications for sulfur, which may need to be given intermittently while recovery is progressing.

Solidago compositum: Provides renal support and drainage during detoxification. It is a phase remedy for the Deposition Phase. There is a connection in Traditional Chinese Medicine between skin disease and the Kidney (Zang Fu organ). Many forms of dermatitis improve when the kidney is treated and supported.

Thyroidea compositum: Provides matrix drainage and neuroendocrine support. It contains a wide variety of glandular support agents such as Glandula thyroidea suis and Thymus suis, as well as Corpus pineale suis, Splen suis, Medulla ossis suis, Funiculus umbilicalis suis, and Hepar suis. Other ingredients support metabolism and drainage. Cortisonum aceticum assists in cases of iatrogenic damage from corticosteroids and chronic stress.

Traumeel S: An anti-inflammatory that repairs blocked enzyme systems to stimulate healing.

Ubichinon compositum: Provides metabolic support.

Authors' suggested protocols

Nutrition
Immune and skin support formulas: 1 tablet for every 25 pounds of body weight BID.

Lecithin/phosphatidyl choline: One-fourth teaspoon for every 25 pounds of body weight BID.

Oil of evening primrose: 1 capsule for every 25 pounds of body weight SID.

Chinese herbal medicine/acupuncture
The author recommends Formula H52 ImmunoDerm and H67 DermGuard at a dose of 1 capsule each for every 10 to 20 pounds. It may be necessary to initially use antibiotics or shampoos to control secondary infections. In addition to the herbs discussed above, these preparations contain scutellaria (Huang Qin), fleece flower root (He shou wu), siler (Fang feng), tokoro (Bi xie), schizonepeta (Jing jie), dandelion (Pu gong ying), oldenlandia (Bai hua she cao), kochia (Di fu zi), xanthium fruit(Cang Er zi), bitter orange (Zhi ke), angelica radix (Dang gui), buffalo horn shavings (Sui Niu jiao), earthworm (Di long), silkworm (Jiang can) and cnidium (Chuan xiong).

The recommended acupuncture points are LI4, LI11, ST36, SP6, GB34, and SP10 (Handbook of TCM Practitioners 1987).

Homotoxicology (Dose: 10 drops PO for 50-pound dog; 5 drops PO small dog or cat)

Symptom formula: Schwef-Heel and/or Graphites homaccord, Psorinoheel, and Abropernol used for 2 to 4 weeks BID.

Detoxification formula (Excretion and Inflammation phase cases): Lymphomyosot, Nux vomica homaccord, and Berberis homaccord BID for 30 days; then re-evaluate case.

Detoxification formula (Deposition, Impregnation, Degeneration, and Dedifferentiation phase cases): Galium-Heel, Lymphomyosot, Hepar compositum, Solidago compositum, and Thyroidea compositum every 3 days for 30 to 120 days or until case change ceases. Then shift to Detox Kit for 30 days. Further use of Deep Detoxification is indicated in chronic cases.

Product sources

Nutrition

Immune and skin support formulas: Animal Nutrition Technologies. **Alternatives:** Immune System Support—Standard Process Veterinary Formulas; Immuno Support—Rx Vitamins for Pets; Immugen—Thorne Veterinary Products; Derma Strength—Vetri Science Laboratories; Canine Dermal Support—Standard Process Veterinary Formulas.

Lecithin/phosphatidyl choline: Designs for Health.

Oil of evening primrose: Jarrow Formulas.

Chinese herbal medicine

Formula H52 ImmunoDerm and H67 DermGuard: Natural Solutions, Inc.

Homotoxicology

BHI/Heel Corporation

REFERENCES

Western medicine references

Mason KV. Malassezia Dermatitis. In: Tilley L, Smith F. The 5-Minute Veterinary Consult: Canine and Feline, 2003Blackwell Publishing.

Scott DW, Miller WH, Griffin CE. Muller and Kirk's small animal dermatology. 5th ed. 1995. Philadelphia: Saunders.

Nutrition references

Brook JG, Linn S, Aviram M. Dietary soya lecithin decreases plasma triglyceride levels and inhibits collagen- and ADP-induced platelet aggregation. *Biochem Med Metab Biol* 1986;35:31–9.

Hanin I, Ansell GB. Lecithin: Technological, Biological, and Therapeutic Aspects, NY: Plenum Press. 1987, 180, 181.

Hederos CA, Berg A. Epogam evening primrose oil treatment in atopic dermatitis and asthma. *Arch Dis Child* 1996; 75(6):494–497.

Humphreys F, Symons J, Brown H, et al. The effects of gamolenic acid on adult atopic eczema and premenstrual exacerbation of eczema. *Eur J Dermatol* 1994;4(598):603.

Morse PF, Horrobin DF, Manku MS, et al. Meta-analysis of placebo-controlled studies of the efficacy of Epogam in the treatment of atopic eczema: relationship between plasma essential fatty acid changes and clinical response. *Br J Dermatol* 1989;121(1):75–90.

Chinese herbal medicine/acupuncture references

Handbook of TCM Practitioners, Hunan College of TCM, Shanghai Science and Technology Press, Oct 1987, p 615.

Kim JH, Han KD, Yamasaki K, Tanaka O. Darutoside, a. diterpenoid from Siegesbeckia pubescens and its structure. *Phytochemistry*, 1979; 18(5):894–895.

Lundesberg T et al. Effect of acupuncture on experimentally induced itch (Abstract). *Am J Acupuncture* 16:275, 1988.

Pi fu Bing Fang Zhi Yan Jiu Tong Xun (*Research Journal on Prevention and Treatment of Dermatological Disorders*), 1972; 3: 215.

Shan Xi Yi Kan (*Shanxi Journal of Medicine*), 1960; (10):32.

Sheng Yao Xue Za Zhi (*Journal of Raw Herbology*), 1979; 33(3): 178.

Schoen A. Veterinary Acupuncture: Ancient Art to Modern Medicine. California: American Vet Pub, Inc., 1994 p.252.

Xin Yi Xue (*New Medicine*), 1975; 6(3): 155.

Xin Zhong Yi (*New Chinese Medicine*), 1989; 21(3):51.

Zhong Cao Yao (*Chinese Herbal Medicine*) 1991; 22 (10):452.

Zhong Cao Yao Xue (*Study of Chinese Herbal Medicine*), 1980;932.

Zhong Guo Yao Ke Da Xue Xue Bao (*Journal of University of Chinese Herbology*), 1990;21 (4):222.

Zhong Guo Zhong Yao Za Zhi (*People's Republic of China Journal of Chinese Herbology*), 1991; 16(9):560.

Zhong Yao Cai (*Study of Chinese Herbal Material*), 1985; (2): 36.

Zhong Yao Cai (*Study of Chinese Herbal Material*), 1991; 14(2):41.

Zhong Yao Xue (*Chinese Herbology*), 1998; 89:91.

Zhong Yao Xue (*Chinese Herbology*), 1998;103:106.

Zhong Yao Xue (*Chinese Herbology*), 1998; 318: 320.

Zhong Yao Yao Li Yu Ying Yong (*Pharmacology and Applications of Chinese Herbs*), 1983: 400.

Zhong Yao Yao Li Yu Ying Yong (*Pharmacology and Applications of Chinese Herbs*), 1983; 866.

Zhong Yao Yao Li Yu Ying Yong (*Pharmacology and Applications of Chinese Herbs*), 1983; 888.

Zhong Yao Zhi (*Chinese Herbology Journal*), 1993:183.

Zhong Yao Zhi (*Chinese Herbology Journal*), 1993; 358.

Homotoxicology references

Boericke W. *Materia Medica with Repertory*, 9th ed. Santa Rosa, CA: Boericke and Tafel, 1927. pp 12–1, 250–1.

Heel. BHI Homeopathic Therapy: Professional Reference. Albuquerque, NM: Heel Inc. 2002. p 96.

Macleod G. A Veterinary Materia Medica and Clinical Repertory with a Materia Medica of the Nosodes. Safron, Walden: CW Daniel Company, LTD. 1983. pp 78, 118–9, 131–2.

Reckeweg H. Biotherapeutic Index: Ordinatio Antihomotoxica et Materia Medica, 5th ed. Baden-Baden, Germany: Biologische Heilmittel Heel GMBH, 2000. pp 285, 343–4, 347–8.

Reinhart E. Liver and Metabolic Diseases. In: Proceedings of 1st Annual Veterinary Congress. Memphis, TN. 2005. Nov 11–13, Heel, pp 22.

MANGE (DEMODECTIC/SARCOPTIC)

Definition and cause

Demodex is a localized or generalized parasitic disease caused by Demodex spp. mites. The underlying cause is believed to be genetic or related to immune deficiency or imbalance. In cats it is most often associated with other systemic disease such as FIV. Sarcoptic mange is a highly pruritic parasitic disease caused by the mite *Sarcoptes scabiei* (Ackerman 1994, Griffin 1993, Medleau 2003, Scott 1995, Rhodes 2003).

Medical therapy rationale, drug(s) of choice, and nutritional recommendations

For demodex the medical therapies of choice are Amitraz, Ivermectin, or Milbemycin, all of which have potential side effects and are potentially toxic. Amitraz is particularly toxic to humans, and proper precautions should be taken to protect humans from exposure to its active ingredient. None of these treatments address the underlying immune imbalance. Therapy for sarcoptic mange involves mitocidal shampoos or dips along with the medications used in demodex, and/or the use of Selamectin. In addition, antipruritic medications such as antihistamines and corticosteroids are often recommended (De Jaham 1995, Griffin 1993, Medleau 2003, Rhodes 2003).

Anticipated prognosis

Localized demodectic mange usually carries a good prognosis. Generalized demodecosis in immune-compromised animals often has a more guarded prognosis. Sarcoptic mange has a good prognosis (Griffin 1993, Medleau 2003, Rhodes 2003).

Integrative veterinary therapies

Mange is a nondescript term meaning infestation with one of several mite ectoparasites. These ectoparasites cause irritation through their waste products and physical injury to the host (burrowing), and by their physical presence on the host, which triggers various responses directed at elimination of the mites (pruritus, grooming, self destructive behavior). Damage directly from the mite's activities and or from the host response leads to a worsening condition.

The integrative approach expands the medical therapy to include the immune system. The integrative approach is cellular protective for the potential toxic effects of medication and mitacidal dips, and helps improve immune function and its ability to rid the body or prevent re-infestation of the mites and lessens inflammation, pruritus, and discomfort.

Nutrition
General considerations/rationale

While medical therapy is focused locally upon destruction of the mite and the skin (inflammation and/or pruritus), the nutritional approach adds gland support for the organs of the immune system as well as nutrients to help decrease local inflammation and improve waste elimination. Because mange, especially demodex, can range in severity from local to generalized and can affect other organs, it is recommended that blood be analyzed both medically and physiologically to determine associated organ involvement and disease. This gives clinicians the ability to formulate therapeutic nutritional protocols to address the skin and organ involvement such as liver inflammation secondary to medication or chemical dips (see Chapter 2, Nutritional Blood Testing, for more information).

Appropriate nutrients

Nutritional/gland therapy: Glandular adrenal, thymus and lymph provide intrinsic nutrients and help neutralize cellular immune organ damage and protect organs from ongoing inflammation and eventual degeneration (See Chapter 2, Gland Therapy, for more information).

Sterols: Plant-derived sterols such as betasitosterol show anti-inflammatory properties, which appear to be similar to corticosteriods (Gupta 1980). A cortisone-like effect without the associated immune suppressing effects is beneficial in inflammatory skin conditions. Bouic (1996) reports on the immune-enhancing and balancing effect that plant sterols have on the body.

Quercetin: Quercetin functions like an antihistamine and an antioxidant, and is beneficial for the skin. In its antihistamine role, quercetin has been shown to inhibit cells from releasing histamines, which makes it helpful in treating inflammatory dermatitis (Middleton 1986, Ogasawara 1985).

Lecithin/phosphatidyl choline: Phosphatidyl choline is a phospholipid that is integral for cellular membranes. It is an essential nutrient required by the skin, which is the body's largest cellular organ (Hanin 1987).

Essential fatty acids: Much research has been conducted on the importance of essential fatty acids on the clinical management of allergic dermatitis. In addition, the importance of the ratio between omega-6 and omega-3 fatty acids has been substantiated. Research on the use of polyunsaturated fatty acids has shown their beneficial and antipruritic effects on skin (Reinhart 1996, Schick 1996).

Vitamin C: De la Fuente (1998) and Penn (1991) showed that vitamin C in combination with other vitamins significantly improved immune function as compared with a placebo.

Chinese herbal medicine/acupuncture
General considerations/rationale

Mange is a result of parasites in both Western and TCM theory. Both modalities have the same treatment objectives: kill the parasite, decrease discomfort, and prevent secondary infections. It may also be prudent in some patients to improve immune function to allow the patient to clear the parasite.

Appropriate Chinese herbs

For topical application:

Alumen (Ming fan): Has been shown to inhibit bacterial growth (Chang Yang Zhong Yao Xian Dai Yan Jiu Yu Lin Chuan 1995), which may help to prevent secondary bacterial infections in lesions caused by scratching.

Cnidium (She chuang zi): Has antibiotic properties (Zhong Yao Xue 1998). It also decreases itching. In a study involving 607 patients with severe pruritis, it stopped itching in 84% of the participants (Lin Chuang Pi Fu Ke Za Zhi 1983).

Prickly ash (Hua jiao): Possesses antibacterial and antidermatophyte properties (Zhong Yao Xue 1998). This may help prevent secondary infections.

Realgar (Xiong huang): Has traditionally been used to kill internal and external parasites by TCM practitioners. It has been shown to treat pinworms and malaria (Zhong Cheng Yao Yan Jiu 1982, He Bei Zhong Ye 1988), which are internal parasites. The efficacy shown against internal parasites suggests that it would also be effective topically against external parasites.

Sulfur (Liu huang): Is commonly used topically in Western medicine for mange, often as a lime sulfur dip. It has been used as a component for the treatment of psoriasis (Liu 1999).

For immunosuppression:

Angelica root (Dang gui): Increases the phagocytic activity of macrophages (Zhong Hua Yi Xue Za Zhi 1978).

Astragalus (Huang qi): Stimulates the cellular and humoral immune systems. It contains astragalan, which enhances phagocytic activity of macrophages and antibody synthesis (Jiao 1999).

Codonopsis (Dang shen): Enhances the immune system by increasing the weight of the spleen and thymus and the total number of white blood cells and lymphocytes. (Huang 1994).

Dioscorea (Shan yao): Enhances both the cellular and humoral immune systems (Miao 1996).

Fleece flower root (He shou wu): Increases the total white cell count, especially the T-cells, and increases the phagocytic activity of macrophages (Zhong Yao Yao Li Yu Lin Chuang 1989).

Licorice (Gan cao): Can enhance the phagocytic activity of macrophages (Zhong Yao Xue 1998).

Lotus seed (Lian zi): Was shown to increase the number of T cells in the thymuses in mice (Ma 1995), which implies that it may be useful in treating immunosuppression.

Poria (Fu ling): Contains pachman, which increases the phagocytic function of macrophage (Lu 1990).

Psoralea (Bu gu zhi): Stimulates the phagocytic actions of macrophages (Wang 1990).

Rehmannia (Shu di huang): Increases the phagocytic activity of macrophages (Cao 1989).

Schizandra (Wu wei zi): Can prevent cyclophosphamide-induced decrease in the white blood count (Li 1995, Qu 1996).

White atractylodes (Bai zhu): Increases the TH cell count and the TH/TS ratio (Xu 1994). It increases the phagocytic function of macrophages (Tang 1998).

Wolfberry (Gou qi zi): Increases the phagocytic activity of macrophage phagocytic and raises the total T cell count (Zhong Cao Yao 19(7).

Zizyphus (Suan zao ren): Enhances cellular and humoral immunity (Lang 1991).

Homotoxicology
General considerations/rationale

A genetic predisposition (Degeneration Phase) is involved with demodectic mange, and affected individuals should not be used for breeding.

Palmquist relies on conventional therapy to treat most of these (lyme dip and Ivermectin in breeds which can tolerate the drug), but in certain cases it may prove helpful to support immune function, detoxification, and repair of tissues injured by homotoxins. Antihomotoxic agents may have a place in therapy in such cases. The authors are unaware of any work reporting single use of homotoxicology in the management of veterinary mange cases.

Appropriate homotoxicology formulas

BHI-Hair and -Skin: May help repair skin and hair in recovery phase and detoxification, provide support in cases of damage from vaccines, and promote vicariation of chronic diseases (Heel 2002).

BHI-Skin: Treats eczema on elbows, scaly scratchy dermatitis, ulcerations, and urticarial reactions (Heel 2002).

Coenzyme compositum: Contains cis-Aconitum acidum for pruritus, skin diseases, and psoriasis (Reckeweg 2002). Several of the active skin catalysts in *Coenzyme compositum* are common to *Cutis compositum*.

Cutis compositum: Provides support of all skin conditions. This is a critical skin remedy, named primarily for Cutis suis, and indicated in allergic reactions, dermatoses, eczema, seborrheic conditions, pemphigus, psoriasis, dermatomycoses, neurodermatitis, and other skin conditions, as well as disturbances of renal excretion. Contains Ichthyolum, which has pustular acne and violent pruritus (facial) as its main indications. Ichthyol ointment serves to soften and clear out abscesses and is a stimulative treatment in inflammations. Sulphur is also a critical component (See *Sulphur-Heel*). The remedy contains Cortisone in homeopathic dilution, which is indicated for diseases manifested in the connective tissue, such as disorders of the skin, blood, and vascular systems. Fumaricum acidum, Alpha ketoglutaricum, and Natrum oxalaceticum included are for pruritus, skin diseases, and psoriasis. These catalysts are also found in *Coenzyme compositum*. Funiculus umbicalis suis is indicated for rehabilitation of tissue. This is a connective tissue remedy indicated in almost all chronic diseases. It repairs damage to connective tissue, and is used for psoriasis, skin eruptions, and dermatitis (Reckeweg 2002).

Echinacea compositum: Used for secondary infections. Arsenicum is indicated for skin eruptions and other symptoms of a stubborn nature that may border on the phase of Degeneration (Reckeweg 2002). It also contains Sulphur (see *Sulphur Heel*) and Cortisonum acidum (see *Cutis compositum*).

Engystol N: Is immune supportive in allergic and viral cases, and contains sulfur, which is indicated in chronic issues.

Graphites homaccord: Treats pigmented, greasy lesions without hair.

Hepar compositum: Improves detoxification status by its action on the liver.

Psorinoheel: A phase remedy in Excretion and Impregnation cases. Psorinum is an extract of scabies mange excretions and has been used in classical homeopathy for many years. This also contains Sulfur, which is indicated in chronic conditions (see *Sulphur-Heel*). May be helpful in so-called constitutional cases.

Schwef-Heel: Works through its higher potency of Sulfur.

Solidago compositum: Used in Deposition phases, this remedy assists the skin by its support of the kidney.

Sulphur-Heel: Primarily named for the contained remedy, Sulphur, known for its use in various skin diseases, especially those of chronic nature, and pruritic eczema and suppurative skin diseases. Sulphur is one of the most important components of tissue in the body. Therefore, Sulphur is the major remedy in practically all cellular phases, particularly in the Impregnation Phase, which still displays a tendency to turn regressive. This also contains Mezereum, which is useful for pruritic skin irritations and skin suppuration, and has several other skin-active remedies as components.

Traumeel S: Treats inflammatory lesions with much inflammation.

Authors' suggested protocols

Nutrition
Skin and immune support formula: 1 tablet for every 25 pounds of body weight BID.

Lymph support formula: One-half tablet for every 25 pounds of body weight BID.

Betathyme: 1 capsule for every 35 pounds of body weight BID. (maximum 2 capsules BID.)

Lecithin/phosphatidyl choline: One-fourth teaspoon for every 25 pounds of body weight BID.

Eskimo fish oil: One-fourth to 1 teaspoon per meal for cats. 1 teaspoon for every 35 pounds of body weight per meal for dogs.

Oil of evening primrose: 1 capsule for every 25 pounds of body weight SID.

Additional vitamin C: 100 mg for every 25 pounds of body weight BID.

Quercetin: 50 mg for every 10 pounds of body weight SID.

Chinese herbal medicine
To kill the mites, the authors use a combination of sulfur (Liu huang), 30g; realgar (Xiong huang), 15g; Alumen dehydratum (Ming fan), 45g; prickly-ash (Hua jiao), 25g; and Cnidium seed (She chuang zi), 25g. Mix well and apply topically daily for 2 to 3 weeks (Yu Chuan, Chen Zi Bin 2000).

The authors also recommended H7 Immune Stimulator for 6 months in conjunction with Mitaban dips, daily Interceptor, Ivermectin, or herbal parasite dips to counteract immunosuppression. The H7 ImmuneStimulator is dosed at 1 capsule for every 10 to 20 pounds twice daily. In addition to the herbs mentioned above, Immune Stimulator contains euryale (Qian shi), longan fruit (Long yan rou), saussurea (Mu xiang), and white peony (Bai shao). These herbs increase the efficacy of the formula.

Homotoxicology (Dose: 10 drops PO for 50-pound dog; 5 drops PO small dog or cat)
Psorinoheel and Schwef-Heel: Mixed and given twice daily orally.

Cutis compositum: Given initially, and then as needed.

Autosanguis Therapy:

1. Traumeel
2. Hepar compositum
3. Galium-Heel
4. Cutis Heel
5. Ubichinon compositum

Oral cocktail: Schwef homaccord, Psorinoheel, and Lymphomyosot, plus the remains of autosanguis in a syringe, taken orally BID to TID.

Echinacea compositum forte tabs: Use if needed.

Ivermectin: Give PO daily in breeds that can tolerate the drug.

Nutraceuticals: AFA Algae, GlutaDMG, vitamin E, fatty acids.

Product sources

Nutrition

Skin, immune and lymph support formula: Animal Nutrition Technologies. **Alternatives:** Immune System Support—Standard Process Veterinary Formulas; Immuno Support—Rx Vitamins for Pets; Immugen—Thorne Veterinary Products; Canine Dermal System Support—Standard Process Veterinary Formulas; Derma Strength—Vetri Science Laboratories.

Betathyme: Best for Your Pet. **Alternative:** Moducare—Thorne Veterinary Products.

Oil of evening primrose: Jarrow Formulas.

Eskimo fish oil: Tyler Encapsulations.

Lecithin/phosphatidyl choline: Designs for Health.

Quercetin: Source Naturals; Quercetone—Thorne Veterinary Products.

Chinese herbal medicine

Formula: H7 Immune Stimulator Natural Solutions, Inc.

Homotoxicology

BHI/Heel Corporation

REFERENCES

Western medicine references

Ackerman L. Skin and Haircoat Problems in Dogs. 1994. Loveland, CO: Alpine Publications.

De Jaham C, Henry CJ. Treatment of canine sarcoptic mange using milbemycin oxime. *Can Vet J* 1995;36;42–43.

Griffin CE. Scabies. In: Griffin CE, Kwochka KW, MacDonald JM, eds. Current veterinary dermatology: the science and art of therapy. St. Louis: Mosby, 1993. 85–89.

Medleau L, Hnilica KA. Sarcoptic Mange. In: Tilley L, Smith F. The 5-Minute Veterinary Consult: Canine and Feline, 2003. Blackwell Publishing.

Scott DW, Miller WH, Griffin CE, eds. Parasitic skin diseases. In: Muller and Kirk's small animal dermatology. 5th ed. Philadelphia: Saunders, 1995: 417–432.

Rhodes KH. Demodicosis. In: Tilley L, Smith F. The 5-Minute Veterinary Consult: Canine and Feline, 2003. Blackwell Publishing.

IVM/nutrition references

Bouic PJD, et al. Beta-sitosterol and beta-sitosterol glucoside stimulate human peripheral blood lymphocyte proliferation: Implications for their use as an immunomodulatory vitamin combination. *International Journal of Immunopharmacology* 1996. 18:693–700.

De la Fuente M, Ferrandez MD, Burgos MS, et al. Immune function in aged women is improved by ingestion of vitamins C and E. *Can J Physiol Pharmacol* 1998;76:373–80.

Gupta MB, Nath R, Srivastava N, et al. Anti-inflammatory and antipyretic activities of β-sitosterol. *Planta Medica* 1980;39:157–163.

Hanin I, Ansell GB. Lecithin: Technological, Biological, and Therapeutic Aspects, NY: Plenum Press, 1987, 180, 181.

Middleton E Jr. Effect of flavonoids on basophil histamine release and other secretory systems. *Prog Clin Biol Res.* 1986;213:493–506.

Ogasawara H, Middleton E Jr. Effect of selected flavonoids on histamine release (HR) and hydrogen peroxide (H2O2) generation by human leukocytes [abstract]. *J Allergy Clin Immunol.* 1985;75(suppl):184.

Penn ND, Purkins L, Kelleher J, et al. The effect of dietary supplementation with vitamins A, C and E on cell-mediated immune function in elderly long-stay patients: a randomized controlled trial. Age Ageing 1991;20:169–74.

Reinhart GA. A Controlled Dietary Omega-6:Omega-3 Ratio Reduces Pruritus in Nonfood Allergic Atopic Dogs, Recent Advances in Canine and Feline Nutritional Research: Iams Proceedings, 1996. p 277,

Schick MP, Schick R, Reinhart G. The Role of Polyunsaturated Fatty Acids in the canine Epidermis, Recent Advances in Canine and Feline Nutritional Research: Iams Proceedings, 1996. p 267.

Chinese herbal medicine/acupuncture references

Cao ZL, et al. Henan Journal of TCM. 1989;9(3):86.

Chang Yang Zhong Yao Xian Dai Yan Jiu Yu Lin Chuan (Recent Study and Clinical Application of Common Traditional Chinese Medicine), 1995;705:707.

He Bei Zhong Ye (*Hebei Chinese Medicine*), 1988;5:17.

Lin Chuang Pi Fu Ke Za Zhi (*Journal of Clinical Dermatology*), 1983;1:15.

Huang TK, et al. Pharmacology research on Ming Dang Shen decoction solution and polysaccharides. *Journal of Chinese Patented Medicine.* 1994;16(7):31–33.

Jiao Y, et al. *China Journal of Integrated Medicine.* 1999;19(6):356–358.

Lang XC, et al. The effects of Suan Zao Ren on immunity and radiation damages of mice. *China Journal of Chinese Medicine.* 1991;16(6):366–368.

Li Y, et al. *Journal of Norman Bethune Medical University.* 1995;21(6):583–385.

Liu SG, et al. Treating psoriasis with Tu Huai Yin. *Shandong Journal of TCM.* 1999;18(12):547–548.

Lu SC, et al. *Journal of No. 1 Military Academy.* 1990;10(3): 267.

Ma ZJ, et al. Experimental research on anti-aging effects of Lian Zi. *Journal of Chinese Materia Medica.* 1995;26(2): 81–82.

Miao MS. *Henan Journal of TCM.* 1996;16(6):349–50.

Qu SC, et al. *Jilin Journal of Chinese Medicine.* 1996;(2): 41–42.

Tang XH. *Journal of Research in Traditional Chinese Medicine.* 1998;11(2):7–9.

Wang BL, et al. *Journal of Bethune Medical University.* 1990; 16(4):325–328.

Xu SC, et al. *Shanghai Journal of Immunology.* 1994;14(1): 12–13.

Yu C and Chen ZB. Modern Complete Works of Traditional Chinese Veterinary Medicine. Guangxi Sci and Tech Press, March 2000 p 632.

Zhong Cao Yao (*Chinese Herbal Medicine*), 19(7):25.

Zhong Cheng Yao Yan Jiu (*Research on Chinese Patent Medicine*), 1982;7:46.

Zhong Hua Yi Xue Za Zhi (*Chinese Journal of Medicine*), 1978;17(8):87.

Zhong Yao Xue (*Chinese Herbology*), 1998; 382:384.

Zhong Yao Xue (*Chinese Herbology*), 1998; 759:766.

Zhong Yao Xue (*Chinese Herbology*), 1998;969:972.

Zhong Yao Yao Li Yu Lin Chuang (*Pharmacology and Clinical Applications of Chinese Herbs*), 1989; 5(1):24.

Homotoxicology references

Heel. BHI Homeopathic Therapy: Professional Reference. Albuquerque, NM: Heel Inc. 2002. pp. 62, 96.

Reckeweg H. Homeopathia Antihomotoxica Materia Medica, 4th ed. Baden-Baden, Germany: Aurelia-Verlag GMBH, 2002. pp. 118, 150–2, 259, 269, 307–8, 310, 354, 373–4, 427, 462, 555–560.

Chapter Eleven

Diseases of the Digestive System

GINGIVITIS

Definition and cause

Gingivitis is an inflammation of the gingival tissues and is common in both dogs and cats. The inciting cause is bacterial accumulation in the gingival space in combination with the animal's immune response and competence. Bacterial growth results in the production of endotoxins, which lead to further inflammation, tissue destruction, and progression of gingivitis to more serious oral pathology. In addition to bacterial accumulation, plaque (a film on the teeth composed of bacteria, saliva, food, and leukocytes) accumulates, causing additional inflammation and deposition of tartar. The result is a progressive irritation and inflammatory process that can lead to periodontal disease if not addressed (Colmery 1986, Harvey 1993, Jensen 1995, Klein 2003, Marretta 2001, West-Hyde 1995, Wiggs 1997).

Medical therapy rationale, drug(s) of choice, and nutritional recommendations

Treatment is multifaceted; prevention is the most effective means of control. Preventive measures include regularly scheduled oral prophylaxis, home brushing with enzymatic products, use of plaque-reducing dentifrices such as lactoperoxidase, cleaning of the periodontal space, use of cortisocoterioids and antibiotics as needed, and proper extraction of diseased teeth, which usually are more properly related to periodontal disease. Improved nutrition and supplemental vitamins and minerals are also recommended (Harvey 1993, Klein 2003, Marretta 2001).

Anticipated prognosis

Gingivitis is reversible if properly treated early in its course. Prognosis is more guarded once periodontal disease begins (see Stomatitis/Periodontal Disease, below).

Integrative veterinary therapies

An integrative approach to gingivitis involves early recognition of the inflammatory process and aggressive institution of preventive measures before the condition progresses to a chronic state, such as generalized stomatitis and/or periodontal disease (see below).

In addition to the local inflammatory process, there is a systemic aspect to ginigivitis, stomatitis, and periodontal disease. The chronic inflammation and localized infection can predispose and cause inflammation and infection in other organ systems such as the heart, kidney, and gastrointestinal tract. It is therefore important in an integrative approach to view the entire body and offer medical therapy when indicated, as well as nutritional, herbal, and homeopathic support systemically. Using early gingivitis as an "alarm" to address the beginning of an inflammatory/degenerative internal process (as opposed to the ginigivitis being an external condition) helps to control the local inflammation and prevent the beginnings of systemic degeneration.

Nutrition
General considerations/rationale
The nutritional approach to oral health consists of reducing inflammation, treating secondary infections, preventing of local, cellular auto-immune processes, and improving immune competency.

Appropriate nutrients
Nutrition/gland therapy: Nutrition and glandular adrenal, thymus, and bone marrow can help to neutralize a cellular immune attack, provide antioxidants to reduce inflammation, and provide specific nutrients to help prevent infection (see Gland Therapy, Chapter 2, for more detailed information).

Coenzyme Q10: Coenzyme Q10 is a strong antioxidant that helps to reduce the associated inflammation that is the precursor to many chronic diseases. CoQ10 has indications in the prevention and treatment of gingivitis and periodontal disease (Gaby 1998, Shigeta 1966).

With regards to periodontal disease, double-blind clinical trials show that people who supplemented with Coenzyme Q10 had improved results as compared to those taking only a placebo (Gaby 1998). Research suggests that periodontal disease is directly linked to a Coenzyme Q 10 deficiency (Nakamura 1973). In addition, double-blind studies show that people who supplemented with 50 mg daily for 3 weeks showed a significant reduction in the symptoms of periodontal disease (Wilkinson 1976).

Vitamin C: Vaananen (1993) showed that people who are vitamin-C-deficient are more prone to periodontal disease. Aurer-Kozelj (1982) showed that increasing the daily dose of vitamin C from 20 mg to 35 mg to 70 mg showed a significant improvement in periodontal disease.

Folic acid: Folic acid, both as a topical rinse and taken systemically, has been clinically proven to be beneficial in reducing inflammation and helping to stop bleeding in people with gingivitis and periodontal disease (Pack 1984; Vogel 1976, 1978).

Sterols: Plant-derived sterols such as betasitosterol show anti-inflammatory properties which appear to be similar to corticosteriods (Gupta 1980). A cortisone-like effect without the associated immune suppressing effects is beneficial in immune mediated conditions (Bouic 1996).

Chinese herbal medicine/acupuncture
General considerations/rationale
Gingivitis is considered to be caused by Heat rising from the Stomach. The Stomach "opens" to the mouth, according to traditional Chinese Medicine. This means that disease processes in the Stomach may be reflected in the mouth. Heat in the Stomach can cause red, irritated, inflamed gingiva. We now know that the "heat" is locally produced by reaction to bacteria in the oral cavity, not in the stomach. Treatment is aimed at relieving the inflammation and irritation and modifying the intraoral bacterial population.

Appropriate Chinese herbs
Cinnamon twig (Gui zhi): Inhibits the formation of plaque on the teeth. One study of 60 human subjects found a 44% decrease in bacterial plaque index. It also decreases pain from oral pathology (Wu 1998).

Dandelion (Pu gong ying): Has demonstrated antibacterial efficacy against a variety of bacteria (Zhong Yi Yao Xue Bao 1991). It may also possess anti-inflammatory actions (Mascolo 1987), which may decrease inflammation in the gingival.

Eclipta (Han lian cao): Has shown antibiotic properties (Xin Hua Ben Cao Gang Mu 1990).

Forsythia (Lian qiao): Inhibits the growth of many types of bacteria. In addition it has anti-inflammatory and analgesic properties (Ma 1982), which may help to decrease bacterial contributions to the stomatitis while soothing the gums.

Gypsum (Shi gao): Was used in a study consisting of 126 human patients with inflammatory diseases. Most showed improvement (Zhong Hua Wai Ke Za Zhi 1960). This may be applicable to gingivitis if the effects are seen on gingival tissue.

Licorice (Gan cao): Contains glycyrrhizin and glycyrrhetinic acid which have anti-inflammatory effects. These components have approximately 10% of the corticosteroid activity of cortisone (Zhong Cao Yao 1991). Many Western practitioners use corticosteroids to decrease the inflammation of the gingiva.

Peach kernel (Tao ren): Has anti-inflammatory effects (Liu 1989, Zhong Yao Tong Bao 1986). It can promote recovery from injury by increasing the partial pressure of oxygen in tissues by increasing blood flow in the microcirculation of ischemic skin (Zhao 1996). In addition, the increased partial pressure of oxygen may inhibit the growth of anaerobic bacteria, which are common oral pathogens.

Rehmannia (Sheng di huang): Reduces swelling and inflammation (Zhong Yao Yao Li Yu Ying Yong 1983).

Scrophularia (Xuan shen): Inhibits many types of bacteria (Chen 1986, Zheng 1960).

Scutellaria (Huang qin): Contains biacalin, which has antibiotic activity against multiple bacteria on its own and is synergistic with penicillin-type antibiotics (Zhong Yao Xue 1988, Liu 2000). Two components, baicalin and biacalein, have been shown to suppress inflammation in mice and rats (Kubo 1984, Cao 1999). It also enhances cellular immunity (Pan 1991), which may help clear any bacterial cause of gingivitis.

Trichosanthes (Tian hua fen): Has been shown to inhibit bacterial growth (Zhong Yao Yao Li Yu Ying Yong 1983).

Viola (Zi hua di ding): Has antibacterial properties (Zhong Hua Yi Xue Za Zhi 1962).

Yi yi ren (coix): Has anti-inflammatory effects. It prevents dimethylbenzene-induced ear swelling and carrageenin-induced foot swelling in mice (Zhang Ming Fa 1998). A study of 26 women with severe menstrual cramps found that treatment with coix was highly effective at decreasing pain (Zhang Yong Luo 1998). This implies that it may be efficacious in treating the pain associated with gingivitis.

Acupuncture
The National Institutes of Health Consensus Panel on Acupuncture has listed dental pain under the category of "well demonstrated evidence of effectiveness" (Sierpina 2005).

Homotoxicology
General considerations/rationale

Gingivitis is an Inflammation Phase homotoxicosis. Gingivitis is usually a reversible condition arising from the accumulation of plaque and tartar on the surface of the tooth. Stomatitis, which is dealt with later in this text, is a more chronic form that can mimic gingivitis but represents phases to the right of the Inflammation Phase. One interesting piece of research indicated that early-age neutered cats may experience reduced incidence of gingivitis (Spain, Scarlett, Houpt 2004).

Homotoxin accumulation on dental surfaces and within dental structures can increase the viscosity and adherence of plaque and lead to alteration of oral health. (Papadimitriou, et al. 2006) It can further alter the character of saliva, which is an important portion of the greater defense mechanism in oral health and disease. Proper diet and gingival hygiene from chewing and at-home dental care can greatly reduce this condition. Chewing hard substances physically removes particles that supply substrate for bacterial growth (Brown, McGenity 2005). It also causes the release of enzymes and immune substances contained in normal salivary secretions.

Regular dental prophylaxis resolves gingivitis and is the treatment of choice. Use of dental sealant is gaining popularity in veterinary dentistry. (Gengler, et al. 2005). Such compounds concern homotoxicologists because the most common product has been shown to decrease accumulation of tartar, but its long-term effects on organs of elimination have not been illustrated. In nutritional supplements, waxes and other agents used for manufacturing tablets have been associated by holistic doctors with aggravation of liver disease and intestinal difficulties.

It is tempting to attempt treating gingivitis with other agents, particularly when clients fear routine dental prophylaxis due to anxiety over anesthesia. Anesthesia-free prophylaxis can be done on some cooperative pets, but the American Veterinary Dental Association frowns on such practices because a full mouth prophylaxis is truly impossible to do on most unsedated animals. However, it may have usefulness in clinical practice and the number of practices offering this service seems to be growing.

Dental rinses may assist in increasing the interval between anesthetized procedures (Girao, et al. 2003). Several products claiming efficacy are available on the Internet and in pet stores. No controlled studies exist for most of these products, and when Palmquist contacted one of these companies he was not welcomed in his efforts to design and implement a study on the product's effectiveness. It may be that these products have great applicability, but for now the evidence is lacking and research would be welcomed. Many companies do not fully disclose ingredients and veterinarians have rightly expressed concern over product quality and safety for this reason.

Antihomotoxic medications can be used to assist gingivitis patients for short periods of time. However, it is important that clients be informed of the importance of proper dental cleaning and home care, and the inevitable progression toward periodontal disease and eventual tooth loss, as well as the potential for disease in other organs such as the heart, liver, renal system, and joints. Most clients who properly understand this opt for proper dental care on a regular basis.

Appropriate homotoxicology formulas

Belladonna homaccord: Used for right-sided intensely red tonsillitis, pharyngitis, poor appetite, nausea and vomiting, stinging rectal pain, and focal and intense inflammatory lesions (Boericke 1927). It is more appropriate for severe gingivitis that probably represents stomatitis changes.

Coenzyme compositum: Contains Citricum acidum, which is useful for dental problems and gingivitis. Also treats scurvy; blackening of teeth and heavy deposits of dental plaque; painful, herpetic vesicles around the lips; nausea; painful cramping in umbilical area; and distension.

Nux vomica homaccord: Treats liver and gastrointestinal disease. Useful in gingivitis (Reckeweg 2002) and after smoke inhalation. Commonly used formula for detoxification as part of the *Detox Kit*.

Traumeel S: An anti-inflammatory agent that promotes healing and modulates inflammation (Reckeweg 2000).

Ubichinon compositum: Contains Anthraquinone for swelling of gums and for GI symptoms such as distention, flatulence, and cramping abdominal pain. Also treats constipation with straining or sudden diarrhea (Reckeweg 2002).

Authors' suggested protocols

Nutrition

Immune and gingival/mouth support formulas: 1 tablet for every 25 pounds of body weight BID.

Betathyme: 1 capsule for every 35 pounds of body weight BID. (maximum 2 capsules BID.)

Coenzyme Q10: 25 mg for every 10 pounds of body weight daily.

Additional vitamin C: 100 mg for every 25 pounds of body weight BID.

Folic acid: 50 micrograms for every 35 pounds of body weight (maximum, 200 micrograms).

Chinese herbal medicine/acupuncture

Formula H59 Ulcerative Gingivitis: 1 capsule per 10 to 20 pounds twice daily to effect. This supplement also contains globe thistle (Luo Lu), imperata (Bai mao gen), and mirabilitum (Mang xiao) to increase the efficacy of the formula.

Recommended acupuncture points include LI11, GB20, KI3, ST6, and ST7 (Handbook of TCM Practitioners, Oct 1987).

Homotoxicology (Dose: 10 drops PO for 50-pound dog; 5 drops PO for cat or small dog)

Belladonna homaccord, Traumeel, and Nux vomica Homaccord: Mix together and give orally TID in conjunction with proper dental hygiene and professional cleaning. Give Ubichinon compositum every other day, in alternation with Coenzyme compositum if more chronic signs occur (see Stomatitis protocol, below).

Product sources

Nutrition

Immune and gingival/mouth support remedies: Animal Nutrition Technologies. **Alternative**: Immuno Support—Rx Vitamins for Pets; Immungen—Thorne Veterinary Products; Immune System Support—Standard Process Veterinary Formulas.

Betathyme: Best for Your Pet. **Alternative**: Moducare Thorne Veterinary Products.

Coenzyme Q10: Vetri Science; Rx Vitamins for Pets; Integrative Therapeutics; Thorne Veterinary Products.

Chinese herbal medicine

Formula H59 Ulcerative Gingivitis: Natural Solutions, Inc.

Homotoxicology

BHI/Heel Corporation

REFERENCES

Western medicine references

Colmery B, Frost P. Periodontal disease: Etiology and pathogenesis, *Vet Clin North Am Small Anim Pract* 1986;16: 817–834.

Bojrab MJ, Tholen M, eds. Small animal medicine and oral surgery, 1990. Philadelphia: Lea and Febiger.

Harvey CE, Emily PP. Small animal dentistry, 1993 St. Louis, MO: Mosby.

Klein T. Gingivitis. In: Tilley L, Smith F. The 5-Minute Veterinary Consult: Canine and Feline, 2003 Blackwell Publishing.

Jensen L, Logan E, et al. Reduction in accumulation of plaque, stain, and calculus in dogs by dietary means. *J Vet Dent* 1995 12(4):161–163.

Marretta, SM. Periodontal Disease in Dogs and Cats, The Atlantic Coast Veterinary Conference, 2001.

West-Hyde L, Floyd M. Dentistry. In: Ettinger SJ, Feldman EC, eds. Textbook of veterinary internal medicine. 4th ed. Philadelphia: Saunders 1995:1097–1121.

Wiggs RB, Lobprise HB. Veterinary dentistry: principles and practice. Philadelphia: Lippincott-Raven, 1997.

Nutrition references

Aurer-Kozelj J, Kralj-Klobucar N, Buzina R, Bacic M. The effect of ascorbic acid supplementation on periodontal tissue ultrastructure in subjects with progressive periodontitis. *Int J Vitam Nutr Res* 1982;52:333–41.

Bouic PJD, et al. Beta-sitosterol and beta-sitosterol glucoside stimulate human peripheral blood lymphocyte proliferation: Implications for their use as an immunomodulatory vitamin combination. International *Journal of Immunopharmacology* 1996 18:693–700.

Gaby AR. Coenzyme Q10. In: Pizzorno JE, Murray MT. A Textbook of Natural Medicine. Seattle: Bastyr University Press, 1998, V:CoQ10-1-8.

Gupta MB, Nath R, Srivastava N, et al. Anti-inflammatory and antipyretic activities of β-sitosterol. *Planta Medica* 1980; 39:157–163.

Nakamura R, Littarru GP, Folkers K. Deficiency of coenzyme Q in gingiva of patients with periodontal disease. *Int J Vitam Nutr Res* 1973;43:84–92.

Pack ARC. Folate mouthwash: effects on established gingivitis in periodontal patients. *J Clin Periodontol* 1984;11:619–28.

Shigeta Y, Izumi K, Abe H. Effect of coenzyme Q7 treatment on blood sugar and ketone bodies of diabetics. *J Vitaminol* 1966; 12:293–8.

Vogel RI, Fink RA, Frank O, Baker H. The effect of topical application of folic acid on gingival health. *J Oral Med* 1978;33(1):20–2.

Vogel RI, Fink RA, Schneider LC, et al. The effect of folic acid on gingival health. *J Periodontol* 1976;47:667–8.

Vaananen MK, Markkanen HA, Tuovinen VJ, et al. Periodontal health related to plasma ascorbic acid. *Proc Finn Dent Soc* 1993;89:51–9.

Wilkinson EG, Arnold RM, Folkers K. Bioenergetics in clinical medicine. VI. Adjunctive treatment of periodontal disease with coenzyme Q10. *Res Commun Chem Pathol Pharmacol* 1976; 14:715–9.

Chinese herbal medicine/acupuncture references

Cao ZS, et al. *Strait Journal of Pharmacology*. 1999;11(3): 53–54.

Chen SY, et al. *Fujian Journal of Chinese Medicine*. 1986; 17(4):57.

Handbook of TCM Practitioners, Hunan College of TCM, Shanghai Science and Technology Press, Oct 1987: 791–792.

Kubo M, Matsuda H, Tanaka M, Kimura Y, Okuda H, Higashino M, Tani T, Namba K, Arichi S. Studies on Scutellariae radix. VII. Anti-arthritic and anti-inflammatory actions of methanolic extract and flavonoid components from Scutellariae radix. *Chem Pharm Bull*, 1984; 32(7):2724–9.

Liu CH, et al. The pharmacology of Tao Ren. *Journal of Pharmacology and Clinical Application of TCM*. 1989;(2):46–47.

Liu IX, Durham DG, Richards RM. Baicalin synergy with beta-lactam antibiotics against methicillin-resistant Staphylococcus aureus and other beta-lactam-resistant strains of S. aureus. *J Pharm Pharmacol*. 2000 Mar;52(3):361–6.

Ma ZY. *Shannxi Journal of Traditional Chinese Medicine and Herbs*. 1982;(4):58.

Mascolo N, Autore G, Capasso F, et al. Biological screening of Italian medicinal plants for anti-inflammatory activity. *Phytotherapy Res* 1987;1(1):28–31.

Pan JF, et al. *Tianjin Journal of Medicine*. 1991;19(8): 468–470.

Sierpina V, Frenkel M. Acupuncture: A Clinical Review. *Southern Medical Journal*. 2005; 98 (3): 330–7.

Wu GH, et al. *Journal of Pharmacy Practice*. 1998;16(6): 337–338.

Xin Hua Ben Cao Gang Mu (*New Chinese Materia Medica*), 1990:415.

Zhang MF, et al. Yi Yi Ren's analgesic, anti-inflammatory, and antithrombotic effects. *Journal of Practical TCM*, 1998; 12(2):36–38.

Zhang YL, et al. Sequential experiments on Yi Yi Ren's analgesic effect in severe functional dysmenorrhea. *Journal of TCM*. 1998;39(10):599–600.

Zhao LG. Tao Ren injection's effect in promoting recovery from ischemia skin incision in rabbits. *China Journal of Integrated External Medicine*. 1996;2(2):112–115.

Zheng QY, et al. *Pharmacy Bulletin*. 1960;8(2):57.

Zhong Cao Yao (*Chinese Herbal Medicine*) 1991;22 (10):452.

Zhong Hua Wai Ke Za Zhi (*Chinese Journal of External Medicine*), 1960;4:366.

Zhong Hua Yi Xue Za Zhi (*Chinese Journal of Medicine*), 1962; 48(3):188.

Zhong Yao Tong Bao (*Journal of Chinese Herbology*), 1986; 11 (11):37.

Zhong Yao Xue (*Chinese Herbology*), 1988; 137:140.

Zhong Yao Yao Li Yu Ying Yong (*Pharmacology and Applications of Chinese Herbs*), 1983: 149.

Zhong Yao Yao Li Yu Ying Yong (*Pharmacology and Applications of Chinese Herbs*), 1983:400.

Zhong Yi Yao Xue Bao (*Report of Chinese Medicine and Herbology*), 1991:(1):41.

Homotoxicology references

Boericke W. Materia Medica with Repertory, 9th ed. Santa Rosa, CA: Boericke and Tafel. 1927 pp 90.

Brown W, McGenity P. Effective periodontal disease control using dental hygiene chews. *J Vet Dent*. 2005 Mar;22(1):pp 16–9.

Gengler W, Kunkle B, Romano D, Larsen D. Evaluation of a barrier dental sealant in dogs. *J Vet Dent*. 2005 Sep;22(3):pp 157–9.

Girao V, Nunes-Pinheiro D, Morais S, Sequeira L, Gioso M. A clinical trial of the effect of a mouth-rinse prepared with Lippia sidoides Cham essential oil in dogs with mild gingival disease. *Prev Vet Med*. 2003 May 30;59(1–2):pp 95–102.

Papadimitriou S, Tsantarliotou M, Makris G, Papaioannou N, Batzios Ch, Kokolis N, Dessiris A. A clinical study of plasminogen activator activity in gingival tissue in dogs with gingivitis and periodontitis. *Res Vet Sci*. 2006 Apr;80(2):pp 189–93.

Reckeweg H. Biotherapeutic Index: Ordinatio Antihomotoxica et Materia Medica, 5th ed. Baden-Baden, Germany: Biologische Heilmittel Heel GMBH, 2000 pp 151.

Reckeweg H. Homeopathia Antihomotoxica Materia Medica, 4th ed. Baden-Baden, Germany: Arelia-Verlag GMBH, 2002 pp. 136–8, 461–3.

Spain C, Scarlett J, Houpt K. Long-term risks and benefits of early-age gonadectomy in cats. *J Am Vet Med Assoc*. 2004 Feb 1;224(3):pp 372–9.

STOMATITIS/PERIODONTAL DISEASE

Definition and cause

Stomatitis represents an inflammatory condition of the oral cavity, and occurs in both dogs and cats. Mucosal inflammation in stomatitis can be generalized or focal involving any region of the mouth. This is a descriptive diagnosis. Successful therapy depends upon an accurate diagnosis, which means that diagnostic processes are usually necessary (Baker 2003, Harvey 1993).

In this text we represent stomatitis and periodontal disease as the more chronic version of gingivitis, whereby the local tissue and the immune system and its response have progressed to the next phase of disease and continual vigilance and a combination of medical and alternative therapies may be required. In addition, because of the chronicity, other organs and systems may be in a similar state of inflammation and degeneration (see Gingivitis, above, for a more detailed description of the inflammatory process).

Medical therapy rationale, drug(s) of choice, and nutritional recommendations

Correction of underlying causes is essential for control. Treatment of periodontal disease (See gingivitis for medical rationale), removal of infected teeth, correction of nutritional deficiencies, and use of antibiotics to control infection and corticosteroids to reduce inflammation are all indicated (Baker 2003, Lyon Wiggs 1997).

Anticipated prognosis

Prognosis is related to the underlying cause, the compliance of treatment, and the animal's immune status. In a chronic condition, there is often associated degeneration secondary to inflammation and or infection in other organ systems, which can affect the prognosis (Baker 2003).

Integrative veterinary therapies

The oral cavity contains a wealth of autonomic nerve fibers and is integrated into the central control centers. Gastrointestinal, immune, neurological, endocrine, musculoskeletal, and vascular elements smoothly coordinate a large number of vital functions.

From a phylogenetic viewpoint this makes sense, as the jaw and tongue appear to originate with the development of bivalves. Neurological supply and coordination through the modern tongue and the bivalve's muscular foot are similar in function. Numerous chemoreceptors exist in the mouth and transmit information to the brain, which in turn coordinates secretion of gastrointestinal organs of digestion, as well as hormonal events and blood supply.

The "DAMN IT" acronym is useful in approaching diagnosis of stomatitis (each letter stands for the following potential categories of disease causation: Degenerative, Anatomic, Metabolic, Nutritional, Neoplastic, Immune-mediated, Idiopathic, Infectious, Traumatic, and Toxic). A careful examination and history are necessary in all cases. Anatomic issues can predispose to development due to failure of the form to function properly. As an example, anatomic errors such as cleft palate, missing teeth, and malocclusion can lead to drying or damage of the mucosa and subsequent alteration of structure. Regional inflammations may reflect localized dental disease such as trauma (injury, electrical injury, foreign bodies, or envenomization), cervical dental lesions in cats, or periodontal disease in both cats and dogs.

Generalized patterns suggest systemic issues such as metabolic problems (diabetes, hypothyroidism, Cushing's disease, hypoparathyroidism, hepatopathies, or renal disease), toxicities (chemotherapy, radiation therapy, caustic chemical exposure, metal poisoning, or phytotoxins), infectious immune disease (periodontal disease, bacterial infection, fungal infection, and viral infection), noninfectious immune disease (pemphigus vulgaris, systemic lupus, and other auto-aggressive conditions), nutritional diseases (poor nutrition or vitamin A toxicity), neoplasia (epulis, squamous cell carcinoma, melanoma, fibrosarcoma and osteosarcoma), and idiopathic issues (eosinophilic stomatitis, plasmocytic stomatitis, and vasculitis of other causes) (White, et al. 1992, Declercq 2004, Baird 2005, Leiva 2005, Lyon 2005).

Laboratory evaluation is suggested in any case that fails to resolve or recurs. Testing for common etiologies can be helpful (FeLV, FIV, Bartonella, Leptospira, etc.).

The integrative approach to stomatitis and periodontal disease is to focus both locally and systemically. The use of therapeutic nutrition, medicinal herbs, and homotoxicology remedies either alone or in combination with medications such as antibiotics and cortisone may be required. The combination of therapies gives the clinician the opportunity to not only control local disease but also to prevent and control secondary disease and auto immune processes that were borne from the inflammatory process in the mouth.

Nutrition
General considerations/rationale
Therapeutic nutrition must be multifaceted and address the inflammatory process in the mouth along with immune system support. Note: Because stomatitis and periodontal disease often act as the nidus for the initiation of inflammation and disease in other organs, it is recommended that the clinician evaluate the blood both medically and physiologically to determine real and impending organ involvement and disease (see Chapter 2, Nutritional Blood Testing, for additional information).

Appropriate nutrients
Nutrition/glandular: In addition to the nutritional remedies recommended in the gingivitis protocol (vitamin C, folic acid, betasitosterol, and coenzyme Q10), the following is recommended:

Colostrum: Colostrum has been shown to improve intestinal health and digestion and help balance intestinal flora. In addition, colostrum can improve the immune status of the intestinal tract, which can, via intestinal production of globulins, help the overall immune competency of the body (Blake 1999). In addition, Giannobile (1994) showed that there is significant improvement in healing from surgery and improved osseous formation and periodontal regeneration in dogs supplemented with a combination product that contained colostrum.

Chinese herbal medicine/acupuncture
General considerations/rationale
According to TCM, stomatitis is caused by Heat rising from the Stomach and Spleen, leading to Yin deficiency. This causes oral mucosal damage. The Stomach opens to the Mouth, in TCM theory. When there is Heat, or inflammation in the Stomach, the Mouth, as the associated organ, may manifest the inflammation. This is revealed as red, swollen gingiva. Long-term inflammation damages the fluids (Yin), which upsets the balance between the Yin and Yang. The decrease in Yin makes the Yang seem excessive. More Yang means more Heat (inflammation). This, in Western terms, can be described as inflammatory mediators creating more inflammation, and worsening rather than resolving the condition. Thus, stomatitis tends to be chronic. Therapy is aimed at decreasing the inflammation and removing or controlling the cause of the inflammation.

Appropriate Chinese herbs
Alisma (Ze xie): Enhances immunity and decreases inflammation (Dai 1991).

Anemarrhena (Zhi mu): Increases the corticosterone level in serum and decreases inflammation (Chen 1999).

Angelica (Dang gui): Has anti-inflammatory action (Yao Xue Za Zhi 1971), yet does not cause immunosuppresion. In fact, it increases phagocytic activity of macrophages (Zhong Hua Yi Xue Za Zhi 1978).

Cinnamon (Rou gui): Normalizes the immune system. It decreases production of nonspecific antibodies (Zeng 1984). At the same time it increases the reticuloendothelial system's ability to phagocytize foreign material (You Tian Zheng Si 1990). It has been proven to have anti-inflammatory effects on both acute and chronic inflammatory conditions (Li 1989).

Crataegus (Shan zha): Enhances immunity. It increases serum lysozyme levels, serum antibody levels, and T cell activity (Jin 1992). It also has direct antibiotic activity on some bacteria (Guang Xi Zhong Yi Yao 1990, Hao 1991).

Forsythia (Lian qiao): Reduces edema and inflammation by decreasing capillary permeability (Ke Yan Tong 1982). It has demonstrated antiviral and antibacterial effects (Zhang 2002, Ma 1982).

Honeysuckle (Jin yin hua): Has antibacterial activity, mainly due to chlorogenic acid and isochlorogenic acid (Xin Yi Xue 1975, Jiang Xi Xin Yi Yao 1960). Anti-inflammatory effects have been demonstrated experimentally in rabbits and mice (Shan Xi Yi Kan 1960).

Isatis root (Ban lan gen): Possesses antiviral activity (Wang 1997, Jiang Xi Yi Yao 1989, Li 2000). In some cases it is as effective as ribavirin (Jiang 1992). It also has antibacterial efficacy (Zhong Cheng Yao Yan Jiu 1987). In addition to direct effects on pathogens, isatis root also stimulates the immune system. It seems to affect both humoral and cellular immunity (Xu 1991).

Licorice (Gan cao): Contains glycyrrhizin and glycyrrhetinic acid. These chemicals have approximately 10% of the steroid effects of cortisone (Zhong Cao Yao 1991). In addition, glycyrrhizin has shown activity against several viruses and therefore may be of use in viral-mediated stomatitis (Zhu 1996).

Ophiopogon (Mai dong): Has demonstrated the ability to inhibit several types of bacteria (Zhong Yao Xue 1998).

Oriental wormwood (Yin chen): Contains capillarin, which has anti-inflammatory properties (Wan 1987, Shan 1982).

Phellodendron (Huang bai): Has antibacterial actions against a variety of bacteria (Zhong Yao Xue 1998, Zhong Yao Da Ci Dien 1977, Zhong Cao Yao 1985).

Plantain seeds (Che qian zi): Decrease inflammation by decreasing capillary permeability (Zhang 1996).

Red peony (Chi shao): Stimulates cellular immunity by enhancing proliferation of T cells (Fan 1992).

Rehmannia (Sheng di huang): Increases the plasma levels of adrenocortical hormone (Zhong Yao Xue 1998). This may increase the amount of cortisol in circulation, and corticosteroids are commonly used to treat stomatitis by Western practitioners. Rehmannia has been shown to

reduce swelling and inflammation (Zhong Yao Yao Li Yu Ying Yong 1983).

Scrophularia (Xuan shen): Inhibits many strains of bacteria (Chen 1986, Zheng 1952).

Sophora root (Shan dou gen): Stimulates the humoral immune system, resulting in increased levels of IgM and IgG (Guo Wai Yi Xue Zhong Yi Zhong Yao Fen Ce 1989). It also has activity against several types of bacteria (Xian Dai Shi Yong Yao Xue 1988).

Homotoxicology
General considerations/rationale

Early presence of homotoxins leads to reaction by the mucosal elements in the form of Inflammation Phase disease. The mucosa recovers rapidly if these homotoxins are removed. This makes a massive case for early and aggressive home care, as well as competent professional prophylaxis. As homotoxins accumulate and are deposited the oral mucosal structure, function becomes altered. In Impregnation Phase homotoxicoses we see chronic and poorly responsive disease forms, which may not recover fully and frequently recur, frustrating client and veterinary professional alike. These conditions can progress into Degeneration Phase disease and resultant tooth loss. Degeneration Phase disorders include congenital malformation of the mouth and associated structures. Some homotoxins may lead to neoplastic changes in Dedifferentiation Phase disease.

Because most cases represent advanced homotoxicoses, management of the chronic condition, rather than cure, is often a realistic treatment goal. Some cases resolve early and represent Excretion or Inflammation phase conditions, but most cases involving cats and elderly pets involve more significant disease. Consultation with an internist or veterinary dentist may prove helpful in cases that are poorly responsive. In addition to good quality dental and internal medicine practices, homotoxicology may assist these pets. Most need long-term detoxification and symptom support. A proper diet consisting of limited antigen diets can assist some cases, and this may be associated with true allergic responses as well as adverse reactions to food ingredients or additives. The author has seen several cases improve when a raw food diet of limited ingredients is fed. Clients opting for biological therapy should be informed that some cases will not respond, while other cases will begin to respond after therapy lasting more than a year, especially when they have been kept on the Deep Detoxification Formula for several months.

Pulsatilla compositum and Traumeel are used in regulation rigidity cases, and stomatitis frequently fits this description of a disorder that is unchanging or poorly responsive. These agents can sometimes shift cases toward healing. Engystol N seems helpful and makes one wonder about impregnated viral particles, which may trigger chronic inflammatory pathways as the immune system attempts eradication of viral elements from chronically infected tissues. Feline immunodeficiency virus, Feline leukemia virus, feline calicivirus, and Feline herpes virus may cause disease in this manner, but their individual roles are unclear (Hargis, Ginn 1999; Addie, et al. 2003; Harley, Gruffydd-Jones, Day 2003; Lommer, Verstraete 2003). Because such viral elements are present in vaccine components, research is warranted into the involvement of vaccinations in this condition, and at least some cases may be adverse reaction to vaccinations. Most holistic doctors advise reduced use of vaccinations when faced with chronic, unresponsive conditions, a practice which is in agreement with most manufacturers' written recommendation to avoid vaccinating unhealthy animals. This seems prudent considering what we currently understand about auto-aggressive pathogenesis.

So-called "Alternative Phase" disease can present as stomatitis. In these cases more severe disease lurks internally and signals its presence through inflammation near the body's exterior. Many homotoxins can damage the GI system's ability to perform its duties. Both toxins and other therapeutic agents can result in progressive vicariation. Corticoids and nonsteroidal anti-inflammatory drugs both damage intestinal mucosal elements. This can result in frank ulcer or in "leaky gut syndrome," which is linked to many other medical syndromes. In leaky gut, antigens are not properly digested into smaller molecular-weight polypeptides before gaining access to the immune system. This issue can lead to chronic inflammatory diseases such as inflammatory bowel disease and allergic syndromes, and, in this discussion, chronic stomatitis.

Successfully treating stomatitis involves providing a nonaggravating diet and clean water, while working at reducing stress, allowing homotoxins to be excreted successfully, supporting organ function, draining homotoxins, and providing metabolic support while repair occurs. Patients will be observed to cycle in and out of inflammatory states, and this is highly desirable. As in other discussions, the position of the patient on the phase table assists in determining proper therapy. In the first two phases, symptomatic treatment is often successful. As homotoxins gain deeper access and do further damage, the use of compositae class antihomotoxic agents becomes necessary to stimulate regressive vicariation.

Appropriate homotoxicology formulas

Anacardium homaccord: The namesake ingredient has been shown to have powerful anti-inflammatory and immunomodulatory effects (Ramprasath, Shanthi, and Sachdanandam 2006). Treats hunger pain, mucosal catarrh including laryngeal and pharyngeal inflammation, duodenal syndrome, constipation, oral vesicles, and gastric/duodenal ulcers (Reckeweg 2000). Anacardium as an herbal extract has been shown to be antiviral against simian rotovirus (Goncalves, et al. 2005).

Arsuraneel: A cellular phase remedy that treats enteritis and diarrhea (*Arsenicum album*). May be useful in arsenic poisoning in areas with contaminated groundwater (Mallick, Mallick, Guha, and Khuda-Bukhsh 2003; Khuda-Bukhsh 2005). Also used in chronic disease, tumors of mucous membranes (*Marsdenia cundurango*), and diabetes mellitus (*Acidum phophoricum*) (Reckeweg 2000).

Belladonna homaccord: Indicated in intensely red and inflamed conditions, especially Inflammation Phase conditions. Supports immune function.

BHI-Nausea: Contains Anacardium orientale, a potent anti-inflammatory agent.

Cantharis compositum: Contains Arsenicum album. Indicated in aphthous stomatitis; when the tongue is dry, red with raised papillae, and possibly coated white, brown, or black; and for violent gastroenteritis with prolonged vomiting and diarrhea, and with unbearable burning stomach-pains after eating. Also indicated for foul-smelling stools. Also contains Mercurius solubilis, indicated in ulcerative lesions of the mucous membranes, and Hepar sulphuris calcareum (Reckeweg 2002).

Coenzyme compositum: Contains Citricum acidum, which is useful for dental problems and gingivitis; scurvy; blackening of teeth and heavy deposits of dental plaque; painful, herpetic vesicles around the lips; nausea; painful cramping in the umbilical area; and distension.

Echinacea compositum: When used in infection, supports the immune reaction, particularly in bacterial infections. It is a phase remedy for Inflammation Phase disease. For more advanced conditions consider *Tonsilla compositum*.

Engystol N: Used for viral origin gastroenteritis (see Parvovirus).

Galium-Heel: Used in all cellular phases, hemorrhoids, and anal fissures, and as a detoxicant.

Hepar compositum: Provides detoxification and drainage of hepatic tissues, organ support, and metabolic support. It is useful in most hepatic and gall bladder pathologies. It is also an important part of Deep Detoxification Formula. Treats duodenitis, pancreatitis, cystic hepatic ducts, cholelithiasis, cholangitis, cholecystitis, vomiting, and diarrhea (Demers 2004, Broadfoot 2004). This combination contains Natrum oxalaceticum (also found in *Coenzyme compositum*, *Ubichinon compositum*, and *Mucosa compositum*) for changes in appetite and stomach distension due to air. Indicated in nausea, stomach pain with a sensation of fullness, gurgling in abdomen, and cramping pain in the hypochondria. Also used for constipation, sudden diarrhea (particularly after eating), and flatus (Reckeweg 2002).

Lymphomyosot: Provides lymph drainage and endocrine support to treat edema. Contains Gentiana for chronic gastritis. Treats flatulence; diarrhea; and distension of stomach with eructations, nausea, retching, and vomiting. The component Geranium robertianum is also useful for nausea, particularly after eating, with distension or sensation of fullness. Myosotis arvensis is also contained, which also has indications for bloat and distension (Reckeweg 2002).

Mercurius-Heel S: Used for viral and bacterial issues, suppuration, and tonsillitis (Reckeweg 2000).

Mucosa compositum: Broadly supportive for repair of mucosal elements. Used in cellular cases and in recovery periods following active disease (Reckeweg 2000). This remedy contains a useful component in Kali bichromicum, indicated for ulcers found on the gums, the tongue, the lips, and even on the gastric mucosa (gastric or duodenal ulcer). The tongue may have a thick, yellow, mucous coating, or in ulcerative stomatitis or tonsillitis it may be dry, smooth, shiny, or fissured. Kali has been used effectively in acute gastroenteritis associated with vomiting of clear, light-colored fluid or quantities of mucous bile, and in cases with hematemesis, flatulent colics, and dysenteric stools with tenesmus (Reckeweg 2002).

It contains Hydrastis, with mucosal support for oral problems such as stomatitis, mucosal suppuration accompanied by ulceration, inflammations and colic of the hepatobiliary system and of the gastrointestinal tract, and polyp formation (Reckeweg 2002).

The Kreosotum component can be used in chronic gastritis with gastric hemorrhages and vomiting of brown masses. It also has a dental implication in cases with spongy gums and carious teeth, neuralgias proceeding from them causing a burning toothache with deep caries, black patches on the teeth, and fetid discharges. The single remedy Phosphorus is broadly useful for dyspepsia and for jaw problems in dental disease (Boericke 1927). Phosphorus is found in many other remedies including *Echinacea compositum* and *Leptandra Homaccord*. It is rich in suis organ preparations for mucosal support, plus a large variety of remedies with indications in the gastrointestinal sphere. Argentum nitricum (also in *Atropinum compositum, Diarrheel, Duodenoheel, Gastricumeel, Momordica compositum, BHI-Nausea*, and several other combinations) is included in this broad remedy for distension in the upper abdomen, gastrocardiac symptom-complex, and amelioration from eructations. It is also used for gastric crises (Reckeweg 2002).

Nux vomica homaccord: Treats liver and gastrointestinal disease. Useful in gingivitis (Reckeweg 2002). It is also used after smoke inhalation, and is a commonly used formula for detoxification as part of the *Detox Kit*.

Osteoheel: Provides support of bony healing and treats periostitis and periodontal disease.

Phosphor homaccord: Treats hepatitis, icterus, tenderness over the liver region, pancreatic diseases, ulcerated gums, thirst but vomiting right after drinking occurs, and pale-clay colored stools (Macleod 1983).

Psorinoheel: Used for chronic illness, and is an Impregnation Phase remedy.

Schwef-Heel: Treats chronic diseases of skin and liver. This remedy should be interposed in most skin and liver cases (Reckeweg 2000). Patients that need this remedy may look dirty and have scruffy skin conditions, red lips, white tongue with red tip, and an itching and burning rectal area with morning diarrhea and prolapsed rectum (Boericke 1927). Sulfur is contained in several other antihomotoxic formulas including *Coenzyme compositum, Echinacea compositum, Engystol, Ginseng compositum, Hepar compositum, Molybdan compositum, Mucosa compositum, Paeonia Heel, Proctheel, Psorinoheel, Sulfur-Heel, Thyroidea compositum*, and *Ubichinon compositum* (Reckeweg 2000).

Solidago compositum: Includes Berberis and other ingredients that support renal function. It is good in Deposition Phase cases.

Thyroidea compositum: A component of the Deep Detoxification Formula; drains matrix and supports endocrine function. It is a phase remedy for Impregnation Phase disease.

Tonsilla compositum: Supports immune organs in Impregnation, Degeneration, and Dedifferentiation phases.

Traumeel S: An anti-inflammatory. It also repairs blocked enzymes. It is used for regulation rigidity patients. Human studies show that it controls pain through speeded healing and homotoxin removal (Zorian, Larentsova, Zorian 1998).

Ubichinon compositum: Contains Anthraquinone for swelling of gums and GI symptoms such as distention, flatulence, and cramping abdominal pain. Also treats constipation with straining or sudden diarrhea (Reckeweg 2002).

Authors' suggested protocols

Nutrition

Immune and gingival/mouth support remedies: 1 tablet for every 25 pounds of body weight BID.

Betathyme: 1 capsule for every 35 pounds of body weight BID. (maximum 2 capsules BID)

Coenzyme Q10: 25 mg for every 10 pounds of body weight daily.

Additional vitamin C: 100 mg for every 25 pounds of body weight BID.

Folic acid: 50 micrograms for every 35 pounds of body weight (maximum, 200 micrograms).

Colostrum: One-third teaspoon of powdered formula for every 25 pounds of body weight BID.

Chinese herbal medicine/acupuncture

Formula H80 Gingival stomatitis/chronic: 1 capsule per 10 to 20 pounds twice daily. This formula is useful for acute or chronic gingival stomatitis of bacterial, viral, or immune-mediated etiology. In addition to the herbs cited above, H80 Gingival stomatitis/chronic contains aurantium fruit (Zhi qiao), dendrobium (Shi hu), imperata (Bai mou gen), malt (Mai ya), melia (Chuan lian zi), polyphorus (Zhu ling), and sweet wormwood (Qing hao). These additional herbs increase the efficacy of the formulation.

Homotoxicology (Dose: 10 drops PO for 50-pound dog; 5 drops PO for cat or small dog)

In addition to proper dental, surgical, and medical management, consider:

Symptom formula: Traumeel S, Echinacea compositum, Mucosa compositum, and Cantharis compositum, mixed together and given TID orally. Consider the following as indicated: BHI-Nausea or Anacardium homaccord (oral vesicles), Osteoheel (periodontal disease and bone loss), Engystol N or Euphorbium compositum (viral conditions), Belladonna homaccord (acute inflammation with intense redness), Mercurius-Heel S (viral or bacterial infections), and Nux vomica homaccord (general gastrointestinal drainage and detoxification).

Deep detoxification formula: Galium-Heel, Lymphomyosot, Hepar compositum, Solidago compositum, Thyroidea compositum (alternate with Tonsilla compositum), Coenzyme compositum, and Ubichinon compositum.

Product sources

Nutrition

Immune and gingival/mouth support remedies: Animal Nutrition Technologies. **Alternatives:** Immuno Support—Rx Vitamins for Pets; Immungen—Thorne Veterinary Products; Immune System Support—Standard Process Veterinary Formulas.

Betathyme: Best for Your Pet. **Alternative:** Moducare Thorne Veterinary Products.

CoEnzyme Q10: Vetri Science—Rx Vitamins for Pets for Pets; Integrative Therapeutics; Thorne Veterinary Products.

Colostrum: New Life Foods, Inc.; Saskatoon Colostrum Company.

Chinese herbal medicine

Gingival Stomatitis (Chronic-H80): Natural Solutions, Inc.

Homotoxicology

BHI/Heel Corporation

REFERENCES

Western medicine references

Baker L. Stomatitis. In: Tilley L, Smith F. The 5-Minute Veterinary Consult: Canine and Feline, 2003. Blackwell Publishing.

Declercq J. Suspected wood poisoning caused by Simarouba amara (marupa/caixeta) shavings in two dogs with erosive stomatitis and dermatitis. *Vet Dermatol.* 2004 Jun;15(3):pp 188–93.

Harvey CE, Emily PP. Oral lesions of soft tissues and bone: differential diagnosis. In: Harvey CE, Emily PP, eds. Small animal dentistry. St. Louis: CV Mosby, 1993:42–88.

Wiggs RB, Lobprise HB. Veterinary dentistry. Philadelphia: Lippincott-Raven. 1997:104–139.

IVM references

Baird K. Lymphoplasmacytic gingivitis in a cat. *Can Vet J.* Jun 2005;46(6):pp 530–2.

Declercq J. Suspected wood poisoning caused by Simarouba amara (marupa/caixeta) shavings in two dogs with erosive stomatitis and dermatitis. *Vet Dermatol.* 2004 Jun;15(3):pp 188–93.

Leiva M, Lloret A, Pena T, Roura X. Therapy of ocular and visceral leishmaniasis in a cat. *Vet Ophthalmol.* 2005 Jan-Feb;8(1):71–5.

Lyon K. Gingivostomatitis. *Vet Clin North Am Small Anim Pract.* 2005 Jul;35(4):pp 891–911, vii.

White S, Rosychuk A, Janik T, Denerole P, Schulteiss P. Plasma cell stomatitis-pharyngitis in cats: 40 cases (1973–1991). *J Am Vet Med Assoc.* 1992;200(9):pp 1377–1380.

Nutrition references

Blake SR. Bovine Colostrum, The Forgotten Miracle, *Journal of the American Holistic Veterinary Medical Association* 1999 July, Volume 18, Number 2, pp 38–39.

Giannobile WV, Finkelman RD, Lynch SE. Comparison of canine and non-human primate animal models for periodontal regenerative therapy: results following a single administration of PDGF/IGF-I. *J Periodontol* 1994, 65:1158–1168.

Chinese herbal medicine/acupuncture references

Chen SY, et al. *Fujian Journal of Chinese Medicine.* 1986; 17(4):57.

Chen WS, et al. *Journal of Second Military Medical College.* 1999;20(10):758–760.

Dai Y, et al. *China Journal of Chinese Medicine.* 1991; 16(10):622.

Fan LQ, et al. *Zhejiang Journal of Traditional Chinese Medicine.* 1992;27(3):123–125.

Guang Xi Zhong Yi Yao (*Guangxi Chinese Medicine and Herbology*), 1990; 13(3):45.

Guo Wai Yi Xue Zhong Yi Zhong Yao Fen Ce (*Monograph of Chinese Herbology from Foreign Medicine*), 1989; 11(2):59.

Hao QG, et al. Study on antibiotic function of ten commonly used herbs. *Shandong Journal of TCM.* 1991;10(3):39–40.

Jiang Xi Xin Yi Yao (Jiangxi New Medicine and Herbology), 1960(1):34.

Jiang Xi Yi Yao (Jiangxi Medicine and Herbology), 1989; 24(5):315.

Jiang XY, et al. Comparison between 50 kinds of Chinese herb that treat hepatitis and suppress in vitro HBAg activity. *Journal of Modern Applied Pharmacy.* 1992;9(5):208–211.

Jin ZC, et al. Effects of Shan Zha injection solution on immune functions. *Journal of Chinese Materia Medica.* 1992;23(11), 592–593.

Ke Yan Tong Xun (*Journal of Science and Research*), 1982;(3):35.

Li JD. *Journal of Foreign Medicine, vol. of Traditional Chinese Medicine.* 1989;11(1):1.

Li S, et al. Various Ban Lan Gen and Da Qing Ye's effect in antagonizing influenza A virus. *Journal of Second Military Medical College.* 2000; 21(3):204–206.

Ma ZY. *Shannxi Journal of Traditional Chinese Medicine and Herbs.* 1982;(4):58.

Shan Xi Yi Kan (*Shanxi Journal of Medicine*), 1960; (10):32.

Shan YTE, et al. *Journal of Pharmacy.* Japan. 1982;102(3): 285.

Wan YD. The antipyretic effects of capillarin. *Pharmacy Bulletin.* 1987;(10):590–593.

Wang SD. Therapeutic observations on treating herpes simplex with Ban Lan Gen Injection. *China Journal of Village Medicine.* 1997;25(10):24–25.

Xian Dai Shi Yong Yao Xue (Practical Applications of Modern Herbal Medicine), 1988; 5(1):7.

Xin Yi Xue (New Medicine), 1975; 6(3):155.

Xu YM, et al. Experimental research on Ban Lan Gen polysaccharide's effect in promoting immune functions. *Journal of Integrated Medicine.* 1991;11(6):357–359, 325.

Yao Xue Za Zhi (*Journal of Medicinals*), 1971;(91):1098.

You TZS, et al. *Journal of Foreign Medicine, vol. of Traditional Chinese Medicine.* 1990;12(6):373.

Zeng XY, et al. *Guangxi Journal of Medicine* 1984;6(2):62.

Zhang G, Song S, Ren J, Xu S. A New Compound from Forsythia suspense (Thunb.) Vahl with Antiviral Effect on RSV. *J of Herbal Pharmacotherapy.* 2002;2(3): 35–39.

Zhang ZQ, et al. Che Qian Zi pharmaceutical effects. *Journal of Traditional Chinese Medicine Material.* 1996;19(2): 87–89.

Zheng WF, et al. *China Journal of Medicine.* 1952;38(4): 315.

Zhong Cao Yao (*Chinese Herbal Medicine*), 1985;16(1):34.

Zhong Cao Yao (*Chinese Herbal Medicine*) 1991;22 (10): 452.

Zhong Cheng Yao Yan Jiu (Research of Chinese patent Medicine), 1987; 12:9.

Zhong Hua Yi Xue Za Zhi (*Chinese Journal of Medicine*), 1978;17(8):87.

Zhong Yao Da Ci Dien (Dictionary of Chinese Herbs), 1977:2032.

Zhong Yao Xue (*Chinese* Herbology), 1998; 144:146.

Zhong Yao Xue (*Chinese Herbology*), 1998; 845:848.

Zhong Yao Yao Li Yu Ying Yong (Pharmacology and Applications of Chinese Herbs), 1983:400.

Zhu LH. *China Journal of TCM Information.* 1996;3(3): 17–20.

Homotoxicology references

Addie D, Radford A, Yam P, Taylor D. Cessation of feline calicivirus shedding coincident with resolution of chronic gingivostomatitis in a cat. *Small Anim Pract.* 2003 Apr;44(4):pp 172–6.

Broadfoot PJ. Inflammation: Homotoxicology and Healing, in proceedings AHVMA/Heel Homotoxicology Seminar. 2004 Denver, CO, p 27.

Boericke W. Materia Medica with Repertory, 9th ed. Santa Rosa, CA: Boericke and Tafel, 1927 pp 90, 408, 497–500.

Demers J. Homotoxicology and Acupuncture, in proceedings of the 2004 Homotoxicology Seminar. AHVMA/Heel. Denver, CO, 2004 p 5, 6.

Goncalves JL, Lopes R, Oliveira D, Costa S, Miranda M, Romanos M, Santos N, Wigg M. 2005. In vitro anti-rotavirus activity of some medicinal plants used in Brazil against diarrhea. *J Ethnopharmacol.* Jul 14;99(3): pp 403–7.

Hargis A, Ginn P. Feline herpesvirus 1-associated facial and nasal dermatitis and stomatitis in domestic cats. *Vet Clin North Am Small Anim Pract.* 1999 Nov;29(6):pp 1281–90.

Harley R, Gruffydd-Jones TJ, Day MJ. 2003. Salivary and serum immunoglobulin levels in cats with chronic gingivostomatitis. *Vet Rec.* Feb 1;152(5):pp 125–9.

Heel. BHI Homeopathic Therapy: Professional Reference. Albuquerque, NM: Heel Inc. 2002 pp 54.

Khuda-Bukhsh AR, Pathak S, Guha B, Karmakar S, Das J, Banerjee P, Biswas S, Mukherjee P, Bhattacharjee N, Choudhury S, Banerjee A, Bhadra S, Mallick P, Chakrabarti J, Mandal B. In vitro anti-rotavirus activity of some medicinal plants used in Brazil against diarrhea. *J Ethnopharmacol.* 2005 Jul 14;99(3): pp 403–7.

Lommer M, Verstraete F. Concurrent oral shedding of feline calicivirus and feline herpesvirus 1 in cats with chronic gingivostomatitis. *Oral Microbiol Immunol.* 2003 Apr;18(2):pp 131–4.

Mallick P, Mallick JC, Guha B, Khuda-Bukhsh AR. Ameliorating effect of microdoses of a potentized homeopathic drug, Arsenicum Album, on arsenic-induced toxicity in mice. *BMC Complement Altern Med.* 2003 Oct 22;3: p 7.

Macleod G. A Veterinary Materia Medica and Clinical Repertory with a Materia Medica of the Nosodes. Safron, Walden: CW Daniel Company, LTD, 1983 pp 50–1, 125–6, 129–30.

Ramprasath V, Shanthi P, Sachdanandam P. Immunomodulatory and anti-inflammatory effects of Semecarpus anacardium LINN. Nut milk extract in experimental inflammatory conditions. *Biol Pharm Bull.* 2006 Apr;29(4): pp 693–700.

Reckeweg H. Biotherapeutic Index: Ordinatio Antihomotoxica et Materia Medica, 5th ed. Baden-Baden, Germany: Biologische Heilmittel Heel GMBH, 2000 pp 290, 294–5, 363–4, 369, 399–400, 538.

Reckeweg H. Homeopathia Antihomotoxica Materia Medica, 4th edition. Arelia-Verlag GMBH, Baden-Baden, 2002 pp. 136–8, 147, 206, 317–19, 345, 366, 461.

Zorian E, Larentsova L, Zorian A. The use of antihomotoxic therapy in dentistry [Article in Russian]. *Stomatologiia (Mosk).* 1998 77(6):pp 9–11.

TOOTH EXTRACTION

Definition and cause

Most common causes that necessitate tooth extraction are secondary to trauma or periodontal disease. Causes of periodontal disease include plaque, tartar, calculus buildup, and bacterial contamination. Underlying causes are related to genetic predisposition, age, and status of the immune system, as well as oral hygiene. Causes secondary to other disease such as neoplasia or parathyroid disease also occur. Signs range from mild redness and halitosis to purulent discharge, anorexia, and bleeding (Andreason 1981; Gorrel 1993, 1995, 2003; Harvey 1993; Wiggs 1997).

Medical therapy rationale, drug(s) of choice, and nutritional recommendations

Tooth extraction is generally curative for local infections and generally requires antimicrobial and possible anti-inflammatory medications post-operative. Dietary recommendations include feeding a soft diet (Andreason 1981, Gorrel 2003, Wiggs 1997).

Anticipated prognosis

Traumatic injuries generally heal well postextraction. Extraction with early periodontal disease usually has a good prognosis, while more advanced periodontal disease has a more guarded prognosis. Oral tumors generally carry a poor prognosis.

Integrative veterinary therapies

An integrative approach to dental care emphasizes prevention. Because the most common cause of tooth extraction is periodontal disease, improvement of oral health directly impacts other organ systems such as the heart and kidney. While extraction is generally curative for the local condition, the integrative approach focuses upon general immune competence, the prevention of future periodonatal disease, and avoiding tooth extractions.

Nutrition
General considerations/rationale
The nutritional approach to oral health consists of reducing inflammation, improving immune competency, and preventing infection.

Appropriate nutrients
Nutrition/gland therapy: Nutrition and glandular adrenal, thymus, and bone marrow can help neutralize a cellular immune attack and provide antioxidants to reduce inflam-

mation and specific nutrients to improve oxygenation (see Gland Therapy, Chapter 2, for additional information)

Coenzyme Q10: CoQ10 is a strong antioxidant and help reduce the associated inflammation that is the predecessor to many chronic diseases. It has indications in the prevention and treatment of chronic diseases such as gingivitis and periodontal disease (Gaby 1998, Shigeta 1966).

With regards to periodontal disease, double-blind clinical trials show that people who supplemented with Coenzyme Q10 had improved results as compared to those taking only a placebo (Gaby 1998). Research suggests that periodontal disease is directly linked to a Coenzyme Q10 deficiency (Nakamura 1973). In addition, double-blind studies show that 50 mg given daily for 3 weeks significantly reduced the symptoms of periodonatal disease (Wilkinson 1976).

Vitamin C: Vaananen (1993) showed that people who are vitamin-C-deficient are more prone to periodontal disease. Aurer-Kozelj (1982) showed that increasing the daily dose of vitamin C from 20 to 35 mg to 70 mg showed a significant improvement in periodontal disease.

Chinese herbal medicine/acupuncture
General considerations/rationale
Periodontal disease is due to Stomach Heat rising, and Qi, Blood, and Yin deficiency in the Kidney. The Stomach "opens" to the Mouth, according to Traditional Chinese Medicine. This means that disease processes in the Stomach may be reflected in the Mouth. Heat in the Stomach can cause red, irritated, inflamed gingiva. (We now know that the "heat" is locally produced by reaction to bacteria in the oral cavity, not in the stomach). The Kidney controls the bones, so when the Kidney suffers from Yin and Blood deficiency it means the bones may not be nourished by the normal fluids. As a result, the bone may degenerate. Deficient Kidney Qi means the bone is not strong enough to hold the teeth in place. The teeth loosen when periodontal bone degenerates.

Treatment is aimed at relieving the inflammation and irritation and modifying the intraoral bacterial population.

Appropriate Chinese herbs
Alisma (Ze xie): Has dual functions of enhancing immunity and decreasing inflammation (Dai 1991). Enhanced immunity controls overgrowth of oral bacteria.

Anemarrhena (Zhi mu): Increases the corticosterone level in serum and decreases inflammation (Chen 1999).

Angelica (Dang gui): Has anti-inflammatory action (Yao Xue Za Zhi 1971), yet does not cause immunosuppresion. In fact, it increases phagocytic activity of macrophages (Zhong Hua Yi Xue Za Zhi 1978).

Cinnamon (Rou gui): Normalizes the immune system. It decreases production of nonspecific antibodies (Zeng 1984). At the same time it increases the reticuloendothelial system's ability to phagocytize foreign material (You Tian Zheng Si 1990). Cinnamon has been proven to have anti-inflammatory effects on both acute and chronic inflammatory conditions (Li 1989). It may help to decrease inflammation, yet not produce immunosuppression which would allow intraoral bacteria to proliferate and cause more destruction.

Crataegus (Shan zha): Enhances immunity. It increases serum lysozyme levels, serum antibody levels, and T cell activity (Jin 1992). In addition to its effects on immunity, it has direct antibiotic activity on some bacteria (Guang Xi Zhong Yi Yao 1990, Hao 1991).

Forsythia (Lian qiao): Reduces edema and inflammation by decreasing capillary permeability (Ke Yan Tong 1982). It has demonstrated antiviral and antibacterial effects (Zhang 2002, Ma 1982).

Honeysuckle (Jin yin hua): Has antibacterial activity mainly due to chlorogenic acid and isochlorogenic acid (Xin Yi Xue 1975, Jiang Xi Xin Yi Yao 1960). Anti-inflammatory effects have been demonstrated experimentally in rabbits and mice (Shan Xi Yi Kan 1960).

Isatis root (Ban lan gen): Possesses antiviral activity (Wang 1997, Jiang Xi Yi Yao 1989, Li 2000). In some cases it is as effective as ribavirin (Jiang 1992). It also has antibacterial efficacy (Zhong Cheng Yao Yan Jiu 1987). In addition to direct effects on pathogens, isatis root stimulates the immune system. It seems to affect both humoral and cellular immunity (Xu 1991).

Licorice (Gan cao): Contains glycyrrhizin and glycyrrhetinic acid. These chemicals have approximately 10% of the steroid effects of cortisone (Zhong Cao Yao 1991). In addition, glycyrrhizin has shown activity against several viruses and therefore may be of use in viral-mediated stomatitis (Zhu 1996).

Ophiopogon (Mai dong): Has demonstrated the ability to inhibit several types of bacteria (Zhong Yao Xue 1998).

Oriental wormwood (Yin chen): Contains capillarin, which has anti-inflammatory properties (Wan 1987, Shan 1982).

Phellodendron (Huang bai): Has antibacterial actions against a variety of bacteria (Zhong Yao Xue 1998, Zhong Yao Da Ci Dien 1977, Zhong Cao Yao 1985).

Plantain seeds (Che qian zi): Decrease inflammation by decreasing capillary permeability (Zhang 1996).

Red peony (Chi shao): Stimulates cellular immunity by enhancing proliferation of T cells (Fan 1992).

Rehmannia (Sheng di huang): Increases the plasma levels of adrenocortical hormone (Zhong Yao Xue 1998,). This may increase the amount of cortisol in circulation

and decrease inflammation in the oral cavity. Rehmannia has been shown to reduce swelling and inflammation (Zhong Yao Yao Li Yu Ying Yong 1983).

Scrophularia (Xuan shen): Inhibits many strains of bacteria (Chen 1986, Zheng 1952).

Sophora root (Shan dou gen): Stimulates the humoral immune system resulting in increased levels of IgM and IgG (Guo Wai Yi Xue Zhong Yi Zhong Yao Fen Ce 1989). It also has activity against several types of bacteria (Xian Dai Shi Yong Yao Xue 1988).

Acupuncture
Liu Zhong, et al. (1996) treated 98 people suffering from chronic periodontitis with a combination of blood letting and acupuncture. The following acupuncture points were used: ST45, LI2, and KI3. After acupuncture, 1 ml of blood was removed from Li dui and Er jian. Sixty-three people had total resolution of signs, 29 people improved, and 6 people did not respond.

Homotoxicology
General considerations/rationale
Tooth extractions become necessary when the condition of the tooth and/or periodontal structures decline to the Degeneration Phase. At this point the best treatment is removal of the tooth because it no longer serves its vital function of mastication and protection and has taken on a toxic quality due to infection and loss of architecture. Good surgical technique, appropriate anesthesia, and pain management are recommended. Following surgery, antihomotoxic drugs can greatly improve patient comfort and surgical outcomes.

Appropriate homotoxicology formulas
Belladonna homaccord: Used for right-sided, intensely red tonsillitis; pharyngitis; poor appetite; nausea and vomiting; stinging rectal pain; and focal and intense inflammatory lesions (Boericke 1927). Also used for cholangitis (Reckeweg 2000).

Coenzyme compositum: Includes Citricum acidum, which is useful for dental problems and gingivitis; scurvy; blackening of teeth and heavy deposits of dental plaque; painful, herpetic vesicles around the lips; nausea; painful cramping in the umbilical area; and distension.

Echinacea compositum: The natural alternative to antibiotics, this formula supports improved immune function and is appropriate in any infection. It is a phase remedy for the Inflammation Phase.

Galium-Heel: Treats all cellular phases, hemorrhoids, and anal fissures, and is a detoxicant.

Gastricumeel: Treats acute gastritis. It includes Antimonium crudum, so it is indicated for tooth decay and toothache, and thus, may be useful when dental work is indicated (Reckeweg 2002).

Lymphomyosot: Provides lymph drainage and endocrine support, and treats edema. Contains Gentiana for chronic gastritis; flatulence; diarrhea; and distension of stomach with eructations, nausea, retching, and vomiting. It also contains Geranium robertianum, which is useful for nausea, particularly after eating, with distension or sensation of fullness. Myosotis arvensis is included and has indications for bloat and distension (Reckeweg 2002).

Mucosa compositum: Broadly supportive for repair of mucosal elements. Used in cellular cases and in recovery periods following active disease (Reckeweg 2000). This remedy contains a useful component in Kali bichromicum, which is indicated for ulcers found on the gums, tongue, lips, and even the gastric mucosa (gastric or duodenal ulcer). The tongue may have a thick, yellow, mucous coating, or, in ulcerative stomatitis or tonsillitis it may be dry, smooth, shiny, or fissured. Kali has been used effectively in acute gastroenteritis associated with vomiting of clear, light-colored fluid or quantities of mucous bile, and in cases with hematemesis, flatulent colics, and dysenteric stools with tenesmus (Reckeweg 2002).

It contains Hydrastis, with mucosal support for oral problems such as stomatitis and mucosal suppuration, accompanied by ulceration, inflammations and colic of the hepatobiliary system and the gastrointestinal tract, and polyp formation (Reckeweg 2002). The Kreosotum component can be used in chronic gastritis with gastric hemorrhages and vomiting of brown masses. Also has a dental implication in cases with spongy gums and carious teeth, neuralgias proceeding from them causing a burning toothache with deep caries, black patches on the teeth, and fetid discharges.

The single remedy Phosphorus is broadly useful for dyspepsia and for jaw problems in dental disease (Reckeweg 2002). Phosphorus is found in many other remedies, including *Echinacea compositum* and *Leptandra homoaccord*. It is rich in suis organ preparations for mucosal support, plus a large variety of remedies with indications in the gastrointestinal sphere. Also contained in this broad remedy is Argentum nitricum (also in *Atropinum compositum*, *Diarrheel*, *Duodenoheel*, *Gastricumeel*, *Momordica compositum*, *BHI-Nausea*, and several other combinations). It is used for distension in the upper abdomen and the gastro-cardiac symptom-complex, and for amelioration from eructations. It is also used for gastric crises (Reckeweg 2002).

Nux vomica homaccord: Used for liver and gastrointestinal disease, and after smoke inhalation. It is useful in gingivitis (Reckeweg 2002). *Nux vomica homaccord* is a commonly used formula for detoxification as part of the *Detox Kit*. Recent research shows that one ingredient (Brucine) affects mitochondria in human hepatoma cells. Further research is needed to determine if homeopathic dilutions are more or less active (Deng, et al. 2006).

Osteoheel: Facilitates healing of bone and reduction of pain involved with surgery and fracture. Contains Asa foetida for stabbing ostealgia and periostitis and Mercurius praecipitatus for bone fistula (Reckeweg 2000).

Traumeel S: Used as an anti-inflammatory and for repairing blocked enzymes and regulating rigidity patients. It provides control of pain through speeded healing and homotoxin removal, according to human studies (Zorian, Larentsova, Zorian 1998).

Ubichinon compositum: Contains Anthraquinone for swelling of the gums and GI symptoms such as distention, flatulence, and cramping abdominal pain. Treats constipation with straining or sudden diarrhea (Reckeweg 2002).

Authors' suggested protocols

Nutrition
Immune and gingival/mouth support formulas: 1 tablet for every 25 pounds of body weight BID.
Coenzyme Q10: 25 mg for every 10 pounds of body weight daily.
Additional vitamin C: 100 mg for every 25 pounds of body weight BID.

Chinese herbal medicine/acupuncture
Formula H80 Gingival stomatitis/chronic: 1 capsule per 10 to 20 pounds twice daily. In addition to the herbs cited above, H80 Gingival stomatitis/chronic contains aurantium fruit (Zhi qiao), dendrobium (Shi hu), imperata (Bai mou gen), malt (Mai ya), melia (Chuan lian zi), polyphorus (Zhu ling), and sweet wormwood (Qing hao). These additional herbs increase the efficacy of the formulation.

Points that may be of benefit include LI4, GB20, LI11, KI3, ST6, ST7, and ST44 (Handbook of TCM 1987).

NOTE: If the condition is due to neoplasia, treatment is aimed at treating the cancer (see the section on neoplastic conditions.)

Homotoxicology (Dose: 10 drops PO for 50-pound dog; 5 drops PO for cat or small dog)
Symptomatic treatment: Mucosa compositum and Echinacea compositum, as a presurgical therapy. Traumeel hourly post-op on surgery day (injection or oral drops), then TID PO for 3 days and BID for 2 more days. Also consider Osteoheel alternated with Traumeel and Gastricumeel for 5 days post-operatively.

Resuscitation therapy: Use to reverse iatrogenic damage from anesthesia, antibiotic, and analgesic medications. Galium-Heel, Nux vomica homaccord, Coenzyme compositum, and Ubichinon compositum mixed together and taken BID orally for 3 to 4 weeks.

Product sources

Nutrition

Immune and gingival/mouth support formulas: Animal Nutrition Technologies. **Alternatives:** Immune System Support—Standard Process Veterinary Formulas; Immuno Support—Rx Vitamins for Pets; Immugen—Thorne Veterinary Products.

   Coenzyme Q10: Vetri Science; Rx Vitamins for Pets; Integrative Therapeutics; Thorne Veterinary Products.

Chinese herbal medicine

Formula H80 Gingival stomatitis/chronic: Natural Solutions, Inc.

Homotoxicology

BHI/Heel Corporation

REFERENCES

Western medicine references

Andreason JO. Traumatic injuries of the teeth. 2nd ed. Philadelphia: WB Saunders, 1981, pp. 71–91, 151–237.

Gorrel C, Penman S, Emily P. Handbook of small animal oral emergencies. New York: Pergamon Press, 1993.

Gorrel C, Robinson J. Endodontic therapy. In: Crossley, Penman, eds. Manual of small animal dentistry. *Br Vet Dent Assoc* 1995:168–181.

Gorrel C. In: Tilley L, Smith F. The 5-Minute Veterinary Consult: Canine and Feline, 2003. Blackwell Publishing.

Harvey CE, Emily PP. Oral surgery. In: Small Animal Dentistry. Philadelphia: Mosby, 1993, pp 316–317.

Wiggs RB, Lobprise HB. Veterinary dentistry: principles and practice. Philadelphia: Lippincott-Raven, 1997, pp 280–350.

Nutrition references

Aurer-Kozelj J, Kralj-Klobucar N, Buzina R, Bacic M. The effect of ascorbic acid supplementation on periodontal tissue ultrastructure in subjects with progressive periodontitis. *Int J Vitam Nutr Res* 1982;52:333–41.

Gaby AR. Coenzyme Q10. In: A Textbook of Natural Medicine, by Pizzorno JE, Murray MT. Seattle: Bastyr University Press, 1998, V:CoQ10-1–8.

Nakamura R, Littarru GP, Folkers K. Deficiency of coenzyme Q in gingiva of patients with periodontal disease. *Int J Vitam Nutr Res* 1973;43:84–92.

Shigeta Y, Izumi K, Abe H. Effect of coenzyme Q7 treatment on blood sugar and ketone bodies of diabetics. *J Vitaminol* 1966;12:293–8.

Wilkinson EG, Arnold RM, Folkers K. Bioenergetics in clinical medicine. VI. Adjunctive treatment of periodontal disease with coenzyme Q10. *Res Commun Chem Pathol Pharmacol* 1976;14:715–9.

Vaananen MK, Markkanen HA, Tuovinen VJ, et al. Periodontal health related to plasma ascorbic acid. *Proc Finn Dent Soc* 1993;89:51–9.

Chinese herbal medicine/acupuncture references

Chen SY, et al. *Fujian Journal of Chinese Medicine.* 1986; 17(4):57.

Chen WS, et al. *Journal of Second Military Medical College.* 1999;20(10):758–760.

Dai Y, et al. *China Journal of Chinese Medicine.* 1991; 16(10):622.

Fan LQ, et al. *Zhejiang Journal of Traditional Chinese Medicine.* 1992;27(3):123–125.

Guang Xi Zhong Yi Yao (Guangxi Chinese Medicine and Herbology), 1990; 13(3):45.

Guo Wai Yi Xue Zhong Yi Zhong Yao Fen Ce (Monograph of Chinese Herbology from Foreign Medicine), 1989; 11(2):59.

Handbook of TCM Practitioners, Hunan College of TCM, Shanghai Science and Technology Press, Oct 1987.

Hao QG, et al. Study on antibiotic function of ten commonly used herbs. *Shandong Journal of TCM.* 1991;10(3):39–40.

Jiang Xi Xin Yi Yao (*Jiangxi New Medicine and Herbology*), 1960(1):34.

Jiang Xi Yi Yao (*Jiangxi Medicine and Herbology*), 1989; 24(5):315.

Jiang XY, et al. Comparison between 50 kinds of Chinese herb that treat hepatitis and suppress in vitro HBAg activity. *Journal of Modern Applied Pharmacy.* 1992;9(5):208–211.

Jin ZC, et al. Effects of Shan Zha injection solution on immune functions. *Journal of Chinese Materia Medica.* 1992;23(11), 592–593.

Ke Yan Tong Xun (*Journal of Science and Research*), 1982;(3):35.

Li JD. *Journal of Foreign Medicine, vol. of Traditional Chinese Medicine.* 1989;11(1):1.

Li S, et al. Various Ban Lan Gen and Da Qing Ye's effect in antagonizing influenza A virus. *Journal of Second Military Medical College.* 2000;21(3):204–206.

Liu Z, et al. Treating chronic periodontitis with combination of acupuncture and pricking method with blood-letting. *Journal of Clinical Acupuncture and Moxibustion.* 1996;12(9): 45–46.

Ma ZY. *Shannxi Journal of Traditional Chinese Medicine and Herbs.* 1982;(4):58.

Shan Xi Yi Kan (*Shanxi Journal of Medicine*), 1960; (10):32.

Shan YTE, et al. *Journal of Pharmacy.* Japan. 1982;102(3): 285.

Wan YD. The antipyretic effects of capillarin. *Pharmacy Bulletin.* 1987;(10):590–593.

Wang SD. Therapeutic observations on treating herpes simplex with Ban Lan Gen Injection. *China Journal of Village Medicine.* 1997;25(10):24–25.

Xian Dai Shi Yong Yao Xue (*Practical Applications of Modern Herbal Medicine*), 1988; 5(1):7.

Xin Yi Xue (New Medicine), 1975; 6(3):155.

Xu YM, et al. Experimental research on Ban Lan Gen polysaccharide's effect in promoting immune functions. *Journal of Integrated Medicine.* 1991;11(6):357–359, 325.

Yao Xue Za Zhi (*Journal of Medicinals*), 1971;(91):1098.

You TZS, et al. *Journal of Foreign Medicine, vol. of Traditional Chinese Medicine.* 1990;12(6):373.

Zeng XY, et al. *Guangxi Journal of Medicine.* 1984;6(2):62.

Zhang G, Song S, Ren J, Xu S. A New Compound from Forsythia suspense (Thunb.) Vahl with Antiviral Effect on RSV. *J of Herbal Pharmacotherapy.* 2002;2(3): 35–39.

Zhang ZQ, et al. Che Qian Zi pharmaceutical effects. *Journal of Traditional Chinese Medicine Material.* 1996;19(2): 87–89.

Zheng WF, et al. *China Journal of Medicine.* 1952;38(4):315.

Zhong Cao Yao (*Chinese Herbal Medicine*), 1985;16(1):34.

Zhong Cao Yao (*Chinese Herbal Medicine*) 1991;22 (10):452.

Zhong Cheng Yao Yan Jiu (Research of Chinese Patent Medicine), 1987; 12:9.

Zhong Hua Yi Xue Za Zhi (*Chinese Journal of Medicine*), 1978;17(8):87.

Zhong Yao Da Ci Dien (Dictionary of Chinese Herbs), 1977:2032.

Zhong Yao Xue (*Chinese Herbology*), 1998; 144:146.

Zhong Yao Xue (*Chinese Herbology*), 1998; 845:848.

Zhong Yao Yao Li Yu Ying Yong (*Pharmacology and Applications of Chinese Herbs*), 1983:400.

Zhu LH. *China Journal of TCM Information.* 1996;3(3): 17–20.

Homotoxicology references

Boericke W. Materia Medica with Repertory, 9th ed. Santa Rosa, CA: Boericke and Tafel, 1927 pp 90, 497–500.

Deng X, Yin F, Lu X, Cai B, Yin W. The apoptotic effect of brucine from the seed of Strychnos nux-vomica on human hepatoma cells is mediated via Bcl-2 and Ca2+ involved mitochondrial pathway. *Toxicol Sci.* 2006 May;91(1):pp 59–69.

Reckeweg H. Biotherapeutic Index: Ordinatio Antihomotoxica et Materia Medica, 5th ed. Baden-Baden, Germany: Biologische Heilmittel Heel GMBH, 2000 pp 269–70, 299–300, 379.

Reckeweg H. Homeopathia Antihomotoxica Materia Medica, 4th ed. Baden-Baden, Germany: Arelia-Verlag GMBH, 2002 pp. 136–8,139–40, 147, 317–19, 345, 366, 461–3, 488–90.

Zorian E, Larentsova L, Zorian A. The use of antihomotoxic therapy in dentistry[Article in Russian]. *Stomatologiia (Mosk).* 1998 77(6):pp 9–11.

DIARRHEA/ENTERITIS

Definition and cause

Diarrhea is classified as acute or chronic and has numerous underlying causes as summarized below. The basic underlying initiating cause and effect, however, is an inflammatory process which alters the functioning of the large intestines. While clinical signs may differ in cats and dogs, both are equally susceptible to the condition (Burrows 1995; Crystal 1998; Dennis 1993; Duval 2003; Grooters 2003; Jergens 1992, 1995; Leib 1991; Sherding 1989; Strombeck 1996). Factors associated with enteritis include:

- Interruption of the motility or absorptive capacity of the large bowel.

- Ingested food that evokes an allergic response such as gluten sensitivity.
- Poor quality food that is poorly digestible or contains food byproducts that are irritating, difficult to digest and assimilate, or contain added chemicals that are foreign, disruptive, or evoke free radical formation (see the nutrition introduction, below).
- Food that contains excessive amounts of non-digestible, irritating fiber.
- A malabsorption condition.
- Parasitic infestation.
- Secondary to other infectious (bacterial or viral such as E. coli or parvovirus), metabolic, or degenerative diseases such as CRF, Addison's disease, or liver disease.
- Reactions to drugs, chemotherapeutics, vaccines, or toxic compounds.
- Foreign body or obstruction.
- Large bowel smooth muscle motility problem.
- An immune-mediated infiltrative process such as IBD (see GI disease protocols).
- Neoplasia.

Medical therapy rationale, drug(s) of choice, and nutritional recommendations

Treatment is dependent upon identifying and addressing the underlying cause; the severity of the bowels' inflammatory state; and complicating factors such as protein loss, dehydration, blood loss, secondary mineral imbalances, the presence of foreign materials, and the presence of underlying primary disease causes.

Medical treatment options are protectant, motility-modifying, anti-secretory, anti-spasmotic, anthelminitic, and antimicrobial in their approach. In addition, secondary issues such as dehydration or blood loss must be simultaneously addressed. Dietary recommendations are most often bland, digestible, easily assimilable, and non-irritating in nature. Fasting and resting are often instituted prior to initiation of therapy depending on the clinical condition (Crystal 1998, Duval 2003, Grooters 2003, Leib 1991).

Anticipated prognosis

The prognosis is dependent upon identifying and addressing the underlying causes. Simple diarrhea generally responds favorably, while acute and recurrent diarrhea require compliance, dietary changes, and perhaps chronic use of medication. Longer standing diarrhea with or without protein loss can progress to immune-mediated infiltrative disease, which along with diarrhea secondary to other chronic disease such as CRF and neoplasia, carry a much more guarded prognosis (Burrows 1995, Duval 2003, Grooters 2003).

Integrative veterinary therapies

Diarrhea can be viewed as acute or chronic, and divided into small intestine versus large intestine types. There is overlap in these systems but they make very useful tools for clinicians when approaching cases and in therapy selection. Small bowel diarrhea originates as larger volume, more liquid stool that tends to come in larger quantities, which is typical of enteritis. Hemorrhage seen in melena from small bowel origin diarrhea is dark to black as the eythrocytes have been digested leaving only iron-containing pigments. Large bowel diarrhea is characterized by urgency and increased frequency of smaller volume stools containing mucus and red blood.

Withholding food and allowing for GI rest and repair constitutes the best approach to most cases of acute diarrhea. After fasting for an appropriate time, a bland diet is instituted. For enteritis this is usually a low-residue, digestible diet that is low in fat. A basic diet consisting of half white potato, half sweet potato, a slice of turnip, and a slice of leek mixed with chicken or lamb can work surprisingly well in mild diarrhea cases (Goldstein 1999). A wide variety of simple and prescription diets exist for treatment of GI diseases, and dietary alteration and therapy may well be the most important part of designing individualized treatment plans for pets suffering with GI disease (Strombeck 1999).

Managing chronic diarrhea requires gaining information so that an understanding of that particular patient's pathophysiology can arise and translate into effective therapeutic and diagnostic actions. Diagnosis of chronic diarrhea is covered in any basic text of gastroenterology and the readers are referred to these for further information.

Recent developments in understanding the psychoneuroendocrine and immune systems reveal that the intestinal system is an important component in endocrine and immune regulation. Many neuroactive substances such as serotonin are produced in the GI system. The immune system is well represented within the digestive system, and it has been estimated that 70% to 80% of the total immune system is located in and around the alimentary tube. Cellular elements of the immune system receive vital coding in this area that consists in large part of instructions regarding tolerance of foreign antigens.

The supplementation of proper prebiotics (such as fiber) and probiotic bacteria may promote or assist in homotoxin removal by binding homotoxins to fiber or through metabolism of toxic material by bacteria, and has been a mainstay of holistic therapy for years. The common practice of treating GI upset by fasting and then giving a bland diet is an excellent approach to mild GI conditions. Use of therapeutic diets higher in fiber may be especially useful for chronic GI disorders, such as colitis, and these diets are also indicated in geriatric patients due to the homotoxins which have been impregnated in their systems. During detoxification and drainage therapy commonly required by these patients, the presence of proper fiber will greatly assist in removal of homotoxins from the body.

Traditional Chinese Medicine (TCM) pairs the Heart and Intestine. This developmental relationship is seen in earthworms and carries forward into the structure of more advanced organisms. The primal heart developed first from circular blood vessels, which surrounded the intestinal tract. The development of a tubular gastrointestinal system was a major evolutionary step that allowed organisms to move further and survive in more varied environments. This relationship can be observed in many conditions (diarrhea in congestive heart disease), and astute clinicians often find that treating one organ system may benefit the other. The immune functions contained within the liver make it a major element in protection against invading organisms as well as other toxins. The Stomach and Spleen are also paired in TCM, as are the Lung and Large Intestine. These relationships are helpful in treating patients with chronic disease, especially when using compositae class remedies such as Mucosa compositum (affects large intestine, lung, small intestine, stomach, and bile duct), and Hepar compositum (affects liver, gallbladder, pancreas, small intestine, colon, and thymus) (Reckeweg 2000).

Corticoids and nonsteroidal anti-inflammatory drugs both damage intestinal mucosal elements. This can result in frank ulcer or "leaky gut syndrome," which is linked to many other medical syndromes. In leaky gut, antigens are not properly digested into smaller molecular weight polypeptides before gaining access to the immune system. This can lead to chronic inflammatory diseases such as inflammatory bowel disease and allergic syndromes. The use of digestive enzymes is suggested in these cases to assist in digestion and reduce the molecular weight of proteins in the digestive system. Further work is needed to determine whether this is helpful or not. Holistic veterinarians frequently recommend digestive enzymes, a prescribing practice that is benign and may have potential for improving the health of the microniches of the bowel. One of the proposed advantages of feeding raw foods is for their content of live and biologically active enzymes.

A wide variety of disease states can occur if the immune elements are negatively affected, and diarrhea is a common symptom. Because 70% of the immune system surrounds the gut in the gut associated lymphatic tissues (GALT), it is apparent why integrative veterinary medicine is so concerned with gut health. Just taking a casual glance at the list of digestive diseases covered in this text gives importance to proper care of our patients' gastrointestinal and immune systems.

Pharmaceutical agents are frequently used and can have adverse reactions associated with diarrhea. Because many drugs are toxins, the body attempts to excrete them, and diarrhea and vomiting are the result. Agents that alter gut flora or function also promote the development of diarrhea (Porras, et al. 2006). Antibiotics, corticoids, nonsteroidal anti-inflammatories, and motility drugs all can be helpful as well as harmful to the body's attempt to eliminate homotoxins and regain homeostasis. Careful consideration of agents administered to any patient should occur prior to use of a product. In gastroenterology, conservative treatment approaches can yield very powerful effects.

Allergy to food and adverse reactions to food additives and food substances are important causes of chronic diarrhea and chronic illness. Food allergy can contribute to medical complications when other agents such as drugs or vaccines are given. A recently published example of this showed that corn-allergic dogs produced more IgE following routine vaccination than non-corn allergic dogs (Tater, et al. 2005). These results demonstrate once again the genetic uniqueness and diversity of each animal we treat. These variations allow for survival in a wide number of circumstances but may leave individuals susceptible to all manner of homotoxin invasions and individual intolerances.

The early identification of the cause of diarrhea and the use of nutrients, nutraceuticals, medicinal herbs, and combination homeopathics that are anti-inflammatory and tissue-sparing and enhance toxin elimination can help control the condition and prevent ongoing or cascading inflammation and progression to more chronic conditions.

Nutrition
General considerations/rationale
The nutritional approach to diarrhea should be multifaceted and prevention oriented. The approach consists of nutrient support of the organs of the gastrointestinal tract; the enhancement of cellular and intestinal elimination and detoxification; dietary adjustment to include beneficial fiber and the removal of chemical additives, preservatives, coloring agent, dyes, byproducts and all other unnatural ingredients; and general support of immune function.

Appropriate nutrients
Nutrition/gland therapy: Nutrients and glandular intestines, adrenal, liver, and thymus can help to neutralize a cellular immune attack and reduce inflammation in an irritated intestinal tract. Support of immune system glands

can be helpful in balancing an exaggerated response toward irritated organs, helping to prevent chronic inflammation and eventual degeneration (see Chapter 2, Gland Therapy, for additional information).

Probiotics: Administration of the proper combination of probiotics has been reported to have a positive impact on the intestines and the digestive process (Goldin 1984, Perdigon 1987). Probiotics have been shown to improve and aid the digestive process by secreting their own source of enzymes (McDonough 1987).

Glutamine: Glutamine has been shown to improve immune function and is beneficial for the cells of the gastro-intestinal tract (Souba 1985, Windmueller 1982, Yoshimura 1993).

Digestive enzymes: Metabolically, enzymes are essential in the conversion of food to meet the energy needs of the body. They are also involved as catalysts in the many biochemical processes. Enzyme deficiency is caused either by a specific organ functioning at a less-than-optimal level, or a deficiency or lack of availability of the proper nutrients required for enzyme production. Minerals, amino acids, and fatty acids are required for the synthesis of various enzymes (Howell 1985). While the use of pancreatic enzyme therapy is controversial it is often beneficial when the digestive process is compromised. The addition of pancreatic enzymes should be part of an overall program to support digestive health.

Colostrum: Colostrum has been shown to improve intestinal health. It helps to balance intestinal flora and improve digestion. One important point raised in the IVM discussion above is the status of the immune system in relationship to the presence of intestinal parasites. Colostrum has been found to improve the immune status of the intestinal tract, which can, via intestinal production of globulins, help the overall immune competency of the body (Blake 1999).

Chinese herbal medicine/acupuncture
General considerations/rationale
Enteritis can result from improper feeding, poor diet, internal or external Cold, Qi or Yang deficiency in the Spleen or Stomach, or vital Yang deficiency in the Kidney. It is understood in Western theory how improper feeding and poor diet contribute to diarrhea. The ancient Chinese physicians recognized other etiologies as well. External Cold can be used to describe a pathogen that enters the body, causing enteritis or ingestion of food that is cold, leading to diarrhea. The Stomach and Spleen are responsible for transforming food into usable energy for the body. If these organs have a Qi deficiency they do not have the energy to perform the necessary functions; if they have a Yang deficiency there is not enough warmth to complete digestive processes. Either leads to improperly digested food entering the intestines and ultimately diar-

rhea. The Kidney is given the responsibility for warming the entire body. If the Kidney has a Yang deficiency it may not be able to send enough warmth to the Spleen and Stomach for those organs to function properly.

Appropriate Chinese herbs

Actractylodes (Bai zhu): Can be used to stop diarrhea (Chang Yong Zhong Yao Cheng Fen Yu Yao Li Shou Ce 1994). At low doses, it has a mild inhibitory effect on the contraction of isolated guinea pig ileum (Ma Xiao Song 1996).

Amomum fruit (Sha ren): Relieves bloating, spasms, and pain (Zhong Yao Xue 1988).

Angelica root (Dang gui): Has antibacterial effects. It has demonstrated inhibitory effects on Salmonelly typhi, E. coli, Corynebacterium diphtheriae, Vibrio cholerae, and a- and b-hemolytic strep (Hou Xue Hua Yu Yan Jia 1981). This may help control bacterial dysentery.

Astragalus (Huang qi): Has antibacterial activity. It has shown efficacy against Bacillus dysenteria, corynebacteria, staphylococci, and others (Zhong Yao Zhi 1949).

Aurantium fruit (Zhi qiao): Was shown to inhibit contraction of isolated rabbit intestinal smooth muscles and to relieve acetylcholine- and BaCl2-induced enterospasm (Ma Ya Bing 1996).

Bamboo shavings (Zhu ru): Inhibits many types of bacteria including E. coli and Salmonella typhi (Zhong Yao Xue 1998).

Bupleurum (Chai hu): Inhibited the effect of dimethyl benzene-induced auricular concha inflammation in mice (Liu Wei 1998). It may also decrease intestinal inflammation.

Cimicifuga (Sheng ma): Inhibits lymphocyte activation. Cimicifuga's inhibitory effect on membrane permeability is greater than that of cortisol and it has been shown to inhibit the formation of antibodies (Zhu Nei Liang Fu 1984). It also suppresses proliferation of immune cells (Huang Yun 1992). These actions may help in cases of diarrhea secondary to immune system abnormalities.

Citrus (Chen pi): Reduces inflammation by decreasing the permeability of blood vessels (Zhong Yao Yao Li Yu Ying Yong 1983).

Coptis (Huang lian): Stops diarrhea (Zhong Yao Xue 1998). In a study of 100 people with acute gastroenteritis there was a 100% improvement in signs (Si Chuan Yi Xue Yuan Xue Bao 1959). One component of coptis, berberine, has been shown to have anti-inflammatory effects in rats (Yao Xue Za Zhi 1981).

Corydalis tuber (Yan hu suo): Increases secretions from adrenal glands in mice (Xi Xue Xue Bao 1988). This may release cortisol and decrease intestinal inflammation.

Immature orange peel (Qing pi): Inhibits smooth muscle contractions in the stomach and thereby relieves cramps (Zhong Yao Zhi 1984).

Licorice (Gan cao): Alleviates intestinal cramping (Zhong Yao Zhi 1993). Two of the components, glycyrrhizin and glycyrrhetinic acid, have anti-inflammatory effects. They have approximately 10% of the corticosteroid activity of cortisone (Zhong Cao Yao 1991). Licorice counteracts food poisoning and enterotoxins. The mechanism by which it has this effect is unknown. Some researchers say licorice binds toxins in the GI tract to prevent absorption; others say it may affect the liver's detoxification system (Zhong Yao Tong Bao 1986).

Peach kernel (Tao ren): Suppresses the immune system in several ways. It was shown to prevent egg-white-induced arthritis in mice (Liu Can Hui 1989). Other studies have shown suppressive effects on fibroblast growth in laboratory cell cultures. It was shown to suppress the proliferation of inflammatory cells and fibroblast hyperplasia in subjects using experimental trabeculae dissection (Wang Su Ping 1993). Another study demonstrated the ability to decrease inflammation in mice with otitis media (Zhong Yao Tong Bao 1986).

Platycodon root (Jie geng): Has been shown to promote the secretion of corticosterone in rats, thereby causing an anti-inflammatory effect (Li Yin Fang 1984, Zhang Shu Chen 1984, Zhou Wen Zheng 1979).

Pulsatilla (Bai tou weng): Has antiamebic properties. It was 100% effective in treating 26 human patients with amoebic dysentery (Wu Han Yi Xue Yuan Xue Bao 1958). In addition, it inhibits many bacteria, including Bacillus dysenterieae and Salmonella typhi (CA, 1948).

Rhubarb (Da huang): In a clinical trial involving 14 human patients with hemorrhagic necrotic enteritis, 12 of the 14 responded after 2 to 6 days (Fu Jian Zhong Yi Yao 1985).

Acupuncture points

Acupuncture has been shown to be effective in controlling or curing diarrhea in many studies. Acupuncture at GV1, ST25 and ST36 was used in a study of 500 infants with diarrhea. 485 were completely cured and 13 improved (Zhonzxin X 1989). In preweaning pigs with experimentally induced E. coli diarrhea, a combination of acupuncture and moxibustion was superior to oral neomycin. Using acupuncture and moxibustion, 82% of the pigs responded as opposed to 71% treated with neomycin (Hwang YC 1988).

Homotoxicology
General considerations/rationale

Diarrhea generally represents an Excretion Phase disorder, but may occur as a consequence of any phase disease process in which the body attempts to remove homotoxins through the gastrointestinal system. Diarrhea is generally a desirable physiologic process, even though it is annoying to client, patient, and veterinarian alike.

However, severe, copious, or chronic diarrhea presents a threat to health as vital fluids and electrolytes are lost to the body and digestion and absorption are negatively affected. In such cases therapy is most definitely indicated.

Nutrient- and homotoxin-laden blood leaves the intestines and proceeds via the portal vein to the liver, where it is directly cleansed and processed. Many GI issues are addressed with remedies that target intestinal and hepatic tissues (i.e., Nux vomica homaccord and Hepar compositum). Enterohepatic circulation provides the opportunity for homotoxins to be reabsorbed after hepatic handling. In this way, homotoxins gain access to the circulatory system again and must be removed. Ancillary excretion and metabolism by other organs (kidney, skin, and lung) may all assist in homotoxin removal.

Antihomotoxic agents that support these organs include Solidago compositum, Berberis homaccord, and Mucosa compositum. Homotoxins that have escaped or bypassed hepatic processing may be deposited into connective tissue and cause disease later as further damage ensues. The health of the bowel and body seem largely determined by a healthy intestinal flora and healthy mucosal barrier (Porras, et al. 2006; Meier, Steuerwald 2005).

Many homotoxins can damage the GI system's ability to perform its duties. Both toxins and other therapeutic agents can result in progressive vicariation.

Food trials with hydrolyzed diets and limited antigen diets can be very helpful in managing chronic diarrhea.

Successfully treating GI disorders involves providing clean food and water, allowing time for repair, reducing stress, allowing homotoxins to be excreted successfully, supporting organ function, providing drainage therapy, and providing metabolic/organelle support while repair occurs. As in other discussions, the position of the patient on the phase table assists in determining proper therapy. In the first 2 phases, symptomatic treatment is often successful. As homotoxins gain deeper access and do further damage, the use of compositae class antihomotoxic agents becomes necessary to stimulate regressive vicariation.

Appropriate homotoxicology formulas

Arsuraneel: A cellular phase remedy that treats enteritis and diarrhea (Arsenicum album). May be useful in arsenic poisoning in areas with contaminated groundwater (Mallick, Mallick, Guha, Khuda-Bukhsh 2003; Khuda-Bukhsh 2005). Also used in chronic disease, tumors of mucous membranes (Marsdenia cundurango), and diabetes mellitus (Acidum phophoricum) (Reckeweg 2000).

Atropinum compositum: Not available in the U.S. market at this time, but is a powerful antispasmodic for biliary, renal, and intestinal colic (Demers 2004). Con-

tains Benzoicum acidum (also common to *Aesculus compositum*, *Arnica-Heel*, *Atropinum compositum*, and *Rhododendroneel*). It is used in inflammatory symptoms which occur throughout the alimentary canal: a slimy coating on the tongue with ulcers at the edges, stomatitis with dysphagia, eructations, retching and vomiting, and flatulent distension below the ribs on both sides. The stools are copious, loose, and white in color, with violent tenesmus and mixed with blood; there are stabbing pains in the rectum, rigors, and a feeling of being seriously ill (Reckeweg 2002).

BHI-Diarrhea: Treats diarrhea in general. A good simple remedy for many cases of diarrhea.

BHI-Intestine: Treats diarrhea, cramping, hard-black stool (*Bryonia alba*); emotional diarrhea, leg spasm and cramps, colitis (Colocynthis); flatulence and liver conditions (Lycopodium); gastroenteritis and colitis (Nux vomica); and mucosal inflammation (Mercurius corrosives). Sulphur activates a blocked metabolism, stimulates regressive vicariation, and promotes healing (Heel 2002).

BHI-Nausea: Treats painful oral vesicles/stomatitis (Anacardium); nausea and vomiting with coughing (Ipecacuanha); and left-sided gastric region pain (Argentum nictricum).

BHI-Pancreas: Treats pancreatitis and related symptomology including diarrhea, vomiting, nausea, and constipation.

BHI-Spasm-Pain: Treats leg cramps, fever, pain and inflammation, sharp pain, colic or intestinal spasm, and colitis.

Cantharis compositum: Contains Arsenicum album, which is indicated in aphthous stomatitis; when the tongue is dry, red with raised papillae, or coated white, brown or black; and for violent gastroenteritis with prolonged vomiting and diarrhea with unbearable burning stomach pains after eating. Also treats foul-smelling stools. Contains Mercurius solubilis, which is indicated in ulcerative lesions of the mucous membranes, and Hepar sulphuris calcareum (Reckeweg 2002).

Ceanothus homaccord: Used for pancreatopathy, epigastric syndrome, tenesmus, diarrhea, and hepatic issues. Splenic enlargement is a primary signalment for this remedy (Macleod 1983).

Chelidonium homaccord: Used for gallbladder conditions such as cholangitis, cholecystitis, obstructive jaundice, hepatic damage, and hepatitis (Demers 2004). Chelidonium contains a substance known as Chelidonine, which has anticancer effects. "Chelidonine turned out to be a potent inducer of apoptosis triggering cell death at concentrations of 0.001 mM," according to Habermehl (2006), a fact that may explain the clinically observed usefulness of this remedy in treating patients with biliary neoplasia.

Chol-Heel: An excellent remedy containing Belladonna, Chelidonium, Carduus marianus, Lycopodium, Veratrum, and Taraxicum, along with some other very useful components, all in potency chords. This can be of great relief in GI discomfort (Broadfoot 2005).

Cinnamomum homaccord: Currently not available in the United States, but used for seeping hemorrhage.

Coenzyme compositum: Contains Citricum acidum, which is useful for dental problems and gingivitis; scurvy; blackening of teeth and heavy deposits of dental plaque; painful, herpetic vesicles around the lips; nausea; painful cramping in the umbilical area; and distension. It is also helpful following anti-inflammatory and antibiotic drug therapy.

Colocynthis homaccord: Treats diarrhea with lower back pain (*Citrullus colocynthis*), colic, pain below the navel, colitis with gelatinous stools.

Diarrheel S: A symptom remedy for acute and chronic diarrhea. It also treats acute gastroenteritis, belching, spurting diarrhea, pancreatopathy, and colitis. This commonly used formula contains Tormentilla, which is used for dysentery, acute gastroenteritis, and mucous and ulcerative colitis with bloody stools (Reckeweg 2002). It is also found in *BHI-Diarrhea* and *Veratrum homaccord*.

Duodenoheel: Treats hunger pains, hyperacidity, gastric and duodenal ulcers, nausea and vomiting, and dysentery with tenesmus (Reckeweg 2000).

Engystol N: Treats viral origin gastroenteritis (see Parvovirus).

Galium-Heel: Treats all cellular phases, hemorrhoids, and anal fissures, and is a detoxicant.

Gingseng compositum: Used for nausea, gastroenteritis, and constitutional support in geriatric or debilitated patients (Reckeweg 2000).

Hepar compositum: Provides detoxification and drainage of hepatic tissues and organ and metabolic support, and is useful in most hepatic and gall bladder pathologies. It is an important part of Deep Detoxification Formula. It treats duodenitis, pancreatitis, cystic hepatic ducts, cholelithiasis, cholangitis, cholecystitis, and vomiting and diarrhea (Demers 2004, Broadfoot 2004). This combination contains Natrum oxalaceticum (also found in *Coenzyme compositum Ubichinon compositum*, and *Mucosa compositum*) for changes in appetite and stomach distension due to air. It treats nausea, stomach pain with a sensation of fullness, gurgling in the abdomen, and cramping pain in the hypochondria. It is also used for constipation, sudden diarrhea, particularly after eating, and flatus (Reckeweg 2002).

Hepeel: Provides liver drainage and detoxification. Used in a wide variety of conditions including cancer of the liver, where *Hepeel* was found to be antiproliferative, hepatoprotective, and an antioxidant when tested in human HepG2 cells (Gebhardt 2003).

Leptandra compositum: Treats epigastric syndrome, portal vein congestion, pancreatopathy, chronic liver disease, and diabetes mellitus (Reckeweg 2000).

Lymphomyosot: Provides lymph drainage and endocrine support, and treats edema. Contains Gentiana for chronic gastritis, flatulence, diarrhea, distension of the stomach with eructations, nausea, retching, and vomiting. Geranium robertianum is useful for nausea, particularly after eating with distension or sensation of fullness. The component Myosotis arvensis has indications for bloat and distension (Reckeweg 2002).

Mercurius-Heel S: Used for viral and bacterial issues, suppuration, and tonsillitis (Reckeweg 2000).

Momordica compositum: Treats pancreatitis, epigastric disease (*Momordica balsamina*), emaciation though good appetite (*Jodum*), and vomiting with collapse (Veratrum album)(Reckeweg 2000).

Mucosa compositum: Broadly supportive for repair of mucosal elements. Used in cellular cases and in recovery periods following active disease (Reckeweg 2000). This remedy contains a useful component in Kali bichromicum, which is indicated for ulcers found on the gums, the tongue, the lips, and even on the gastric mucosa (gastric or duodenal ulcer). The tongue may have a thick, yellow, mucous coating, or, in ulcerative stomatitis or tonsillitis, it may be dry, smooth, shiny, or fissured. Kali has been used effectively in acute gastroenteritis associated with vomiting of clear, light-colored fluid or quantities of mucous bile, and in cases with hematemesis, flatulent colics, and dysenteric stools with tenesmus (Reckeweg 2002). It contains Hydrastis as well, with mucosal support for oral problems such as stomatitis, and mucosal suppuration, which are also accompanied by ulceration, inflammations, colic of the hepatobiliary system and the gastrointestinal tract, and polyp formation (Reckeweg 2002).

The Kreosotum component can be used in chronic gastritis with gastric hemorrhages and vomiting of brown masses. Also has a dental implication in cases with spongy gums and carious teeth, neuralgias proceeding from them causing a burning toothache with deep caries, black patches on the teeth, and fetid discharges. The single remedy Phosphorus is broadly useful for dyspepsia and for jaw problems in dental disease (Reckeweg 2002.) Phosphorus is found in many other remedies including *Echinacea compositum* and *Leptandra homaccord*. It is rich in suis organ preparations for mucosal support, plus a large variety of remedies with indications in the gastrointestinal sphere. Argentum nitricum is also contained in this broad remedy, (it is also in *Atropinum compositum*, *Diarrheel*, *Duodenoheel*, *Gastricumeel*, *Momordica compositum*, *BHI-Nausea*, and several other combinations) for distension in the upper abdomen, gastro-cardiac symptom-complex, and amelioration from eructations. It is used for gastric crises (Reckeweg 2002).

Nux vomica homaccord: Used for liver and gastrointestinal disease and after smoke inhalation. Useful in gingivitis (Reckeweg 2002). It is a commonly used formula for detoxification as part of the *Detox Kit*. Recent research shows that one ingredient (Brucine) affects mitochondria in human hepatoma cells. Further research is needed to determine if homeopathic dilutions are more or less active (Deng, et al. 2006).

Paeonia-Heel: Used for anal region issues such as hemorrhoids, anal fissures, colitis, spasmodic constipation, weeping anal lesions, anal pruritus, and painful defecation (Reckeweg 2000). A topical cream is useful.

Podophyllum homaccord: Treats chronic gastroenteritis, gastroenteritis in juvenile dogs and cats, dyspepsia, catarrhal colitis, hemorrhoids, and watery-green diarrhea alternating with constipation (Macleod 1983).

Procteel: Contains Lycopodium, Sulfur, Phosphorus, and Aluminum oxydatum. It may be useful for megacolon and rectal atony, hemorrhoids, sore body orifices, alternating diarrhea and constipation, hepatic disease with cystic ducts, and intestinal stasis (Reckeweg 2000).

Psorinoheel: Used for chronic illness, and is an Impregnation Phase remedy.

Schwef-Heel: Treats chronic diseases of the skin and liver. This remedy should be interposed in most skin and liver cases (Reckeweg 2000). Patients that need this remedy may look dirty and have scruffy skin conditions, red lips, a white tongue with red tip, an itching and burning rectal area with morning diarrhea, or a prolapsed rectum (Boericke 1927). Sulfur is contained in several other antihomotoxic formulas including *Coenzyme compositum*, *Echinacea compositum*, *Engystol*, *Ginseng compositum*, *Hepar compositum*, *Molybdan compositum*, *Mucosa compositum*, *Paeonia-Heel*, *Proctheel*, *Psorinoheel*, *Sulfur-Heel*, *Thyroidea compositum*, and *Ubichinon compositum* (Reckeweg 2000).

Syzygium compositum: Treats chronic gastritis, chronic enteritis, diabetes mellitus, and hepatic disorders.

Tanacet-Heel: Used for complications following removal of helminths. Also treats gastroenteritis, dysentery, and gas and pain following ascarids, especially in juvenile pets.

Ubichinon compositum: Contains Anthraquinone for swelling of gums, and GI symptoms such as distention, flatulence, and cramping abdominal pain. Also treats constipation with straining or sudden diarrhea (Reckeweg 2002).

Veratrum homaccord: Treats gastritis, intense vomiting with blood, collapse (pale mucous membranes), psychosis, dysentary, fecal incontinence, and intestinal spasm. It is used widely by the authors for general vomiting cases. Consider its use in cases of gastritis following general

anesthesia. Classical provings were recently repeated and found consistent with earlier work (Van Wassenhoven 2004).

Vomitusheel S: Treats nausea and vomiting with a cough (Ipecacuanha), liver and gastrointestinal issues (*Nux vomica*), eructation, and possibly anxiety or depression (Ignatia) (Reckeweg 2000). Also treats irritable bowel syndrome with stress-related issues. No known adverse reactions have occurred and it is extremely safe to use in pediatric patients. This remedy contains Aethusa for vomiting obviously originating in the nervous system. In serious cases, capillary paralysis, hematemesis, stomach cramps, and tympanitic distension may occur, with an irresistible urge to pass stool. The nervous vomiting is characterized by spasmodic contractions of the esophageal muscles and violent pains which shoot upwards from the cardiac sphincter (Reckeweg 2002). In more severe vomiting consider *Veratrum homaccord* instead or in combination.

Authors Suggested Protocol

Nutrition
Immune and intestinal support formulas: 1 tablet for every 25 pounds of body weight BID.

Liver support formula: One-half tablet for every 25 pounds of body weight BID.

Glutamine: One-fourth scoop per 25 pounds of body weight daily.

Colostrum: One-third teaspoon powdered formula for every 25 pounds of body weight BID.

Probiotic: One-half capsule per 25 pounds of body weight with food.

Pan 5 Plus: 1 capsule opened and mixed with food per every 25 pounds of body weight (maximum, 4 capsules).

Chinese herbal medicine/acupuncture
Any specific etiology should be addressed. In most cases, the authors use Formula ColonGuard at a dose of 1 capsule per 10 to 20 pounds twice daily. In addition to the herbs mentioned above, ColonGuard also contains codonopsis (Dang shen), lindera (Wu yao), pueraria (Ge gen), and raw white lotus seed (Lian zi), which help increase the efficacy of the formula.

The authors use the following acupuncture points: BL20, ST36, BL26, and Baihui.

Homotoxicology (Dose: 10 drops PO for 50-pound dog; 5 drops PO for cat or small dog)
Also see the vomiting protocol as needed.

BHI-Diarrhea: Use as a simple starting place, given hourly until effect is noted. Or use Nux vomica, Veratrum homaccord, and Diarrheel mixed together and given hourly until conditions improve. Consider Mercurius-Heel in watery diarrhea with bacterial or protozoan causes.

Product sources

Nutrition

Immune, intestinal, and liver support formulas: Animal Nutrition Technologies. **Alternatives:** NutriGest—Rx Vitamins for Pets; Canine and Feline Enteric Support—Standard Process Veterinary Formulas; Acetylator—Vetri Science; Immune System Support—Standard Process Veterinary Formulas; Immuno Support—Rx Vitamins for Pets; Immugen—Thorne Veterinary Products; Hepatic Support—Standard Process Veterinary Formulas; Hepato Support—Rx Vitamins for Pets; Hepagen—Thorne Veterinary Products.

Glutimmune: Well Wisdom. **Alternative:** L-glutamine powder—Thorne Veterinary Products.

Colostrum: New Life Foods, Inc.; Saskatoon Colostrum Company.

Probiotic: Progressive Labs; Biotic—Rx Vitamins for Pets.

Pan 5 Plus: Progressive Labs.

Chinese herbal medicine
Colon Guard: Natural Solutions, Inc.

Homotoxicology
BHI/Heel Corporation

REFERENCES

Western medicine references

Burrows CF, Batt RM, Sherding RG. Disease of the small intestine. In: Ettinger SJ, Feldman EC, eds. Textbook of veterinary internal medicine. Philadelphia: Saunders, 1995:1169–1232.

Crystal MA. Diarrhea, In: The feline patient. Essentials of diagnosis and treatment. Baltimore: Williams and Wilkins 1998: 42–46.

Dennis JS, Kruger JM, Mullaney TP. Lymphocytic/plasmacytic colitis in cats: 14 cases (1985–1990). *J Am Vet Med Assoc* 1993;202:313–318.

Duval DS. Acute Diarrhea. In: Tilley L, Smith F. The 5-Minute Veterinary Consult: Canine and Feline, 2003. Blackwell Publishing.

Grooters AM. Chronic Diarrhea in the Dog. In: Tilley L, Smith F. The 5-Minute Veterinary Consult: Canine and Feline, 2003. Blackwell Publishing.

Grooters AM. Chronic Diarrhea in the Cat, In: Tilley L, Smith F. The 5-Minute Veterinary Consult: Canine and Feline, 2003. Blackwell Publishing.

Jergens AE. Acute diarrhea. In: Bonagura JD, ed. Kirk's current veterinary therapy XII. Philadelphia: Saunders, 1995:701–705.

Jergens AE. Feline idiopathic inflammatory bowel disease. *Comp Contin Educ Pract Vet* 1992;14:509–518.

Leib MS, Monroe WE, Codner EC. Management of chronic large bowel diarrhea in dogs. *Vet Med* 1991;86:922–929.

Sherding RG. Diseases of the intestines. In: Sherding RG, ed. The cat: diseases and clinical management. New York: Churchill Livingstone, 1989:955–1006.

Strombeck DR, Guilford WG. Strombeck's small animal gastroenterology. 3rd ed. Philadelphia: Saunders, 1996.

Integrative veterinary medicine references

Goldstein, M. The Nature of Animal Healing. New York: Ballantine Books. 1999. pp 184, 198.

Porras M, Martin M, Yang P, Jury J, Perdue M, Vergara P. Correlation Between Cyclical Epithelial Barrier Dysfunction and Bacterial Translocation in the Relapses of Intestinal Inflammation. *Inflamm Bowel Dis.* 2006. Sep;12(9):pp 843–852.

Strombeck D. Home-Prepared Dog and Cat Diets: The Healthful Alternative. 1999. Ames, Iowa: Iowa State University Press.

Tater K, Jackson H, Paps J, Hammerberg B. Effects of routine prophylactic vaccination or administration of aluminum adjuvant alone on allergen-specific serum IgE and IgG responses in allergic dogs. *Am J Vet Res.* 2005 Sep;66(9):pp 1572–7.

Reckeweg H. Biotherapeutic Index: Ordinatio Antihomotoxica et Materia Medica, 5th ed. Baden-Baden, Germany: Biologische Heilmittel Heel GMBH, 2000. pp 290, 294–5, 300, 329–30, 358–9, 363–4, 366–7, 369, 381, 390, 399–400, 432, 538.

Nutrition references

Blake SR. Bovine Colostrum, The Forgotten Miracle. *Journal of the American Holistic Veterinary Medical Association.* July 1999, Volume 18, Number 2, pp 38–39.

Golden BR, Gorbach SL. The Effect of Milk and Lactobacillus Feeding on Human Intestinal Bacteria Activity. *Am. J. of Clin. Nutr.*, 1984. 39: 756–61.

Howell E. Enzyme Nutrition, The Food Enzyme Concept. 1985. Garden City, NY. Avery Publ.

McDonough FE, Hitchins AD, Wong NP, et al. Modification of sweet acidophilus milk to improve utilization by lactose-intolerant persons. Am J Clin Nutr 1987;45:570–4.

Perdigon GN, de Masius N, Alvarez S, et al. Enhancement of Immune Response in Mice fed with S. Thermophilus and L. Acidophilus. *J. of Dairy Sci.*, 1987.70: 919–926.

Souba W et al. Glutamine metabolism in the intestinal tract: invited review, *JPEN* 1985;9:608–617.

Windmueller HG. Glutamine utilization by the small intestine, *Adv. Enzymol* 1982;53:201–237.

Yoshimura K, et al. Effects of enteral glutamine administration on experimental inflammatory bowel disease, *JPEN* 1993;17: 235.

Chinese herbal medicine/acupuncture references

CA, 1948; 42:4228a.

Chang Yong Zhong Yao Cheng Fen Yu Yao Li Shou Ce (A Handbook of the Composition and Pharmacology of Common Chinese Drugs), 1994; 739:742.

Fu Jian Zhong Yi Yao (*Fujian Chinese Medicine and Herbology*), 1985;1:36.

Hou Xue Hua Yu Yan Jia (*Research on Blood-Activating and Stasis-Eliminating Herbs*), 1981:335.

Huang Y. Sheng Ma's effects on advanced inflammation. *Journal of Chinese Materia Medica.* 1992;23(6):288.

Hwang YC and Jenkins EM: Effect of acupuncture on young pigs with induced enterpathogenic Escherichia coli diarrhea. *Am J Vet Res* 1988.49:1641–1643.

Li YF (translator). Foreign Medicine, vol. of TCM. 1984;6(1): 15–18.

Liu CH, et al. The pharmacology of Tao Ren. *Journal of Pharmacology and Clinical Application of TCM.* 1989;(2):46–47.

Liu W, et al. *Henan Journal of TCM Pharmacy.* 1998;13(4): 10–12.

Ma XS, et al. *New Journal of Digestive Diseases.* 1996;4(11): 603–604.

Ma YB. Zhi Qiao's effects on gastroinstestinal movement. *Journal of Pharmacology of Clinical Application of TCM.* 1996;12(6): 28–29.

Si Chuan Yi Xue Yuan Xue Bao (*Journal of Sichuan School of Medicine*), 1959;1:102.

Wang SP, et al. Tao Ren extract's effect in suppressing filter bed fibroblasts hyperplasia in subjects of experimental trabeculae dissection. *Journal of Shanghai Medical University.* 1993;20(1): 35–381.

Wu Han Yi Xue Yuan Xue Bao (*Journal of Wuhan University School of Medicine*), 1958;(1):1.

Xi Xue Xue Bao (*Academic Journal of Medicine*), 1988; 23(10):721.

Yao Xue Za Zhi (*Journal of Medicinals*), 1981, 101(10):883.

Zhang SC, et al. *Journal of Chinese Patent Medicine Research.* 1984;(2):37.

Zhong Cao Yao(*Chinese Herbal Medicine*) 1991;22 (10):452.

Zhong Yao Tong Bao (*Journal of Chinese Herbology*), 1986; 11 (11):37.

Zhong Yao Tong Bao (*Journal of Chinese Herbology*), 1986; 11(10):55.

Zhong Yao Xue (*Chinese Herbology*), 1988; 326:327.

Zhong Yao Xue (*Chinese Herbology*), 1998;140:144.

Zhong Yao Xue (*Chinese Herbology*), 1998; 623:625.

Zhong Yao Yao Li Yu Ying Yong (*Pharmacology and Applications of Chinese Herbs*), 1983; 567.

Zhong Yao Zhi (*Chinese Herbology Journal*), 1949;(12):648.

Zhong Yao Zhi (*Chinese Herbology Journal*), 1984;37.

Zhong Yao Zhi (*Chinese Herbology Journal*), 1993;358.

Zhonzxin X. Clinical observation of 500 cases with pediatric diarrhea treated by acupuncture. *Chinese Acupuncture and Moxibustion* 1989.9:10.

Zhou WZ, et al. *Pharmacy Bulletin.* 1979;14(5):202–203.

Zhu NLF, et al. Chinese Herbs and Immunity. Foreign Medicine (TCM vol). 1984;(1):47.

Homotoxicology references

Broadfoot PJ. Inflammation: Homotoxicology and Healing, in proceedings AHVMA/Heel Homotoxicology Seminar. 2004. Denver, CO, p 27.

Boericke W. Materia Medica with Repertory, 9th edition. Santa Rosa, CA: Boericke and Tafel, 1927. pp 90, 497–500.

Deng X, Yin F, Lu X, Cai B, Yin W. The apoptotic effect of brucine from the seed of Strychnos nux-vomica on human hepatoma cells is mediated via Bcl-2 and Ca2+ involved mitochondrial pathway. *Toxicol Sci.* 2006. May;91(1):pp 59–69.

Gebhardt R. Antioxidative, antiproliferative and biochemical effects in HepG2 cells of a homeopathic remedy and its constituent plant tinctures tested separately or in combination. *Arzneimittelforschung.* 2003. 53(12): pp 823–30.

Goncalves JL, Lopes R, Oliveira D, Costa S, Miranda M, Romanos M, Santos N, Wigg M. In vitro anti-rotavirus activity of some medicinal plants used in Brazil against diarrhea. *J Ethnopharmacol.* 2005. Jul 14;99(3): pp 403–7.

Habermehl D, Kammerer B, Handrick R, Eldh T, Gruber C, Cordes N, Daniel PT, Plasswilm L, Bamberg M, Belka C, Jendrossek V. Proapoptotic activity of Ukrain is based on Chelidonium majus L. alkaloids and mediated via a mitochondrial death pathway. *BMC Cancer.* 2006. Jan 17;6: p 14.

Heel. BHI Homeopathic Therapy: Professional Reference. Albuquerque, NM: Heel Inc. 2002. pp 43, 47, 73.

Khuda-Bukhsh AR, Pathak S, Guha B, Karmakar S, Das J, Banerjee P, Biswas S, Mukherjee P, Bhattacharjee N, Choudhury S, Banerjee A, Bhadra S, Mallick P, Chakrabarti J, Mandal B. In vitro anti-rotavirus activity of some medicinal plants used in Brazil against diarrhea, *J Ethnopharmacol.* 2005. Jul 14;99(3): pp 403–7.

Mallick P, Mallick JC, Guha B, Khuda-Bukhsh AR. Ameliorating effect of microdoses of a potentized homeopathic drug, Arsenicum Album, on arsenic-induced toxicity in mice. *BMC Complement Altern Med.* 2003. Oct 22;3: p 7.

Macleod G. A Veterinary Materia Medica and Clinical Repertory with a Materia Medica of the Nosodes. Safron, Walden: CW Daniel Company LTD, 1983. pp 50–1, 125–6, 129–30.

Meier R, Steuerwald M. Place of probiotics. *Curr Opin Crit Care.* 2005. Aug;11(4):pp 318–25.

Reckeweg H. Homeopathia Antihomotoxica Materia Medica, 4th ed. Baden-Baden, Germany: Arelia-Verlag GMBH, 2002. pp. 136–8, 139–40, 125–6, 147, 150–3, 179, 206, 241–2, 317–19, 345, 366, 461–3, 488–90, 578–80.

Shamsa F, Ahmadiani A, Khosrokhavar R. Antihistaminic and anticholinergic activity of barberry fruit (Berberis vulgaris) in the guinea-pig ileum. *J Ethnopharmacol.* 1999. Feb;64(2):pp 161–6.

Van Wassenhoven M. Towards an evidence-based repertory: clinical evaluation of Veratrum album. *Homeopathy.* 2004. Apr;93(2): pp 71–7.

Zhu B, Ahrens FA. Effect of berberine on intestinal secretion mediated by Escherichia coli heat-stable enterotoxin in jejunum of pigs. *Am J Vet Res.* 1982. Sep;43(9): pp 1594–8.

IRRITABLE BOWEL SYNDROME

Definition and cause

Irritable bowel syndrome (IBS) is an idiopathic disorder involving the large intestine. Patients have intermittent bouts of colitis with no apparent structural alternations. IBS is much less severe than IBD. This diagnosis is "backed into," by ruling out other causes of colitis. It might also be referred to as idiopathic colitis. IBS is also known as mucous colitis, spastic colitis, and nervous colitis. The reader is referred to the colitis protocol below for a more complete discussion of large bowel inflammation. Potential underlying causes include inflammation, impaired motility, food allergy, low-fiber food, and behavioral plus stress (Grooters 2003, Tams 1992).

Medical therapy rationale, drug(s) of choice, and nutritional recommendations

Dietary adjustment to a higher fiber food or the addition of fiber supplementation such as psyllium often helps. In addition, motility modifiers such as Lomotil and antispasmotics such as Darbazine are beneficial. Addressing the anxiety which often accompanies IBS often helps the overall response. Anti-anxiety drugs such as amitriptyline have proven beneficial in some cases (Leib 1991, Grooters 2003, Strombeck 1996, Tams 1992).

Anticipated prognosis

Response to dietary changes, stress reduction, and slowing down the colon often controls the condition. Long-term prognosis is most often very good (Grooters 2003).

Integrative veterinary therapies

Conventional medicine relies on diet and medical therapy with a combination of drugs aimed at motility modification, inflammation control, infection control, and antiemetics. Integrative therapies address both the physical inflammation in the GI tract as well as the emotional component and stressors that may bring on the clinical symptoms. Use of nutraceutical, herbal, and homeopathic remedies that can help balance the emotions as well as the colitis without the inherent side effects of chronic medication represents a good option for the client and the animal.

Dietary recommendations are an important part of therapy for all types of colitis. A highly digestible diet with higher fiber is generally preferred. In some cases the symptoms nearly disappear. Fiber can be supplemented using pumpkin or psyllium-type laxatives. Psyllium has been shown to help some people with IBS (Hotz 1994, Manning 1977).

Stress is thought to play a part in this condition, so use of biological agents that assist mood may be helpful. Bach Flower remedies such as Rescue Remedy or Anaflora Recovery are another idea for stress management with far less potential for neurological damage than some psychotropic drugs (see Product Sources).

Early identification of the cause and the use of nutrients, nutraceuticals, medicinal herbs, and combination homeopathics that are anti-inflammatory and tissue-sparing can help control the condition and prevent ongoing inflammation and progression to more chronic conditions.

Nutrition
General considerations/rationale
The nutritional approach consists of nutrient support of the stomach and intestines, reducing inflammation, and addressing the animal's emotions and behavior traits.

Appropriate nutrients
Nutrition/gland therapy: Glandular brain, pineal, intestines, and stomach supply intrinsic nutrients required by these organs. They also help to neutralize stress-induced inflammation (see Chapter 2, Gland Therapy, for additional information).

Glutamine: Glutamine has been shown to improve immune function and is beneficial for the cells of the gastrointestinal tract (Souba 1985, Windmueller 1982, Yoshimura 1993).

Phosphatidyl serine: Phosphatidyl serine is a phospholipid, which is essential for the integrity of cell membranes, particularly of nerve and brain cells. It has been studied extensively in people with altered mental functioning and degeneration with positive results (Cenacchi 1993).

Lecithin/phosphatidyl choline: Phosphatidyl choline is a phospholipid that is integral to cellular membranes and particularly of nerve and brain cells. It helps to move fats into the cells, and is involved in acetylcholine uptake, neurotransmission, and cellular integrity. As part of the cell membranes, lecithin is an essential nutrient required by all cells of the body for general health and wellness (Hanin 1987).

Probiotics: Administration of the proper combination of probiotics has been reported to have a positive impact on the intestines and the digestive process (Goldin 1984, Perdigon 1987). Probiotics have been shown to improve and aid the digestive process by secreting their own source of enzymes, which is beneficial for animals that are pancreatic enzyme deficient (McDonough 1987).

Evening primrose oil (EPO): In a double blind study, Cotterell (1990) showed that more than 50% of the women taking evening primrose oil with mentally related irritable bowel syndrome improved, while none in the non-EPO group showed a benefit.

Fiber: In a study of people with IBS, Manning (1977) and Hotz (1994) showed improvement by adding psyllium to the diet.

Chinese herbal medicine/acupuncture
General considerations/rationale
According to TCM, irritable bowel syndrome is due to Qi and Yang deficiency in the Spleen and Stomach with

Heat and Damp accumulation in the Lower Burner. There may be accompanying Qi and Blood stagnation. The Spleen and Stomach are charged with converting food and water to usable substances in the body. Inability of these organs to perform this function leads to gastrointestinal signs. Without enough Qi or Yang (energy and warmth), the Stomach and Spleen are unable to transform food into usable substances in the body. The Lower Burner is the lower aspect of the trunk, namely the Intestines. When the Stomach and Spleen do not process the food properly, the intestines receive abnormal chyle. The intestines must then work on undigested foodstuffs. In this condition the stool contains mucus (Damp). Heat refers to the inflammatory cells and toxins in the stool as a result of improper digestion. Stagnation leads to pain. Blood or Qi stagnation can lead to pain and cramping. Treatment is aimed at stopping diarrhea and cramping and controlling the underlying cause of the disorder.

Appropriate Chinese herbs

Atractylodes (Bai zhu): Can treat both diarrhea and constipation, depending on the doses administered (Chang Yong Zhong Yao Cheng Fen Yu Yao Li Shou Ce 1994).

Coptis (Huang lian): A broad-spectrum antibiotic. It contains berberine, which is well suited for gastrointestinal infections. It is not well absorbed so is unlikely to cause systemic side effects, but works synergistically with other herbs to inhibit pathogenic gastrointestinal bacteria (The Merck Index 12th edition 2000). Berberine has the added benefit of having anti-inflammatory properties (Yao Xue Za Zhi 1981). In a trial of 100 people with acute gastroenteritis who were treated with coptis and white cardamon (Bai dou kou), there was 100% response (Si Chuan Yi Xue Yuan Xue Bao 1959). In another study, more than 1,000 people with acute bacterial dysentery were treated with coptis, either alone or along with other herbs, with excellent results and few side effects (Zhong Hua Nei Ke Za Zhi 1976).

Dry ginger (Gan jiang): Can increase peristalsis and has protective effects on the GI system (Zhong Cao Yao 1988).

Magnolia bark (Hou po): Has been shown experimentally to prevent toxin-induced diarrhea in mice (Zhu 1997). It can decrease contractions in the small intestine (Konoshima 1991). It also inhibits bacterial proliferation (Namba 1982, Yao Jian Gong Zuo Tong Xun 1980).

Pulsatilla root (Bai tou weng): Can inhibit bacterial growth (CA 1948). Interestingly, in Western thought, anxiety or stress may precipitate a bout of diarrhea with this condition. Pulsatilla has sedative effects (Zhong Yao Xue 1998).

Sanguisorba (Di yu): Helps control diarrhea. In a trial of 91 human patients suffering from bacterial dysentery, 87 responded well (Hu Nan Yi Yao Za Zhi 1978).

Saussurea (Mu xiang): Inhibits bacteria, including those that tend to overgrow in the intestines, i.e. E. coli and corynebacteria (Zhong Yao Yao Li Yu Ying Yong 1983).

Acupuncture

Acupuncture has been used for colitis with some reports of excellent results. In one trial, 33 people with ulcerative colitis were treated with a combination of herbal supplements and acupuncture (Bl 18, Bl20, St36, Sp6, CV6, St 25, Bl25, and ST37. Twenty-eight people experienced complete resolution of signs while another 3 people had improvement in symptoms. Two people did not respond (Zhong 1998).

Homotoxicology
General considerations/rationale
Patients with IBS who have no detectible structural lesions likely are placed near the Deposition and Impregnation phases on the Six-Phase Table of Homotoxicology. Regressive vicariation takes them to the Inflammation Phase and clinical conditions of colitis and progressive vicariation drive them into worsening states. Because of the connection between the psychoneuorendocrine and immune systems, stress and strong emotions can release homotoxins and result in an altered GI condition. This especially applies to microfloral populations and bowel mobility.

The results can be excellent when antihomotoxic therapy is aimed at symptoms and phases. Because dietary changes may improve these cases substantially, therapy begins there. Symptom remedies for colitis include Podophyllum compositum, Colcynthis homaccord, Nux vomica Homaccord, and Veratrum homaccord. Other agents may be helpful as well, depending upon other signs and medical history. Injection therapy can be used in acute flare-ups with good results. The liver is involved in repair of colonic mucosal defects, and so the use of Hepar compositum is commonly recommended. Because stress seems to be involved, it seems prudent to select remedies supportive of adrenal function. Tonsilla compositum and Thyroidea compositum should be considered. Berberis homaccord and Solidago compositum (which contain Berberis) are recommended. Other formulas such as Nervoheel, Ignatia homaccord, and BHI-Calming can be used to reduce stress and anxiety responses. Mucosa compositum supports the colonic mucosa strongly and should be given intermittently.

There are no studies on probiotics for IBS, but their use may assist in recovery and is considered safe according to generally regarded as safe (GRAS) legislation. The authors do not prescribe probiotics in all such cases, but do consider their use. Ulceration and immune suppression are conditions in which probiotics may have harmful effects.

Proper training that helps the pet predict and understand its role in the home reduces stress. Palmquist has seen dogs that have repeated bouts of colitis in response to emotional issues such as owner absence and familial disharmony. Colitis vanishes quickly in these cases when attention is given to the emotional issue.

Appropriate homotoxicology formulas

Berberis homaccord: Berberis has major actions on the liver and gallbladder (Reckeweg 2000), and has been shown to have effects in diarrhea (Zhu, Ahrens 1982; Shamsa, Ahmadiani, Khosrokhavar 1999). It also treats colic, collapse, and bloody vomitus, and is supportive of adrenal and renal function. It is part of the basic *Detox Kit*.

BHI-Calming: Includes a wide variety of commonly used homeopathic remedies for anger, resentment, fear, depression, nervousness, and mania.

BHI-Diarrhea: Treats diarrhea in general. It is a good simple remedy for many cases of diarrhea.

BHI-Intestine: Treats diarrhea, cramping, hard-black stool (Bryonia alba); emotional diarrhea, leg spasm and cramps, colitis (Colocynthis); flatulence and liver conditions (Lycopodium); gastroenteritis and colitis (Nux vomica); and mucosal inflammation (Mercurius corrosives). Sulphur activates a blocked metabolism, stimulates regressive vicariation, and promotes healing (Heel 2002).

BHI-Spasm-Pain: Treats leg cramps, fever, pain and inflammation, sharp pain, colic or intestinal spasm, and colitis.

BHI-Stomach: Used for stomach distress relieved by eructation, stomach pain, heartburn, chalky white tongue, flatulence, and tendency to collapse.

Chol-Heel: An excellent remedy that contains Belladonna, Chelidonium, Carduus marianus, Lycopodium, Veratrum, and Taraxicum, along with some other very useful components, all in potency chords. This can be of great relief in GI discomfort (Broadfoot 2005).

Coenzyme compositum: Contains Citricum acidum, which is useful for dental problems and gingivitis; scurvy; blackening of teeth and heavy deposits of dental plaque; painful, herpetic vesicles around the lips; nausea; painful cramping in the umbilical area; and distension.

Colocynthis homaccord: Treats diarrhea with lower back pain (Citrullus colocynthis), colic, pain below the navel, and colitis with gelatinous stools.

Diarrheel S: A symptom remedy for acute and chronic diarrhea. Treats acute gastroenteritis, belching, spurting diarrhea, pancreatopathy, and colitis. This commonly used formula contains Tormentilla, which is used for dysentery, acute gastroenteritis, and mucous and ulcerative colitis with bloody stools (Reckeweg 2002). It is also found in *BHI-Diarrhea* and *Veratrum homaccord*.

Duodenoheel: Treats hunger pains, hyperacidity, gastric and duodenal ulcers, nausea and vomiting, and dysentery with tenesmus (Reckeweg 2000).

Galium-Heel: Used for all cellular phases, hemorrhoids, and anal fissures, and as a detoxicant.

Hepar compositum: Provides detoxification and drainage of hepatic tissues and organ and metabolic support, and is useful in most hepatic and gall bladder pathologies. It is an important part of Deep Detoxification Formula. It treats duodenitis, pancreatitis, cystic hepatic ducts, cholelithiasis, cholangitis, cholecystitis, vomiting, and diarrhea (Demers 2004, Broadfoot 2004). This combination contains Natrum oxalaceticum (also found in *Coenzyme compositum*, *Ubichinon compositum*, and *Mucosa compositum*) for changes in appetite and stomach distension due to air. Treats nausea, stomach pain with a sensation of fullness, gurgling in the abdomen, and cramping pain in the hypochondria. Also used for constipation, sudden diarrhea (particularly after eating), and flatus (Reckeweg 2002).

Hepeel: Provides liver drainage and detoxification. It is used in a wide variety of conditions including cancer of the liver, where *Hepeel* was found to be antiproliferative, hepatoprotective, and an antioxidant when tested in human HepG2 cells (Gebhardt 2003).

Lymphomyosot: Provides lymph drainage and endocrine support, and treats edema. Contains Gentiana for chronic gastritis. It treats flatulence, diarrhea, distension of the stomach with eructations, nausea, retching, and vomiting. It contains Geranium robertianum for nausea, particularly after eating, with distension or sensation of fullness. Myosotis arvensis is contained for bloat and distension (Reckeweg 2002).

Mucosa compositum: Broadly supportive for repair of mucosal elements. Used in cellular cases and in recovery periods following active disease (Reckeweg 2000). This remedy contains a useful component in Kali bichromicum, which is indicated for ulcers found on the gums, the tongue, the lips, and even on the gastric mucosa (gastric or duodenal ulcer). The tongue may have a thick, yellow, mucous coating, or, in ulcerative stomatitis or tonsillitis it may be dry, smooth, shiny, or fissured. Kali has been used effectively in acute gastroenteritis associated with vomiting of clear, light-colored fluid or quantities of mucous bile, and in cases with hematemesis, flatulent colics, and dysenteric stools with tenesmus (Reckeweg 2002). It contains Hydrastis with mucosal support for oral problems such as stomatitis, mucosal suppuration that is accompanied by ulceration, inflammations and colic of the hepatobiliary system and the gastrointestinal tract, and polyp formation (Reckeweg 2002).

The Kreosotum component is for chronic gastritis with gastric hemorrhages and vomiting of brown masses. It also has a dental implication in cases with spongy gums and carious teeth, neuralgias proceeding from them causing a burning toothache with deep caries, black patches on the teeth, and fetid discharges. The single remedy Phosphorus is broadly useful for dyspepsia and for jaw problems in dental disease (Reckeweg 2002).

Phosphorus is found in many other remedies including *Echinacea compositum* and *Leptandra Homaccord*. It is rich in suis organ preparations for mucosal support, plus a large variety of remedies with indications in the gastrointestinal sphere. Also contained in this broad remedy is Argentum nitricum (also in *Atropinum compositum*, *Diarrheel*, *Duodenoheel*, *Gastricumeel*, *Momordica compositum*, *BHI-Nausea*, and several other combinations). It is included for distension in the upper abdomen, gastrocardiac symptom-complex, and amelioration from eructations. It is used for gastric crises (Reckeweg 2002).

Nervoheel: A first-choice agent for reducing stress and nervousness. It is useful in people with psychosomatic issues and it covers signs including restlessness, depression, mental exhaustion, neuralgia, and restless hands.

Nux vomica homaccord: Treats liver and gastrointestinal disease, and is used after smoke inhalation. Useful in gingivitis (Reckeweg 2002). It is a commonly used formula for detoxification as part of the *Detox Kit*. Recent research shows that the ingredient Brucine affects mitochondria in human hepatoma cells. Further research is needed to determine if homeopathic dilutions are more or less active (Deng, et al 2006).

Paeonia-Heel: Treats anal region issues such as hemorrhoids, anal fissures, colitis, spasmodic constipation, weeping anal lesions, anal pruritus, and painful defecation (Reckeweg 2000). A topical cream is useful.

Podophyllum homaccord: Treats chronic gastroenteritis, gastroenteritis in juvenile dogs and cats, dyspepsia, catarrhal colitis, hemorrhoids, and watery-green diarrhea alternating with constipation (Macloed 1983).

Tonico-Heel: Treats nervous exhaustion, depression, anger and gastrointestinal disorders associated with stress and anxiety, anorexia, asthma, and hyperactivity.

Traumeel S: An anti-inflammatory that activates blocked enzymes.

Ubichinon compositum: Contains Anthraquinone for swelling of gums and GI symptoms such as distention, flatulence, and cramping abdominal pain. Also treats constipation with straining or sudden diarrhea (Reckeweg 2002).

Valerianaheel: Used for oversensitivity, sleeplessness, irritability, and anger. Assists in sleep and has a sedative effect.

Veratrum homaccord: Treats gastritis, intense vomiting with blood, collapse (pale mucous membranes), and psychosis. Symptoms include tearing up paper and clothes, and mania and sadness. Treats dysentary, fecal incontinence, and intestinal spasm. This very useful remedy is used widely by the authors for general vomiting cases.

Consider its use in cases of gastritis following general anesthesia. Classical provings were recently repeated and found consistent with earlier work (Van Wassenhoven 2004).

Vomitusheel S: Treats nausea and vomiting with a cough (*Ipecacuanha*), liver and gastrointestinal issues (*Nux vomica*), eructation, and possibly anxiety or depression (*Ignatia*) (Reckeweg 2000). No known adverse reactions have occurred, so this is extremely safe to use in pediatric patients.

This remedy contains Aethusa for vomiting obviously originating in the nervous system. In serious cases capillary paralysis, hematemesis, stomach cramps, and tympanitic distension may occur, with an irresistible urge to pass stool. The nervous vomiting is characterized by spasmodic contractions of the esophageal muscles and violent pains that shoot upwards from the cardiac sphincter (Reckeweg 2002). In more severe vomiting cases consider *Veratrum homaccord* instead or in combination.

Authors' suggested protocols

Nutrition

Intestine/IBD and/or esophagus/stomach support formulas: 1 tablet for every 25 pounds of body weight BID.

Brain/nerve support formula: One-half tablet for every 25 pounds of body weight BID.

Glutimmune: One-fourth scoop for every 25 pounds of body weight daily.

Lecithin/phosphatidyl choline: One-fourth teaspoon for every 25 pounds of body weight BID.

Phosphatidyl serine: 25 mg for every 25 pounds of body weight BID.

Evening primrose oil: 1 capsule (500 mg) per 25 pounds of body weight daily.

Psyllium: 1 teaspoon per 25 pounds of body weight per meal.

Probiotic: 1/2 capsule per 25 pounds of body weight with food.

Chinese herbal medicine/acupuncture

Formula Colitis/chronic-ulcerative: 1 capsule per 10 to 20 pounds twice daily. In addition to the herbs mentioned above, Colitis/chronic-ulcerative contains cooked aconite (Zhi fu zi)and immature bitter orange (Zhi shi) to help increase the efficacy of the formula.

The authors commonly use the following points in the treatment of irritable bowel syndrome: CV12, ST25, BL25, ST36, BL20, CV4, and GV4.

Homotoxicology (Dose: 10 drops PO for 50-pound dog; 5 drops PO for cat or small dog)

Treatment must be individualized, but the following represent good starting therapies. They can be readily adapted based upon clinical response.

Traumeel-S, Galium-Heel, Duodenoheel, Podophyllum compositum, Veratrum homaccord, Hepar compositum and/or Hepeel, Atropinum compositum, and Mucosa compositum: Mixed together and given orally BID to TID.

Tonico-Heel, Valerianaheel, BHI-Calming, Ignatia homaccord, or others: For stress-related issues. Sometimes one can choose just 1 or 2 remedies and have excellent results, while in other cases more individual products must be combined.

Product sources

Nutrition
Brain/nerve, intestine/IBD, and esophagus/stomach support formulas: Animal Nutrition Technologies. Alternatives: Enteric Support—Standard Process Veterinary Formulas; NutriGest—Rx Vitamins for Pets; Composure—Vetri Science Laboratories.

Glutimmune: Well Wisdom. Alternative: L-Glutamine powder—Thorne Veterinary Products.

Phosphatidyl serine: Integrative Therapuetics.

Lecithin/phosphatidyl choline: Designs for Health.

Psyllium seed powder: Progressive Labs.

Probiotic MPF: Progressive Labs.

Chinese herbal medicine
Formula Colitis/chronic-ulcerative: Natural Solutions, Inc.

Homotoxicology
BHI/Heel Corporation

REFERENCES

Western medicine references
Leib MS, Monroe WE, Codner EC. Management of chronic large bowel diarrhea in dogs, Vet Med 1991;86:922–929.

Grooters AM. Irritable Bowel Syndrome. In: Tilley L, Smith F. The 5-Minute Veterinary Consult: Canine and Feline, 2003Blackwell Publishing.

Strombeck DR, Guilford WG. Strombeck's small animal gastroenterology. 3rd ed. 1996.Philadelphia: Saunders.

Tams TR. Irritable Bowel Syndrome. In: Kirk RW, Bonagura JD, eds. Current veterinary therapy XI. Philadelphia: Saunders, 1992:604–608.

IVM/nutrition references
Cenacchi T, Bertoldin T, Farina C, et al. Cognitive decline in the elderly: a double-blind, placebo-controlled multicenter study on efficacy of phosphatidylserine administration. Aging (Milano) 1993;5:123–33.

Cotterell CJ, Lee AJ, Hunter JO. Double-blind cross-over trial of evening primrose oil in women with menstrually-related irritable bowel syndrome. In: Omega-6 Essential Fatty Acids:

Pathophysiology and roles in clinical medicine, Alan R Liss, New York, 1990, 421–6.

Golden BR, Gorbach SL. The Effect of Milk and Lactobacillus Feeding on Human Intestinal Bacteria Activity. Am. J. of Clin. Nutr., 1984.39: 756–61.

Hanin IG, Ansell B. Lecithin: Technological, Biological, and Therapeutic Aspects, NY: Plenum Press, 1987. 180, 181.

Hotz J, Plein K. Effectiveness of plantago seed husks in comparison with wheat bran on stool frequency and manifestations of irritable colon syndrome with constipation. Med Klin 1994; 89:645–51.

Manning AP, Heaton KW, Harvey RF, Uglow P. Wheat fibre and irritable bowel syndrome. Lancet 1977;ii:417–8.

McDonough FE, Hitchins AD, Wong NP, et al. Modification of sweet acidophilus milk to improve utilization by lactose-intolerant persons. Am J Clin Nutr 1987;45:570–4.

Perdigon GN, de Masius N, Alvarez S, et al. Enhancement of Immune Response in Mice fed with S. Thermophilus and L. Acidophilus, J. of Dairy Sci., 198;770: 919–926.

Souba W, et al. Glutamine metabolism in the intestinal tract: invited review, JPEN 1985;9:608–617.

Windmueller HG. Glutamine utilization by the small intestine, Adv. Enzymol 1982;53:201–237.

Yoshimura K, et al. Effects of enteral glutamine administration on experimental inflammatory bowel disease, JPEN 1993; 17:235.

Chinese herbal medicine/acupuncture references
CA, 1948; 42:4228a.

Chang Yong Zhong Yao Cheng Fen Yu Yao Li Shou Ce (A Handbook of the Composition and Pharmacology of Common Chinese Drugs), 1994; 739:742.

Hu Nan Yi Yao Za Zhi (Hunan Journal of Medicine and Herbology), 1978;3:18.

Konoshima T, Kozuka M, Tokuda H, Nishino H, Washima A, Hiruna M, Ito K, Tanabe M. J of Nat Prod, 1991; 54(3): 816.

The Merck Index 12th edition, 2000. Chapman and Hall/CRCnetBASE/Merck.

Namba T, Tsunezuka M, Hattori M. Dental caries prevention by traditional Chinese medicines. Part II. Potent antibacterial action of Magnoliae cortex extracts against Streptococcus mutans. Planta Med, 1982; 44(2):100.

Si Chuan Yi Xue Yuan Xue Bao (Journal of Sichuan School of Medicine), 1959;1:102.

Yao Jian Gong Zuo Tong Xun (Journal of Herbal Preparations), 1980;10(4):209.

Yao Xue Za Zhi (Journal of Medicinals), 1981, 101(10):883.

Zhong BL, et al. Treating nonspecific ulcerative colitis with combination of acupuncture and herbs. China Journal of Acupuncture. 1998;18(5):312.

Zhong Cao Yao (Chinese Herbal Medicine), 1988; 13(11):17.

Zhong Hua Nei Ke Za Zhi (Chinese Journal of Internal Medicine), 1976;4:219.

Zhong Yao Xue (Chinese Herbology), 1998; 195:197.

Zhong Yao Yao Li Yu Ying Yong (Pharmacology and Applications of Chinese Herbs), 1983;169.

Zhu ZP, et al. Hou Pu's effect on the digestive system. China Journal of Chinese Medicine. 1997;22(11):686–688.

Homotoxicology references

Broadfoot PJ. Inflammation: Homotoxicology and Healing, in proceedings AHVMA/Heel Homotoxicology Seminar. 2004. Denver, CO, p 27.

Demers, J., Homotoxicology and Acupuncture, in proceedings of the 2004 Homotoxicology Seminar. AHVMA/Heel. Denver, CO, p 5,6.

Deng X, Yin F, Lu X, Cai B, Yin W. The apoptotic effect of brucine from the seed of Strychnos nux-vomica on human hepatoma cells is mediated via Bcl-2 and Ca2+ involved mitochondrial pathway. *Toxicol Sci.* 2006. May;91(1):pp 59–69.

Gebhardt R. Antioxidative, antiproliferative and biochemical effects in HepG2 cells of a homeopathic remedy and its constituent plant tinctures tested separately or in combination. *Arzneimittelforschung.* 2003.53(12): pp 823–30.

Heel. BHI Homeopathic Therapy: Professional Reference. Albuquerque, NM: Heel Inc, 2002. pp 43, 47, 73.

Reckeweg H. Biotherapeutic Index: Ordinatio Antihomotoxica et Materia Medica, 5th ed. 2000. Baden-Baden, Germany: Biologische Heilmittel Heel GMBH, pp 290, 294–5, 300, 329–30, 358–9, 363–4, 366–7, 369, 381, 390, 399–400, 432, 538.

Reckeweg H. Homeopathia Antihomotoxica Materia Medica, 4th ed. Baden-Baden, Germany: Arelia-Verlag GMBH, 2002. pp. 136–8, 139–40, 125–6, 147,150–3, 179, 206, 241–2, 317–19, 345, 366, 461–3, 488–90, 578–80.

Shamsa F, Ahmadiani A, Khosrokhavar R. Antihistaminic and anticholinergic activity of barberry fruit (Berberis vulgaris) in the guinea-pig ileum. *J Ethnopharmacol.* 1999. Feb;64(2):pp 161–6.

Van Wassenhoven M. Towards an evidence-based repertory: clinical evaluation of Veratrum album. *Homeopathy.* 2004. Apr;93(2): pp 71–7.

Zhu B, Ahrens FA. Effect of berberine on intestinal secretion mediated by Escherichia coli heat-stable enterotoxin in jejunum of pigs. *Am J Vet Res.* 1982. Sep;43(9): pp 1594–8.

COLITIS

Definition and cause

Colitis is an inflammatory process of the colon that leads to cellular inflammation and a decrease in the ability to reabsorb water, resulting in diarrhea. Long-standing colitis is often complicated with bloody diarrhea, discomfort, and weight loss. Common causes are intestinal parasites, allergic reaction (often to food), an immune-mediated reaction focused in the colon, and infections. It also can be secondary to other diseases such as CRF, liver disease, anal sac disease, perianal fistulae, and neoplasia (Burrows 2003, Guilford 1996, Leib 1995, Sherding 1992).

Medical therapy rationale, drug(s) of choice, and nutritional recommendations

The medications of choice are antibiotics such as metronidazole or drugs such as sulfasalazine and corticosteroids to reduce inflammation and suppress the immune response in combination with azothiaprine if necessary. Dietary support involves feeding a bland, low-fat, digestible, hypoallergenic diet along with the addition of fiber to increase stool bulk and improve intestinal motility. Surgical intervention is required for strictures and granulomatous inflammatory response (Dimski 1992, Burrows 2003, Guilford 1996).

Anticipated prognosis

The prognosis is often good with dietary and medical treatment and client compliance. Colitis that is longstanding or secondary to other diseases such as neoplasia carries a more guarded prognosis (Burrows 2003).

Integrative veterinary therapies

The colon and its associated microflora constitute an amazingly complex and effective mechanism for waste excretion, vital nutrient manufacturing, and immune defense for the body. Probiotic bacteria and fungi are vital to proper digestion and homotoxin elimination. These diverse components of the large intestine work in perfect concert to achieve these goals and thereby promote survival of the organism. Conditions which imbalance this system can readily lead to disease signs.

A wide variety of exogenous homotoxins can be associated with disease of the gastrointestinal system. Of particular importance are food additives such as carrageenan, a waxy substance derived from seaweed and used to bind dry food together. While listed as a GRAS food additive, this compound has received large amounts of attention in the literature (Tobacman 2001). Carrageenan is actually used in laboratories to induce colitis in experimental models. Watt and Marcus (1981) discuss carnageenan's proposed association with neoplastic change. Cohen and Ito (2002) reviewed the toxicologic effects of carrageenan and found it safe. However, veterinarians may wish to note cases of colitis presenting on diets containing this ingredient. Food dyes can also lead to inflammation of the intestinal tract in susceptible individuals, and no one knows the extent that such chemicals may form haptens and otherwise assist in the development of auto-aggressive pathologies.

Medical drugs can also lead to colon disease. Some drugs cause entero-colitis as a direct adverse reaction, and professionals are well aware of these issues. More than 700 medications list diarrhea as a potential side effect: "Those most frequently involved are antimicrobials, laxatives, magnesium-containing antacids, lactose- or sorbitol-containing products, nonsteroidal anti-inflammatory drugs, prostaglandins, colchicine, antineoplastics, antiarrhythmic drugs and cholinergic agents" (Chassany, Michaux, Bergmann 2000).

Stress and emotional issues can contribute to endogenous homotoxins as the psychoneuroendocrine-immune (PNEI) responds to the condition. Because minor changes in bowel conditions may cause drastic disturbances in bowel microflora, it is not uncommon to see stress associated with the presence of colitis. Palmquist has seen colitis strongly associated with stressful divorce, and other practitioners no doubt have similar stories to convey. Providing colitis patients with safe, nonstressful environments is simply practicing good medicine.

The inclusion of proper prebiotics (such as fiber) and probiotic bacteria may promote or assist in homotoxin removal by binding homotoxins to fiber or through metabolism of toxic material by bacteria. The common practice of treating GI upset by fasting and then giving a bland diet is an excellent approach to mild GI conditions. Use of therapeutic diets higher in fiber may be especially useful for colitis, and these diets are also indicated in geriatric patients due to the homotoxins, which have been impregnated in their systems. Many cases of mild colitis can be treated exclusively by altering the diet to a high-fiber, low-fat prescription product or homemade diet.

During the detoxification and drainage therapy that is commonly required by these patients, the presence of proper fiber greatly assists in removal of homotoxins from the body. Such diets are also tolerated well by geriatric patients and for that reason alone concerned healthcare professionals may recommend them as part of a geriatric nutritional program.

The early identification of the underlying cause(s) and the use of nutrients, nutraceuticals, medicinal herbs and combination homeopathics that are anti-inflammatory and tissue-sparing can help control the condition and prevent ongoing inflammation and progression to more chronic conditions.

Nutrition
General considerations/rationale

The nutritional approach to colitis is multifaceted and prevention oriented. The approach consists of nutrient support of colon cells; the enhancement of cellular elimination and detoxification; dietary adjustment to include beneficial fiber, removal of chemical additives, preservatives, coloring agent, dyes, byproducts and other unnatural ingredients, and support of overall immune function.

Appropriate nutrients

Nutritional/gland therapy: Nutrients and glandular intestine, adrenal, lymph, and thymus supply intrinsic nutrients that improve organ function and reduce cellular inflammation. This helps to spare these organs from cascading inflammation and eventual degeneration (see Chapter 2, Gland Therapy, for a more detailed explanation).

Glutamine: Glutamine has been shown to improve immune function and is beneficial for the cells of the gastro-intestinal tract (Souba 1985, Windmueller 1982, Yoshimura 1993).

Probiotics: Administration of the proper combination of probiotics has been reported to have a positive impact on the intestines and the digestive process (Goldin 1984, Perdigon (1987). Probiotics have been shown to improve and aid the digestive process by secreting their own source of enzymes, which is beneficial for animals that are pancreatic enzyme deficient (McDonough 1987).

Colostrum: Colostrum has been shown to improve intestinal health. It helps to balance intestinal flora and improves digestion. Colostrum has been found to improve the immune status of the intestinal tract, which can, via intestinal production of globulins, help the overall immune competency of the body (Blake 1999).

Enzymes: Metabolically, enzymes are essential in the conversion of foods to meet the energy needs of the body. They are also involved as catalysts in the many biochemical processes. Enzyme deficiency is caused by underactive organ production or a deficiency or lack of availability of the proper nutrients required for enzyme production. Minerals, amino acids, and fatty acids are required for the synthesis of various enzymes (Howell (1985).

Fiber: In a study of people with IBS, Manning (1977) and Hotz (1994) showed improvement by adding psyllium to the diet.

Chinese herbal medicine/acupuncture
General considerations/rationale

Colitis is described as a Qi and Yang deficiency in the Spleen and Stomach, with Heat and Damp accumulation in the Lower Burner. Qi and Blood may become stagnant. The Stomach and Spleen function to promote digestion. With Qi and Yang deficiency there is not enough energy and heat, respectively, to complete this process. When digestion is disrupted, abnormal digesta fills the Lower Burner, or intestines in Western parlance. This abnormal chyle contains mucus in most cases (Damp) and there may be bacterial overgrowth leading to inflammation (Heat). Without proper movement in the intestinal tract, Blood and Qi may become stagnant. Stagnation leads to pain, in this case intestinal cramping.

Treatment is aimed at decreasing diarrhea and controlling secondary bacterial overgrowth, inflammation, and cramping.

Appropriate Chinese herbs

Atractylodes (Bai zhu): Treats both diarrhea and constipation, depending on the doses administered

(Chang Yong Zhong Yao Cheng Fen Yu Yao Li Shou Ce 1994).

Coptis (Huang lian): A broad-spectrum antibiotic. It contains berberine, which is well suited for gastrointestinal infections. It is not well absorbed so is unlikely to cause systemic side effects, but works synergistically with other herbs to inhibit pathogenic gastrointestinal bacteria (The Merck Index 12th edition 2000). Berberine has the added benefit of having anti-inflammatory properties (Yao Xue Za Zhi 1981). In a trial of 100 people with acute gastroenteritis who were treated with coptis and white cardamon (Bai dou kou), there was 100% response (Si Chuan Yi Xue Yuan Xue Bao 1959). In another study more than 1,000 people with acute bacterial dysentery were treated with coptis, either alone or along with other herbs, with excellent results and few side effects (Zhong Hua Nei Ke Za Zhi 1976).

Dry ginger (Gan jiang): Can increase peristalsis and has a protective effects on GI system (Zhong Cao Yao 1988).

Magnolia bark (Hou po): Has been shown experimentally to prevent toxin-induced diarrhea in mice (Zhu 1997). It can decrease contractions in the small intestine (Konoshima 1991). It also inhibits bacterial proliferation (Namba 1982, Yao Jian Gong Zuo Tong Xun 1980).

Pulsatilla root (Bai tou weng): Can inhibit bacterial growth (CA 1948). Interestingly, in Western thought, anxiety or stress may precipitate a bout of diarrhea with this condition. Pulsatilla has sedative effects (Zhong Yao Xue 1998).

Sanguisorba (Di yu): Helps control diarrhea. In a trial of 91 human patients suffering from bacterial dysentery, 87 responded well (Hu Nan Yi Yao Za Zhi 1978).

Saussurea (Mu xiang): Inhibits bacteria, including those that tend to overgrow in the intestines, i.e. E. coli and corynebacteria (Zhong Yao Yao Li Yu Ying Yong 1983).

Acupuncture has been used for colitis with some reports of excellent results. In one trial, 33 people with ulcerative colitis were treated with a combination of herbal supplements and acupuncture (Bl18, Bl20, St36, Sp6, CV6, St25, Bl25, and ST37). Twenty-eight people experienced complete resolution of signs while another 3 people had improvement in symptoms. Two people did not respond (Zhong 1998).

Homotoxicology
General considerations/rationale
Colitis is an Inflammation Phase disorder in acute disease and an Impregnation Phase disease in more chronic conditions. It is a commonly seen gastrointestinal condition in dogs and cats.

Homotoxins alter the complex tissues and environment of the colon and the body reacts through an inflammatory response to result in colitis. Inflammation in organs lying in close proximity can occur, as in pancreatitis and renal disease, which can lead to irritation and inflammation of the colon and resulting signs of colitis. When homotoxins are excreted via the gastrointestinal system, Excretion Phase, Inflammation Phase, Deposition Phase, Impregnation Phase, Degeneration Phase, and Dedifferentiation Phase diseases can appear in the colon itself.

The normal condition of the colon is the Excretion Phase, which results after it has completed its work on the final stages of digestion and absorption. The rate of transit through the colon is a critical determinant of health, as putrefaction, bacterial overgrowth, and resulting accumulation of homotoxins are undesirable to general health. Voiding the bowels removes homotoxins from the body in large quantities.

A more insidious situation comes from Deposition Phases caused by drug residues and their combination, interaction, or reaction with other agents at later periods of time (Reckeweg 1989). Many idiopathic conditions may be associated with such reactions, and further research is indicated but is difficult to perform. Therefore, it may be a long time before this area of medicine is fully understood.

Antihomotoxic drugs are generally safe and well tolerated and can be used to assist patients with colitis. Before selecting drugs that may have more potential harm, it may be helpful to first treat with biological therapies. Dietary change and antihomotoxic agents work well together. Some cases may be more severe and require pharmaceutical agents, and in these cases the veterinarian should remember pertinent side effects and drug residue issues.

Appropriate homotoxicology formulas
Atropinum compositum: Not available in vials on the U.S. market at this time, but a powerful antispasmodic for biliary, renal, and intestinal colic (Demers 2004). Tablets can be given separately or in a mixture with other antihomotoxic agents. Contains Benzoicum acidum (common also to *Aesculus compositum*, *Arnica-Heel*, *Atropinum compositum*, and *Rhododendroneel*). It is used in inflammatory symptoms which occur throughout the alimentary canal (Contains Cantharis for dysentery and ulcerative colitis): a slimy coating on the tongue with ulcers at the edges, stomatitis with dysphagia, eructations, retching, vomiting, and flatulent distension below the ribs on both sides. The stools are copious, loose, and white in color, with violent tenesmus and mixed with blood; there are stabbing pains in the rectum, rigors, and a feeling of being seriously ill (Reckeweg 2002).

BHI-Intestine: Used for diarrhea, cramping, hard-black stool (Bryonia alba); emotional diarrhea, leg spasm and cramps, colitis (Colocynthis); flatulence and liver conditions (Lycopodium); gastroenteritis and colitis (Nux vomica); and mucosal inflammation (Mercurius corrosives). Sulphur activates a blocked metabolism, stimulates regressive vicariation, and promotes healing (Heel 2002).

BHI-Spasm-Pain: Used for leg cramps, fever, pain and inflammation, sharp pain, colic or intestinal spasm, and colitis.

Coenzyme compositum: Contains *Citricum acidum*, which is useful for dental problems and gingivitis; scurvy; blackening of teeth and heavy deposits of dental plaque; painful, herpetic vesicles around the lips; nausea; painful cramping in the umbilical area; and distension.

Colocynthis homaccord: Treats diarrhea with lower back pain (Citrullus colocynthis), colic, pain below the navel, and colitis with gelatinous stools.

Diarrheel S: A symptom remedy for acute and chronic diarrhea. Treats acute gastroenteritis, belching, spurting diarrhea, pancreatopathy, and colitis. This commonly used formula contains Tormentilla, which is used for dysentery, acute gastroenteritis, and mucous and ulcerative colitis with bloody stools (Reckeweg 2002). It is also found in *BHI-Diarrhea* and *Veratrum homaccord*.

Galium-Heel: Used for all cellular phases, hemorrhoids, and anal fissures, and as a detoxicant.

Hepar compositum: Provides detoxification and drainage of hepatic tissues and organ and metabolic support, and is useful in most hepatic and gall bladder pathologies. It is an important part of the Deep Detoxification Formula. Treats duodenitis, pancreatitis, cystic hepatic ducts, cholelithiasis, cholangitis, cholecystitis, vomiting, and diarrhea (Demers 2004, Broadfoot 2004). This combination contains Natrum oxalaceticum (also found in *Coenzyme compositum*, *Ubichinon compositum*, and *Mucosa compositum*) for changes in appetite and stomach distension due to air. Also treats nausea, stomach pain with a sensation of fullness, gurgling in the abdomen, and cramping pain in the hypochondria. It is also used for constipation, sudden diarrhea (particularly after eating), and flatus (Reckeweg 2002).

Lymphomyosot: Provides lymph drainage and endocrine support, and treats edema. Contains Gentiana for chronic gastritis. Treats flatulence, diarrhea, distension of stomach with eructations, nausea, retching, and vomiting. Contains Geranium robertianum for nausea, particularly after eating with distension or sensation of fullness. Myosotis arvensis is contained for bloat and distension (Reckeweg 2002).

Mucosa compositum: Broadly supportive for repair of mucosal elements. Used in cellular cases and in recovery periods following active disease (Reckeweg 2000). This remedy contains a useful component in Kali bichromicum, which is indicated for ulcers found on the gums, the tongue, the lips, and even on the gastric mucosa (gastric or duodenal ulcer). The tongue may have a thick, yellow,

mucous coating, or in ulcerative stomatitis or tonsillitis it may be dry, smooth, shiny, or fissured. Kali has been used effectively in acute gastroenteritis associated with vomiting of clear, light-colored fluid or quantities of mucous bile, and in cases with hematemesis, flatulent colics, and dysenteric stools with tenesmus (Reckeweg 2002). It contains Hydrastis, with mucosal support for oral problems such as stomatitis and mucosal suppuration accompanied by ulceration, inflammations and colic of the hepatobiliary system and the gastrointestinal tract, and polyp formation (Reckeweg 2002)

The Kreosotum component can be used in chronic gastritis with gastric hemorrhages and vomiting of brown masses. Also has a dental implication in cases with spongy gums and carious teeth, neuralgias proceeding from them causing a burning toothache with deep caries, black patches on the teeth, and fetid discharges. The single remedy Phosphorus is broadly useful for dyspepsia and for jaw problems in dental disease (Reckeweg 2002). Phosphorus is found in many other remedies including Echinacea compositum and Leptandra Homoaccord. It is rich in suis organ preparations for mucosal support, plus a large variety of remedies with indications in the gastrointestinal sphere. Also contained in this broad remedy is Argentum nitricum (also in *Atropinum compositum*, *Diarrheel*, *Duodenoheel*, *Gastricumeel*, *Momordica compositum*, *BHI-Nausea*, and several other combinations), which is used for distension in the upper abdomen, gastro-cardiac symptom-complex, and amelioration from eructations. It is also used for gastric crises (Reckeweg 2002).

Nux vomica homaccord: Treats liver and gastrointestinal disease and is used after smoke inhalation. It is useful in gingivitis (Reckeweg 2002). This commonly used formula for detoxification is part of the *Detox Kit*. Recent research shows that 1 ingredient (Brucine) affects mitochondria in human hepatoma cells. Further research is needed to determine whether homeopathic dilutions are more or less active (Deng, et al. 2006).

Podophyllum homaccord: Used for chronic gastroenteritis, gastroenteritis in juvenile dogs and cats, dyspepsia, catarrhal colitis, hemorrhoids, and watery-green diarrhea alternating with constipation (Macloed 1983).

Ubichinon compositum: Contains Anthraquinone for swelling of gums, and GI symptoms such as distention, flatulence, and cramping abdominal pain. It also treats constipation with straining or sudden diarrhea (Reckeweg 2002).

Veratrum homaccord: Treats gastritis, intense vomiting with blood, collapse (pale mucous membranes), psychosis, dysentery, fecal incontinence, and intestinal spasm. This very useful remedy is used widely by the authors for general vomiting cases. Consider its use in cases of gastritis following general anesthesia. Classical provings were recently repeated and found consistent with earlier work (Van Wassenhoven 2004).

Authors Suggested Protocol

Nutrition

Intestinal/IBD and immune support formulas: 1 tablet for every 25 pounds of body weight BID.

Glutimmune: One-fourth scoop per 25 pounds of body weight daily.

Probiotic: One-half capsule per 25 pounds of body weight with food.

Colostrum: One-third teaspoon powdered formula for every 25 pounds of body weight BID.

Pan 5 Plus: 1 capsule opened and mixed with food per every 25 pounds of body weight (maximum, 4 capsules).

Psyllium: 1 teaspoon per every 25 pounds of body weight per meal.

Chinese herbal medicine/acupuncture

Colitis/chronic-ulcerative: 1 capsule per 10 to 20 pounds twice daily. In addition to the herbs mentioned above, Colitis/chronic-ulceritive contains cooked aconite (Zhi fu zi)and immature bitter orange (Zhi shi).

The authors use the following points for colitis: CV12, ST25, BL25, ST36, BL20, CV4, and GV4.

Homotoxicology (Dose: 10 drops PO for 50-pound dog; 5 drops PO for cat or small dog)

Nux vomica homaccord, Galium-Heel, Mercurius-Heel S, Veratrum compositum, and Podophyllum compositum mixed together and taken TID orally. BHI-Diarrhea or Diarrheel, as needed, along with BHI-Spasm-Pain, or Atropinum compositum for spastic pains if present. A high-fiber, low-fat diet is important in most cases.

Product sources

Nutrition

Intestinal/IBD and immune support formulas: Animal Nutrition Technologies. **Alternatives:** Enteric Support—Standard Process Veterinary Formulas; Nutrigest—Rx Vitamins for Pets; Immune System Support—Standard Process Veterinary Formulas; Immuno Support—Rx Vitamins for Pets; Immugen—Thorne Veterinary Products.

Glutimmune: Well Wisdom. **Alternative:** L-Glutamine powder—Thorne Veterinary Products.

Probiotic: Progressive Labs. **Alternative:** Biotic—Rx Vitamins for Pets.

Colostrum: New Life Foods, Inc., The Saskatoon Colostrum Company Ltd.

Pan 5 Plus: Progressive Labs.

Psyllium seed powder: Progressive Labs.

Chinese herbal medicine

Colitis/chronic-ulcerative: Natural Solutions, Inc.

Homotoxicology

BHI/Heel Corporation

REFERENCES

Western medicine references

Burrows CF, Moore LE. Colitis and Proctitis. In: Tilley L, Smith F. The 5-Minute Veterinary Consult: Canine and Feline, 2003. Blackwell Publishing.

Dimski DS. Dietary fiber in the management of gastro-intestinal disease. In Kirk RW, Bonagura JD, eds. Current Veterinary Therapy XI. Philadelphia: WB Saunders, 1992, pp 592–595.

Guilford WG. Approach to clinical problems in gastroenterology. In Guilford WG, Center SA, Strombeck DR, Williams DA, Meyer DJ, eds. Strombeck's Small Animal Gastroenterology. 3rd ed. Philadelphia: WB Saunders, 1996, pp 50–76.

Leib MS, Matz ME. Diseases of the large intestine. In: Ettinger SJ, Feldman EC, eds. Textbook of veterinary internal medicine. Philadelphia: Saunders, 1995:1232–1260.

Sherding RG, Burrows CF. Diarrhea, In: Anderson NV, ed. Veterinary gastroenterology. Philadelphia: Lea and Febiger, 1992:455–477.

IVM references

Chassany O, Michaux A, Bergmann JF. Drug-induced diarrhoea. *Drug Saf.* 2000. Jan;22(1):pp 53–72.

Onderdonk AB. The carrageenan model for experimental ulcerative colitis. *Prog Clin Biol Res.* 1985. 186:pp 237–245.

Tobacman J. Review of harmful gastrointestinal effects of carrageenan in animal experiments. *Environ Health Perspect.* 2001. Oct;109(10):pp 983–94.

Watt J, Marcus R. Harmful effects of carrageenan fed to animals. *Cancer Detect Prev.* 1981. 4(1–4):pp 129–34.

Nutrition references

Blake SR. Bovine Colostrum, The Forgotten Miracle. *Journal of the American Holistic Veterinary Medical Association.* July 1999, Volume 18, Number 2, pp 38–39.

Golden BR, Gorbach SL, The Effect of Milk and Lactobacillus Feeding on Human Intestinal Bacteria Activity. *Am. J. of Clin. Nutr.,* 1984.39: 756–61.

Howell E. Enzyme Nutrition, The Food Enzyme Concept. 1985. Garden City, NY: Avery Publ.

McDonough FE, Hitchins AD, Wong NP, et al. Modification of sweet acidophilus milk to improve utilization by lactose-intolerant persons. *Am J Clin Nutr* 1987;45:570–4.

Manning AP, Heaton KW, Harvey RF, Uglow P. Wheat fibre and irritable bowel syndrome. *Lancet* 1977;ii:417–8.

Perdigon GN, de Masius, N, Alvarez S, et al. Enhancement of Immune Response in Mice fed with S. Thermophilus and L. Acidophilus, *J. of Dairy Sci.,* 1987.70: 919–926.

Souba W, et al, Glutamine metabolism in the intestinal tract: invited review, *JPEN* 1985;9:608–617.

Windmueller HG. Glutamine utilization by the small intestine, *Adv. Enzymol* 1982. 53:201–237.

Yoshimura K, et al. Effects of enteral glutamine administration on experimental inflammatory bowel disease, *JPEN* 1993; 17:235.

Chinese herbal medicine/acupuncture references

CA, 1948; 42:4228a.

Chang Yong Zhong Yao Cheng Fen Yu Yao Li Shou Ce (A Handbook of the Composition and Pharmacology of Common Chinese Drugs), 1994; 739:742.

Hu Nan Yi Yao Za Zhi (Hunan Journal of Medicine and Herbology), 1978;3:18.

Konoshima T, Kozuka M, Tokuda H, Nishino H, Washima A, Hiruna M, Ito K, Tanabe M. *J of Nat Prod*, 1991; 54(3): 816.

The Merck Index 12th edition, Chapman and Hall/CRCnet-BASE/Merck, 2000.

Namba T, Tsunezuka M, Hattori M. Dental caries prevention by traditional Chinese medicines. Part II. Potent antibacterial action of Magnoliae cortex extracts against Streptococcus mutans. *Planta Med*, 1982; 44(2):100.

Si Chuan Yi Xue Yuan Xue Bao (*Journal of Sichuan School of Medicine*), 1959;1:102.

Yao Jian Gong Zuo Tong Xun (*Journal of Herbal Preparations*), 1980;10(4):209.

Yao Xue Za Zhi (*Journal of Medicinals*), 1981, 101(10): 883.

Zhong BL, et al. Treating nonspecific ulcerative colitis with combination of acupuncture and herbs. *China Journal of Acupuncture*. 1998;18(5):312.

Zhong Cao Yao (*Chinese Herbal Medicine*), 1988; 13(11):17.

Zhong Hua Nei Ke Za Zhi (*Chinese Journal of Internal Medicine*), 1976;4:219.

Zhong Yao Xue (*Chinese Herbology*), 1998; 195:197.

Zhong Yao Yao Li Yu Ying Yong (*Pharmacology and Applications of Chinese Herbs*), 1983;169.

Zhu ZP, et al. Hou Pu's effect on the digestive system. *China Journal of Chinese Medicine*. 1997;22(11):686–688.

Homotoxicology references

Broadfoot PJ. Inflammation: Homotoxicology and Healing, in proceedings AHVMA/Heel Homotoxicology Seminar. 2004. Denver, CO, p 27.

Demers, J. Homotoxicology and Acupuncture, in proceedings of the 2004 Homotoxicology Seminar. AHVMA/Heel. Denver, CO, p 5,6.

Deng X, Yin F, Lu X, Cai B, Yin W. The apoptotic effect of brucine from the seed of Strychnos nux-vomica on human hepatoma cells is mediated via Bcl-2 and Ca2+ involved mitochondrial pathway. *Toxicol Sci*. 2006. May;91(1):pp 59–69.

Heel. BHI Homeopathic Therapy: Professional Reference. Albuquerque, NM: Heel Inc. 2002. pp 43, 47, 73.

Reckeweg H. Homotoxicology—Illness and Healing through Anti-homotoxic Therapy, 3rd ed. Albuquerque, NM: Menaco Publishing Company. pp. 1989. 62–84.

Reckeweg H. Biotherapeutic Index: Ordinatio Antihomotoxica et Materia Medica, 5th ed. Baden-Baden, Germany: Biologische Heilmittel Heel GMBH, 2000. pp 369–71.

Reckeweg H. Homeopathia Antihomotoxica Materia Medica, 4th ed. Baden-Baden, Germany: Arelia-Verlag GMBH, 2002. pp. 136–8, 206, 241–2, 345, 366, 446–8, 461–3, 488–90, 578–80.

Van Wassenhoven M. Towards an evidence-based repertory: clinical evaluation of Veratrum album. *Homeopathy*. 2004. Apr;93(2): pp 71–7.

VOMITING

Definition and cause

If the cause of vomiting is determined to be gastritis, please refer to gastritis disease protocol in this section of the book. Vomiting can be acute or chronic with many underlying causes (Guilford 1996, DeNovo 2003, Hart 2003, Strombeck 1990, Willard 1995).

Some of the more common underlying causes are:

- Allergic reactions to foods and allergens.
- Adverse reactions to chemicals including drugs, toxins, pesticides, herbicides, vaccines, etc.
- Infectious agents—bacteria, viruses, protozoan parasites.
- Foreign bodies.
- Secondary to local or systemic diseases—chronic renal disease (CRD), liver disease.
- Intestinal parasites.
- Physiological and endocrines disease and imbalances.
- Anatomical disorders.
- Neoplasia.
- Immune-mediated diseases—IBD.
- Neurological diseases.

Medical therapy rationale, drug(s) of choice, and nutritional recommendations

Besides withdrawal from food and resting the system, the following medications are commonly recommended for vomiting:

- Antiemetics—chlorpromazine, metoclopramide.
- H2 receptor antagonists such as rantidine, cimetidine.
- Mucosal protectants such as sucralfate.
- Antibiotics such as metronidazole.
- Fluid therapy for dehydration
- Potassium supplementation.
- Corticosteroids to reduce inflammation and suppress the immune response.
- Chemotherapeutics for immune suppression and neoplasia.

Anticipated prognosis

The prognosis is dependent upon diagnosing and correcting the underlying causes (DeNovo 2003, Hart 2003, Strombeck 1990).

Integrative veterinary therapies

Proper diagnostics and a working diagnosis are needed in approaching vomiting patients. Blood chemistries, complete blood count, urinalysis, urine culture, fecal examination, fecal culture, radiographs, ultrasound, MRI, and CT scan, as well as surgery and endoscopy, are all commonly performed procedures that may be required to determine the underlying cause in chronic or persistent, nonresponsive cases. Because vomiting can originate from local or more distant issues in the body, clinicians must remember to evaluate all systems so that the underlying cause is not missed. Food allergies, adverse reactions to food or food ingredients, drug reactions, occult neoplasia, seizure disorders, subclinical or occult infections, scarring from traumatic incidents, and a wide variety of issues can make diagnosis of chronic vomiting difficult.

Vomiting that does not readily resolve, that is severe and unrelenting in nature, or that is associated with rapid patient decline or pain warrants immediate professional involvement. The reader is referred to any gastroenterology text for a full discussion of these factors. A complete history of things ingested and chemical exposure is warranted. This includes a drug history as well as topical agents and insecticides. Inquiring about missing toys or possessions can give a clue in cases involving foreign body ingestion, and severe vomiting requiring surgical intervention has been reported from use of chew treats sold in many pet stores. In this case the obstruction is caused by a "homotoxin" that will not dissolve and digest properly, leading to blockage. Changes in treats and food types and use of pet treats containing dyes and preservatives can all be involved (see Homotoxicology in this section for a more detailed discussion).

With the early identification of the underlying inflammatory process, the use of nutrients, nutraceuticals, medicinal herbs, and combination homeopathics that are anti-inflammatory and tissue-protective can help to re-establish balance and prevent ongoing symptoms and organ degeneration.

Nutrition
General considerations/rationale
Medical therapy is often required to control the vomiting. The use of nutritional therapies if often limited to avoid initiating or increasing vomiting episodes. However, vomiting is often secondary to other conditions, diseases, or organ system involvement; and therefore, it is recom-mended that blood be analyzed both medically and physiologically to determine associated organ involvement and disease. This information gives clinicians the ability to formulate therapeutic nutritional protocols that address the stomach as well as other underlying conditions (see Chapter 2, Nutritional Blood Testing, for additional information).

Appropriate nutrients
Nutritional/gland therapy: Glandular stomach provides the intrinsic nutrients to help reduce cellular inflammation and damage and to help protect the stomach from ongoing inflammation and eventual degeneration. The addition of other gland and nutrient support should be considered if the underlying cause is related to other organ systems such as those secondary to kidney disease and azotemia (see other related disease protocols and Gland Therapy in Chapter 2 for more information).

Chinese herbal medicine/acupuncture
General considerations/rationale
Vomiting is caused by rebellious Stomach Qi. It can be due to external Cold, overeating, Phlegm accumulation, Cold and Yang deficiency in the Spleen and Stomach, Stomach Yin deficiency, or a combination of factors. The Qi of the Stomach descends. It ascends when it rebels, bringing stomach contents with it, and thus resulting in the vomiting. Vomiting, in TCM as in Western medicine, is not a diagnosis, but a symptom. The etiology varies. External Cold refers to an external pathogen that in effect interferes with the ability of the stomach to digest the food.

One can think of digestion as a chemical process. Back in chemistry class we were taught that when the environment cools, chemical transformations are slowed. This thought process could be used here. Overeating is recognized in Western medicine as a cause of vomition and requires no explanation. Phlegm accumulation refers to a thick material that interferes with digestion. In this case, the vomitus may well contain a lot of mucus or phlegm. Cold or Yang deficiency in the Stomach refer to internal disease processes that interfere with digestion. The Stomach lacks sufficient heat or energy to digest the food. With Stomach Yin deficiency there are not enough fluids (digestive enzymes) in the Stomach for digestion. Treatment is aimed at decreasing vomition and treating the underlying cause.

Appropriate Chinese herbs
Auranium fruit (Zhi qiao): Promotes gastric emptying and decreases enterospasm in mice and rabbits (Ma 1996).

Citrus (Chen pi): Increases intestinal peristalsis and may help to decrease vomiting (Jiang Su Zhong Yi Za Zhi 1981).

Codonopsis (Dang shen): Improves peristalsis in injured intestines. This effect was investigated in mice after scalding (Wang 1999).

Ginger (Gan jiang): Has been widely used as an antiemetic herb in TCM. Experiments in induced vomiting in dogs have confirmed the efficacy of this herb (Zhong Yao Xue 1998).

Inula flower (Xuan fu hua): Has antibiotic efficacy against multiple strains of bacteria (Zhong Yao Yao Li Yu Ying Yong 1983). This may be of use in bacteria-mediated vomition.

Licorice (Gan cao): Helps to reduce gastrointestinal toxicity from a variety of causes including drug ingestion, food poisoning, bacterial enterotoxins, and pesticides. Some investigators have theorized that it works by binding the offending chemical in the gastrointestinal tract; others feel it may enhance the liver's ability to detoxify the substance after absorption (Zhong Yao Tong Bao 1986).

Pinellia (Ban xia): Has an antiemetic effect. It decreased apomorphine-induced vomiting in cats (Gui 1998).

Saussurea (Mu xiang): Has demonstrated antibiotic actions against several bacterial strains (Zhong Yao Yao Li Yu Ying Yong 1983). This may be beneficial in cases of bacterial gastritis. Experiments in mice and rats have shown that saussurea helps protect the gastric mucosa from damage induced by NSAIDs, ethyl alcohol, and hydrochloric acid (Qu 1999, Ying 1999).

Acupuncture

Acupuncture has been studied in regard to nausea and vomiting of various etiologies and found to be efficacious. A review of 26 separate studies involving 3,347 patients with postoperative vomiting found that acupuncture at PC6 was as effective as Western antiemetics (Wrist acupuncture 2004).

In another study, 39 patients were treated with ondansetron with acupuncture at PC6 or ondansetron alone to control cyclophosphamide-induced vomiting. Twenty percent of the ondansetron group had severe vomiting, versus 8% of the acupuncture-plus-ondansetron group (Josefson 2003).

Homotoxicology
General considerations/rationale

Vomiting is a common clinical sign. Strictly speaking, vomiting represents an Excretion Phase change that occurs as the body attempts to rid itself of agents perceived to be in opposition to survival. It can occur in any phase on the Six-Phase Table of Homotoxicology (both regressive and progressive vicariations) as a wide variety of factors enter into control and initiation of the vomiting reaction.

The excretion of homotoxins through the GI system is an important mechanism for homotoxin removal. In many conditions, after hepatic conjugation and biliary excretion, homotoxins pass rapidly through the GI tract to be removed through vomiting and/or diarrhea. It is generally advisable not to interfere with this important process, and the practice of giving medications that alter gut motility and secretion may actually allow homotoxins to regain access, and thereby cause more severe or deeper homotoxicoses to result.

Simple vomiting resolves rapidly upon allowing the gastrointestinal system to empty and repair itself through Excretion Phase actions. Seventy percent to 80% of all vomiting resolves within 72 hours with conservative management (withholding food and water for a few hours and then gradually reintroducing fluids first and then a low-residue, low-fat, highly digestible diet). Patients with no serious imbalances can be approached in this manner and there is good agreement for this process in both conventional and alternative veterinary practices. A precise diagnosis is often not necessary in treatment of these patients, and the doctor can record them as simply "gastritis," or "gastroenteritis," depending upon the case specifics.

The use of motility modifiers or centrally acting antiemetics in these cases may be unnecessary, and theoretically could create a Deposition or Impregnation phase condition, which could threaten future health. Use of acupuncture or biopuncture (giving antihomotoxic agents into acupuncture points or regions) seems to be extremely helpful in such cases and provides little danger to the patient (Broadfoot, Demers, Palmquist 2004; Streitberger, Ezzo, Schneider 2006; Yi 2006).

The authors have seen several cases of chronic vomiting disappear or improve markedly with simple acupuncture, biopuncture, or chiropractics, and it should be remembered that interruption of communication and control can lead to homotoxin accumulation, chemoreceptor irritation, and ultimately vomiting as a clinical sign. A note of caution is advised here, in that antihomotoxic agents can improve a patient's apparent condition but may fail to address the causative issue. Patients in Dedifferentiation Phase, for example, often have great resurgences in energy and vitality on support with antihomotoxic drugs; however, if their primary, inciting disease pathology continues, sudden death or sudden worsening may occur. This is seen in many patients under palliative therapy for tumors. This means that disappearance of vomiting is not always synonymous with cure of the primary condition. Veterinarians need to communicate this fact clearly to owners who may think differently and then be surprised at a sudden decline in their pet's condition.

If a diagnosis is evident the clinician can then design the treatment program around the specific pathology so that homotoxins that are present can be reduced or eliminated and their resulting damage repaired over time. If a diagnosis is not readily evident, the clinician must begin therapy to protect and preserve fluid and electrolyte levels. Intravenous fluids are critical in this stage of treatment. The patient's immune and myoneural function is improved by improving hydration and electrolyte status, and recovery may follow.

Other pharmaceutical agents are used as required. The reader should note that throughout this text, discussion of adverse reactions from pharmaceuticals is not meant to direct the clinician away from these medications, but rather to serve as an effort to remind veterinarians that drugs are potent agents and often have strong effects on the body. A clinician must be free to select the best therapeutic options for their patients and pharmaceuticals do assist many patients in recovery. H-2 blockers are commonly recommended for vomiting patients and can be useful, but they do alter the microenvironment and give the possibility of future homotoxicoses. Palmquist prefers absorptive and protective agents such as sucralfate to H-2 blockers, but uses whatever agent is needed for patient recovery. These cannot be given in severe vomiting because oral alimentation may exacerbate vomiting.

Centrally acting antiemetics such as chlorapromazine are popular but can cause hypotension in dehydrated patients. There is some question as to their value, and their use may prolong hospitalization and delay recovery in certain conditions such as canine parvovirus diarrhea (Mantione, Otto 2005). An assessment must be made regarding patient comfort and recovery periods when selecting antiemetic therapy, and in some cases a trade-off may be made. Metaclopramide, an antiemetic, promotility drug that is frequently used, but whose mechanism of action is unclear, should not be used in patients with suspected obstruction because it can lead to interruption of normal protective body reflects and resultant viscous perforation. In humans, metaclopramide is also associated with central nervous system, gastrointestinal, endocrine, cardiovascular, hepatic, renal, hematologic, and allergic adverse reactions, which seem to be associated with dosage and duration of therapy. These reactions generally have not been observed or noted in veterinary medicine, but should be considered (Kerstan, Seitz, Brocker, Trautmann 2006). The package insert states that it has been associated with fatal neuroleptic malignant syndrome in human patients.

The clinician should carefully consider the use of antibiotics in these cases because they often exacerbate vomiting and gastrointestinal upset through their actions on the nervous system, gastrointestinal mucosa, cellular organelles, and microflora. Antibiotics can cause a large die off of normal intestinal gram-negative bacteria and the resultant flooding of endotoxins into the circulation can cause widespread difficulty including pancreatitis, hepatic upset, and even shock. Once again, we see Reckeweg's advice that antibiotics are valuable but must be properly used

and respected if we are to avoid shifting our patients into progressive vicariation.

Nutrient- and homotoxin-laden blood leaves the intestines and proceeds via the portal vein to the liver, where it is directly cleansed and processed. Many GI issues are addressed with remedies that target intestinal and hepatic tissues (i.e., Nux vomica Homaccord, Berberis homaccord, and Hepar compositum). Enterohepatic circulation provides the opportunity for homotoxins to be reabsorbed after hepatic handling. This gives homotoxins access to the circulatory system, where they can trigger centrally mediated chemoreceptors and emesis. Ancillary excretion and metabolism by other organs (kidney, skin, and lung) may all assist in homotoxin removal. Antihomotoxic agents that support these organs include Solidago compositum, Berberis homaccord, and Mucosa compositum. Catalysts (Glyoxal compositum, Coenzyme compositum, and Ubichinon compositum) assist in repair and reactivation of receptors and energy metabolism in the cytosol and mitochondria. Many chronic diseases have the decline in mitochondrial health as a common issue, and these agents cause a clinically evident improvement in energy and metabolism of patients suffering from chronic diseases.

Homotoxins that have escaped or bypassed hepatic processing may be deposited into connective tissue and cause disease later as further damage ensues. The inclusion of proper prebiotics (such as fiber) and probiotic bacteria may promote or assist in homotoxin removal by binding homotoxins to fiber or through metabolism of toxic material by bacteria. The common practice of treating GI upset by fasting and then giving a bland, low-fiber diet is an excellent initial approach to mild GI conditions. Later use of therapeutic diets higher in fiber may be especially useful for chronic GI disorders, such as colitis, which may be associated with vomiting as a secondary sign. These diets are also indicated in geriatric patients due to the homotoxins that have been impregnated in their systems. During the detoxification and drainage therapy that is commonly required by these patients, the presence of proper fiber will greatly assist in removal of homotoxins from the body.

Traditional Oriental Medicine pairs the Heart and Intestine. This developmental relationship is seen in earthworms and carries forward into the structure of more advanced organisms. The primal heart developed first from circular blood vessels, which surrounded the intestinal tract and assisted the movement of blood throughout the body. The development of a tubular gastrointestinal system was a major evolutionary step that allowed organisms to move further and survive in more varied environments. This relationship can be observed in many conditions (diarrhea in congestive heart disease), and astute clinicians often find that treating one organ system may benefit the other. The immune functions contained within the liver make it a major element in protection against invading organisms as well as other toxins. The Stomach and Spleen are also paired in TOM, as are the Lung and Large Intestine. These relationships are helpful in treating patients with chronic disease, especially when using compositae class remedies such as Mucosa compositum (affects the large intestine, lung, small intestine, stomach, and bile duct), Hepar compositum (affects the liver, gallbladder, pancreas, small intestine, colon, and thymus), and Tonsilla compositum (affects the spleen and immune elements) (Reckeweg 2000).

Recent developments in understanding the psychoneuroendocrine and immune systems reveal that the intestinal system is an important component in endocrine and immune regulation. Many neuroactive substances such as serotonin are produced in the GI system. The immune system is well represented within the digestive system, and it has been estimated that 70% to 80% of the total immune system is located in and around the alimentary tube. Cellular elements of the immune system receive vital coding in this area that consists in large part of instructions regarding tolerance of foreign antigens.

Many homotoxins can damage the GI system's ability to perform its duties. Both toxins and other therapeutic agents can result in undesirable progressive vicariation. Corticoids and nonsteroidal anti-inflammatory drugs both damage intestinal mucosal elements. This can result in frank ulceration and/or "leaky gut syndrome," which is linked to many other medical syndromes such as allergy and inflammation, malnutrition, bacterial dysbiosis, and hepatic overload (Broadfoot 2003, Silver 2003). In leaky gut, antigens are not properly digested into smaller molecular weight polypeptides before gaining access to the immune system. This issue can lead to chronic inflammatory diseases such as inflammatory bowel disease and allergic syndromes.

If the immune elements are negatively affected, then a wide variety of disease states can occur, and vomiting can emerge as a sign of the underlying homotoxicosis. Table 11.1 provides a simple illustration of how gastrointestinal diseases are often associated with vomiting in many different phases.

Successfully treating many GI disorders involves providing clean diet and water, reducing stress, allowing homotoxins to be excreted successfully; supporting organ function; and providing drainage therapy, organ support, and metabolic support while repair occurs. As in other discussions, the position of the patient on the phase table assists in determining proper therapy. Symptomatic treatment is often successful in the first 2 phases. As homotoxins gain deeper access and do further damage, the use of compositae class antihomotoxic agents becomes necessary to stimulate regressive vicariation.

Table 11.1. Common gastrointestinal conditions associated with vomiting or diarrhea and their relative position on the Six-Phase Table of Homotoxicology.

Condition	Phase Table Position
Anal gland sacculitis, acute	Inflammation
Anal gland saccultitis, chronic	Impregnation
Cholangiohepatitis, acute	Inflammation
Cholangiohepatitis, chronic	Impregnation
Chronic active hepatitis	Impregnation/Degeneration
Colitis, acute	Excretion/Inflammation
Colitis, chronic	Impregnation/Degeneration
Diarrhea	Excretion
Enteritis	Excretion
Eosinophilic granuloma	Impregnation/Degeneration
Exocrine pancreatic insufficiency	Degeneration
Food allergy	Impregnation
Gastric dilatation/bloat	Degeneration
Gastritis/vomiting	Excretion/Inflammation
Gingivitis	Inflammation
Hepatic cirrhosis	Degeneration
Hepatic lipidosis	Deposition to Degeneration
Inflammatory bowel disease	Impregnation/Degeneneration
Internal parasites	Deposition
Irritable bowel syndrome	Impregnation
Malabsorption syndrome	Degeneration
Megacolon	Degeneration
Megaesophagus	Degeneration
Pancreatitis, acute	Inflammation
Pancreatitis, chronic	Impregnation
Periodontal disease	Inflammation/Deposition/ Degeneration
Stomatitis, acute	Inflammation
Stomatitis, chronic	Deposition/Impregnation/ Degeneration

Appropriate homotoxicology formulas

Anacardium homaccord: The namesake ingredient has been shown to have powerful anti-inflammatory and immunomodulatory effects (Ramprasath, Shanthi, and Sachdanandam 2006). Treats hunger pain, mucosal catarrh including laryngeal and pharyngeal inflammation, duodenal syndrome, constipation, and gastric/duodenal ulcers (Reckeweg 2000). Anacardium as an herbal extract has been shown to be antiviral against simian rotovirus (Goncalves, et al. 2005).

Berberis homaccord: Berberis has major actions on the liver and gallbladder (Reckeweg 2000), and has been shown to have effects in diarrhea (Zhu, Ahrens 1982; Shamsa, Ahmadiani, and Khosrokhavar 1999). Also treats colic, collapse, and bloody vomitus, and is supportive of adrenal and renal function. It is part of the basic *Detox Kit*.

BHI-Nausea: Used for painful oral vesicles/stomatitis (Anacardium), nausea and vomiting with coughing (Ipecacuanha), and left-sided gastric region pain (Argentum nictricum).

Cantharis compositum: Contains Arsenicum album, which is indicated in aphthous stomatitis; when the tongue is dry, red with raised papillae, and possibly coated white, brown, or black; for violent gastroenteritis with prolonged vomiting and diarrhea; with unbearable burning stomachpains after eating; and for foul-smelling stools. Also contains Mercurius solubilis, which is indicated in ulcerative lesions of the mucous membranes, and Hepar sulphuris calcareum (Reckeweg 2002).

Chol-Heel: An excellent remedy that contains Belladonna, Chelidonium, Carduus marianus, Lycopodium, Veratrum, and Taraxicum, along with some other very useful components, all in potency chords. This can be of great relief in GI discomfort (Broadfoot 2005).

Cinnamomum homaccord: Off the U.S. market at this time but used for seeping hemorrhage.

Cocculus homaccord: Treats motion sickness and vestibular syndromes with nausea (Claussen, et al. 1984).

Coenzyme compositum: Contains Citricum acidum, which is useful for dental problems and gingivitis; scurvy; blackening of teeth; heavy deposits of dental plaque; painful, herpetic vesicles around the lips; nausea; painful cramping in the umbilical area; and distension.

Colchicum compositum: Treats cachexia and neoplastic conditions.

Colocynthis homaccord: Treats diarrhea with lower back pain (Citrullus colocynthis), colic, pain below the navel, and colitis with gelatinous stools.

Diarrheel S: A symptom remedy for acute and chronic diarrhea. Treats acute gastroenteritis, belching, spurting diarrhea, pancreatopathy, and colitis. This commonly used formula contains Tormentilla for dysentery, acute gastroenteritis, and mucous and ulcerative colitis with bloody stools (Reckeweg 2002). Tormentilla is also found in *BHI-Diarrhea* and *Veratrum homaccord*.

Duodenoheel: Treats hunger pains, hyperacidity, gastric and duodenal ulcers, nausea and vomiting, and dysentery with tenesmus (Reckeweg 2000).

Engystol N: Treats viral origin gastroenteritis (see Parvovirus).

Erigotheel: Treats gastric catarrh, hepatic diseases, and duodenal ulcers with spasm. Has antipyretic effects (Demers 2004).

Galium-Heel: Used for all cellular phases, hemorrhoids, and anal fissures, and as a detoxicant.

Gastricumeel: Used for acute gastritis. Contains Antimonium crudum, which is indicated for tooth decay and toothache, and thus may be useful when dental work is indicated (Reckeweg 2002).

Ginseng compositum: Used for nausea, gastroenteritis, and constitutional support in geriatric or debilitated patients (Reckeweg 2000).

Hepar compositum: Provides detoxification and drainage of hepatic tissues and organ and metabolic support, and is useful in most hepatic and gallbladder pathologies. It is an important part of Deep Detoxification Formula. Treats duodenitis, pancreatitis, cystic hepatic ducts, cholelithiasis, cholangitis, cholecystitis, vomiting, and diarrhea (Demers 2004, Broadfoot 2004). This combination contains Natrum oxalaceticum (also found in *Coenzyme compositum*, *Ubichinon compositum*, and *Mucosa compositum*) for changes in appetite and stomach distension due to air. Treats nausea, stomach pain with a sensation of fullness, gurgling in the abdomen, and cramping pain in the hypochondria. It is also used for constipation, sudden diarrhea (particularly after eating), and flatus (Reckeweg 2002).

Hepeel: Provides liver drainage and detoxification. Used in a wide variety of conditions including cancer of the liver, where Hepeel was found to be antiproliferative, hepatoprotective, and an antioxidant when tested in human HepG2 cells (Gebhardt 2003).

Leptandra compositum: Treats epigastric syndrome, portal vein congestion, pancreatopathy, chronic liver disease, and diabetes mellitus (Reckeweg 2000).

Lymphomyosot: Provides lymph drainage and endocrine support, and treats edema. Contains Gentiana for chronic gastritis. Used for flatulence, diarrhea, distension of the stomach with eructations, nausea, retching and vomiting, contains Geranium robertianum for nausea, particularly after eating, with distension or sensation of fullness. The ingredient Myosotis arvensis has indications for bloat and distension (Reckeweg 2002).

Mercurius-Heel S: Used for viral and bacterial issues, suppuration, and tonsillitis (Reckeweg 2000).

Momordica compositum: Treats pancreatitis, epigastric disease (Momordica balsamina), emaciation though good appetite (Jodum), and vomiting with collapse (Veratrum album)(Reckeweg 2000). Combines well with *Hepar compositum* and *Tonsilla compositum* in conditions involving the triad areas (liver, pancreas, and small intestine).

Mucosa compositum: Broadly supportive for repair of mucosal elements. Used in cellular cases and in recovery periods following active disease (Reckeweg 2000). This remedy contains a useful component in Kali bichromicum, which is indicated for ulcers found on the gums, tongue, lips, and even on the gastric mucosa (gastric or duodenal ulcer). The tongue may have a thick, yellow, mucous coating, or in ulcerative stomatitis or tonsillitis it may be dry, smooth, shiny, or fissured. Kali has been used effectively in acute gastroenteritis associated with vomiting of clear, light-colored fluid or quantities of mucous bile, and in cases with hematemesis, flatulent colics, and dysenteric stools with tenesmus (Reckeweg 2002).

It also contains Hydrastis, with mucosal support for oral problems such as stomatitis, and mucosal suppuration that is accompanied by ulceration, inflammations and colic of the hepatobiliary system and of the gastrointestinal tract, and polyp formation (Reckeweg 2002). The Kreosotum component can be used in chronic gastritis with gastric hemorrhages and vomiting of brown masses. Also has a dental implication in cases with spongy gums and carious teeth, neuralgias proceeding from them causing a burning toothache with deep caries, black patches on the teeth, and fetid discharges.

The single remedy Phosphorus is broadly useful for dyspepsia and for jaw problems in dental disease (Reckeweg 2002). Phosphorus is found in many other remedies including *Echinacea compositum* and *Leptandra homaccord*. It is rich in suis organ preparations for mucosal support, plus a large variety of remedies with indications in the gastrointestinal sphere. The component Argentum nitricum (also in *Atropinum compositum*, *Diarrheel*, *Duodenoheel*, *Gastricumeel*, *Momordica compositum*, *BHI-Nausea*, and several other combinations) is indicated for distension in the upper abdomen, gastrocardiac symptom-complex, and amelioration from eructations. It is also used for gastric crises (Reckeweg 2002).

Nux vomica homaccord: Used for liver and gastrointestinal disease and after smoke inhalation. It is useful in gingivitis (Reckeweg 2002). This is a commonly used formula for detoxification that is part of the *Detox Kit*. Recent research shows that one ingredient (Brucine) affects mitochondria in human hepatoma cells. Further research is needed to determine if homeopathic dilutions are more or less active (Deng, et al. 2006). Calves treated with Nux vomica 30cc had fewer incidents of stomach and intestinal disease than controls (Schutte 2005).

Podophyllum homaccord: Treats chronic gastroenteritis, gastroenteritis in juvenile dogs and cats, dyspepsia, catarrhal colitis, hemorrhoids, and watery-green diarrhea alternating with constipation (Macloed 1983).

Syzygium compositum: Treats chronic gastritis, chronic enteritis, diabetes mellitus, and hepatic disorders.

Tanacet-Heel: Used for complications following removal of helminths, gastroenteritis, dysentery, and gas and pain following ascarids, especially in juvenile pets.

Veratrum homaccord: Treats gastritis, intense vomiting with blood, collapse (pale mucous membranes), psychosis, dysentery, fecal incontinence, and intestinal spasm. This very useful remedy is used widely by the authors for general vomiting cases. Consider its use in cases of gastritis following general anesthesia. Classical provings were recently repeated and found consistent with earlier work (Van Wassenhoven 2004).

Vomitusheel S: Used for nausea and vomiting with a cough (Ipecacuanha), liver and gastrointestinal issues (Nux vomica), eructation, and possibly anxiety or depression (Ignatia) (Reckeweg 2000). No known adverse reactions have occurred and this is extremely safe to use in pediatric patients. This remedy contains Aethusa for vomiting that obviously originates in the nervous system. In serious cases, capillary paralysis, hematemesis, stomach cramps, and tympanitic distension may occur, with an irresistible urge to pass stool. The nervous vomiting is characterized by spasmodic contractions of the esophageal muscles and violent pains that shoot upwards from the cardiac sphincter (Reckeweg 2002). In more severe vomiting consider *Veratrum homaccord* instead or in combination.

Authors' suggested protocols

Nutrition
Esophagus and stomach support formula: 1 tablet for every 25 pounds of body weight BID.

Chinese herbal medicine/acupuncture
Formula H102 Vomiting/chronic: 1 capsule per 10 to 20 pounds twice daily as a basic formula for vomiting. Additional herbs may be used or substituted by practitioners who are familiar with TCM pattern diagnosis. This formula was designed for chronic vomiting due to gastritis (bacterial, viral dietary, IBD, or idiopathic). In addition to the herbs cited above, H102 Vomiting/chronic also contains atractylodes (Bai zhu), brucea fruit (Ya dan zi), hematite (Dai zhe shi), and jujube (Da zao).

The authors use the following points: CV12, PC6, ST36, BL21, CV25, BL20, and GB34 as basic points. Other points may be added by experienced acupuncturists based upon TCM pattern diagnosis.

Homotoxicology (Dose: 10 drops PO for 50-pound dog; 5 drops PO for cat or small dog)
Treatment must be individualized but the following represent good starting therapies, which can be readily adapted based upon clinical response.

Veratrum homaccord and Gastricumeel: Combined and taken orally once per hour for 5 hours, and then TID as needed.

Product sources

Nutrition
Esophagus and stomach support formula: Animal Nutrition Technologies.

Chinese herbal medicine
Formula H102 Vomiting/chronic: Natural Solutions, Inc.

Homotoxicology
BHI/Heel Corporation

REFERENCES

Western medicine references
Guilford WG, Strombeck DR. Acute gastritis. In: Guilford WG, et al., eds., Small animal gastro-enterology. Philadelphia: Saunders, 1996:261–274.

DeNovo RC, Jenkins, CC. Chronic vomiting. In: Tilley L, Smith F. The 5-Minute Veterinary Consult: Canine and Feline, 2003. Blackwell Publishing.

Hart JR. Acute Vomiting. In: Tilley L, Smith F. The 5-Minute Veterinary Consult: Canine and Feline, 2003. Blackwell Publishing.

Strombeck DR, Guilford WG. Small animal gastroenterology. 2nd ed. Davis, CA: Stronegate Publishing 1990:186–207.

Willard M. Disease of the stomach. In: Ettinger SJ, Feldman ED, eds. Textbook of veterinary internal medicine. 4th ed. Philadelphia: Saunders, 1995:1143–1167.

Chinese herbal medicine/acupuncture
Gui CQ, et al. *Journal of Pharmacology and Clinical Application of TCM.* 1998;14(4):27–28.

Jiang Su Zhong Yi Za Zhi (*Jiangsu Journal of Chinese Medicine*), 1981;(3):61.

Josefson A, Kreuter M. Acupuncture to reduce nausea during chemotherapy treatment for rheumatic diseases. *Rheumatology* 2003;42:1149–54.

Ma YB. Zhi Qiao's effects on gastroinstestinal movement. *Journal of Pharmacology of Clinical Application of TCM.* 1996;12(6):28–29.

Qu H, et al. *Inner Mongolia Journal of TCM.* 1999;18(2):45.

Wang SG, et al. Dang Shen's effect on gastrointestinal motility in mice at early stage of third degree burn. *Journal of Anhui College of TCM.* 1999;18 (6):50–51.

Wrist Acupuncture Reduces Incidence of Post-Op Nausea and Vomiting. Review Finds Treatment Works as Well as Anti-Nausea Medications. *Acupuncture Today* October, 2004, Volume 05, Issue 10.

Ying J, et al. *Journal of TCM Medicinal Materials.* 1999;22(10):526–627.

Zhong Yao Tong Bao (*Journal of Chinese Herbology*), 1986; 11(10):55.

Zhong Yao Xue (*Chinese Herbology*), 1998;378–380.

Zhong Yao Yao Li Yu Ying Yong (*Pharmacology and Applications of Chinese Herbs*), 1983;169.

Zhong Yao Yao Li Yu Ying Yong (*Pharmacology and Applications of Chinese Herbs*), 1983;1080.

Homotoxicology references
Broadfoot PJ. Introduction to Homotoxicology: The Matrix and Inflammation. In: Proceedings of the American Holistic Veterinary Medical Association annual meeting, 2003. September 20–23, pp 1–11.

Broadfoot PJ. Inflammation: Homotoxicology and Healing. In Proceedings AHVMA/Heel Homotoxicology Seminar. Denver, CO, 2004. p 27.

Broadfoot P, Demers J, Palmquist R. Clinical Case Studies. In: Homotoxicology Seminar, Heel/AHVMA sponsored, Denver Colorado, appendix 2004. May 15–16.

Claussen CF, Bergmann J, Bertora G, Claussen E. Clinical experimental test and equilibrimetric measurements of the therapeutic action of a homeopathic drug consisting of ambra, cocculus, conium and mineral oil in the diagnosis of vertigo and nausea [Article in German]. *Arzneimittelforschung.* 1984. 34(12): pp 1791–8.

Demers J. Homotoxicology and Acupuncture. In: Proceedings of the 2004 Homotoxicology Seminar. AHVMA/Heel. Denver, CO, 2004. p 5, 6.

Deng X, Yin F, Lu X, Cai B, Yin W. The apoptotic effect of brucine from the seed of Strychnos nux-vomica on human hepatoma cells is mediated via Bcl-2 and Ca2+ involved mitochondrial pathway. *Toxicol Sci.* 2006. May;91(1): pp 59–69.

Gebhardt R. Antioxidative, antiproliferative and biochemical effects in HepG2 cells of a homeopathic remedy and its constituent plant tinctures tested separately or in combination. *Arzneimittelforschung.* 2003. 53(12): pp 823–30.

Goncalves JL, Lopes R, Oliveira D, Costa S, Miranda M, Romanos M, Santos N, Wigg M. In vitro anti-rotavirus activity of some medicinal plants used in Brazil against diarrhea. *J Ethnopharmacol.* 2005. Jul 14;99(3): pp 403–7.

Habermehl D, Kammerer B, Handrick R, Eldh T, Gruber C, Cordes N, Daniel PT, Plasswilm L, Bamberg M, Belka C, Jendrossek V. Proapoptotic activity of Ukrain is based on Chelidonium majus L. alkaloids and mediated via a mitochondrial death pathway. *BMC Cancer.* 2006. Jan 17;6: p 14.

Heel. BHI Homeopathic Therapy: Professional Reference. Albuquerque, NM: Heel Inc: 2002. p 26.

Kerstan A, Seitz C, Brocker E, Trautmann A. Anaphylaxis During Treatment of Nausea and Vomiting: IgE-Mediated Metoclopramide Allergy (October). *Ann Pharmacother.* 2006. Aug 29; [Epub ahead of print]

Khuda-Bukhsh AR, Pathak S, Guha B, Karmakar S, Das J, Banerjee P, Biswas S, Mukherjee P, Bhattacharjee N, Choudhury S, Banerjee A, Bhadra S, Mallick P, Chakrabarti J, Mandal B. In vitro anti-rotavirus activity of some medicinal plants used in Brazil against diarrhea. *J Ethnopharmacol.* 2005. Jul 14;99(3): pp 403–7.

Ramprasath V, Shanthi P, Sachdanandam P. Immunomodulatory and anti-inflammatory effects of Semecarpus anacardium LINN. Nut milk extract in experimental inflammatory conditions. *Biol Pharm Bull.* 2006. Apr;29(4): pp 693–700.

Reckeweg H. Biotherapeutic Index: Ordinatio Antihomotoxica et Materia Medica, 5th ed. Baden-Baden, Germany: Biologische Heilmittel Heel GMBH, 2000 pp 290, 294–5, 300, 329–30, 358–9, 363–4, 366–7, 369, 381, 390, 399–400, 432, 538.

Reckeweg H. Homeopathia Antihomotoxica Materia Medica, 4th ed. Baden-Baden: Arelia-Verlag GMBH, 2002. pp. 136–8, 139–40, 125–6, 147, 150–3, 179, 206, 241–2, 317–19, 345, 366, 461–3, 488–90, 578–80.

Schutte A. Clinical Research in Veterinary Homeopathy—A review of veterinary publications, in proceedings of LIGA-Congress 2005, May 6, Berlin, Germany, p 39.

Shamsa F, Ahmadiani A, Khosrokhavar R. Antihistaminic and anticholinergic activity of barberry fruit (Berberis vulgaris) in the guinea-pig ileum. *J Ethnopharmacol.* 1999. Feb;64(2): pp 161–6.

Silver R. Leaky Gut Syndrome. In: Proceedings of the annual meeting of the American Holistic Veterinary Medical Association, Durham, North Carolina, 2003. pp 97–110.

Streitberger K, Ezzo J, Schneider A. Acupuncture for nausea and vomiting: An update of clinical and experimental studies. *Auton Neurosci.* 2006. Aug 31; [Epub ahead of print].

Van Wassenhoven M. Towards an evidence-based repertory: clinical evaluation of Veratrum album. *Homeopathy.* 2004. Apr;93(2): pp 71–7.

Yi SX, Yang R, Yan J, Chang X, Ling Y. Effect of electro-acupuncture at Foot-Yangming Meridian on somatostatin and expression of somatostatin receptor genes in rabbits with gastric ulcer. *World J Gastroenterol.* 2006. Mar 21;12(11):pp 1761–5.

Zhu B, Ahrens FA. Effect of berberine on intestinal secretion mediated by Escherichia coli heat-stable enterotoxin in jejunum of pigs. *Am J Vet Res.* 1982. Sep;43(9): pp 1594–8.

GASTRITIS

Definition and cause

Generally defined as inflammation of the stomach associated with vomiting. The cause of the inflammation ranges from secondary reactions to toxins, chemicals, medications, infections, ulcerations, immune-mediated conditions, allergens, food, and neoplasia. More common causes are chemically preserved foods; NSAIDS; infectious agents such as Heliobacter; and toxins such as pesticides, cleaning agents, fertilizers, and herbicides. Gastritis is common in both dogs and cats (Guilford 1996, Hart 2003, Webb 2003, Willard 1995).

Medical therapy rationale, drug(s) of choice, and nutritional recommendations

Therapy for gastritis is directed at the primary or secondary cause. Early gastritis is often managed with gastric coating and protective medication such as Pepto-Bismol or sucralfate. Antisecretory drugs such as cimetidine, famotidine, and ranitidine are often prescribed for the vomiting and for gastric ulcers, and are effective depending upon the underlying cause. Antibiotics for the treatment of heliobacter, corticosteroids, immune-suppressive drugs for immune-mediated diseases such as IBD, and prokinetic drugs such as Cisapride to increase gastric emptying time are often prescribed. Surgery is indicated for granulomatous reaction, foreign bodies, ulcerations, and neoplasia (Guilford 1996, Hart 2003, Happonen 1998, Liptak 2002, Webb 2003).

Dietary recommendations are a short fasting period followed by a bland diet of soft, low-fat food such as cottage cheese, boiled rice, or pasta, along with tofu, boiled chicken, or beef as the norm.

Anticipated prognosis

The prognosis depends upon identifying and addressing the underlying cause. Simple gastritis responds well to treatment and dietary changes. Acute and chronic gastritis often has a more guarded prognosis (Guilford 1996, Hart 2003, Willard 1995).

Integrative veterinary therapies

For a general discussion of vomiting the reader is referred to vomiting or related diseases for a more in-depth discussion and protocol recommendations.

Nutrition
General considerations/rationale

Medical therapy is often required to control gastritis. Nutritional therapies are often limited to avoid initiating or increasing episodes of vomiting. Gastritis may be secondary to other conditions, diseases, or organ system involvement; and therefore, it is recommended that blood be analyzed both medically and physiologically to determine associated organ involvement and disease. This allows clinicians to formulate therapeutic nutritional protocols that address the stomach as well as other underlying conditions (see Chapter 2, Nutritional Blood Testing, for additional information).

Appropriate nutrients

Nutritional/gland therapy: Glandular stomach provides the intrinsic nutrients to reduce cellular inflammation and damage and help protect the stomach from ongoing inflammation and eventual degeneration. The addition of other gland and nutrient support should be considered if the underlying cause is related to other organ systems secondary to kidney disease and azotemia (see other related disease protocols and Gland Therapy in Chapter 2 for more information).

Chinese herbal medicine/acupuncture
General considerations/rationale

Improper feeding, stress, external Cold, Qi or Yang deficiency in Stomach or Spleen, Qi stagnation and Yin deficiency in Stomach can all lead to gastritis.

Improper feeding and stress are commonly recognized causes of gastritis in Western medicine. External cold can refer to the ingestion of cold food, which may cause cramping. The Spleen and Stomach are responsible for the transformation of food into usable energy. If these organs suffer from a Qi deficiency, they do not have enough energy to digest. If there is a Yang deficiency, there is not enough heat to accomplish the chemical reactions needed to break down food. Yin is fluid; a Stomach Yin deficiency can be thought of as a deficiency of gastric acid. Again, the Stomach cannot properly digest.

Treatment is aimed at controlling cramping and vomiting and improving digestion. When treating gastritis, the clinician must stop the vomiting, improve digestion, and treat any underlying causes of vomiting, i.e., viruses, bacteria, immune-mediated inflammation, ulceration, neoplasia, etc.

Appropriate Chinese herbs

Bamboo (Zhu ru): Has antibiotic effects (Zhong Yao Xue 1998). This may be efficacious in cases of bacterial gastritis.

Corydalis tuber (Yan hu suo): Decreases the secretion of gastric acid and helps prevent gastric ulcers (Zhong Cao Yao Xue 1976). It also inhibits histamine release and formation of edema in rats, and has been shown to control both acute and chronic inflammation (Kubo 1994). This suggests it may play a role in controlling inflammatory gastritis.

Cuttle bone (Hai piao xiao): Neutralizes gastric acid (Zhong Yao Xue 1998). This may help decrease gastric ulceration.

Cyperus (Xiang fu zi): Can stop stomach cramps and pain (Zhong Cao Yao Fang Ji De Ying Yong 1976).

Dandelion (Pu gong ying): May possess anti-inflammatory actions (Mascolo 1987), which may be useful in inflammatory causes of gastritis.

Evodia (Wu zhu yu): Inhibits the formation of ulcers by decreasing secretion of gastric acid, and decreases vomiting (Zhong Yao Yao Li Du Li Yu Lin Chuan 1988).

Licorice (Gan cao): Can inhibit immersion-induced stress and hydrochloride-acid-induced ulcers (Zhu 1998, Wu 1998).

Melia (Chuan lian zi): Inhibits parasites (Zhong Yao Yao Li Yu Lin Chuan 1983). This may be of use when gastritis is due to inflammation caused by gastric parasites.

Pinellia (Ban xia): Seems to have a central nervous system effect to decrease chemical-mediated vomition (Zhong Yao Yao Li Yu Ying Yong 1983). It can inhibit the development of hydrochloric acid and indolmycin-alchohol-induced ulcers in mice (Shen 1998). In addition, it has been shown to have efficacy against some tumor cell lines. It prevented the growth of K562 tumor cells experimentally (Wu 1996), which indicates that it may have some inhibitory effect on neoplastic causes of vomiting.

White peony (Bai shao): Contains paeoniflorin, which is a strong antipyretic anti-inflammatory. It also inhibits the secretion of gastric acid and helps to treat peptic ulcers (Zhong Yao Zhi 1993).

Acupuncture

One study examined the effect of acupuncture verses medication in the treatment of chronic gastritis. Fifty people were treated with acupuncture and 50 were treated with medication. The response rate was 98% with acupuncture and 88% with medication (Huang 2005).

Homotoxicology
General considerations/rationale

Gastritis is extremely common. Acute gastritis is an Inflammation Phase condition, whereas chronic gastritis represents Impregnation and/or Degeneration phases. General remarks about homotoxin accumulation and therapy in the enteritis protocol apply here as well, and the reader is referred to that protocol for a more in-depth discussion.

Appropriate homotoxicology formulas

Anacardium homaccord: The namesake ingredient has been shown to have powerful anti-inflammatory and immunomodulatory effects (Ramprasath, Shanthi, and Sachdanandam 2006). Treats hunger pain, mucosal catarrh including laryngeal and pharyngeal inflammation, duodenal syndrome, constipation, and gastric/duodenal ulcers (Reckeweg 2000). Anacardium as an herbal extract has been shown to be antiviral against simian rotovirus (Goncalves, et al. 2005).

Berberis homaccord: Berberis has major actions on the liver and gallbladder (Reckeweg 2000), and has been shown to have effects in diarrhea (Zhu, Ahrens 1982; Shamsa, Ahmadiani, and Khosrokhavar 1999). Treats colic, collapse, and bloody vomitus, and is supportive of adrenal and renal function. It is part of the basic *Detox Kit*.

BHI-Nausea: Used for painful oral vesicles/stomatitis (Anacardium), nausea and vomiting with coughing (Ipecacuanha), and left-sided gastric region pain (Argentum nictricum) (Heel 2002).

BHI-Stomach: Used for stomach distress relieved by eructation, stomach pain, heartburn, chalky white tongue, flatulence, and tendency to collapse.

Cantharis compositum: Contains Arsenicum album, which is indicated in aphthous stomatitis; when the tongue is dry, red with raised papillae, and possibly coated white, brown, or black; and for violent gastroenteritis with prolonged vomiting, diarrhea, and unbearable burning stomach-pains after eating. It also is used for foul-smelling stools. Contains Mercurius solubilis for ulcerative lesions of the mucous membranes and Hepar sulphuris calcareum (Reckeweg 2002).

Coenzyme compositum: Contains Citricum acidum, which is useful for dental problems and gingivitis; scurvy; blackening of teeth; heavy deposits of dental plaque; painful, herpetic vesicles around the lips; nausea; painful cramping in the umbilical area; and distension.

Duodenoheel: Treats hunger pains, hyperacidity, gastric and duodenal ulcers, nausea and vomiting, and dysentery with tenesmus (Reckeweg 2000).

Engystol N: Used for viral origin gastroenteritis (see Parvovirus).

Erigotheel: Used for gastric catarrh, hepatic diseases, duodenal ulcers with spasm, and for its antipyretic actions (Demers 2004).

Galium-Heel: Used for all cellular phases, hemorrhoids, and anal fissures, and as a detoxicant.

Gastricumeel: Treats acute gastritis. Contains Antimonium crudum, which is indicated for tooth decay and toothache, and thus may be useful when dental work is indicated (Reckeweg 2002).

Ginseng compositum: Used for nausea, gastroenteritis, and constitutional support in geriatric or debilitated patients (Reckeweg 2000).

Lymphomyosot: Provides lymph drainage and endocrine support, and treats edema. Contains Gentiana for chronic gastritis. Treats flatulence, diarrhea, distension of the stomach with eructations, nausea, retching, and vomiting. is the component Geranium robertianum, and is useful for nausea, particularly after eating with distension or sensation of fullness. Myosotis arvensis is contained for bloat and distension (Reckeweg 2002).

Mucosa compositum: Broadly supportive for repair of mucosal elements. Used in cellular cases and in recovery periods following active disease (Reckeweg 2000). This remedy contains a useful component in Kali bichromicum, which is indicated for ulcers found on the gums, tongue, lips, and even on the gastric mucosa (gastric or duodenal ulcer). The tongue may have a thick, yellow, mucous coating, or in ulcerative stomatitis or tonsillitis it may be dry, smooth, shiny, or fissured. Kali has been used effectively in acute gastroenteritis associated with vomiting of clear, light-colored fluid or quantities of mucous bile, and in cases with hematemesis, flatulent colics, and dysenteric stools with tenesmus (Reckeweg 2002).

It also contains Hydrastis, with mucosal support for oral problems such as stomatitis, and mucosal suppuration that is accompanied by ulceration, inflammations and colic of the hepatobiliary system and of the gastrointestinal tract, and polyp formation (Reckeweg 2002). The Kreosotum component can be used in chronic gastritis with gastric hemorrhages and vomiting of brown masses. Also has a dental implication in cases with spongy gums and carious teeth, neuralgias proceeding from them causing a burning toothache with deep caries, black patches on the teeth, and fetid discharges.

The single remedy Phosphorus is broadly useful for dyspepsia and for jaw problems in dental disease (Reckeweg 2002). Phosphorus is found in many other remedies including *Echinacea compositum* and *Leptandra homaccord*. It is rich in suis organ preparations for mucosal support, plus a large variety of remedies with indications in the gastrointestinal sphere. The component Argentum nitricum (also in *Atropinum compositum, Diarrheel, Duodenoheel, Gastricumeel, Momordica compositum, BHI-Nausea,* and several other combinations) is indicated for distension in the upper abdomen, gastrocardiac symptom-complex, and amelioration from eructations. It is also used for gastric crises (Reckeweg 2002).

Nux vomica homaccord: Used for liver and gastrointestinal disease and after smoke inhalation. Useful in gingivitis (Reckeweg 2002). Commonly used formula for detoxification as part of the *Detox Kit*. Recent research shows that one ingredient (Brucine) affects mitochondria in human hepatoma cells. Further research is needed to determine whether homeopathic dilutions are more or less active (Deng, et al. 2006).

Ubichinon compositum: Contains Anthraquinone for swelling of gums, and GI symptoms such as distention, flatulence, and cramping abdominal pain. Treats constipation with straining or sudden diarrhea (Reckeweg 2002).

Veratrum homaccord: Treats gastritis, intense vomiting with blood, collapse (pale mucous membranes), psychosis, dysentary, fecal incontinence, and intestinal spasm. This very useful remedy is used widely by the authors for general vomiting cases. Consider its use in cases of gastritis following general anesthesia. Classical provings were recently repeated and found consistent with earlier work (van Wassenhoven 2004).

Vomitusheel S: Treats nausea and vomiting with a cough (Ipecacuanha), liver and gastrointestinal issues (Nux vomica), eructation, and possibly anxiety or depression (Ignatia) (Reckeweg 2000). No known adverse reactions have occurred and this is extremely safe to use in pediatric patients. This remedy contains Aethusa for vomiting that obviously originates in the nervous system. In serious cases, capillary paralysis, hematemesis, stomach cramps, and tympanitic distension may occur, with an irresistible urge to pass stool. The nervous vomiting is characterized by spasmodic contractions of the esophageal muscles and violent pains that shoot upwards from the cardiac sphincter (Reckeweg 2000). In more severe vomiting consider *Veratrum homaccord* instead or in combination.

Authors' suggested protocols

Nutrition
Esophagus and stomach support formula: 1 tablet for every 25 pounds of body weight BID.

Chinese herbal medicine/acupuncture
H35 Gastritis: 1 capsule per 10 to 20 pounds as needed. In addition to the herbs mentioned above, H35 Gastritis

also contains aquilaria (Chen xiang) and lindera (Wu yao), which increase efficacy of the formula.

The points the authors use are CV12, ST36, PC6, GB34, BL20, BL21, CV25, BL25, BL18, and BL22.

Homotoxicology (Dose: 10 drops PO for 50-pound dog; 5 drops PO for cat or small dog)

Gastricumeel: TID orally as beginning therapy. Duodeno-heel, Erigotheel, or BHI-Stomach are also often very effective.

Product sources

Nutrition
Esophagus and stomach support formulas: Animal Nutrition Technologies.

Chinese herbal medicine
Formula Gastritis (H35): Natural Solutions, Inc.

Homotoxicology
BHI/Heel Corporation

REFERENCES

Western medicine references

Guilford WG, Strombeck DR. Chronic gastric diseases. In: Guilford WG, Center SA, Strombeck DR, et al., eds. Small animal gastroenterology. Philadelphia: Saunders, 1996. 275–302.

Hart JR, Chronic Gastritis. In: Tilley L, Smith F. The 5-Minute Veterinary Consult: Canine and Feline, 2003. Blackwell Publishing.

Happonen I, Linden J, Saari S, Karjalainen M, et al. Detection and effects of Helicobacters in healthy dogs and dogs with signs of gastritis. *J Am Vet Med Assoc*, 1998. 213: 1767–1774.

Liptak JM, Hunt GB, Barrs VRD, Foster SF, et al. Gastroduodenal ulceration in cats: eight cases and a review of the literature. *J Fel Med Surg*, 2002. 4: 27–42.

Webb C, Twedt DC. Canine gastritis. *Vet Clin N Am*, 2003. 33: 969–985.

Willard MD. Diseases of the stomach. In: Ettinger SJ, Feldman EC, eds. Textbook of veterinary internal medicine. Philadelphia: Saunders, 1995. 1143–1168.

Chinese herbal medicine/acupuncture references

Huang H. Comparison of Efficacy Between Acupuncture and Drug Treatment of Chronic Gastritis. *J of Acup and Tuina Science* 2005 vol 3(2):12–13.

Kubo M, Matsuda H, Toluoka K, Ma S, Shiomoto H. Anti-inflammatory activities of methanolic extract and alkaloidal components from Corydalis tuber. *Biol Pharm Bull*, 1994: Feb; 17(2):262–5.

Mascolo N, Autore G, Capasso F, et al. Biological screening of Italian medicinal plants for anti-inflammatory activity. *Phytotherapy Res* 1987;1(1):28–31.

Shen YQ, et al. *China Journal of Biochemical Products.* 1998;19(3):141–143.

Wu H, et al. *Journal of Chinese Patented Medicine.* 1996; 18(5):20–22.

Wu XH, et al. *Xinjiang Journal of Traditional Chinese Medicine.* 1998;16(1):42–43.

Zhong Cao Yao Fang Ji De Ying Yong (*Applications of Chinese Herbal Formulas*), 1976. 101.

Zhong Cao Yao Xue (*Study of Chinese Herbal Medicine*), 1976. 34.

Zhong Yao Xue (*Chinese Herbology*), 1998. 623:625.

Zhong Yao Xue (*Chinese Herbology*), 1998. 903:904.

Zhong Yao Yao Li Du Li Yu Lin Chuan (*Pharmacology, Toxicology and Clinical Applications of Chinese Herbs*), 1988. 4(3):9.

Zhong Yao Yao Li Yu Lin Chuan (*Pharmacology and Clinical Applications of Chinese Herbs*), 1983. 648.

Zhong Yao Yao Li Yu Ying Yong (*Pharmacology and Applications of Chinese Herbs*), 1983. 383.

Zhong Yao Zhi (*Chinese Herbology Journal*), 1993. 183.

Zhu ZP, et al. *China Journal of Integrated Splenico-Gastrology.* 1998;16(1):42–43.

Homotoxicology references

Demers J. Homotoxicology and Acupuncture. In: Proceedings of the 2004 Homotoxicology Seminar. AHVMA/Heel. Denver, CO, 2004. p 5, 6.

Deng X, Yin F, Lu X, Cai B, Yin W. The apoptotic effect of brucine from the seed of Strychnos nux-vomica on human hepatoma cells is mediated via Bcl-2 and Ca2+ involved mitochondrial pathway. *Toxicol Sci.* 2006. May;91(1):pp 59–69.

Gebhardt R. Antioxidative, antiproliferative and biochemical effects in HepG2 cells of a homeopathic remedy and its constituent plant tinctures tested separately or in combination. *Arzneimittelforschung.* 2003. 53(12): pp 823–30.

Goncalves JL, Lopes R, Oliveira D, Costa S, Miranda M, Romanos M, Santos N, Wigg M. In vitro anti-rotavirus activity of some medicinal plants used in Brazil against diarrhea. *J Ethnopharmacol.* 2005. Jul 14;99(3): pp 403–7.

Habermehl D, Kammerer B, Handrick R, Eldh T, Gruber C, Cordes N, Daniel PT, Plasswilm L, Bamberg M, Belka C, Jendrossek V. Proapoptotic activity of Ukrain is based on Chelidonium majus L. alkaloids and mediated via a mitochondrial death pathway. *BMC Cancer.* 2006. Jan 17;6: p 14.

Heel. BHI Homeopathic Therapy: Professional Reference. Heel Albuquerque, NM: Inc. 2002. p 14.

Ramprasath V, Shanthi P, Sachdanandam P. Immunomodulatory and anti-inflammatory effects of Semecarpus anacardium LINN. Nut milk extract in experimental inflammatory conditions. *Biol Pharm Bull.* 2006. Apr;29(4): pp 693–700.

Reckeweg H. Biotherapeutic Index: Ordinatio Antihomotoxica et Materia Medica, 5th ed. Baden-Baden, Germany: Biologische Heilmittel Heel GMBH, 2000. pp 329–30, 340–1, 432.

Reckeweg H. Homeopathia Antihomotoxica Materia Medica, 4th ed. Baden-Baden, Germany: Arelia-Verlag GMBH, 2002. pp. 136–8, 139–40, 345, 366, 461–3, 488–90.

Shamsa F, Ahmadiani A, Khosrokhavar R. Antihistaminic and anticholinergic activity of barberry fruit (Berberis vulgaris) in the guinea-pig ileum. *J Ethnopharmacol.* 1999. Feb;64(2):pp 161–6.

van Wassenhoven M. Towards an evidence-based repertory: clinical evaluation of Veratrum album. *Homeopathy.* 2004. Apr;93(2): pp 71–7.

Zhu B, Ahrens FA. Effect of berberine on intestinal secretion mediated by Escherichia coli heat-stable enterotoxin in jejunum of pigs. *Am J Vet Res.* 1982. Sep;43(9): pp 1594–8.

ACUTE GASTRIC DILATATION/BLOAT

Definition and cause

Acute gastric dilatation—volvulus (GDV) is suspected to be caused by a number of different factors such as a stomach filled with ingested food, water, and air; a blockage of the pylorus; or nervous innervation abnormalities to the wall of the stomach. GDV occurs most commonly in deep-chested dogs such as Great Danes, St. Bernards, Weimaraners, German Shepherds, and Irish and Gordon Setters. It is also felt that there is a genetic predisposition tied to the width and depth of the chest (Broome 2003, Guilford 1996, Matthiesen 1993, Simpson 2005, Waschak 2003).

Risk factors have been reviewed elsewhere (Glickman, et al. 2000; Broome, Walsh 2003). Diet may have some effect on this condition and "findings suggest that the feeding of dry dog foods that list oils or fats among the first four label ingredients predispose a high-risk dog to GDV" (Raghavan, Glickman 1997, 2006).

Medical therapy rationale, drug(s) of choice, and nutritional recommendations

Acute gastric dilation is classified as an emergency. Medical therapy for shock as well as supportive care and client education are important factors in the treatment of GDV. The treatment of choice is gastric decompression via intubation or trocharization followed by surgical gastroplexy. After medical stability, restricted exercise along with small, multiple feedings of a high-quality, highly digestible and assimilated diet is recommended. Reducing gastric secretion with famotidine or ranitidine is often recommended (Guilford 1996, Simpson 2005, Waschak 2003).

Anticipated prognosis

The prognosis depends upon the timing of the surgery and decompression along with post-surgical recovery, dietary adjustments and feeding schedule, and the status of secondary organ system involvement or complications. The prognosis for recurrence is often good post-surgery and there are little or no post-operative complications (Simpson 2005, Waschak 2003).

Integrative veterinary therapies

Successfully treating gastric dilatation and GDV requires rapid and proper conventional surgical and medical support. Efficient patient evaluation and imaging assist in determining if volvulus and/or splenic torsion are present. Immediate surgery and decompression may be required. Due to excessive homotoxin levels, shock and cardiac events are commonplace and may occur several hours or days following initial presentation. Following decompression, the patient is stabilized and surgery is performed as indicated.

Providing clean diet and water, reducing stress, allowing toxins to be excreted successfully, supporting organ function, enhancing elimination, and offering organ and metabolic support while repair occurs constitute the steps of integrative therapies. The controlled introduction of nutrients, nutraceuticals, medicinal herbs, and combination homeopathics that are anti-inflammatory, cellular-protective, and regenerating are beneficial in supporting stability and preventing recurrences.

Nutrition
General considerations/rationale

Therapeutic nutrition is focused upon improved cellular function of the nerves and muscles of the stomach. Because gastric dilation is a serious and often life-threatening condition that affects all organ systems, it is recommended that blood be analyzed both medically and physiologically to determine underlying organ involvement and disease. This allows clinicians to formulate therapeutic nutritional protocols that specifically address the stomach and other underlying organ weaknesses and nutrient and mineral deficiencies (see Chapter 2, Nutritional Blood Testing, for additional information).

Appropriate nutrients

Nutritional/gland therapy: Glandular stomach and brain/nerves supply the intrinsic nutrients to reduce cellular inflammation, help prevent cellular degeneration, and improve stomach muscle and organ function (see Gland Therapy in Chapter 2 for a more detailed explanation).

Phospholipids found in glandular brain are a source of unsaturated omega-3 fatty acids, which are now thought to play a vital role in the development and maintenance of the central nervous system. High concentrations of phosphatidyl choline and serine are found in brain tissue. Horrocks (1986) reported on the potential clinical use of these nutrients in chronic neurological conditions.

Glutamine: Glutamine has been shown to improve immune function and is beneficial for the cells of the gastro-intestinal tract (Souba 1985).

Lecithin/phosphatidyl choline: Phosphatidyl choline is a phospholipid that is integral to cellular membranes, particularly those of nerve and brain cells. It helps to move fats into the cells, and is involved in acetylcholine uptake, neurotransmission, and cellular integrity. As part of the cell membranes, lecithin is an essential nutrient required by all cells for general health and wellness (Hanin 1987).

Magnesium: Physiologically, magnesium activates adenosine triphosphatase, which is required for the proper functioning of the nerve cell membranes and fuels the sodium potassium pump. Magnesium has also been associated with neuromuscular function and dysfunction. Magnesium is recommended for weakening muscle function (Bibley 1996, Levin 2002).

Chinese herbal medicine/acupuncture
General considerations/rationale
Gastric dilation is a condition of Spleen and Stomach Qi deficiency secondary to improper feeding, overeating, or drinking when the patient is stressed or nervous. When the Spleen and Stomach have a Qi deficiency they do not have sufficient strength to digest properly and the stomach can fill with food. Alternatively, the stomach may not have sufficient energy to contract properly and this can lead to smooth muscle weakness and dilation with air accumulation.

Appropriate Chinese herbs
Bitter orange (zhi qiao): Increases gastric motility (Ma Ya Bing 1996), which may help propel gas and ingesta out of the stomach, making bloat and torsion less likely.

Citrus (Chen pi): Increases peristalsis (Jiang Su Zhong Yi Za Zhi 1981).

Magnolia bark (Zhi hou po): Improves gastric motility (Ci 1999). In a trial involving 36 women who underwent hysterectomy, the women who received the magnolia bark were less likely to experience bloating (Xin Yi Yai Xue Za Zhi 1973).

Malt (Chao mai ya): Facilitates digestion of starches and carbohydrates (Zhong Yao Yao Li Yu Ying Yong 1983), which may help to move food more quickly through the intestinal tract and make bloating less likely.

Medicated leaven (Chao shen qu): Facilitates digestion (Zhong Yao Xue 1998). Again, the faster ingesta passes through, the less likely bloat is to occur.

Unripe bitter orange (Zhi shi): Has been shown to increase the motility of the small intestines and uterus (Kuang 1997, Lu 1986). It may have similar effects on the stomach.

White atractylodes (Bai zhu): Can increase the contractions of guinea pig ileum smooth muscles (Ma Xiao Song 1996). It may have a similar effect on the stomach.

Acupuncture
Gastric dilation and volvulus is a condition of altered gastric motility. Acupuncture has been shown to be as effective as Western medicine in improving gastric motility (Zhang 1996). There have been reports of treatment of gastric volvulus using acupuncture (Wan 1981, Lining 1997).

Homotoxicology
General considerations/rationale
The gastrointestinal system is commonly affected by homotoxins owing to its important position as intermediary between the outside environment and the body itself. Both gastric dilatation and gastric dilatation with volvulus (GDV) are Degenerative Phase conditions. Degeneration Phase homotoxicoses, particularly those with a genetic predisposition, represent more serious issues wherein cure is not possible. Concurrent use of compositae class agents is necessary. The reader is referred to other appropriate sections such as cardiovascular protocols and other gastrointestinal protocols for ideas regarding therapy of gastric dilatation dogs and the many complications that may arise while these patients are undergoing care.

Appropriate homotoxicology formulas
Atropinum compositum: Not available on the U.S. market at this time, but is a powerful antispasmodic for biliary, renal, and intestinal colic (Demers 2004). It is also for gastritis pain and spasm. Contains Benzoicum acidum (common also to *Aesculus compositum*, *Arnica-Heel*, *Atropinum compositum*, and *Rhododendroneel*). It is used in inflammatory symptoms which occur throughout the alimentary canal: a slimy coating on the tongue with ulcers at the edges, stomatitis with dysphagia, eructations, retching and vomiting, and flatulent distension below the ribs on both sides. The stools are copious and loose and white in color, with violent tenesmus and mixed with blood; there are stabbing pains in the rectum, rigors, and a feeling of being seriously ill (Reckeweg 2002).

BHI-Nausea: Treats painful oral vesicles/stomatitis (Anacardium), nausea and vomiting with coughing (Ipecacuanha), and left-sided gastric region pain (Argentum nictricum).

BHI-Stomach: Used for stomach distress relieved by eructation, stomach pain, heartburn, chalky white tongue, flatulence, and tendency to collapse.

Cantharis compositum: Contains Arsenicum album, which is indicated in aphthous stomatitis; when the tongue is dry, red with raised papillae, and possibly coated white, brown, or black; for violent gastroenteritis with prolonged vomiting and diarrhea and unbearable burning stomach-pains after eating; and for foul-smelling stools. Also contains Mercurius solubilis, which is indicated in ulcerative lesions of the mucous membranes, and Hepar sulphuris calcareum (Reckeweg 2002).

Coenzyme compositum: Contains Citricum acidum, which is useful for dental problems and gingivitis; scurvy; blackening of teeth and heavy deposits of dental plaque; painful, herpetic vesicles around the lips; nausea, painful cramping in the umbilical area; and distension.

Galium-Heel: Used for all cellular phases, hemorrhoids, and anal fissures, and as a detoxicant.

Gastricumeel: Treats acute gastritis. Contains Antimonium crudum, which is indicated for tooth decay and toothache, and thus may be useful when dental work is indicated (Reckeweg 2002).

Ginseng compositum: Used for nausea, gastroenteritis, and constitutional support in geriatric or debilitated patients (Reckeweg 2000).

Hepar compositum: Provides detoxification and drainage of hepatic tissues and organ and metabolic support, and is useful in most hepatic and gall bladder pathologies. It is an important part of the Deep Detoxification Formula. Treats duodenitis, pancreatitis, cystic hepatic ducts, cholelithiasis, cholangitis, cholecystitis, vomiting, and diarrhea (Demers 2004, Broadfoot 2004). This combination contains Natrum oxalaceticum (also found in *Coenzyme compositum*, *Ubichinon compositum*, and *Mucosa compositum*) for changes in appetite and stomach distension due to air. Treats nausea, stomach pain with a sensation of fullness, gurgling in the abdomen, and cramping pain in the hypochondria. It is also used for constipation, sudden diarrhea (particularly after eating), and flatus (Reckeweg 2002).

Hepeel: Provides liver drainage and detoxification and is used in a wide variety of conditions including cancer of the liver, where *Hepeel* was found to be antiproliferative, hepatoprotective and an antioxidant when tested in human HepG2 cells (Gebhardt 2003).

Lymphomyosot: Used for lymph drainage and endocrine support, and edema. Contains Gentiana for chronic gastritis. Treats flatulence, diarrhea distension of the stomach with eructations, nausea, retching, and vomiting. Contains Geranium robertianum for nausea, particularly after eating, with distension or sensation of fullness. Myosotis arvensis is included for bloat and distension (Reckeweg 2002).

Mucosa compositum: Broadly supportive for repair of mucosal elements. Used in cellular cases and in recovery periods following active disease (Reckeweg 2000). This remedy contains a useful component in Kali bichromicum, which is indicated for ulcers found on the gums, tongue, lips, and even on the gastric mucosa (gastric or duodenal ulcer). The tongue may have a thick, yellow, mucous coating, or in ulcerative stomatitis or tonsillitis it may be dry, smooth, shiny, or fissured. Kali has been used effectively in acute gastroenteritis associated with vomiting of clear, light-colored fluid or quantities of mucous bile, and in cases with hematemesis,

flatulent colics, and dysenteric stools with tenesmus (Reckeweg 2002).

It also contains Hydrastis, with mucosal support for oral problems such as stomatitis, and mucosal suppuration that is accompanied by ulceration, inflammations and colic of the hepatobiliary system and of the gastrointestinal tract, and polyp formation (Reckeweg 2002). The Kreosotum component can be used in chronic gastritis with gastric hemorrhages and vomiting of brown masses. Also has a dental implication in cases with spongy gums and carious teeth, neuralgias proceeding from them causing a burning toothache with deep caries, black patches on the teeth, and fetid discharges.

The single remedy Phosphorus is broadly useful for dyspepsia and for jaw problems in dental disease (Reckeweg 2002). Phosphorus is found in many other remedies including *Echinacea compositum* and *Leptandra homaccord*. It is rich in suis organ preparations for mucosal support, plus a large variety of remedies with indications in the gastrointestinal sphere. The component Argentum nitricum (also in *Atropinum compositum*, *Diarrheel*, *Duodenoheel*, *Gastricumeel*, *Momordica compositum*, *BHI-Nausea*, and several other combinations) is indicated for distension in the upper abdomen, gastrocardiac symptom-complex, and amelioration from eructations. It is also used for gastric crises (Reckeweg 2002).

Spascupreel: Useful in cases of smooth muscle spasm and pain.

Ubichinon compositum: Contains Anthraquinone for swelling of gums and GI symptoms such as distention, flatulence, and cramping abdominal pain. Treats constipation with straining or sudden diarrhea (Reckeweg 2002).

Authors' suggested protocols

Nutrition

Esophagus/stomach and brain/nerve support formulas: 1 tablet for every 25 pounds of body weight BID.

Glutimmune: One-fourth scoop per 25 pounds of body weight daily.

Lecithin/phosphatidyl choline: One-fourth teaspoon for every 25 pounds of body weight BID.

Magnesium: 10 mg for every 10 pounds of body weight SID.

Chinese herbal medicine/acupuncture

The following only applies to primary gastric dilation without torsion. Torsion is a surgical condition.

In the acute stage use the patent formula Zhi Shi Xiao Pi Wan, which contains unripe bitter orange (Zhi shi), bitter orange (zhi qiao), blue citrus (Qing pi), citrus (Chen pi), dolomiaea root (Chuan mu xiang), hawthorn fruit(Shan zha), magnolia bark (Zhi hou po), malt (Mai ya), mirabilite (Mang xiao), radish seeds (lai fu zi), rhubarb (Da huang), and white atractylodes (Bai zhu).

In the chronic stage use the patent formula Jian Pi San at the manufacturer's recommended dose. It contains areca (Bing lang), hawthorn fruit (Shan zha), licorice (Gan cao), malt (Chao mai ya), medicated leaven (Chao shen qu), radish seed (Lai fu zi), rhubarb (Da huang), and unripe bitter orange (Zhi shi).

These formulas are recommended in Modern Complete Works of Traditional Chinese Veterinary Medicine (Yu Chuan 2000).

Acupuncture
Schoen (1994) recommends the following points for gastric dilation: ST36, BL21, CV12, CV10, St21 and BL18. For torsion he recommends ST36, St44, PC6, CV12, BL17, BL20 and BL21.

Homotoxicology (Dose: 10 drops PO for 50-pound dog; 5 drops PO for cat or small dog)
Spascupreel and Hepeel: Mix together or give separately IV and in acupuncture points.

Hepar compositum, Lymphomyosot, Gastricumeel, Atropinum compositum, Spascupreel, and Hepeel: All have components useful for bloat, and may be given every 10 to 15 minutes in a crisis.

Product sources
Nutrition
Esophagus/stomach and brain/nerve support formulas: Animal Nutrition Technologies. **Alternative:** Composure—Vetri Science Laboratories.

Glutimmune: Well Wisdom. **Alternative:** L-Glutamine powder—Thorne Veterinary Products.

Lecithin/phosphatidyl choline: Designs for Health.
Magnesium: Over the counter.

Chinese herbal medicine
Patent formulas Zhi Shi Xiao Pi Wan and Jian Pi San: Mayway Company.

Homotoxicology
BHI/Heel Corporation

REFERENCES

Western medicine references
Broome C, Walsh V. Gastric dilatation-volvulus in dogs. *N Z Vet J.* 2003, Dec;51(6):275–83.

Ellison GW. Gastric dilatation volvulus: An update. Presented at the Western Veterinary Conference, 2004. Las Vegas, NV.

Glickman LT, Glickman NW, Schellenberg DB, et al. Multiple risk factors for the GDV syndrome in dogs: A practitioner/owner case control study. *Journal of the American Animal Hospital Association,* 1997, 33: 197–204.

Glickman L, Glickman N, Schellenberg D, Raghavan M, Lee T. Incidence of and breed-related risk factors for gastric dilation-volvulus in dogs. *J Am Vet Med Assoc.* 2000, Jan 1;216(1):pp 40–5.

Guilford WG. Gastric dilatation, gastric dilatation—volvulus, and chronic gastric volvulus. In: Guilford WG, Center SA, Stombeck, et al., eds. Strombeck's small animal gastroenterology. 3rd ed. Philadelphia: Saunders, 1996:303–317.

Matthiesen DT. Pathophysiology of gastric dilatation volvulus. In: Bojrab MJ, ed. Disease mechanisms in small animal surgery. 2nd ed. Philadelphia: Lea and Febiger, 1993:220–231.

Simpson KW. Diseases of the stomach. In Ettinger, SJ, Feldman, EC. Textbook of Veterinary Internal Medicine. Philadelphia: WB Saunders Co. 2005. 1319–1321

Raghavan M, Glickman N, Glickman L. The effect of ingredients in dry dog foods on the risk of gastric dilatation—volvulus in dogs. *J Am Anim Hosp Assoc.* 2006, Jan-Feb;42(1):pp 28–36.

Waschak MJ. Gastric Dilation and Volvulus Syndrome (GDV), In: Tilley L, Smith F. The 5-Minute Veterinary Consult: Canine and Feline, 2003. Blackwell Publishing.

IVM/nutrition references
Bilbey DLJ, Prabhakaran VM. Muscle cramps and magnesium deficiency: case reports. *Canadian Family Physician,* Vol. 42, 1996, July, pp. 1348–51.

Hanin IG, Ansell B. Lecithin: Technological, Biological, and Therapeutic Aspects. NY: Plenum Press, 1987. 180, 181.

Horrocks LA, et al. Phosphatidyl Research and the Nervous System, 1986. Berlin: Springer Verlach.

Levin C. Canine Epilepsy. Oregon City, OR: Lantern Publication. 2002. p 18–19.

Souba W, et al. Glutamine metabolism in the intestinal tract: invited review, *JPEN* 1985, 9:608–617.

Chinese herbal medicine/acupuncture references
Ci XL, et al. Hou Pu's effect on gastrointestine electric activity in normal and endotoxin-shocked rats. *China Journal of TCM Science and Technology.* 1999;6(3):154–156.

Journal of Pharmacology of Clinical Application of TCM. 1996;12(6): 28–29.

Jiang Su Zhong Yi Za Zhi (*Jiangsu Journal of Chinese Medicine*), 1981; (3): 61.

Kuang L. The effect of Zhi Shi on the myoelectric activity of sheep ileum. *Journal of Chinese Medicine Research.* 1997; 13(3):49–50.

Lining H. Case report on the use of acupuncture for treatment of chronic gastric volvulus. *Am J Acupunct* 1997;25(1): 17–9.

Lu YMH, et al. The chemistry and pharmacology of Zhi Shi, Shan Jiao, and Gua Lou Ren. *Foreign Medicine* (vol. of TCM). 1986;8(6):17–20.

Ma XS, et al. *New Journal of Digestive Diseases.* 1996;4(11): 603–604.

Ma YB. Zhi Qiao's effects on gastroinstestinal movement. *Journal of Pharmacology of Clinical Application of TCM.* 1996;12(6): 28–29.

Schoen A. Veterinary Acupuncture Ancient Art to Modern Medicine. American Veterinary Publications, Inc, Ca, 1994 p 228.

Wan YG, Yu LY. Volvulus of the stomach successfully treated with acupuncture report of 9 cases. *J Tradit Chin Med* 1981 Sep;1(11):39–42.

Xin Yi Yai Xue Za Zhi (*New Journal of Medicine and Herbology*), 1973; 4:25.

Zhang AL et al. Clinical effect of acupuncture in the treatment of gastrokinetic disturbance. *World Journal of Acupuncture—Moxibustion*, 1996, 6(1):3–8.

Zhong Yao Xue (Chinese Herbology), 1998, 436: 437.

Zhong Yao Yao Li Yu Ying Yong (*Pharmacology and Applications of Chinese Herbs*), 1983; 473.

Homotoxicology references

Broadfoot PJ. Inflammation: Homotoxicology and Healing. In: Proceedings AHVMA/Heel Homotoxicology Seminar. Denver, CO, 2004. p 27.

Demers J. Homotoxicology and Acupuncture. In: Proceedings of the 2004 Homotoxicology Seminar. AHVMA/Heel. Denver, CO, 2004. p 5, 6.

Gebhardt R. Antioxidative, antiproliferative and biochemical effects in HepG2 cells of a homeopathic remedy and its constituent plant tinctures tested separately or in combination. *Arzneimittelforschung.* 2003. 53(12): pp 823–30.

Reckeweg H. Biotherapeutic Index: Ordinatio Antihomotoxica et Materia Medica, 5th ed. Baden-Baden, Germany: Biologische Heilmittel Heel GMBH, 2000. pp 340–1, 369.

Reckeweg H. Homeopathia Antihomotoxica Materia Medica, 4th ed. Baden-Baden, Germany: Arelia-Verlag GMBH, 2002. pp. 136–8, 139–40, 147, 150–3, 179, 317–19, 345, 488–90.

INFLAMMATORY BOWEL DISEASE—IMMUNE-MEDIATED

Definition and cause

Inflammatory bowel disease (IBD) is a complex group of inflammatory disorders of the large and small intestine. Cellular infiltrates are present in the lamina propria. Signs of vomiting and/or diarrhea with various other GI manifestations can occur. Breed prevalence is noted, indicating at least some genetic predisposition. The current thought is that several factors predispose the disease: genetic factors, an exaggerated immune response and immune cell infiltrate, infectious agents, altered normal flora, reactions to food substances and environmental chemicals or toxins, therapeutic damage, and other unidentified issues which affect the integrity and function of the mucosa and related immune system elements (Allenspach 2006a, Diehl 2003, Dimski 1995, German 2001, Sherding 1994, Strombeck 1996). IBD is common in both dogs and cats (Sherding 1994, Tams 1993).

Medical therapy rationale, drug(s) of choice, and nutritional recommendations

The primary focus of treatment is a combination of dietary adjustments, anti-inflammatories, antimicrobials, and immune suppressing medications. Dietary adjustments are focused on hypoallergenic, novel proteins and low-gluten carbohydrates (such as rice, duck, potato, fish, rabbit, venison, etc). Both high-fiber and low-residue diets have been used with success, but this depends upon the individual animal. The addition of omega-3 fatty acids that are high in both eicosapentanoic acid (EPA) and docosahaenoic acid (DHA) have been beneficial (Dimski 1995, Leib 1995, Marks 1998).

Medications include corticosteroids, sulfa drugs such as sulfasalazine, or antibiotics such as metronidazole, along with antispasmotics. In animals with overly reactive immune responses, immunosuppressants such as azathioprine and cyclophosphamide may be required to quiet the immune attack (Strombeck 1996).

Anticipated prognosis

IBD is a controllable disease that requires client compliance and special attention to diet and medication. Because of the immune-mediated nature and the possibility of other underlying disease, the prognosis becomes somewhat guarded, especially if the disease has progressed to a protein-losing enteritis (Diehl 2003, Strombeck 1996).

Integrative veterinary therapies

A complete history, physical examination, and appropriate testing are necessary to rule out other conditions. While these patients may benefit from limited antigen or hydrolyzed diets, they are not truly food allergy patients. Patients that respond totally to food changes more properly have food allergy and not IBD. Such discussions may seem academic but are relevant when examining response to treatment and disease response patterns. Definitive diagnosis is by biopsy.

Leaky gut syndrome (LGS) becomes a large part of understanding the events leading up to chronic inflammation and cellular infiltration in IBD. The functions of a normal intestinal system include the barrier function of the mucosal elements (keeps bad things out and lets good things in), the absorption function (digestion, transformation by enzymes and flora), and the immunological cellular and humoral components (the gut-associated lymph tissue and antibody production) (Silver 2003).

Genetic issues can manifest as missing or inactive genes. These lead to deficiencies in protein synthesis and absence of needed enzymes and receptors. Any genetic alteration or omission can cause dysfunctional digestion, mucus production, receptor activity, and injury to the mucosal surface, which in turn leads to antigen access to the immune system due to improper digestion and absorption. The initial result is Excretion Phase disease as cells activate mechanisms which release fluid and electrolytes into the bowel to flush the area clean for repair. If this is ineffective, or if genetic coding prevents that repair from occurring, then chronic inflammatory changes ensue with the onset of diarrhea, vomiting, constipation, and nausea.

Enzymes and receptors can be missing if genetic errors occur, or they can be injured and blocked in their production or function by other homotoxins. Damage by homotoxins to enzymes leads to dysfunction and potential degradation. The development of IBD then proceeds.

LGS is aggravated ultimately by increased gut permeability to which a host of things contribute. Trauma, emotional stress, toxins, drugs, exercise, radiation, and malnutrition are commonly known factors that lead to increased gut permeability. Such changes cause extra stress and increased homotoxin levels in the liver, general circulation, and other organs of excretion (kidney, skin, and lung). Fibrosis can result as homotoxins and inflammation give rise to altered connective tissue structure.

Therapy for LGS involves removing causative agents when possible (anaerobic bacterial overgrowth, giardia, coccidia, nematode parasites, fungal overgrowths); resting the bowel by providing an easily digested and absorbed form of nutrition; removing toxins and abnormal microflora, parasites, and pathogens; replacing and repopulating the microflora with appropriate probiotic cultures and digestive enzymes; and beginning the process of repairing the matrix, cells, organelles, tissues, and organs damaged in the process. Further intoxication or genetic defects may block total recovery, but these four Rs (Rest, Remove, Replace, Repair) provide a path toward helpful treatment plans for LGS patients. These actions are frequently helpful for managing IBD cases.

Because fasting can actually increase intestinal permeability, it is important to feed something during the resting period. Silver's method for addressing LGS, as outlined in his presentation, is well worth reviewing (Silver 2003).

Therapeutic agents are necessary in most cases of confirmed IBD, and these drugs can cause widespread, subclinical damage leading to increased intestinal permeability, as well as damage to immune elements and their functioning. It can be very difficult in some situations to decide whether a drug is useful or not. In treating IBS, many patients require medications such as anti-inflammatories (corticosteroids), antiparasitic agents, immunomodulators such as cyclosporin, and antibiotics such as metronidazole (Allenspach, et al. 2006b). A particularly interesting study that was just released shows no change in intestinal permeability before or after treatment (Allenspach 2006c).

It may be that the increase in intestinal permeability in these cases is a foundational issue upon which the remaining pathogenesis depends. In any case, integrative techniques allow for lower doses to be used and in some cases, for the need of drugs to be reduced. Because these patients often have or develop other health challenges, such as allergies, arthritis, diabetes, immunosuppression, obesity, etc., several medications may be used simultaneously, and the possibility for drug interactions rises dramatically. The clinician may be able to repair damage and return a patient to a higher level of health, as well as reduce the therapeutic damage done with other medications, by using coordinated integrative processes. It is also important to reduce unpleasant and difficult side effects, such as polyuria and polydyspea, which aggravate and upset clients who own these pets and cause them to seek professional care elsewhere.

Clients and professionals both desire to use fewer harmful medications in treating their animal charges. Therefore, there has been great interest in complementary treatments for IBD from both consumers and clinicians (Joos, et al. 2006). In human patients and animal patients, the interest in alternative options increases with the corticosteroid dose needed to manage IBD symptoms (Langhorst, et al. 2005). The connection between unpleasant and dangerous adverse reactions and a desire for gentler, more effective therapy is obvious.

Nutrition
General considerations/rationale

Therapeutic nutrition focuses upon the body's cellular autoimmune reaction against the chronically inflamed GI tract as well as minimizing the potential side effects of chronically required medications such as corticosteroids. Continual ingestion of chemical preservatives, additives, dyes, contaminated byproducts, and highly cooked and processed foods can lead to high free radical production, associated cellular inflammation, and intestinal cell death. Cellular debris can evoke the production of autoantibodies, which sets up an autoimmune cellular reaction. Left unchecked, this cellular process can cascade and spread throughout the intestinal tract, leading first to chronic inflammation and eventually to inflammatory bowel disease (Goldstein 2005) (see Chapter 2, Free Radicals and Inflammation, for additional information). Also, because IBD has an immune component that can affect all organ systems, it is recommended that blood be analyzed both medically and physiologically to determine underlying organ involvement and disease. This allows clinicians to formulate therapeutic nutritional protocols that specifically address the stomach or intestines and other associated organ weaknesses and nutrient and mineral deficiencies (see Chapter 2, Nutritional Blood Testing, for additional information).

Appropriate nutrients

Gland therapies: Glandular adrenal, thymus, intestines, and stomach supply intrinsic nutrients and can help protect and reduce inflammation in gastrointestinal cells. The adrenal and thymus glands are integral to the immune response and are important in all autoimmune diseases (see Chapter 2, Gland Therapy, for more details).

Probiotics: Administration of the proper combination of probiotics has been reported to have a positive impact on the intestines and the digestive process (Goldin 1984, Perdigon 1987). Probiotics have been shown to improve and aid the digestive process by secreting their own source of enzymes, which is beneficial for animals with compromised GI function (McDonough 1987).

Sterols: Plant-derived sterols such as betasitosterol show anti-inflammatory properties that appear to be similar to corticosteriods (Gupta 1980). They have a cortisone-like effect without the associated immune-suppressing effects. Bouic (1996) reports on the immune-enhancing and balancing effect of plant sterols, which are also beneficial to animals with immune-mediated diseases.

Glutamine: Glutamine has been shown to improve immune function and is beneficial for the cells of the gastro-intestinal tract (Souba 1985, Windmueller 1982, Yoshimura 1993).

Essential fatty acids: It has been clinically proven that people suffering from colitis and Crohn's disease who supplement their diet with EPA and DHA, the two omega-3 fatty acids that are found in fish oil, had significantly fewer recurrences over a 1- to 2-year period (Belluzzi 1996, Mate 1991).

Chinese herbal medicine/acupuncture
General considerations/rationale

Inflammatory bowel disease is considered to be Qi and Blood stagnation with Heat and Damp affecting the Stomach and Spleen. The Stomach and Spleen (which includes the pancreas in TCM) are responsible for digestion. When they do not have the nourishment (Blood) or the free-flowing energy (Qi) to perform their functions, digestive disorders follow. In the case of IBD, the digestive disorder manifests as diarrhea and/or vomiting, especially in cats. The Heat refers to the Blood in the stool and the Damp to the mucus and white blood cells. The inflammation and bleeding in the bowels must be decreased and the diarrhea stopped to treat inflammatory bowel disease.

Appropriate Chinese herbs

Actractylodes (Bai zhu): Can be used to stop diarrhea (Chang Yong Zhong Yao Cheng Fen Yu Yao Li Shou Ce 1994). At low doses, it has a mild inhibitory effect on the contraction of isolated guinea pig ileum (Ma Xiao Song 1996).

Amomum fruit (Sha ren): Relieves bloating, spasms, and pain. It also relieves nausea (Zhong Yao Xue 1988).

Aurantium fruit (Zhi qiao): Was shown to inhibit contraction of isolated rabbit intestinal smooth muscles and relieve acetylcholine- and BaCl2-induced enterospasm (Ma Ya Bing 1996).

Bupleurum (Chai hu): Inhibited the effect of dimethyl benzene-induced auricular concha inflammation in mice (Liu Wei 1998).

Cimicifuga (Sheng ma): Inhibits lymphocyte activation. Cimicifuga's inhibitory effect on membrane permeability is greater than that of cortisol and it has been shown to inhibit the formation of antibodies (Zhu 1984). It also suppresses proliferation of immune cells (Huang 1992).

Citrus (Chen pi): Reduces inflammation by decreasing the permeability of blood vessels (Zhong Yao Yao Li Yu Ying Yong 1983).

Coptis (Huang lian): Stops diarrhea (Zhong Yao Xue 1998). There was a 100% improvement in signs in a study of 100 people with acute gastroenteritis (Si Chuan Yi Xue Yuan Xue Bao 1959). One component of coptis, berberine, has been shown to have an anti-inflammatory effect in rats (Yao Xue Za Zhi 1981).

Corydalis tuber (Yan hu suo): Increases secretions from adrenal glands in mice (Xi Xue Xue Bao 1988). This may release cortisol and decrease intestinal inflammation.

Immature orange peel (Qing pi): Inhibits smooth muscle contractions in the stomach, and thereby relives cramps (Zhong Yao Zhi 1984).

Licorice (Gan cao): Alleviates intestinal cramping (Zhong Yao Zhi 1993). Two of the components, glycyrrhizin and glycyrrhetinic acid, have anti-inflammatory effects. They have approximately 10% of the corticosteroid activity of cortisone (Zhong Cao Yao 1991).

Peach kernel (Tao ren): Suppresses the immune system in several ways. It was shown to prevent egg-white-induced arthritis in mice (Liu 1989). Other studies have shown suppressive effects on fibroblast growth in laboratory cell cultures. It was shown to suppress the proliferation of inflammatory cells and fibroblast hyperplasia in subjects using experimental trabeculae dissection (Wang 1993). Another study demonstrated the ability to decrease inflammation in mice with otitis media (Zhong Yao Tong Bao 1986).

Platycodon root (Jie geng): Has been shown to promote the secretion of corticosterone in rats, and thereby cause an anti-inflammatory effect (Li 1984, Zhang 1984, Zhou 1979).

Rhubarb (Da huang): In a clinical trial involving 14 human patients with hemorrhagic necrotic enteritis, 12 responded after 2 to 6 days (Fu Jian Zhong Yi Yao 1985).

Acupuncture points

Acupuncture has been shown to be effective in controlling or curing diarrhea in many studies. Acupuncture at GV1, St25, and ST36 was used in a study of 500 infants with diarrhea. 485 were completely cured and 13 improved (Zhonzxin 1989). In preweaning pigs with experimentally induced E. coli diarrhea, a combination of acupuncture and moxibustion was superior to oral neomycin. Using acupuncture and moxibustion, 82% of the pigs responded as opposed to 71% treated with neomycin (Hwang YC 1988).

Homotoxicology
General considerations/rationale

Because this condition consists of a recurring inflammatory reaction, it represents an Impregnation Phase disorder, which progresses to Degeneration Phase and even Dedifferentiation Phase as the patient ages. The development of GI lymphoma in cats with IBD is well documented. Homotoxicologists view this as a continuum of damage and degeneration related to homotoxins. Homotoxins also include the concept of psychical elements, meaning that negative or stressful emotional conditions can result in damage to the body through endogenous homotoxins and altered circulation.

Homotoxins can also injure the important tight junctions of the GI mucosal barriers, which compromises gut function and leads to inflammatory changes as antigens gain access to deeper layers of the gut. If either genetic or homotoxin damage occurs, the lymphoid system may fail to properly produce immunoglobulins, which bind with antigens to be excreted in the stool or present data to the GALT system. Proper gut motility is needed for intestinal health, and peristalsis is needed to properly move material out of the gut in a coordinated fashion. Gut motility is also related to normal populations of microflora. Homotoxins can block or even reverse this process, leading to putrefaction and static gut syndrome, a condition that increases the workload and the levels of potentially damaging homotoxins. This can lead to damage and invasion in patients with other issues, aggravating their intestinal permeability (Simpson, et al. 2006).

Clients requesting alternative therapies tend to have higher personal income and higher levels of education. They also tend to be willing to make a larger commitment to the recovery of their pets. These people read and understand material and seek other ways of accomplishing their goals. Antihomotoxic agents are well-suited for integrating into the care of inflammatory bowel syndrome patients. Clinicians are treating patients with success, but more formal research is needed in this area.

Many of these pets have been treated in the authors' offices with good success. Cure is rare, and when it occurs it may well represent incorrect diagnosis (food allergy diagnosed as inflammatory bowel disease), but in many cases the common thread to the chronic nature of the disease is the leaky bowel syndrome and veterinary medicine would do well to pay considerable attention to this condition.

Appropriate homotoxicology formulas

Please refer to the Diarrhea, Vomiting, and Colitis protocols for more formulas and details.

Atropinum compositum: Not available on the U.S. market at this time, but it is a powerful antispasmodic for biliary, renal, and intestinal colic (Demers 2004). Contains Benzoicum acidum (also common to *Aesculus compositum*, *Arnica-Heel*, *Atropinum compositum*, and *Rhododendroneel*). It is used in inflammatory symptoms which occur throughout the alimentary canal: a slimy coating on the tongue with ulcers at the edges, stomatitis with dysphagia, eructations, retching and vomiting, and flatulent distension below the ribs on both sides. The stools are copious, loose, and white in color, with violent tenesmus and mixed with blood; there are stabbing pains in the rectum, rigors, and a feeling of being seriously ill (Reckeweg 2002).

BHI-Intestine: Treats diarrhea, cramping, hard-black stool (Bryonia alba); emotional diarrhea, leg spasm and cramps, colitis (Colocynthis); flatulence and liver conditions (Lycopodium); gastroenteritis and colitis (Nux vomica); and mucosal inflammation (Mercurius corrosives). Sulphur activates a blocked metabolism, stimulates regressive vicariation, and promotes healing (Heel 2002).

Coenzyme compositum: Contains Citricum acidum, which is useful for dental problems and gingivitis; scurvy; blackening of teeth and heavy deposits of dental plaque; painful, herpetic vesicles around the lips; nausea; painful cramping in the umbilical area, and distension.

Colocynthis homaccord: Treats diarrhea with lower back pain (Citrullus colocynthis), colic, pain below the navel, and colitis with gelatinous stools.

Diarrheel S: A symptom remedy for acute and chronic diarrhea. Treats acute gastroenteritis, belching, spurting diarrhea, pancreatopathy, and colitis. This commonly used formula contains Tormentilla for dysentery, acute gastroenteritis, and mucous and ulcerative colitis with bloody stools (Reckeweg 2002). It is also found in *BHI-Diarrhea* and *Veratrum homaccord*.

Duodenoheel: Treats hunger pains, hyperacidity, gastric and duodenal ulcers, nausea and vomiting, and dysentery with tenesmus (Reckeweg 2000).

Engystol N: Used for viral-origin gastroenteritis (see Parvovirus).

Erigotheel: Used for gastric catarrh, hepatic diseases, and duodenal ulcers with spasm; has antipyretic indications (Demers 2004).

Galium-Heel: Treats all cellular phases, hemorrhoids, and anal fissures, and is a detoxicant.

Ginseng compositum: Treats nausea and gastroenteritis, and provides constitutional support in geriatric or debilitated patients (Reckeweg 2000).

Hepar compositum: Used for detoxification and drainage of hepatic tissues, provides organ and metabolic support, and is useful in most hepatic and gallbladder pathologies. It is an important part of Deep Detoxification Formula. It is used to treat duodenitis, pancreatitis, cystic hepatic ducts, cholelithiasis, cholangitis, cholecystitis, vomiting, and diarrhea (Demers 2004, Broadfoot 2004). This combination contains Natrum oxalaceticum (also found in *Coenzyme compositum*, *Ubichinon compositum*, and *Mucosa compositum*) for changes in appetite and stomach distension due to air. Treats nausea and stomach pain with a sensation of fullness, gurgling in the abdomen, and cramping pain in the hypochondria. It is also used for constipation, sudden diarrhea (particularly after eating), and flatus (Reckeweg 2002).

Hepeel: Provides liver drainage and detoxification. Used in a wide variety of conditions including cancer of the liver, where Hepeel was found to be antiproliferative, hepatoprotective, and an antioxidant when tested in human HepG2 cells (Gebhardt 2003).

Lymphomyosot: Provides lymph drainage and endocrine support, and treats edema. Contains Gentiana for chronic gastritis. Treats flatulence, diarrhea, distension of the stomach with eructations, nausea, retching, and vomiting. Contains Geranium robertianum for nausea, particularly after eating with distension, or sensation of fullness. Myosotis arvensis is included for bloat and distension (Reckeweg 2002).

Mucosa compositum: Broadly supportive for repair of mucosal elements. Used in cellular cases and in recovery periods following active disease (Reckeweg 2000). This remedy contains a useful component in Kali bichromicum, which is indicated for ulcers found on the gums, tongue, lips, and even on the gastric mucosa (gastric or duodenal ulcer). The tongue may have a thick, yellow, mucous coating, or in ulcerative stomatitis or tonsillitis it may be dry, smooth, shiny, or fissured. Kali has been used effectively in acute gastroenteritis associated with vomiting of clear, light-colored fluid or quantities of mucous bile, and in cases with hematemesis, flatulent colics, and dysenteric stools with tenesmus (Reckeweg 2002).

It also contains Hydrastis, with mucosal support for oral problems such as stomatitis, and mucosal suppuration that is accompanied by ulceration, inflammations and colic of the hepatobiliary system and of the gastrointestinal tract, and polyp formation (Reckeweg 2002). The Kreosotum component can be used in chronic gastritis with gastric hemorrhages and vomiting of brown masses. Also has a dental implication in cases with spongy gums and carious teeth, neuralgias proceeding from them causing a burning toothache with deep caries, black patches on the teeth, and fetid discharges.

The single remedy Phosphorus is broadly useful for dyspepsia and for jaw problems in dental disease (Reckeweg 2002). Phosphorus is found in many other remedies including *Echinacea compositum* and *Leptandra homaccord*. It is rich in suis organ preparations for mucosal support, plus a large variety of remedies with indications in the gastrointestinal sphere. The component Argentum nitricum (also in *Atropinum compositum*, *Diarrheel*, *Duodenoheel*, *Gastricumeel*, *Momordica compositum*, *BHI-Nausea*, and several other combinations) is indicated for distension in the upper abdomen, gastro-cardiac symptom-complex, and amelioration from eructations. It is also used for gastric crises (Reckeweg 2002).

Nux vomica homaccord: Used for liver and gastrointestinal disease and after smoke inhalation. Useful in gingivitis (Reckeweg 2002). This commonly used formula is part of the *Detox Kit*. Recent research shows that one ingredient (*Brucine*) affects mitochondria in human hepatoma cells. Further research is needed to determine whether homeopathic dilutions are more or less active (Deng, et al. 2006).

Podophyllum homaccord: Treats chronic gastroenteritis, gastroenteritis in juvenile dogs and cats, dyspepsia, catarrhal colitis, hemorrhoids, and watery-green diarrhea alternating with constipation (Macloed 1983).

Procteel: Combines Lycopodium, Sulfur, Phosphorus, and Aluminum oxydatum to make a formula that may be useful for megacolon and rectal atony, hemorrhoids, sore body orifices, alternating diarrhea and constipation, hepatic disease with cystic ducts, and intestinal stasis (Reckeweg 2000).

Psorinoheel: Treats chronic illness, and is an Impregnation Phase remedy.

Schwef-Heel: Treats chronic diseases of the skin and liver. This remedy should be interposed in most skin and liver cases (Reckeweg 2000). Patients that need this remedy may look dirty and have scruffy skin conditions, red lips, a white tongue with red tip, itching and burning rectal area with morning diarrhea, or a prolapsed rectum (Boericke 1927). Sulfur is contained in several other antihomotoxic formulas including *Coenzyme compositum*, *Echinacea compositum*, *Engystol*, *Ginseng compositum*, *Hepar compositum*, *Molybdan compositum*, *Mucosa compositum*, *Paeonia-Heel*, *Proctheel*, *Psorinoheel*, *Sulfur-Heel*, *Thyroidea compositum*, and *Ubichinon compositum* (Reckeweg 2000).

Ubichinon compositum: Contains Anthraquinone for swelling of the gums and GI symptoms such as distention, flatulence, and cramping abdominal pain. Treats constipation with straining or sudden diarrhea (Reckeweg 2002).

Veratrum homaccord: Treats gastritis, intense vomiting with blood, collapse (pale mucous membranes), psychosis, dysentary, fecal incontinence, and intestinal spasm. This very useful remedy is used widely by the authors for general vomiting cases. Consider its use in cases of gastritis following general anesthesia. Classical provings were recently repeated and found consistent with earlier work (Van Wassenhoven 2004).

Vomitusheel S: Treats nausea and vomiting with a cough (*Ipecacuanha*), liver and gastrointestinal issues (*Nux vomica*), eructation, and possibly anxiety or depression (*Ignatia*) (Reckeweg 2000). No known adverse reactions have occurred and it is extremely safe to use in pediatric patients. This remedy contains Aethusa for vomiting, that obviously originates in the nervous system. In serious cases, capillary paralysis, hematemesis, stomach cramps, and tympanitic distension may occur, with an irresistible urge to pass stool. The nervous vomiting is characterized by spasmodic contractions of the esophageal muscles and violent pains which shoot upwards from the cardiac sphincter (Reckeweg 2002). In more severe vomiting, consider *Veratrum homaccord* instead or in combination.

Authors' suggested protocols

Nutrition

For upper GI—Esophagus, stomach, and immune support formulas: 1 tablet for every 25 pounds of body weight BID.

For lower GI—Intestines/IBD and immune support formulas: 1 tablet for every 25 pounds of body weight BID.

Probiotic: One-half capsule for every 25 pounds of body weight with food.

Betathyme: 1 capsule for every 35 pounds of body weight BID.

Glutimmune: One-fourth scoop for every 25 pounds of body weight daily.

Eskimo fish oil: One-half to 1 teaspoon per meal for cats; 1 teaspoon for every 35 pounds of body weight for dogs.

Chinese herbal medicine/acupuncture

ColonGuard: 1 capsule per 10 to 20 pounds twice daily. It can be used in conjunction with conventional medicine, but is often not needed. In addition to the herbs mentioned above, ColonGuard also contains angelica radix (Dang gui), astragalus (Huang qi), bamboo shavings (Zhu ru), codonopsis (Dang shen), lindera (Wu yao), pueraria (Ge gen), pulsatilla root (Bai tou weng), and raw white lotus seed (Lian zi).

The authors use BL20, ST36, BL26, Baihui, ST25, BL21, CV12, and CV4 in various combinations for inflammatory bowel disease.

Homotoxicology (Dose: 10 drops PO for 50-pound dog; 5 drops PO for cat or small dog)

Treatment must be individualized and continue for long periods of time. The following represent good starting therapies, which can be readily adapted based upon clinical response.

Starting symptom formula: Traumeel, Podophyllum compositum, Veratrum homaccord, Hepeel, and Atropinum compositum (if available) mixed together and given BID to TID orally.

Deep detoxification formula: Galiumheel, Lymphomyosot, Hepar compositum, Solidago compositum, Thyroidea compositum, and Mucosa compositum mixed together and given every 3 days until patient response is seen, then 1 to 3 times weekly for 30 to 120 days minimum.

Product sources

Nutrition

Intestines/IBD, esophagus/stomach, and immune support formulas: Animal Nutrition Technologies. **Alternatives:** Immune System Support—Standard Process Veterinary Formulas; Immuno Support—Rx Vitamins for Pets; Immugen—Thorne Veterinary Products; Enteric Support—Standard Process Veterinary Formulas; NutriGest—Rx Vitamins for Pets.

Probiotic MPF: Progressive Labs.

Betathyme: Best for Your Pet. **Alternative:** Moducare—Thorne Veterinary Products.

Glutimmune: Well Wisdom. Alternative: L-Glutamine powder—Thorne Veterinary Products.

Eskimo fish oil: Tyler Encapsulations.

Chinese herbal medicine

Formula ColonGuard: Natural Solutions, Inc.

Homotoxicology

BHI/Heel Corporation

REFERENCES

Western medicine references

Allenspach K, Bergman P, Sauter S, Grone A, Doherr M, Gaschen F. P-glycoprotein expression in lamina propria lymphocytes of duodenal biopsy samples in dogs with chronic idiopathic enteropathies. *J Comp Pathol.* 2006a; Jan;134(1):pp 1–7.

Allenspach K, Rufenacht S, Sauter S, Grone A, Steffan J, Strehlau G, Gaschen F. Pharmacokinetics and clinical efficacy of cyclosporine treatment of dogs with steroid-refractory inflammatory bowel disease. *J Vet Intern Med.* 2006b; Mar-Apr;20(2): pp 239–44.

Allenspach K, Steiner JM, Shah BN, Berghoff N, Ruaux C, Williams DA, Blum JW, Gaschen F. Evaluation of gastrointestinal permeability and mucosal absorptive capacity in dogs with chronic enteropathy. *Am J Vet Res.* 2006c; Mar;67(3): pp 479–83.

Diehl KJ. Inflammatory Bowel Disease (IBD). In: Tilley L, Smith F. The 5-Minute Veterinary Consult: Canine and Feline, 2003. Blackwell Publishing.

Dimski DS. Therapy of inflammatory bowel disease. In Bonagura, JD, ed. Current Veterinary Therapy XII. Philadelphia: WB Saunders Co. 1995;723–8.

German A, Hall E, Day M. Immune cell populations within the duodenal mucosa of dogs with enteropathies. *J Vet Intern Med.* 2001; Jan-Feb; 15(1):pp 14–25.

Leib MA, Matz ME. Diseases of the large intestine. In: Ettinger SJ, Feldman EC, eds. Textbook of Veterinary Internal Medicine. Philadelphia: WB Saunders Co. 1995;1241–48.

Marks SL. Management of canine inflammatory bowel disease. The Compendium on Continuing Education for the Practicing Veterinarian. 1998;317–32.

Sherding RG. Lymphocytic-plasmacytic inflammatory bowel disease of cats. *Veterinary International.* 1994;11–20.

Sherding RG, Johnson SE. Diseases of the intestines. In: Birchard SJ, Sherding RG, eds. Saunders Manual of Small Animal Practice. Philadelphia: WB Saunders Co. 1994;704–9.

Strombeck DR, Guilford WG. Idiopathic inflammatory bowel diseases. In: Guilford WG, Center SA, Strombeck DR, et al., eds. Strombeck's small animal gastroenterology. 3rd ed. Philadelphia: Saunders, 1996:451–486.

Tams TR. Feline inflammatory bowel disease. *Vet Clin North Am* 1993;23.

IVM references

Joos S, Rosemann T, Szecsenyi J, Hahn E, Willich S, Brinkhaus B. Use of complementary and alternative medicine in Germany—a survey of patients with inflammatory bowel disease. *BMC Complement Altern Med.* 2006; May 22;6:p 19.

Langhorst J, Anthonisen IB, Steder-Neukamm U, Ludtke R, Spahn G, Michalsen A, Dobos GJ. Amount of systemic steroid medication is a strong predictor for the use of complementary and alternative medicine in patients with inflammatory bowel disease: results from a German national survey. *Inflamm Bowel Dis.* 2005 Mar;11(3):pp 287–95.

Silver R. Leaky Gut Syndrome. In: Proceedings of the American Holistic Veterinary Medical Association annual meeting, Durham, NC, 2003. pp 97–110.

Nutrition references

Belluzzi A, Brignola C, Campieri M, et al. Effect of an enteric-coated fish-oil preparation on relapses in Crohn's disease. *N Engl J Med* 1996;334:1557–60.

Bouic PJD, et al. Beta-sitosterol and beta-sitosterol glucoside stimulate human peripheral blood lymphocyte proliferation: Implications for their use as an immunomodulatory vitamin combination. *International Journal of Immunopharmacology,* 1996;18:693–700.

Golden BR, Gorbach SL. The Effect of Milk and Lactobacillus Feeding on Human Intestinal Bacteria Activity. *Am. J. of Clin. Nutr.,* 1984;39: 756–61.

Goldstein R, Goldstein S. The Goldstein Wellness and Longevity Program, 2005. Neptune City, NJ: TFH Publication .

Gupta MB, Nath R, Srivastava N, et al. Anti-inflammatory and antipyretic activities of β-sitosterol. *Planta Medica* 1980; 39:157–163.

Mate J, Castanos R, Garcia-Samaniego J, Pajares JM. Does dietary fish oil maintain the remission of Crohn's disease: a case control study. *Gastroenterology* 1991;100:A228 [abstract].

McDonough FE, Hitchins AD, Wong NP, et al. Modification of sweet acidophilus milk to improve utilization by lactose-intolerant persons. *Am J Clin Nutr* 1987;45:570–4.

Perdigon GN, de Masius N, Alvarez S, et al. Enhancement of Immune Response in Mice fed with S. Thermophilus and L. Acidophilus, *J. of Dairy Sci.,* 1987;70: 919–926.

Souba W, et al. Glutamine metabolism in the intestinal tract: invited review, *JPEN,* 1985 9:608–617.

Windmueller HG. Glutamine utilization by the small intestine, *Adv. Enzymol,* 1982 53:201–237.

Yoshimura K, et al. Effects of enteral glutamine administration on experimental inflammatory bowel disease, *JPEN,* 1993; 17:235.

Chinese herbal medicine/acupuncture references

Chang Yong Zhong Yao Cheng Fen Yu Yao Li Shou Ce (A Handbook of the Composition and Pharmacology of Common Chinese Drugs), 1994; 739:742.

Fu Jian Zhong Yi Yao (*Fujian Chinese Medicien and Herbology*), 1985;1:36.

Huang Y. Sheng Ma's effects on advanced inflammation. *Journal of Chinese Materia Medica.* 1992;23(6):288.

Hwang YC, Jenkins EM. Effect of acupuncture on young pigs with induced enterpathogenic Escherichia coli diarrhea. *Am J Vet Res,* 1988 49:1641–1643.

Li YF (translator). *Foreign Medicine, vol. of TCM.* 1984;6(1): 15–18.

Liu CH, et al. The pharmacology of Tao Ren. *Journal of Pharmacology and Clinical Application of TCM.* 1989;(2):46–47.

Liu W, et al. *Henan Journal of TCM Pharmacy.* 1998;13(4): 10–12.

Ma XS, et al. *New Journal of Digestive Diseases.* 1996; 4(11):603–604.

Ma YB. Zhi Qiao's effects on gastroinstestinal movement. *Journal of Pharmacology of Clinical Application of TCM.* 1996;12(6): 28–29.

Si Chuan Yi Xue Yuan Xue Bao (*Journal of Sichuan School of Medicine*), 1959;1:102.

Wang SP, et al. Tao Ren extract's effect in suppressing filter bed fibroblasts hyperplasia in subjects of experimental trabeculae dissection. *Journal of Shanghai Medical University.* 1993; 20(1):35–381.

Xi Xue Xue Bao (*Academic Journal of Medicine*), 1988;23(10): 721.

Yao Xue Za Zhi (*Journal of Medicinals*), 1981, 101(10):883.

Zhang SC, et al. *Journal of Chinese Patent Medicine Research.* 1984;(2):37.

Zhong Cao Yao (*Chinese Herbal Medicine*) 1991;22 (10): 452.

Zhong Yao Tong Bao (*Journal of Chinese Herbology*), 1986; 11 (11):37.

Zhong Yao Xue (*Chinese Herbology*), 1988; 326:327.

Zhong Yao Xue (*Chinese Herbology*), 1998;140:144.

Zhong Yao Yao Li Yu Ying Yong (*Pharmacology and Applications of Chinese Herbs*), 1983;567.

Zhong Yao Zhi (*Chinese Herbology Journal*), 1984;37.

Zhong Yao Zhi (*Chinese Herbology Journal*), 1993;358.

Zhonzxin X: Clinical observation of 500 cases with pediatric diarrhea treated by acupuncture. *Chin Acupuncture and Moxibustion* 9:10, 1989.

Zhou WZ, et al. *Pharmacy Bulletin.* 1979;14(5):202–203.

Zhu NLF, et al. Chinese Herbs and Immunity. *Foreign Medicine (TCM vol).* 1984;(1):47.

Homotoxicology references

Broadfoot PJ. Inflammation: Homotoxicology and Healing. In: Proceedings AHVMA/Heel Homotoxicology Seminar. Denver, CO, 2004. p 27.

Boericke W. Materia Medica with Repertory, 9th ed. Santa Rosa, CA: Boericke and Tafel, 1927. pp 90, 497–500.

Demers J. Homotoxicology and Acupuncture. In: Proceedings of the 2004 Homotoxicology Seminar. AHVMA/Heel. Denver, CO, 2004. p 5, 6.

Deng X, Yin F, Lu X, Cai B, Yin W. The apoptotic effect of brucine from the seed of Strychnos nux-vomica on human hepatoma cells is mediated via Bcl-2 and Ca2+ involved mitochondrial pathway. *Toxicol Sci.* 2006;May;91(1):pp 59–69.

Gebhardt R. Antioxidative, antiproliferative and biochemical effects in HepG2 cells of a homeopathic remedy and its constituent plant tinctures tested separately or in combination. *Arzneimittelforschung.* 2003. 53(12): pp 823–30.

Heel. BHI Homeopathic Therapy: Professional Reference. Albuquerque, NM: Heel Inc., 2002. pp 43, 47, 73.

Macleod G. A Veterinary Materia Medica and Clinical Repertory with a Materia Medica of the Nosodes. Safron, Walden: CW Daniel Company, LTD., 1983. pp 50–1, 125–6, 129–30.

Reckeweg, H. Biotherapeutic Index: Ordinatio Antihomotoxica et Materia Medica, 5th ed. Baden-Baden, Germany: Biologische Heilmittel Heel GMBH, 2000 pp 290, 294–5, 300, 329–30, 358–9, 363–4, 366–7, 369, 381, 390, 399–400, 432, 538.

Reckeweg H. Homeopathia Antihomotoxica Materia Medica, 4th edition. Baden-Baden, Germany: Arelia-Verlag GMBH, , 2002 pp. 136–8, 139–40, 125–6, 147, 150–3, 179, 206, 241–2, 317–19, 345, 366, 461–3, 488–90, 578–80.

Simpson K, Dogan B, Rishniw M, Goldstein R, Klaessig S, McDonough P, German A, Yates R, Russell D, Johnson S, Berg DE, Harel J, Bruant G, McDonough S, Schukken Y. Adherent and invasive Escherichia coli is associated with granulomatous colitis in boxer dogs. *Infect Immun.* 2006;Aug;74(8):pp 4778–92.

Van Wassenhoven M. Towards an evidence-based repertory: clinical evaluation of Veratrum album. *Homeopathy.* 2004; Apr;93(2): pp 71–7.

INTERNAL PARASITES: COCCIDIA/GIARDIA/ROUNDWORM/HOOKWORM/WHIPWORM/TAPEWORM

Definition and cause

This section covers the more common intestinal parasitic conditions: ancylostomiasis, ascariasis, cestodiasis, coccidiosis, giardiasis, and tricuriasis. Predisposing causes include eating infested rodents, transmission via flea bites or from maternal passage, egg-contaminated environment, and ingestion of fecal-contaminated food or water. Stress and immune system status play a part in the clinical signs associated with the infestation. Hemorrhagic enteritis, bronchial coughing, malabsorption, weight loss, and death are associated with immunosuppressed puppies and kittens (Barr 1994, Bowman 1992, Corwin 2003, Georgi 1992, Sherding 1994, Soulsby 1982).

Medical therapy rationale, drug(s) of choice, and nutritional recommendations

Therapy includes hygiene, flea control, and parasiticides such as albendazole, dichlorvos, fenbendazole, ivermectin, metronidazole, milbemycin oxime, pyrantel pamoate, and sulfadimethoxine. In addition, fluid replacement therapy as well as medication to help stop intestinal hemorrhage and diarrhea are often necessary (Barr 1998, Bowman 1992, Corwin 2003, Sherding 1994).

Anticipated prognosis

Prognosis is dependent upon the dog or cat's clinical state. In most instances repeated medical treatment is curative. The prognosis is more guarded with immunosuppressed animals.

Integrative veterinary therapies

Mucosal surface immunity is important, and parasitism may become harder to eliminate in cases of immunosuppression. This is seen commonly in coccidiosis. Because medication does not kill the parasite directly, but rather slows its reproductive rate while the immune system eradicates the infection, clinicians should suspect either environmental cleanliness issues and reinfection or immune suppression in cases that fail normal therapy. Addressing the immune system and gut terrain may cause the parasite to disappear without treatment in some cases, indicating the importance of normal host defenses, but in clinical practice it is usually desirable to simply treat the parasite and the terrain, and then allow the body to repair and heal.

Both treatment and prevention are needed. Prevention involves practicing good animal husbandry. Proper hygiene, proper diet, and environmental cleanliness are critical to prevention of parasites. Clients benefit from instruction in the zoonotic nature of parasites and may clean up after their pets more conscientiously if they understand the health issues of routine parasitism. Routinely deworming dams and queens prior to delivery may help, and regular parasite evaluations and treatment are indicated for juveniles as part of the pediatric healthcare program. Modern medications are quite safe and effective in handling most simple parasitic issues. Drugs need to be repeated at appropriate intervals according to good medical practice and clients must clean up the home environment and treat other animals in the household to reduce repeated infection. The efficacy of some medications may be enhanced through integrative practice. For example, metronidazole against Giardia has improved efficacy when it is used in combination with milk thistle extract (silymarin) (Chon 2005).

Some drugs, such as metronidazole and sulfa types, are more likely to cause adverse reactions. These can encompass many different presentations and they are often missed as causative agents in other disease syndromes. Human medicine is beginning to document reactions that occur later in life and are associated with hypersensitivities to other drugs. Veterinarians need to become more aware of this situation and carefully observe the pharmaceutical histories of their patients. Such reactions may appear suddenly, as in pancreatitis and polyarthritis, and may not be associated with the correct causation during initial diagnostic evaluation (Juang 2006). Reckeweg warned of sulfa drugs' potential to damage the body many years ago and included homeopathically diluted pharmaceuticals in his therapy recommendations.

Side effects can occur from conventional drugs as well as from herbal preparations, and clinicians should become well versed in adverse effects associated with antiparasitic agents commonly prescribed in their offices. Reference materials and poison control should be consulted if an interaction or adverse effect is suspected.

A final note concerns the increasingly common practice of feeding raw meat to pets. Miraculous therapeutic results can occur in pets fed raw meat diets; however, clients need to be carefully instructed on their selection and preparation. Many meats are parasite-contaminated, especially wild fish and game, and should be avoided (Martini 1992). In endemic areas, Echinococcus infection and disease results from feeding raw viscera to pets. Appropriate care should be used in feeding raw diets, and routinely deworming pets on these diets is a sensible strategy. If a pet is doing well on a raw diet and suddenly

begins to destabilize, routine deworming with a broad-spectrum agent is advised and can cause a remarkable improvement. Because both processed, commercial diets and homemade diets can contain homotoxins, clinicians should know what diet their patients are eating and keep this in mind when diagnosing current health issues.

The integration of nutrients, nutraceuticals, medicinal herbs, and combination homeopathics that are anti-inflammatory and cell-protective can help improve immunity as well as cellular function after parasite removal.

Nutrition
General considerations/rationale
See the IVM explanation above for more in-depth information. Because worming medications are generally safe and effective, nutritional support focuses on reducing intestinal inflammation as well as general support of the immune system.

Appropriate nutrients
Nutrition/gland therapy: Glandular intestine, adrenal, thymus, and lymph help to neutralize a cellular immune attack, and protect and spare the intestines from ongoing inflammation and eventual degeneration (see Chapter 2, Gland Therapy, for additional information).

Colostrum: Colostrum has been shown to improve intestinal health. It helps to balance intestinal flora and improve digestion. One important point raised in the IVM discussion above is the status of the immune system in relation to the presence of intestinal parasites. Colostrum has been found to improve the immune status of the intestinal tract which can, via intestinal production of globulins, help the overall immune competency of the body (Blake 1999).

Probiotics: Administration of the proper combination of probiotics has been reported to have a positive impact on the intestines and the digestive process (Goldin 1984, Perdigon 1987). Probiotics have been shown to improve and aid the digestive process by secreting their own source of enzymes (McDonough 1987).

Chinese herbal medicine/acupuncture
General considerations/rationale
Intestinal parasites are considered external pathogens by practitioners of TCM, just as they are by Western-trained doctors.

Appropriate Chinese herbs
Betel nut (Bing Lang): Was shown to be 61% successful in expelling roundworms from 26 human patients when given along with omphalia (Lei wan) (Jiang Su Zhong Yi Za Zhi 1960). It also was shown to clear hookworms in 24 patients when given along with pumpkin seed (Nan

gua zi) (Zhong Hua Yi Xue Za Zhi 1957). The efficacy against tapeworms in dogs, cows, and pigs was proven in a more recent study (Zhe Jiang Yi Ke Da Xue Xue Bao 1980, Zhong Hua Yi Xue Za Zhi 1956).

Brucea seed (Ya Dan zi): Contains 2 compounds, bruceantin and burceine C, which have demonstrated efficacy against the protozoa Entamoeba histolitica in humans (Wright 1986). It was used in 65 patients with amoebic dysentery with a 94% success rate (Zhong Yi Za Zhi 1956).

Dichroa root (Chang Shan): Has significant antiamoebic effects (Wu Han Yi Xue Yuan Xue Bao 1958).

Garlic (Da Suan): Prevents the eggs of intestinal parasites from developing into larvae (Bastidas 1969).

Melia root (Ku lian pi): Paralyzes intestinal parasites. Once the parasites can no longer move, normal intestinal peristalsis removes them from the body (Sheng Li Xue Bao 1958). As an additional benefit, melia also increases intestinal peristalsis (Zhong Yao Yao Li Yu Ying Yong 1983). In one study, 94% of 4,757 people with roundworms were successfully treated with melia root. However, at high levels (1.8 g to 3.6 g), one-third reported side effects which were unpleasant but not fatal, and included headaches, nausea, vomiting, diarrhea, abdominal pain, blurry vision, dizziness, and numb extremities (Zhong Hua Nei Ke Za Zhi 1962).

Mume (Wu Mei): Inhibits the movement of roundworms (Chang Yong Zhong Yao Xian Dai Yan Jiu Yu Lin Chuan 1995), which may make it easier for the body to eliminate the parasites. 70% of treated patients cleared hookworms in one study (Zhong Yi Za Zhi 1959).

Omphalia (Lei wan): Clears tapeworms and roundworms as demonstrated in multiple trials (Zhong Hua Yi Xue Za Zhi 1956, Zhong Yao Yao Li Yu Ying Yong 1983). In addition, omphalia (Lei wan) was 100% effective for treating hookworm in 188 human patients when given along with Da Huang and Qian niu zi (Zhong Ji Yi Kan 1960). Lie wan powder was 85% effective (Shang Hai Zhong Yi Yao Za Zhi 1957).

Pulsatilla (Bai tou Weng): Demonstrated 100% efficacy in treating 26 human patients with amoebic dysentery (Wu Han Yi Xue Yuan Xue Bao 1958).

Rhubarb (Da huang): Contains sennoside A, aloeemodin, and rhein, which cause defecation to help eliminate the parasites the other herbs paralyze. It increases peristalsis in the large intestine, but does not interfere with absorption of nutrients in the small intestine (Zhong Yao Xue 1998).

Homotoxicology
General considerations/rationale
Internal parasitism is a common veterinary condition and constitutes Deposition Phase disease, which may rapidly undergo regressive vicariation to Inflammation and Excre-

tion phases in some instances (Miro 2006). Some parasites may cause severe disruption, leading to a Degeneration Phase (*Echinococcus*), and recovery following these diseases may be negatively affected by damage to functional tissues. The majority of puppies have ascarids, and coccidia are commonly encountered in both cats and dogs (Hoskins, Malone, Smith 1982).

Acariasis may potentiate canine parvovirus morbidity and mortality in puppies through immunosuppression caused by the release of homotoxins (Faquim-Mauro, Macedo 1998). In this situation, an unknown, subclinical Deposition Phase homotoxicosis undergoes progressive vicariation after exposure to the virus. Many parasites constitute zoonotic diseases, and every veterinary clinic should institute effective preventative strategies for the parasites that are commonly seen in their locale. To fail to properly perform this function leaves a large percentage of patients in the Deposition Phase; it is a short trip to the other side of the biological divide and the Impregnation Phase, where natural recovery is less likely. Both humans and animals benefit from such programs.

Parasites produce agents that are harmful to local cellular function and inhibit local immunity (Troeger, et al. 2006). These homotoxins and the body's response generate a wide array of pathology. Upon the death or removal of parasites, Excretion Phase diarrhea may result as the body attempts elimination of these undesirable materials. Such cases of diarrhea are generally handled by simple methods as discussed in the Diarrhea protocol section of this text. Chronic parasitism can damage vital GI function, as in the case of Giardia, which is well known to create a thickening of the small intestine with correspondingly poor absorption (Scott, et al. 2003).

Malabsorptive diarrhea can result. Heavy infestations of ascarids can decrease bowel wall integrity and lead to "leaky gut syndrome." Trichuris vulpis, the whipworm, is frequently associated with colitis signs. Because this parasite damages the colon by inserting itself into the wall, it creates a mild Impregnation Phase disease and compromises mucosal integrity. These cases generally return to normal after eliminating the parasites and allowing time to heal the damage. Finally, parasites can be associated with intestinal obstruction and static bowel syndrome, and may contribute to the development of intussusception in juveniles, a Degeneration Phase disorder requiring surgical repair.

Appropriate homotoxicology formulas
Nux vomica homaccord: Treats liver and gastrointestinal disease. It is a commonly used formula for detoxification as part of the Detox Kit.

Tanacet-Heel: Treats complications following removal of helminths, gastroenteritis, dysentery, gas, and pain following ascarids, especially in juvenile pets.

Traumeel: Has an anti-inflammatory effect and activates blocked enzymes.

Authors' suggested protocols

Nutrition

Intestinal/IBD and immune support formulas: 1 tablet for every 25 pounds of body weight BID.

Colostrum: One-third teaspoon of powdered formula for every 25 pounds of body weight BID.

Probiotic MPF: One-half capsule per 25 pounds of body weight with food.

Chinese herbal medicine/acupuncture

For roundworms, whipworms, tapeworms, and coccidian, the veterinarian may choose H92 Dewormer—round, whip, tape, coccidian. This formula contains betel nut (Bing Lang), melia root (Ku lian pi), mume fruit (Wu Mei), omphalia (Lei wan), and rhubarb (Da huang). It also contains coptis (Huang lian) and saussurea (Mu xiang) to increase efficacy.

For tapeworms or hookworms, the veterinarian may use H93 Dewormer—tapeworm, hookworm, which contains garlic (Da suan) and betel nut (Bing lang).

For coccidian and giardia, H94 Dewormer—coccidia, giardia is appropriate. This formula contains brucea seed (Ya dan zi), dichroa root (Chang Shan), and pulsatilla (Bai tou weng). In addition, it contains bupleurum (Chai hu), citrus (Chen pi), sargentodoxa vine (Hong teng) and saussurea (Mu xiang) to increase the efficacy of the cited herbs.

The dose of these herbs is 1 capsule per 10 pounds a day for 10 to 14 days.

Homotoxicology (Dose: 10 drops PO for 50-pound dog; 5 drops PO for cat or small dog)

For intestinal parasites (coccidia, giardia, roundworms, hookworms, whipworms, and tapeworms), deworm with proper conventional drugs. Treat symptoms according to the condition that is manifested (see protocols for vomiting, enteritis, diarrhea, colitis, etc.). Tanacet, Traumeel S, and Nux vomica homaccord mixed together and used orally TID is useful for parasitic colic and difficulties following removal of parasites.

Product sources

Nutrition

Intestinal/IBD and immune support formulas: Animal Nutrition Technologies. **Alternatives**: Immune System Support—Standard Process Veterinary Formulas; Immuno Support—Rx Vitamins for Pets; Immugen—Thorne Veterinary Products; Enteric Support—Standard Process Veterinary Formulas; NutriGest—Rx Vitamins for Pets.

Colostrum: New Life Foods, Inc., Saskatoon Colostrum Company.

Probiotic MPF: Progressive Labs.

Chinese herbal medicine

Formula H92, 93, 94: Natural Solutions, Inc.

Homotoxicology

BHI/Heel Corporation

REFERENCES

Western medicine references

Barr SC, Bowman DD. Giardiasis in dogs and cats. Compendium on Continuing Education for the Practicing Veterinarian. 1994;16(5):603–614.

Barr SC, Bowman DD, Frongillo MF, Joseph SL. Efficacy of a drug combination of praziquantel, pyrantel pamoate, and febental against giardiasis in dogs. *American Journal of Veterinary Research*. 1998;59(1):1134–1136.

Bowman DD. Hookworm parasites of dogs and cats. *Comp Contin Educ Pract Vet* 1992;14(5):585–595.

Corwin RM. In: Tilley L, Smith F. The 5-Minute Veterinary Consult: Canine and Feline, 2003. Blackwell Publishing.

Barr JR, Georgi ME. Canine Clinical Parasitology. Philadelphia: Lea and Febiger. 1992;59–61.

Georgi JR, Georgi ME. Canine Clinical Parasitology. Philadelphia: Lea and Febiger. 1992;153–160.

Sherding RG, Johnson SE. Diseases of the intestine. In Birchard SJ, Sherding RG., eds. Saunders Manual of Small Animal Practice. Philadelphia: WB Saunders Co. 1994;699–700.

Soulsby EJL. Helminths, arthropods and protozoa of domesticated animals. Philadelphia: Lea and Febiger. 1982;577–580.

IVM references

Chon S, Kim N. Evaluation of silymarin in the treatment on asymptomatic Giardia infections in dogs. *Parasitol Res.* 2005 Dec;97(6):pp 445–51.

Juang P, Page RL 2nd, Zolty R. Probable loop diuretic-induced pancreatitis in a sulfonamide-allergic patient. *Ann Pharmacother.* 2006 Jan;40(1):128–34.

Martini M, Poglayen G, Minerva N, Zanangeli A. A study of factors influencing intestinal parasites in dogs. *Ann 1st Super Sanita.* 1992;28(4):pp 477–84.

Troeger H, Epple HJ, Schneider T, Wahnschaffe U, Ullrich R, Burchard GD, Jelinek T, Zeitz M, Fromm M, Schulzke JD. Effect of chronic Giardia lamblia infection on epithelial transport and barrier function in human duodenum. *Gut.* 2006 Aug 25; [Epub abstract ahead of print].

Nutrition references

Blake SR. Bovine Colostrum, The Forgotten Miracle. *Journal of the American Holistic Veterinary Medical Association.* July 1999, Volume 18, Number 2, pp 38–39.

Golden BR, Gorbach SL. The Effect of Milk and Lactobacillus Feeding on Human Intestinal Bacteria Activity. *Am. J. of Clin. Nutr.*, 1984 39: 756–61.

McDonough FE, Hitchins AD, Wong NP, et al. Modification of sweet acidophilus milk to improve utilization by lactose-intolerant persons. *Am J Clin Nutr* 1987;45:570–4.

Perdigon GN, de Masius N, Alvarez S, et al. Enhancement of Immune Response in Mice fed with S. Thermophilus and L. Acidophilus, *J. of Dairy Sci.*, 1987 70: 919–926.

Chinese herbal medicine/acupuncture references

Bastidas GJ. Effect of ingested garlic on Necator americanus and Ancylostoma caninum. *Am. J. Trop. Med. Hyg.* 1969 18(6): 920–923.

Chang Yong Zhong Yao Xian Dai Yan Jiu Yu Lin Chuan (*Recent Study and Clinical Application of Common Traditional Chinese Medicine*), 1995; 669:672.

Jiang Su Zhong Yi Za Zhi (*Jiangsu Journal of Chinese Medicine*), 1960;(5):30.

Shang Hai Zhong Yi Yao Za Zhi (*Shanghai Journal of Chinese Medicine and Herbology*), 1957;5:22.

Sheng Li Xue Bao (*Physiology News*), 1958; 22(1):18.

Wright CW, O'Neill MJ, Phillipson, JD and Warhurst DC. Use of microdilution to assess in vitro antiamoebic activities of Brucea javanica fruits, Simarouba amara stem, and a number of quassinoids. *Antimicrob Agents Chemother.* 1988 November; 32(11): 1725–1729.

Wu Han Yi Xue Yuan Xue Bao (*Journal of Wuhan University School of Medicine*), 1958;1:11.

Zhe Jiang Yi Ke Da Xue Xue Bao (*Journal of Zhejiang Province School of Medicine*),1980;9(1):1.

Zhong Hua Nei Ke Za Zhi (*Chinese Journal of Internal Medicine*), 1962;8:491.

Zhong Hua Yi Xue Za Zhi (*Chinese Journal of Medicine*), 1956;6:556.

Zhong Hua Yi Xue Za Zhi (*Chinese Journal of Medicine*), 1956;42(2):138.

Zhong Hua Yi Xue Za Zhi (*Chinese Journal of Medicine*), 1957;43(5):371.

Zhong Ji Yi Kan (*Medium Medical Journal*), 1960;7:35.

Zhong Yao Xue (*Chinese Herbology*), 1998; 251:256.

Zhong Yao Yao Li Yu Ying Yong (*Pharmacology and Applications of Chinese Herbs*); 1983;648.

Zhong Yao Yao Li Yu Ying Yong (*Pharmacology and Applications of Chinese Herbs*); 1983;1184.

Zhong Yi Za Zhi (*Journal of Chinese Medicine*), 1956;1:16.

Zhong Yi Za Zhi (*Journal of Chinese Medicine*), 1959;(3):153.

Homotoxicology references

Faquim-Mauro E, Macedo M. The immunosuppressive activity of Ascaris suum is due to high molecular weight components. *Clin Exp Immunol.* 1998 Nov;114(2):pp 245–51.

Hoskins J, Malone J, Smith P. Prevalence of parasitism diagnosed by fecal examination in Louisiana dogs. *Am J Vet Res.* 1982 Jun;43(6):pp 1106–9.

Miro G, Mateo M, Montoya A, Vela E, Calonge R. Survey of intestinal parasites in stray dogs in the Madrid area and comparison of the efficacy of three anthelmintics in naturally infected dogs. *Parasitol Res.* 2006 Aug 17; [Epub ahead of print].

Scott K, Meddings J, Kirk D, Lees-Miller S, Buret A. Intestinal infection with Giardia spp. reduces epithelial barrier function in a myosin light chain kinase-dependent fashion. *Gastroenterology.* 2002 Oct;123(4):pp 1179–90.

MEGAESOPHAGUS

Definition and cause

Megaesophagus is a dilation of the esophagus, which may be inherited and primary or secondary to other conditions such as myasthenia gravis or a primary neuropathy. The causes may be secondary to esophageal obstruction (foreign body, neoplasia etc.), inflammation, an infectious condition affecting the esophagus, or secondary to other primary diseases such as hypothyroid or hypoadrenocorticism (Guilford 1990, Twedt 1995). The loss of neuromuscular control leads to hypomotility and a ballooning of the esophagus.

Medical therapy rationale, drug(s) of choice, and nutritional recommendations

The underlying cause should be determined once megaesophagus has been diagnosed. While no specific therapy exists for the condition, control can be achieved via feeding calorically dense food from an elevated position. If the underlying cause is determined to be genetic, then advising against further breeding is indicated. Surgery is indicated for blockages and to improve tone; however, motility is not improved surgically. Drugs to quiet inflammation, such as sucralfate, may be recommended. Medication may also be required for secondary conditions such as treating myasthenia gravis or neuropathies with corticosteroids (Jenkins 1996).

Anticipated prognosis

Control can often be achieved with dietary and feeding support. Prognosis is often poor or guarded when no support is given or when there are serious underlying disease causes (Leib 1993, Longshore 2003).

Integrative veterinary therapies

Most cases involve dogs, but feline cases are reported (van Geffen, et al. 2006). Several issues can lead to esophageal dysfunction, and these include hereditary disease and acquired conditions involving the muscle or nerve constituents of the esophagus. A full medical evaluation should be recommended. Once a complete diagnosis has been reached, the client can be informed of recommended treatment options (Wray, Sparkes 2006). In most cases there are only limited options such as feeding a gruel-consistency diet from a raised tray and keeping the head elevated for 10 minutes following feeding, or using parental feeding through external feeding tubes. Aspiration pneumonia is a common complication due to esophageal reflux of material.

While no clinical trials exist, a combination of therapeutic nutrients along with acupuncture and herbal and biological therapies can often improve the animal's condition and day-to-day quality of life.

Nutrition
General considerations/rationale
Besides dietary support (as listed above), nutrition is focused upon improving smooth muscle function, nerve function, and muscle contractibility, as well as reducing the secondary symptoms and inflammation often associated with the disease.

Appropriate nutrients
Nutritional/gland therapy: Glandular esophagus/stomach and nerve can help improve functions and neutralize cellular immune-mediated inflammation in spinal nerves, esophagus, and stomach. In addition, gland therapy supplies specific intrinsic nutrients required for stomach and esophageal cellular health (see Chapter 2, Gland Therapy, for more detailed information).

Note: Because megaesophagus can affect the entire body, it is recommended that blood be analyzed both medically and physiologically to determine associated organ involvement or disease. This allows for a more specific gland and nutritional support protocol for the patient (see Nutritional Blood Testing, Chapter 2).

Glutamine: Glutamine has been shown to improve immune function and is beneficial for the cells of the gastro-intestinal tract (Souba 1985, Windmueller 1982, Yoshimura 1993).

Magnesium: Magnesium has also been associated with neuromuscular function and conditions such as muscle cramping, weakness, and neuromuscular dysfunction. Magnesium is recommended for weakening muscle function (Bibley 1996, Levin 2002).

Lecithin/phosphatidyl choline: Phosphatidyl choline is a phospholipid that is integral to cellular membranes particularly those of nerve and brain cells. It helps to move fats into the cells, and is involved with acetylcholine uptake, neurotransmission, and cellular integrity. As part of the cell membranes, lecithin is an essential nutrient required by all cells of the body for general health and wellness (Hanin 1987).

Chinese herbal medicine/acupuncture
General considerations/rationale
According to TCM, megaesophagus is the result of Qi deficiency and Stagnation with Phlegm accumulation in the Middle Burner, affecting the Stomach and Spleen. Megaesophagus is a deficiency of energy or strength (Qi).

In terms of gastrointestinal signs, the animal does not have the strength to digest food, leading to the accumulation of Phlegm. In this case the term Phlegm refers to the liquid ingesta in the gastrointestinal tract as well as the interference with normal digestion. According to the traditional Chinese medicine system, the Stomach and Spleen are both involved with digestion. The Spleen is easily obstructed by excess liquid (or Phlegm) and becomes unable to function correctly. The normal flow of ingesta through the gastrointestinal tract is disrupted, resulting in vomiting.

Appropriate Chinese herbs
Atractylodes (Bai zhu): Was shown to exhibit excellent antineoplastic effects against esophageal cancer in vitro studies (Zhong Liu Yu Zhi Tong Xun 1976).

Astragalus (Huang qi): Has been shown to inhibit some tumors (Shi 1999). It may be of use in neoplastic etiologies of megaesophagus.

Cyperus seeds (Xiang fu zi): Stops stomach cramping (Zhong Cao Yao Fang Ji De Ying Yong 1976).

Ginseng (Ren shen): May be effective in treating megaesophagus secondary to hypoadrenocorticism or hypothyroidism. As rats age, their plasma T3, T4 cortisol levels decrease. Ginseng is able to reverse this trend (Shi 1998).

Licorice (Gan cao): Contains glycyrrhizin and glycyrrhetinic acid, which have anti-inflammatory effects. They have approximately 10% of the corticosteroid activity of cortisone (Zhong Cao Yao 1991). This may be equivalent to using low-dose steroid therapy. It may be especially useful for megaesophagus secondary to hypoadreoncoriticism.

Pinellia (Ban xia): Can inhibit the growth of tumor cell strain K_{562} (Wu 1996). If it has efficacy against other neoplasias it may be useful for cancerous causes of megaesophagus.

Poria (Fu ling): Contains pachman, which has antineoplastic activity (Zhou 1982). In one experiment it was shown to be very effective at inhibiting Sarcoma 180 tumors in mice (Chen 1986), which suggests that it may help control tumors leading to megaesophagus.

Pueraria (Ge gen): Has anticancer effects. It has been shown to inhibit HL-60, an acute myeloid leukemia cell line (Modern TCM Pharmacology 1997).

Acupuncture
Chang et al. (1996) demonstrated that acupuncture could affect the muscular contraction of the normal esophagus. It may be of use in promoting the contraction in patients with megaesophagus.

Homotoxicology
General considerations/rationale
Megaespophagus represents a Degeneration Phase homotoxicosis that is often frustrating to treat, and not generally curable.

No written record could be located of any successful antihomotoxic treatment, but Broadfoot reports treating one case with apparent clinical improvement. Because these agents are generally safe, it makes sense to try a course of therapy and see what response, if any, occurs. Professionals are encouraged to share their experiences in this regard with the authors.

Appropriate homotoxicology formulas

Coenzyme compositum: Contains Citricum acidum, which is useful for dental problems and gingivitis; scurvy; blackening of teeth and heavy deposits of dental plaque; painful, herpetic vesicles around the lips; nausea; painful cramping in the umbilical area, and distension.

Galium-Heel: Used for all cellular phases, hemorrhoids, and anal fissures, and as a detoxicant.

Gastricumeel: Treats acute gastritis. Contains Antimonium crudum, which is indicated for tooth decay and toothache, and thus, may be useful when dental work is indicated (Reckeweg 2002).

Gelsemium homaccord: Used for muscle weakness and in support of cervical and cranial neural issues.

Lymphomyosot: Provides lymph drainage and endocrine support, and treats edema.

Myelin Sheath Nosode: Provides direct support of tissues involved in neurological weakness.

Neuro-Injeel: Contains broadly active ingredients that are supportive of neurological tissues (Reckeweg 2000).

Placenta compositum: Contains Plumbum metalicum, which is indicated for atonic paresis and muscular atrophy, particularly in megaesophagus.

Ubichinon compositum: Contains Anthraquinone for swelling of the gums and GI symptoms such as distention, flatulence, and cramping abdominal pain. Treats constipation with straining or sudden diarrhea (Reckeweg 2002).

Authors' suggested protocols

Nutrition

Esophagus/stomach support formula: 1 tablet for every 25 pounds of body weight BID.

Glutimmune: One-fourth scoop per 25 pounds of body weight daily.

Lecithin/phosphatidyl choline: One-fourth teaspoon for every 25 pounds of body weight BID.

Magnesium: 10 mg for every 10 pounds of body weight SID.

Chinese herbal medicine/acupuncture

The patent formula Ding Chen Tou Ge Tang may be used for the regurgitation. In addition to the herbs cited above, this formula contains agaste (Huo xiang), amomum fruit (Sha ren), aquilaria (Chen xiang), blue citrus (Qing pi), Chinese eaglewood (Chen xiang), citrus (Chen pi), cloves (Ding xiang), leaven (Shen qu), lindera (Wu yao), magnolia bark (Hou po), malt (Mai ya), massa fermentata (Shen qu), nutmeg seeds (Rou dou kou), ophiopogon (Mai men dong), round cardamon (Bai dou kou), tsaoko fruit (Cao guo), and white peony (Bai shao). These additional herbs increase the efficacy of the formula. The supplement is dosed to the supplier's directions.

Acupuncture points: The authors are not aware of any well-controlled studies to evaluate the efficacy of acupuncture in patients with megaesophagus. The following points are suggested points based upon TCM theory: PC6, BL17, CV22, CV23, and CV17.

Homotoxicology (Dose: 10 drops PO for 50-pound dog; 5 drops PO for cat or small dog)

This advanced degenerative condition is not generally responsive to therapy. Consider the following after advising clients of its experimental nature:

Injection therapy: Placenta compositum, Coenzyme compositum, Neuro-Injeel vials given by injection twice weekly.

Oral therapy: Lymphomyosot, Galium-Heel, Myelin Sheath nosode, Gastricumeel, and Spascupreel mixed together and given orally BID to TID. Consider Gelsemium homaccord orally BID in addition to the above.

Product sources

Nutrition

Esophagus/stomach support formulas: Animal Nutrition Technologies.

Glutimmune: Well Wisdom. **Alternative**: L-Glutamine powder—Thorne Veterinary Products.

Lecithin/phosphatidyl choline: Designs for Health.

Magnesium: Over the counter.

Chinese herbal medicine

Ding Chen Tou Ge Tang: May be special ordered through Mayway Company.

Homotoxicology

BHI/Heel Corporation

REFERENCES

Western medicine references

Guilford WG. Megaesophagus in the dog and cat. *Semin Vet Med Surg (Small Anim)* 1990;5:37–45.

Jenkins CC, Mears EA. What's new in the diagnosis and management of megaesophagus. ACVIM. Proceedings of the 14th Annual Vet. Med. Forum, 1996, p. 585–586.

Leib MS. Megaesophagus. In: Bojrab MJ, ed. Disease mechanisms in small animal surgery. 2nd ed. Philadelphia: Lea and Febiger, 1993, 205–209.

Longshore RC. Megaesophagus. In: Tilley L, Smith F. The 5-Minute Veterinary Consult: Canine and Feline, 2003. Blackwell Publishing.

Twedt DC. Diseases of the esophagus. In: Ettinger EJ, Feldman EC, eds. Textbook of Veterinary Internal Medicine. Toronto: WB Saunders Co. 1995 pp.1124–1142.

IVM references

van Geffen C, Saunders JH, Vandevelde B, Van Ham L, Hoybergs Y, Daminet S. Idiopathic megaoesophagus and intermittent gastro-oesophageal intussusception in a cat. *J Small Anim Pract.* 2006 Aug;47(8):pp 471–5.

Wray JD, Sparkes AH. Use of radiographic measurements in distinguishing myasthenia gravis from other causes of canine megaoesophagus. *J Small Anim Pract.* 2006 May;47(5):pp 256–63.

Nutrition references

Bilbey DLJ, Prabhakaran VM. Muscle cramps and magnesium deficiency: case reports. *Canadian Family Physician*, Vol. 42, July 1996, pp. 1348–51.

Hanin I, Ansell GB. Lecithin: Technological, Biological, and Therapeutic Aspects, 1987, NY: Plenum Press, 180, 181.

Levin C. Caninie Epilepsy. Oregon City, OR: Lantern Publication, 2002 P 18–19.

Souba WW. Glutamine physiology, biochemistry, and nutrition in critical illness. Austin, TX: RG Landes Co.; 1992.

Souba W et al, Glutamine metabolism in the intestinal tract: invited review, *JPEN* 1985 9:608–617.

Windmueller HG. Glutamine utilization by the small intestine, *Adv. Enzymol* 1982. 53:201–237.

Yoshimura K, et al. Effects of enteral glutamine administration on experimental inflammatory bowel disease, *JPEN*, 1993 17:235.

Chinese herbal medicine/acupuncture references

Chang FY, Chey WY, Ouyang A. Effect of transcutaneous nerve stimulation on esophageal function in normal subjects—evidence for a somatovisceral reflex. *Am J Chin Med* 1996;24(2):185–92.

Chen CX. *Journal of Chinese Materia Medica.* 1986;16(4):40.

Modern TCM Pharmacology. 1997. Tianjin: Science and Technology Press.

Shi RB. *Journal of Beijing University of TCM.* 1999;22(2): 63–64.

Shi RR, et al. *Journal of Traditional Chinese Medicine.* 1998; 26(3):56–57.

Wu H, et al. *Journal of Chinese Patented Medicine.* 1996; 18(5):20–22.

Zhong Cao Yao (*Chinese Herbal Medicine*) 1991;22 (10): 452.

Zhong Cao Yao Fang Ji De Ying Yong (*Applications of Chinese Herbal Formulas*), 1976;101.

Zhong Liu Yu Zhi Tong Xun (*Journal of Prevention and Treatment of Cancer*), 1976; 2:40.

Zhou MX. *Fujian Journal of Medicine.* 1982;4(4):back cover.

Homotoxicology references

Reckeweg H. Biotherapeutic Index: Ordinatio Antihomotoxica et Materia Medica, 5th ed. Baden-Baden, Germany: Biologische Heilmittel Heel GMBH, 2000 pp 374–5.

Reckeweg H. Homeopathia Antihomotoxica Materia Medica, 4th edition. Baden-Baden, Germany: Arelia-Verlag GMBH, 2002 pp. 136–8, 139–40.

MEGACOLON

Definition and cause

An enlarged, impaired-motility, lower bowel along with chronic constipation. Genetic loss of nervous enervation is seen in humans. Hirchsprung's disease has not been reported in animals. It is believed that in animals (common in cats, rare in dogs) it is a neurological interruption of smooth muscle contraction. Acquired megacolon is secondary to chronic constipation leading to permanent damage to the smooth muscle of the bowel. Trauma, fractured pelvis and blockage of the colon, spinal nerve insult or disease, foreign body, stricture of the colon, anal sac disease, and/or perianal fistulas are all common causes (Dixon 2003, Bertoy 2002, Washabau 1999).

Medical therapy rationale, drug(s) of choice, and nutritional recommendations

Removal of the underlying cause often requires surgery (foreign body, neoplasia, anal sac problem, fracture). The surgical treatment of choice is a subtotal colectomy. Medical therapy of stool softeners such as Lactulose or Metamucil and improved motility (Cisapride) can be beneficial. Fluid replacement therapy along with antibiotics are often used. A low-residue diet is also recommended (Hasler 1997, Rosin 1993, Washabau 1999).

Anticipated prognosis

In general, medical management can be helpful in the short-term but not in the long-term. Surgical correction has proven beneficial in the long-term (Dixon 2003, Washabau 1999).

Integrative veterinary therapies

Colonic dilation occurs due to lack of proper motility. The idiopathic form is most commonly seen in clinical practice involving cats, and there may be some breed-related predisposition to megacolon in Manx cats. A wide variety of causative events can contribute to the condition and any condition which blocks the outflow of stool or negatively impacts myoneural function can ultimately lead to megacolon in both dogs and cats.

A thorough physical examination and history are indicated. Blood work is useful in determining health status (hydration and electrolytes as well as organ condition) and evaluating thyroid levels. Imaging may show the presence of neoplastic processes or traumatic incidents.

The initial treatment involves rehydrating and balancing electrolytes, treating static bowel syndrome, and removing the offending stool impaction or outflow tract issues. This may be adequate in early cases, particularly if the obstruction is not long-lived. Such cases may represent with obstipation and eventual development of megacolon. Exercise and play assist colon function, as does proper diet. A high-fiber diet is helpful in some cats, but in others this may cause aggravation and more rapid constipation, so the clinician must seek the diet that is most effective for each individual. Because fiber (soluble and insoluble) assists in homotoxin removal, the authors favor these initially. Dry food removes water from the system and may promote constipation through dehydration. Meat-based and canned diets may provide additional hydration and assist in colon function in obstipation cases. Canned pumpkin is readily accepted by many patients and can be very helpful. Other commonly bulking laxatives may prove helpful as well, but often cause worsening of constipation. A soluble fiber laxative such as lactulose is preferred.

Surgical solutions should be discussed with the client in advanced cases. Surgery does not cure the colonic atony, but can be particularly helpful in cases with colon outflow tract issues. Subtotal colectomy has been shown helpful in many cats, and while these cats may have loose stools for a time after surgery they eventually tend to form more normal stool with time.

The integration of nutrients, nutraceuticals, medicinal herbs, and combination homeopathics that are anti-inflammatory and cell-protective can help improve cellular function.

Nutrition
General considerations/rationale
Besides dietary support (as listed above), nutrition is focused upon improving smooth muscle function, nerve innervation, and contractibility as well as reducing the secondary inflammation associated with the disease.

Appropriate nutrients
Nutritional/gland therapy: Glandular intestines and nerve help to improve muscle function and neutralize cellular immune-mediated inflammation on both spinal nerves and the large bowel. Gland therapy also supplies specific intrinsic nutrients required for intestinal cellular health (see Chapter 2, Gland Therapy, for more detailed information).

Note: Because megacolon can affect the entire body, it is recommended that blood be analyzed both medically and physiologically to determine associated organ involvement or disease. This allows for a more specific gland and nutritional support protocol for the patient (see Chapter 2, Nutritional Blood Testing, for additional information).

Glutamine: Glutamine has been shown to improve immune function and is beneficial for the intestinal tract. It helps to improve cellular integrity and permeability, especially in inflamed conditions (Souba 1985, Windmueller 1982, Yoshimura 1993).

Probiotics: Administration of the proper combination of probiotics has been reported to have a positive impact on the intestines and the digestive process (Goldin 1984, Perdigon 1987). Probiotics have been shown to improve and aid the digestive process by secreting their own source of enzymes, which is beneficial for animals that are pancreatic-enzyme-deficient (McDonough 1987).

Magnesium: Magnesium has also been associated with neuromuscular function and conditions such as muscle cramping and weakness and neuromuscular dysfunction. Magnesium is recommended for weakening muscle function (Bibley 1996, Levin 2002).

Lecithin/phosphatidyl choline: Phosphatidyl choline is a phospholipid that is integral to cellular membranes particularly those of nerve and brain cells. It helps to move fats into the cells, and is involved in acetylcholine uptake, neurotransmission, and cellular integrity. As part of the cell membranes, lecithin is an essential nutrient required by the cells of the body for general health and wellness (Hanin 1987).

Fiber: In a study involving people with IBS, Manning (1977) and Hotz (1994) showed improvement by adding psyllium to the diet.

Chinese herbal medicine/acupuncture
General considerations/rationale
Megacolon is a condition of Qi deficiency. There is concurrent Blood deficiency and Qi stagnation. The Intestines need Qi, or energy, to move the stool. When this energy is not sufficient, constipation results. In this condition, Blood deficiency precludes normal nourishment of the Intestine. The result is dryness of the Large Intestine, which in turn leads to dry stool. The Qi stagnation causes the discomfort associated with this condition.

Appropriate Chinese herbs
Apricot seed (Xing ren): Has an analgesic effect (Zhu 1994) and may help decrease discomfort associated with the constipation.

Areca peel (Da fu pi): Increases intestinal contraction (Xin Yi Yao Xue Za Zhi 1974).

Citrus (Chen pi): Has been shown to improve the intestine's digestive function in sheep (Kuang 1996). It increases peristalsis (Jiang Su Zhong Yi Za Zhi 1981).

Hemp seed (Huo ma ren): Has laxative properties. It increases peristalsis (Zhong Yao Xue 1998; 265:266).

Immature bitter orange (Zhi shi): Increases peristalsis and promotes defecation (Zhong Guo Yi Yao Xue Bao 1991).

Rhubarb (Da huang): Contains sennoside A, aloe-emodin, and rhein, which cause defecation. It also increases peristalsis in the large intestine, but does not interfere with absorption of nutrients in the small intestine (Zhong Yao Xue 1998).

Saussurea (Mu xiang): Contains multiple compounds that affect the intestines. Some inhibit cramping; some enhance peristalsis (Zhong Yao Yao Li Yu Ying Yong 1983).

Trichosanthes seed (Gua lou ren): Has a laxative effect (Chang Yong Zhong Yao Cheng Fen Yu Yao Li Shou Ce 1994).

White peony (Bai shao): Has been used for constipation. In one trial, 60 human patients with chronic constipation were treated with an herbal supplement consisting of peony (Bai shao) and licorice (Gan cao). Other herbs were added as needed according to the TCM disease pattern of the patient. Almost all patients responded within 2 to 7 days (Zhong Yi Za Zhi 1983).

Acupuncture

Acupuncture has been shown in multiple trials to have positive results when used for habitual constipation, especially when combined with herbal therapy. One study investigated the use of a combined patent herbal supplement consisting of Ma Zi Ren (Huo ma ren, Xing ren, Shao yao, Zhi shi, Huo po and Da huang) and modified Zeng Ye Teng (Xuan shen, Mai men dong, Sheng di huang and Bai shao) and acupuncture. Fifty-five people with chronic constipation participated in the trial. After 2 weeks 65% resolved and 27% improved (Wu 2000). A second trial involved 31 people with habitual constipation. These patients received a variety of herbal supplements based upon the TCM diagnosis along with acupuncture therapy. All patients received acupuncture therapy at Bl25, St25, and St37. Then, based upon the TCM diagnosis, various combinations of the following points were used: LI4, LI11, St36, St40, Sp3, Sp6, Sp15, Liv2, Bl20, and/or Bl21. Seventy-seven percent resolved and another 16% experienced significant improvement (Guo 1999).

Homotoxicology
General considerations/rationale

Megacolon represents a Degeneration Phase condition. In early cases, there may still be time to salvage vital systems before their total demise, and antihomotoxic drugs may greatly assist patients. These can be used integratively or on their own. Palmquist has used cisapride alone and in combination with antihomotoxic drugs and they seem compatible.

As in all disorders, regressive vicariation may come unexpectedly and the clinician should be pleased if other inflammatory conditions suddenly arise, because this may mark the beginning of homotoxin removal and excretion accompanying organ repair and revitalization. These events are not always startling and in many cases gentle, gradual improvement is noted and improved function gradually manifests. It should be remembered that Degeneration Phase diseases may be too far advanced for biological therapy to succeed, but because this type of therapy is very gentle, it is well worth considering.

Appropriate homotoxicology formulas

Berberis homaccord: Supportive of adrenal function, drains kidneys, and supports liver function. Contains Citrullis colocynthis for support of the lumbosacral area.

BHI-Constipation: Used for constipation, constipation altering with diarrhea, and incomplete stool (Heel 2002).

BHI-Neuralgia: Used for its complement of Silicea, which may assist in cases of constipation in which the patient's stool moves in and out before finally passing.

Coenzyme compositum: Contains Citricum acidum, which is useful for dental problems and gingivitis; scurvy; blackening of teeth and heavy deposits of dental plaque; painful, herpetic vesicles around the lips; nausea; painful cramping in the umbilical area, and distension.

Colocynthis homaccord: Used for diarrhea with lower back pain (Citrullus colocynthis), colic, pain below the navel, and colitis with gelatinous stools.

Cruroheel S: Contains Silicea for "bashful stool" (stool that moves in and out before passing). Also used for support of degenerate connective tissue. This remedy can bring about a strong regressive vicariation in some cases.

Galium-Heel: Used for all cellular phases, hemorrhoids, and anal fissures, and as a detoxicant.

Ginseng compositum: Used for nausea, gastroenteritis, and constitutional support in geriatric or debilitated patients (Reckeweg 2000).

Hepar compositum: Provides detoxification and drainage of hepatic tissues, organ and metabolic support, and is useful in most hepatic and gall bladder pathologies. It is an important part of Deep Detoxification Formula. Treats duodenitis, pancreatitis, cystic hepatic ducts, cholelithiasis, cholangitis, cholecystitis, vomiting, and diarrhea (Demers 2004, Broadfoot 2004). This combination contains Natrum oxalaceticum (also found in *Coenzyme compositum, Ubichinon compositum,* and *Mucosa compositum*) for changes in appetite and stomach distension due to air. Used for nausea, stomach pain with a sensation of fullness, gurgling in the abdomen, and cramping pain in the hypochondria. Also used for constipation, sudden diarrhea (particularly after eating), and flatus. (Reckeweg 2002) Calcarea carbonica is included for constipation in which the patient has no urge to pass stool.

Hepeel: Provides liver drainage and detoxification. Used in a wide variety of conditions including cancer of the liver, in which *Hepeel* was found to be antiproliferative, hepatoprotective, and an antioxidant when tested in human HepG2 cells (Gebhardt 2003).

Lymphomyosot: Provides lymph drainage and endocrine support, and treats edema. Contains Gentiana for chronic gastritis. Treats flatulence, diarrhea, distension of the stomach with eructations, nausea, retching, and vomiting. Contains Geranium robertianum for nausea, particularly after eating with distension or sensation of fullness.

Mucosa compositum: Broadly supportive for repair of mucosal elements. Used in cellular cases and in recovery periods following active disease (Reckeweg 2000). This remedy contains a useful component in Kali bichromicum, which is indicated for ulcers found on the gums, tongue, lips, and even on the gastric mucosa (gastric or duodenal ulcer). The tongue may have a thick, yellow, mucous coating, or in ulcerative stomatitis or tonsillitis it may be dry, smooth, shiny, or fissured. Kali has been used effectively in acute gastroenteritis associated with vomiting of clear, light-colored fluid or quantities of mucous bile, and in cases with hematemesis, flatulent colics, and dysenteric stools with tenesmus (Reckeweg 2002).

It also contains Hydrastis, with mucosal support for oral problems such as stomatitis, and mucosal suppuration that is accompanied by ulceration, inflammations and colic of the hepatobiliary system and of the gastrointestinal tract, and polyp formation (Reckeweg 2002). The Kreosotum component can be used in chronic gastritis with gastric hemorrhages and vomiting of brown masses. Also has a dental implication in cases with spongy gums and carious teeth, neuralgias proceeding from them causing a burning toothache with deep caries, black patches on the teeth, and fetid discharges.

The single remedy Phosphorus is broadly useful for dyspepsia and for jaw problems in dental disease (Reckeweg 2002). Phosphorus is found in many other remedies including *Echinacea compositum* and *Leptandra homaccord*. It is rich in suis organ preparations for mucosal support, plus a large variety of remedies with indications in the gastrointestinal sphere. The component Argentum nitricum (also in *Atropinum compositum, Diarrheel, Duodenoheel, Gastricumeel, Momordica compositum, BHI-Nausea*, and several other combinations) is indicated for distension in the upper abdomen, gastrocardiac symptom-complex, and amelioration from eructa-

tions. It is also used for gastric crises (Reckeweg 2002).

Neuralgo-Rheum-Injeel: Contains Citrullus colocynthis for neuralgia, stabbing pains, and sciatica. Gnaphalium polycephalum is included for numbness in the back and paresthesia and twinges in the lower back (Reckeweg 2000).

Nux vomica homaccord: Used for liver and gastrointestinal disease and after smoke inhalation. Useful in gingivitis (Reckeweg 2002). This commonly used formula for detoxification is part of the *Detox Kit*. Recent research shows that 1 ingredient (Brucine) affects mitochondria in human hepatoma cells. Further research is needed to determine whether homeopathic dilutions are more or less active (Deng, et al. 2006).

Paeonia-Heel: Used for anal region issues such as hemorrhoids, anal fissures, colitis, spasmodic constipation, weeping anal lesions, anal pruritus, and painful defecation (Reckeweg 2000). A topical cream is useful.

Podophyllum homaccord: Treats chronic gastroenteritis, gastroenteritis in juvenile dogs and cats, dyspepsia, catarrhal colitis, hemorrhoids, and watery-green diarrhea alternating with constipation.

Procteel: Contains Lycopodium, Sulfur, Phosphorus, and Aluminum oxydatum to make a formula that may be useful for megacolon and rectal atony, hemorrhoids, sore body orifices, alternating diarrhea and constipation, hepatic disease with cystic ducts, and intestinal stasis (Reckeweg 2000).

Solidago compositum: Provides drainage and support of the adrenal and urinary organs and is part of the Deep Detoxification Formula.

Thyroidea compositum: Provides matrix drainage and support of endocrine function. It is part of the Deep Detoxification Formula.

Ubichinon compositum: Contains anthraquinone for swelling of gums, and GI symptoms such as distention, flatulence, and cramping abdominal pain. Treats constipation with straining or sudden diarrhea (Reckeweg 2002).

Veratrum homaccord: Treats gastritis, intense vomiting with blood, collapse (pale mucous membranes), psychosis, dysentary, fecal incontinence, and intestinal spasm. This very useful remedy has been used widely by the authors for general vomiting cases. Consider its use in cases of gastritis following general anesthesia. Classical provings were recently repeated and found consistent with earlier work (Van Wassenhoven 2004).

Authors' suggested protocols

Nutrition

Intestine and brain/nerve support formulas: 1 tablet for every 25 pounds of body weight BID.

Glutimmune: One-fourth scoop per 25 pounds of body weight daily.

Probiotic MPF: One-half capsule per 25 pounds of body weight with food.

Magnesium: 10 mg for every 10 pounds of body weight SID.

Lecithin/phosphatidyl choline: One-fourth teaspoon for every 25 pounds of body weight BID.

Psyllium: 1 teaspoon per 25 pounds of body weight per meal.

Chinese herbal medicine/acupuncture

H11 Megacolon: 1 capsule per 10 to 20 pounds twice daily as needed for optimal results. It can be combined with conventional medicines for better results. In addition to the herbs described above, H11 Megacolon contains astragalus root (Huang qi), cimicifuga (Sheng ma), ginseng (Ren shen), magnolia bark (Hou pu), and pinellia (Ban xia). These herbs increase efficacy of the formula.

Acupuncture points: BL25, ST25, TH6, ST36, ST37, LI11, BL20, BL21, CV4, and CV6 (Handbook of TCM Practitioners 1987).

Homotoxicology (Dose: 10 drops PO for 50-pound dog; 5 drops PO for cat or small dog)

Megacolon is an advanced degenerative condition poorly responsive to therapy.

For chronic atonies and megacolon: Broadfoot has experienced some success with autosanguis using Nux vomica homaccord, Lymphomyosot plus Colocynthis homaccord, Mucosa compositum, and Coenzyme compositum plus Ubichinon compositum. Give half by injection to the patient and add the other half to an oral cocktail of Berberis homaccord and Colocynthis Homaccord, success the mixture, and administer BID to TID orally.

For cases of spinal origin: Combine Veratrum homaccord, Podophyllum compositum, Nux vomica homaccord, Berberis homaccord, Mucosa compositum, Neuralgo-Rheum-Injeel, Hepeel, BHI Enzyme, Chelidonium homaccord, and BHI-Constipation tabs and administer orally BID to TID.

For refractory cases: Consider the following for long-term use after advising clients of its experimental nature: Proctheel, Nux vomica homaccord, and Lymphomyosot mixed together and given TID orally. Also consider Deep Detoxification Formula consisting of Galium-Heel, Hepar compositum, Solidago compositum, Thyroidea compositum, Ubichinon compositum, and Coenzyme compositum mixed together and given orally twice weekly. Proper diet and use of laxatives and enemas are essential.

Product sources

Nutrition

Intestine and brain/nerve support formulas: Animal Nutrition Technologies. **Alternatives:** Enteric Support—

Standard Process Veterinary Formulas; NutriGest—Rx Vitamins for Pets.

Glutimmune: Well Wisdom. **Alternative:** L-Glutamine powder—Thorne Veterinary Products.

Probiotic: Progressive Labs.

Lecithin/phosphatidyl choline: Designs for Health.

Magnesium: Over the counter.

Psyllium seed powder: Progressive Labs.

Chinese herbal medicine

H11 Megacolon: Natural Solutions, Inc.

Homotoxicology

BHI/Heel Corporation

REFERENCES

Western medicine references

Bertoy RW. Megacolon in the cat, *Vet Clin North Am Small An Pract.* 2002 Jul;32(4):901–15.

Dixon BC. Megacolon, In: Tilley L, Smith F. The 5-Minute Veterinary Consult: Canine and Feline, Blackwell Publishing, 2003.

Hasler AH, Washabau RJ. Cisapride stimulates contraction of idiopathic megacolonic smooth muscle in cats. *J Vet Intern Med* 1997 Nov-Dec;11(6):313–8.

Rosin E. Megacolon in cats. The role of colectomy, *Vet Clin North Am Small Anim Pract.* 1993 May;23(3):587–94.

Washabau RJ, Holt D. Pathogenesis, diagnosis, and therapy of feline idiopathic megacolon, *Vet Clin North Am Small Anim Pract.* 1999, Mar;29(2) : 589–603.

IVM/nutrition references

Bilbey DLJ, Prabhakaran, VM. Muscle cramps and magnesium deficiency: case reports. *Canadian Family Physician*, Vol. 42, July 1996, pp. 1348–51.

Golden BR, Gorbach SL. The Effect of Milk and Lactobacillus Feeding on Human Intestinal Bacteria Activity. *Am. J. of Clin. Nutr.* 1984 39: 756–61.

Hanin I, Ansell GB. Lecithin: Technological, Biological, and Therapeutic Aspects, (1987), NY: Plenum Press, 180, 181.

Levin C. Caninie Epilepsy. Oregon City, OR: Lantern Publication, 2002 P 18–19.

Manning AP, Heaton KW, Harvey RF, Uglow P. Wheat fibre and irritable bowel syndrome. *Lancet* 1977;ii:417–8.

McDonough FE, Hitchins AD, Wong NP, et al. Modification of sweet acidophilus milk to improve utilization by lactose-intolerant persons. *Am J Clin Nutr* 1987;45:570–4.

O'Dwyer S, et al. Maintenance of small bowel mucosa with glutamine-enriched parenteral nutrition, *Journal of Parenteral and Enteral Nutrition*, 1989 13:579.

Perdigon GN, de Masius N, Alvarez S, et al. Enhancement of Immune Response in Mice fed with S. Thermophilus and L. Acidophilus, *J. of Dairy Sci.*, 1987 70: 919–926.

Souba WW. Glutamine physiology, biochemistry, and nutrition in critical illness. Austin, TX: RG Landes Co. 1992.

Souba W, et al. Glutamine metabolism in the intestinal tract: invited review, *JPEN* 9:608–617,1985.

Windmueller HG. Glutamine utilization by the small intestine, *Adv. Enzymol*, 1982 53:201–237.

Yoshimura K, et al. Effects of enteral glutamine administration on experimental inflammatory bowel disease, *JPEN*, 1993 17:235.

Chinese herbal medicine/acupuncture references

Chang Yong Zhong Yao Cheng Fen Yu Yao Li Shou Ce (A Handbook of the Composition and Pharmacology of Common Chinese Drugs), 1994; 768:769.

Guo CY, et al. Treating constipation with Chinese herbs and acupuncture. *Journal of Clinical Acupuncture.* 1999;15(11): 12–13.

Handbook of TCM Practitioners. Hunan College of TCM. Oct 1987 p.268.

Jiang Su Zhong Yi Za Zhi (*Jiangsu Journal of Chinese Medicine*), 1981; (3):61.

Kuang L, et al. *Journal of Traditional Chinese Medicine Research.* 1996;(1):49–50.

Wu ZX. 55 cases of senile constipation treated with Ma Zi Ren Wan and modified Zeng Ye Tang. *Journal of New TCM.* 2000;32(1):18.

Xin Yi Yao Xue Za Zhi (*New Journal of Medicine and Herbology*), 1974; 12:39.

Zhong Guo Yi Yao Xue Bao (*Chinese Journal of Medicine and Herbology*), 1991; 6(1):39.

Zhong Yao Xue (*Chinese Herbology*), 1998; 251:256.

Zhong Yao Xue (*Chinese Herbology*), 1998; 265:266.

Zhong Yao Yao Li Yu Ying Yong (*Pharmacology and Applications of Chinese Herbs*), 1983;169.

Zhu YP, et al. Amygdalin's analgesic effect. *China Journal of Chinese Medicine.* 1994;19(2):105–107.

Zhong Yi Za Zhi (*Journal of Chinese Medicine*), 1983; 8:79.

Homotoxicology references

Broadfoot PJ. Inflammation: Homotoxicology and Healing. In: Proceedings AHVMA/Heel Homotoxicology Seminar. Denver, CO, 2004 p 27.

Demers J. Homotoxicology and Acupuncture. In: Proceedings of the 2004 Homotoxicology Seminar. AHVMA/Heel. Denver, CO, 2004 p 5, 6.

Deng X, Yin F, Lu X, Cai B, Yin W. The apoptotic effect of brucine from the seed of Strychnos nux-vomica on human hepatoma cells is mediated via Bcl-2 and Ca2+ involved mitochondrial pathway. *Toxicol Sci.* 2006 May;91(1):pp 59–69.

Gebhardt R. Antioxidative, antiproliferative and biochemical effects in HepG2 cells of a homeopathic remedy and its constituent plant tinctures tested separately or in combination. *Arzneimittelforschung.* 2003 53(12): pp 823–30.

Habermehl D, Kammerer B, Handrick R, Eldh T, Gruber C, Cordes N, Daniel PT, Plasswilm L, Bamberg M, Belka C, Jendrossek V. Proapoptotic activity of Ukrain is based on Chelidonium majus L. alkaloids and mediated via a mitochondrial death pathway. *BMC Cancer.* 2006 Jan 17;6: p 14.

Heel. BHI Homeopathic Therapy: Professional Reference. Albuquerque, NM: Heel Inc. 2002 pp 47, 73, 124.

Reckeweg H. Biotherapeutic Index: Ordinatio Antihomotoxica et Materia Medica, 5th ed. Baden-Baden, Germany: Biologische Heilmittel Heel GMBH, 2000 pp 300, 369, 374, 382, 390.

Reckeweg H. Homeopathia Antihomotoxica Materia Medica, 4th ed. Baden-Baden, Germany: Arelia-Verlag GMBH, 2002 pp. 136–8, 147, 317–19, 340–1, 345, 366, 446–449, 461–3, 488–90.

Van Wassenhoven M. Towards an evidence-based repertory: clinical evaluation of Veratrum album. *Homeopathy.* 2004 Apr;93(2): pp 71–7.

CHRONIC ACTIVE HEPATITIS

Definition and cause

Chronic active hepatitis is chronic inflammation of the liver, often resulting in an elevation of both serum alanine aminotransferase (ALT) and serum aspartate aminotransferase (AST), and leading to cellular infiltration (most commonly lymphocytic), liver cell death, and fibrosis. Commonly suspected sources of the chronic inflammation include toxins, copper, adverse reactions to drugs such as anticonvulsants, and infections. The condition is suspected but not proven to be associated with an immune-mediated process (Center 1996; Dill-Macky 1995; Doige 1981; Hardy 1975, 2003).

Medical therapy rationale, drug(s) of choice, and nutritional recommendations

Commonly recommended drugs include corticosteroids or immunosuppressing medications such as azathioprine along with antibiotics such as metronidazole. In addition to dietary support with restricted protein diets, there is some suggestion that polyunsaturated phosphatidylcholine may be beneficial but there is no definitive proof that this is so. Vitamins E and K are recommended along with liver-protective remedies such as SAMe (S-adenosyl-L-methionine) and milk thistle (silymarin). There is no definitive proof of their effectiveness, but they are given because they are believed to be liver-protective and help to reduce inflammation. Zinc acetate is often recommended to help control plasma copper levels, which are found in copper hepatopathy (Hardy 2003, Magne 1986, Meyer 2000, Neuberg 1983).

The use of immunomodulators such as prednisone and azothioprine along with antifibrotic and protective drugs such as ursodeoxycholic acid are typically part of the therapy plan. The dietary recommendation is usually protein-restricted diets that use vegetable sources of protein (Gitlin 1884, Hardy 2003, Laflamme 2000, Leveille-Webster 1995).

Anticipated prognosis

Prognosis is dependent upon correction of the underlying cause. If the cause, such as toxicity, is determined and corrected, the prognosis is good. Immune-mediated and chronic longstanding conditions have a more guarded prognosis (Magne 1986, Sevelius 1995).

Integrative veterinary therapies

A complete history with regard to toxin and drug exposures (both systemic and topical agents, as well as vaccinations), physical examination, and laboratory testing are needed in all cases. The clinician should also take a careful history of alternative medicine agents such as herbal, nutraceutical, and homeopathic agents, because these can be associated with increased liver enzymes and hepatotoxicity as well. Specialized testing such as bile acid determination may be helpful in the decision to conduct a biopsy, a step that is often needed for the most complete diagnosis of chronic hepatitis patients. Imaging with radiographs or ultrasound is often indicated, and ultrasound is a valuable tool in diagnosis of hepatitis in clinical practice.

Chronic active hepatitis is conventionally viewed as a disease that often requires lifetime management. When treated with integrative veterinary approaches, a surprising number of these patients may make slow progress and show improvement. Evidence now supports several long-used holistic therapies such as antioxidant vitamins, milk thistle and its extracts, and SAMe.

Dietary therapy is very important in all gastrointestinal and hepatic disorders. A highly digestible diet that has reduced protein levels that are high in biological value is recommended. Diets for liver patients should also contain appropriate copper levels, and may have additional nutraceutical agents such as vitamin E, zinc, milk thistle, SAMe, and others as detailed in the nutritional therapy section of this text. Glandular therapy is particularly helpful in chronic, nonresponsive cases.

Antibiotics, corticosteroids, choleretics, diuretics, intravenous or subcutaneous fluid administration, and immunosuppressive and soluble-fiber laxative drugs may also be required. Many pharmaceutical agents are toxins; while they may be vitally important in preserving the patient's life, clinicians need to exercise caution in selecting these agents and determining proper dosing for patients with altered liver function. If possible, drugs that require hepatic metabolism should be avoided. The clinician needs to know common side effects of all agents in use, so that appropriate actions can be taken if adverse reactions arise (gastrointestinal toxicity with azothiaprine, vestibular/neurological issues with metronidazole, hepatoencephalopathy following steroid administration, etc.). Complementary therapeutic agents may be harmful to patients with compromised liver function as well, and generally care is warranted in designing treatment programs for all liver patients (Miele 2004).

Clients should be encouraged to inform the clinician of all agents they are administering or considering using to avoid side effects and toxic interactions. Proper integration of therapies to reduce disease pathology, eliminate toxins, support organ repair, reduce necessary drug intervals and dosing quantities, and prevent adverse interactions is a laudable goal of all medical treatment plans. Well-meaning but improperly informed individuals can create situations which threaten treatment success; however, with proper understanding, a wide variety of agents can be used to assist a patient in coordinating healing in chronic liver disease.

Use of high-soluble and insoluble fiber diets assists in trapping and moving these toxins out of the system, and probiotics may further assist in removing toxic agents from the bowel by converting them to other less toxic agents. Soluble fiber laxatives are routinely used in treatment of hepatoencephalopathy for their ability to bind ammonia in the intestinal contents. A new veterinary probiotic product called Azodyl® (Vetoquinol) selectively removes ammonia and other nitrogen wastes from the blood and is used in reducing azotemia in renal failure patients.

Clinical application of Azodyl® may prove helpful in these cases, but research is needed to see if evidence supports the theoretical application of this particular probiotic product, since urease activity by the organism could potentially worsen conditions in hepatitis.

The use of nutrients, nutraceuticals, medicinal herbs, and combination homeopathics that are anti-inflammatory and tissue-sparing and that enhance cellular elimination of toxins can improve cellular health and enhance liver cell regeneration.

Nutrition
General considerations/rationale

Chronic liver disease has a similar nutritional focus as more acute inflamed conditions: reducing toxins and metabolic wastes as well as increasing antioxidant and phytonutrient levels can help neutralize compounds that the liver must deal with in its role as the body's filter and detoxifier. Because of the more chronic nature of liver disease, additional nutraceuticals should be added to further help protect liver cells and reduce scarring.

Note: Because liver disease can be severe and involve multiple organ disease, it is recommended that blood be analyzed both medically and physiologically to determine real and impending organ involvement and disease. This allows for a more specific gland and nutritional support protocol (see Chapter 2, Nutritional Blood Testing, for additional information).

Appropriate nutrients

Nutrition/gland therapy: Clinical trials using thymus extract have shown that it is beneficial in people with hepatitis B (Skotnicki 1989). Additional clinical studies with oral thymus extract showed that blood values related to liver function as well as the blood immune markers all improved. Civereira (1989) showed similar results with hepatitis C (Galli 1985, Bortolotti 1988).

Glandular liver: Helps neutralize a cellular immune response and spare liver cells (see Gland Therapy in Chapter 2).

Lecithin/phosphatidyl choline: Lecithin/phosphatidyl choline has been shown to help break down scar tissue in the liver and prevent cirrhosis by reversing the cellular changes that lead to cirrhotic cell formation (Ma 1996). Phosphatidyl choline has been shown to reverse the progression of alcohol induced cirrhosis in humans (Lieber 1994).

Alpha-lipoic acid: Alpha-lipoic acid is a potent antioxidant that is proven to reduce oxidative stress and inflammation. It has also been shown to increase the effectiveness of other antioxidants, such as vitamins C and E, Co-Enzyme Q10, and glutathione, making them more readily available for bodily function (Busse 1992, Lykkesfeldt 1998, Scholich 1989). There was significant improvement of liver function in a study of people with cirrhosis who received a combination antioxidant-rich supplement that contained 300 mg of alpha-lipoic acid (Berkson 1999).

S-adenosylmethionine (SAMe): SAMe is an antioxidant and has anti-inflammatory effects on the liver (Center 2000). SAMe has been shown to significantly improve survival and decrease the need for liver transplantation in people with liver disease. It has also been shown to improve liver function in less severe cases of cirrhosis (Gorbakov 1998, Mato 1999, Miglio 1975).

Vitamin E: Vitamin E was shown to decrease liver damage and immune imbalances that may contribute to the disease progression; however, further clinical work is required to definitively confirm this because another clinical trial failed to confirm these results (Ferro 1999, de la Maza 1995).

Zinc: Clinical trials have confirmed that zinc deficiencies are associated with cirrhosis in people (Scholmerich 1983, Taniguchi 1995). In double-blind testing with zinc acetate supplementation, Reding (1984) and Marchesini (1996) showed a significant improvement in portal systemic encephalopathy.

Chinese herbal medicine/acupuncture
General considerations/rationale
Traditional Chinese Medicine considers chronic active hepatitis to be a condition of Heat and Damp in the Liver and Gallbladder. There is concurrent Qi and Blood stagnation, which leads to indigestion, inappetance, mid-abdominal discomfort, and possible icterus or fever.

Heat is Inflammation. We now know that this inflammation may be due to bacteria, toxins, or immune-mediated causes. Heat can also be used to describe the yellow seen in icteric patients. This concept of yellow as a warm color continues today. Fever is an obvious manifestation of Heat. Damp can describe purulent debris in the case of bacterial etiologies or bile accumulation if the gallbladder becomes involved.

When there is Qi stagnation in the Liver and Gallbladder there is weakness in the body. This leaves insufficient energy to digest the food. Blood stagnation causes pain, so when there is Blood stagnation in the Liver, there is epigastric pain. The Blood is also responsible for nourishing the body.

Appropriate Chinese herbs
Angelica root (Dang gui): Is hepatoprotective. It promotes generation of hepatocytes (Chong Qing Yi Yao 1989). In one study, 17 patients with chronic hepatitis and 10 with liver cirrhosis had reductions in clinical signs (Zhong Yi Yao Xin Xie 1985). Chronic active hepatitis may be due to bacteria. Angelica root has antibacterial action against different strains of bacteria, including E. coli (Hou Xue Hua Yu Yan Jia 1981).

Astragalus (Huang qi): Was used in 29 humans with chronic hepatitis for 1 to 3 months with good results (Zhe Jiang Zhong Yi Za Zhi 1983). Another 174 human patients who tested positive for hepatitis B antibodies were treated by injection every third day for 3 months; 75% became seronegative for hepatitis B. (Ji Lin Zhong Yi 1985).

Atractylodes (Bai zhu): Has been used in cases of infectious hepatitis with good results (An Hui Zhong Yi Xue Yuan Xue Bao 1984).

Blue citrus (Qing pi): Has hepatoprotective properties. In CCl4-treated rats and mice, there was a 10% decrease in ALT and AST over controls when curcuma was given (Zhong Guo Mian Yi Xue Za Zhi 1989).

Bupleurum (Chai hu): Is well suited for use in chronic active hepatitis. It contains saikosaponin which has analgesic and antipyretic properties (Shen Yang Yi Xue Yuan Bao 1984). Furthermore, it has anti-inflammatory effects (Liu 1998). Studies have shown that it inhibits various bacteria (Zhong Yao Xue 1988).

Curcuma root (Yu jin): Can protect the liver by increasing the amount of superoxide dismutase, increasing serum albumin, and decreasing the ALT in cases of CCL4 toxicity (Liu 1999). In CCl4-treated rats and mice, there was a 10% decrease in ALT and AST over controls when curcuma was given (Zhong Guo Mian Yi Xue Za Zhi 1989). This hepatoprotective effect may extend to bacterial or inflammatory cell mediator toxins.

Cyperus (Xiang fu zi): Relieves pain and decreases fevers. The antipyretic activity in rats is 6 times stronger than aspirin (Gui Yang Yi Xue Yuan Xue Bao 1959, Indian J Med Res 1971).

Forsythia (Lian qiao): Contains an antiviral compound called rengynic acid (Zhang 2002), which may make it helpful in viral etiologies. It also inhibits many bacteria and possesses anti-inflammatory, analgesic, and antipyretic effects (Ma 1982). Other studies show that forsythia has hepatoprotective activity in cases of hepatotoxins (Group of Liver Diseases 1973).

Gentian root (Qin jiao): Is an anti-inflammatory herb. It causes the adrenal glands to secrete corticosteroids (Chang Yong Zhong Yao Cheng Fen Yu Yao Li Shou Ce 1994). In one trial 20 people with either hepatitis or neonatal jaundice were treated with gentiana along with Huang qin and Lian qiao, or with Cang zhu, Bai zhu, and Hou po for 14 days. Both groups improved (Shang Hai Zhong Yi Yao Za Zhi 1965).

Licorice (Gan cao): Has several functions that are beneficial in cases of chronic active hepatitis. It contains glycyrrhizin and glycyrrhetinic acid, which have anti-inflammatory effects. They have approximately 10% of the corticosteroid activity of cortisone (Zhong Cao Yao 1991). Glycyrrhizin also has antiviral activity (Zhu 1996). In one study it was 77% effective in treating 330 human patients with hepatitis B. It reduced inflammation, increased regeneration of hepatic cells, and decreased hepatic necrosis and cirrhosis (Zhong Yao Tong Bao 1987).

Ophiopogon (Mai men dong): Inhibits bacteria including E. coli (Zhong Yao Xue 1998).

Oriental wormwood (Yin chen hao): Is an excellent herb to use in cases of hepatitis. It can relieve fevers. It has a duration of 3 to 4 hours in rats with experimentally induced pyrexia (Planta Med 1984). The compound responsible for this effect seems to be capillarin. Another compound, 6, 7-dimethoxy coumarin, has analgesic and anti-inflammatory effects (Wan Yao De 1987, Shan 1982). Oriental wormwood is also hepatoprotective in that it can induce the activity of microsomal cholesterol esterase, thereby increasing the metabolism of toxic substances (Hu Yi Qiao 1999, He Ping 1990). It can promote bile secretion, enhance bile flow, and protect the functions of hepatocytes (He Ping 1990, Sui Yan Hua 1993). It possesses antibacterial properties against multiple bacteria including E. coli (Zhong Yao Yao Li Yu Ying Yong 1990). Thirty-two people with acute hepatitis were treated with oriental wormwood 3 times a day for 3 to 15 days. There was significant decrease in hepatomegaly, icterus, and pyrexia (Fu Jian Zhong Yi Yao 1959).

Peach kernel (Tao ren): Prevents the depletion of glutathione in the liver caused by toxic chemicals, and increases the activity of superoxide dismutase (Sun Wei Qiang, 1993, Jiang 1995). It decreases hepatic fibrosis caused by CCl_4, allowing the recovery of hepatic tissues (Xu 1993). This may help the liver recover from inflammatory damage.

Poria (Fu ling): Protects the liver (Han 1977). It inhibits some bacteria (Nanjing College of Pharmacy 1976).

Salvia (Dan shen): Protects the liver. It improves hepatic circulation and promotes regeneration of liver cells (Zhong Yi Za Zhi 1982, Zhong Xi Yi Jie He Za Zhi 1988). It has been shown to reduce the amount of fibrosis in rats given CCl4 or DMN (dimethylnitrosamine) (Hu Yi Yang 1999). This action may help prevent the formation of fibrosis in cases of chronic active hepatitis. In one study involving 22 human patients with chronic active hepatitis, all 11 patients who received injections of salvia and 6 of the 11 who took the salvia orally had normal liver enzymes within 3 months (Zhong Xi Yi Jie He Za Zhi 1984).

Schisandra (Wu wei zi): Has been shown experimentally to lower ALT in laboratory animals with toxin-induced hepatic damage. It seems to alter the liver cell membrane to prevent toxins from entering the cell. It also increases blood flow to the liver and promotes the regeneration of hepatic cells (Nagai 1989, Takeda 1986). This herb promotes bile secretion in healthy mice, and promotes liver regeneration in mice whose liver has been partially removed (Gao 1996, Wu 1987). Thirty-four human patients with chronic active hepatitis were treated with a formula containing Wu wei zi, Ling zhi, Dan shen, and Chai hu for 3 months. Thirty-three patients responded (Shan Xi Zhong Yi 1988).

White peony (Bai shao): Contains paeoniflorin, which is a strong antipyretic and has anti-inflammatory efficacy (Zhong Yao Zhi 1993). Additionally, it has demonstrated antibacterial actions against various bacteria including E. coli (Xin Zhong Yi 1989).

Acupuncture

Some acupuncturists have felt that this modality can be used to enhance liver function and decrease inflammation by reducing the toxins (infectious agents, inflammatory mediators) (Handbook of Traditional Chinese Medicine Practitioners 1987).

Homotoxicology
General considerations/rationale

Chronic active hepatitis is a descriptive diagnosis that is useful in categorizing pathology of the liver. It is not a specific or causal diagnosis, and as such has limited usefulness. This diagnosis is usually applied to canine patients, and as the name implies, pathology consists of an ongoing pathological process with the presence of inflammatory cells and development of fibrosis (Watson 2004). Human and canine conditions are similar and can serve as treatment and disease models for one another (Spee, et al. 2006). Such changes are viewed in homotoxicology as originating from the body's attempted handling of homotoxins generally in the Impregnation and Degeneration phases.

Homotoxins can manifest in many ways. Damage to the genome results in genetic causes, which are suspected in several breed-related hepatopathies (Doberman pinschers, Cocker spaniels, Labradors, Skye terriers, Bedlington terriers, and West highland white terriers, for example). Toxins (environmental and pharmaceutical, particularly anticonvulsants, heartworm preventatives, and nonsteroidal anti-inflammatory drugs), bacteria (leptospirosis), and viruses (infectious canine hepatitis virus) all can play a part in the development of chronic liver disease (Watson 2004).

Homotoxicology agents can cause homotoxin off-load from cells and the matrix. While this is desirable, the clinician must carefully supervise it. Homotoxin off-load results in increased circulating levels of homotoxins that can further irritate a weakened or diseased liver. Monitoring of hepatic enzymes is recommended, and a reduction in detoxifying products is advised when more marked increases in hepatic enzyme levels occur. Some minor rise in ALT and SAP may be desirable and simply indicate that the liver is working. For instance, Galium-Heel is a very effective cellular detoxifying agent that can cause increased enzyme levels (Miele, et al 2004). It is frequently required in treating chronic diseases. When liver enzymes rise in patients on Galium-Heel or other antihomotoxic agents, the product should be used at lower levels or given at longer intervals, and in some cases must to be discontinued for short periods of time while the body catches up with homotoxin elimination.

Concentrating on liver support with Hepar compositum and catalysts during these times is helpful. When liver enzymes increase during therapy, the veterinary clinician should assist the patient by moving homotoxins out through other elimination organs, such as the kidney (Solidago compositum, Berberis homaccord), and support of the gastrointestinal system is of utmost importance due to the entero-hepatic recycling of homotoxins (Mucosa compositum, Nux homaccord).

Appropriate homotoxicology formulas

Oral drop combinations may contain alcohol. In most cases this is such a small quantity that it is well tolerated, but when possible, selecting oral vials and tablets may reduce the workload on the liver (Reckeweg 2000). See also specific protocols for enteritis, colitis, pancreatitis, and other applicable gastrointestinal conditions for more information and remedy selection ideas.

Arsuraneel: A cellular phase remedy that treats enteritis and diarrhea (Arsenicum album). May be useful in arsenic poisoning in areas with contaminated ground water (Mallick, Mallick, Guha, and Khuda-Bukhsh 2003; Khuda-Bukhsh 2005). Also used in chronic disease, tumors of mucous membranes (Marsdenia cundurango), and diabetes mellitus (Acidum phophoricum) (Reckeweg 2000).

Atropinum compositum: Not available on the U.S. market at this time, but a powerful antispasmodic for biliary, renal, and intestinal colic (Demers 2004). Contains Benzoicum acidum (common also to *Aesculus compositum, Arnica-Heel, Atropinum compositum*, and *Rhododendroneel*). It is used in inflammatory symptoms which occur throughout the alimentary canal: a slimy coating on the tongue with ulcers at the edges, stomatitis with dysphagia, eructations, retching and vomiting, and flatulent distension below the ribs on both sides. The stools are copious, loose, and white in color, with violent tenesmus and mixed with blood; there are stabbing pains in the rectum, rigors, and a feeling of being seriously ill (Reckeweg 2002).

Berberis homaccord: Berberis has major actions on the liver and gallbladder (Reckeweg 2000), and has been shown to have effects in diarrhea (Zhu, Ahrens 1982; Shamsa, Ahmadiani, and Khosrokhavar 1999). Treats colic, collapse, and bloody vomitus, and is supportive of adrenal and renal function. Part of the basic *Detox Kit*. Berberis is also contained in *Solidago compositum*.

BHI-Chelidonium complex: Used for abdominal distention and flatulence (Lycopodium, Calcarea carbonica); Gastralgia and yellow-clay-colored stools (Chelidonium majus); painful, distended abdomen, spasmodic hiccup, and epigastric pain (Belladonna) (Heel 2002).

Ceanothus homaccord: Treats pancreatopathy, epigastric syndrome, tenesmus, diarrhea, and hepatic issues. Splenic enlargement is a primary signalment for this remedy (Macleod 1983).

Chelidonium homaccord: A commonly used agent in hepatic damage and hepatitis, and gallbladder conditions such as cholangitis, cholecystitis, and obstructive jaundice (Demers 2004). Chelidonium contains a substance known as Chelidonine that has anticancer effects. "Chelidonine turned out to be a potent inducer of apoptosis triggering cell death at concentrations of 0.001 mM," according to Habermehl (2006), a fact that may explain the clinically observed usefulness of this remedy in treating patients with biliary neoplasia.

Chol-Heel: An excellent remedy containing Belladonna, Chelidonium, Carduus marianus, Lycopodium, Veratrum, and Taraxicum, along with some other very useful components, all in potency chords. This can be of great relief in GI discomfort (Broadfoot 2005).

Coenzyme compositum: Contains Citricum acidum, which is useful for dental problems and gingivitis; scurvy; blackening of teeth and heavy deposits of dental plaque; painful, herpetic vesicles around the lips; nausea; painful cramping in the umbilical area, and distension. Used as an agent to repair mitochondrial damage resulting from antibiotic therapy (also with *Ubichinon compositum* and *Galium-Heel* for that purpose).

Colchicum compositum: Used for cachexia and neoplastic conditions. Cholichicine has been used in hepatitis patients to reduce cirrhosis. The use of *Colchicum compositum* should be considered but has no clinical evidence at this time. Reports of its use are welcomed by the authors.

Engystol N: Used for viral-origin gastroenteritis and hepatitis (see Parvovirus).

Erigotheel: Used for gastric catarrh, hepatic diseases, and duodenal ulcers with spasm, and as an antipyretic (Demers 2004).

Galium-Heel: Used for all cellular phases, hemorrhoids, and anal fissures, and as a detoxicant. See notes above for proper use.

Hepar compositum: The main remedy for chronic hepatitis cases. Provides detoxification and drainage of hepatic tissues, organ and metabolic support, and is useful in most hepatic and gall bladder pathologies. It is an important part of Deep Detoxification Formula. Treats duodenitis, pancreatitis, cystic hepatic ducts, cholelithiasis, cholangitis, cholecystitis, vomiting, and diarrhea (Demers 2004, Broadfoot 2004). This combination contains Natrum oxalaceticum (also found in *Coenzyme compositum*, *Ubichinon compositum*, and *Mucosa compositum*) for changes in appetite and stomach distension due to air. Used for nausea, stomach pain with a sensation of fullness, gurgling in the abdomen, and cramping pain in the hypochondria. Also used for constipation, sudden diarrhea (particularly after eating), and flatus (Reckeweg 2002).

Hepeel: Provides liver drainage and detoxification. Used in a wide variety of conditions including cancer of the liver, where *Hepeel* was found to be antiproliferative, hepatoprotective, and an antioxidant when tested in human HepG2 cells (Gebhardt 2003).

Leptandra compositum: Used for epigastric syndrome, portal vein congestion, pancreatopathy, chronic liver disease, and diabetes mellitus (Reckeweg 2000).

Lymphomyosot: Provides lymph drainage and endocrine support, and treats edema. Contains Gentiana for chronic gastritis. Treats flatulence, diarrhea, distension of the stomach with eructations, nausea, retching, and vomiting. Also contains Geranium robertianum for nausea, particularly after eating with distension or sensation of fullness. Myosotis arvensis is included for bloat and distension (Reckeweg 2002).

Mucosa compositum: Broadly supportive for repair of mucosal elements. Used in cellular cases and in recovery periods following active disease (Reckeweg 2000). This remedy contains a useful component in Kali bichromicum, which is indicated for ulcers found on the gums, tongue, lips, and even on the gastric mucosa (gastric or duodenal ulcer). The tongue may have a thick, yellow, mucous coating, or in ulcerative stomatitis or tonsillitis it may be dry, smooth, shiny, or fissured. Kali has been used effectively in acute gastroenteritis associated with vomiting of clear, light-colored fluid or quantities of mucous bile, and in cases with hematemesis, flatulent colics, and dysenteric stools with tenesmus (Reckeweg 2002).

It also contains Hydrastis, with mucosal support for oral problems such as stomatitis, and mucosal suppuration that is accompanied by ulceration, inflammations and colic of the hepatobiliary system and of the gastrointestinal tract, and polyp formation (Reckeweg 2002). The Kreosotum component can be used in chronic gastritis with gastric hemorrhages and vomiting of brown masses. Also has a dental implication in cases with spongy gums and carious teeth, neuralgias proceeding from them causing a burning toothache with deep caries, black patches on the teeth, and fetid discharges.

The single remedy Phosphorus is broadly useful for dyspepsia and for jaw problems in dental disease (Reckeweg 2002). Phosphorus is found in many other remedies including *Echinacea compositum* and *Leptandra homaccord*. It is rich in suis organ preparations for mucosal support, plus a large variety of remedies with indications in the gastrointestinal sphere. The component Argentum nitricum (also in *Atropinum compositum*, *Diarrheel*, *Duodenoheel*, *Gastricumeel*, *Momordica compositum*, *BHI-Nausea*, and several other combinations) is indicated for distension in the upper abdomen, gastro-cardiac symptom-complex, and amelioration from eructations. It is also used for gastric crises (Reckeweg 2002).

Nux vomica homaccord: Used for liver and gastrointestinal disease and after smoke inhalation. Useful in gingivitis (Reckeweg 2002). This commonly used formula for detoxification is part of the *Detox Kit*. Recent research shows that one ingredient (Brucine) affects mitochondria in human hepatoma cells. Further research is needed to determine whether homeopathic dilutions are more or less active (Deng, et al. 2006).

Phosphor homaccord: Treats hepatitis, icterus, tenderness over the liver region, pancreatic diseases, ulcerated gums, thirst but vomiting right after drinking occurs, and pale-clay-colored stools (Macleod 1983).

Schwef-Heel: Treats chronic diseases of the skin and liver. This remedy should be interposed in most skin and liver cases (Reckeweg 2000). Patients that need this remedy may look dirty and have scruffy skin conditions, red lips, a white tongue with red tip, itching and burning rectal area with morning diarrhea, or a prolapsed rectum (Boericke 1927). Sulfur is contained in several other antihomotoxic formulas including *Coenzyme compositum*, *Echinacea compositum*, *Engystol*, *Ginseng compositum*, *Hepar compositum*, *Molybdan compositum*, *Mucosa compositum*, *Paeonia-Heel*, *Proctheel*, *Psorinoheel*,

Sulfur-Heel, Thyroidea compositum, and *Ubichinon compositum* (Reckeweg 2000).

Syzygium compositum: Used for chronic gastritis, chronic enteritis, diabetes mellitus, and hepatic disorders.

Ubichinon compositum: Contains Anthraquinone for swelling of the gums, and GI symptoms such as distention, flatulence, and cramping abdominal pain. Treats constipation with straining or sudden diarrhea (Reckeweg 2002).

Authors' suggested protocols

Nutrition

Liver and immune support formulas (thymus-enriched): 1 tablet for every 25 pounds of body weight BID.

Alpha-lipoic acid: 20 mg per 10 pounds of body weight daily.

S-adenosylmethionine SAMe: 10 to 20 mg/kg SID or follow manufacturer's dosing directions.

Lecithin/phosphatidyl choline: One-fourth teaspoon for every 25 pounds of body weight BID.

Zinc: 15 mg for every 25 pounds of body weight SID.

Additional vitamin E: 50 IU for every 25 pounds of body weight.

Chinese herbal medicine/acupuncture

LiverGuard: 1 capsule per 10 to 20 pounds twice daily based upon response. In addition to the herbs cited above, LiverGuard also contains amomum fruit (Sha ren), hawthorn fruit (Shan zha), immature bitter orange (Zhi qiao), lindera root (Wu yao), massa fermentata (Shen qu), mastic (Ru xiang), melia (Chuan lian zi), myrrh (Mo yao), rehmannia (Sheng di huang), and tortoise shell (Bie jia).

The authors commonly choose from the following acupuncture points: LI3, GB34, BL18, BL19, BL20, PC6, CV12, and GB34.

Homotoxicology (Dose: 10 drops PO for 50-pound dog; 5 drops PO for cat or small dog)

In addition to the necessary conventional therapy:

Phosphor homaccord, Chelidonium homaccord, Nux homaccord, Duodenoheel: Mixed together and give BID.

Alternate: Hepeel and BHI-Enzyme—BID PO.

Gastricumeel: If vomiting.

Engystol N: For viral hepatitis.

Galium-Heel, Lymphomyosot, Hepar compositum, Solidago compositum: Give every 3 days. If diarrhea, consider adding Coenzyme compositum and Ubichinon compositum twice weekly.

Product sources

Nutrition

Liver and immune support formulas: Animal Nutrition Technologies. **Alternatives:** Immune System Support—Standard Process Veterinary Formulas; Immuno Support—Rx Vitamins for Pets; Immugen—Thorne Veterinary Products; Hepatic Support—Standard Process Veterinary Formulas; Hepato Support—Rx Vitamins for Pets; Hepagen—Thorne Veterinary Products.

Alpha-lipoic acid: Source Naturals.

SAMe: Nutramax Labs.

Lecithin/phosphatidyl choline: One-quarter teaspoon for each 25 pounds of body weight BID

Chinese herbal medicine

Liver Guard: Natural Solutions, Inc.

Homotoxicology

BHI/Heel Corporation

REFERENCES

Western medicine references

Center SA. Chronic liver disease. In: Guilford WG, Center SA, Strombeck DR, et al., eds. Strombeck's small animal gastroenterology. 3rd ed. Philadelphia: Saunders, 1996:705–765.

Dill-Macky E. Chronic hepatitis in dogs. *Vet Clin North Am Small Anim Pract* 1995;25:387–398.

Doige CE, Lester S. Chronic active hepatitis in dogs: A review of fourteen cases. *J Am Anim Hosp Assoc* 1981.17:725.

Gitlin N. Corticosteroid therapy for chronic active hepatitis. *Am J Gastroenterol* 1984.79:573.

Hardy, RM. In: Tilley L, Smith F. The 5-Minute Veterinary Consult: Canine and Feline, 2003. Blackwell Publishing.

Hardy RM, et al. Chronic progressive hepatitis in Bedlington terriers associated with elevated liver copper concentrations. *Minn Vet* 1975.15:13.

Laflamme DP. Nutritional management of liver disease. In: Bonagura JD, ed. Kirk's Current Veterinary Therapy XIII. Philadelphia: WB Saunders, 2000, pp 693–697.

Leveille-Webster CR, Center SA. Chronic hepatitis: therapeutic considerations. In: Bonagura JD, ed. Kirk's current veterinary therapy XII. Philadelphia: Saunders, 1995:749–756.

Magne ML, Chiapella AM. Medical management of canine chronic active hepatitis. *Comp Contin Educ Small Anim Pract* 1986.8:915.

Meyer D, Twedt D. Current Vet Therapy XIII, 2000.pp. 668–671.

Neuberg J, et al. Effect of polyunsaturated phosphatidylcholine immune mediated hepatocyte damage. *Gut* 1983.24:751.

Sevelius E. Diagnosis and prognosis of chronic hepatitis and cirrhosis in dogs, *J Small Anim Pract* 1995;36:521–528.

IVM/nutrition references

Berkson BM. A conservative triple antioxidant approach to the treatment of hepatitis C. Combination of Alpha lipoic acid (thioctic acid), silymarin, and selenium: three case histories. *Med Klin* 1999;94 Suppl 3:84–9.

Bortolotti F, Cadrobbi P, Crivellaro C, et al. Effect of an orally administered thymic derivative, thymomodulin, in chronic type B hepatitis in children. *Curr Ther Res* 1988;43:67–72.

Busse E, Zimmer G, Schorpohl B, et al. Influence of alpha-lipoic acid on intracellular glutathione in vitro and in vivo. *Arzneimittelforschung* 1992;42:829–31.

Civeira MP, Castilla A, Morte S, et al. A pilot study of thymus extract in chronic non-A, non-B hepatitis. *Aliment Pharmacol Ther* 1989;3:395–401.

Galli M, Crocchiolo P, Negri C, et al. Attempt to treat acute type B hepatitis with an orally administered thymic extract (thymomodulin): Preliminary results. *Drugs Exp Clin Res* 1985;11:665–9.

Center SA. S-adenosyl-methionine: an antioxidant and anti-inflammatory nutraceutical. Proceedings of the 18th ACVIM, 2000.Seattle, WA:550–552.

de la Maza MP, Petermann M, Bunout D, Hirsch S. Effects of long-term vitamin E supplementation in alcoholic cirrhotics. *J Am Coll Nutr* 1995;14:192–6.

Ferro D, Basili S, Practico D, et al. Vitamin E reduces monocyte tissue factor expression in cirrhotic patients. *Blood* 1999;93:2945–50.

Gorbakov VV, Galik VP, Kirillov SM. Experience in heptral treatment of diffuse liver diseases. *Ter Arkh* 1998;70:82–6 [in Russian].

Lieber CS, Robins SJ, Li J, et al. Phosphatidylcholine protects against fibrosis and cirrhosis in the baboon. *Gastroenterology* 1994;106:152–9.

Lykkesfeldt J, Hagen TM, Vinarsky V, Ames BN. Age-associated decline in ascorbic acid concentration, recycling, and biosynthesis in rat hepatocytes—reversal with (R)-alpha-lipoic acid supplementation. *FASEB J* 1998;12:1183–9.

Ma X, Zhao J, Lieber CS. Polyenylphosphatidylcholine attenuates non-alcoholic hepatic fibrosis and accelerates its regression. *J Hepatol* 1996;24:604–13.

Marchesini G, Fabbri A, Bianchi G, et al. Zinc supplementation and amino acid-nitrogen metabolism in patients with advanced cirrhosis. *Hepatology* 1996;23:1084–92.

Mato JM, Camara J, Fernandez de Paz J, et al. S-adenosylmethionine in alcoholic liver cirrhosis: a randomized, placebo-controlled, double-blind, multicenter clinical trial. *J Hepatol* 1999;30:1081–9.

Miglio F, Stefanini GF, Corazza GR, et al. Double-blind studies of the therapeutic action of S-Adenosylmethionine (SAMe) in oral administration, in liver cirrhosis and other chronic hepatitides. *Minerva Med* 1975;66:1595–9 [in Italian].

Reding P, Duchateau J, Bataille C. Oral zinc supplementation improves hepatic encephalopathy. Results of a randomised controlled trial. *Lancet* 1984;2(8401):493–5.

Scholmerich J, Lohle E, Kottgen E, Gerok W. Zinc and vitamin A deficiency in liver cirrhosis. *Hepatogastroenterology* 1983;30:119–25.

Scholich H, Murphy ME, Sies H. Antioxidant activity of dihydrolipoate against microsomal lipid peroxidation and its dependence on alpha-tocopherol. *Biochem Biophys Acta* 1989;1001:256–61.

Taniguchi S, Kaneto K, Hamada T. Acquired zinc deficiency associated with alcoholic liver cirrhosis. *Int J Dermatol* 1995;34:651–2.

Chinese herbal medicine/acupuncture references

An Hui Zhong Yi Xue Yuan Xue Bao (*Journal of Anhui University School of Medicine*), 1984;2:25.

Chang Yong Zhong Yao Cheng Fen Yu Yao Li Shou Ce (A Handbook of the Composition and Pharmacology of Common Chinese Drugs), 1994; 1479: 1482.

Chong Qing Yi Yao (*Chongching Medicine and Herbology*), 1989;18(4):39.

Fu Jian Zhong Yi Yao (*Fujian Chinese Medicine and Herbology*), 1959;7:42.

Gao PJ, et al. *Journal of Norman Bethune Medical University.* 1996;22(1):23–24.

Group of Liver Diseases. Shanxi College of Traditional Chinese Medicine. *Journal of Modern Medicine.* 1973;(9):21.

Gui Yang Yi Xue Yuan Xue Bao (*Journal of Guiyang Medical University*), 1959: 113.

Han DW, et al. *China Journal of Internal Medicine.* 1977;2(1):13.

Handbook of Traditional Chinese Medicine Practitioners. Hunan College of Traditional Chinese Medicine. Shanghai Science and Technology Publishing Oct 1987 p 275.

He P, et al. Yin Chen's effect on antipyrin metabolism in humans and rabbits. *China Journal of Hospital Pharmacy.* 1990; 10(10):459–460.

He P, et al. Yin Chen's effect on drug-metabolizing enzymes in mice. *China Journal of Chinese Medicine.* 1990;15(6):372.

Hou Xue Hua Yu Yan Jia (Research on Blood-Activating and Stasis-Eliminating Herbs), 1981:335.

Hu YQ, et al. The extraction and separation of Yin Chen polypeptides and their liver-protecting effects in mice. *Journal of Chinese Materia Medica.* 1999;30(12):894–896.

Hu YY, et al. Dan Shen extract's effect on CCl4- and DMN-induced liver fibrosis in rats. *Shanghai Journal of Traditional Chinese Medicine and Herbs.* 1999;(10):7–10.

Indian J Med Res; 1971; 59(1):76.

Ji Lin Zhong Yi Yao (*Jilin Chinese Medicine and Herbology*), 1985; 5:24.

Jiang CM, et al. Tao Ren's effect on in vitro and in vivo rat lipid peroxidation. *Journal of Bengbu Medical College.* 1995; 20(2):81–82.

Liu J, et al. Blood stasis-removing herbs' effect on CC14-induced mild liver damages. *Journal of Chinese Patented Medicine.* 1999;21(8):422–425.

Liu W, et al. *Henan Journal of TCM Pharmacy.* 1998; 13(4):10–12.

Ma ZY. *Shannxi Journal of Traditional Chinese Medicine and Herbs.* 1982;(4):58.

Nagai, H. et al. *Planta Medica.* 1989.55(1): 13–17.

Nanjing College of Pharmacy. Materia Medica, vol.2. Jiangsu: People's Press; 1976.

Planta Med, 1984; 46(1):84.

Rui J. *Journal of Chinese Materia Medica.* 1999;30(1):43–45.

Shan Xi Zhong Yi (*Shangxi Chinese Medicine*), 1988;3:106.

Shan YTE, et al. *Journal of Pharmacy.* Japan. 1982;102(3): 285.

Shang Hai Zhong Yi Yao Za Zhi (*Shanghai Journal of Chinese Medicine and Herbology*), 1965; 7:10.

Shen Yang Yi Xue Yuan Bao (*Journal of Shenyang University of Medicine*), 1984; 1(3):214.

Sui YH, et al. A comparative study of Xiang Fu, Qing Pi, Ci Li, Yin Chen, Xi Nan Zhang Ya Cai: Their effects on bile secretion. *Henan Journal of TCM.* 1993;13(1):19–20,44.

Sun WQ, et al. Tao Ren's effect in counteracting liver damages due to lipid peroxidation. *Hunan Journal of Medicine.* 1993;9(6):47–48.

Takeda, S. et al. Nippon Yakurigaku Zasshi. 88(4):321–30. 1986.

Wan YD. The antipyretic effects of capillarin. *Pharmacy Bulletin.* 1987;(10):590–593.

Wu BC, et al. *Journal of Chinese Medicine.* 1987;(3):32–33.

Xin Zhong Yi (*New Chinese Medicine*), 1989; 21(3):51.

Xu LM, et al. Tao Ren extract's effect in counteracting experimental liver fibrosis—an immunohistochemistry and collagen metabolism research. *Journal of Pharmacology and Clinical Application of TCM.* 1993;9(5):14–16.

Zhang G, Song S, Ren J, Xu S. A New Compound from Forsythia suspense (Thunb.) Vahl with Antiviral Effect on RSV. *J of Herbal Pharmacotherapy.* 2002;2(3): 35–39.

Zhe Jiang Zhong Yi Za Zhi (*Zhejiang Journal of Chinese Medicine*), 1983;3:103.

Zhong Cao Yao (*Chinese Herbal Medicine*) 1991;22 (10): 452.

Zhong Guo Mian Yi Xue Za Zhi (*Chinese Journal of Immunology*), 1989; 5(2):121.

Zhong Xi Yi Jie He Za Zhi (*Journal of Integrated Chinese and Western Medicine*), 1984;2:86.

Zhong Xi Yi Jie He Za Zhi (*Journal of Integrated Chinese and Western Medicine*), 1988;8(3):p 161 and 180.

Zhong Yao Tong Bao (*Journal of Chinese Herbology*), 1987;9:60.

Zhong Yao Xue (*Chinese Herbology*) 1988;103:106.

Zhong Yao Zhi (*Chinese Herbology Journal*), 1993:183.

Zhong Yao Xue (*Chinese Herbology*), 1998; 845:848.

Zhong Yao Yao Li Yu Ying Yong (*Pharmacology and Applications of Chinese Herbs*), 1990; 15(6):52.

Zhong Yi Yao Xin Xie (Information on Chinese Medicine and Herbology), 1985;3:18.

Zhong Yi Za Zhi (*Journal of Chinese Medicine*), 1982; (1): 67.

Zhu LH. *China Journal of TCM Information.* 1996;3(3): 17–20.

Homotoxicology references

Broadfoot PJ. Inflammation: Homotoxicology and Healing. In: Proceedings AHVMA/Heel Homotoxicology Seminar. Denver, CO, 2004. p 27.

Demers, J. Homotoxicology and Acupuncture. In: Proceedings of the 2004 Homotoxicology Seminar. AHVMA/Heel. Denver, CO, 2004. p 5, 6.

Deng X, Yin F, Lu X, Cai B, Yin W. The apoptotic effect of brucine from the seed of Strychnos nux-vomica on human hepatoma cells is mediated via Bcl-2 and Ca2+ involved mitochondrial pathway. *Toxicol Sci.* 2006. May;91(1):pp 59–69.

Gebhardt R. Antioxidative, antiproliferative and biochemical effects in HepG2 cells of a homeopathic remedy and its constituent plant tinctures tested separately or in combination. *Arzneimittelforschung.* 2003. 53(12): pp 823–30.

Habermehl D, Kammerer B, Handrick R, Eldh T, Gruber C, Cordes N, Daniel PT, Plasswilm L, Bamberg M, Belka C, Jendrossek V. Proapoptotic activity of Ukrain is based on Chelidonium majus L. alkaloids and mediated via a mitochondrial death pathway. *BMC Cancer.* 2006. Jan 17;6: p 14.

Heel. BHI Homeopathic Therapy: Professional Reference. Albuquerque, NM: Heel Inc., 2002.pp 43, 47, 73.

Khuda-Bukhsh AR, Pathak S, Guha B, Karmakar S, Das J, Banerjee P, Biswas S, Mukherjee P, Bhattacharjee N, Choudhury S, Banerjee A, Bhadra S, Mallick P, Chakrabarti J, Mandal B. In vitro anti-rotavirus activity of some medicinal plants used in Brazil against diarrhea. *J Ethnopharmacol.* 2005. Jul 14;99(3): pp 403–7.

Mallick P, Mallick JC, Guha B, Khuda-Bukhsh AR. Ameliorating effect of microdoses of a potentized homeopathic drug, Arsenicum Album, on arsenic-induced toxicity in mice. *BMC Complement Altern Med.* 2003. Oct 22;3: p 7.

Macleod G. 1983. A Veterinary Materia Medica and Clinical Repertory with a Materia Medica of the Nosodes. Safron, Walden: CW Daniel Company, LTD., pp 50–1, 125–6, 129–30.

Miele L, Vero V, Gasbarrini G, Grieco A. Braised liver with herbs: the risks of naturopathic hepatoprotection. *J Clin Gastroenterol.* 2004. Apr;39(4):p 344.

Reckeweg H. Biotherapeutic Index: Ordinatio Antihomotoxica et Materia Medica, 5th ed. Baden-Baden, Germany: Biologische Heilmittel Heel GMBH, 2000. pp 157, 294–5, 300, 358–9, 369, 399–400.

Reckeweg H. Homeopathia Antihomotoxica Materia Medica, 4th ed. Baden-Baden, Germany: Arelia-Verlag GMBH, 2002., pp. 136–8, 139–40, 125–6, 147,150–3, 179, 206, 241–2, 317–19, 345, 366, 461–3, 488–90, 578–80.

Shamsa F, Ahmadiani A, Khosrokhavar R. Antihistaminic and anticholinergic activity of barberry fruit (Berberis vulgaris) in the guinea-pig ileum. *J Ethnopharmacol.* 1999. Feb;64(2):pp 161–6.

Spee B, Arends B, van den Ingh TS, Brinkhof B, Nederbragt H, Ijzer J, Roskams T, Penning L, Rothuizen J. Transforming growth factor beta-1 signaling in canine hepatic diseases: new models for human fibrotic liver pathologies. *Liver Int.* 2006. Aug;26(6):pp 716–25.

Watson PJ. Chronic hepatitis in dogs: a review of current understanding of the aetiology, progression, and treatment. *Vet J.* 2004. May;167(3):228–41.

Zhu B, Ahrens FA. Effect of berberine on intestinal secretion mediated by Escherichia coli heat-stable enterotoxin in jejunum of pigs. *Am J Vet Res.* 1982. Sep;43(9): pp 1594–8.

CHOLANGIOHEPATITIS

Definition and cause

An inflammatory process of the liver and bile ducts that can manifest as suppurative or infiltrative (lymphocytic or plasmalymphocytic). In cats, it is very commonly associated with pancreatitis and inflammatory bowel disease (Triad disease) as well as kidney disease. The initiating cause of the inflammation is commonly infection or a pre-existing condition such as extrahepatic bile duct obstruction (EHBDO). An immunological response is also suspected (Bunch 1992; Center 1994, 1996, 2003; Johnson 1994).

Medical therapy rationale, drug(s) of choice, and nutritional recommendations

Medical therapy is broad-spectrum antibiotics, usually clavamox in combination with metronidazole and glucocorticoids. In more resistant cases immunosuppressing drugs such as azathioprine or chlorambucil in combination with prednisone are suggested. Liver protectants such as ursodeoxycholic acid (Actigall) are recommended along with water-soluble antioxidant vitamins such as vitamins E and B. Dietary recommendations are a low-fat, high-protein diet to prevent hepatic lipidosis (Bunch 1992, Center 2003).

Anticipated prognosis

More acute disease often responds well to medication and dietary changes. Chronic disease requires ongoing medication and care and can be controlled well for long periods of time (Center 2003, Johnson 1994).

Integrative veterinary therapies

The integrative approach to liver disease focuses upon the inciting inflammatory process that results in liver cell destruction. Early identification, addressing the cause, and instituting integrative measures, along with medical therapy when necessary, often gives the best prognosis.

Liver cell regeneration may be improved if the underlying cause is identified early and nutrients, nutraceuticals, medicinal herbs, and combination homeopathics that are anti-inflammatory and organ sparing are used. It is possible to prevent progressive inflammation, cell death, and scarring that leads to cirrhotic conditions if integrative therapies are instituted early in the treatment of hepatitis or at early signs of liver issues such as chronic elevation of ALT, AST, or GGTP levels (Goldstein 2005).

Nutrition
General considerations/rationale

Liver health depends upon reducing toxins and metabolic wastes and increasing antioxidants and phytonutrients that help neutralize compounds that the liver must deal with in its role as the body's filter and detoxifier. Glutathione is a compound that is composed of three amino acids: glutamic acid, glysine, and cysteine. Glutathione binds and neutralizes various chemicals, toxins, herbicides, pesticides, heavy metals, etc. so they can pass through the liver and be excreted via the bile into the intestines, or pass to the kidneys to be excreted in the urine (Sen 1997).

Body glutathione levels can be raised by other nutrients such as vitamin C, whey protein, glutamine, methionine, S-adenosyl-L-methionine (SAMe), and alpha-lipoic acid (Amores-Sanchez 1999, Bounous 1989, Vendemiale 1989, Wang 1997).

Appropriate nutrients

Nutrition/gland therapy: Clinical trials using thymus extract have shown that they are beneficial in people with hepatitis B (Skotnicki 1989). Additional clinical studies with oral thymus extract showed that blood values related to liver function as well as blood immune markers improved. Civereira (1989) showed similar results with hepatitis C (Galli 1985, Bortolotti 1988). Glandular liver helps to neutralize a cellular immune response and helps spare liver cells (see Chapter 2, Gland Therapy, for additional information).

Note: Because liver disease can be severe and involve multiple organ disease, it is recommended that blood be analyzed both medically and physiologically to determine real and impending organ involvement and disease. This allows for a more specific gland and nutritional support protocol (see Chapter 2, Nutritional Blood Testing, for additional information).

Lecithin/phosphatidyl choline: Has been shown to help break down scar tissue in the liver and prevent cirrhosis by reversing the cellular changes that lead to cirrhotic cell formation (Ma 1996). Phosphatidyl choline has been shown to reverse the progression of alcohol-induced cirrhosis in humans (Lieber 1994).

Alpha-lipoic acid is a potent antioxidant, proven to reduce oxidative stress and inflammation. It has also been shown to increase the effectiveness of other antioxidants, such as vitamins C and E, CoEnzyme Q10, and glutathione, making them more readily available for bodily function (Busse 1992, Lykkesfeldt 1998, Scholich 1989). There was significant improvement of liver function in a study of people with cirrhosis who received a combination antioxidant-rich supplement that contained 300 mg of alpha-lipoic acid (Berkson 1999).

S-adenosylmethionine (SAMe): SAMe is an antioxidant that has anti-inflammatory effects on the liver (Center 2000). SAMe has been shown to significantly improve survival and decrease the need for liver transplantation in people with liver disease. It has also been shown to improve liver function in less severe cases of cirrhosis (Gorbakov 1998, Mato 1999, Miglio 1975).

Vitamin E: Was shown to decrease liver damage and immune imbalances that may contribute to the disease progression; however, further clinical work is required to definitively confirm this because another clinical trial failed to confirm these results (Ferro 1999, de la Maza 1995).

Chinese herbal medicine/acupuncture
General considerations/rationale
Cholangiohepatitis is a disorder of Heat and Damp in the Stomach and Spleen. There is a cleansing disorder in the Liver and Gallbladder. Heat is infection or inflammation. Damp refers to purulent debris or accumulation of sludged bile in the Gallbladder. The ancient Chinese attributed the condition to the Stomach and Spleen because the signs presented, such as vomiting or in more chronic cases ascites, are categorized as Stomach and Spleen signs. The Liver and Gallbladder are said to clean the Blood at night. Toxins can build up in the blood if they are not functioning well. This concept is similar to the Western idea in which hepatoencephalopathy may result if the liver does not detoxify compounds in the body.

Treatment is aimed at decreasing the Heat (infection or inflammation), moving the Damp (increasing bile flow), and controlling signs such as ascites, anorexia, nausea, etc.

Appropriate Chinese herbs
Alisma (Ze xie): Has been used to treat hepatic lipidosis (Chinese Journal of Modern Developments in Traditional Medicine 1981). In addition it has diuretic properties (Sheng Yao Xue Za Zhi 1982).

Atractylodes (Bai zhu): Has immunomodulatory effects. It can increase the T helper cell count and increase the ratio of helper to suppressor cells (Xu 1994). It has a diuretic effect and has been used for ascites from infectious hepatitis (An Hui Zhong Yi Xue Yuan Xue Bao 1984).

Barley sprouts (Mai ya): Syrup was used in patients with hepatitis, and symptoms improved in 85% of the cases of acute hepatitis and 57% of the cases of chronic hepatitis. Positive effects were defined as improved appetite, decreased pain, and decreased liver enzyme levels (Xin Yi Yao Tong Xun 1972).

Cinnamon twigs (Gui zhi): Have demonstrated antibiotic properties against several bacteria and viruses (Zhong Yao Xue 1998). They also have diuretic actions (Zhong Yao Xue 1998).

Crataegus (Shan zha): Counteracts nausea (Zhong Xi Yi Jie He Za Zhi 1984). Nausea is most commonly seen in chronic suppurative cholangiohepatitis, but may be present in other forms of this disease.

Ginger (Gan jiang): Helps relieve signs of abdominal fullness and epigastric pain (Zhong Yi Za Zhi 1965).

Licorice (Gan cao): Can play many roles in a supplement designed for cholangiohepatitis. Corticosteroids are often part of the therapeutic protocol in Western therapy. Licorice contains glycyrrhizin and glycyrrhetinic acid, which enhance the action of endogenous corticosteroids in the body (Zhong Yao Zhi 1993). Licorice is hepatoprotective and has antibacterial and antiviral properties. It has efficacy against E. coli and adenovirus II, among other pathogens (Zhong Yao Zhi 1993, Zhu 1996). It was 77% effective in treating 330 human patients with hepatitis B. It reduced inflammation, increased regeneration of hepatic cells, and decreased hepatic necrosis and cirrhosis (Zhong Yao Tong Bao 1987).

Oriental wormwood (Yin chen hao): Ideally suited for use in an herbal supplement designed for cholangiohepatitis. It has hepatoprotective properties. It can increase the phagocytic action of macrophages and has been shown experimentally to enhance the ability of the liver to detoxify drugs in both humans and rabbits (Hu 1999, He 1990). It has cholagogic effects (Sheng Yao Xue Za Zhi 1978). Furthermore, it has antibacterial activity against a variety of bacteria, including E. coli (Zhong Yao Yao Li Yu Ying Yong 1990). It also has analgesic and anti-inflammatory effects (Wan 1987, Shan 1982). Oriental wormwood was used in a trial involving 32 people with acute hepatitis. After 3 to 15 days of treatment there was significant decrease in hepatomegaly, icterus, and pyrexia (Fu Jian Zhong Yi Yao 1959). Cats with cholangiohepatitis often have concurrent pancreatitis. When wormwood was administered to rats with deoxydium-induced acute hemorrhagic necrotic pancreatitis, it decreased the death rate (Li 1996).

Pinella (Ban xia): Seems to affect the central nervous system to decrease chemical-mediated vomiting (Zhong Yao Yao Li Yu Ying Yong 1983). It may decrease nausea and vomiting secondary to hepatic failure.

Polyporus (Zhu ling): Has been shown to be hepatoprotective in studies involving the administration of CCl4 to rats (Zhong Guo Yao Li Xue Tong Bao 1988). In addition, it is a diuretic (Yao Xue Xue Bao 1964) and may help decrease ascites. It inhibits E. coli, a common hepatic pathogen (Zhong Yao Xue 1998).

Poria (Fu ling): Protects the liver. It has been shown experimentally to decrease damage induced by CCl4 (Han 1977). It has a diuretic effect as demonstrated in rabbits (Lu 1987, Lu 1988). It also inhibits bacteria (Nanjing College of Pharmacy 1976).

Acupuncture

Acupuncture may help protect the liver. In one experiment 36 rats were treated with CCl4. The efficacy of acupuncture at St36 and LI3 for hepatoprotection was investigated. The rats treated after exposure to CCl4 had lower AST and ALT levels, suggesting that acupuncture can protect the liver (Hsu-Jan Liu 2001).

Homotoxicology
General considerations/rationale

The liver and gallbladder are crucial organs in the body's defense against both endogenous and exogenous homotoxins. Homotoxins originating in the gastrointestinal system are absorbed and presented to the liver for handling via the portal vein system. The liver has an effective system for defense, but disease can result if homotoxins accumulate and damage the tissues associated with the liver. Disease involving the bile ducts is called cholangitis, while conditions involving both liver and bile ducts are known as cholangiohepatitis. Both conditions represent homotoxicoses of either the Inflammation Phase (in acute disease states) or the Impregnation Phase (in more chronic or recurring disease). Cellular infiltrates of immune cells may consist of neutrophils, lymphocytes, or plasmacytes.

Concurrent diseases of the gallbladder, liver, pancreas, or gastrointestinal system can result in cholangiohepatitis, particularly if the bile becomes thickened and sludged, a change commonly seen during ultrasound examination of the abdomen (Weiss, Gagne, Armstrong 1996; McCaw 1997; Newell, et al. 1998). Such abnormal terrain favors the development of bacterial invasion, and biliary ducts respond by hyperplasia, which further compromises the area. Bacterial invasion often results in suppurative infiltrates. More chronic pathologies may lead to antigenic stimulation that can result in lymphocytic and lymphoplasmacytic infiltrates.

Successfully treating cholangiohepatitis involves providing clean diet and water, reducing stress, allowing homotoxins to be excreted successfully, supporting organ function, and providing drainage therapy, organ support, and metabolic support while repair occurs.

Antibiotic agents are frequently necessary in more severe or chronic cases, and selection of agents that inhibit or kill both aerobic and anaerobic bacteria is advised. Amoxicillin and metronidazole are frequently chosen, but other medications may be needed in resistant bacterial infections. Clearing the bacterial infection may not resolve the cholangiohepatitis (Pressel, et al. 2005). Treatment goals include liquefying biliary sludge, promoting bile flow, controlling existing infection, and protecting associated tissues from further harm as homotoxins are removed and drained from the area. Ursodeoxycholic acid is commonly used to thin bile in conventional practice. *Chelido-nium* is well known in homotoxicology practices for its ability to perform similarly, and this herb figures prominently in treatment plans for cholangiohepatitis. As is the case in treating all homotoxicoses, proper nutrition and fluid intake are helpful as well.

Regressive vicariation in these patients frequently involves some degree of gastrointestinal dysfunction, which usually consists of mild to moderate diarrhea or constipation. Stool character can vary between these two extremes as autoregulation is reinstated. Stool color may vary greatly as homotoxins clear the system. Because homotoxins can be recycled from reabsorption of gastrointestinal contents, the addition of adequate fiber can greatly assist in binding homotoxins and moving them out of the system. Supporting other excretion organs, particularly the kidney, is advised as well.

Appropriate homotoxicology formulas

Because gastrointestinal disease plays prominently in the pathogenesis of liver disease, the reader is referred to the more complete list of remedies at the end of the gastrointestinal chapter.

Atropinum compositum: Currently only available in the U.S. market in tablet form, this agent functions as a powerful antispasmodic for biliary, renal, and intestinal colic (Demers 2004). Contains Benzoicum acidum (common also to *Aesculus compositum*, *Arnica-Heel*, *Atropinum compositum*, and *Rhododendroneel*). It is used in inflammatory symptoms which occur throughout the alimentary canal: a slimy coating on the tongue with ulcers at the edges, stomatitis with dysphagia, eructations, retching and vomiting, and flatulent distension below the ribs on both sides. The stools are copious, loose, and white in color, with violent tenesmus and mixed with blood; there are stabbing pains in the rectum, rigors, and a feeling of being seriously ill (Reckeweg 2002).

Belladonna homaccord: Treats right-sided intensely red tonsillitis, pharyngitis, poor appetite, nausea and vomiting, stinging rectal pain, and focal and intense inflammatory lesions (Boericke 1927). Also treats cholangitis, cholecystitis, and cholelithiasis (Reckeweg 2000).

BHI-Chelidonium complex: Treats abdominal distention and flatulence (Lycopodium, Calcarea carbonica); gastralgia and yellow-clay colored stools (Chelidonium majus); painful, distended abdomen, spasmodic hiccup, and epigastric pain (Belladonna).

BHI-Gall Bladder Rx: Used for disorders of the gallbladder, gallstones, gallbladder colic, abdominal bloating, and discomfort.

Chelidonium homaccord: A major remedy that is used for gallbladder conditions such as cholangitis, cholecystitis, cholelithiasis, obstructive jaundice, hepatic damage, and hepatitis (Demers 2004). Chelidonium contains a substance known as Chelidonine, which has anticancer effects. "Chelidonine turned out to be a potent inducer of apoptosis triggering cell death at concentrations of 0.001 mM," according to Habermehl (2006), a fact that may explain the clinically observed usefulness of this remedy in treating patients with biliary neoplasia. Chelidonium also affects choleresis, increasing bile acid independent bile flow, and Celadine reduces formation of bile calculi and has a spasmolytic effect on biliary ducts (Vahlensieck, et al. 1995; Wynn, Marsden 2003).

Coenzyme compositum: Contains Citricum acidum, which is useful for dental problems and gingivitis; scurvy; blackening of teeth and heavy deposits of dental plaque; painful, herpetic vesicles around the lips; nausea; painful cramping in the umbilical area; and distension.

Engystol N: Used for viral origin and allergic gastroenteritis (see Parvovirus).

Galium-Heel: Used for all cellular phases, hemorrhoids, and anal fissures; and as a detoxicant.

Hepar compositum: Provides detoxification and drainage of hepatic tissues and organ and metabolic support, and is useful in most hepatic and gallbladder pathologies. It is an important part of Deep Detoxification Formula. Treats duodenitis, pancreatitis, cystic hepatic ducts, cholelithiasis, cholangitis, cholecystitis, vomiting, and diarrhea (Demers 2004, Broadfoot 2004). This combination contains Natrum oxalaceticum (also found in *Coenzyme compositum*, *Ubichinon compositum*, and *Mucosa compositum*) for changes in appetite and stomach distension due to air. It treats nausea, stomach pain with a sensation of fullness, gurgling in the abdomen, and cramping pain in the hypochondria. It is also used for constipation, sudden diarrhea (particularly after eating), and flatus (Reckeweg 2002).

Hepeel: Used for liver drainage and detoxification. *Hepeel* is also used in a wide variety of conditions including cancer of the liver, where *Hepeel* was found to be antiproliferative, hepatoprotective, and an antioxidant when tested in human HepG2 cells (Gebhardt 2003).

Lymphomyosot: Provides lymph drainage and endocrine support, and treats edema. Contains Gentiana for chronic gastritis. Treats flatulence, diarrhea, distension of the stomach with eructations, nausea, retching and vomiting. Contains Geranium robertianum for nausea, particularly after eating, with distension or sensation of fullness. Myosotis arvensis is included for bloat and distension (Reckeweg 2002).

Mucosa compositum: Broadly supportive for repair of mucosal elements. Used in cellular cases and in recovery periods following active disease (Reckeweg 2000). This remedy contains a useful component in Kali bichromicum, which is indicated for ulcers found on the gums, tongue, lips, and even on the gastric mucosa (gastric or duodenal ulcer). The tongue may have a thick, yellow, mucous coating, or in ulcerative stomatitis or

tonsillitis it may be dry, smooth, shiny, or fissured. Kali has been used effectively in acute gastroenteritis associated with vomiting of clear, light-colored fluid or quantities of mucous bile, and in cases with hematemesis, flatulent colics, and dysenteric stools with tenesmus (Reckeweg 2002).

It also contains Hydrastis, with mucosal support for oral problems such as stomatitis, and mucosal suppuration that is accompanied by ulceration, inflammations and colic of the hepatobiliary system and of the gastrointestinal tract, and polyp formation (Reckeweg 2002). The Kreosotum component can be used in chronic gastritis with gastric hemorrhages and vomiting of brown masses. Also has a dental implication in cases with spongy gums and carious teeth, neuralgias proceeding from them causing a burning toothache with deep caries, black patches on the teeth, and fetid discharges.

The single remedy Phosphorus is broadly useful for dyspepsia and for jaw problems in dental disease (Reckeweg 2002). Phosphorus is found in many other remedies including *Echinacea compositum* and *Leptandra homaccord*. It is rich in suis organ preparations for mucosal support, plus a large variety of remedies with indications in the gastrointestinal sphere. The component Argentum nitricum (also in *Atropinum compositum*, *Diarrheel*, *Duodenoheel*, *Gastricumeel*, *Momordica compositum*, *BHI-Nausea*, and several other combinations) is indicated for distension in the upper abdomen, gastro-cardiac symptom-complex, and amelioration from eructations. It is also used for gastric crises (Reckeweg 2002).

Nux vomica homaccord: Used for liver and gastrointestinal disease and after smoke inhalation. Useful in gingivitis (Reckeweg 2002). This commonly used formula is part of the Detox Kit. Recent research shows that one ingredient (Brucine) affects mitochondria in human hepatoma cells. Further research is needed to determine whether homeopathic dilutions are more or less active (Deng, et al. 2006).

Spascupreel: Used for spasm and pain from smooth muscle spasm (Reckeweg 2000).

Ubichinon compositum: Contains Anthraquinone for swelling of gums, and GI symptoms such as distention, flatulence, and cramping abdominal pain. Treats constipation with straining or sudden diarrhea (Reckeweg 2002).

Authors' suggested protocols

Nutrition

Liver and immune support formulas (thymus-enriched): 1 tablet for every 25 pounds of body weight BID.

Alpha-lipoic acid: 20 mg per 10 pounds of body weight daily.

SAMe: 10 to 20 mg/kg SID or follow manufacturer's dosing directions.

Vitamin E: 50 IU for every 20 pounds of body weight SID.

Lecithin/phosphatidyl choline: One-fourth teaspoon for every 25 pounds of body weight BID.

Chinese herbal medicine/acupuncture

Formula H 77 Cholangiohepatitis/Chronic: 1 capsule per 10 to 20 pounds twice daily. This supplement is indicated for acute or chronic cholangiohepatitis. In most of the cases, it needs to be combined with conventional medicine such as antibiotics, prednisone, cyproheptadine to stimulate the appetite, fluid therapy, and/or ursodiol. Once the acute phase is over many pets can be maintained on the herb alone to prevent recurrence of symptoms or progression of the disease.

In addition to the herbs discussed above, H 77 Cholangiohepatitis/Chronic also contains aconite (Fu zi) and leaven (Shen qi), which help to increase the efficacy of the formula.

The authors recommend using the following acupuncture points: CV12, ST36, PC6, BL19, Li3,SP6, GB34, and BL20.

Homotoxicology (Dose: 10 drops PO for 50-pound dog; 5 drops PO for cat or small dog)

Chelidonium homaccord, Echinacea compositum, and Nux vomica homaccord: Mix together and give orally BID to TID. Give Hepar compositum weekly to biweekly. Give Spascupreel (if spasmodic pain) TID with Coenzyme compositum if diarrhea is present. Use Engystol N if viral etiology is suspected. Administer Hepeel BID PO.

Deep detoxification formula (in chronic cases): Mix together the following and give orally 1 to 3 times weekly for long periods of time: Galium-Heel, Lymphomyosot, Hepar compositum, Solidago compositum, Thyroidea compositum (alternated with Tonsilla compositum in difficult infections), Coenzyme compositum, and Ubichinon compositum.

Product sources

Nutrition

Liver and immune support formulas: Animal Nutrition Technologies. **Alternatives:** Hepatic Support—Standard Process Veterinary Formulas; Hepato Support—Rx Vitamins for Pets; Hepagen—Thorne Veterinary Products; Immune System Support—Standard Process Veterinary Formulas; Immuno Support—Rx Vitamins for Pets; Immugen—Thorne Veterinary Products.

Alpha-lipoic acid: Source Naturals.

SAMe: Nutramax Laboratories, Inc.

Vitamin E: Over the counter.

Lecithin/phosphatidyl choline: Designs for Health.

Chinese herbal medicine

Formula H 77-Cholangiohepatitis/Chronic: Natural Solutions, Inc.

Homotoxicology

BHI/Heel Corporation

REFERENCES

Western medicine references

Bunch SE. Hepatobiliary diseases of the cat. In: Nelson RW, Couto CG, eds. Essentials of small animal internal medicine. St. Louis: Mosby Year Book, 1992;398–411.

Center SA, Rowland PH. The cholangitis/cholangiohepatitis complex in the cat. Proceedings 12th Annual Forum Am Col Vet Int Med 1994;766771.

Center SA. In: Tilley L, Smith F. The 5-Minute Veterinary Consult: Canine and Feline, 2003. Blackwell Publishing.

Center SA. Diseases of the gallbladder and biliary tree. In: Guilford WG, Center SA, Strombeck DR, et al., eds. Strombeck's small animal gastroenterology. 3rd ed. Philadelphia: Saunders, 1996:860–888.

Johnson SE, Sherding RG. Diseases of the liver and biliary tract. In: Birchard SJ, Sherding RG, eds. Saunders manual of small animal practice. Philadelphia: WB Saunders, 1994;722–767.

IVM/nutrition references

Amores-Sanchez MI, Medina MA. Glutamine, as a precursor of glutathione, and oxidative stress. *Mol Genet Metab* 1999;67:100–5.

Berkson BM. A conservative triple antioxidant approach to the treatment of hepatitis C. Combination of Alpha lipoic acid (thioctic acid), silymarin, and selenium: three case histories. *Med Klin* 1999;94 Suppl 3:84–9.

Bortolotti F, Cadrobbi P, Crivellaro C, et al. Effect of an orally administered thymic derivative, thymomodulin, in chronic type B hepatitis in children. *Curr Ther Res* 1988;43:67–72.

Busse E, Zimmer G, Schorpohl B, et al. Influence of alpha-lipoic acid on intracellular glutathione in vitro and in vivo. *Arzneimittelforschung* 1992;42:829–31.

Bounous G, Gervais F, Amer V, et al. The influence of dietary whey protein on tissue glutathione and the diseases of aging. *Clin Invest Med* 1989;12:343–9.

Center SA. S-adenosyl-methionine an antioxidant and anti-inflammatory nutraceutical. Proceedings of the 18th ACVIM, Seattle, WA. 2000.550–552,

Civeira MP, Castilla A, Morte S, et al. A pilot study of thymus extract in chronic non-A, non-B hepatitis. Aliment *Pharmacol Ther* 1989;3:395–401.

de la Maza MP, Petermann M, Bunout D, Hirsch S. Effects of long-term vitamin E supplementation in alcoholic cirrhotics. *J Am Coll Nutr* 1995;14:192–6.

Ferro D, Basili S, Practico D, et al. Vitamin E reduces monocyte tissue factor expression in cirrhotic patients. *Blood* 1999; 93:2945–50.

Galli M, Crocchiolo P, Negri C, et al. Attempt to treat acute type B hepatitis with an orally administered thymic extract (thymomodulin): Preliminary results. *Drugs Exp Clin Res* 1985;11:665–9.

Goldstein R, Goldstein S. The Goldstein Wellness and Longevity Program, Neptune City, NJ: 2005. TFH Publication.

Gorbakov VV, Galik VP, Kirillov SM. Experience in heptral treatment of diffuse liver diseases. *Ter Arkh* 1998;70:82–6 [in Russian].

Lieber CS, Robins SJ, Li J, et al. Phosphatidylcholine protects against fibrosis and cirrhosis in the baboon. *Gastroenterology* 1994;106:152–9.

Lykkesfeldt J, Hagen TM, Vinarsky V, Ames BN. Age-associated decline in ascorbic acid concentration, recycling, and biosynthesis in rat hepatocytes—reversal with (R)-alpha-lipoic acid supplementation. *FASEB J* 1998;12:1183–9.

Ma X, Zhao J, Lieber CS. Polyenylphosphatidylcholine attenuates non-alcoholic hepatic fibrosis and accelerates its regression. *J Hepatol* 1996;24:604–13.

Mato JM, Camara J, Fernandez de Paz J, et al. S-adenosylmethionine in alcoholic liver cirrhosis: a randomized, placebo-controlled, double-blind, multicenter clinical trial. *J Hepatol* 1999;30:1081–9.

Miglio F, Stefanini GF, Corazza GR, et al. Double-blind studies of the therapeutic action of S-Adenosylmethionine (SAMe) in oral administration, in liver cirrhosis and other chronic hepatitides. *Minerva Med* 1975;66:1595–9 [In Italian].

Sen CK. Nutritional biochemistry of cellular glutathione. *Nutr Biochem* 1997;8:660–72.

Scholich H, Murphy ME, Sies H. Antioxidant activity of dihydrolipoate against microsomal lipid peroxidation and its dependence on alpha-tocopherol. *Biochem Biophys Acta* 1989;1001:256–61.

Skotnicki AB. Therapeutic application of calf thymus extract (TFX). *Med Oncol Tumor Pharmacother* 1989;6: 31–43.

Vendemiale G, Altomare E, Trizio T, et al. Effects of oral S-adenosyl-L-methionine on hepatic glutathione in patients with liver disease. *Scand J Gastroenterol* 1989;24:407–15.

Wang ST, Chen HW, Sheen LY, Lii CK. Methionine and cysteine affect glutathione level, glutathione-related enzyme activities and the expression of glutathione S-transferase isozymes in rat hepatocytes. *J Nutr* 1997;127:2135–41.

Chinese herbal medicine/acupuncture references

An Hui Zhong Yi Xue Yuan Xue Bao (*Journal of Anhui University School of Medicine*), 1984;2:25.

Chinese Journal of Modern Developments in Traditional Medicine. Oct. 1981. 1(2): 114–7.

Fu Jian Zhong Yi Yao (*Fujian Chinese Medicine and Herbology*), 1959;7:42.

Han DW, et al. *China Journal of Internal Medicine.* 1977; 2(1):13.

He Ping, et al. Yin Chen's effect on antipyrin metabolism in humans and rabbits. *China Journal of Hospital Pharmacy.* 1990;10(10):459–460.

Hsu-Jan Liu, Sheng-Feng Hsu, Chang-Chi Hsieh, Tin-Yun Ho, Ching-Liang Hsieh, Chin-Chuan Tsai, Jaung-Geng Lin. The Effectiveness of Tsu-San-Li and Tai-Chung Acupoints for Treatment of Acute Liver Damage in Rats, *American Journal of Chinese Medicine*, Spring, 2001.

Hu YQ, et al. The extraction and separation of Yin Chen polypeptides and their liver-protecting effects in mice. *Journal of Chinese Materia Medica.* 1999;30(12):894–896.

Li DD, et al. Yin Chen Hao Tang's preventive and therapeutic effects on acute hemorrhagic necrotic pancreatitis. *China Journal of Integrated Splenico-Gastrology.* 1996;4(3): 163–165.

Lu D, et al. *Journal of China Medical Academy.* 1987; 9(6):433.

Lu D, et al. *Journal of China Medical Academy.* 1988; 10(4):294.

Nanjing College of Pharmacy. Materia Medica, vol. 2. 1976. Jiangsu: People's Press;

Shan YTE, et al. *Journal of Pharmacy.* Japan. 1982;102(3):285.

Sheng Yao Xue Za Zhi (*Journal of Raw Herbology*), 1978; 32(2):177.

Sheng Yao Xue Za Zhi (*Journal of Raw Herbology*), 1982; 36(2):150.

Wan YD. The antipyretic effects of capillarin. *Pharmacy Bulletin.* 1987;(10):590–593.

Xin Yi Yao Tong Xun (*Journal of New Medicine and Herbology*), 1972; 1:21.

Xu SC, et al. *Shanghai Journal of Immunology.* 1994;14(1): 12–13.

Yao Xue Xue Bao (*Journal of Herbology*), 1964; 11(12):815.

Zhong Guo Yao Li Xue Tong Bao (*Journal of Chinese Herbal Pharmacology*), 1988; 9(4):345.

Zhong Xi Yi Jie He Za Zhi (*Journal of Integrated Chinese and Western Medicine*), 1984; 5:315.

Zhong Yao Tong Bao (*Journal of Chinese Herbology*), 1987;9:60.

Zhong Yao Xue (*Chinese Herbology*), 1998;65:67.

Zhong Yao Xue (*Chinese Herbology*), 1998; 334:336.

Zhong Yao Yao Li Yu Ying Yong (*Pharmacology and Applications of Chinese Herbs*), 1983:383.

Zhong Yao Yao Li Yu Ying Yong (*Pharmacology and Applications of Chinese Herbs*), 1990; 15(6):52.

Zhong Yao Zhi (*Chinese Herbology Journal*), 1993;358.

Zhong Yi Za Zhi (*Journal of Chinese Medicine*), 1965; 11:6.

Zhu LH. *China J of TCM Information.* 1996;3(3):17–20.

Homotoxicology references

Broadfoot PJ. Inflammation: Homotoxicology and Healing. In: Proceedings AHVMA/Heel Homotoxicology Seminar. 2004. Denver, CO, p 27.

Demers, J. Homotoxicology and Acupuncture. In: Proceedings of the 2004 Homotoxicology Seminar. 2004. AHVMA/Heel. Denver, CO, p 5, 6.

Deng X, Yin F, Lu X, Cai B, Yin W. The apoptotic effect of brucine from the seed of Strychnos nux-vomica on human hepatoma cells is mediated via Bcl-2 and Ca2+ involved mitochondrial pathway. *Toxicol Sci.* 2006. May; 91(1):pp 59–69.

Gebhardt R. Antioxidative, antiproliferative and biochemical effects in HepG2 cells of a homeopathic remedy and its constituent plant tinctures tested separately or in combination. *Arzneimittelforschung.* 2003. 53(12): pp 823–30.

Habermehl D, Kammerer B, Handrick R, Eldh T, Gruber C, Cordes N, Daniel PT, Plasswilm L, Bamberg M, Belka C, Jendrossek V. Proapoptotic activity of Ukrain is based on Chelidonium majus L. alkaloids and mediated via a mitochondrial death pathway. *BMC Cancer.* 2006. Jan 17;6: p 14.

Heel. BHI Homeopathic Therapy: Professional Reference. Albuquerque, NM: Heel Inc. 2002. pp 43, 59.

McCaw D. Cholangitis/Cholangiohepatitis. In: The 5 Minute Veterinary Consult: Canine and Feline, Tilley L, Smith F, eds. Baltimore, MD: Williams and Wilkins. 1997pp442–443.

Newell S, Selcer B, Girard E, Roberts G, Thompson J, Harrison J. Correlations between ultrasonographic findings and specific hepatic diseases in cats: 72 cases (1985–1997). *J Am Vet Med Assoc.* 1998. Jul 1;213(1):pp 94–8.

Pressel M, Fox L, Apley M, Simutis F. Vancomycin for multidrug resistant Enterococcus faecium cholangiohepatitis in a cat. *J Feline Med Surg.* 2005. Oct;7(5):pp 317–21.

Reckeweg H. Biotherapeutic Index: Ordinatio Antihomotoxica et Materia Medica, 5th ed. Baden-Baden, Germany: Biologische Heilmittel Heel GMBH, 2000. pp 106, 310–11, 330–32, 347–8, 349–50, 369–70, 402–3.

Reckeweg H. Homeopathia Antihomotoxica Materia Medica, 4th ed. Baden-Baden, Germany: Arelia-Verlag GMBH, 2002. pp. 136–8, 147, 179, 317–19, 345, 366, 461–3, 488–90.

Vahlensieck U, Hahn R, Winterhoff H, Gumbinger H, Nahrstedt A, Kemper F. The effect of Chelidonium majus herb extract on choleresis in the isolated perfused rat liver. *Planta Med.* 1995. Jun;61(3):pp 267–71.

Weiss D, Gagne J, Armstrong P. Relationship between inflammatory hepatic disease and inflammatory bowel disease, pancreatitis, and nephritis in cats. *J Am Vet Med Assoc.* 1996.Sep 15;209(6):pp 1114–6.

Wynn S, Marsden S. Manual of Natural Veterinary Medicine: Science and Tradition. St Louis: Mosby: 2003. p 325.

CIRRHOSIS OF THE LIVER

Definition and cause

Cirrhosis is characterized by chronic inflammation leading to hepatic fibrosis loss of normal liver cell architecture, often resulting in end-stage liver disease. The causes include infections; chronic injury; chronic exposure to medications such as corticosteroids, anticonvulsants, and fungal agents; exposure to toxins or metabolites; or it can result from chronic liver disease. Animals that are genetically prone to chronic active hepatitis or copper storage disease are more susceptible to hepatic cirrhosis. It is believed that there is an immune-mediated component to the chronic inflammatory process (Center 1986, 1999; Hardy 1985; Twedt 2003).

Medical therapy rationale, drug(s) of choice, and nutritional recommendations

Medical therapy is directed toward the underlying cause as listed above. Common therapies include corticosteroids, immunosuppressants, zinc acetate, and anti-fibrotic medications. Dietary recommendations include high-quality, digestible protein sources in food that contains normal levels of protein fat, and carbohydrates such as Hill L/D. Antioxidant vitamins, specifically vitamin E and S-adenosylmethionine, should be included to help prevent oxidative stress (Center 1989, 1996; Laflamme 2000; Twedt 2003).

Anticipated prognosis

Prognosis is dependent upon the severity of the fibrosis, the underlying cause that led to the fibrosis, and the secondary effects of the fibrosis such as ascites, icterus, weight loss, low serum protein levels, etc. (Center 1989, 1996; Laflamme 2000; Twedt 2003).

Integrative veterinary therapies

Cirrhosis is the end result of a chronic inflammatory process leading to fibrosis and loss of functional liver cells. The integrative approach focuses upon the inciting inflammatory process which leads to liver cell destruction, cellular infiltration, and scarring. Identifying and removing the underlying cause, if possible, gives the best results. The most prudent approach is becoming aware of liver issues early on and instituting integrative measures along with medical therapy as a method of: (1) identifying and eliminating the cause, (2) instituting a dietary and supplemental program that supports liver metabolism and reduces metabolic and toxic wastes, and (3) monitoring that therapy is cellular-protective to both the initiating cause and the potential side effects of medications.

Liver cell regeneration may be enhanced by early identification of the underlying inflammatory response, and the use of nutrients, nutraceuticals, medicinal herbs, and combination homeopathics that are anti-inflammatory and tissue-sparing. If integrative therapies are instituted early, such as during the treatment for hepatitis or at early signs of liver issues such as chronic elevation of ALT, AST, or GGTP levels, then it is possible to prevent progressive inflammation, cell death, and scarring that precede cirrhosis (Goldstein 2005).

Nutrition
General considerations/rationale

The key to liver health is reducing toxins and metabolic wastes and increasing antioxidants and phytonutrients that can help neutralize compounds that the liver must deal with in its role as the body's filter and detoxifier. Glutathione is a compound that is composed of 3 amino acids: glutamic acid, glysine, and cysteine. Glutathione binds and neutralizes various chemicals, toxins, herbicides, pesticides, heavy metals, etc. so they can pass through the liver and be excreted via the bile into the intestines or pass to the kidneys to be excreted in the urine (Sen 1997).

Body glutathione levels can be raised by other nutrients such as vitamin C, whey protein, glutamine, methionine, S-adenosyl-L-methionine (SAMe), and alpha-lipoic acid (Amores-Sanchez 1999, Bounous 1989, Vendemiale 1989, Wang 1997).

Appropriate nutrients

Nutrition/gland therapy: Glandular liver and kidney can help improve organ function, reduce inflammation, protect liver and kidney cells, and enhance metabolic elimination of toxins and wastes (See Chapter 2, Gland Therapy, for additional information).

Note: Because cirrhosis can result from liver and associated multiple organ conditions, it is recommended that blood be analyzed both medically and physiologically to determine real and impending organ involvement and disease. This allows for a more specific gland and nutritional support protocol (See Chapter 2, Nutritional Blood Testing, for additional information).

Lecithin/phosphatidyl choline: Has been shown to help break down scar tissue in the liver and prevent cirrhosis by reversing the cellular changes that lead to cirrhotic cell formation (Ma 1996). Phosphatidyl choline has been shown to reverse the progression of alcohol-induced cirrhosis in people (Lieber 1990, 1994).

Vitamin E: Was shown to decrease liver damage and immune imbalances that may contribute to the disease progression; however, further clinical work is required to definitively confirm this because another clinical trial failed to confirm these results (Ferro 1999, de la Maza 1995).

Zinc: Clinical trials have confirmed that zinc deficiencies are associated with cirrhosis in people (Scholmerich 1983, Taniguchi 1995). In double-blind testing with zinc acetate supplementation, Reding (1984) and Marchesini (1996) showed a significantly improved portal systemic encephalopathy.

Alpha-lipoic acid: A potent antioxidant that is proven to reduce oxidative stress and inflammation. It has also been shown to increase the effectiveness of other antioxidants, such as vitamins C and E, CoEnzyme Q10, and glutathione, making them more readily available for bodily function (Busse 1992, Lykkesfeldt 1998, Scholich 1989). In a study of people with cirrhosis who received a combination antioxidant-rich supplement that contained 300 mg of alpha-lipoic acid, there was significant improvement of liver function (Berkson 1999).

S-adenosylmethionine (SAMe): SAMe is an antioxidant and has anti-inflammatory effects on the liver (Center 2000). It has been shown to significantly improve survival and decrease the need for liver transplantation in people with liver disease. It has also been shown to improve liver function in less severe cases of cirrhosis (Gorbakov 1998, Mato 1999, Miglio 1975).

Chinese herbal medicine/acupuncture
General considerations/rationale
Cirrhosis is a result of Qi and Blood Stagnation and Qi and Yang Deficiency in the Spleen. There may be Water and Phlegm retention. The Spleen is responsible for regulating the Water, especially in the abdomen. The Spleen also regulates the digestive system. The Spleen cannot perform these functions because of the Qi (energy) and Yang (heat) deficiency. Without proper digestion, weight loss ensues. The inability to regulate the Water leads to Water retention known as ascites in Western terminology. Qi and Blood stagnation in the abdomen describe the pain associated with the distension of the abdomen.

We now know that this condition is truly a liver pathology. Interestingly, many of the herbs the traditional Chinese practitioners used have now been shown to have hepatoprotective effects. Treatment for cirrhosis is aimed at protecting the liver from further damage, relieving ascites, and normalizing liver function.

Appropriate Chinese herbs
Alisma (Ze xie): Increases the excretion of sodium and urine, and therefore has a diuretic effect (Shi 1962, Xu 1963, Deng 1961).

Atractylodes(Cang zhu): Is hepatoprotective. Experimentally, it was shown to protect against CCL4-induced hepatic damage in mice (Guo 1985).

Ginger (Sheng jiang): Has been shown to be hepatoprotective. It decreases the amount of liver damage induced by experimental administration of CCl4 to rats and mice as evidenced by lower AST levels and sulfobromophthalein sodium (BSP) retention values (Zhang 1989).

Jujube (Da zao): Also protects the liver. Rabbits given jujube prior to being treated with CCl4 recovered faster than those that did not receive jujube (Guang Dong Zhong Yi 1962).

Licorice (Gan cao): Is hepatoprotective. It increases the cytochrome p-450 levels in the liver (Zhong Yao Tong Bao 1986). In one trial, it was 77% effective in treating 330 human patients with hepatitis B. It reduced inflammation, increased regeneration of hepatic cells, and decreased hepatic necrosis and cirrhosis (Zhong Yao Tong Bao 1987).

Polyporus (Zhu ling): Increases excretion of water, sodium chloride, and potassium in dogs (Yao Xue Xue Bao 1964). This diuretic effect may help decrease ascites.

It has also proven to be hepatoprotective in experiments involving hepatotoxicity of CCl4 in rats (Zhong Guo Yao Li Xue Tong Bao 1988).

Poria (Fu ling): Has been shown to be hepatoprotective in CCl4 toxicity experiments (Han 1977). It also has a diuretic effect (Lu 1988).

White atractylodes (Bai zhu): Has been used successfully for ascites from cirrhosis (An Hui Zhong Yi Xue Yuan Xue Bao 1984). In mice it was shown to control ascites via its regulatory effects on peritoneal pores (Lu 1996).

Acupuncture

Some practitioners have claimed to cure cirrhosis using acupuncture alone (Cheng 1959). However, most people now combine herbs and/or Western therapy to treat cirrhosis.

Homotoxicology
General considerations/rationale

Cirrhosis represents an end-stage disease of the liver. Normal architecture and functionality of the liver are severely compromised. This represents Degeneration Phase disease. Cure of these cases is unlikely due to the excessive damage that has already occurred. Treatment and management are similar to chronic active hepatitis; however, the clinician must emphasize support of remaining liver tissue while carefully guarding against increased release or ingestion of homotoxins. Detoxification of Degeneration Phase patients must be done extremely slowly and with much care to avoid progressive vicariation. Likewise, use of any therapeutic agent needs to be carefully considered so that the chosen agent improves patient condition with a minimum chance of aggravation or worsening. In cirrhosis, it is often much better to design very simple programs and then to implement those changes gradually. For more details about management see Chronic Active Hepatitis in this chapter.

Appropriate homotoxicology formulas

Oral drop combinations may contain alcohol. In most cases this is such a small quantity that it is well tolerated, but when possible, selecting oral vials and tablets may reduce the workload on the liver (Reckeweg 2000). Also see the list of gastrointestinal remedies at the end of chapter 23, as well as protocols for enteritis, colitis, pancreatitis, and other applicable gastrointestinal conditions for more information and remedy selection ideas.

BHI-Enzyme: Supportive of metabolism and similar to *Coenzyme compositum*. Contains water-soluble vitamins (Niacin, B_1, B_2, B_6, B_{12}, and C) and other components and cofactors of the Krebs cycle. Sulphur activates a blocked metabolism and promotes detoxification. Pulsatilla is

useful in regulation rigidity and for pain in the legs with restlessness and difficult sleep (Heel 2002).

Chelidonium homaccord: Commonly used agent in hepatic damage and hepatitis, and gallbladder conditions such as cholangitis, cholecystitis, and obstructive jaundice (Demers 2004). Chelidonium contains a substance known as Chelidonine, which has anticancer effects. "Chelidonine turned out to be a potent inducer of apoptosis triggering cell death at concentrations of 0.001 mM," according to Habermehl (2006), a fact that may explain the clinically observed usefulness of this remedy in treating patients with biliary neoplasia.

Coenzyme compositum: Contains Citricum acidum, which is useful for dental problems and gingivitis; scurvy; blackening of teeth; heavy deposits of dental plaque; painful, herpetic vesicles around the lips; nausea; painful cramping in the umbilical area; and distension. Used as an agent to repair mitochondrial damage resulting from antibiotic therapy (also used with *Ubichinon compositum* and *Galium-Heel* for that purpose).

Colchicum compositum: Used for cachexia and neoplastic conditions. Colchicine has been used in hepatitis patients to reduce cirrhosis (Honeckman 2003, Nikolaidis et al. 2006). The use of *Colchicum compositum* should be considered but has no clinical evidence at this time. The authors welcome reports of its use.

Galium-Heel: Used for all cellular phases, hemorrhoids, and anal fissures, and as a detoxicant. Monitor liver enzymes and if SAP and/or ALT show marked increases, adjust use accordingly (Miele, et al. 2005). Interrupt therapy and restart as needed. Many patients benefit from a month on *Galium-Heel* 3 to 4 times per year. Another method is to use *Galium-Heel* 1 to 3 times weekly.

Hepar compositum: The main remedy for chronic hepatitis cases. Provides detoxification and drainage of hepatic tissues and organ and metabolic support, and is useful in most hepatic and gallbladder pathologies. An important part of Deep Detoxification Formula. Treats duodenitis, pancreatitis, cystic hepatic ducts, cholelithiasis, cholangitis, cholecystitis, vomiting, and diarrhea (Demers 2004, Broadfoot 2004). This combination contains Natrum oxalaceticum (also found in *Coenzyme compositum*, *Ubichinon compositum*, and *Mucosa compositum*) for changes in appetite and stomach distension due to air. Treats nausea, stomach pain with a sensation of fullness, gurgling in the abdomen, and cramping pain in the hypochondria. Also used for constipation, sudden diarrhea (particularly after eating), and flatus (Reckeweg 2002).

Hepeel: Used for liver drainage and detoxification. Used in a wide variety of conditions including cancer of the liver, where *Hepeel* was found to be antiproliferative, hepatoprotective, and an antioxidant when tested in human HepG2 cells (Gebhardt 2003).

Lymphomyosot: Provides lymph drainage and endocrine support, and treats edema. Contains Gentiana for chronic gastritis. Treats flatulence, diarrhea, distension of the stomach with eructations, nausea, retching, and vomiting. Also contains Geranium robertianum for nausea, particularly after eating with distension or sensation of fullness. Myosotis arvensis is included for bloat and distension (Reckeweg 2002).

Mucosa compositum: Broadly supportive for repair of mucosal elements. Used in cellular cases and in recovery periods following active disease (Reckeweg 2000). This remedy contains a useful component in Kali bichromicum, which is indicated for ulcers found on the gums, tongue, lips, and even on the gastric mucosa (gastric or duodenal ulcer). The tongue may have a thick, yellow, mucous coating, or in ulcerative stomatitis or tonsillitis it may be dry, smooth, shiny, or fissured. Kali has been used effectively in acute gastroenteritis associated with vomiting of clear, light-colored fluid or quantities of mucous bile, and in cases with hematemesis, flatulent colics, and dysenteric stools with tenesmus (Reckeweg 2002).

It also contains Hydrastis, with mucosal support for oral problems such as stomatitis, and mucosal suppuration that is accompanied by ulceration, inflammations and colic of the hepatobiliary system and of the gastrointestinal tract, and polyp formation (Reckeweg 2002). The Kreosotum component can be used in chronic gastritis with gastric hemorrhages and vomiting of brown masses. Also has a dental implication in cases with spongy gums and carious teeth, neuralgias proceeding from them causing a burning toothache with deep caries, black patches on the teeth, and fetid discharges.

The single remedy Phosphorus is broadly useful for dyspepsia and for jaw problems in dental disease (Reckeweg 2002). Phosphorus is found in many other remedies including *Echinacea compositum* and *Leptandra homaccord*. It is rich in suis organ preparations for mucosal support, plus a large variety of remedies with indications in the gastrointestinal sphere. The component Argentum nitricum (also in *Atropinum compositum*, *Diarrheel*, *Duodenoheel*, *Gastricumeel*, *Momordica compositum*, *BHI-Nausea*, and several other combinations) is indicated for distension in the upper abdomen, gastro-cardiac symptom-complex, and amelioration from eructations. It is also used for gastric crises (Reckeweg 2002).

Phosphor homaccord: Treats hepatitis, icterus, tenderness over the liver region, pancreatic diseases, ulcerated gums, thirst but vomiting right after drinking occurs, and pale-clay colored stools (Macleod 1983).

Ubichinon: Contains Anthraquinone for swelling of the gums, and GI symptoms such as distention, flatulence, and cramping abdominal pain. Treats constipation with straining or sudden diarrhea (Reckeweg 2002). *Ubichinon compositum* is a Degeneration Phase remedy.

Authors' suggested protocols

Nutrition

Liver support formula: 1 tablet for every 25 pounds of body weight BID.

Kidney support formula: One-half tablet for every 25 pounds of body weight BID.

Alpha-lipoic acid: 20 mg per 10 pounds of body weight daily.

SAMe: 10 to 20 mg/kg SID or follow manufacturer's dosing directions.

Vitamin E: 50 IU for every 20 pounds of body weight SID.

Zinc: 15 mg for every 25 pounds of body weight SID.

Lecithin/phosphatidyl choline: One-fourth teaspoon for every 25 pounds of body weight BID.

Chinese herbal medicine/acupuncture

H75 Hepatic cirrhosis/ascites: 1 capsule per 10 to 20 pounds twice daily. In addition to the herbs cited above, H75 Hepatic cirrhosis contains cinnamon bark (Rou gui), citrus (Chen pi), magnolia bark (Hou po), plantain leaves (Che qian cao), pinellia (Ban xia), and verbena (Ma bian cao).

The following acupuncture points are used by the authors to treat cirrhosis: CV12, ST36, PC6, BL19, Li3, SP6, GB34, and BL20.

Homotoxicology (Dose: 10 drops PO for 50-pound dog; 5 drops PO for cat or small dog)

Be extremely careful not to overload a cirrhotic liver with toxins.

Galium-Heel and Phosphor homaccord: BID orally initially. Adjust dosage and frequency according to patient response.

Hepar compositum: Weekly to twice weekly. Hepeel and BHI-Enzyme (or Coenzyme compositum) given orally BID.

Product sources

Nutrition

Liver support formula: Animal Nutrition Technologies. **Alternatives**: Hepatic Support—Standard Process Veterinary Formulas; Hepato Support—Rx Vitamins for Pets; Hepagen—Thorne Veterinary Products.

Alpha-lipoic acid: Source Naturals.

SAMe: Nutramax Laboratories, Inc.

Lecithin/phosphatidyl choline: Designs for Health.

Vitamin E: Over the counter.

Chinese herbal medicine
H75 Hepatic Cirrhosis: Natural Solutions, Inc.

Homotoxicology
BHI/Heel Corporation

REFERENCES

Western medicine references
Center SA. Chronic hepatitis, cirrhosis, breed-specific hepatopathies, copper storage hepatopathy, suppurative hepatitis, granulomatous hepatitis, and idiopathic hepatic fibrosis. In: Guilford WG, Center SA, Strombeck DR, et al., eds. Strombeck's small animal gastroenterology. Philadelphia: Saunders, 1996:705–765.

Center SA. Pathophysiology and Laboratory Diagnosis of Liver Disease. In: Textbook of Veterinary Internal Medicine, 1989, Philadelphia: WB Saunders and Company.

Hardy RM. Diseases of the Liver. In: Textbook of Veterinary Internal Medicine. Disease of Dog and Cat. Ettinger SJ, ed. 1985, Philadelphia: WB Saunders Company.

Laflamme DP. Nutritional management of liver disease. In: Bonagura JD, ed. Kirk's Current Veterinary Therapy XIII. Philadelphia: WB Saunders, 2000, pp 693–697.

Twedt DC. Cirrhosis/Fibrosis of the Liver. In: Tilley L, Smith F. The 5-Minute Veterinary Consult: Canine and Feline, 2003. Blackwell Publishing.

IVM/nutritional references
Amores-Sanchez MI, Medina MA. Glutamine, as a precursor of glutathione, and oxidative stress. *Mol Genet Metab* 1999; 67:100–5.

Berkson BM. A conservative triple antioxidant approach to the treatment of hepatitis C. Combination of Alpha lipoic acid (thioctic acid), silymarin, and selenium: three case histories. *Med Klin* 1999;94 Suppl 3:84–9.

Busse E, Zimmer G, Schorpohl B, et al. Influence of alpha-lipoic acid on intracellular glutathione in vitro and in vivo. *Arzneimittelforschung* 1992;42:829–31.

Bounous G, Gervais F, Amer V, et al. The influence of dietary whey protein on tissue glutathione and the diseases of aging. *Clin Invest Med* 1989;12:343–9.

Center SA. S-adenosyl-methionine an antioxidant and anti-inflammatory nutraceutical. Proceedings of the 18th ACVIM, Seattle, WA: 2000. 550–552.

de la Maza MP, Petermann M, Bunout D, Hirsch S. Effects of long-term vitamin E supplementation in alcoholic cirrhotics. *J Am Coll Nutr* 1995;14:192–6.

Ferro D, Basili S, Practico D, et al. Vitamin E reduces monocyte tissue factor expression in cirrhotic patients. *Blood* 1999; 93:2945–50.

Gorbakov VV, Galik VP, Kirillov SM. Experience in heptral treatment of diffuse liver diseases. *Ter Arkh* 1998;70:82–6 [in Russian].

Lieber CS, Robins SJ, Li J, et al. Phosphatidylcholine protects against fibrosis and cirrhosis in the baboon. *Gastroenterology* 1994;106:152–9.

Lieber CS, DeCarli LM, Mak KM, et al. Attenuation of alcohol-induced hepatic fibrosis by polyunsaturated lecithin. *Hepatology* 1990;12:1390–8.

Lykkesfeldt J, Hagen TM, Vinarsky V, Ames BN. Age-associated decline in ascorbic acid concentration, recycling, and biosynthesis in rat hepatocytes—reversal with (R)-alpha-lipoic acid supplementation. *FASEB J* 1998;12:1183–9.

Ma X, Zhao J, Lieber CS. Polyenylphosphatidylcholine attenuates non-alcoholic hepatic fibrosis and accelerates its regression. *J Hepatol* 1996;24:604–13.

Marchesini G, Fabbri A, Bianchi G, et al. Zinc supplementation and amino acid-nitrogen metabolism in patients with advanced cirrhosis. *Hepatology* 1996;23:1084–92.

Mato JM, Camara J, Fernandez de Paz J, et al. S-adenosylmethionine in alcoholic liver cirrhosis: a randomized, placebo-controlled, double-blind, multicenter clinical trial. *J Hepatol* 1999;30:1081–9.

Miglio F, Stefanini GF, Corazza GR, et al. Double-blind studies of the therapeutic action of S-Adenosylmethionine (SAMe) in oral administration, in liver cirrhosis and other chronic hepatitides. *Minerva Med* 1975;66:1595–9 [In Italian].

Reding P, Duchateau J, Bataille C. Oral zinc supplementation improves hepatic encephalopathy. Results of a randomised controlled trial. *Lancet* 1984;2(8401):493–5.

Sen CK. Nutritional biochemistry of cellular glutathione. *Nutr Biochem* 1997;8:660–72.

Scholmerich J, Lohle E, Kottgen E, Gerok W. Zinc and vitamin A deficiency in liver cirrhosis. *Hepatogastroenterology* 1983; 30:119–25.

Scholich H, Murphy ME, Sies H. Antioxidant activity of dihydrolipoate against microsomal lipid peroxidation and its dependence on alpha-tocopherol. *Biochem Biophys Acta* 1989;1001:256–61.

Taniguchi S, Kaneto K, Hamada T. Acquired zinc deficiency associated with alcoholic liver cirrhosis. *Int J Dermatol* 1995;34:651–2.

Vendemiale G, Altomare E, Trizio T, et al. Effects of oral S-adenosyl-L-methionine on hepatic glutathione in patients with liver disease. *Scand J Gastroenterol* 1989;24:407–15.

Wang ST, Chen HW, Sheen LY, Lii CK. Methionine and cysteine affect glutathione level, glutathione-related enzyme activities and the expression of glutathione S-transferase isozymes in rat hepatocytes. *J Nutr* 1997;127:2135–41.

Chinese herbal medicine/acupuncture references
An Hui Zhong Yi Xue Yuan Xue Bao (*Journal of Anhui University School of Medicine*), 1984;2:25.

Cheng, BC and Wang BH. Experience in 9 case of liver cirrhosis cured by acupuncture. *Shandong Yi Kan* 1959 Jan 1617–8.

Deng ZP, et al. *China Journal of Medicine*. 1961;47(1):7–11.

Guang Dong Zhong Yi (*Guangdong Chinese Medicine*), 1962; 5:1.

Guo Wai Ti Tao Zhi Wu Yao Fen Ce (*Monograph of Foreign Botanical Medicine*), 1985; (2):54.

Han DW, et al. *China Journal of Internal Medicine*. 1977;2(1): 13.

Lu D, et al. *Journal of China Medical Academy*. 1988;10(4): 294.

Lu ZL, et al. *Journal of Chinese Materia Medica.* 1996;37(9): 560–561.

Shi JL, et al. *Haerbin Journal of Traditional Chinese Medicine.* 1962;(1):60–61.

Xu WF. *Fujian Journal of Chinese Medicine.* 1963;8(1):42–44.

Yao Xue Xue Bao (*Journal of Herbology*), 1964; 11(12):815.

Zhang ZX, et al. *Journal of Chinese Patent Medicine.* 1989; 11(8):25–26.

Zhong Guo Yao Li Xue Tong Bao (*Journal of Chinese Herbal Pharmacology*), 1988; 9(4):345.

Zhong Yao Tong Bao (*Journal of Chinese Herbology*), 1986; 11(10):55.

Zhong Yao Tong Bao (*Journal of Chinese Herbology*), 1987; 9:60.

Homotoxicology references

Broadfoot PJ. Inflammation: Homotoxicology and Healing. In: Proceedings AHVMA/Heel Homotoxicology Seminar. 2004. Denver, CO, p 27.

Demers, J. Homotoxicology and Acupuncture. In: Proceedings of the 2004 Homotoxicology Seminar. 2004. AHVMA/Heel. Denver, CO, p 5, 6.

Gebhardt R. 2003. Antioxidative, antiproliferative and biochemical effects in HepG2 cells of a homeopathic remedy and its constituent plant tinctures tested separately or in combination. *Arzneimittelforschung.* 53(12): pp 823–430.

Habermehl D, Kammerer B, Handrick R, Eldh T, Gruber C, Cordes N, Daniel PT, Plasswilm L, Bamberg M, Belka C, Jendrossek V. Proapoptotic activity of Ukrain is based on Chelidonium majus L. alkaloids and mediated via a mitochondrial death pathway. *BMC Cancer.* 2006. Jan 17;6: p 14.

Heel. BHI Homeopathic Therapy: Professional Reference. Albuquerque, NM: Heel Inc. 2002. p 54.

Honeckman A. Current concepts in the treatment of canine chronic hepatitis. *Clin Tech Small Anim Pract.* 2003 Nov;18(4): pp 239–44

Macleod G. A Veterinary Materia Medica and Clinical Repertory with a Materia Medica of the Nosodes. Safron, Walden: CW Daniel Company, LTD, 1983. pp 50–1, 125–6, 129–30.

Miele L, Vero V, Gasbarrini G, Grieco A. Braised liver with herbs: the risks of naturopathic hepatoprotection. *J Clin Gastroenterol.* 2004. Apr;39(4):p 344.

Nikolaidis N, Kountouras J, Giouleme O, Tzarou V, Chatzizisi O, Patsiaoura K, Papageorgiou A, Leontsini M, Eugenidis N, Zamboulis C. Colchicine treatment of liver fibrosis. *Hepatogastroenterology.* 2006. Mar-Apr;53(68):pp 281–5.

Reckeweg H. Homeopathia Antihomotoxica Materia Medica, 4th ed. Baden-Baden, Germany: Arelia-Verlag GMBH, 2002. pp 136–8, 147, 179, 317–19, 345, 366, 461–3, 488–90.

FATTY LIVER SYNDROME (HEPATIC LIPIDOSIS)

Definition and cause

Hepatic lipidosis, defined as fatty accumulation in liver cells, is common in cats and rare in dogs. It is a progressive disease and as more liver cells become affected, the functioning of the liver decreases accordingly. The condition can lead to liver failure and death (Center 2003).

Chronic liver disease can progress to lipidosis. It can also be secondary to other chronic diseases such as diabetes, IBD, CRD, or infectious diseases such as FIP or toxoplasmosis. Vitamin B$_{12}$ deficiency has also been implicated (Day 1994, Johnson 1994).

Fatty liver syndrome begins long before the patient presents in acute disease. Changes accumulate slowly over time as the hepatocyte becomes overburdened with adipose tissue and ultrastructural alterations occur, which affect proper cellular metabolism (Center 1993).

Medical therapy rationale, drug(s) of choice, and nutritional recommendations

Treatment of these cases can proceed on an outpatient basis if the cat is eating. Hospitalization is warranted in anorectic patients. Attention should be given to reducing the patient's stress as much as is feasible because stress leads to cortisol release, which aggravates the condition.

Dietary recommendations and administration are important to treatment because many cats are off food and may require an esophageal or nasogastric feeding tube. Food should be a high-caloric, highly digestible, and high-protein. While no clinical proof exists for supplementation, adding amino acids (taurine and l-carnitine), essential fatty acids (fish oil), and vitamins (vitamins B, K) appears to be beneficial. Antibiotics are recommended for infections (Cornelius 2000, Day 1994).

Anticipated prognosis

Early correction of underlying liver disease improves prognosis. The prognosis can be good with early attention to diet, feeding tube, and supplementation. Prognosis is more guarded when secondary diseases are present or intensive therapy is not instituted early on (Center 1996, 2003, 2005).

Integrative veterinary therapies

Routine monitoring of patient condition and handling these cases long before they cross the biological divide is the preferred route (Center 2005). Proper diet, exercise, and maintenance of a favorable body condition are extremely helpful. Many cases present to the veterinarian after another mild illness surfaces and the cat fails to eat for a few days. As obligate carnivores, cats need protein on a daily basis. Failure to handle this dietary requirement leaves the hepatocyte unable to function properly and hepatic disease occurs. In mild cases it may be possible to simply feed the cat by natural means or stomach tube and see a total recovery. In such cases the incident of hepatopathy should serve as a wake-up call to both client and veterinarian and serious steps should be taken at once to control weight and reduce homotoxin levels in the patient.

Fatty infiltration of the liver can be worsened by drug therapy, most notably corticosteroids, but also drugs such as anticonvulsants. Genetics may also play a role because some cats seem more prone to weight gain, obesity, and pancreatopathies.

Proper diet and exercise are the cornerstones of prevention of this condition. Maintaining proper body weight is proven to extend life, a goal common to all veterinarians and clients. The use of nutraceuticals, medicinal herbs, and combination homeopathics that improve lipid metabolism and have tissue-protective and regenerative effects on liver cells is beneficial for long-term liver health.

Nutrition
General considerations/rationale
While hepatic lipidosis is a well-known clinical condition in cats, the underlying mechanism is unknown, although it is believed to be a nutritional and biochemical peculiarity (Buckner 1998). The focus of therapeutic nutrition is upon the improvement of lipid metabolism, the addition of specific antioxidants and nutraceuticals that improve fat metabolism, and glandular support for the primary organs, i.e., the intestines, pancreas, and liver.

Appropriate nutrients
Nutritional/gland therapy: Glandular liver, pancreas, intestines, and pituitary supply the intrinsic nutrients that improve organ function (see Gland Therapy in Chapter 2 for a more detailed explanation).

Note: Because lipid metabolism can be influenced by many organs, a medical and physiological blood evaluation is recommended to assess glandular health. This helps clinicians formulate therapeutic nutritional protocols that address the underlying liver or other organ conditions that may be ultimately responsible for the excessive deposition of fat (see Chapter 2, Nutritional Blood Testing, for additional information).

L-carnitine and taurine: L-carnitine is required in the metabolism of fatty acids for the release of energy by the cells. Supplementing the diet with L-carnitine has a direct lowering effect on the blood trigylcene levels (Sachan 1984). In studies conducted by the Iams Company, the addition of carnitine to the diet of dogs was shown to reduce body weight by 6.4%, compared to 1.8% without supplementation (Sunvold 1998). Similar research in cats also suggests weight loss (Center 1998). Evangeliou (2003) showed that the addition of carnitine to the diet also helps to lower both cholesterol and triglyceride levels. Taurine's role and importance in feline health have been widely reported (Monson 1989).

Essential fatty acids: Fish oil has been reported to lower triglyceride levels in double-blind studies (Prichard 1995). Blue-green algae has also been reported to lower triglyceride levels in people (Iwata 1990, Gonzalez de Rivera 1993).

Lecithin/phosphatidyl choline: Phosphatidyl choline is a phospholipid that assists in lipid digestion and helps to move fats into the cells (Hanin 1987).

Enzymes: Required for the proper and efficient digestion of fats and fatty acids (Howell 1985).

Chinese herbal medicine/acupuncture
General considerations/rationale
Hepatic lipidosis is considered to be a condition of Phlegm and accumulation of Damp. There is Qi and Blood Stagnation in the Liver and Gallbladder. Phlegm and Damp refer to the fatty accumulation in the Liver and hypercholesterolemia, which is often seen with liver disorders. Qi and Blood stagnation in the Liver and Gallbladder refer to epigastric pain. There also may be bile accumulation in the Gallbladder when there is insufficient Qi in this organ. Treatment objectives include protecting the liver, decreasing the fatty accumulation, and improving the appetite.

Appropriate Chinese herbs
Alisma (Ze xie): Has been shown to inhibit the development of hepatic lipidosis secondary to high-fat diets (Institute of Pharmacy 1976).

Bupleurum (Chai hu): Protects the liver from various insults. It was shown to decrease hepatic damage caused by reperfusion injuries (Tang 1998). It also protects the liver from toxic insults such as CCl4 administration (Chen 1994). One component of bupleurum, saikosaponin, has demonstrated protective effects on hepatic cells (Chen 1999).

Cassia seed (Cao jue ming): Helps to normalize the blood lipid profile. It lowers total cholesterol, but raises HDL levels (Zhong Yao Zhi 1984, Zhong Cao Yao 1991).

Crataegus (Shan zha): Was shown to decrease serum cholesterol in hyperlipidemic quail by 34% to 63% (Chu 1988). Another study suggests that crataegus may prevent deposition of lipids on vascular walls (Cai 2000). It also may help prevent lipid deposition in the liver; however, this supposition requires further study.

Fleece flower root (He shou wu): Helps to protect the liver. In one experiment it was shown to prevent lipid deposition in mice treated with prednisone (Liu 1992).

Oriental wormwood (Yin chen): Was shown to increase the activity of microsomal cholesterol esterase in rat liver. This indicates that it can improve hydrolytic reactions in the liver and protect it from toxic substances. It can also increase the phagocytic activity of hepatic macrophages

(Hu 1999, He 1990). Wormwood has cholagogic efficacy, as demonstrated in the rat model (Sui 1993).

Polygonatum root (Huang jing): Decreases serum cholesterol and triglyceride levels (Jiang Su Zhong Yi 1988).

Rhubarb (Da huang): Is hepatoprotective. In one experiment it decreased the degree of hepatic necrosis the liver of mice given CCl4 (Zhong Guo Zhong Yao Za Zhi 1989). It was used in 80 people with acute hepatitis causing jaundice, with improvement in 76 patients (Zhong Xi Yi Jie He Za Zhi 1983). It has been shown to increase the secretion of bile in dogs and cats (Xin Yi Yao Xue Za Zhi 1974).

Salvia (Dan shen): Has hepatoprotective properties. In experiments in which mice were give CCl4, salvia had the effect of reducing liver enzymes. It improves hepatic circulation and promotes regeneration of liver cells (Zhong Yi Za Zhi 1982, Zhong Xi Yi Jie He Za Zhi 1988).

Acupuncture

Acupuncture may help protect the liver. In one experiment 36 rats were treated with CCl4. The efficacy of acupuncture at St36 and LI3 for hepatoprotection was investigated. The rats treated after exposure to CCl4 had lower AST and ALT levels, suggesting that acupuncture can protect the liver (Hsu-Jan 2001).

Homotoxicology
General considerations/rationale

Asymptomatic Deposition Phase pathology progresses to Impregnation Phase disease. This suddenly appears as liver dysfunction, which can rapidly progress into the Degeneration Phase (Tsochatzis, Papatheodoridis, Archimandritis 2006).

From a biological therapy viewpoint, we try to get adequate calories into the patient, assist the liver and gastrointestinal systems with digestion and absorption, and allow for homotoxin (fat) removal and organ repair. As proper nutrition is obtained and support for the hepatocyte occurs, these patients gradually recover their abilities and improve. The agents used are similar for other forms of hepatic disease, and remarks under chronic active hepatitis treatment are applicable with the following exception: cats must have significantly higher protein in their diets. The use of long-term feeding tubes may be needed, and recovery is slower with this condition. Coordination with a veterinary internist may be helpful, especially during the acute onset of more serious cases.

Appropriate homotoxicology formulas

Oral drop combinations may contain alcohol. In most cases this is such a small quantity that it is well tolerated, but when possible, selecting oral vials and tablets may reduce the workload on the liver (Reckeweg 2000). The authors recommend making dilutions of the remedies by combining 10 drops of each formula with 1 ounce of water. This solution is succussed 10 times and then dispensed with instructions to keep the mixture refrigerated. It should be remembered that nutritional support is the most important aspect of therapy, and homotoxicology formulas support that effort.

Berberis homaccord: Berberis has major actions on the liver and gallbladder (Reckeweg 2000), and has been shown to have effects in diarrhea (Zhu, Ahrens 1982; Shamsa, Ahmadiani, and Khosrokhavar 1999). It treats colic, collapse, and bloody vomitus, and is supportive of adrenal and renal function. It is part of the basic *Detox Kit* and is contained in *Solidago compositum*.

BHI-Chelidonium complex: Treats abdominal distention and flatulence (Lycopodium, Calcarea carbonica); gastralgia, yellow-clay colored stools (Chelidonium majus); and painful, distended abdomen, spasmodic hiccup, and epigastric pain (Belladonna) (Heel 2002).

Ceanothus homaccord: Used for pancreatopathy, epigastric syndrome, tenesmus, diarrhea, and hepatic issues. Splenic enlargement is a primary signalment for this remedy (Macleod 1983).

Chelidonium homaccord: This is a commonly used agent in hepatic damage and hepatitis, and gallbladder conditions such as cholangitis, cholecystitis, and obstructive jaundice (Demers 2004). Chelidonium contains a substance known as Chelidonine, which has anticancer effects. "Chelidonine turned out to be a potent inducer of apoptosis triggering cell death at concentrations of 0.001 mM," according to Habermehl (2006), a fact that may explain the clinically observed usefulness of this remedy in treating patients with biliary neoplasia.

Chol-Heel: An excellent remedy containing Belladonna, Chelidonium, Carduus marianus, Lycopodium, Veratrum, and Taraxicum, along with some other very useful components, all in potency chords. This can be of great relief in GI discomfort (Broadfoot 2005).

Coenzyme compositum: Contains Citricum acidum, which is useful for dental problems and gingivitis; scurvy; blackening of teeth; heavy deposits of dental plaque; painful, herpetic vesicles around the lips; nausea; painful cramping in the umbilical area; and distension. Used as an agent to repair mitochondrial damage resulting from antibiotic therapy (also used with *Ubichinon compositum* and *Galium-Heel* for that purpose).

Engystol N: Used for viral origin gastroenteritis and hepatitis (see Parvovirus).

Erigotheel: Used for gastric catarrh, hepatic diseases, duodenal ulcers with spasm, and has antipyretic properties (Demers 2004).

Galium-Heel: Used for all cellular phases, hemorrhoids, anal fissures, and as a detoxicant. See notes above for proper use.

Hepar compositum: The main remedy for chronic hepatitis cases. Provides detoxification and drainage of hepatic tissues and organ and metabolic support, and is useful in most hepatic and gallbladder pathologies. It is an important part of Deep Detoxification Formula. Treats duodenitis, pancreatitis, cystic hepatic ducts, cholelithiasis, cholangitis, cholecystitis, vomiting, and diarrhea (Demers 2004, Broadfoot 2004). This combination contains Natrum oxalaceticum (also found in *Coenzyme compositum*, *Ubichinon compositum*, and *Mucosa compositum*) for changes in appetite and stomach distension due to air. Treats nausea, stomach pain with a sensation of fullness, gurgling in the abdomen, and cramping pain in the hypochondria. Also used for constipation, sudden diarrhea (particularly after eating), and flatus (Reckeweg 2002).

Hepeel: Provides liver drainage and detoxification. Used in a wide variety of conditions including cancer of the liver, where *Hepeel* was found to be antiproliferative, hepatoprotective, and an antioxidant when tested in human HepG2 cells (Gebhardt 2003).

Leptandra compositum: Used for epigastric syndrome, portal vein congestion, pancreatopathy, chronic liver disease, diabetes mellitus (Reckeweg 2000).

Lymphomyosot: Provides lymph drainage and endocrine support, and treats edema. Contains Gentiana for chronic gastritis. Used for flatulence, diarrhea, distension of stomach with eructations, nausea, retching, and vomiting. Contains Geranium robertianum for nausea, particularly after eating with distension or sensation of fullness. Myosotis arvensis is contained for bloat and distension (Reckeweg 2002).

Mucosa compositum: Broadly supportive for repair of mucosal elements. Used in cellular cases and in recovery periods following active disease (Reckeweg 2000). This remedy contains a useful component in Kali bichromicum, which is indicated for ulcers found on the gums, tongue, lips, and even on the gastric mucosa (gastric or duodenal ulcer). The tongue may have a thick, yellow, mucous coating, or in ulcerative stomatitis or tonsillitis it may be dry, smooth, shiny, or fissured. Kali has been used effectively in acute gastroenteritis associated with vomiting of clear, light-colored fluid or quantities of mucous bile, and in cases with hematemesis, flatulent colics, and dysenteric stools with tenesmus (Reckeweg 2002).

It also contains Hydrastis, with mucosal support for oral problems such as stomatitis, and mucosal suppuration that is accompanied by ulceration, inflammations and colic of the hepatobiliary system and of the gastrointestinal tract, and polyp formation (Reckeweg 2002). The Kreosotum component can be used in chronic gastritis with gastric hemorrhages and vomiting of brown masses. Also has a dental implication in cases with spongy gums and carious teeth, neuralgias proceeding from them causing a burning toothache with deep caries, black patches on the teeth, and fetid discharges.

The single remedy Phosphorus is broadly useful for dyspepsia and for jaw problems in dental disease (Reckeweg 2002). Phosphorus is found in many other remedies including *Echinacea compositum* and *Leptandra homaccord*. It is rich in suis organ preparations for mucosal support, plus a large variety of remedies with indications in the gastrointestinal sphere. The component Argentum nitricum (also in *Atropinum compositum*, *Diarrheel*, *Duodenoheel*, *Gastricumeel*, *Momordica compositum*, *BHI-Nausea*, and several other combinations) is indicated for distension in the upper abdomen, gastrocardiac symptom-complex, and amelioration from eructations. It is also used for gastric crises (Reckeweg 2002).

Nux vomica homaccord: Used for liver and gastrointestinal disease and after smoke inhalation. Useful in gingivitis (Reckeweg 2002). This commonly used formula is part of the *Detox Kit*. Recent research shows that one ingredient (Brucine) affects mitochondria in human hepatoma cells. Further research is needed to determine whether homeopathic dilutions are more or less active (Deng, et al. 2006).

Phosphor homaccord: Treats hepatitis, icterus, tenderness over the liver region, pancreatic diseases, ulcerated gums, thirst but vomiting right after drinking occurs, pale-clay-colored stools (Macleod 1983).

Schwef-Heel: Treats chronic diseases of skin and liver; should be interposed in most skin and liver cases (Reckeweg 2000). Patients that need this remedy may look dirty and have scruffy skin conditions, red lips, white tongue with red tip, itching and burning rectal area with morning diarrhea, and prolapsed rectum (Boericke 1927). Sulfur is contained in several other antihomotoxic formulas including *Coenzyme compositum*, *Echinacea compositum*, *Engystol*, *Ginseng compositum*, *Hepar compositum*, *Molybdan compositum*, *Mucosa compositum*, *Paeonia Heel*, *Proctheel*, *Psorinoheel*, *Sulfur-Heel*, *Thyroidea compositum*, and *Ubichinon compositum* (Reckeweg 2000).

Syzygium compositum: Treats chronic gastritis, chronic enteritis, diabetes mellitus, and hepatic disorders.

Ubichinon compositum: Contains Anthraquinone for swelling of gums, and GI symptoms such as distention, flatulence, and cramping abdominal pain. Treats constipation with straining or sudden diarrhea (Reckeweg 2002).

Authors' suggested protocols

Use in addition to conventional therapy and nutraceuticals as in other sections of this text.

Nutrition

Liver and pancreas support formulas: One-half tablet BID.

Intestine and pituitary support formulas: One-half tablet SID.

Megaliptrophic: 1 capsule for every 20 pounds of body weight.

Taurine: 250 mg SID.

L-Carnitine: 150 mg SID.

Eskimo fish oil: One-half to 1 teaspoon per meals for cats or blue-green algae: one-fourth teaspoon for every 25 pounds of body weight daily.

Lecithin/phosphatidyl choline: One-fourth teaspoon for every 25 pounds of body weight BID.

Chinese herbal medicine/acupuncture

Hepatic Lipidosis: 1 capsule per 10 to 20 pounds twice daily. As in Western medicine, dietary support is critical. Underlying causes of the anorexia must be addressed.

In addition to the herbs cited above, hepatic lipidosis also contains cyperus (Xiang fu zi), pueraria (Ge gen), raphanus (Lai fu zi), and white peony (Bai shao) to help improve the efficacy of the formula.

The authors recommend the acupuncture points ST36 and LI3 as noted above.

Homotoxicology (Dose: 10 drops PO for 50-pound dog; 5 drops PO for cat or small dog)

Echinacea compositum: TID. Chelidonium Homaccord, twice daily. Hepar compositum twice weekly. Galium-Heel every other day. Ubichinon compositum and Coenzyme compositum given every other day. Hepeel BID alternated with Hepar therapy.

Product sources

Nutrition

Liver, pancreas, intestine, and pituitary support formulas: Animal Nutrition Technologies. **Alternatives:** Hepatic Support—Standard Process Veterinary Formulas; Hepato Support—Rx Vitamins for Pets; Hepagen—Thorne Veterinary Products; Enteric Support—Standard Process Veterinary Formulas; NutriGest—Rx Vitamins for Pets.

Megaliptrophic: Best For Your Pet.

L-Carnitine and taurine: Over the counter.

Eskimo fish oil: Tyler Encapsulations.

Blue-green algae: Simplexity.

Lecithin/phosphatidyl choline: Designs for Health.

Chinese herbal medicine

Hepatic Lipidosis: Natural Solutions, Inc.

Homotoxicology

BHI/Heel Corporation

REFERENCES

Western medicine references

Center SA. Hepatic Lipidosis, glucocorticoid hepatopathy, vacuolar hepatopathy, storage disorders, amyloidosis, and iron toxicity. In: Guilford WG, Center SA, Strombeck DR, et al., eds., Strombeck's small animal gastroenterology. 3rd ed. Philadelphia: Saunders, 1996:766–801.

Center SA. Hepatic Lipidosis. In: Tilley L, Smith F. The 5-Minute Veterinary Consult: Canine and Feline, 2003. Blackwell Publishing.

Center SA, Guida L, Zanelli MJ, Dougherty E, Cummings J, King J. Ultrastructural hepatocellular features associated with severe hepatic lipidosis in cats. *Am J Vet Res.* 1993. May;54(5): pp 724–31.

Cornelius LM, Bartges JW, Miller CC. CVT Update: Therapy for hepatic lipidosis. In: Bonagura, JD, ed. Current Veterinary Therapy XIII. Philadelphia: WB Saunders Co. 2000:686–90.

Day DG. Diseases of the liver. In: Sherding RG, ed. The Cat: Diseases and Clinical Management. New York: Churchill Livingstone. 1994: 1312–16.

Johnson SE, Sherding RG. Diseases of the liver and biliary tract. In: Birchard SJ,; Sherding RG, eds. Saunders Manual of Small Animal Practice. Philadelphia: WB Saunders Co. 1994: 749–51.

IVM reference

Center SA. Feline hepatic lipidosis. *Vet Clin North Am Small Anim Pract.* 2005, Jan;35(1):pp 225–69.

Nutrition references

Buckner GG, Szabo J, Sunvold GD. Implications of Nutrition on Feline Hepatic Fatty Acid Metabolism, In: Reinhart GA, Carey DP, eds. Recent Advances in Canine and Feline Nutrition, Volume II, 1998. Iams Nutrition Symposium Proceeding.

Center SA. Safe weight loss in cats. In: Reinhart GA, Carey DP, eds. Recent Advances in Canine and Feline Nutrition Volume II: 1998 Iams Nutrition Symposium Proceedings. Wilmington, Ohio: Orange Frazer Press, 1998; 165–181.

Evangeliou A, Vlassopoulos D. Carnitine metabolism and deficit—when is supplementation necessary? *Curr Pharm Biotechnol.* 2003 Jun;4(3):211–9.

Gonzalez de Rivera C, Miranda-Zamora R, Diaz-Zagoya JC, et al. Preventive effect of Spirulina maxima on the fatty liver induced by a fructose-rich diet in the rat, a preliminary report. *Life Sci* 1993;53:57–61.

Hanin IG, Ansell B. Lecithin: Technological, Biological, and Therapeutic Aspects, NY: Plenum Press, 1987. 180, 181.

Howell E. Enzyme Nutrition, The Food Enzyme Concept. 1985. Garden City, NY: Avery Publ.

Iwata K, Inayama T, Kato T. Effects of Spirulina platensis on plasma lipoprotein lipase activity in fructose-induced hyperlipidemic rats. *J Nutr Sci Vitaminol (Tokyo)* 1990;36: 165–71.

Monson W. Taurine's Role in the Health of Cats. *Vet. Med.*, Oct. 1989.84(10): 1013–105.

Prichard BN, Smith CCT, Ling KLE, Betteridge DJ. Fish oils and cardiovascular disease. *BMJ* 1995;310:819–20.

Sachan DH, Rhew TH, Ruark RA. Ameliorating Effects of Carnitine and its Precursors on Alcohol-Induced Fatty Liver. *Amer. J. of Clin. Nut.*, 1984.38, 738–744,

Sunvold GD, Tetrick MA, Davenport GM, Bouchard GF. Carnitine supplementation promotes weight loss and decreased adiposity in the canine. Proceedings of the XXIII World Small Animal Veterinary Association. October, 1998.p.746.

Chinese herbal medicine/acupuncture references

Cai L, et al. Research on the therapeutic effects and mechanisms of exercise and Shan Zha on rat hyperlipidemia. *China Journal of Sports Medicine.* 2000;19(1):29–32.

Chen QL, et al. *Journal of Chinese Patented Medicine.* 1994; 16(3):22–23.

Chen S, et al. *China Journal of TCM Theories.* 1999;5(5): 21–25.

Chu YF, et al. Effects of Shan Zha core alcohol soluble extracts on quail blood serum and cholesterol level on artery walls. *Journal of Chinese Materia Medica.* 1988; 19(1):25–27.

He P, et al. Yin Chen's effect on antipyrin metabolism in humans and rabbits. *China Journal of Hospital Pharmacy.* 1990; 10(10):459–460.

Hsu JL, Sheng-Feng Hsu, Chang-Chi Hsieh, Tin-Yun Ho, Ching-Liang Hsieh, Chin-Chuan Tsai, Jaung-Geng Lin. The Effectiveness of Tsu-San-Li and Tai-Chung Acupoints for Treatment of Acute Liver Damage in Rats. Spring, 2001.*American Journal of Chinese Medicine.*

Hu YQ, et al. The extraction and separation of Yin Chen polypeptides and their liver-protecting effects in mice. *Journal of Chinese Materia Medica.* 1999;30(12):894–896.

Institute of Pharmacy. People's Experiment Hospital of Zhejiang. *Chinese Materia Medica Bulletin.* 1976;(7):26–30.

Jiang Su Zhong Yi (*Jiangsu Chinese Medicine*), 1988; (7):41.

Liu CJ, et al. *China Journal of Chinese Medicine.* 1992; 17(10):595.

Sui YH, et al. A comparative study of Xiang Fu, Qing Pi, Ci Li, Yin Chen, Xi Nan Zhang Ya Cai: Their effects on bile secretion. *Henan Journal of TCM.* 1993;13(1):19–20, 44.

Tang B, et al. *Journal of Chinese Materia Medica.* 1998; 29(12):814–817.

Xin Yi Yao Xue Za Zhi (*New Journal of Medicine and Herbology*), 1974; (5):34.

Zhong Cao Yao (*Chinese Herbal Medicine*), 1991;22(2):72.

Zhong Guo Zhong Yao Za Zhi (*People's Republic of China Journal of Chinese Herbology*), 1989; 14(10):46.

Zhong Xi Yi Jie He Za Zhi (*Journal of Integrated Chinese and Western Medicine*), 1983;1:19.

Zhong Xi Yi Jie He Za Zhi (*Journal of Integrated Chinese and Western Medicine*), 1988;8(3):p 161, 180.

Zhong Yao Zhi (*Chinese Herbology Journal*), 1984:352.

Zhong Yi Za Zhi (*Journal of Chinese Medicine*), 1982; (1):67.

Homotoxicology references

Broadfoot PJ. Inflammation: Homotoxicology and Healing. In: Proceedings AHVMA/Heel Homotoxicology Seminar. 2004. Denver, CO, p 27.

Demers, J. Homotoxicology and Acupuncture. In: Proceedings of the 2004 Homotoxicology Seminar. 2004. AHVMA/Heel. Denver, CO, p 5, 6.

Deng X, Yin F, Lu X, Cai B, Yin W. The apoptotic effect of brucine from the seed of Strychnos nux-vomica on human hepatoma cells is mediated via Bcl-2 and Ca2+ involved mitochondrial pathway. *Toxicol Sci.* May; 2006. 91(1):pp 59–69.

Gebhardt R. Antioxidative, antiproliferative and biochemical effects in HepG2 cells of a homeopathic remedy and its constituent plant tinctures tested separately or in combination. *Arzneimittelforschung.* 2003. 53(12): pp 823–30.

Habermehl D, Kammerer B, Handrick R, Eldh T, Gruber C, Cordes N, Daniel PT, Plasswilm L, Bamberg M, Belka C, Jendrossek V. Proapoptotic activity of Ukrain is based on Chelidonium majus L. alkaloids and mediated via a mitochondrial death pathway. *BMC Cancer.* 2006. Jan 17;6: p 14.

Heel. BHI Homeopathic Therapy: Professional Reference. Albuquerque, NM: Heel Inc. 2002. pp 43, 47, 73.

Khuda-Bukhsh AR, Pathak S, Guha B, Karmakar S, Das J, Banerjee P, Biswas S, Mukherjee P, Bhattacharjee N, Choudhury S, Banerjee A, Bhadra S, Mallick P, Chakrabarti J, Mandal B. In vitro anti-rotavirus activity of some medicinal plants used in Brazil against diarrhea. *J Ethnopharmacol.* 2005. Jul 14;99(3): pp 403–7.

Macleod G. A Veterinary Materia Medica and Clinical Repertory with a Materia Medica of the Nosodes. Safron, Walden: CW Daniel Company, LTD. 1983. pp 50–1, 125–6, 129–30.

Miele L, Vero V, Gasbarrini G, Grieco A. Braised liver with herbs: the risks of naturopathic hepatoprotection. *J Clin Gastroenterol.* 2004. Apr;39(4):p 344.

Reckeweg H. Biotherapeutic Index: Ordinatio Antihomotoxica et Materia Medica, 5th ed. Baden-Baden, Germany: Biologische Heilmittel Heel GMBH, 2000. pp 157, 294–5, 300, 358–9, 369, 399–400.

Reckeweg H. Homeopathia Antihomotoxica Materia Medica, 4th ed. Baden-Baden, Germany: Arelia-Verlag GMBH, 2002. pp. 136–8, 146–8, 344–5, 365–6, 447–9, 488–90. 136–8, 139–40, 125–6, 147, 150–3, 179, 206, 241–2, 317–19, 345, 366, 461–3, 446–49, 488–90, 578–80.

Shamsa F, Ahmadiani A, Khosrokhavar R. Antihistaminic and anticholinergic activity of barberry fruit (Berberis vulgaris) in the guinea-pig ileum. *J Ethnopharmacol.* 1999. Feb;64(2):pp 161–6.

Spee B, Arends B, van den Ingh TS, Brinkhof B, Nederbragt H, Ijzer J, Roskams T, Penning L, Rothuizen J. Transforming growth factor beta-1 signaling in canine hepatic diseases: new models for human fibrotic liver pathologies. *Liver Int.* 2006. Aug;26(6):pp 716–25.

Tsochatzis E, Papatheodoridis G, Archimandritis A. The Evolving Role of Leptin and Adiponectin in Chronic Liver Diseases. *Am J Gastroenterol.* 2006. Sep 4. [Epub ahead of print].

Watson PJ. Chronic hepatitis in dogs: a review of current understanding of the aetiology, progression, and treatment. *Vet J.* 2004.May;167(3):228–41.

Zhu B, Ahrens FA. Effect of berberine on intestinal secretion mediated by Escherichia coli heat-stable enterotoxin in jejunum of pigs. *Am J Vet Res.* 1982. Sep;43(9): pp 1594–8.

ACUTE AND CHRONIC PANCREATITIS

Definition and cause

Pancreatitis is an inflammation of the pancreas. Acute pancreatitis occurs rapidly, often with serious clinical secondary signs. Acute pancreatitis is distinguished from a chronic inflammatory process of the pancreas in that the cellular integrity of the pancreas is changed in chronic episodes. Causes of pancreatitis include infectious agents; nutrition (high-fat diets); secondary inflammation to toxins, medications, vaccination, and inflammatory producers such as excessive free radicals and reactive oxygen species; and are secondary to other conditions such as hyperlipidemia and hypercalcemia (Jergens 2003, Simpson 1993, Stewart 1994, Williams 2000).

Medical therapy rationale, drug(s) of choice, and nutritional recommendations

Resting of pancreatic function is essential because of the potential damage from excessive production of digestive enzymes. Withdrawal of food and water stops the digestive process and the production of enzymes. Pain and anti-inflammatory medications in combination with fluid therapy for rehydration are essential, especially in acute episodes (Jergens 2003, Williams 2000).

The diet should be low in protein and fat, such as boiled carbohydrates (oatmeal or rice), and contain low levels of lean protein, such as boiled chicken or beef. Medical therapy includes corticosteroids to reduce inflammation, antiemetics to prevent or stop vomiting, and painkillers for comfort.

Anticipated prognosis

Acute and chronic pancreatitis often responds to medication. The prognosis depends on damage to the pancreas and associated other organ damage. Intense medical therapy with acute pancreatitis often quiets the condition and helps to achieve stability. Chronic episodes are less intense; however, the risk of pancreatic cell destruction secondary to chronic inflammation makes the prognosis more guarded (Jergens 2003, Stewart 1994).

Integrative veterinary therapies

Acute pancreatitis is a medical emergency. Withdrawal of food and water and resting of the gastrointestinal system greatly assists these patients. Parenteral fluids and electrolyte maintenance are important aspects. Pharmaceutical agents can be used as needed for pain and nausea, but many patients do very nicely with antihomotoxic medications (see Homotoxicology in this protocol). Because such

medications have fewer adverse reactions, they may be preferred in these cases. Canine patients can be fasted for longer periods of time, while feline patients may require assistance with alimentation to prevent the development of other complications such as hepatic lipidosis.

The inclusion of proper prebiotics (such as fiber) and probiotic bacteria may promote or assist in homotoxin removal by binding homotoxins to fiber or through metabolism of toxic material by bacteria. Probiotic bacteria assist with the health of the mucosal lining and may prevent pancreatitis from occurring. The common practice of treating GI upset by fasting is important in treating pancreatitis, but in chronic disease it may not be feasible or possible to withhold feeding until pancreatic inflammation ceases. Giving a bland diet that is low in fat is an excellent approach. Some patients do better on low-residue diets, while others make great strides while eating higher fiber foods. A clinician should be prepared to try both dietary types in managing chronic pancreatitis. Providing digestive enzymes in supplemental amounts may help the digestive processes and reduce the workload of the pancreas.

Successfully treating chronic pancreatitis involves providing clean diet and water, reducing stress, allowing toxins to be excreted successfully, supporting organ function, and providing drainage therapy and metabolic support while repair occurs.

The properly timed addition of nutrients, nutraceuticals, medicinal herbs, and combination homeopathics that have anti-inflammatory, tissue-protective, and regenerative effects on the cells of the pancreas, liver, stomach, and intestine tissue can help control the clinical signs, reduce pain, shorten recovery time, and prevent recurrences.

Nutrition
General considerations/rationale

Medical therapy if often essential to control pain, vomiting, and organ inflammation. The nutritional approach of adding gland support and anti-inflammatory nutrients often speeds up stability and recovery.

Note: Pancreatitis often has systemic effects upon other organ systems, and therefore it is recommended that blood be analyzed both medically and physiologically to determine overall organ involvement. This helps clinicians to formulate therapeutic nutritional protocols that specifically address all involved organ systems (See Chapter 2, Nutritional Blood Testing, for more specific information). Also, with acute pancreatitis and related vomiting, the timing and use of oral nutraceuticals should be properly selected so as not to exacerbate vomiting.

Appropriate nutrients

Nutritional/gland therapy: Glandular pancreas, intestines, stomach, and liver supply the intrinsic nutrients to reduce cellular inflammation and improve organ function and healing (see Gland Therapy in Chapter 2 for a more detailed explanation).

Probiotics: Have been shown to reduce intestinal pain, inflammation, and other gastrointestinal symptoms such as excessive gas production (Niedzielin 2001, Nobaek 2000).

Colostrum: Has been shown to improve intestinal health. It helps to balance intestinal flora and improves digestion (Blake 1999).

Fiber: In a study with people with IBS, Manning (1977) and Hotz (1994) showed improvement by adding psyllium to the diet.

Chinese herbal medicine/acupuncture
General considerations/rationale

Pancreatitis is due to Qi stagnation in the Liver with excessive Heat in the Stomach and Spleen. Qi stagnation in the Liver leads to abdominal pain. Any time there is stagnation there is an accumulation. Think of a flowing stream of water. If the flow is stopped, i.e., by a dam, the water accumulates. The Western-trained doctor is used to addressing this concept with substantive materials. For example, if the accumulation is pus, it is intuitive that there will be pain because abscesses are painful. To those trained in TCM, excessive accumulation of Qi can lead to pain even though these practitioners cannot point to a pocket of "Qi" to show the stagnation. Heat in the Stomach and Spleen refers to the inflammation. This Heat may manifest as fever, purulent debris, redness, and swelling.

Treatment is aimed at decreasing the inflammation (Heat) and the cause of the inflammation (bacteria, viruses, hyperlipidemia). This may be accomplished by directly attacking the inciting cause or by enhancing the immune system to allow the body to ameliorate the condition. The pain, fever, and vomiting caused by the disorder must also be controlled.

Appropriate Chinese herbs

Bupleurum (Chai hu): Contains saikosaponin A and D, which have several functions in an herbal supplement designed for pancreatitis. They have analgesic and antipyretic properties (Shen Yang Yi Xue Yuan Bao 1984). In terms of treating potential causes of pancreatitis, these compounds decrease triglyceride levels, and to a lesser extent cholesterol levels (Zhong Yao Xue 1988). In addition, bupleurum enhances both humoral and cellular immunity (Shang Hai Yi Ke Da Xue Xue Bao 1986) and has antiviral and antibacterial properties (Wang 1998, Liao 1999, Zhong Yao Xue 1988).

Cinnamon twig (Gui zhi): Has analgesic properties (Zhong Yao Xue 1998) as well as antibacterial and antiviral activity (Zhong Yao Xue 1998, Chu 1998).

Codonopsis (Dang shen): Helps stimulate the immune system (Zhong Xi Yi Jie He Za Zhi 1985). It also decreases blood cholesterol and triglyceride levels and improves the ratio of high density lipoproteins to low density lipoproteins (Hua 1994).

Coptis (Huang lian): Decreases serum lipid concentrations (Song 1992). One of the components, berberine, has anti-inflammatory effects (Yao Xue Za Zhi 1981). Coptis can also be used to lower fevers (Zhong Guo Bing Li Sheng Li Za Zhi 1991).

Evodia (Wu zhu yu): An effective antiemetic (Zhong Yao Yao Li Du Li Yu Lin Chuan 1988).

Ginger (Sheng jiang): Has strong antiemetic effects (Xi Ye Shi Lang 1990).

Licorice (Gan cao): Has antibiotic and antiviral effects (Zhong Yao Zhi 1993, Zhu 1996) and analgesic properties (Zhong Yao Xue 1998). Furthermore, it lowers serum cholesterol levels (Zhong Yao Xue 1998). Two components, glycyrrhizin and glycyrrhetinic acid, decrease inflammation (Zhong Cao Yao 1991).

Pinellia (Ban xia): Lowers serum total cholesterol and LDL-C levels (Hong 1995) and has analgesic and anti-inflammatory effects (Shen Ya Qin 1998, Shen Ya Qin 1998). In terms of symptomatic relief, it can inhibit vomiting (Gui 1998).

Saussurea (Mu xiang): Has antibacterial effects against several bacteria, including E. coli (Zhong Yao Yao Li Yu Ying Yong 1983).

Scutellaria (Huang qin): Contains baicalin, which has antibiotic activity against many bacteria including E. coli (Zhong Yao Xue 1988). In addition, 2 compounds in scutellaria, baicalin and baicalein, have anti-inflammatory effects (Kubo 1984). Scutellaria can help decrease fevers (Zhong Hua Yi Xue Za Zhi 1956), and it enhances the cellular immune system (Pan 1991).

White peony (Bai shao): Inhibits various bacteria, including E coli (Xin Zhong Yi 1989). It contains paeoniflorin, which is a strong antipyretic and anti-inflammatory (Zhong Yao Zhi 1993:183). It also can help control pain (Shang Hai Zhong Yi Yao Za Zhi 1983).

The use of acupuncture in pancreatitis is controversial. One study of 23 people found that acupuncture did not preclude the use of medication for pain relief (Ballegaard 1985). Others feel that acupuncture may be helpful (Su 1987).

Homotoxicology—acute pancreatitis
General considerations/rationale

Pancreatitis can occur as a manifestation of many different phases on the Six-Phase Table of Homotoxicology. Acute pancreatitis is most often due to reactions by the pancreas that result from Inflammation Phase homotoxicoses. Anything that directly traumatizes the pancreas can result in pancreatitis. Pancreatitis can arise suddenly as a component of regressive or progressive vicariation, in which pancreatic enzymes are activated outside the normal gastrointestinal system. Activated enzymes attack normal body structures, creating irritating compounds such as soap from digestion of lipids, and these substances cause further inflammatory changes, pain, and metabolic imbalance. Rapid changes in serum calcium from soap formation can result in cardiac irregularities and sudden death. Release of substances from an inflamed pancreas, such as myocardial depressant factor, can also lead to severe complications.

Many homotoxins can damage the pancreas' ability to function normally. Both toxins and other therapeutic agents can result in progressive vicariation. Corticoids and nonsteroidal anti-inflammatory drugs both damage intestinal mucosal elements. This can result in frank ulcer or "leaky gut syndrome," which is linked to many other medical syndromes. In leaky gut, antigens are not properly digested into smaller molecular weight polypeptides before gaining access to the immune system. This issue can lead to chronic inflammatory diseases such as inflammatory bowel disease and allergic syndromes. Chronic pancreatitis is sometimes due to incomplete treatment and monitoring, and there are no good results in some cases regardless of what the clinician attempts (see Inflammatory Bowel Disease protocol, above, for further discussion of leaky gut syndrome).

Appropriate homotoxicology formulas

Gastrointestinal diseases may require a wide variety of antihomotoxic agents. A more complete list of these is included at the end of the gastrointestinal chapter, chapter 24.

Atropinum compositum: Not available on the U.S. market at this time as oral vial or injection, but available as tablets, this agent is a powerful antispasmodic for biliary, renal, and intestinal colic (Demers 2004). Contains Benzoicum acidum (also common to *Aesculus compositum*, *Arnica-Heel*, *Atropinum compositum*, and *Rhododendroneel*). It is used in inflammatory symptoms which occur throughout the alimentary canal: a slimy coating on the tongue with ulcers at the edges, stomatitis with dysphagia, eructations, retching and vomiting, and flatulent distension below the ribs on both sides. The stools are copious, loose, and white in color, with violent tenesmus and mixed with blood; there are stabbing pains in the rectum, rigors, and a feeling of being seriously ill (Reckeweg 2002).

BHI-Pancreas: Treats pancreatitis and related symptomology including diarrhea, vomiting, nausea, and constipation.

BHI-Spasm-Pain: Treats leg cramps, fever, pain and inflammation, sharp pain, colic or intestinal spasm, and colitis.

Bryaconeel: Treats inflammation of serosal surfaces, and is a geriatric medicant.

Chelidonium homaccord: A commonly used formula for problems including gallbladder conditions such as cholangitis, cholecystitis, obstructive jaundice, hepatic damage and hepatitis (Demers 2004). Chelidonium contains a substance known as Chelidonine, which has anticancer effects. "Chelidonine turned out to be a potent inducer of apoptosis triggering cell death at concentrations of 0.001 mM," according to Habermehl (2006), a fact that may explain the clinically observed usefulness of this remedy in treating patients with biliary neoplasia.

Coenzyme compositum: Contains Citricum acidum, which is useful for dental problems and gingivitis; scurvy; blackening of teeth; heavy deposits of dental plaque; painful, herpetic vesicles around the lips; nausea; painful cramping in the umbilical area; and distension.

Duodenoheel: Treats hunger pains, hyperacidity, gastric and duodenal ulcers, nausea and vomiting, and dysentery with tenesmus (Reckeweg 2000).

Hepar compositum: Provides detoxification and drainage of hepatic tissues and organ and metabolic support, and is useful in many common gastrointestinal pathologies, such as duodenitis, pancreatitis, cystic hepatic ducts, cholelithiasis, cholangitis, cholecystitis, vomiting, and diarrhea (Demers 2004, Broadfoot 2004). Contains Pancreas suis for glandular support. *Hepar compositum* is an important part of Deep Detoxification Formula. This combination contains Natrum oxalaceticum (also found in *Coenzyme compositum*, *Ubichinon compositum*, and *Mucosa compositum*) for changes in appetite and stomach distension due to air. Treats nausea, stomach pain with a sensation of fullness, gurgling in the abdomen, and cramping pain in the hypochondria. It is also used for constipation, sudden diarrhea (particularly after eating), and flatus (Reckeweg 2002). Veratrum album is included for vomiting and bloody diarrhea (Van Wassenhoven 2004).

Hepeel: Treats liver drainage and detoxification. Used in a wide variety of conditions including cancer of the liver, where Hepeel was found to be antiproliferative, hepatoprotective, and an antioxidant when tested in human HepG2 cells (Gebhardt 2003).

Leptandra compositum: Indicated for epigastric syndrome, portal vein congestion, pancreatopathy, chronic liver disease, and diabetes mellitus (Reckeweg 2000).

Lymphomyosot: Provides lymph drainage and endocrine support, and treats edema. Contains Gentiana for chronic gastritis. Treats flatulence, diarrhea, distension of stomach with eructations, nausea, retching, and vomiting. Also contains Geranium robertianum for nausea, particularly after eating with distension or sensation of fullness. Myosotis arvensis is included for bloat and distension (Reckeweg 2002).

Momordica compositum: Treats pancreatitis, epigastric disease (Momordica balsamina), emaciation though good appetite (Jodum), and vomiting with collapse (Veratrum album)(Reckeweg 2000).

Mucosa compositum: Broadly supportive for repair of mucosal elements. Used in cellular cases and in recovery periods following active disease (Reckeweg 2000). This remedy contains a useful component in Kali bichromicum, which is indicated for ulcers found on the gums, tongue, lips, and even on the gastric mucosa (gastric or duodenal ulcer). The tongue may have a thick, yellow, mucous coating, or, in ulcerative stomatitis or tonsillitis it may be dry, smooth, shiny, or fissured. Kali has been used effectively in acute gastroenteritis associated with vomiting of clear, light-colored fluid or quantities of mucous bile, and in cases with hematemesis, flatulent colics, and dysenteric stools with tenesmus (Reckeweg 2002).

It also contains Hydrastis, with mucosal support for oral problems such as stomatitis, and mucosal suppuration that is accompanied by ulceration, inflammations and colic of the hepatobiliary system and of the gastrointestinal tract, and polyp formation (Reckeweg 2002). The Kreosotum component can be used in chronic gastritis with gastric hemorrhages and vomiting of brown masses. Also has a dental implication in cases with spongy gums and carious teeth, neuralgias proceeding from them causing a burning toothache with deep caries, black patches on the teeth, and fetid discharges.

The single remedy Phosphorus is broadly useful for dyspepsia and for jaw problems in dental disease (Reckeweg 2002). Phosphorus is found in many other remedies including *Echinacea compositum* and *Leptandra homaccord*. It is rich in suis organ preparations for mucosal support, plus a large variety of remedies with indications in the gastrointestinal sphere. The component Argentum nitricum (also in *Atropinum compositum, Diarrheel, Duodenoheel, Gastricumeel, Momordica compositum, BHI-Nausea*, and several other combinations) is indicated for distension in the upper abdomen, gastrocardiac symptom-complex, and amelioration from eructations. It is also used for gastric crises (Reckeweg 2002).

Syzygium compositum: Used for chronic gastritis, chronic enteritis, diabetes mellitus, and hepatic disorders.

Ubichinon compositum: Contains Anthraquinone for swelling of gums, and GI symptoms such as distention, flatulence, and cramping abdominal pain. Treats constipation with straining or sudden diarrhea (Reckeweg 2002).

Homotoxicology—chronic pancreatitis
General considerations/rationale
Chronic pancreatitis represents an Impregnation Phase to Degeneration Phase homotoxicosis. Chronic bouts of inflammation lead to gradual loss of pancreatic function

as both endocrine and exocrine pancreatic functions are damaged. Conventional therapy is aimed at reducing dietary stressors and inflammation. Biological therapy also works toward reducing stress and managing diet. Draining homotoxins and supporting organ repair are additional strategies in the battle with chronic disease.

As in hepatic diseases, pancreatic pathologies can result from leaky gut syndrome as antigens gain access to areas that they normally could not reach. Inflammation results and immune elements injure normal tissue and negatively affect its function. Inflammatory elements can activate normally quiescent digestive enzymes in the inactive, proenzymatic form. Once activated, these pancreatic enzymes can begin to digest normal tissues instead of nutritional substrates. Continuing inflammation from calcium soap formation aggravates the condition further. Inflammatory cascades result in fibrotic changes. Amyloid is also deposited, furthering the degeneration of the pancreas.

Removal of homotoxins and organ support are essential. Because the pancreas has an endocrine function, it is advisable to support the general endocrine system as well. Several common antihomotoxic drugs such as Lymphomyosot, Thyroidea compositum, Hepar compositum, and Tonsilla compositum all support endocrine and neurological function in addition to their primary target organs. Homotoxins bound to proteins alter their function, leaving cell membrane receptors blocked and less active. Organelle degeneration occurs rapidly once cellular communication is damaged. This can lead to damage of the DNA as the condition progresses. Theoretically, this is one mechanism for the development of neoplasia. Some repair is possible as homotoxins are removed, and the matrix components are repaired through the process of physiological inflammation and gelification. Regressive vicariation may occur of fibrosis is not too severe.

In chronic pancreatitis the mediation and causation of chronic inflammation may result from pathology elsewhere in the body. A septic condition from an abscessed tooth or tumor can be seen as causal conditions. Many forms of homotoxicoses are occult and unknown to owner and veterinarian alike. The cause of this condition may not be found, and it may surface as a vicariation reaction. The body speaks to the biological therapist with every sign and symptom manifest, and astute clinicians learn this language as they handle cases over time.

Nutrient- and homotoxin-laden blood leaves the intestines and proceeds via the portal vein to the liver, where it is directly cleansed and processed. Many GI issues are addressed with remedies that target intestinal and hepatic tissues (i.e., Nux vomica homaccord and Hepar compositum). Enterohepatic circulation provides the opportunity for homotoxins to be reabsorbed after hepatic handling. As a result, homotoxins gain access to the circulatory system again and must be removed. Ancillary excretion and metabolism by other organs (kidney, skin, and lung) may all assist in homotoxin removal. Antihomotoxic agents that support these organs include Solidago compositum, Berberis homaccord, and Mucosa compositum. Tonsilla compositum supports other immune system functions and is useful in this condition. Homotoxins that have escaped or bypassed hepatic processing may be deposited into connective tissue and cause disease later as further damage ensues.

As in other discussions, the position of the patient on the phase table assists in determining proper therapy. Because chronic disease is more difficult to handle, the use of compositae class antihomotoxic agents becomes necessary to stimulate regressive vicariation.

Appropriate homotoxicology formulas

BHI-Pancreas: Treats pancreatitis and related symptomology including diarrhea, vomiting, nausea, and constipation.

Chelidonium homaccord: Gallbladder conditions such as cholangitis, cholecystitis, obstructive jaundice, hepatic damage and hepatitis commonly used (Demers 2004). Chelidonium contains a substance known as Chelidonine, which has anticancer effects. "Chelidonine turned out to be a potent inducer of apoptosis triggering cell death at concentrations of 0.001 mM," according to Habermehl (2006), a fact that may explain the clinically observed usefulness of this remedy in treating patients with biliary neoplasia.

Coenzyme compositum: Contains Citricum acidum, which is useful for dental problems and gingivitis; scurvy; blackening of teeth; heavy deposits of dental plaque; painful, herpetic vesicles around the lips; nausea; painful cramping in the umbilical area; and distension.

Diarrheel S: A symptom remedy for acute and chronic diarrhea. Treats acute gastroenteritis, belching, spurting diarrhea, pancreatopathy, and colitis.

Galium-Heel: Used for all cellular phases, hemorrhoids, and anal fissures, and as a detoxicant.

Hepar compositum: Provides detoxification and drainage of hepatic tissues and organ and metabolic support, and is useful in most hepatic and gallbladder pathologies. It is an important part of Deep Detoxification Formula. Treats duodenitis, pancreatitis, cystic hepatic ducts, cholelithiasis, cholangitis, cholecystitis, vomiting, and diarrhea (Demers 2004, Broadfoot 2004). This combination contains Natrum oxalaceticum (also found in *Coenzyme compositum*, *Ubichinon compositum*, and *Mucosa compositum*) for changes in appetite and stomach distension due to air. Treats nausea, stomach pain with a sensation of fullness, gurgling in the abdomen, and cramping pain in the hypochondria. It is also used for constipation, sudden diarrhea (particularly after eating), and flatus (Reckeweg 2002).

Leptandra compositum: Treats epigastric syndrome, portal vein congestion, pancreatopathy, chronic liver disease, and diabetes mellitus (Reckeweg 2000).

Lymphomyosot: Provides lymph drainage and endocrine support, and treats edema.

Momordica compositum: Used for pancreatitis, epigastric disease (Momordica balsamina), emaciation though good appetite (Jodum), and vomiting with collapse (Veratrum album) (Reckeweg 2000).

Mucosa compositum: Broadly supportive for repair of mucosal elements. Used in cellular cases and in recovery periods following active disease (Reckeweg 2000). This remedy contains a useful component in Kali bichromicum, which is indicated for ulcers found on the gums, tongue, lips, and even on the gastric mucosa (gastric or duodenal ulcer). The tongue may have a thick, yellow, mucous coating, or in ulcerative stomatitis or tonsillitis it may be dry, smooth, shiny, or fissured. Kali has been used effectively in acute gastroenteritis associated with vomiting of clear, light-colored fluid or quantities of mucous bile, and in cases with hematemesis, flatulent colics, and dysenteric stools with tenesmus (Reckeweg 2002).

It also contains Hydrastis, with mucosal support for oral problems such as stomatitis, and mucosal suppuration that is accompanied by ulceration, inflammations and colic of the hepatobiliary system and of the gastrointestinal tract, and polyp formation (Reckeweg 2002). The Kreosotum component can be used in chronic gastritis with gastric hemorrhages and vomiting of brown masses. Also has a dental implication in cases with spongy gums and carious teeth, neuralgias proceeding from them causing a burning toothache with deep caries, black patches on the teeth, and fetid discharges.

The single remedy Phosphorus is broadly useful for dyspepsia and for jaw problems in dental disease (Reckeweg 2002). Phosphorus is found in many other remedies including *Echinacea compositum* and *Leptandra homaccord*. It is rich in suis organ preparations for mucosal support, plus a large variety of remedies with indications in the gastrointestinal sphere. The component Argentum nitricum (also in *Atropinum compositum*, *Diarrheel*, *Duodenoheel*, *Gastricumeel*, *Momordica compositum*, *BHI-Nausea*, and several other combinations) is indicated for distension in the upper abdomen, gastro-cardiac symptom-complex, and amelioration from eructations. It is also used for gastric crises (Reckeweg 2002).

Ubichinon compositum: Contains Anthraquinone for swelling of gums, and GI symptoms such as distention, flatulence, and cramping abdominal pain. Treats constipation with straining or sudden diarrhea (Reckeweg 2002).

Authors' suggested protocols

Nutrition

Pancreas support formula: 1 tablet for every 25 pounds of body weight BID.

Esophagus/stomach and intestines/IBD formulas: One-half tablet for every 25 pounds of body weight SID.

Probiotic: One-half capsule for every 25 pounds of body weight with food.

Psyllium: 1 teaspoon per 25 pounds of body weight per meal.

Colostrum: One-third teaspoon of powdered formula for every 25 pounds of body weight BID.

Chinese herbal medicine/acupuncture

Herbal Formula Pancreatitis: 1 capsule per 10 to 20 pounds twice daily. Depending upon the severity of the condition, in acute cases supportive therapy in the form of IV fluids, fresh frozen plasma for disseminated intravascular coagulation (DIC), and other Western therapies may be indicated.

Acupuncture points are: ST36, PC6, CV13, CV12, GB34, and ST37 (Handbook of TCM Practitioner 1987).

Homotoxicology—acute pancreatitis (Dose: 10 drops PO for 50-pound dog; 5 drops PO for cat or small dog)

In addition to proper medical care, consider the following antihomotoxic agents. Injection is recommended until the acute phase of the disease is completed, and then oral therapy can proceed.

Acute pancreatitis: Traumeel, IV. Leptandra compositum alternated with Momordica compositum daily by injection. Hepar compositum injected subcutaneously every other day. Leptandra compositum, Bryaconeel, Spascupreel, Duodenoheel mixed together and given BID orally if possible (not in NPO patients). Give Chelidonium homaccord at intervals for biliary drainage. If intense abdominal pain, consider Atropinum compositum (where available). Cardiacum-Heel if cardiac issues arise (3 to 6 times/day in acute issues).

Homotoxicology—chronic pancreatitis (Dose: 10 drops PO for 50-pound dog; 5 drops PO for cat or small dog)

Chelidonium homaccord, Diarrheel, and BHI-Pancreas: Mixed together and taken BID orally. Mucosa compositum twice weekly. Ubichinon compositum and Coenzyme compositum given twice weekly. As the case responds and stabilizes, consider the Deep Detoxification Formula given orally 1 to 3 times weekly.

Product sources

Nutrition

Pancreas, esophagus/stomach, and intestines/IBD formulas: Animal Nutrition Technologies. **Alternatives:** Enteric Support—Standard Process Veterinary Formulas; NutriGest—Rx Vitamins for Pets.

Colostrum: New Life Foods, Inc., the Saskatoon Colostrum Company Ltd.

Probiotic: Progressive Labs, Biotic—Rx Vitamins for Pets.

Psyllium seed powder: Progressive Labs.

Chinese herbal medicine

Herbal Pancreatitis: Natural Solutions, Inc.

Homotoxicology

BHI/Heel Corporation

REFERENCES

Western medicine references

Jergens AE. In: Tilley L, Smith F. The 5-Minute Veterinary Consult: Canine and Feline, 2003. Blackwell Publishing.

Simpson KW. Current concepts of the pathogenesis and pathophysiology of acute pancreatitis in the dog and cat. *Comp Contin Ed Pract Vet* 1993;15:247–253.

Stewart AF. Pancreatitis in dogs and cats: Cause, pathogenesis, diagnosis and treatment. The Compendium on Continuing Education for the Practicing Veterinarian. 1994;16(11): 1423–1431.

Williams DA. Exocrine pancreatic disease. In: Ettinger SJ, Feldman EC, eds. Textbook of Veterinary Internal Medicine. Philadelphia: WB Saunders Co. 2000;1347–1355.

IVM/nutrition references

Blake SR. Bovine Colostrum, The Forgotten Miracle. *Journal of the American Holistic Veterinary Medical Association*—July 1999, Volume 18, Number 2, pp 38–39.

Manning AP, Heaton KW, Harvey RF, Uglow P. Wheat fibre and irritable bowel syndrome. *Lancet* 1977;ii:417–8.

Niedzielin K, Kordecki H, Birkenfeld B. A controlled, double-blind, randomized study on the efficacy of *Lactobacillus plantarum* 299V in patients with irritable bowel syndrome. *Eur J Gastroenterol Hepatol.* 2001;13:1143–1147.

Nobaek S, Johansson M-L, Molin G, et al. Alteration of intestinal microflora is associated with reduction in abdominal bloating and pain in patients with irritable bowel syndrome. *Am J Gastroenterol.* 2000;95:1231–1238.

Chinese herbal medicine/acupuncture references

Ballegaard S, Christophersen SJ, Dawids SG, Hesse J, Olsen NV. Acupuncture and transcutaneous electric nerve stimulation in the treatment of pain associated with chronic pancreatitis. A randomized study. *Scand J Gastroenterol* 1985 Dec;20(10): 1249–54.

Chu XH, et al. *China Journal of New Herbal Medicine and Clinical Practice.* 1998;17(60):327–328.

Gui CQ, et al. *Journal of Pharmacology and Clinical Application of TCM.* 1998;14(4):27–28.

Handbook of TCM Practitioner, Hunan College of Traditional Chinese Medicine October 1987 p 568.

Hong XQ, et al. *Journal of Zhejiang College of TCM.* 1995; 19(2):28–29.

Hua YL, et al. Experimental research on Ming Dang Shen's effect in lowering blood lipid level. *Journal of Nanjing College of TCM.* 1994;10(4):31–32.

Kubo M, Matsuda H, Tanaka M, Kimura Y, Okuda H, Higashino M, Tani T, Namba K, Arichi S. Studies on Scutellariae radix. VII. Anti-arthritic and anti-inflammatory actions of methanolic extract and flavonoid components from Scutellariae radix. *Chem Pharm Bull*, 1984; 32(7):2724–9.

Liao CS, et al. *Shenzhen Journal of Integrated Medicine.* 1999; 9(2):20–21.

Pan JF, et al. *Tianjin Journal of Medicine.* 1991;19(8): 468–470.

Shang Hai Yi Ke Da Xue Xue Bao (*Journal of Shanghai University of Medicine*), 1986; 13(1):20.

Shang Hai Zhong Yi Yao Za Zhi (*Shanghai Journal of Chinese Medicine and Herbology*), 1983; 4:14.

Shen YQ, et al. *China Journal of Biochemical Products.* 1998;19(3):141–143.

Shen YQ, et al. *Journal of Pharmacology and Clinical Application of TCM.* 1998;14(2):29–31.

Shen Yang Yi Xue Yuan Bao (*Journal of Shenyang University of Medicine*), 1984; 1(3):214.

Song LC, et al. Huang Lian's effects on lipid peroxidation and MDA in rats. *Journal of Integrated Traditional Chinese and Western Medicine.* 1992;12(7):421–423, 390.

Su XM. The treatment of acute pancreatitis by acupuncture. *J Chin Med* 1987;No26:24–25.

Wang SC, et al. *Journal of Shizhen Medicine.* 1998; 9(5):418–419.

Xi Ye Shi Lang. *Journal of Nanjing College of TCM.* 1990; 6(2):60.

Xin Zhong Yi (*New Chinese Medicine*), 1989; 21(3):51.

Yao Xue Za Zhi (*Journal of Medicinals*), 1981, 101(10):883.

Zhong Cao Yao (*Chinese Herbal Medicine*) 1991;22 (10):452.

Zhong Guo Bing Li Sheng Li Za Zhi (*Chinese Journal of Pathology and Biology*), 1991; 7(3):264.

Zhong Hua Yi Xue Za Zhi (*Chinese Journal of Medicine*), 1956; 42(10):964.

Zhong Xi Yi Jie He Za Zhi (*Journal of Integrated Chinese and Western Medicine*), 1985; 5(8):487.

Zhong Yao Xue (*Chinese Herbology*), 1988;103:106.

Zhong Yao Xue (*Chinese Herbology*), 1988; 137:140.

Zhong Yao Xue (*Chinese Herbology*), 1998; 65:67.

Zhong Yao Xue (*Chinese Herbology*), 1998;759:765.

Zhong Yao Yao Li Du Li Yu Lin Chuan (*Pharmacology, Toxicology and Clinical Applications of Chinese Herbs*), 1988; 4(3):9.

Zhong Yao Yao Li Yu Ying Yong (*Pharmacology and Applications of Chinese Herbs*), 1983;169.

Zhong Yao Zhi (*Chinese Herbology Journal*), 1993;183.

Zhong Yao Zhi (*Chinese Herbology Journal*), 1993;358.

Zhu Li Hong. *China Journal of TCM Information.* 1996;3(3): 17–20.

Homtoxicology references—chronic

Broadfoot PJ. Inflammation: Homotoxicology and Healing. In: Proceedings AHVMA/Heel Homotoxicology Seminar. 2004. Denver, CO, p 27.

Demers, J. Homotoxicology and Acupuncture. In: Proceedings of the 2004 Homotoxicology Seminar. 2004. AHVMA/Heel. Denver, CO, p 5, 6.

Habermehl D, Kammerer B, Handrick R, Eldh T, Gruber C, Cordes N, Daniel PT, Plasswilm L, Bamberg M, Belka C, Jendrossek V. 2006. Proapoptotic activity of Ukrain is based on Chelidonium majus L. alkaloids and mediated via a mitochondrial death pathway. *BMC Cancer.* Jan 17;6: p 14.

Heel. BHI Homeopathic Therapy: Professional Reference. Albuquerque, NM: Heel Inc. 2002. pp 43, 47, 73.

Reckeweg H. Biotherapeutic Index: Ordinatio Antihomotoxica et Materia Medica, 5th ed. Baden-Baden, Germany: Biologische Heilmittel Heel GMBH, 2000. pp 358–9, 367–8, 369–71.

Reckeweg H. Homeopathia Antihomotoxica Materia Medica, 4th ed. Baden-Baden, Germany: Arelia-Verlag GMBH, 2002. pp. 136–8, 147, 345, 366, 446–9, 488–90.

Homtoxicology references—acute

Broadfoot PJ. Inflammation: Homotoxicology and Healing. In: Proceedings AHVMA/Heel Homotoxicology Seminar. Denver, CO, 2004. p 27.

Demers J. Homotoxicology and Acupuncture. In: Proceedings of the 2004 Homotoxicology Seminar. AHVMA/Heel. Denver, CO, 2004. pp 5–6.

Gebhardt R. Antioxidative, antiproliferative and biochemical effects in HepG2 cells of a homeopathic remedy and its constituent plant tinctures tested separately or in combination. *Arzneimittelforschung.* 2003. 53(12): pp 823–30.

Habermehl D, Kammerer B, Handrick R, Eldh T, Gruber C, Cordes N, Daniel PT, Plasswilm L, Bamberg M, Belka C, Jendrossek V. Proapoptotic activity of Ukrain is based on Chelidonium majus L. alkaloids and mediated via a mitochondrial death pathway. *BMC Cancer.* 2006. Jan 17;6: p 14.

Reckeweg H. Biotherapeutic Index: Ordinatio Antihomotoxica et Materia Medica, 5th ed. Baden-Baden, Germany: Biologische Heilmittel Heel GMBH, 2000. pp 367–8, 369, 538.

Reckeweg H. Homoeopathia Antihomotoxica Materia Medica, 4th ed. Baden-Baden, Germany: Arelia-Verlag GMBH, 2002. pp. 136–8, 146–8, 344–5, 365–6, 447–9, 488–90.

Shamsa F, Ahmadiani A, Khosrokhavar R. Antihistaminic and anticholinergic activity of barberry fruit (Berberis vulgaris) in the guinea-pig ileum. *J Ethnopharmacol.* 1999. Feb;64(2):pp 161–6.

Van Wassenhoven M. Towards an evidence-based repertory: clinical evaluation of Veratrum album. *Homeopathy.* 2004. Apr;93(2): pp 71–7.

Zhu B, Ahrens FA. Effect of berberine on intestinal secretion mediated by Escherichia coli heat-stable enterotoxin in jejunum of pigs. *Am J Vet Res.* 1982. Sep;43(9): pp 1594–8.

EXOCRINE PANCREATIC INSUFFICIENCY (EPI)

Definition and cause

Exocrine pancreatic insufficiency is the loss of exocrine pancreatic function resulting in a decrease in the production of digestive enzymes and lack of absorption and assimilation. Underlying causes are a degeneration of the pancreatic acinar tissue and failure to produce pancreatic enzymes. The second common reason for loss of acinar function is secondary to chronic episodes of pancreatitis (Jergens 2003; Simpson 2003; Williams 1996, 2000). EPI can occur in both dogs and cats (Steiner 1999, Westermarck 2003).

Medical therapy rationale, drug(s) of choice, and nutritional recommendations

The dietary approach to therapy often controls the condition. Switching to a highly digestible, low-fat, low-fiber diet is suggested. Longstanding, unthrifty animals should also receive vitamin supplementation (vitamins A, E, and B_{12}). Replacement therapy with pancreatic enzymes (Viokase) is the recommended therapy of choice (Jergens 2003, Simpson 2003, Williams 2000).

Anticipated prognosis

Most cases of EPI, if detected early, respond well to enzyme replacement therapy. However, pancreatic cellular changes are often permanent and require lifelong replacement therapy. The prognosis is more guarded when the condition is secondary to chronic bouts of pancreatitis or neoplasia (Jergens 2003, Williams 2000).

Integrative veterinary therapies

The loss of pancreatic acinar cells and the decreased production of enzymes are usually the result of an inflammatory process. This inflammation can be secondary to chronic infection or free radical damage causing a cellular autoimmune response against the target pancreatic cells. The integrative approach is aimed at reducing inflammation before cell destruction, death, infiltration, and scarring occur.

In human allergic conditions, autoimmune disorders such as systemic lupus (SLE) and immune-mediated arthritis have been implemented in the development of EPI (D'Ambrosi 1997, Dreiling 1976, Watts 1989).

Considering this inflammatory response, the use of nutrients, nutraceuticals, medicinal herbs, and combination homeopathics that have anti-inflammatory and regenerative effects on the acinar cells is indicated. If instituted early, such as during the treatment of pancreatitis, or when pancreatic enzyme symptoms such as voluminous stools first occur, it is possible to prevent the progressive inflammation, cell death, and scarring that leads to EPI (Goldstein 2005).

Nutrition
General considerations/rationale

Nutritional therapies are more beneficial when they are administered early in the treatment of the disease. Besides pancreatic enzyme replacement, nutritional therapy is directed toward reducing inflammation, enhancing enzyme production as well as improving the diet, digestion and assimilation. The dietary approach to therapy often helps to control the condition. Switching to a highly digestible, higher protein lower fat diet is recommended (Strombeck 1999).

Appropriate nutrients

Nutritional/gland therapy: Glandular pancreas and intestine can be helpful in neutralizing a cellular autoimmune reaction that can lead to cell destruction, infiltration, and scarring (see Gland Therapy in Chapter 2).

Pancreatic enzyme replacement: While the use of pancreatic enzyme therapy is controversial, it is often beneficial when the digestive process is compromised. The addition of pancreatic enzymes should be part of an overall program to reduce pancreatic inflammation and improve cellular function.

Probiotics: The addition of the proper combination of probiotics has a reported positive impact on the intestines and the digestive process (Goldin 1984, Perdigon 1987). Probiotics have been shown to improve and aid the digestive process by secreting their own source of enzymes, which is beneficial for animals that are pancreatic-enzyme-deficient (McDonough 1987).

Vitamins A, E, C, and B_{12}: Beneficial for animals with longstanding digestion problems that are unable to assimilate nutrients and vitamins required for health and the maintenance of wellness.

Chinese herbal medicine/acupuncture
General considerations/rationale

Exocrine pancreatic insufficiency is a result of Yang and Qi deficiency in the Spleen and Stomach. The Spleen and Stomach are responsible for changing the food and drink ingested into usable energy sources for the body. When there is not enough heat (Yang) or energy (Qi) to do so, the food remains partially digested. Treatment is aimed at improving digestive functions and decreasing uncomfortable gastrointestinal signs such as cramping and bloating.

Appropriate Chinese herbs

Amomum (Sha ren): Relieves bloating, spasms, and pain (Zhong Yao Xue 1988).

Atractylodes (Bai zhu): Can treat diarrhea or constipation, depending upon the dose (Chang Yong Zhong Yao Cheng Fen Yu Yao Li Shou Ce 1994).

Dioscorea (Shan yao): Has anti-diarrhea effects in mice with diarrhea of multiple etiologies that fall under the diagnosis of spleen deficiency in TCM (Li 1999).

Licorice (Gan cao): Stops intestinal cramping (Zhong Yao Zhi 1993).

Acupuncture

Some practitioners report success treating chronic diarrhea with acupuncture. In one human trial, 30 infants with chronic diarrhea who did not respond to Western medicine or herbs were treated with acupuncture. All were cured within 3 courses of treatment (Wenling 1989).

Homotoxicology
General considerations/rationale

German shepherd dogs are afflicted by an autosomal recessive gene, which results in pancreatic decline and maldigestion in younger dogs. Genetic disturbances such as this represent a Degeneration or Dedifferentiation phase disorder. Such conditions are generally viewed as incurable/irreversible, and clinicians are advised to concentrate on the more important treatment strategies of enzyme supplementation and dietary therapy to assist patients. The use of antihomotoxic agents may benefit these patients in other ways and may be appropriate as part of a whole patient management system. A complete discussion with the client should precede such therapy.

Exocrine pancreatic insufficiency can result from injury to the pancreatic acinar cells and such damage may be treatable via homotoxicology. This is occasionally seen as a temporary condition following pancreatitis in dogs and cats. Early treatment may assist these patients but further research is indicated. Chronic pancreatitis can be associated in some dogs and more commonly in cats. Diabetes mellitus can result from chronic pancreatitis. By the time glandular insufficiency manifests in signs of maldigestion, the disease must be fairly advanced and may not respond clinically to antihomotoxic therapy.

Autoimmune pancreatitis can lead to exocrine pancreatic insufficiency in humans, and this may well explain refractory veterinary cases as well (Van Buuren, et al. 2006). Such cases represent Impregnation Phase disorders in their origins and are often asymptomatic as they progress to more serious dysfunction.

There are no studies regarding this condition and antihomotoxic medications, so the following discussion should be viewed as experimental or theoretical in nature.

Appropriate homotoxicology formulas

Also see pancreatitis protocols.

Echinacea compositum: Used in acquired cases involving infectious damage to the pancreas and as a phase remedy in Inflammation and Impregnation phase disease conditions.

Galium-Heel: A phase remedy in Deposition, Impregnation, Degeneration, and Dedifferentiation phase disorders. Provides cellular detoxification and matrix drainage.

Glyoxal compositum: Depolymerizes homotoxins and activates blocked enzymes and receptors. It is a phase remedy in Degeneration and Dedifferentiation phase disorders.

Hepar compositum: Provides drainage, detoxification, and organ support of the liver. Contains Pankreas suis.

Leptandra homaccord: Used for pancreatic repair and drainage in cases of pancreatopathy (Leptandra, Podophyllum, Niccolum metalicum, Arsenicum album, and Phosphorus). This remedy is more helpful in pancreatitis cases but has not been researched for this purpose in animals (Reckeweg 2000).

Lymphomyosot: Provides lymphatic drainage and detoxification.

Molybdan compositum: Provides replacement of the cofactors needed in chronic cases. It is a Degeneration Phase remedy.

Momordica compositum: Provides pancreatic support and drainage. Contains Momordica, Jodam, Podophyllum, Lycopodium, Lachesis, and Veratrum, which are helpful in cases of diarrhea (Reckeweg 2000).

Mucosa compositum: Provides repair and support of mucosal elements following insult or injury. Contains Pankreas suis (Reckeweg 2000).

Placenta compositum: A phase remedy for difficult cases. Used experimentally to assist repair and activation of blood vessels. May activate stem cell action. Its use would be intermittent in pulses.

Psorinoheel: A remedy useful in deep homotoxicoses that are refractory to therapy.

Solidago compositum: Provides drainage and support of the urinary system. Part of the deep detoxification program.

Syzygium compositum: A classical remedy for diabetes and more advanced pancreatic diseases.

Thryoidea compositum: A part of the deep detoxification formula. Drains the matrix and supports the endocrine system.

Tonsilla compositum: Provides endocrine support and is an Impregnation and Dedifferentiation phase medicant. In Oriental medicine, disease of the pancreas is part of Spleen organ disease, and as such, this remedy may prove helpful in supporting immune functions (Reckeweg 2000).

Authors' suggested protocols

Nutrition

Pancreas and intestinal support formulas: 1 tablet for every 25 pounds of body weight BID.

Pan 5 Plus: 1 capsule opened and mixed with food for every 25 pounds of body weight (maximum, 4 capsules).

Probiotic MPF: One-half capsule for every 25 pounds of body weight with food.

Chinese herbal medicine/acupuncture

The authors recommend the patent formula shen ling bai zhu Tang at the manufacturer's labeled dose. In addition to the herbs mentioned above, shen ling bai zhu tang also contains coix (Yi yi ren), dolichos nut (Bai bian dou), ginseng (Ren shen), lotus seed (Lian zi), platycodon (Jie geng), and poria (Fu ling). These herbs increase the efficacy of the herbs cited above.

Shen ling bai zhu tang has undergone multiple trials in human medicine and has demonstrated efficacy in controlling diarrhea of various etiologies. In one trial 36 people with chronic diarrhea were treated with shen ling bai shu tang, with modifications depending upon classic TCM diagnosis. Seventy-eight percent had complete response, and another 17% showed improvement (Zhang 1998).

The author suggests the following points to help decrease diarrhea in cases of exocrine pancreatic insufficiency: BL20, ST36, Baihui, and ST25 (Yu 2000).

Homotoxicology—acquired cases (Dose: 10 drops PO for 50-pound dog; 5 drops PO for cat or small dog)

Pancreatic enzyme and glandular supplements are essential in treating this Degeneration Phase disorder. Prognosis is guarded.

A modified deep detoxification formula: Galium-Heel, Hepar compositum, Solidago compositum, Thyroidea compositum, Mucosa compositum, Ubichinon compositum, and Coenzyme compositum mixed together and taken orally; give twice weekly.

Podophyllum compositum: Has shown to be valuable in pancreatic issues, and should be given BID to TID. Also consider Syzygium compositum for the regulation of blood sugar.

Product sources

Nutrition

Pancreas and intestinal support formulas: Animal Nutrition Technologies. **Alternatives:** Enteric Support—Standard Process Veterinary Formulas; NutriGest—Rx Vitamins for Pets.

Pan 5 Plus and Probiotic MPF: Progressive Labs.

Chinese herbal medicine

Shen Ling Bai Zhu Tang: Mayway Company of Bluelight Inc.

Homotoxicology

BHI/Heel Corporation

REFERENCES

Western medicine references

Jergens AE. Exocrine pancreatic insufficiency (EPI). In: Tilley L, Smith F. The 5-Minute Veterinary Consult: Canine and Feline, 2003. Blackwell Publishing.

Simpson M. Diseases of the pancreas. In: Tam's Small Animal Gastroenterology, 2nd ed, Saunders, 2003, 365–368.

Steiner J, Williams D. Feline exocrine pancreatic disorders: insufficiency, neoplasia and uncommon condition. *Compendium in Continuing Education*, 1997, 19(7), 836–848.

Westermarck E, Wiberg M. Exocrine pancreatic insufficiency in dogs. *The Veterinary Clinics of North America, Small Animal Practice*, 2003, 33, 1165–1179.

Williams DA. Exocrine pancreatic disease. In: Ettinger SJ, Feldman EC, eds. Textbook of veterinary internal medicine. 5th ed. Philadelphia: Saunders, 2000:1345–1367.

Williams D. The pancreas. In: Guilford WG, et al., eds. Strombeck's Small Animal Gastroenterology. Philadelphia: Saunders, 1996, 381–410.

IVM/nutrition references

D'Ambrosi A, Verzola A, Gennaro P, et al. Functional reserve of the exocrine pancreas in Sjögren's syndrome. *Recenti Prog Med* 1997;88:21–5

Dreiling DA, Soto JM. The pancreatic involvement in disseminated "collagen" disorders. *Am J Gastroenterology* 1976; 66:546–53.

Golden BR, Gorbach SL. The Effect of Milk and Lactobacillus Feeding on Human Intestinal Bacteria Activity. *Am. J. of Clin. Nutr.*, 1984.39: 756–61.

Goldstein R, Goldstein S. The Goldstein Wellness and Longevity Program, 2005 Neptune City, NJ: TFH Publication.

McDonough FE, Hitchins AD, Wong NP, et al. Modification of sweet acidophilus milk to improve utilization by lactose-intolerant persons. *Am J Clin Nutr* 1987;45:570–4.

Perdigon GN, de Masius N, Alvarez S, et al., Enhancement of Immune Response in Mice Fed with S. Thermophilus and L. Acidophilus, *J. of Dairy Sci.*, 1987.70: 919–926.

Strombeck DR. Home-Prepared Dog and Cat Diets: the Healthful Alternative, 1st ed. January 15, 1999.Iowa State Press.

Watts RA, Isenberg DA. Pancreatic disease in the autoimmune rheumatic disorders. *Semin Arthritis Rheum* 1989;19: 158–65

Chinese herbal medicine/acupuncture references

Chang Yong Zhong Yao Cheng Fen Yu Yao Li Shou Ce (A Handbook of the Composition and Pharmacology of Common Chinese Drugs), 1994; 739:742).

Li QH, et al. *Journal of Traditional Chinese Medicine Material.*
1999;22(11):587–588.

Wenling F: Acupuncture treatment for 30 cases of infantile diarrhea. *J Trad Chin Med* 9:106–106, 1989.

Yu C and Chen Zi Bin. Modern Complete Works of Traditional
Chinese Veterinary Medicine Guang Xi Sci and Tech Press,
March 2000:469.

Zhang HY. Treating 36 cases of chronic diarrhea with modified
Shen Ling Bai Zhu Tang. *Journal of Applied TCM.* 1998;
14(10):22.

Zhong Yao Xue (*Chinese Herbology*), 1988; 326:327.

Zhong Yao Zhi (*Chinese Herbology Journal*), 1993; 358.

Homotoxicology references

Reckeweg H. 2000. Biotherapeutic Index: Ordinatio Antihomotoxica et Materia Medica, 5th ed. Baden-Baden, Germany:
Biologische Heilmittel Heel GMBH, pp 358–9, 367–71,
418–20.

Van Buuren HR, Vleggaar FP, Willemien Erkelens G, Zondervan
PE, Lesterhuis W, Van Eijck CH, Puylaert JB, Van Der Werf
SD. Autoimmune pancreatocholangitis: A series of ten patients.
Scand J Gastroenterol Suppl. 2006. May;(243):pp 70–8.

MALABSORPTION SYNDROME

Definition and cause

Severe alterations are needed before the bowel loses its
ability to absorb nutrients. Often these patients have
genetic factors, which may be aggravated by dietary
intake or other environmental factors (Garden 2000,
Battersby 2005). Celiac disease, a genetic-based intolerance to wheat gluten in Irish setters and humans, is
an important cause of malabsorption syndrome (Stazi
2005). The enzymatic digestion of food occurs in malabsorption, but nutrients cannot be properly imported inside
the body due to defects in absorptive mechanisms. A wide
variety of signs develop from malabsorption such as
diarrhea, vomiting, weight loss, malnutrition, and flatulence based upon the body's inability to get nutrients
into the correct sphere for growth, development, and
maintenance.

Medical therapy rationale, drug(s) of choice, and nutritional recommendations

Therapy depends upon the type of disease present and the
underlying cause(s) (Rodriguez-Franco, et al. 1999).

Anticipated prognosis

The prognosis depends upon the type of change and the
severity. Intestinal parasites are generally reversible.
Colitis and inflammatory bowel disease often require
ongoing medical therapy (See the following disease protocols for more detailed information: diarrhea, vomiting,
inflammatory bowel disease, colitis, and intestinal
parasites).

Integrative veterinary therapies

It is important to determine the underlying cause of the
malabsorption. Once diagnosed, the integrative approach
can help control local inflammation, improve organ function and absorption, and help prevent cellular degeneration. The addition of nutrients, nutraceuticals, medicinal
herbs, and combination homeopathics, even in genetically
induced malabsorption, can help reduce inflammation,
help with regenerative cellular integrity, and improve
function.

Nutrition
General considerations/rationale

Therapeutic nutrition adds gland support, antioxidants,
and nutrient support for the key digestive organs (liver,
intestine, and pancreas) with the goal of reducing cellular
inflammation and improving cellular function and
assimilation.

Appropriate nutrients

Nutritional/gland therapy: Glandular liver, intestines,
and pancreas supply the intrinsic nutrients that improve
organ function and reduce cellular inflammation (see
Gland Therapy in Chapter 2 for a more detailed
explanation).

Enzymes: Metabolically, enzymes are essential in the
conversion of foods to meet the energy needs of the body
(Howell 1985).

Glutamine: Has been shown to improve immune
function and is beneficial for the cells of the gastrointestinal tract (Souba 1985, Windmueller 1982, Yoshimura
1993).

Probiotics: Administration of the proper combination
of probiotics has been reported to have a positive impact
on the intestines and the digestive process (Goldin 1984,
Perdigon (1987).

Colostrum: Has been shown to improve intestinal
health. It helps to balance intestinal flora and improves
digestion (Blake 1999).

Chinese herbal medicine/acupuncture
General considerations/rationale

Malabsorption syndrome is considered Qi and Blood
stagnation with Heat and Damp affecting Stomach and
Spleen. The Stomach and Spleen are given the tasks of
digestion. When they do not have the nourishment (Blood)
or the free-flowing energy (Qi) to perform their functions,
digestive disorders follow. In the case of malabsorption,
the digestive disorder manifests as diarrhea. The Heat
refers to Inflammation, possibly in the intestinal walls in

Western terminology, and the Damp can be thought of as the mucus and undigested intestinal contents. One must decrease the inflammation in the bowels and stop the diarrhea to treat malabsorption.

Appropriate Chinese herbs

Actractylodes (Bai zhu): Can be used to stop diarrhea (Chang Yong Zhong Yao Cheng Fen Yu Yao Li Shou Ce 1994). At low doses, it has a mild inhibitory effect on the contraction of isolated guinea pig ileum (Ma Xiao Song 1996).

Amomum fruit (Sha ren): Relieves bloating, spasms, and pain (Zhong Yao Xue 1988).

Aurantium fruit (Zhi qiao): Was shown to inhibit contraction of isolated rabbit intestinal smooth muscles and to relieve acetylcholine- and BaCl2-induced enterospasm (Ma Ya Bing 1996).

Bupleurum (Chai hu): Inhibited the effect of dimethyl benzene-induced ear swelling in mice (Liu 1998). This anti-inflammatory action may help with inflammation in the intestines, allowing better absorption of nutrients.

Cimicifuga (Sheng ma): Inhibits lymphocyte activation. Cimicifuga's inhibitory effect on membrane permeability is greater than that of cortisol and it has been shown to inhibit the formation of antibodies (Zhu Nei Liang Fu 1984).

Citrus (Chen pi): Reduces inflammation by decreasing the permeability of blood vessels (Zhong Yao Yao Li Yu Ying Yong 1983). The anti-inflammatory action may decrease intestinal swelling. Citrus also can increase the activity of amylase in the saliva (Zhang 1989). If the citrus can improve digestion, absorption may be improved.

Codonopsis (Dang shen): Seems to protect the intestine. In experiments in which third-degree burns were induced in the small intestine of mice, codonopsis increased the rate of peristalsis as compared to untreated mice (Wang 1999). It may have similar protective effects from other causes of intestinal damage.

Coptis (Huang lian): Stops diarrhea (Zhong Yao Xue 1998). There was a 100% improvement in signs in a study of 100 people with acute gastroenteritis (Si Chuan Yi Xue Yuan Xue Bao 1959). One component of coptis, berberine, has been shown to have anti-inflammatory effects in rats (Yao Xue Za Zhi 1981). Berberine also increases the production of bile acids (Zhong Yao Xue 1998). This may help the body to more completely digest the food, making it easier to absorb.

Corydalis tuber (Yan hu suo): Increases secretions from adrenal glands in mice (Xi Xue Xue Bao 1988). This may release cortisol and decrease intestinal inflammation.

Immature orange peel (Qing pi): Inhibits smooth muscle contractions in the stomach and thereby relives cramps (Zhong Yao Zhi 1984).

Licorice (Gan cao): Alleviates intestinal cramping (Zhong Yao Zhi 1993). Two of the components, glycyrrhizin and glycyrrhetinic acid, have anti-inflammatory effects. They have approximately 10% of the corticosteroid activity of cortisone (Zhong Cao Yao 1991). Licorice can increase bile production (Zhu 1998, Wu 1998).

Lindera (Wu yao): Increases the secretion of gastric acid (Zhong Yao Yao Li Yu Ying Yong 1983). This may help improve digestion.

Peach kernel (Tao ren): Suppresses the immune system in several ways. It was shown to prevent egg-white-induced arthritis in mice (Liu Can Hui 1989). Other studies have shown suppressive effects on fibroblast growth in laboratory cell cultures. It was shown to suppress the proliferation of inflammatory cells and fibroblast hyperplasia in subjects using experimental trabeculae dissection (Wang 1993). Another study demonstrated the ability to decrease inflammation in mice with otitis media (Zhong Yao Tong Bao 1986).

Platycodon root (Jie geng): Has been shown to promote the secretion of corticosterone in rats, thereby causing an anti-inflammatory effect (Li 1984, Zhang 1984, Zhou 1979).

Rhubarb (Da huang): Has been shown to increase the secretion of bile in dogs and cats (Xin Yi Yao Xue Za Zhi 1974). It helps maintain a healthy intestine. Experimentally, it has been shown to prevent endotoxins from injuring the intestines, prevent viruses and bacterial translocation from damaged intestines, and maintain the intestinal mucous membrane barrier (Yang 1998, Liu 1998).

Acupuncture

Acupuncture has been shown to be effective in controlling or curing diarrhea in many studies. Acupuncture at GV1, St25, and ST-36 was used in a study of 500 infants with diarrhea; 485 were completely cured and 13 improved (Zhonzxin 1989). In preweaning pigs with experimentally induced E. coli diarrhea, a combination of acupuncture and moxibustion was superior to oral neomycin. Using acupuncture and moxibustion, 82% of the pigs responded as opposed to 71% treated with neomycin (Hwang 1988).

Homotoxicology
General considerations/rationale

Malabsorption syndrome indicates Deposition, Impregnation, Degeneration, or Dedifferentiation phase disease. Homotoxicology deals with malabsorption by determining the cause and pathological change present, and then addressing the area with appropriate formulas to remove homotoxins and attempt tissue repair.

The prognosis depends upon the type of change and the severity. Deposition Phase conditions (such as intestinal parasites) are generally reversible with proper therapy and time, while Impregnation (inflammatory bowel disease), Degeneration (parvovirus enteritis), and Dedifferentiation (intestinal lymphoma) phase diseases may only be managed and not cured due to the extensive damage to normal structure and function of the organism's systems. Notes from the protocol sections on diarrhea, vomiting, inflammatory bowel disease, and intestinal parasites apply.

Many antihomotoxic formulas may be needed, but the most important ones support the liver, intestine, and pancreatic tissues. Hepar compositum is one of the most important in this regard, followed by Mucosa compositum for its action on the mucosal lining. Catalysts (Glyoxal compositum, Coenzyme compositum, BHI-Enzyme, and Ubichinon compositum) are critical in the repair of chronically damaged cellular elements due to their ability to rehabilitate energy metabolism.

Appropriate homotoxicology formulas

BHI-Enzyme: A catalyst similar to *Coenzyme compositum*. Contains Sulphur at the 30X dilution and cysteinum for detoxification and activation of blocked sulfide enzymes. Pulsatilla is useful in chronic diseases. Other components support energy metabolism and reduce free radical damage. Indicated for nutritional insufficiency and exhaustion (Heel 2002).

BHI-Stomach: Used for stomach distress relieved by eructation, stomach pain, heartburn, chalky white tongue, flatulence, and tendency to collapse.

Coenzyme compositum: Contains Citricum acidum, which is useful for dental problems and gingivitis; scurvy; blackening of teeth and heavy deposits of dental plaque; painful, herpetic vesicles around the lips; nausea; painful cramping in the umbilical area; and distension.

Galium-Heel: Used for all cellular phases, hemorrhoids, and anal fissures, and as a detoxicant.

Gastricumeel: Treats acute gastritis, diseases of the stomach, and nausea.

Glyoxal compositum: Methyglyoxal and glyoxal are methylators. They assist in unblocking receptors and other proteins whose actions become blocked by binding of homotoxins. It is used intermittently and not repeated until signs of detoxification and excretion abate.

Hepar compositum: Provides detoxification and drainage of hepatic tissues and organ and metabolic support, and is useful in most hepatic and gallbladder pathologies. An important part of Deep Detoxification Formula. Treats duodenitis, pancreatitis, cystic hepatic ducts, cholelithiasis, cholangitis, cholecystitis, vomiting, and diarrhea (Demers 2004, Broadfoot 2004). Factors generated in the liver assist in healing of the bowel. This combination contains Natrum oxalaceticum (also found in *Coenzyme compositum, Ubichinon compositum*, and *Mucosa com-*

positum) for changes in appetite and stomach distension due to air. Used for nausea, stomach pain with a sensation of fullness, gurgling in the abdomen, and cramping pain in the hypochondria. It is also used for constipation, sudden diarrhea (particularly after eating), and flatus (Reckeweg 2002).

Hepeel: Provides liver drainage and detoxification. Used in a wide variety of conditions including cancer of the liver, where Hepeel was found to be antiproliferative, hepatoprotective, and an antioxidant when tested in human HepG2 cells (Gebhardt 2003).

Lymphomyosot: Provides lymph drainage and endocrine support, and treats edema. Contains Gentiana for chronic gastritis. Treats flatulence, diarrhea, distension of the stomach with eructations, nausea, retching, and vomiting. Also contains Geranium robertianum for nausea, particularly after eating, with distension or sensation of fullness. Myosotis arvensis is included for bloat and distension (Reckeweg 2002).

Molybdan compositum: A trace mineral formula for supplementation of Degeneration Phase cases. This formula can be overdosed, and it should be kept out of reach of children. While no adverse reactions are known when it is used at recommended doses, Reckeweg (2000) advises that therapy be interrupted for 5 days if untoward or unexpected signs appear. Therapy can be restarted at a lower dose upon their resolution (Reckeweg 2000).

Mucosa compositum: Broadly supportive for repair of mucosal elements. Used in cellular cases and in recovery periods following active disease (Reckeweg 2000). This remedy contains a useful component in Kali bichromicum, which is indicated for ulcers found on the gums, tongue, lips, and even on the gastric mucosa (gastric or duodenal ulcer). The tongue may have a thick, yellow, mucous coating, or in ulcerative stomatitis or tonsillitis it may be dry, smooth, shiny, or fissured. Kali has been used effectively in acute gastroenteritis associated with vomiting of clear, light-colored fluid or quantities of mucous bile, and in cases with hematemesis, flatulent colics, and dysenteric stools with tenesmus (Reckeweg 2002).

It also contains Hydrastis, with mucosal support for oral problems such as stomatitis, and mucosal suppuration that is accompanied by ulceration, inflammations and colic of the hepatobiliary system and of the gastrointestinal tract, and polyp formation (Reckeweg 2002). The Kreosotum component can be used in chronic gastritis with gastric hemorrhages and vomiting of brown masses. Also has a dental implication in cases with spongy gums and carious teeth, neuralgias proceeding from them causing a burning toothache with deep caries, black patches on the teeth, and fetid discharges.

The single remedy Phosphorus is broadly useful for dyspepsia and for jaw problems in dental disease (Reckeweg 2002). Phosphorus is found in many other remedies including *Echinacea compositum* and *Leptandra Homaccord*. It is rich in suis organ preparations for mucosal support, plus a large variety of remedies with indications in the gastrointestinal sphere. The component Argentum nitricum (also in *Atropinum compositum*, *Diarrheel*, *Duodenoheel*, *Gastricumeel*, *Momordica compositum*, *BHI-Nausea*, and several other combinations) is indicated for distension in the upper abdomen, gastro-cardiac symptom-complex, and amelioration from eructations. It is also used for gastric crises (Reckeweg 2002).

Nux vomica homaccord: Used for liver and gastrointestinal disease and after smoke inhalation. Useful in gingivitis (Reckeweg 2002). This commonly used formula for detoxification is part of the *Detox Kit*. Recent research shows that one ingredient *(Brucine)* affects mitochondria in human hepatoma cells. Further research is needed to determine whether homeopathic dilutions are more or less active (Deng, et al. 2006).

Syzygium compositum: Used for chronic gastritis, chronic enteritis, diabetes mellitus, and hepatic disorders.

Tanacet-Heel: Treats complications following the removal of helminths. Used for gastroenteritis, dysentery, gas, and pain following ascarids, especially in juvenile pets.

Ubichinon compositum: Contains Anthraquinone for swelling of gums, and GI symptoms such as distention, flatulence, and cramping abdominal pain. Treats constipation with straining or sudden diarrhea (Reckeweg 2002).

Authors' suggested protocols

Nutrition
Intestines/IBD and pancreas support formulas: 1 tablet for every 25 pounds of body weight BID.

Liver support formula: One-half tablet for every 25 pounds of body weight BID.

Pan 5 Plus: 1 capsule opened and mixed with food for every 25 pounds of body weight (maximum, 4 capsules).

Glutimmune: One-fourth scoop for every 25 pounds of body weight SID.

Probiotic: One-half capsule for every 25 pounds of body weight with food.

Colostrum: One-third teaspoon powdered formula for every 25 pounds of body weight BID.

Chinese herbal medicine/acupuncture
Formula ColonGuard: 1 capsule per 10 to 20 pounds twice daily. It can be used in conjunction with conventional medicine, but that is often not needed. In addition to the herbs mentioned above, ColonGuard also contains angelica radix (Dang gui), astragalus (Huang qi), bamboo shavings (Zhu ru), pueraria (Ge gen), pulsatilla root (Bai tou weng), and raw white lotus seed (Lian zi). In some severe cases, the practitioner may need to use conventional medicine (steroids, metronidazole, dietary restrictions, pancreatic enzymes) along with the herbal supplement. However, if drug therapy is needed, it should be at a lower dose than was needed before herbal therapy was instituted.

The authors use BL20, ST36, BL26, Baihui, ST25, BL21, CV12, and CV4 in various combinations for intestinal malabsorption.

Homotoxicology (Dose: 10 drops PO for 50-pound dog; 5 drops PO for cat or small dog)
Treatment must be individualized but the following represent good starting therapies that can be readily adapted based upon clinical response.

Find and treat the primary condition (neoplasia, giardiasis, chronic fibrosis, lymphangiectasia, inflammation).

Hepar compositum, Mucosa compositum, and the catalysts (Coenzyme compositum and Ubichinon compositum): Give on a rotating basis once to 3 times weekly.

Syzygium compositum, Hepeel, and BHI-Enzyme BID, Gastricumeel or BHI-Stomach BID: Mixed together and give orally BID.

Molybdan compositum: Use for the loss of critical nutrients. Give 1 tablet daily for 3 to 4 days, then 1 tablet every other to every third day orally.

Product sources

Nutrition
Intestines/IBD, pancreas, and liver support formulas: Animal Nutrition Technologies. **Alternatives**: Enteric Support—Standard Process Veterinary Formulas; NutriGest—Rx Vitamins for Pets.

Pan 5 Plus: Progressive Labs.

Glutimmune: Well Wisdom. **Alternative**: L-Glutamine powder—Thorne Veterinary Products.

Probiotic: Progressive Labs, Biotic Rx Vitamins for Pets.

Colostrum: New Life Foods, Inc., The Saskatoon Colostrum Company Ltd.

Chinese herbal medicine
Formula ColonGuard: Natural Solutions, Inc.

Homotoxicology
BHI/Heel Corporation

REFERENCES

Western medicine references

Battersby I, Giger U, Hall E. Hyperammonaemic encephalopathy secondary to selective cobalamin deficiency in a juvenile Border collie. *J Small Anim Pract*. 2005. Jul;46(7):pp 339–44.

Garden O, Pidduck H, Lakhani K, Walker D, Wood J, Batt R. Inheritance of gluten-sensitive enteropathy in Irish Setters. *Am J Vet Res*. 2000. Apr;61(4):pp 462–8.

Rodriguez-Franco F, Sainz A, Tesouro MA, Amusategui I, Cortes O. Pharmacological and dietary treatment of canine malabsorption syndrome: a retrospective study of 17 clinical cases. *Zentralbl Veterinarmed A*. 1999. Sep;46(7):pp 439–52.

Stazi A. Coeliac disease and reproduction: possible in vivo models[Article in Italian], *Ann Ist Super Sanita*. 2005. 41(4): pp 523–31.

IVM/nutrition references

Blake SR. Bovine Colostrum, The Forgotten Miracle. *Journal of the American Holistic Veterinary Medical Association*. July 1999, Volume 18, Number 2, pp 38–39.

Golden BR, Gorbach SL. The Effect of Milk and Lactobacillus Feeding on Human Intestinal Bacteria Activity. *Am. J. of Clin. Nutr.*, 1984.39: 756–61.

Howell E. Enzyme Nutrition, The Food Enzyme Concept. 1985. Garden City, NY: Avery Publ.

Perdigon GN, de Masius N, Alvarez S, et al. Enhancement of Immune Response in Mice Fed with S. Thermophilus and L. Acidophilus, *J. of Dairy Sci.*, 1987.70: 919–926.

Souba W, et al. Glutamine metabolism in the intestinal tract: invited review, *JPEN* 1985.9:608–617.

Windmueller HG. Glutamine utilization by the small intestine, *Adv. Enzymol* 1982.53:201–237.

Yoshimura K, et al. Effects of enteral glutamine administration on experimental inflammatory bowel disease, *JPEN* 1993. 17:235.

Chinese herbal medicine/acupuncture references

Chang Yong Zhong Yao Cheng Fen Yu Yao Li Shou Ce (A Handbook of the Composition and Pharmacology of Common Chinese Drugs), 1994; 739:742.

Hwang YC and Jenkins EM. Effect of acupuncture on young pigs with induced enterpathogenic Escherichia coli diarrhea. *Am J Vet Res* 1988.49:1641–1643.

Li YF (translator). Foreign Medicine, vol. of TCM. 1984;6(1):15–18.

Liu CH, et al. The pharmacology of Tao Ren. *Journal of Pharmacology and Clinical Application of TCM*. 1989;(2):46–47.

Liu CZ, et al. *Journal of Bengbu Medical College*. 1998; 23(6):380–381.

Liu W, et al. *Henan Journal of TCM Pharmacy*. 1998;13(4): 10–12.

Ma XS, et al. *New Journal of Digestive Diseases*. 1996;4(11): 603–604.

Ma YB. Zhi Qiao's effects on gastroinstestinal movement. *Journal of Pharmacology of Clinical Application of TCM*. 1996;12(6): 28–29.

Si Chuan Yi Xue Yuan Xue Bao (*Journal of Sichuan School of Medicine*), 1959;1:102.

Wang SG, et al. Dang Shen's effect on gastrointestinal motility in mice at early stage of third degree burn. *Journal of Anhui College of TCM*. 1999;18 (6):50–51.

Wang SP, et al. Tao Ren extract's effect in suppressing filter bed fibroblasts hyperplasia in subjects of experimental trabeculae dissection. *Journal of Shanghai Medical University*. 1993;20(1):35–381.

Wu XH, et al. *Xinjiang Journal of Traditional Chinese Medicine*. 1998;16(1):42–43.

Xi Xue Xue Bao (*Academic Journal of Medicine*), 1988; 23(10)721.

Xin Yi Yao Xue Za Zhi (*New Journal of Medicine and Herbology*), 1974; (5):34.

Yang JD, et al. *China Journal of TCM Emergency Treatment*. 1998;7(3):131–132.

Yao Xue Za Zhi (*Journal of Medicinals*), 1981, 101(10):883.

Zhang SC, et al. *Journal of Chinese Patent Medicine Research*. 1984;(2):37.

Zhang WZ, et al. *Liaoning Journal of Traditional Chinese Medicine*. 1989;13(4):30.

Zhong Cao Yao(*Chinese Herbal Medicine*) 1991;22 (10):452.

Zhong Yao Tong Bao (*Journal of Chinese Herbology*), 1986; 11(11):37.

Zhong Yao Xue (*Chinese Herbology*), 1988; 326:327.

Zhong Yao Xue (*Chinese Herbology*), 1998;140:144.

Zhong Yao Yao Li Yu Ying Yong (*Pharmacology and Applications of Chinese Herbs*), 1983: 217.

Zhong Yao Yao Li Yu Ying Yong (*Pharmacology and Applications of Chinese Herbs*), 1983;567.

Zhong Yao Zhi (*Chinese Herbology Journal*), 1984;37.

Zhong Yao Zhi (*Chinese Herbology Journal*), 1993;358.

Zhonzxin X: Clinical observation of 500 cases with pediatric diarrhea treated by acupuncture. *Chin Acupuncture and Moxibustion* 9:10, 1989.

Zhou WZ, et al. *Pharmacy Bulletin*. 1979;14(5):202–203

Zhu NLF, et al. Chinese Herbs and Immunity. Foreign Medicine (TCM vol). 1984;(1):47.

Zhu ZP, et al. *China Journal of Integrated Splenico-Gastrology*. 1998;16(1):42–43.

Homotoxicology references

Broadfoot PJ. Inflammation: Homotoxicology and Healing. In: Proceedings AHVMA/Heel Homotoxicology Seminar. 2004. Denver, CO, p 27.

Boericke W. Materia Medica with Repertory, 9th edition. Santa Rosa, CA: Boericke and Tafel. 1927. pp 90, 497–500.

Brooks T. Case study in canine intestinal lymphangiectasia. *Can Vet J*. 2005. Dec;46(12):pp 1138–42.

Demers J. Homotoxicology and Acupuncture. In: Proceedings of the 2004 Homotoxicology Seminar. 2004. AHVMA/Heel. Denver, CO, p 5, 6.

Deng X, Yin F, Lu X, Cai B, Yin W. The apoptotic effect of brucine from the seed of Strychnos nux-vomica on human hepatoma cells is mediated via Bcl-2 and Ca2+ involved mitochondrial pathway. *Toxicol Sci*. 2006. May;91(1):pp 59–69.

Gebhardt R. Antioxidative, antiproliferative and biochemical effects in HepG2 cells of a homeopathic remedy and its constituent plant tinctures tested separately or in combination. *Arzneimittelforschung*. 2003. 53(12): pp 823–30.

Heel. BHI Homeopathic Therapy: Professional Reference. Albuquerque, NM: Heel Inc. 2002. pp 54.

Reckeweg H. Biotherapeutic Index: Ordinatio Antihomotoxica et Materia Medica, 5th ed. Baden-Baden, Germany: Biologische Heilmittel Heel GMBH, 2000. pp 290, 294–5, 300, 329–30, 358–9, 363–4, 366–7, 369, 381, 390, 399–400, 432, 538.

Reckeweg H. Homeopathia Antihomotoxica Materia Medica, 4th ed. Baden-Baden, Germany: Arelia-Verlag GMBH, 2002. pp. 136–8, 139–40, 125–6, 147, 150–3, 179, 206, 241–2, 317–19, 345, 366, 461–3, 488–90, 578–80.

Chapter Twelve

Diseases of the Eye and Ear

ANTERIOR UVEITIS

Definition and cause

Anterior uveitis is an inflammation of the iris that can arise from multiple causes. Common underlying causes include infectious agents such as blastomycosis, ehrlichiosis, leptospirosis in the dog and FIV in cats, immune-mediated reaction, trauma, and neoplasia. The underlying inflammatory process causes the cellular damage and the resultant cellular infiltration (Collins 1999, Davidson 1991, Glaze 1999, Ringle 2003).

Medical therapy rationale, drug(s) of choice, and nutritional recommendations

Because this condition is inflammatory and often immune-mediated, the treatment of choice is often topical and systemic corticosteroids along with immunosuppressant drugs such as azathioprine, covered by antibiotics.

Anticipated prognosis

As with most immune-mediated inflammatory processes, the results depend upon the initial autoimmune process and the degree of secondary cellular damage.

Integrative veterinary therapies

Inflammation of the uveal tissues of the anterior chamber of the eye can occur from many causes. Eighty percent of these cases are idiopathic. An attempt should be made to identify the correct cause, and a complete medical work-up is recommended in these animals.

An integrative approach takes into consideration local inflammation in the eye, the exaggerated immune response, and the prevention of ongoing degeneration. Nutrients, nutraceuticals, medicinal herbs, and combination homeopathics that have anti-inflammatory, tissue-sparing, and regenerative effects on the cells of the eye can often control the pain and discomfort, help reduce inflammation, and improve healing time.

Nutrition
General considerations/rationale
Therapeutic nutritional therapy early in the treatment can help to reduce and control the underlying inflammatory process, nourish cells, and help to balance the immune response to the tissues of the eye (target organ).

Appropriate nutrients
Nutritional/gland therapy: Glandular eye, adrenal, thymus, and spleen supply the intrinsic nutrients that reduce cellular inflammation and improve general immune organ function and balance. This helps to spare the eye from further immune attack, cascading inflammation, and eventual degeneration (see Gland Therapy, Chapter 2, for a more detailed explanation).

Note: Anterior uveitis can be a severe autoimmune reaction that can involve multiple organ systems. It is recommended that blood be analyzed both medically and physiologically to determine associated organ involvement and disease. This will allow for a more specific gland and nutritional support protocol (see Chapter 2, Nutritional Blood Testing, for more information).

The following nutrients have shown a beneficial effect on the eyes.

Essential fatty acids: Proper levels of essential fatty acids, particularly DHA and EPA, are essential for healthy eye function and retinal development (Pawlosky 1997). Hemp oil is a plant-derived oil that is high in both linoleic (LA) and linolenic (LNA) fatty acids, which are the building blocks for the longer chained eicosapentaenoic (EPA) and docosahexaenoic acid (DHA). The analysis of hemp oil shows that it is extremely low in saturated fats. More than 70% of its composition is polyunsaturated fatty acids, and less than 20% is saturated fats (Kralovansky 1994, Weil 1993). Because of its high level of gamma linolenic acid (GLA), it is being investigated for its beneficial effects on immune function (Horrobin 1992).

Lutein: Lutein is in the carotenoid family and is a potent antioxidant, which is beneficial for the health of the eye. Seddon (1994) showed the beneficial effects of lutein in people, including a decreased risk of macular degeneration and protection of eye tissue. Hankinson (1992) showed that lower levels of lutein are associated with an increased risk of cataract formation. In another study, Dagnelie (2000) found that people with retinitis pigmentosa (RP) showed a significant improvement in visual acuity and the prevention of degeneration with lutein supplementation.

Flavonoids: Quercetin has been shown to lessen the progression of diabetic retinopathy (Varma 1986). Another group of flavonoids, **Proanthocyanidans** (POCs), which come from grape seeds or pine bark, have also been shown to limit the progression of retinopthy (Fromantin 1981, Verin 1978).

Chinese herbal medicine
General considerations/rationale
According to Traditional Chinese Medicine theory, anterior uveitis is a disorder caused by Wind, Heat, and toxins in the Liver, along with a Liver Yin deficiency. According to the Western interpretation, Wind is the pathogen that "blows" the condition into the eyes. Wind can also cause pruritis. Heat is the inflammation, and toxins are the inflammatory mediators produced by the body as well as the etiologic cause—virus, bacteria, immune-mediated reaction, fungus, etc. In TCM, the Liver controls the Eyes. When there is a Yin or fluid deficiency in the Liver, the eyes may not receive the normal nourishment and they may become diseased. Treatment of anterior uveitis, therefore, involves decreasing the inflammation, controlling the etiologic cause, and decreasing discomfort.

Appropriate Chinese herbs
Bupleurum (Chai hu): Contains saikosaponin, which has analgesic and antipyretic properties (Shen Yang Yi Xue Yuan Bao 1984), as well as anti-inflammatory properties (Liu Wei 1998). Bupleurum has also demonstrated efficacy against several viruses (Wang 1998, Liao 1999, Zhong Yao Xue 1988).

Coptis (Huang lian): Contains berberine, an anti-inflammatory component. Its effects have been demonstrated in rats (Yao Xue Za Zhi 1981).

Dendrobium (Shi hu): Contains dendrobine, which has an analgesic effect only slightly weaker than phenacetin (Borch 1977).

Gardenia (Zhi zi): Can decrease inflammation by counteracting increases in capillary permeability (Zhang 1994).

Gentiana (Long Dan cao): Contains gentiopicroside and gentianine, which have marked anti-inflammatory effects. Gentiopicroside has anti-histamine activity and

can help decrease capillary permeability in inflammatory conditions (Xu Qiang 1993). It also has mild antibiotic and antifungal effects (Zhong Yao Yao Li Yu Ying Yong 1983, Wang 1983).

Honeysuckle (Jin yin hua): Has been shown to have anti-inflammatory and antipyretic properties in rabbits and mice (Shan Xi Yi Kan 1960).

Licorice (Gan cao): Contains both glycyrrhizin and glycyrrhetinic acid. These compounds prolong the effect of cortisones in the body, either by decreasing their metabolism in the liver or by decreasing the protein-binding, thereby raising cortisone plasma concentration. This exerts an anti-inflammatory effect (Zhong Yao Zhi 1993). Additionally, licorice has an analgesic effect (Zhong Yao Xue 1998). Glycyrrhizin has demonstrated some antiviral effects (Zhu 1996).

Ligustrum (Nu zhen zi): Has been demonstrated to decrease inflammation, swelling, and capillary permeability in mice (Zhong Guo Zhong Yao Za Zhi 1989).

Red peony (Chi shao): Can decrease ocular inflammation. It reduces redness, swelling, and pain (Bao 1999). It also has demonstrated antiviral effects in several experiments (Yang 1994, Liu 1999).

Rehmannia (Sheng di huang): Reduces swelling and inflammation (Zhong Yao Yao Li Yu Ying Yong 1983).

Rhubarb (Da huang): Has analgesic and anti-inflammatory efficacy (Chang Yong Zhong Yao Cheng Fen Yu Yao Li Shou Ce 1994).

Schizonepeta (Jing jie): Can help to relieve discomfort. It has demonstrated analgesic effects (Zhong Yao Cai 1989).

Scutellaria (Huang qin): Contains biacalein, which has been shown to suppress inflammation in mice (Kubo 1984). The total flavone component has shown anti-inflammatory effects in mice and rats (Cao 1999). It also contains biacalin, which has demonstrated antibacterial effects against multiple bacteria (Wang 1999, Zhong Yao Xue 1988). Additionally, scutellaria has been shown to increase cellular immunity by promoting the production of IL2 (Pan 1991).

Vitex fruit (Man jing zi): Has analgesic properties (Zhong Yao Xue 1998).

Homotoxicology
General considerations/rationale
Trauma (Inflammation Phase), viral infections (Impregnation Phase), metabolic diseases (Deposition Phase), and tumors (Degeneration Phase) can all be associated with anterior uveitis. Therapy depends upon the precise phase of the patient's homotoxicosis as well as other concurrent signs of disease. Intraocular and blood pressures should be determined in these pets. Consultation with an ophthalmologist should be considered.

Appropriate homotoxicology formulas

Apis homaccord: Reduces swelling.

Belladonna homaccord: Treats acute cases and red eyes.

BHI-Eye: Used for red, swollen eyes with irritation.

Galium-Heel: Used in cellular and matrix phases for detoxification and drainage, and support of glomeruli.

Hepar compositum: Provides liver support, and drainage and detoxification.

Hepeel: Provides liver detoxification and support.

Kalmia compositum: Treats connective tissue vessels, ostealgia, periostitis, and neuralgia.

Lymphomyosot: Provides drainage of lymphatics, and reduces pain and swelling.

Mucosa compositum: Supports ocular tissues through *Ocularis suis*.

Oculoheel: Treats periocular swelling and inflammation and keratitis.

Reneel: Supports the kidney.

Solidago compositum: Drains kidney and associated urogenital tissues.

Thyroidea compositum: Provides deep detoxification of matrix and support of endocrine tissues.

Tonsilla compositum: Modulates chronic immune responses.

Traumeel S: Has anti-inflammatory effects, supports ocular tissues in vasculitis, and reactivates sulfur-containing enzymes.

Authors' suggested protocols

Nutrition

Eye and immune support formulas (contains vitamins A and E): 1 tablet for every 25 pounds of body weight BID.

Quercetin: 35 mg for every 10 pounds of body weight SID.

Lutein: 5 mg for every 50 pounds of body weight.

Proanthocyanidans (PCO): 20 mg for every 10 pounds of body weight daily.

Hemp oil: 1 teaspoon for every 25 pounds of body weight with food BID.

Chinese herbal medicine

Chronic uveitis is the recommended formula for this condition. It is dosed at a rate of 1 capsule for every 10 to 20 pounds twice daily. In addition to the herbs cited above, Chronic uveitis contains cassia seed (Jue ming zi), chrysanthemum (Ju hua), dianthus (Qu mai), siler (Fang feng), and wolfberry (Gou qi zi) to help increase the efficacy of the formula.

Homotoxicology

BHI-Eye or Oculoheel, Kalmia compositum, Lymphomyosot, Traumeel: Mix together and given 3 to 5 times daily the first day, and then TID to BID as needed. Add Engystol N BID if a viral cause is suspected. Add Echinacea compositum if bacterial or protozoal disease is suspected.

Pure Eye Drops: Alternate with Pure Ear Drops (or Traumeel oral vials), topically.

Veratrum homaccord: Use for eye diseases tending toward degeneration.

Product sources

Nutrition

Eye and immune support formulas: Animal Nutrition Technologies. Alternatives: Immune System Support—Standard Process Veterinary Formulas; Immuno Support—Rx Vitamins for Pets; Immugen—Thorne Veterinary Products.

Quercetin: Source Naturals; Quercitone—Thorne Veterinary Products.

Antiox (PCO): Vetri Science.

Lutein: Progressive Labs.

Hemp oil: Nature's Perfect Oil.

Chinese herbal medicine

Chronic Uveitis—Natural Solutions, Inc.

Homotoxicology remedies

BHI/Heel Corporation

REFERENCES

Western medicine references

Collins BK, Moore CP. Diseases and surgery of the canine anterior uvea. In: Gelatt KN, ed., Veterinary ophthalmology. 3rd ed. Philadelphia: Lippincott Williams and Wilkins. 1999:755–775.

Davidson MG, Nasisse MP, English RV, et al. Feline anterior uveitis: a study of 53 cases. *J Am Anim Hosp Assoc* 1991;27:77–83.

Glaze MB, Gelatt KN. Feline ophthalmology. In: Gelatt KN, ed. Veterinary ophthalmology. 3rd ed. Philadelphia: Lippincott Williams and Wilkins, 1999:997–1052.

Ringle MJ. Anterior Uveitis—Dogs. In: Tilley L, Smith F. The 5-Minute Veterinary Consult: Canine and Feline, 2003, Blackwell Publishing.

Ringle MJ. Anterior Uveitis—Cats. In: Tilley L, Smith F. The 5-Minute Veterinary Consult: Canine and Feline, 2003, Blackwell Publishing.

Slatter D. Fundamentals of veterinary ophthalmology. 2nd ed. Philadelphia: Saunders, 1990:304–337.

IVM/nutrition references

Dagnelie G, Zorge IS, McDonald TM. Lutein improves visual function in some retinal degeneration patients: a pilot study via Internet. *Optometry* 2000;71:147–64.

Dagnelie G. Lutein supplements may improve vision, *Optometry: Journal of the American Optometric Association* 2000;71:147–64.

Fromantin M. Procyanidolic oligomers in the treatment of fragile capillaries and diabetic retinopathy. *Med Int* 1981;16:432–4 [in French].

Hankinson SE, Stampfer MJ, Seddon JM, et al. Nutrient intake and cataract extraction in women: a prospective study. *Br Med J* 1992;305(6849):335–9.

Horrobin DF. Nutritional and medical importance of gamma-linolenic acid. *Prog. Lipid Res.* 1992.31(2): 163–94.

Kralovansky UP, Marthné-Schill J. Data composition and use value of hemp seed (Hungarian with English summary). *Novenytermeles* 1994. 43(5): 439–446.

Pawlosky RJ, et al. Retinal and brain accretion of long-chain polyunsaturated fatty acids in developing felines: the effects of corn-based maternal diets. *Am J Clin Nutr* 1997;65:465–72.

Semba RD, Dagnelie G. Are lutein and zeaxanthin conditionally essential nutrients for eye health? *Med Hypoth* 2003;61, 465–72.

Seddon JM, Ajani UA, Sperduto RD, et al. Dietary carotenoids, vitamins A, C, and E, and advanced age-related macular degeneration. *JAMA* 1994;272:1413–20.

Varma SD. Inhibition of aldose reductase by flavonoids: Possible attenuation of diabetic complications. *Progr Clin Biol Res* 1986;213:343–58.

Verin MM, Vildy A, Maurin JF. Retinopathies and OPC. *Bordeaux Medicale* 1978;11:1467–74 [in French].

Weil A. Therapeutic hemp oil. *Natural Health*, 1993. March/April, pps. 10–12.

Chinese herbal medicine/acupuncture references

Bao GY, et al. Treating 32 cases of retinal vein obstruction with Xue Fu Zhu Yu Tang. 1999. *Henan Journal of TCM.*

Borch RF, Evans AJ, Wade JJ. Synthesis of 8-epi-Dendrobine. *J Am Chem Soc.* 1977; 99(3):1612.

Cao ZS, et al. *Strait Journal of Pharmacology.* 1999;11(3): 53–54.

Chang Yong Zhong Yao Cheng Fen Yu Yao Li Shou Ce (A Handbook of the Composition and Pharmacology of Common Chinese Drugs), 1994; 226:323.

Kubo M, Matsuda H, Tanaka M, Kimura Y, Okuda H, Higashino M, Tani T, Namba K, Arichi S. Studies on Scutellariae radix. VII. Anti-arthritic and anti-inflammatory actions of methanolic extract and flavonoid components from Scutellariae radix. *Chem Pharm Bull*, 1984; 32(7):2724–9.

Liao CS, et al. *Shenzhen Journal of Integrated Medicine.* 1999;9(2):20–21.

Liu N, et al. *Journal of Guangzhou University of TCM.* 1999;16(4):308–310.

Liu W, et al. *Henan Journal of TCM Pharmacy.* 1998;13(4):10–12.

Pan JF, et al. *Tianjin Journal of Medicine.* 1991;19(8): 468–470.

Shan Xi Yi Kan (*Shanxi Journal of Medicine*), 1960; (10):32.

Shen Yang Yi Xue Yuan Bao (*Journal of Shenyang University of Medicine*), 1984; 1(3):214.

Wang SC, et al. *Journal of Shizhen Medicine.* 1998;9(5): 418–419.

Wang YP, et al. *Shanghai Journal of Medical Inspection.* 1999;14(4):206–207.

Wang YS, et al. TCM Pharmacology and Application. Beijing: People's Health Press; 1983.

Xu Q, et al. Long Dan Cao's inhibitory effect on delayed allergic reaction. *Journal of Pharmacology and Clinical Application of TCM.* 1993;9(5):25.

Yang DG. Comparison of pre- and post-treatment hepatohistology with heavy dosage of Paeonia rubra on chronic active hepatitis caused liver fibrosis. *Chung Kuo Chung His I Chieh Ho Tsa Chih* 1994; 14:195, 207–09.

Yao Xue Za Zhi (*Journal of Medicinals*), 1981, 101(10):883.

Zhang XL, et al. *Journal of Shandong College of TCM.* 1994;18(6):416–417.

Zhong Guo Zhong Yao Za Zhi (*People's Republic of China Journal of Chinese Herbology*), 1989; 14(7):47.

Zhong Yao Cai (Study of Chinese Herbal Material), 1989; 12(6):37.

Zhong Yao Xue (*Chinese Herbology*)1988;103:106.

Zhong Yao Xue (*Chinese Herbology*), 1988; 137:140.

Zhong Yao Xue (*Chinese Herbology*), 1998; 759: 765.

Zhong Yao Xue (*Chinese Herbology*), 1998; 99:100.

Zhong Yao Yao Li Yu Ying Yong (*Pharmacology and Applications of Chinese Herbs*), 1983; 295.

Zhong Yao Yao Li Yu Ying Yong (*Pharmacology and Applications of Chinese Herbs*), 1983:400.

Zhong Yao Zhi (*Chinese Herbology Journal*), 1993;358.

Zhu LH. *China Journal of TCM Information.* 1996;3(3): 17–20.

CATARACTS

Definition and cause

Cataracts are defined as any loss of transparency, or opacity of the lens. Causes include genetic predisposition, nutritional imbalances, reaction to environmental or toxic chemicals, related disease of the eye such as iriditis, retinal degeneration or uveitis, and trauma, or they can be secondary to other diseases such as diabetes. It is believed that there is an interruption in the normal lens metabolism between the water and protein levels that starts the formation of the cataract (Gelatt 1991, 1992; Nasisse 2003).

Medical therapy rationale, drug(s) of choice, and nutritional recommendations

The recommended treatment for cataracts is the surgical removal of the lens. Medical options for cataracts are usually used for secondary conditions such as the use of topical corticosteroids to reduce the inflammation of uveitis before cataract surgery is performed. (Gelatt 1991, 1992; Nasisse 1994; Slatter 1990).

Anticipated prognosis

The prognosis for returned vision is good post surgically. This depends upon the involvement or influence of other disease processes such as diabetes, autoimmune disease, or uveitis. Untreated cataracts are a progressive disease which result in impaired or complete loss of vision (Gelatt 1992, Nasisse 2003).

Integrative veterinary therapies

An integrative approach to cataract formation and prevention focuses upon reducing cellular inflammation, nourishing the tissues of the eye, and improving waste elimination. Nutrients, nutraceuticals, medicinal herbs and combination homeopathics that have anti-inflammatory, tissue-sparing, and regenerative effects can help to prevent waste accumulation and cataract formation.

Nutrition
General considerations/rationale

Cataract therapy is most often surgical removal, and does not focus upon prevention. The nutritional approach adds nutrients, antioxidants, and gland support to help reduce initiating inflammation and improve waste elimination.

Appropriate nutrients

Nutritional/gland therapy: Glandular eye and liver supply the intrinsic nutrients to help control free radical build-up, reduce cellular inflammation, and improve elimination of metabolic wastes, all of which are beneficial for lens health (see Gland Therapy, Chapter 2, for a more detailed description).

Lutein: Lutein is in the carotenoid family and is a potent antioxidant, which is beneficial for the health of the eye. Hankinson (1992) showed that lower levels of lutein were associated with increased risk of cataract.

Vitamin E: Vitamin E is associated with decreased risk and the prevention of cataract formation (Lyle 1999, Rouhiainen 1996, Seddon 1994, Teikari 1997, Trevithick 1981). Leske (1998), in a 5-year study, showed that people who took vitamin E had 50% less risk of developing cataracts.

Vitamin C: Vitamin C is an important antioxidant for the health of the eye. Packer (1979) reported that vitamin C is required to activate vitamin E, which is important for decreased risk of cataract formation. Supplementing the diet with vitamin C has been associated with decreased cataract formation in people (Hankinson 1992; Jacques 1988, 1991, 1997; Robertson 1991).

Quercetin: Quercetin has been shown to block the accumulation of sorbitol in the eye, which may be beneficial in people with diabetic cataracts (Varma 1977). Similarly, people who consume fruit and vegetables that are rich in antioxidants such as flavonoids are less at risk of developing cataracts (Jacques 1991, Knekt 1992).

Chinese herbal medicine/acupuncture

According to TCM, cataracts are caused by Blood and Yin deficiency in the Liver, Kidney, and Spleen. In the Western interpretation, the Liver controls the Eyes. The Eyes are not nourished when there is a Blood and/or Yin deficiency in the Liver, leading to blurry vision in most cases. The Spleen is charged with transforming food into Blood and Yin, so a deficiency in the Spleen leads to deficiency in the Liver. The Kidney is responsible for the aging process because it houses the Essence, or genetic blueprint. Degenerative changes take place as the Kidney ages, which explains why cataracts are more common in older patients.

Appropriate Chinese herbs

Because cataracts are considered a surgical disease in Western medicine, there are no studies in Western journals describing the treatment of cataracts with herbs. Some of the following herbs treat conditions that lead to cataracts in Western thought, i.e. hyperglycemia.

Ophiopogon (Mai men dong): Can lower blood glucose levels (Wan 1998).

Sage tangle (Kun bu): Has been shown to decrease blood glucose levels in mice (Zhong Cao Yao, 1987).

White atractylodes (Bai zhu): Lowers blood glucose levels (Zhong Hua Yi Xue Za Zhi, 1958).

Homotoxicology
General considerations/rationale

Cataracts result from Degenerative Phase homotoxicoses (Reckeweg 2000). There is no known medical cure for cataracts, and a complete medical work-up and early consultation with an ophthalmologist to evaluate medical and surgical modalities is indicated. When clients are not interested in pursuing surgical therapy, anti-inflammatory treatment (topical 1% prednisone) is recommended to minimize protein-leakage-induced anterior uveitis.

The classical homeopathic literature contains references to using Cineraria for cataracts. Boericke (1927) states that this is most effective when done for several months for traumatic cataracts. The authors have not experienced measurable success with such topical ophthalmic products in our veterinary patients. Clients should be advised of this before embarking on homeopathic treatment of cataracts in animals.

While antihomotoxic drugs cannot cure cataracts, treating the correct phase homotoxicosis may provide numerous other benefits to the patient, and ocular function and comfort may improve as a result. A full diagnostic evaluation is appropriate, with particular attention paid to breed, familial history, traumatic events, drug history, intraocular pressure, and metabolic diseases (such as diabetes mellitus).

Appropriate homotoxicology formulas

Causticum compositum: Given for classical homeopathic indications for cataracts of Causticum and Sulphur.

Cerebrum compositum: Given for classical homeopathic indications for Sulphur and Conium. It is helpful in many geriatric patients and worth consideration for its other CNS benefits.

Cutis compositum: Contains Calc fluor and Sulphur.

Discus compositum: Contains Silica, Sulphur, and Kali carb. It is used classically for some cases of cataract, but it is particularly effective in other areas of geriatric medicine and could be considered as part of an overall program.

Engystol N: Used in chronic diseases; supports enzyme activation through Sulfur.

Galium-Heel: Used in cellular phases, provides matrix drainage, and reduces swelling and pain.

Lymphomyosot: A phase remedy for Degeneration Phase disorders.

Oculoheel: Treats ocular inflammation.

Phosphor homaccord: Intermittent use may support organ function.

Spigelia: Contains Sulphur and Kali carb, and is used in classical homeopathic prescribing for cataracts. If the remedy pattern matches the patient, consider this as a trial.

Syzygium compositum: Used to treat diabetic-induced cataracts.

Thyroidea compositum: Contains Calc fluor, Sulphur, and Conium. Provides deep matrix flushing and detoxification in advanced cases.

Authors' suggested protocols

Nutrition

Eye and liver support formulas (contain vitamins C and E): 1 tablet for every 25 pounds of body weight BID.

Lutein: 5 mg for every 50 pounds of body weight.

Quercetin: 35 mg for every 10 pounds of body weight SID.

Vitamin C: 100 mg for every 15 pounds of body weight BID.

Vitamin E: 50 IU for every 20 pounds of body weight SID.

Chinese herbal medicine/acupuncture

The authors recommend Complex 88 at a dose of 1 capsule per 10 to 20 pounds twice daily. In the authors' experience this formula helps to clear the opacity in the lens. In addition to the herbs listed above, Complex 88 contains apricot seed (Xing ren), arisaema (Dan nan xing), asparagus (Tian men dong), astragalus(Huang qi), barbat skull cap (Ban zhi lian), centipede (Wu gong), Chinese sage (Shi jian chuan), codonopsis (Dang shen), corydalis (Yan hu suo), glehnia root (Sha shen), houttuynia (Yu xing cao), lily bulb (Bai he), oldenlandia (Bai hua she cao), oyster shell (Mu li), peucedanum (Qian hu), prunella (Xia ku cao), pseudotellaria (Tai zi shen), rehmania (Sheng di huang), sargassum (Hai zao), scorpion (Quan xie), scrophularia (Xuan shen), selaginella (Shi shang bai), sophera root (Shan dou gen), stemoma (Bai bu), tortoise shell (Bie jie), and trichosanthes (Gua lou).

Homotoxicology (Dose: 10 drops PO for 50-pound dog; 5 drops PO for small dog or cat)

The following protocols are not expected to cure cataracts but are used to address the Degeneration Phase state of the patient. Readers should take notice of any positive effects seen in patients so treated, and are advised to seek publication of their experience.

Symptom formula: Galium-Heel, Lymphomyosot, and Oculoheel mixed together and given BID. Engystol given twice weekly PO. If anterior uveitis is present consider Traumeel intermittently.

Deep detoxification formula: Should be considered. Contains Galium-Heel, Lymphomyosot, Thyroidea compositum, Hepar compositum, Solidago compositum, Coenzyme compositum, Ubichinon compositum, and Testes compositum OR Ovarium compositum (depending upon the patient's sex) mixed together and given orally every 3 days for 60 to 120 days.

Product sources

Nutrition

Eye and liver support formulas: Animal Nutrition Technologies. **Alternatives**: Hepatic Support—Standard Process Veterinary Formulas; Hepato Support—Rx Vitamins for Pets; Hepagen—Thorne Veterinary Products.

Lutein: Progressive Labs.

Quercetin: Source Naturals; Quercitone: Thorne Veterinary Products.

Vitamins C and E: Over the counter.

Chinese herbal medicine

Complex 88: Natural Solutions Inc.

Homotoxicology remedies

BHI/Heel Corporation

REFERENCES

Western medicine references

Gelatt KN. The canine lens. In: Gelatt KN, ed. Veterinary ophthalmology. 2nd ed. Philadelphia: Lea and Febiger, 1992:429–460.

Gelatt KN. Veterinary Ophthalmology. Lea and Febiger. Malvern, PA; 1991.

Glover TL, Constantinescu GM. Surgery for Cataracts, *Vet Clin North Am* 1997;27:1143–1173.

Nasisse MP. Innovations in cataract surgery. In: Kirk RW, ed. Current veterinary therapy XII. Philadelphia: Saunders, 1994:1261–1264.

Nasisse MP. In: Tilley L, Smith F. The 5-Minute Veterinary Consult: Canine and Feline, Blackwell Publishing, 2003.

Slatter D. Fundamentals of Veterinary Ophthalmology. Philadelphia: WB Saunders Co. 1990.

IVM/nutrition references

Hankinson SE, Stampfer MJ, Seddon JM, et al. Nutrient intake and cataract extraction in women: a prospective study. *Br Med J* 1992;305(6849):335–9.

Jacques PF, Chylack LT Jr. Epidemiologic evidence of a role for the antioxidant vitamins and carotenoids in cataract prevention. *Am J Clin Nutr* 1991;53:352S–5S.

Jacques PF, Chylack LT, McGandy RB, Hartz SC. Antioxidant status in persons with and without senile cataract. *Arch Ophthalmol* 1988;106:337–40.

Jacques PF, Taylor A, Hankinson SE, et al. Long-term vitamin C supplement use and prevalence of early age-related lens opacities. *Am J Clin Nutr* 1997;66:911–6.

Knekt P, Heliovaara M, Rissanen A, et al. Serum antioxidant vitamins and risk of cataract. *BMJ* 1992;305:1392–4.

Leske MC, Chylack LT Jr, He Q, et al. Antioxidant vitamins and nuclear opacities. The Longitudinal Study of Cataract. *Ophthalmology* 1998;105:831–6.

Lyle BJ, Mares-Perlman JA, Klein BE, et al. Serum carotenoids and tocopherols and incidence of age-related nuclear cataract. *Am J Clin Nutr* 1999;69:272–7.

Lyle BJ, Mares-Perlman JA, Klein BE, et al. Antioxidant intake and risk of incident age-related nuclear cataracts in the Beaver Dam Eye Study. *Am J Epidemiol* 1999;149:801–9.

Robertson J McD, Donner AP, Trevithick JR. A possible role for vitamins C and E in cataract prevention. *Am J Clin Nutr* 1991;53:346S–51S.

Rouhiainen P, Rouhiainen H, Salonen JT. Association between low plasma vitamin E concentration and progression of early cortical lens opacities. *Am J Epidemiol* 1996;144:496–500.

Seddon JM, Christen WG, Manson JE, et al. The use of vitamin supplements and the risk of cataract among US male physicians. *Am J Public Health* 1994;84:788–92.

Teikari JM, Virtamo J, Rautalahti M, et al. Long-term supplementation with alpha-tocopherol and beta-carotene and age-related cataract. *Acta Ophthalmol Scand* 1997;75:634–40.

Trevithick JR, Creighton MO, Ross WM, et al. Modelling cortical cataractogenesis: 2. In vitro effects on the lens of agents preventing glucose- and sorbitol-induced cataracts. *Can J Ophthalmol* 1981;16:32–8.

Varma SD, Mizuno A, Kinoshita JH. Diabetic cataracts and flavonoids. *Science* 1977;195:205.

Chinese herbal medicine/acupuncture references

Wan HJ, et al. *China Journal of TCM Science and Technology.* 1998;5(4):218–219.

Zhong Cao Yao (*Chinese Herbal Medicine*), 1987; 18(2): 15.

Zhong Hua Yi Xue Za Zhi (*Chinese Journal of Medicine*), 1958;44(22):150.

Homotoxicology references

Boericke W. Materia Medica with Repertory, 9th edition. Santa Rosa, CA: Boericke and Tafel; 1927. p 168.

Reckeweg H. Biotherapeutic Index: Ordinatio Antihomotoxica et Materia Medica, 5th ed. Baden-Baden, Germany: Biologische Heilmittel Heel GMBH, 2000. p 102.

CONJUNCTIVITIS

Definition and cause

Conjunctivitis is any inflammation of the conjunctiva. The causes are allergy, infection with bacteria, chlamydia, fungi, viral organisms, environmental, immune-mediated (follicular in dogs and eosinophilic in cats), and mechanical (lash issues), or can be secondary to other diseases such as glaucoma, uveitis, keratoconjunctivitis sicca, or cancer. Conjunctivitis in cats is commonly caused secondary to calici or herpes viral infection. It is common in both dogs and cats (Angarano 1989, Champagne 2003, Gelatt 1999, Gilger 2000, Morgan 1996, Narfstrom 1999, Ramsey 2000, Stiles 2000, Whitley 2000).

Medical therapy rationale, drug(s) of choice, and nutritional recommendations

Treatment is focused on the condition and dependent upon the underlying cause(s). Surgery, antibiotics, antiviral drugs such as Trifluridine, corticosteroids, and hypoallergenic diets for allergic causes are commonly used (Bedford 1999, Champagne 2003, Gilger 2000, Hendrix 1999, Larocca 2000).

Anticipated prognosis

The response to medication depends upon the underlying cause. Simple bacterial infections offer good prognosis, while immune-mediated cases and those secondary to other diseases are more often controlled rather than cured. Viral infections often can be controlled and also may lead to chronic conjunctivitis that requires chronic use of medication for control. Surgery is often curative for mechanical issues (Champagne 2003).

Integrative veterinary therapies

In most instances conjunctivitis is an inflammatory process that responds well to medication. Chronic recurrent and allergic conjunctivitis often has underlying causes that are related to the glandular immune system and its response against its own tissue. Reducing inciting inflammation and supporting and balancing the immune response can help control future outbreaks in chronic recurrent conditions.

Nutrition
General considerations/rationale

Conjunctivitis that is non-responsive or requires chronic medication for its control benefits from nutritional and biological remedies. The reduction of inflammation as well as immune system balance often results in an improved prognosis.

Appropriate nutrients

Nutritional gland therapy: Eye and adrenal gland support have anti-inflammatory and cellular-protective benefits and can help reduce allergic reactions (see Gland Therapy in Chapter 2 for more details).

Quercetin: Quercetin is in the flavonoid family (see Phytonutrients in Chapter 2). It has an antihistamine effect and is beneficial in the treatment of allergically incited conditions (Middleton 1986, Ogasawara 1985).

Betasitosterol: Animal studies have demonstrated that phytosterols have anti-inflammatory and antipyretic activity (Gupta 1980) as well as immune-modulating activity (Bouic 1996).

Chinese herbal medicine/acupuncture
General considerations/rationale

Traditional Chinese Medicine views conjunctivitis as a disorder involving Damp, Heat, and toxins. Heat refers to the reddened, inflamed conjunctiva. The Damp element is manifested by the discharge that is seen in many cases. The term "toxins" refers to the etiologic cause of the condition. In modern terms, this means viruses, fungi, bacteria, and immune-mediated inflammation. To treat conjunctivitis with one general formula, the supplement must have anti-inflammatory, analgesic, antibacterial, and antiviral functions.

Appropriate Chinese herbs

Atractylodes (Cang zhu): Effective against bacteria, dermatophytes, and some viruses (Zhong Yao Xue 1998). This suggests that it may be effective in treating conjunctivitis of bacterial, fungal, and viral etiology. In addition, it has anti-inflammatory effects and can prevent inflammatory increases in capillary permeability (Zhang 1998).

Cassia seed (Jue Ming zi): Demonstrates antibiotic effects against Staphylococcus aureus, E. coli, and other bacteria and fungi (Zhi Wu Yao You Xiao Cheng Fen Shou Ce 1986).

Chrysanthemum (Ju hua): Has antibacterial actions (Yi Xue Ji Shu Zi Liao 1974).

Equisetum (Mu zei): Has anti-inflammatory effects (Zhong Yao Xue 1998).

Eriocaulis (Gu jing cao): Has demonstrated efficacy against Pseudomonas aeruginosa and some dermatophytes and pathogenic fungi (Zhong Yao Xue 1998, Xiu Hua Ben Cao Gang Mu 1991).

Gardenia (zhi zi): An anti-inflammatory herb that can decrease capillary permeability (Zhang 1994). Zhi Zi has a rather pronounced inhibitory effect on Staphylococcus aureus (Meng 1996, Song 1997). It has demonstrated antibacterial and antifungal efficacy (Zhong Yao Zhi 1984).

Gentianna root (Long dan cao): Has antibacterial activity against multiple bacteria including Pseudomonas aeruginosa, Bacillus proteus, and Staphylococcus aureus. It also has antifungal efficacy (Zhong Yao Yao Li Yu Ying Yong 1983, Wang 1983). One of the components, swertiamarin, has been demonstrated to have analgesic effects in mice. It can be as effective as morphine (Lei 1982). This action may decrease discomfort associated with the condition. Two other components, gentiopicroside and gentianine, have significant anti-inflammatory effects. Gentiopicroside can block histamine effects and reduce capillary permeability (Xu 1993).

Isatis root (Ban lan gen): Has been used to treat conjunctivitis of both viral and bacterial etiologies. Isatis root has been shown to have antibacterial effects in multiple studies (Xu 1987, Cao 1999, Zhong Cheng Yao Yan Jiu 1987). Other studies have demonstrated antiviral effects (Jiang 1992, Li 1994 (1), Li 1994 (2), Zhu 1999, Li 2000). In one trial 25 people with conjunctivitis were treated with isatis root eye drops 4 times daily while 73 received 0.25% chloramphenicol 4 times a day. Symptoms resolved in 3 days in the isatis eye drop group but took 7 days to resolve in the chloramphenicol-treated group (Li 1990). Isatis root has also been used to treat viral ocular lesions. Sixty-one people with herpes simplex viral keratitis were treated with either isatis or virazole. In the isatis root group, 95% of shallow and 75% of the deep ulcers resolved. In the virazole group the success rates were 83.3% and 58.3%, respectively (Li 1998).

Moutan (Mu dan pi): Exerts an anti-inflammatory effect by interfering with prostaglandin synthesis and decreasing the permeability of blood vessels (Sheng Yao Xue Za Zhi 1979, Zhong Guo Yao Ke Da Xue Xue Bao 1990). However, despite the anti-inflammatory effect of moutan, one of its components, paeonol, can enhance phagocytosis of peripheral neutrophils of Staphylococcus aureus, thereby augmenting immunity (Li Feng Chun 1994). Additionally, moutan has shown antibiotic effects against multiple strains of bacteria (Zhong Yao Cai 1991).

Rhubarb (Da huang): Inhibits many species of bacteria including staphylococci and streptococci (Zhao 1999, Yang 1997). Rhubarb also demonstrates antiviral activity (Xie 1996). In addition, it possesses antipyretic, analgesic, and anti-inflammatory effects (Chang Yong Zhong Yao

Cheng Fen Yu Yao Li Shou Ce 1994). Rhubarb has an immunostimulant effect. It is able to increase macrophage phagocytosis and phytohemagglutinin-induced lymphocyte transformation reaction in mice (Zhang Bing Sheng 1997).

Scutellaria (Huang qin): Possesses antibiotic efficacy against various species of bacteria, fungi, and viruses. It contains biacilin, which seems to provide much of this effect. Biacilin can have synergistic effects with ampicillin, amoxicillin, methacillin, and cefotaxime (Wang 1999, Cao 1999, **Liu 2000**). In addition, the flavone component demonstrates anti-inflammatory effects. Baicalin and biacalein suppress inflammation in mice (Kubo 1984, Cao 1999). Scutellaria also stimulates the cellular immune system (Pan 1991).

Siler (Fang feng): Has demonstrated antibacterial effects against Shigella, Pseudomonas aeruginosa, and *Staphylococcus aureus* and shows efficacy against some influenza viruses (Zhong Yao Tong Bao 1988).

A combination of buddleja (Mi meng hua), schizonepeta (Jing jie), cassia seed (Ju ming zi), and celosia argentea seed (Qing xiang zi) resolved conjunctivitis in 9 of 10 humans after 2 to 6 treatments. The combination also contained Dang gui, Chi shao, Chai hu, Niu xi, Hong hua, Chuan xiong, Tao ren, and Sheng di huang (Hu Bei Yi Sheng 1976).

Homotoxicology
General considerations/rationale
Conjunctivitis can represent Inflammation Phase disorders or Impregnation Phase conditions. Acute bacterial conjunctivitis is usually simple to deal with, but if homotoxins have penetrated or altered the natural defenses, then it can become a recurrent or chronic condition. Such is commonly the case in allergic conditions, which always represent Impregnation Phase homotoxicoses.

Appropriate homotoxicology formulas
Belladonna homaccord: Used for focal, intense redness and inflammatory issues, and dry burning eyes.

BHI-Eye: Used for support of periocular tissues, conjunctivitis, and dacryocystitis.

Mercurius-Heel: Antiviral.

Mucosa compositum: Provides support of ocular repair through Ocularis suis.

Oculoheel: Used for conjunctivitis.

Oculoheel eye drops: Prescribed for conjunctivitis.

Traumeel S: Anti-inflammatory.

Authors' suggested protocols
Nutrition
Eye and adrenal support formulas: 1 tablet for every 25 pounds of body weight twice daily.

Quercetin: 35 mg for every 10 pounds of body weight SID.

Betathyme: 1 capsule for every 35 pounds of body weight BID (maximum, 2 capsules BID).

Chinese herbal medicine/acupuncture
H45 Conjunctivitis: 1 capsule for every 10 to 20 pounds twice daily as needed to control signs. In addition to the herbs mentioned above, H45 Conjunctivitis also contains leonuris fruit (Chong wei zi).

Homotoxicology
See also Herpes Virus.

Oculoheel or BHI-Eye, Belladonna homaccord, and Traumeel S: Mix together and give BID. Use Oculoheel eye drops BID in affected eyes. Add Mercurius-Heel in suppurative conjunctivitis and Apis homaccord with Lymphyomyosot in cases with marked swelling.

Echinacea compositum: Use for infectious etiologies.

Product sources
Nutrition
Eye and adrenal support formulas: Animal Nutrition Technologies. **Alternatives:** Canine Adrenal Support—Standard Process Veterinary Formulas.

Quercetin: Source Naturals; Quercitone—Thorne Veterinary Products.

Betathyme: Best for Your Pet. **Alternative:** Thorne Veterinary Products.

Chinese herbal medicine
Formula H45 Conjunctivitis: Natural Solutions, Inc.

Chinese herbal medicine
BHI/Heel Corporation

REFERENCES

Western medicine references
Angarano DW. Dermatologic disorders of the eyelid and periocular region. In: Kirk RW, ed: Current Veterinary Therapy X. Philadelphia: WB Saunders, 1989, pp. 678–681.
Bedford PGC. Diseases and surgery of the canine eyelid. In: Gelatt KN, ed: Veterinary Ophthalmology 3rd ed. Philadelphia: Lea and Febiger, 1999, pp.535–568.
Champagne ES. In: Tilley L, Smith F. The 5-Minute Veterinary Consult: Canine and Feline, Blackwell Publishing, 2003.
Gelatt KN. Veterinary Ophthalmology 3rd ed. Philadelphia: Lea and Febiger, 1999, pp.535–568.
Gilger BC. Diagnosis and treatment of canine conjunctivitis. In: Bonagura JD, ed. Kirk's Current Veterinary Therapy XIII Small Animal Practice. Philadelphia: WB Saunders, 2000, pp.1053–1054.

Hendrix DVH. Diseases and surgery of the canine conjunctive. In: Gelatt KN, ed. Veterinary ophthalmology 3rd ed. Philadelphia: Lippincott Williams and Wilkins 1999:619–634.

Larocca RD. Eosinophilic conjunctivitis, herpes virus and mast cell tumor of the third eyelid in a cat. *Vet Ophthalmol* 2000;3:221–225.

Morgan RV, Abrams KL, Kern TJ. Feline eosinophilic keratitis; A retrospective study of 54 cases (1989–1994). *Vet Comp Ophthalmol* 1996;6:131–134.

Narfstrom K. Hereditary and congenital ocular disease in the cat. *J Fel Med Surg* 1999;1:135–141.

Ramsey DT. Feline chlamydia and calicivirus infections. *Vet Clin N Am Small Anim Prac* 30(5):1015–1028, 2000.

Stiles J. Feline Herpesvirus. *Vet Clin N Am Small Anim Prac* 2000;30(5):1001–1014.

Whitley RD. Canine and feline primary ocular bacterial infections. *Vet Clin N Am Small Anim Prac* 2000; 30(5):1151–1167.

IVM/nutrition references

Bouic PJD. Plant sterols and sterolins: a review of their immune-modulating properties. *Altern Med Rev* 1999;4:170–177.

Gupta MB, Nath R, Srivastava N, et al. Anti-inflammatory and antipyretic activities of Beta sitosterol. *Planta Medica* 1980; 39: 157–163.

Middleton E Jr. Effect of flavonoids on basophil histamine release and other secretory systems. *Prog Clin Biol Res.* 1986;213:493–506.

Ogasawara H, Middleton E Jr. Effect of selected flavonoids on histamine release (HR) and hydrogen peroxide (H2O2) generation by human leukocytes [abstract]. *J Allergy Clin Immunol.* 1985;75(suppl):184.

Chinese herbal medicine/acupuncture references

Cao ZS, et al. Research on antibacterial effects against pyloric helicobacterium in 50 kinds of Chinese herbs. *Strait Journal of Pharmacy.* 1999;11(3):53–54.

Chang Yong Zhong Yao Cheng Fen Yu Yao Li Shou Ce (A Handbook of the Composition and Pharmacology of Common Chinese Drugs), 1994; 226:323.

Hu Bei Yi Sheng (Hubei Doctor), 1976;(5:42).

Jiang XY, et al. Comparison between 50 kinds of Chinese herbs that treat hepatitis and suppress in vitro HBAg activity. *Journal of Modern Applied Pharmacy.* 1992;9(5):208–211.

Kubo M, Matsuda H, Tanaka M, Kimura Y, Okuda H, Higashino M, Tani T, Namba K, Arichi S. Studies on Scutellariae radix. VII. Anti-arthritic and anti-inflammatory actions of methanolic extract and flavonoid components from Scutellariae radix. *Chem Pharm Bull*, 1984; 32(7):2724–9.

Lei WY, et al. Swertiamarin's central inhibitory effects. *Journal of Chinese Materia Medica.* 1982;13(8):368.

Li WW. Ban Lan Gen's effect on nephritic syndrome. Hunan *Journal of Medicine.* 1994(1);11(3):168.

Li WW. Experimental research on Ban Lan Gen and Xi Shu Guo's effect in counteracting HFRSV and HSV-2. *Journal of Hunan University of Medicine.* 1994(2);19(4):309–311.

Li FC, et al. *China Journal of Integrated Medicine.* 1994;14(1):37–38.

Li RY, et al. Therapeutic observation of treating 62 cases of chronic pharyngitis with Ban Lan Gen Injection. *Journal of Integrated Medicine.* 1990;10(12):739.

Li S, et al. Various Ban Lan Gen and Da Qing Ye's effect in antagonizing influenza A virus. *Journal of Second Military Medical College.* 2000;21(3):204–206.

Li SF, et al. Clinical observations on treating herpes simplex viral keratitis with Ban Lan Gen Injection. *Journal of Hebei Medical University.* 1998;19(4):215–217.

Liu IX, Durham DG, Richards RM. Baicalin synergy with beta-lactam antibiotics against methicillin-resistant Staphylococcus aureus and other beta-lactam-resistant strains of S. aureus. *J Pharm Pharmacol.* 2000 Mar;52(3):361–6.

Meng JH, et al. *Journal of Hebei College of TCM.* 1996;11(3): 31–33.

Pan JF, et al. *Tianjin Journal of Medicine.* 1991;19(8): 468–470.

Sheng Yao Xue Za Zhi (*Journal of Raw Herbology*), 1979; 33(3):178.

Song ZQ, et al. *China Journal of Dermatology.* 1997;11(3): 143–144.

Wang YP, et al. *Shanghai Journal of Medical Inspection.* 1999;14(4):206–207.

Wang YS, et al. TCM Pharmacology and Application. Beijing: People's Health Press; 1983.

Xi Shu Guo's effect in countering HFRSV and HSV-2. *Journal of Hunan University of Medicine.* 1994;19(4):309–311.

Xie YY, et al. *Journal of Shandong Medical University.* 1996;34(2):166–169.

Xiu Hua Ben Cao Gang Mu (New Chinese Materia Medica), 1991;579.

Xu Q, et al. Long Dan Cao's inhibitory effect on delayed allergic reaction. *Journal of Pharmacology and Clinical Application of TCM.* 1993;9(5):25.

Xu ZC, et al. Assessment of antibacterial effects of the Chinese herb Ban Lan Gen. *Journal of Chinese Patented Medicine Research.* 1987;11(12):9–11.

Yang SZ, et al. *Liaoning Journal of Traditional Chinese Medicine.* 1997;24(4):187.

Yi Xue Ji Shu Zi Liao (Resource of Medical Techniques), 1974;(1:2):113.

Zhang BS, et al. *Journal of Traditional Chinese Medicine Material.* 1997;20(2):85–88.

Zhang MF, et al. *Journal of Pharmacology and Clinical Application of TCM.* 1998;14(6):12–16.

Zhang XL, et al. *Journal of Shandong College of TCM.* 1994;18(6):416–417.

Zhao MJ, et al. *Zhejiang Journal of Traditional Chinese Medicine.* 1999;34(12):544.

Zhi Wu Yao You Xiao Cheng Fen Shou Ce (Manual of Plant Medicinals and Their Active Constituents), 1986; 41,212,384,829.

Zhong Cheng Yao Yan Jiu (Research of Chinese Patent Medicine), 1987; 12:9.

Zhong Guo Yao Ke Da Xue Xue Bao (*Journal of University of Chinese Herbology*), 1990;21(4):222.

Zhong Yao Cai (Study of Chinese Herbal Material), 1991; 14(2):41.

Zhong Yao Tong Bao (*Journal of Chinese Herbology*), 1988:13(6):364.

Zhong Yao Xue (*Chinese Herbology*), 1998; 109:110.

Zhong Yao Xue (*Chinese Herbology*), 1998;133:134.

Zhong Yao Xue (*Chinese Herbology*), 1998; 318:320.

Zhong Yao Yao Li Yu Ying Yong (Pharmacology and Applications of Chinese Herbs), 1983; 295.

Zhong Yao Zhi (*Chinese Herbology Journal*), 1984;578.

Zhu LA, et al. Research on Ban Lan Gen's preventive effects on cardiac cells in experimental cyocarditis models. *China Journal of Cardiovascular Disease*. 1999;27(6):467–468.

CORNEAL ULCERS

Definition and cause

Corneal ulcers are classified as either superficial or deep and more commonly are caused secondary to injury or self-trauma. Other causes are chronic eyelash irritation, exposure to foreign or environmental irritants, and bacterial or viral infections. They also can be secondary to other diseases such as KCS. The pain and inflammation associated with corneal ulcers often disappears when the healing is completed. Non-healing and deep ulcers often involve other tissue of the eye, such as the iris, or result in desmetoceles. Indolent ulcers result when nonvital tissues mechanically block the eyes' ability to heal (Glaze 1999; Nasisse 1982, 1997; Slatter 1990; Whitley 1999).

Medical therapy rationale, drug(s) of choice, and nutritional recommendations

Superficial corneal ulcers generally respond well to topical ointments or drops. Deep corneal ulcers often require surgical intervention such as a third eyelid flap, corneal graft, or keratotomy. Topical and systemic antibiotics, topical anesthetics, and medical dilating agents such as atropine along with an Elizabethan collar are often recommended (Champagne 1992; Gilger 1999; Gelatt 1982, 2000; Kirschner 1990).

Anticipated prognosis

Superficial corneal ulcers, especially those secondary to trauma, heal well. Deep corneal ulcers also heal well with both longstanding medical therapy and surgical intervention. Ulcers secondary to other conditions such as viral infection, KCS, and continual irritation have a poorer prognosis and often require ongoing medication, surgical correction, and client compliance (Slatter 1990, Whitley 1999).

Integrative veterinary therapies

It is essential to define and address the underlying cause of the corneal ulceration. Medical therapy and prevention of the self-trauma is often needed to allow for proper healing. The normal cornea heals so quickly and easily that generally accepted medical modalities are sufficient in most cases. Most cases heal in 3 to 7 days. All cases should be stained with an agent capable of identifying corneal undermining, because these cases require special handling. It is also important to evaluate the patient's tear production.

The integrative approach is often needed in recurrent, nonhealing, and indolent ulcers. Along with appropriate medical therapy, nutritional support of the cornea and the use of remedies that are designed to reduce inflammation and improve blood flow often promote and enhance healing.

Nutrition
General considerations/rationale

Nutritional support of the eye helps to reduce inflammation and improve circulation to the cornea. In addition, support of related organs such as the liver often has a positive effect on the healing process.

Appropriate nutrients

Nutritional/gland therapy: Glandular eye can help reduce inflammation (see Gland Therapy in Chapter 2).

Lutein: Lutein, a member of the carotenoid family, is a potent antioxidant that benefits eye health. Seddon (1994) showed that people treated with lutein had a decreased risk of macular degeneration and increased protection of the eye. Hankinson (1992) showed that lower levels of lutein were associated with increased risk of cataract. Dagnelie (2000) found that people with retinitis pigmentosa (RP) showed a significant improvement in visual acuity with lutein supplementation.

Chinese herbal medicine/acupuncture
General considerations/rationale

Corneal ulcers are a result of excessive Heat in the Liver and Gallbladder, accompanied by Yin and Blood deficiency. The Liver is reflected in the Eyes. When there is Heat in the Liver the Eyes may become red, inflamed, and painful. This Heat may be a result of infection, i.e. bacterial, viral, or fungal. The Yin and Blood deficiency are reflected in a dry, unnourished cornea. The ulcer develops when the cornea is dry, and the lack of nourishment makes it susceptible to colonization by bacteria and fungi.

The herbs in formulas developed to treat corneal ulcers must stop pain, decrease inflammation, repel pathogens, and help heal the cornea.

Appropriate Chinese herbs

Angelica (Bai zhi): Has demonstrated anti-inflammatory effects in mice (Zhong Guo Zhong Yao Za Zhi 1991).

Angelica root (Dang gui): Has antibacterial effects (Hou Xue Hua Yu Yan Jia 1981), and is as strong as aspirin at decreasing inflammation and is 1.7 times as strong as aspirin for pain relief (Yao Xue Za Zhi 1971). Despite its effect on inflammation, it has immunostimulant effects (Zhong Hua Yi Xue Za Zhi 1978).

Astragalus (Huang qi): Improves both the humoral and cellular immune systems (Jiao 1999) and demonstrates antibacterial properties (Zhong Yao Zhi 1949). It also has analgesic effects (Zhong Yao Tong Bao 1986).

Chrysanthemum (Ju hua): Has antibacterial efficacy (Yi Xue Ji Shu Zi Liao 1974).

Dandelions (Pu gong ying): May possess anti-inflammatory actions (Mascolo 1987). Dandelions also inhibit bacteria (Zhong Yi Yao Xue Bao 1991).

Forsythia (Lian qiao): Has multiple functions in a supplement for cornea ulcers. It possesses anti-inflammatory properties. It can reduce inflammation by decreasing capillary permeability (Ke Yan Tong Xun 1982). Forsythia decreases edema and inflammatory exudate (Ma 1982). In addition, it has anti-inflammatory and analgesic effects (Rui 1999). Finally, it inhibits both viruses and bacteria (Zhang 2002, Ma 1982).

Honeysuckle (Jin yin hua): A strong antibiotic that also has activity against Candida albicans (Wang 1998, Liu 1998, Cao 1999, Feng 1996). It may be useful for bacterial and fungal causes of ulceration.

Plantain (Che qian cao): Has anti-inflammatory effects (*Journal of Traditional Chinese Medicine Material* 1996).

Red peony (Chi shao): Has been shown to diminish ocular inflammation. It decreases the redness, swelling, and pain in the eyes (Bao 1999). In addition, red peony has antiviral activity; it has shown efficacy against herpesviruses (Liu 1999).

Rhubarb (Da huang): Has been proven to inhibit many viruses including herpesvirus (Xie 1996). It contains emodin, rhein, and aloe-emodin, which have antibiotic effects (Zhong Yao Xue 1998). Furthermore, it has analgesic and anti-inflammatory effects (Chang Yong Zhong Yao Cheng Fen Yu Yao Li Shou Ce 1994).

Scutellaria (Huang qin): Contains biacalin, which has antibiotic activity on its own and has synergistic effects with some penicillins. Additionally, it can help overcome B lactam resistance (Zhong Yao Xue 1988, **Liu** 2000). Baicalin and another component of scutellaria, biacalein, have been shown to suppress inflammation in mice and rats (Kubo 1984, Cao 1999). Finally, scutellaria enhances cellular immunity and may help to clear corneal pathogens (Pan 1991).

Thlaspi (Bai jiang cao): Inhibits bacteria and viruses (Zhong Yao Xue 1998).

Viola (Zi hua di ding): Has antibacterial and antiviral effects, including activity against herpesvirus (Zhong Hua Yi Xue Za Zhi 1962).

Vitex fruit (Man jing zi): Contains vitexicarpin, which inhibits bacteria (Zhong Cao Yao Xue 1980). It has analgesic effects (Zhong Yao Xue 1998).

Homotoxicology
General considerations/rationale
Traumatic and other acute onset corneal ulcerations represent Inflammation Phase disorders. Ulceration can also result from deeper homotoxicoses and represent Degenerative Phase lesions. Changes in the state of health can result in corneal ulceration as both regressive and progressive vicariation. It is important for the clinician to identify the correct phase so that appropriate therapeutic entities are selected.

In recurrent or indolent conditions involving corneal ulceration, the clinician should recall the relationship between the eye and the liver in Traditional Chinese Medicine. Some cases resolve upon the addition of antihomotoxic medicines directed at supporting liver function and drainage. Nonhealing ulcers may also require assistance in activating blocked enzyme systems and in repairing errors in energy metabolism through use of catalyst agents. In difficult cases, autosanguis therapy may move a patient toward healing, especially when used in conjunction with autogenous serum therapy topically. Surgery is needed in some cases.

Referral of non-healing corneal ulcerations to a veterinary ophthalmologist is strongly advised because multiple entities may be involved in such cases (Reckeweg 2000).

Appropriate homotoxicology formulas
There are no veterinary studies on the use of antihomotoxic agents in the healing of corneal ulceration. Appropriate remedies commonly used include:

Belladonna homaccord: Treats localized, suppurative Inflammation Phase disorders.

BHI-Eye: Contains Belladonna and Euphrasia, which have strong indications for eye pathologies, including spasmodic photophobia, pain and pressure in the eyes, acute conjunctivitis, coryza with lachrymation, chemosis, blepharitis, corneal ulcers, and iritis. (Stoss, et al. 2000, Reckeweg 2002).

BHI-Inflammation: Used for generalized inflammatory conditions. Contains Belladonna, which has strong indicators for eye pain, or irritations of the conjunctiva with photophobia, lachrymation, and engorgement of the blood vessels (Reckeweg 2002). This is also common to many other remedies that may be used, including *Belladonna homaccord, Mercurius-Heel, Mucosa compositum, Traumeel, Viburcol, BHI-Bladder, BHI-Bronchitis, BHI-Eye, and BHI-Injury.*

Coenzyme compositum: Supports energy production.

Discus compositum: Used for long-term repair of deep connective tissue elements. This remedy contains several helpful ingredients, including Ranunculus, Funiculus umbicalis suis, Mercurius precipitatus ruber, Glandula suprarenalis suis, Medulla ossis suis, and Zincum metallicum (Reckeweg 2002).

Flu Plus: Used for viral ulcers, based on the components Bryonia, Mercurius sublimates corrosives, and Zincum metallicum (Reckeweg 2002).

Galium-Heel: Provides general cellular support. Contains Aurum for corneal ulcers as well as Nitricum acidum and Conium (Reckeweg 2002).

Ginseng compositum: Contains several excellent remedies for ulceration or conjunctivits, including Kreosotum, Hydrastis, and Conium (Reckeweg 2002).

Glyoxal compositum: Used for depolymerization of homotoxin polymers that can block enzyme function.

Hepar compositum: Provides hepatic drainage and support in chronic cases.

Lamioflur: Includes Nitricum acidum, Hydrastis candensis, Kreosotum, and Mezereum (Reckeweg 2002).

Lymphomyosot: Treats corneal edema and swelling, and is immune-supportive.

Mercurius-Heel S: Provides antibacterial effects and support of localized ulcerative processes (Vestweber, et al. 1995, Reckeweg 2000).

Mucosa compositum: Provides drainage and support of mucosal surfaces, and support of ocular tissues. Contains several excellent remedies, including Hydrastis, Kali bichromicum, Belladonna, and Kreosotum (Reckeweg 2002).

Nasoheel: Contains Hydrastis canadensis, Kali bichromicum, Aurum muriaticum natronatum, Mercurius sulphuratus ruber, and Mercurius iodatus ruber, and provides strong support for corneal tissue that is ulcerated (Reckeweg 2002).

Oculoheel: Used for conjuctival irritation and ocular pain.

Pure eye drops: The topical form of Oculoheel.

Traumeel S: Activates blocked enzyme systems, and has anti-inflammatory effects.

Ubichinon compositum: Provides mitochondrial repair. Contains the eye remedies Conium, Hydrastis canadensis, and Ubiquinon.

Authors' suggested protocols

Nutrition

Eye support formula: 1 tablet for every 25 pounds of body weight BID.

Lutein: 5 mg for every 50 pounds of body weight.

Chinese herbal medicine/acupuncture

Formula Corneal Ulcer: 1 capsule for every 10 to 20 pounds, twice daily. Underlying causes such as ectopic cilia must be addressed or the condition will not respond well or will recur when the supplement is discontinued.

Homotoxicology

Acute ulcerations: Traumeel S BID for 3 days orally, Oculoheel BID for 5 days PO, Topical drops (Pure Eye Drops), BHI-Eye, Ginseng compositum, Coenzyme and Ubichinon. Use Nasoheel, Lamioflur, and Flu Plus for viral ulcers.

Chronic ulcers: Traumeel S once weekly, Mucosa compositum, Galium Heel, Discus compositum, and Oculoheel BID PO, Deep Detoxification Formula every 3 days for 30 to 120 days to stimulate regressive vicariation.

Deep detoxification formula: Galium-Heel, Lymphomyosot, Hepar compositum, Solidago compositum plus UriCleanse, Coenzyme compositum, Ubichinon compositum PO every 3 days.

Product sources

Nutrition

Eye support formula: Animal Nutrition Technologies.
    Lutein: Progressive Labs.

Chinese herbal medicine

Formula Corneal Ulcer: Natural Solutions, Inc.

Chinese herbal medicine

BHI/Heel Corporation

REFERENCES

Western medicine references

Champagne E, Munger R. Multiple punctuate keratotomy for the treatment of recurrent epithelial erosions in dogs. *J Am Anim Hosp Assoc* 1992; 28: 213–216.

Gilger BC, Whitley RD. Surgery of the Cornea and Sclera. In: Gelatt KN, ed. Veterinary Ophthalmology, Third ed. Philadelphia: Lippincott Williams and Wilkins. 1999:675–700.

Glaze MB, Gelatt KN. Feline Ophthalmology. In: Veterinary Ophthalmology, Third ed. Philadelphia: Lippincott Williams and Wilkins. 1999:997–1052.

Gelatt K, Samuelson D. Recurrent corneal erosions and epithelial dystrophy in the boxer dog. *J Am Anim Hosp Assoc* 1982; 18: 453–460.

Gelatt KN. Essentials of Veterinary Ophthalmology. Philadelphia: Lippincott Williams and Wilkins. 2000. 125–164.

Kirschner SE. Persistent corneal ulcers. What to do when ulcers won't heal. *Vet Clin North Am Small Anim Pract* 1990; 20:627–642.

Nasisse MP, Weigler BJ. The Diagnosis of Ocular Feline Herpesvirus Infection. *Vet Comp Ophthalmol* 1997: 7: 44.

Nasisse MP. Manifestations, diagnosis, and treatment of ocular herpesvirus infection in the cat. *Comp Cont Educ Pract Vet* 1982:4:962.

Slatter D. Fundamentals of Veterinary Ophthalmology, Vol 1, 2nd ed. Philadelphia: WB Saunders Co. 1990:257–303.

Whitley R, Gilger BC. Diseases of Canine Cornea and Sclera. In: Gelatt KN, ed. Veterinary Ophthalmology, third ed. Philadelphia: Lippincott Williams and Wilkins. 1999:635–673.

Nutrition references

Dagnelie G. Lutein supplements may improve vision. *Optometry: Journal of the American Optometric Association* 2000;71: 147–64.

Hankinson SE, Stampfer MJ, Seddon JM, et al. Nutrient intake and cataract extraction in women: a prospective study. *Br Med J* 1992;305(6849):335–9.

Miller W. Using polysulfated glycoaminoglycans to treat persistent corneal erosions in dogs. *Vet Med* 1996; 71: 916–922.

Seddon JM, Ajani UA, Sperduto RD, et al. Dietary carotenoids, vitamins A, C, and E, and advanced age-related macular degeneration. *JAMA* 1994;272:1413–20.

Chinese herbal medicine/acupuncture references

Bao GY, et al. Treating 32 cases of retinal vein obstruction with Xue Fu Zhu Yu Tang. *Henan Journal of TCM.* 1999.

Cao ZS, et al. *Strait Journal of Pharmacy.* 1999;11(3):53–54.

Chang Yong Zhong Yao Cheng Fen Yu Yao Li Shou Ce (A Handbook of the Composition and Pharmacology of Common Chinese Drugs), 1994; 226:323.

Feng YM, et al. *Journal of Norman Bethune Medical University.* 1996;22(2):150–151.

Hou Xue Hua Yu Yan Jia (Research on Blood-Activating and Stasis-Eliminating Herbs), 1981:335.

Jiao Y, et al. *China Journal of Integrated Medicine.* 1999;19(6): 356–358.

Journal of Traditional Chinese Medicine Material. 1996;19(2): 87–89.

Ke Yan Tong Xun (*Journal of Science and Research*), 1982;(3):35.

Kubo M, Matsuda H, Tanaka M, Kimura Y, Okuda H, Higashino M, Tani T, Namba K, Arichi S. Studies on Scutellariae radix. VII. Anti-arthritic and anti-inflammatory actions of methanolic extract and flavonoid components from Scutellariae radix. *Chem Pharm Bull*, 1984; 32(7):2724–9.

Liu N, et al. *Journal of Guangzhou University of TCM.* 1999;16(4):308–310.

Liu TF, et al. *China Journal of Modern Medicine.* 1998;8(6): 38–39.

Liu IX, Durham DG, Richards RM. Baicalin synergy with beta-lactam antibiotics against methicillin-resistant Staphylococcus aureus and other beta-lactam-resistant strains of S. aureus. *J Pharm Pharmacol.* 2000 Mar;52(3):361–6.

Ma ZY. *Shannxi Journal of Traditional Chinese Medicine and Herbs.* 1982;(4):58.

Mascolo N, Autore G, Capasso F, et al. Biological screening of Italian medicinal plants for anti-inflammatory activity. *Phytotherapy Res* 1987;1(1):28–31.

Pan JF, et al. *Tianjin Journal of Medicine.* 1991;19(8): 468–470.

Rui J. *Journal of Chinese Materia Medica.* 1999;30(1):43–45.

Wang SP, et al. *Journal of Popular Medicine of Chinese Ethnic Minorities.* 1998;(5):40–41.

Xie YY, et al. *Journal of Shandong Medical University.* 1996;34(2):166–169.

Yao Xue Za Zhi (*Journal of Medicinals*), 1971;(91):1098.

Yi Xue Ji Shu Zi Liao (*Resource of Medical Techniques*), 1974;(1:2):113.

Zhang G, Song S, Ren J, Xu S. A New Compound from Forsythia suspense (Thunb.) Vahl with Antiviral Effect on RSV. *J of Herbal Pharmacotherapy.* 2002;2(3):35–39.

Zhong Cao Yao Xue (Study of Chinese Herbal Medicine), 1980;915.

Zhong Guo Zhong Yao Za Zhi (*People's Republic of China Journal of Chinese Herbology*), 1991; 16(9):560.

Zhong Hua Yi Xue Za Zhi (*Chinese Journal of Medicine*), 1962; 48(3): 188.

Zhong Hua Yi Xue Za Zhi (*Chinese Journal of Medicine*), 1978;17(8):87.

Zhong Yao Tong Bao (*Journal of Chinese Herbology*), 1986; 11(9):47.

Zhong Yao Xue (*Chinese Herbology*), 1988; 137:140.

Zhong Yao Xue (*Chinese Herbology*), 1998; 202:203.

Zhong Yao Xue (*Chinese Herbology*), 1998; 99:100.

Zhong Yao Xue (*Chinese Herbology*), 1998; 251: 256.

Zhong Yao Zhi (*Chinese Herbology Journal*), 1949;(12):648.

Zhong Yi Yao Xue Bao (Report of Chinese Medicine and Herbology), 1991;(1):41.

Homotoxicology references

Reckeweg H. Biotherapeutic Index: Ordinatio Antihomotoxica et Materia Medica, 5th ed. Baden-Baden, Germany: Biologische Heilmittel Heel GMBH, 2000. p 272, 364–5.

Reckeweg H. Homeopathia Antihomotoxica Materia Medica, 4th edition. Aurelia-Verlag GMBH, Baden-Baden, 2002. pp 162, 172–5, 187, 254, 294, 322, 344–5, 366, 378, 410, 416–420, 424, 459, 610.

Stoss M, Michels C, Peter E, Beutke R, Gorter RW. 2000. Prospective cohort trial of Euphrasia single-dose eye drops in conjunctivitis. *J Altern Complement Med.* 2000 Dec;6(6):pp 499–508.

Vestweber AM, Beuth J, Ko HL, Tunggal L, Buss G, Pulverer G. 1995. In vitro activity of Mercurius cyanatus complex against relevant pathogenic bacterial isolates. [Article in German]. *Arzneimittelforschung.* Sep;45(9):pp 1018–20.

GLAUCOMA

Definition and cause

Glaucoma's complex, multifactorial pathogenesis eventually results in increased intraocular pressure, and is characterized by optic nerve damage resulting in pain and progressive visual loss. Affected veterinary patients are usually asymptomatic until late in the disease's course. Oxidative DNA damage in the trabecular meshwork of glaucoma patients has been recently linked to glaucoma, as well as nitrous oxide alterations (Morgan 1999, Sacca 2005). Primary glaucoma is characterized by elevated intraocular pressure without concurrent ocular disease, often involving narrow angle glaucoma, with obstruction of aqueous outflow through the iridocorneal angle. Primary open angle glaucoma is characterized by a more insidious onset, and is seen almost solely in beagles. Primary glaucoma is seen bilaterally and is most common in dogs. Glaucoma is rare in cats, and is most commonly seen as a complication of chronic anterior uveitis. Intraocular neoplasia can lead to secondary glaucoma and represents a Dedifferentiation Phase disorder, which is usually addressed by surgical removal of the affected eye.

Secondary glaucoma is characterized by elevated intraocular pressure associated with concurrent ocular disease, e.g., uveitis and/or intraocular hemorrhage (seen as a sequelae to diseases such as ehrlichiosis), neoplasia, and lens displacement. In uveitis, inflammatory mediators are liberated into the eye and alter the iridocorneal angle. Standard treatment attempts to control inflammation through the use of topical corticosteroids, along with other medications to reduce intraocular pressure. Dogs with anterior uveitis should not receive miotic agents (Picket 1997). Lens luxation has many of the characteristics of primary glaucoma, and is breed related, with a preponderance of cases involving Sharpeis and terriers. Surgical repair of lens luxation by removal of the luxated lens carries one of the best prognoses for managing longterm glaucoma.

The clinical signs of glaucoma, in addition to increased intraocular pressure, vary greatly by stage. In early glaucoma, episcleral venous congestion and conjunctival hyperemia are present, resulting in a red, painful eye (episcleral vascular congestion) with variations in vision. The pupil may be normal or slightly dilated with sluggish to normal papillary reflexes. Mild corneal edema may be present. Vomiting and a general feeling of sickness can occur in humans but is frequently missed as a significant sign in animals suffering from glaucoma. In more advanced stages, glaucoma signs include buophthalmos, corneal striae, optic disc cupping, and retinal degeneration, and possibly exposure keratitis and lens luxation. Pupillary reflex is often missing in advanced cases. Iritis, conjunctivitis, episcleritis, panophthalmitis, and trigeminal neuralgia are some differential diagnoses to be considered. Tonometry is needed to accurately diagnose this condition.

The goals of medical management of glaucoma include reducing intraocular pressure, improving blood flow to the optic nerve and retina, and decreasing the damage caused by toxic metabolites such as glutamate. In humans, risk factors include cardiovascular disease, diabetes mellitus (sugar diabetes), myopia (nearsightedness), high blood pressure, and migraine headache. Diseases of the sensory organs and of the nervous system may be induced by mercury toxicity. Retinal detachment may occur when the lymph system in the area of the eyes has been afflicted by an auto-aggressive immune system. Cataracts and disorders of the vitreous body can also demonstrate a similar etiology. Hindrance of the outward flow of the intraocular fluid produced by the ciliary body, i.e., glaucoma, is induced at a certain percentage level by mercury (Nolte 1988).

A recent study in dogs suggested that collars and leashes could be implicated in a steep rise in intraocular pressure, which is similar to a human study that found a positive relationship in men who wore tight neckties (Pauli, et al. 2006). Thyroid disease has also been positively linked to glaucoma, as have other medical problems such as hypertension (Glaucoma Study Group C, 2006).

Medical therapy rationale, drug(s) of choice, and nutritional recommendations

A thorough ocular evaluation including intraocular pressure determination is indicated, and early referral to a veterinary ophthalmologist may be appropriate. Because certain medical conditions such as lens luxation and uveitis are associated with higher incidents of glaucoma, patients in these risk groups should be screened more frequently for glaucoma (Johnsen, Maggs, Kass 2006).

Surgery to improve the fluid flow through the eye or to decrease fluid production is generally the therapy of choice. With progressive painful disease, enucleation is often recommended (Picket 2003).

Anticipated prognosis

Glaucoma is a chronic progressive disease, and even with medical therapy blindness often occurs. Surgical intervention often improves the prognosis; however, progression of the disease often continues.

Integrative veterinary therapies

An integrative approach to glaucoma includes the addition of nutrients, medicinal herbs, and combination homeopathics to conventional medical therapy. These natural ingredients have anti-inflammatory, tissue-sparing, and regenerative effects on the eyes, and help to improve circulation and reduce intraocular pressure.

Nutrition
General considerations/rationale
While medical therapy is focused on stabilizing the intraocular pressure, therapeutic nutrition adds nutrients, antioxidants, and gland support to help reduce inflammation and improve circulation and function.

Appropriate nutrients
Nutritional/gland therapy: Glandular adrenal, thymus, and eye provide intrinsic nutrients and also help reduce

inflammation, improve organ function, and slow cellular degeneration (see Gland Therapy in Chapter 2).

Vitamin C: Vitamin C has been shown to help lower intraocular pressure in patients who did not respond well to conventional medical therapies (Fishbein 1972, Virno 1967).

Omega-3 fatty acids: In a study with animals, fish oil significantly reduced intraocular pressure as compared to other animals whose diet was supplemented with lard (McGuire 1991).

Chromium: Deficiencies of chromium and vitamin C are associated with higher intraocular pressure in people (Lane 1991).

Magnesium: Magnesium has been shown to act similar to a calcium channel blocker. Gaspar (1995) showed that magnesium improved blood supply and the visual field in people with glaucoma.

Chinese herbal medicine/acupuncture
General considerations/rationale

Glaucoma is due to stress, Liver stagnation leading to fire formation, and Wind and Fire rising up to the Eyes. In the author's interpretation, stagnation can lead to Heat or, in more severe cases, Fire. This can be likened to grass packed in a pile. It eventually becomes warm and under the right circumstances may even combust. This Heat or Fire in the Liver can manifest as ocular pathology as the Liver opens to the eyes in TCM theory. This Heat or inflammation can increase intraocular pressure. If it is severe, there may be retinal detachment and bleeding. Treatment is aimed at decreasing the intraocular pressure and protecting the vision.

Appropriate Chinese herbs

Angelica root (Dang gui): As strong as aspirin at decreasing inflammation and 1.7 times as strong as aspirin for pain relief (Yao Xue Za Zhi 1971). It may help decrease the ocular inflammation and discomfort associated with glaucoma.

Cnidium (Chuan xiong): Has anti-neoplastic effects (Liu 1993). It may be useful in cases of glaucoma secondary to neoplasia.

Cyperus (Xiang fu zi): Has demonstrated analgesic effects in mice (Gui Yang Yi Xue Yuan Xue Bao 1959). This may help control the discomfort of glaucoma. Note: This effect is mild. Western pain killers must be given if indicated.

Haliotis (Shi jue ming): Has been shown to protect the eye. It prevents D-galactose-induced lens damage in rats and prevented the formation of cataracts (Huang 1997).

Licorice (Gan cao): Can improve the general condition of blood vessels (Xu 1997). It may also preserve intraocular blood vessels damaged by high pressures.

Oyster shell (Mu li): Has demonstrated anti-neoplastic activity (Wang 1997). It may be beneficial in glaucoma of neoplastic etiology.

Peach kernel (Tao ren): Decreases inflammation (Liu 1989). In one experiment it was shown to inhibit the proliferation of inflammatory cells and fibroblast hyperplasia in subjects of experimental trabeculae dissection (Wang 1993). It also has anti-oxidation effects. It can increase the activity of SOD (Jiang 1995). As mentioned above, oxidative damage may be linked to the development of glaucoma.

Plantain seeds (Che qian zi): Can decrease intraocular pressure, as was demonstrated experimentally in rabbits (Li 1990).

Prunella (Xia ku cao): Can reduce blood glucose in normal mice as well as in mice with alloxan-induced diabetes, and can improve glucose tolerance (Liu 1995). Open angle glaucoma is linked to type II diabetes in humans (Bonovas 2004). Similar factors may occur in animals.

Salvia (Dan shen): Inhibits neoplastic cells (Li 1999).

Siler (Fang feng): Has demonstrated some efficacy against neoplastic cells (Li Li, et al. 1999). It may be of use in glaucoma secondary to neoplasia.

Skullcap (Huang qin): Contains baicalein, which has anti-neoplastic effects (Zi 2005). Again, this herb may be helpful in cases of neoplastic etiology.

Acupuncture

Acupuncture has been shown to affect the eye. In one study using Doppler flow ultrasonography, acupuncture at BL2, TH23, SI6, and GB37 was shown to increase the blood flow through the supratrochlear artery, which is the inner end branch of the ophthalmic artery (Litscher 1998). It has been reported to be useful in treating glaucoma (Ralston 1977).

Homotoxicology
General considerations/rationale

Glaucoma is a complex medical condition and can encompass Inflammation Phase through Degeneration Phase homotoxicoses. Generally speaking, most cases presented to veterinarians are in the Impregnation or Degeneration phases, and carry a correspondingly poor prognosis for long-term success with only medical therapy.

Homotoxicology therapy may be attempted after emergency management of ocular pressure in an attempt to reduce damages from homotoxins. Further research is needed to determine how effective biological therapy is in altering the disease course and in improving patient conditions.

The reader should note that, as for other areas of homotoxicology, many symptoms that are useful in prescribing classical homeopathic remedies are hard to verify in animals. Therefore, the clinician choosing to use anti-homotoxic medicines must make every effort to observe his patients carefully and may need to make certain educated guesses when choosing therapeutic agents. Fortunately, antihomotoxic medicines are generally safe when taken for short periods of time, so it is unlikely that any serious conditions would arise from selecting an incorrect agent.

Appropriate homotoxicology formulas
Standard medical therapy should be initiated and emergency steps taken to stabilize intraocular pressure. Antihomotoxic drugs to consider for augmenting therapy are:

Barijodeel: Used as an alternating remedy in cases involving arteriosclerotic causation (Reckeweg 1996). This remedy contains several useful therapeutics, including Aconitum, which repertorizes in the classic homeopathy realm, and Calc iodatum, which is used for activating mesenchymal processes and is useful for corneal disease such as conjunctivitis and corneal ulcers. It also contains Ignatia for eye symptoms that may include optical illusions, e.g., white, flickering, shining zigzags at the periphery of the field of vision, as occurs in detachment of the retina. Another strong component is Stramonium for dilated pupils in every affection and diseases accompanied by impairment of emotional and/or psychological functions, as well as inflammations of the eyes (Reckeweg 2002).

Belladonna homaccord: Belladonna's typical action on the eyes is characterized by symptoms referable to atropine poisoning, such as cramps in the muscles of the eyes and eyelids, enlargement of the pupils, and an inflammatory condition of the conjunctiva with photophobia, lachrymation, and pain. This is linked with engorgement of the inner blood vessels, weakness and dimness of vision, and disturbances of vision including sparks, fire, fog and diplopia, all pointing to the retina being affected. There may be a right-sided ciliary neuralgia, which is also seen with Kalmia, Sanguinaria, Chelidonium, etc. (Reckeweg 2002). A published clinical report involves the reversal of canine glaucoma in a 10-year-old Shih Tzu with previously unresponsive glaucoma, using twice weekly injections of *Belladonna homaccord* in combination with Euphrasia Eye drops (Bidarte 1997).

BHI-Eye: Contains Belladonna and Euphrasia, which has strong indications for eye pathologies, including spasmodic photophobia, pains and pressure in the eyes, acute conjunctivitis, coryza with lachrymation, chemosis, blepharitis, corneal ulcers, and iritis (Reckeweg 2002).

BHI-Inflammation: Used for generalized inflammatory conditions. Contains Belladonna, which has strong indicators for eye pain or irritations of the conjunctiva with photophobia, lachrymation, and engorgement of the blood vessels (see above) (Reckeweg 2002). This is also common to many other remedies that may be used, including: *Belladonna compositum*, *Belladonna homaccord*, *Mercurius*, *Mucosa compositum*, *Traumeel*, *BHI-Eye*, and *BHI-Injury*.

BHI-Perspiration: Contains Cedron, which is reported to have a beneficial effect on neural origin pain that accompanies iritis and glaucoma. It has been used in malaria with tumor of the spleen, anemia, and dropsical symptoms, and particularly in recurrent fevers. Thus, it might be useful in a disease such as ehrlichiosis. Jaborandi, which contains pilocarpine, is known for its qualities as a diaphoretic, which promotes sweating, and as a myotic (i.e. causing the pupils to contract).

Heinigke, in Meilman and Krayer (1950), describes the action of Jaborandi in the form of an infusion containing 6 grams of the leaves as follows: "The face immediately flushes, the temporal arteries begin to throb, and a strange sensation of heat occurs in the mouth and face—an agreeable feeling of warmth predominates." In patients poisoned by this agent, there are also palpitations and an irregular pulse. This symptom picture of the effects of pilocarpine, which is the main active ingredient of Jaborani, can be used to good effect according to reversal effect and the Law of Similars in visual disorders, such as difficulties in accommodation and spasms of the eyelids. This is similar to a clinical picture seen in a study on Veratrum alkaloids, in which specific extracts were injected intravenously (Meilman Krayer 1950).

A 1% to 2% solution of pilocarpine is used in ophthalmology to contract the pupils, e.g., in injuries to the iris and in glaucoma. Pilocarpine has a less powerful action than eserine, so the accommodation is affected to a lesser degree and there is a decreased tendency toward the enhancement of iritis.

The component of nitric acid is indicated in classical homeopathy for inflammations of the eye, with specks on the cornea, corneal ulcers, photophobia, and constant lachrymation. Sulphuricum acidum is indicated for numerous symptoms anywhere from the Reaction Phase to the Degeneration Phase. There is a typical taut feeling in the facial skin and ptosis of the upper eyelids, which may be accompanied by conjunctivitis with photophobia and dimness of vision. Petroleum is included for patients with skin conditions that may extend to the mucosa of the eyes, with dacryocystitis, lachrymation, easy tiredness of the eyes, weakness of vision, and floaters (Reckeweg 2002).

Coenzyme compositum: Supports energy production.

Cruroheel: Suggested in the Biotherapeutic Index as an initial therapeutic along with *Veratrum homaccord*. It contains several remedies with homeopathic indications for glaucoma: Lycopodium clavatum, Hamamelis virginiana, Apis mellifica, and Pulsatilla pratensis (Smit 2006).

Galium-Heel: Used for general cellular support. Contains Aurum, which is indicated for corneal ulcers and visual disturbances such as hemianopia. Also contains Nitricum acidum and Conium. The component Saponaria is useful in elevations in intraocular pressure (Reckeweg 2002).

Gelsemium homaccord: Particularly useful for iritis, retinitis, and accompanying headaches (Reckeweg 2000). Consider its use in cases showing violent congestions in the head. These are associated with headaches and neuralgias, particularly migraines, in which the pains may be dull or sudden or shooting. Nausea may also be linked with the headache. *Gelsemium homaccord* is also indicated in nervous insomnia and in glaucoma (Reckeweg 2002). Practitioners are advised to administer frequent small doses in the sense of cumulative stimulation therapy to achieve radical and speedy effects. This is useful for treating painful conditions, particularly headaches and cervical migraines. The ampoule form can be used to better and more radically influence the defense mechanisms (Reckeweg 1987). It can be administered in acute cases to initiate regulation (Reckeweg 1998).

Paralytic symptoms, diplopia, double vision, and ptosis may be present in cases benefiting from this agent. Double vision is very characteristic; giddiness and pains in the eyeballs are sure indications for the remedy in human patients. Intra-ocular inflammations in which serous exudations occur, dull pains, double vision, and vertigo, as well as serous iritis and choroiditis where there is a gradual impairment of vision are other indications for its use. Another symptom that may direct use of Gelsemium is the inability to accommodate quickly. *Gelsemium homaccord* has been used for detachment of the retina and in strabismus from weakening of the muscles. Gelsemium is one of the most valuable remedies in glaucoma, often palliating the severe pains and improving the neurotic symptom of the disease. It dilates the pupil through its paralyzing effect on the third cranial nerve (Hpathy 2006).

Glonoin homaccord: Nitroglycerin (Glonoinum) can be used harmlessly in low dilutions for long durations as an auxiliary remedy in glaucoma (Reckeweg 1996). The main indications for nitroglycerin include hypertension, migraine, cranial congestion, and glaucoma (Hamalcik 1992). *Glonoin homaccord* is currently unavailable in the United States, but Glonoinum is common to other remedies, including *Cactus compositum*, *Cor compositum*, *Strophanthus compositum*, and *Ypsiloheel* (Reckeweg 2000). *Ypsiloheel* is a fairly logical selection (see below).

Glyoxal compositum: Used for depolymerization of homotoxin polymers that can block enzyme function.

Hepar compositum: Includes Pancreas suis for dryness of the eyes; burning pain in the eyeballs; and dim, distorted, or loss of vision. Veratrum, Lycopodium, and Sulfur are also included in this valuable drainage agent. Hepar compositum can have surprising effects on a wide variety of ocular issues in dogs, cats, and humans. Many patients who undergo desirable regressive vicariation resulting from antihomotoxic drugs manifest ocular changes such as increased redness and mucous discharge. This clinical observation is in agreement with information first reported in Traditional Chinese Medicine concerning a relationship between the Zang fu organ (Liver) and the Eye (Maciocia, 1989).

Hepeel: Used for detoxification of the liver. It contains Veratrum, Lycopodium, and Phosphorus.

Kalmia compositum: Treats accompanying iritis.

Lymphomyosot: Used for corneal edema and swelling, and is immune supportive. The ingredient Equisetum is particularly indicated in cases of kidney disorders and can also be very effectively applied in cases of glaucoma, owing to its diuretic and "channeling" actions (John 1991).

Mucosa compositum: Provides drainage and support of mucosal surfaces, and support of ocular tissues. It contains several excellent remedies, including Hydrastis for mucosal suppuration that is accompanied by ulceration. Kali bichromicum, Belladonna (see *Belladonna homaccord*), and Kreosotum are included for when the eyelids are also inflamed, for conjunctivitis, and for severe reddening and swelling. It possibly treats Meibomian cysts and styes. The ingredient Pancreas suis is indicated in dryness of the eyes; burning pain in the eyeballs; and dim, distorted, or loss of vision. Phosphorus (see *Phosphor homaccord*)and Sulphur (see *Spigelion*) are also included.

Nasoheel: This remedy, which includes Hydrastis canadensis, Kali bichromicum, Aurum muriaticum natronatum, Mercurius sulphuratus ruber, and Mercurius iodatus ruber, has strong support for corneal tissue that is ulcerated (Reckeweg 2002). In addition, the Mercurius components may be valuable if the intraocular pressure is in response to an elevated level of mercury in the body (Nolte 1988).

Oculoheel: Works by way of constituents specific for eye complaints. It contains the following remedies, with their indications: Apis mellifica for conjunctivitis and edema of the eyelids; Natrium muriaticum for dacrocystitis and burning, acrid epiphora; Rhus toxicodendron for conjunctivitis with a tendency toward suppuration, edema of the eyelids, and epiphora; Hepar sulfuris for tendency toward suppurations, chalazions, and hordeolums; Spigelia for neuritis, ciliary neuralgia, and trigeminal neuralgia; Staphisagria for hordeolums, chalazions, blepharoconjunctivitis, and dacrocystitis; and Aethiops mineralis for ophthalmia and keratitis (Reckeweg 1996). Also contains Sulphur, a critical agent in mesenchymal therapy.

Phosphorus homaccord: Phosphorus is a component that is useful in eye problems, such as those in which there is hypersensitivity of the sensory organs, and in eye diseases in which there are black spots dancing in front of the eyes or the patient may see as if through a mist with momentary states of blindness (Reckeweg 2002). Phosphorus cases may have hyperemia of the choroid and retina, and also amblyopia and asthenopia (Hpathy 2006). Also contains Paris quadrifolia (see *Ypsiloheel*).

Psorinoheel: Used for chronic phase diseases.

Pure eye drops: The topical form of *Oculoheel*.

Spigelon: Spigelia is included for neuritis, ciliary neuralgia, and trigeminal neuralgia (Reckeweg 2002). This valuable remedy contains Bryonia, which is useful for symptoms of increased tension of the eyeballs, lachrymation, and photophobia. Also contains Gelsemium, (see *Gelsemium homaccord*). Ranunculus is included for attacks of vertigo; swimming in the head; a sensation of heaviness; stabbing, tearing headaches with congestion of blood; and burning and itching of the eyelids with redness. Sulphur is useful because synthetic drugs and heavy metals easily block the SH-groups that are present in receptors and enzymes, and this forms the basis for the iatrogenic damage that follows the use of many drugs. Thus, Sulphur may be valuable in conditions following toxicity with these compounds (Reckeweg 2002). It can be used in scrofulous inflammation of the eyes with tendency to congestion, when the eyes are red and injected, when there are opacities and ulcerations of the cornea, and when there is extreme sensitivity to light The eyeballs are painful, and the remedy is not useful when the external coats of the eyes are involved (Hpathy 2006). Spigelon may be indicated in Impregnation Phases, which attempt a regressive transformation into the Inflammation Phase. It has appeared in classic repertories for glaucoma (Shelton 2006).

Traumeel S: Can be used intermittently for its anti-inflammatory effects and to activate blocked enzyme systems. Contains Mercurius, which is useful in the hindrance of the outward flow of the intraocular fluid, i.e., glaucoma. (Nolte 1988).

Ubichinon compositum: Provides mitochondrial repair. Contains Benzochinon, which has parabenzoquinone for use in degenerative diseases of the eyes (retina) and ears, and also in diabetes mellitus. It also contains Conium for atypical ophthalmia with an unusually intensive photophobia, which bears no relationship to the actual degree of ophthalmia and which is only relieved in the dark and by pressure; corneal ulcers may also be present. Hydrastis canadensis is included for corneal ulceration. Sulfur, which when defined in physiological, chemical, or enzymological terms, achieves its effects by the reactivation of enzyme-based detoxifying procedures that have been destroyed. It is used for connective tissue lesions and numerous illnesses that are characterized as iatrogenic. Reddened mucosa, especially at orifices of the body, strik-

ingly red eyelids with tendency towards tubercular inflammations, styes, and blepharitis are also indications for Sulfur. Also contained is Ubiquinone (Coenzyme Q-10), which has special affinities for the eyes, e.g., conjunctivitis, but it is also indicated in toxoplasmosis, corneal erosions, paralysis of the eye muscles, and in infantile glaucoma. It may be used successfully in many cases of glaucoma and retinal disease, because it is a phase remedy in Degeneration Phase diseases (Reckeweg 2002).

Veratrum homaccord: This remedy contains *Veratrum album*, a remedy known in TCM for its treatment of "cold," stagnation conditions (Ben Jacob 2006). It is listed in *the Clarke Dictionary of Practical Materia Medica, vol. 3*, for loss of sight and headache with nausea and vomiting. The *Allen Encyclopaedia of Homeopathic Materia Medica* notes pressing pain in the eyes, with loss of appetite, vanishing vision and complete blindness, and Schroyen's synthesis notes loss of colors and loss of vision to be prescribing characteristics (Smit 2006). Veratrum is noted as a therapy for circulatory insufficiency and collapse. Veratrum homaccord acts favorably in various eye affections, especially when there is a tendency toward hemorrhage (Reckeweg 1996). In this regard, it may be a very valuable adjunct in diseases such as ehrlichiosis, which have a bleeding component in the initial causative mechanism of the glaucoma.

Ypsiloheel: Contains Glonoinum (see Glonoin homaccord). Also contains Paris quadrifolia with indications for a sensation that the eyeballs feel too large. It is a valuable remedy in certain forms of asthenopia with inability to fix the eyes on anything steadily. A peculiar symptom of asthenopia is a sensation as if a string were drawing the eye back into the head, as if the optic nerve were too short. *Ypsiloheel* is very useful for the sharp shooting and sticking pains accompanying glaucoma, which are worse at night and on motion (Hpathy 2006). This remedy also contains Ignatia for eye symptoms which may include optical illusions, e.g. white, flickering, shining zigzags at the periphery of the field of vision, as occurs in detachment of the retina (Reckeweg 2002). The ingredient Pulsatilla has specific indications for glaucoma in many of the classical repertories.

Authors' suggested protocols

Nutrition

Eye and immune support formulas: 1 tablet for every 25 pounds of body weight BID.

Vitamin C: 100 mg for every 15 pounds of body weight BID.

Eskimo fish oil: 1 teaspoon for each 20 pounds of body weight with meals.

Chromium: 25 mcg for every 25 pounds of body weight SID (maximum, 200 mcg).

Magnesium: 10 mg for every 10 pounds of body weight SID.

Chinese herbal medicine/acupuncture

Acute glaucoma is a medical emergency. It may be prudent to send the patient to a board certified ophthalmologist for initial treatment. In addition, it may be necessary to use Western medications initially to preserve sight. Some patients may require concurrent Western medications, but the dose of the Western medications should be lower.

The authors use the herbal formula Glaucoma at a dose of 1 capsule per 10 to 20 pounds twice daily as needed. In addition to the herbs discussed above, Glaucoma contains chrysanthemum (Ju hua), leonurus (Yi mu cao), lepidium (Ting li zi), phragmites (Lu gen), platycodon (Jie geng), and safflower (Hong hua). These herbs help increase the efficacy of the formula.

Commonly selected acupuncture points include ST36, tai yang, and TH5 (Handbook of TCM Practitioners 1987).

Homotoxicology

Always treat conventionally to normalize the intraocular pressure. Many approaches may be needed to best manage these patients. The following are suggested for starting therapy only. Adjust therapy to patient response.

Initial emergency homotoxicology approach: Phosphorus homaccord, Belladonna homaccord, and Galium-Heel mixed together and given orally every 15 minutes initially until pressure reduces, and then BID to TID.

Injection therapy: Belladonna homaccord plus Spigelon as an injection, preferably an autosanguis, twice weekly initially, then once weekly. These may also be given as a subconjunctival injection, using a 30-gauge needle.

Cruroheel plus Oculoheel: 1 tablet each TID PO.

Oral cocktail: Veratrum homaccord, Traumeel, Glonoin-homaccord, and Gelsemium homaccord, or possibly Spigelon. Ypsiloheel may be added, if indicated.

BHI Pure eye drops mixed with Mucosa compositum: Instilled in the eyes as often as possible.

An unlikely candidate at first glance, but one with some very useful components is BHI Perspiration, which may be given BID or interposed.

In addition, treatment with *suis*-organ preparations is useful, but we do not currently have single injeels in the United States. The recommended remedies are *Funiculus umbicalis suis, Oculus totalis suis, Corpus Vitreum suis, and Retina suis.* The former remedy is in several combinations, including Cutis compositum, Discus compositum, Placenta compositum, Thyroidea compositum, Tonsilla compositum, and Zeel. Because of the embryological origin of eye tissue, we suggest Cutis compositum in alternation with Placenta compositum for circulatory support.

The remaining suis preparations, with specific eye dilutions, may be obtained from Europe, because they are not currently available in the United States.

Conventional drug therapy should be initiated at once and may be reduced if a response to therapy occurs. Careful monitoring of intraocular pressure is recommended. Surgical therapy has a higher success in many cases and should be discussed with the owner. Surgical repair of lens luxation has the best prognosis.

Psorinoheel: Recommended intercurrently, on an intermittent basis.

Deep detoxification formula: Consider this formula because these are most often Degeneration Phase cases. The formula contains Galium-Heel, Lymphomyosot, Hepar compositum, Solidago compositum, Thyroidea compositum, Coenzyme compositum, Ubichinon compositum, and Mucosa compositum mixed together and taken twice weekly orally. If strong detoxification starts, reduce or eliminate this step until the initial crisis is abated.

Product sources

Nutrition

Eye and immune support formulas: Animal Nutrition Technologies. **Alternatives:** Immune System Support—Standard Process Veterinary Formulas; Immuno Support—Rx Vitamins for Pets; Immugen—Thorne Veterinary Products.

Eskimo fish oil: Tyler Encapsulations.

Vitamin C, chromium, and magnesium: Over the counter.

Chinese herbal medicine

Herbal Formula Glaucoma: Natural Solutions, Inc.

Chinese herbal medicine

BHI/Heel Corporation

REFERENCES

Western medicine references

Glaucoma Study Group C. 2006. Canadian Glaucoma Study: 1. Study design, baseline characteristics, and preliminary analyses. *Can J Ophthalmol.* Oct;41(5):pp 566–575.

Johnsen D, Maggs D, Kass P. 2006. Evaluation of risk factors for development of secondary glaucoma in dogs: 156 cases (1999–2004). *JAVMA.* 229(8):PP 1270-4.

Miller PE. Glaucoma, In: Bonagura JD, ed. Kirk's current veterinary therapy XII. Philadelphia: Saunders, 1995:1265–1272.

Picket J. Glaucoma. In: Tilley L, Smith F. The 5-Minute Veterinary Consult: Canine and Feline. Baltimore: Williams and Wilkins, 1997. pp 630–631.

Morgan J, Caprioli J, Koseki Y. Nitric oxide mediates excitotoxic and anoxic damage in rat retinal ganglion cells. *Arch Ophthalmol.* 1999. 117:pp 1524–1529.

Nolte, H. The pathogenic multipotency of mercury. *Bio Ther.* 1988.6(3):p 64.

Pauli A, Bentley E, Diehl K, Miller P. Effects of the application of neck pressure by a collar or harness on intraocular pressure in dogs. *J Am Anim Hosp Assoc.* May-Jun; 2006. 42(3):pp 207–11.

Picket J. Glaucoma. In Tilley L, Smith F. The 5-Minute Veterinary Consult: Canine and Feline. Baltimore: Williams and Wilkins, 1997. pp 630–631.

Sacca S, Pascotto A, Camicione P, Capris P, Izzotti A. Oxidative DNA damage in the human trabecular meshwork: Clinical correlations in patients with primary open-angle glaucoma. *Arch Ophthalmol.* 2005.Apr;123(4):pp 458–63.

IVM/nutrition references

Fishbein S, Goodstein S. The Pressure Lowering Effect of Ascorbic Acid, *Annal Opthalmol.* 4:1972, 487–491.

Gaspar AZ, Gasser P, Flamer, J. The Influence of Magnesium on Visual Field and Peripheral Vasospasm in Glaucoma, *Opthalmoligica* 209: 1995, 11.

Lane BC. Diet and Glaucoma, *J of Amer College of Nutrition,* 10/abstract 11:1991, 536.

McGuire R. Fish Oil Cuts Lower Ocular Pressure, *Medical Tribune,* 1991: 25.

Virno M, Bucci M, Pecorin-Giraldi J, Missiroli A. Oral Treatment of Glaucoma with Vitamin C. *Eye, Ear, Nose and Throat Monthly* 46:1967, 1502–15–8.

Chinese herbal medicine/acupuncture references

Bonovas S, Peponis V, Filioussi K. Diabetes mellitus as a risk factor for primary open-angle glaucoma: a meta-analysis. *Diabetic Medicine* June 2004 21(6) p 609.

Gui Yang Yi Xue Yuan Xue Bao (*Journal of Guiyang Medical University*), 1959:113.

Handbook of TCM Practitioners, Hunan College of TCM, Shanghai Science and Technology Press, Oct 1987, p 712–713.

Huang SW, et al. *Journal of Chinese Patented Medicine.* 1997;19(9):30–31.

Jiang CM, et al. Tao Ren's effect on in vitro and in vivo rat lipid peroxidation. *Journal of Bengbu Medical College.* 1995;20(2): 81–82.

Li L, et al. *Journal of Beijing Medical University.* 1999;22(3): 38–40.

Li WM, et al. The effects of Si Zi Tang's constituent herbs on rabbits' intraocular pressure. *Yunan Journal of TCM.* 1990;11(4):27–28:36.

Li XF, et al. In vitro anti-tumor effects of Dan Shen and Dan Shen compound injection. *Zhejiang Journal of Integrated Medicine.* 1999;9(5):291–292.

Litscher G, Yang N, Wang L. Ultrasound-controlled Acupuncture. *The Internet Journal of Anesthesiology.* 1998 volume 2 number 4.

Liu BL, et al. *Journal of University of Pharmacy of China.* 1995;26(1):44–46.

Liu CH, et al. The pharmacology of Tao Ren. *Journal of Pharmacology and Clinical Application of TCM.* 1989;(2):46–47.

Liu JR, et al. *China Journal of Pharmacology and Toxicology.* 1993;7(2):149.

Ralston NC. Successful treatment and management of acute glaucoma using acupuncture. *American Journal of Acupuncture* 1977; 5(3):283.

Wang SP, et al. Tao Ren extract's effect in suppressing filter bed fibroblasts hyperplasia in subjects of experimental trabeculae dissection. *Journal of Shanghai Medical University.* 1993; 20(1):35–381.

Xu L, et al. *Journal of Research in Chinese Medicine.* 1997;10(2):31–32.

Yao Xue Za Zhi (*Journal of Medicinals*), 1971;(91):1098.

Zi M, Ken-ichiro Otsuyama, Shangqin Liu, Saeid Abroun, Hideaki Ishikawa, Naohiro Tsuyama, Masanori Obata, Fu-Jun Li, Xu Zheng, Yasuko Maki, Koji Miyamoto, Michio M. Kawano. Baicalein, a component of *Scutellaria radix* from Huang-Lian-Jie-Du-Tang (HLJDT), leads to suppression of proliferation and induction of apoptosis in human myeloma cells, *Blood.* 2005; 105:3312–3318.

Homotoxicology references

ben-Jacob I. Personal communication in October 2006.

Bidarte, A. Summaries of reports in veterinary medicine: homeopathic treatment of glaucoma (reprinted from *Biomedicina Veterinaria* (June 1997):p 64). *Biomed Ther.* 1998. 16(1): p 146.

Hamalcik P. The biological therapy of cardiac, circulatory, and vascular disorders. *Biol Ther J Nat Med.* 1992. April,20(2): p 217.

Heel. Veterinary Guide, 3rd English edition. Biologische Baden-Baden, Germany: Heilmettel Heel GmbH, 2003. p 40.

Hpathy. Homeopathy for Everyone, Eye Diseases. 2006. http://www.hpathy.com/diseases/eyes-symptoms-treatment-cure.asp.

John J. The pharmacology and application of Lymphomyosot, (reprint, taken from the German medical journal *Biologische Medizin*; 1975(4): pp. 374–386) *Bio Ther J Nat Med.* April, 1991. 9(2):pp 121–126.

Maciocia G. The Foundations of Chinese Medicine: A comprehensive text for acupuncturists and herbalists. London: Churchill Livingstone, 1989. p 80.

Meilman E, Krayer O. Clinical studies on veratrum alkaloids I. The action of protoveratrine and veratridine in hypertension. *Circulation.* 1950. 1:pp 204–213.

Reckeweg H. Biotherapeutic Index, pdf version. 1996. pp. 199, 287.

Reckeweg H. Biotherapeutic Index: Ordinatio Antihomotoxica et Materia Medica, 5th ed. Baden-Baden, Germany: Biologische Heilmittel Heel GMBH, 2000. p 272, 364–5, 532.

Reckeweg H. Homeopathia Antihomotoxica Materia Medica, 4th ed. Baden-Baden, Germany: Aurelia-Verlag GMBH, 2002. pp. 162, 172–5, 177, 187, 198, 221, 254, 294, 315–16, 322, 344–5, 358, 362, 366, 378, 410, 416–420, 424, 458–60, 478, 484, 488–90, 508–9, 535, 541, 547, 555–60, 561, 584–5, 610.

Reckeweg H. Gelsemium sempervirens (jasmine) homeopathic single remedy. *Bio Ther.* 1987. 5(2): pp 35–36.

Shelton B. Personal communication in October 2006.

Smit A. Personal communication regarding Reckeweg repertory in October 2007.

KERATOCONJUCTIVITIS SICCA

Definition and cause

Keratoconjuctivitis sicca is deficient tear production, dry eye, and corneal irritation. The condition can be congenital or secondary to trauma, viral infections, metabolic conditions such as diabetes, immune-mediated, or from exposure to medications or toxic substances. Breeds that are more prone are Boston terriers, English bulldogs, Lhasa apsos, Shih tzus, Pekingese, and Pugs. Secondary irritation often leads to corneal and conjunctival irritation, ulceration, edema, vascularization, and pigmentation, and can lead to blindness (Champagne 2003, Salisbury 1995).

Medical therapy rationale, drug(s) of choice, and nutritional recommendations

Medical therapy includes cyclosporine for immune-mediated conditions in combination with artificial tears, or drugs that promote tear formation such as pilocarpine. Topical antibiotics and corticosteroids are recommended with secondary inflammation and infection when no ulceration is present. Surgical transplantation of the parotid salivary duct is now recommended less frequently because of the success of cyclosporine therapy (Champagne 2003, Moore 1999, Salisbury 1995).

Anticipated prognosis

Prognosis is often good; however, lifelong medical therapy may be required (Champagne 2003, Moore 1999, Salisbury 1995).

Integrative veterinary therapies

Damage to the tear glands can occur from many causes such as trauma, pharmaceutical exposure, and viral infections. Loss of adequate tear secretion leads to ocular pain and compromise of the general defense system. Pigmentary deposition and corneal thickening can occur as the body attempts to protect the delicate ocular tissues. Auto-aggressive lymphyocytic attack of lacrimal glandular tissue may lead to reduced tear film formation.

Cyclosporine suppresses the immune response and increases tear production; however, it does not address the inciting or underlying cause(s). An integrative approach uses nutrients, nutraceuticals, medicinal herbs, and combination homeopathics that are anti-inflammatory and tissue-sparing to the cells of the tear duct and the eye and immune-modulating effects on the glands of the immune system.

Nutrition
General considerations/rationale

Therapeutic nutritional therapy can help to reduce and control the underlying inflammatory process, help to balance the immune response, and improve tear production and flow.

Appropriate nutrients

Nutritional/gland therapy: Glandular eye, adrenal, and thymus supply the intrinsic nutrients that help balance immune function, reduce cellular inflammation, and improve tear production and flow (see Gland Therapy, Chapter 2, for a more detailed explanation).

Betasitosterol: Betasitosterol is a plant sterol and immune-modulating agent that has immune-enhancing and anti-inflammatory effects (Bouic 1996, Gupta 1980).

Lutein: A member of the carotenoid family, lutein is a potent antioxidant that is beneficial for eye health (Dagnelie 2000, Seddon 1994).

Chinese herbal medicine/acupuncture
General considerations/rationale

Keratoconjunctivitis sicca is Dryness and Heat in the Lung and Liver. There may be a deficiency of Essence. According to the Western interpretation, the Liver opens to the Eyes in TCM, so Heat or Dryness in the Liver is evident from the signs of keratoconjunctivitis sicca. The Lung is given the task of distributing water, so Dryness and Heat in the Lung can manifest anywhere on the body. Essence is your basic being. It is what you are born with and the potential you have to grow. Western practitioners translate this concept into genetic potential. Animals with a genetic predisposition to develop KCS or congenital KCS are considered to have deficient Essence or a weak genetic constitution.

Appropriate Chinese herbs

Anemarrhena (Zhi mu): Inhibits bacteria and fungi (Yao Xue Qing Bao Tong Xun 1987). Anemarrhena also decreases inflammation. It was shown to increase the level of corticosterone in rat plasma (Chen 1999). This may make it beneficial in decreasing the inflammation in the eye.

Arctium (Niu bang zi): Has anti-inflammatory effects (Zhong Yao Xue 1998). It may help to decrease the inflammation associated with KCS. It also has demonstrated efficacy against some bacteria and fungi (Group of Internal Medicine 1960, Cao 1957).

Chrysanthemum (Ju hua): Has antibiotic activity (Yi Xue Ji Shu Zi Liao 1974). It may be helpful in cases of KCS due to bacterial infections.

Equisetum (Mu zei): Has anti-inflammatory properties (Zhong Yao Xue 1998).

Gypsum (Shi gao): Decreases inflammation. In one study, 126 human patients with inflammatory disease processes were treated with gypsum, and most showed improvement (Zhong Hua Wai Ke Za Zhi 1960).

Platycodon (Jie geng): Has anti-inflammatory properties by virtue of its ability to promote the secretion of corticosterone (Li 1984, Zhang 1984, Zhou 1979).

Prunella (Xia ku cao): Can enlarge the adrenal glands and increase the plasma cortisol level (Jiang 1988). This property may make it effective in counteracting ocular inflammation.

Red peony (Chi shao): Reduces ocular inflammation. It has been shown to reduce redness, swelling, and pain in the eyes (Bao 1999).

Rhubarb (Da huang): Inhibits both aerobic and anaerobic bacteria (Zhao 1999, Yang 1997). It has also shown efficacy against various viruses (Xie 1996). In addition, it has both anti-inflammatory and analgesic properties (Chang Yong Zhong Yao Cheng Fen Yu Yao Li Shou Ce 1994).

Scrophularia (Xuan shen): Inhibits bacteria and some fungi (Chen 1986, Zheng 1960, Cao 1957).

Scutellaria (Huang qin): Contains biacalin, which has antibiotic activity against many bacteria and a few viruses (Zhong Yao Xue 1988, Liu 2000). Biacalin along with a second component of Scutellaria, biacalein, suppress inflammation (Kubo 1984). This suggests that it may have efficacy on the inflammation associated with KCS.

Acupuncture

There are conflicting reports concerning the efficacy of acupuncture for the treatment of KCS. Gronlund et al. (2004) studied a group of 25 people with KSC. The participants were randomly assigned to the acupuncture group or a control group. This study concluded that acupuncture decreased discomfort but did not change any parameters that could be measured, such as tear quantity or quality. The conclusion of the researchers was that acupuncture may be useful as a complement to Western medicine. Niemtzow, et al. (2006) presented case reports of 4 people with KCS of various etiologies and found that the patients who were treated with acupuncture had positive responses. These patients had been receiving Western therapy with little response. When acupuncture was added to the regimen, the number of times the participants needed to apply eye drops decreased significantly.

Homotoxicology
General considerations/rationale

There are no documented antihomotoxic protocols or case reports for treatment of keratoconjunctivitis sicca in animals, but general biological treatment principles can be applied to this disease, which often represents Impregnation to Degeneration phase homotoxicoses. Palmquist has recently seen a German Shepherd dog reverse chronic KCS following deep detoxification therapy. Theoretically, if such cases were caught early in their pathogenesis, it might be possible to reverse the changes before they became permanent. Use of homotoxicology remedies in this fashion should be viewed as experimental, and they may benefit a patient in other ways while failing to cure the keratoconjunctivitis sicca. Use of appropriate pharmaceutical agents is indicated to reduce pain and reverse disease signs in those patients that respond. Artificial tear replacement or surgical transplantation of salivary ducts may be needed in advanced cases.

Appropriate homotoxicology formulas

Classical homeopathy texts list many remedies that may be useful for the complaint of dry eye. Among these are major remedies such as *Aconitum, Aluminum, Arsenicum album, Belladona, Lycopodium, Mezereum, Nux moschata, Opium, Pulsatilla,* and *Nux vomica* (Kent 1999). Antihomotoxic medicants that contain these agents, or that might be useful in such cases, include:

Aconitum homaccord: Used to treat red skin and fever that historically accompanies the dry eye. Fearful pets are another indication for this remedy.

Apis compositum: Contains Apis (see BHI-Eye). Also contains Mercurius sublimates corrosives for keratitis, iritis, and highly acute inflammations of the mucosae of the eyes (Reckeweg 2002).

Arsuraneel: Works through the action of Arsenicum album, (which is also in *Traumeel*), a remedy known to be associated with dry eye in people. It is useful for excoriating discharges, burning coryza, and conjunctivitis with burning secretion (Reckeweg 2002).

Belladonna homaccord: Treats dry eyes (see Mucosa compositum).

BHI-Eye: Useful for ocular fatigue, ocular irritation, and dry and red conjunctivae (Heel 2002). Useful components include Apis, which is indicated in inflammation of the eyes with intense photophobia and increased secretions, and in keratitis with intense chemosis of the conjunctiva. Rhus toxicodendron helps with conjunctivitis, in serious cases of keratitis, and possibly when attempts to open the eyelids are accompanied by a thick, purulent discharge with lacrimation. Aethiops antimonialis is included for scrofulous conjunctivitis with marked photophobia and keratitis (Reckeweg 2002). Belladonna (see *Mucosa compositum*) is also included.

BHI-Lymphatic: Not currently available. Tuberculinum, a useful nosode in conjunctivitis, styes, keratitis, and photophobia, was a component of this remedy (Reckeweg 2002).

BHI-Sinus: Contains Kali iodatum, which has been indicated in keratitis, photophobia, lachrymation, and burning in the eyes. Also contains Cinnabaris (see Nasoheel) (Reckeweg 2002).

Echinacea compositum: An antibacterial. This is indicated in Impregnation Phase disorders; its components include Aconitum, Sulphur, Influenzeum nodode, and Arsenicum album (Reckeweg 2000).

Galium-Heel: A cellular phase remedy that provides support of Deposition and Impregnation phase cases.

Gripp-Heel: Used when viral impregnation is suspected.

Hepar compositum: Contains *Lycopodium*, supports of the liver, and provides detoxification and drainage of hepatic tissues. In Traditional Chinese Medicine, the Eyes and Liver organs are connected, so liver support may benefit ocular conditions.

Lamioflur: Indications include photophobia and sharp, burning secretions. This remedy has an affinity for mucocutaneous junctions. It contains Mezereum (see *Mezereum homaccord*).

Lymphomyosot: Provides lymphatic drainage.

Mezereum homaccord: This remedy is known to assist in the sensation of dry eye and might be considered if other symptom pictures in the case match.

Mucosa compositum: Belladonna can be used in cases of dry eye. Belladonna's typical action on the eyes is well known. It is characterized by special symptoms that arise from atropine poisoning, such as cramps in the muscles of the eyes and eyelids, enlargement of the pupils and, in particular, an inflammatory or irritative condition of the conjunctiva with great photophobia, lachrymation, and pain linked with engorgement of the inner blood vessels. *Mucosa oculi suis* also supports ocular mucosal elements. "*Mucosa compositum®* consists of suis-mucosal extracts from various parts of the body combined with dilutions (8X to 10X) of pancreas and Belladonna, which stimulate the cornea and conjunctiva in specific ways that promote the secretory function, stabilizing it rather than replacing it. The stimuli sent by these substances are a kind of code that helps initiate neuronal stimulation, both locally and centrally" (Sradj 1996).

Nasoheel: Contains Cinnabaris (also in found in *BHI-Sinus*), which has a special reputation in corneal affections, syphilitic iritis, ulcerative destruction of the nasal septum, and chronic blepharitis (Reckeweg 2002).

Oculoheel: Contains the following remedies, and their indications: *Apis mellifica* for conjunctivitis, edema of the eyelids, and hordeolums; Natrium muriaticum for dacrocystitis and burning, and acrid epiphora; Rhus toxicodendron for conjunctivitis with a tendency toward suppurations, edema of the eyelids, and epiphora; Hepar sulfuris for cases with a tendency toward suppurations, chalazions, and hordeolums; Spigelia neuritis for ciliary neuralgia and trigeminal neuralgia; Staphisagria hordeolums in chalazions, blepharoconjunctivitis, and dacrocystitis; and Aethiops mineralis for scrofulous ophthalmia and keratitis (Heel 1996). Palmquist has seen chronic keratoconjunctivitis cases reverse on this formula when used long-term and in conjunction with deep detoxification.

Solidago compositum: The component Arsenicum album is indicated in some cases of dry eye. It also supports renal tissue and provides elimination, which is helpful in Deposition, Impregnation, and Degeneration phase cases. Also contains Mercurius sublimatus corrosives (see *Apis compositum*).

Thyroidea compositum: A phase remedy in Impregnation and Deposition phases.

Tonsilla compositum: Indicated in autoimmune disorders to regulate immune response.

Traumeel S: Used as an anti-inflammatory agent.

Authors' suggested protocols

Nutrition

Eye and immune support formulas: 1 tablet for every 25 pounds of body weight BID.

Betathyme: 1 capsule for every 35 pounds of body weight BID (maximum, 2 capsules BID)

Lutein: 5 mg for every 50 pounds of body weight.

Chinese herbal medicine

Herbal KCS: 1 capsule for every 10 to 20 pounds twice daily. In addition to the herbs mentioned above, Herbal KCS also contains cassia seed (Jue ming zi), lycium bark (Di gu pi), and mulberry bark (Sang bai pi), which help to increase the efficacy of the formula.

The recommended acupuncture points are ST36, SP6, PC6, LI3, LI11, and tai yang.

Homotoxicology

Symptom remedy: BHI-Eye and/or Oculoheel, given orally BID for several weeks. Recently, subconjunctival administration of Mucosa compositum ampules has been successful in treating dry eye (keratoconjunctivitis sicca). Also, Mucosa compositum, Traumeel, and Pure Eye Drops can be mixed and used as eye drops BID to TID topically They can possibly mixed with the patient's own serum.

Psorinoheel: Used as an autosanguis in refractory cases, along with Lamioflur and BHI-Sinus and/or Nasoheel.

Product sources

Nutrition

Eye and immune support formulas: Animal Nutrition Technologies. **Alternatives:** Immune System Support—Standard Process Veterinary Formulas; Immuno Support—Rx Vitamins for Pets; Immugen—Thorne Veterinary Products.

Betathyme: Best for Your Pet. **Alternative:** Moducare—Thorne Veterinary Products.

Lutein (6-mg capsules): Progressive Labs.

Chinese herbal medicine
Formula KCS: Natural Solutions, Inc.

Chinese herbal medicine
BHI/Heel Corporation

REFERENCES

Western medicine references
Champagne ES. Keratoconjunctivits Sicca (KCS), In: Tilley L, Smith F. The 5-Minute Veterinary Consult: Canine and Feline, 2003. Blackwell Publishing.

Moore CP. Diseases and surgery of the lacrimal system. In: Gelatt KN, ed. Veterinary Ophthalmology. Philadelphia: Lippincott Williams and Wilkins 1999:583–607.

Salisbury MA. Keratoconjuctivitis sicca. In: Bonagura JD, Kirk RW, eds. Kirk's Current Veterinary Therapy XII. Small Animal Practice. Toronto: WB Saunders Co. 1995. p. 1231–1239.

IVM/nutrition references
Bouic PJD, et al. Beta-sitosterol and beta-sitosterol glucoside stimulate human peripheral blood lymphocyte proliferation: Implications for their use as an immunomodulatory vitamin combination. *International Journal of Immunopharmacology* 1996; 18:693–700.

Dagnelie G, Zorge IS, McDonald TM. Lutein improves visual function in some retinal degeneration patients: a pilot study via Internet. *Optometry* 2000, 71, 147–64.

Gupta MB, Nath R, Srivastava N, et al. Anti-inflammatory and antipyretic activities of β-sitosterol. *Planta Medica* 1980;39:157–163.

Seddon JM, Ajani UA, Sperduto RD, et al. Dietary carotenoids, vitamins A, C, and E, and advanced age-related macular degeneration. *JAMA* 1994;272:1413–20.

Chinese herbal medicine/acupuncture references
Bao GY, et al. Treating 32 cases of retinal vein obstruction with Xue Fu Zhu Yu Tang. *Henan Journal of TCM.* 1999.

Cao RL, et al. *China Journal of Dermatology.* 1957;(4):286.

Chang Yong Zhong Yao Cheng Fen Yu Yao Li Shou Ce (A Handbook of the Composition and Pharmacology of Common Chinese Drugs), 1994; 226:323.

Chen SY, et al. *Fujian Journal of Chinese Medicine.* 1986; 17(4):57.

Chen WS, et al. *Journal of Second Military Medical College.* 1999;20(10):758–760.

Gronlund MA, Stenevi U, Lundeberg T. Acupuncture treatment in patients with keratoconjunctivitis sicca: a pilot study. *Acta Ophthalmol Scand* 2004;82(3 Pt 1):283–90.

Group of Internal Medicine, Chongqing Medical University Hospital, No. 1. *Journal of Microbiology.* 1960;8(1):52.

Jiang Y, et al. *Gansu Journal of TCM.* 1988;7(4):4–7.

Kubo M, Matsuda H, Tanaka M, Kimura Y, Okuda H, Higashino M, Tani T, Namba K, Arichi S. Studies on Scutellariae radix. VII. Anti-arthritic and anti-inflammatory actions of methanolic extract and flavonoid components from Scutellariae radix. *Chem Pharm Bull*, 1984; 32(7):2724–9.

Li YF (translator). Foreign Medicine, vol. of TCM. 1984;6(1): 15–18.

Liu IX, Durham DG, Richards RM. Baicalin synergy with beta-lactam antibiotics against methicillin-resistant Staphylococcus aureus and other beta-lactam-resistant strains of S. aureus. *J Pharm Pharmacol.* 2000 Mar;52(3):361–6.

Niemtzow RC, Kempf KJ, Johnstone, PAS. *Medical Acupuncture Online Journal* Volume 13 Number 3. http://www. medicalacupuncture.org/aama_maf/journal/vol13_3/case3. html Accessed 10/22/2006.

Xie YY, et al. *Journal of Shandong Medical University.* 1996;34(2):166–169.

Yang SZ, et al. *Liaoning Journal of Traditional Chinese Medicine.* 1997;24(4):187.

Yao Xue Qing Bao Tong Xun (*Journal of Herbal Information*), 1987; 5(4):62.

Yi Xue Ji Shu Zi Liao (*Resource of Medical Techniques*), 1974;(1:2):113.

Zhang SC, et al. *Journal of Chinese Patent Medicine Research.* 1984;(2):37.

Zhao MJ, et al. *Zhejiang Journal of Traditional Chinese Medicine.* 1999;34(12):544.

Zheng QY, et al. *Pharmacy Bulletin.* 1960;8(2):57.

Zhong Hua Wai Ke Za Zhi (*Chinese Journal of External Medicine*), 1960;4:366.

Zhong Yao Xue (*Chinese Herbology*), 1988; 137:140.

Zhong Yao Xue (*Chinese Herbology*), 1998; 91:92.

Zhong Yao Xue (*Chinese Herbology*), 1998; 109:110.

Zhou WZ, et al. *Pharmacy Bulletin.* 1979;14(5):202–203.

Homotoxicology references
Heel. BHI Homeopathic Therapy: Professional Reference. Albuquerque, NM: Heel Inc. 2002. p 56.

Kent J. Repertory of the Homeopathic Materia Medica and a Word Index. Paharganj, New Delhi: B. Jain, LTD, 1921. p 238.

Heel. 1996. Biotherapeutic Index on CD in pdf format.

Reckeweg H. Biotherapeutic Index: Ordinatio Antihomotoxica et Materia Medica, 5th ed. Baden-Baden, Germany: Biologische Heilmittel Heel GMBH, 2000. pp 330–2.

Reckeweg H. Homeopathia Antihomotoxica Materia Medica, 4th ed. Baden-Baden, Germany: Arelia-Verlag GMBH, 2002. pp. 125, 150–2, 172–3, 419,420, 512–14, 583.

Sradj N. The Neuropsychoimmunology of Kerato-conjunctivitis Sicca and its Treatment with a Homeopathic Preparation. Reprinted from *Biologische Medizin.* 1998. 6 (1996 Deczember):264–67, *Biomedical Therapy.*

PROGRESSIVE RETINAL ATROPHY/ RETINAL DEGENERATION

Definition and cause

Progressive Retinal Atrophy (PRA) is an inherited group of diseases of the retina. It usually begins early on as retinal dysplasia, or it can occur after the retina has fully matured (usually after 12 weeks of age). PRA can be related to a physical change in the retina or a nutritional deficiency or metabolic defect, or it can be secondary to a local, diffuse, or cellular autoimmune inflammatory process. In dogs it can be an inherited (autosomal recessive) disease that commonly affects collies, Irish setters, miniature poodles, cocker spaniels, and Labrador retrievers. In cats it can be autosomal dominant or recessive and more commonly affects Abyssinians.

Other causes of PRA can have a nutritional component. Experimental deficiencies of vitamins A and E can cause a partial degeneration of the retina. In cats, a taurine deficiency can cause retinal degeneration. Most veterinary ophthalmologists do not recommend nutritional supplementation because there have been no studies to substantiate their effectiveness or benefit (Glaze 1999, Narfström 1999, Smith 2003).

Medical therapy rationale, drug(s) of choice, and nutritional recommendations

No medical therapies have been proven effective. Pyridoxine supplementation in cats for ornithine aminotransferase deficiency may increase the activity of the enzyme; however, it has not been proven to reverse the degeneration. Supplementing cats' daily diets with proper levels of taurine may halt the progression in taurine-deficient retinopathy.

Anticipated prognosis

Inherited PRA progresses to complete blindness. The progression is often slow enough for the patient to adapt to visual loss and is most often nonpainful, unless complicated with other conditions such as cataract formation or glaucoma. A degenerative process from previous inflammation or trauma usually does not progress unless a systemic disease such as uveodermatologic syndrome, blastomycosis, or toxoplasmosis causes persistent inflammation.

Integrative veterinary therapies

PRA appears to be a progressive degenerative process that is related to a local/cellular autoimmune reaction. There is often a genetic predisposition to the retina as the target organ. As such, the initial free-radical-induced inflammation occurs locally in the retina, followed by a cascading, diffuse inflammatory process, leading to destruction of the rods and cones of the retina and finally loss of sight. Although the literature clearly states that there is no treatment for retinal degeneration and that blindness is inevitable, some veterinary ophthalmologists believe that nutritional antioxidant supplementation may slow the degeneration of the retina. In addition, specific herbal and homeopathic remedies may add to the neutralizing of the cellular inflammation with a slowing of the autoimmune attack of the retinal tissue.

Nutrition
General considerations/rationale

Early nutritional therapy can help to reduce free radical production, control the underlying inflammatory process, and nourish the cells of the retina in an attempt to slow down the degenerative process and preserve cellular integrity.

Appropriate nutrients

Nutritional/gland therapy: Glandular eye and liver supply the intrinsic nutrients to reduce cellular inflammation, improve organ function, and slow degeneration (see Gland Therapy in Chapter 2 for a more detailed explanation).

Taurine: Dietary supplementation with taurine has led to clinical improvement in cats with retinal and cardiac disease (Kramer 1995, Monson 1989, Pion 1987).

Essential fatty acids: Proper levels of essential fatty acids, particularly DHA and EPA, are essential for healthy eye function and retinal development (Pawlosky 1997). Hemp oil is a plant-derived oil that is high in both linoleic (LA) and linolenic (LNA) fatty acids, which are the building blocks for the longer chained eicosapentaenoic (EPA) and docosahexaenoic acid (DHA). The analysis of hemp oil shows that more than 70% is polyunsaturated fatty acids and less than 20% saturated fats, making it extremely low in saturated fats (Kralovansky 1994, Weil 1993). Because of its high level of gamma linolenic acid (GLA), hemp oil is being investigated for it beneficial effects on immune function (Horrobin 1992).

Lutein: A member of the carotenoid family, lutein is a potent antioxidant that is beneficial for eye health. Seddon (1994) showed that people who received lutein showed a decreased risk of macular degeneration and had increased protection of the eye. Hankinson (1992) showed that lower levels of lutein were associated with increased risk of cataract. Dagnelie (2000) found that people with retinitis pigmentosa (RP) showed a significant improvement in visual acuity with lutein supplementation.

Flavonoids: Quercetin has been shown to lessen the progression of diabetic retinopathy (Varma 1986).

Another group of flavonoids, proanthocyanidans (POCs), which come from grape seeds or pine bark, have also been shown to limit the progression of retinopathy (Fromantin 1981, Verin 1978).

Chinese herbal medicine
General considerations/rationale
Traditional Chinese Medicine theory holds that retinal degeneration is due to Blood and Yin deficiency of the Liver and Kidney. There may also be some Liver Qi stagnation involved. The Liver opens to the Eyes and the Kidney nourishes the Liver. If the Kidney and Liver are not nourished, the Eyes show pathology. Liver Qi stagnation may describe pain if it is present. The Western understanding of herbal supplements has shown that herbs can be used to increase circulation, improve cellular nourishment, and help to reduce inflammation of the retina. Chinese herbal remedies for retinal degeneration may include some of the herbs listed below. Some of these herbs have been shown to improve circulation, thereby improving nourishment of the retina, while others have been shown to decrease inflammation and swelling. Studies have shown improvement in vision, even though the specific chemical component(s) of the herbs was not identified as being responsible for the effect.

Appropriate Chinese herbs
Astragalus (Huang qi): Increases red blood cell production to increase nutrition to the retina (Nan Jiang Zhong Yi Xue Yuan Xue Bao 1989). It also decreases immune disorders (Yun Nan Zhong Yi Za Zhi (1980).

Dendrobium (Shi hu): Nourishes the retina. Several studies have shown improvement in vision in diabetics with retinal degeneration who are given formulas containing dendrobium (Wang 1999, Ling 1999, Yang 2001).

Red peony (Chi shao): Reduces redness, swelling, and pain in the eyes. It is a component of formulas used to decrease retinal vein occlusion (Bao 1999).

Chinese wolfberry (Gou ji zi): Has more betacarotene than carrots. It contains zeaxanthin, which is related to lutein. It protects the retina by neutralizing free radicals from sunlight (Cheng 2005).

Ophiopogon (mai men dong): Shows a marked decrease in blurred vision, as was seen in elderly people given ophiopogon (Zhong Gou Zhong Yao Za Zhi 1992).

The following herbs have been shown to decrease inflammation: prinsepia (Rui ren rou), angelica root (Dang gui) (Yao Xue Za Zhi, 1971), White peony (Bai shao) (Zhong Yao Zhi 1993), peach kernel (Tao ren) (Zhong Yao Tong Bao 1986), cimicifuga (Sheng ma) (Zhong Yao Xue 1998), fresh rehmannia root (Sheng di huang) (Zhong Yao Yao Li Yu Ying Yong 1983), and ligustrum (Nu zhen zi) (Zhong Guo Zhong Yao Za Zhi, 1989).

Homotoxicology
General considerations/rationale
Retinal degeneration is a Degeneration Phase disorder with an Inflammation or Impregnation phase early in the onset. Improvement of circulation and reduction in reactive oxygen species are critical to slowing the progress of such disorders. Placenta compositum, Aesculus compositum, Secale compositum, and/or Cerebrum compositum may be helpful but have not been researched for this condition. These are general support remedies for the circulatory function of the eye, and have been used clinically by European practitioners, but there is no current research data that defines their use.

Appropriate homotoxicology remedies
As noted earlier, there are no reports documenting successful use of homotoxicology to reverse retinal atrophy. Therapy depends upon the primary pathological processes involved. Once a primary diagnosis is made, every attempt should be made to determine which conditions are causal. Based upon primary causation the following options are available for consideration:

Lymphomyosot: Use if the condition is inflammatory or autoaggressive in nature.

Oculoheel or BHI-Eye: Used for general ocular support.

For most cases, use:

Psorinoheel, Lymphomyosot, Galium-Heel: Use if the conditions hereditary. (There are not many options for hereditary cases except those that offer general support and detoxification).

Traumeel, Spigelon, Gelsemium, Phosphor homaccord, Galium-Heel, Ubichinon compositum, Phosphor homaccord, Coenzyme compositum: Use if the condition is due to metabolic/mitochondrial defects.

Veratrum homaccord, Scwef-Heel, Ubichinon compositum, Coenzyme compositum: Use for Degeneration Phase disorders.

Authors' suggested protocols
Nutrition
Eye and liver support formulas: 1 tablet for every 25 pounds of body weight BID.

Eskimo fish oil: One-half to 1 teaspoon per meal for cats. 1 teaspoon for every 35 pounds of body weight for dogs.

Taurine: 500 mg for every 20 pounds of body weight daily.

Lutein: 5 mg for every 50 pounds of body weight.

Quercetin: 35 mg for every 10 pounds of body weight SID.

Proanthocyanidans (PCOs): 20 mg for every 10 pounds of body weight daily.

Chinese herbal medicine

Retinal degeneration: 1 capsule for every 10 pounds of body weight BID.

Note for Chinese herbal formulation: In addition to the herbs listed above, the authors suggest an herbal preparation that contains the following herbs: codonopsis (dang shen), tribulus (bai ji li), carthamus (hong hua), leeches (shui zhi), eriocaulis (gu jing cao), equisetum (mu zhi), earthworm (di long), mugwort (liu ji nu), liquid amber (lu lu tong), scorpion (quan xie), and centipede (wu gong). These herbs help balance the formula, making it more specific for the intended clinical condition while minimizing potential side effects that are inherent in some multiple herbal formulations.

Homotoxicology

BHI-Eye, Traumeel, and Lymphomyosot: Mixed together; 1 dropper given BID.

Product sources

Nutrition

Eye and liver support formulas: Animal Nutrition Technologies. **Alternatives:** Hepatic Support—Standard Process Veterinary Formulas; Hepato Support—Rx Vitamins for Pets; Hepagen—Thorne Veterinary Products.

Lutein: Progressive Labs.

Eskimo fish oil: Tyler Encapsulations.

Quercetin: Source Naturals; Quercitone—Thorne Veterinary Products.

Antiox (PCO): Vetri Science.

Chinese herbal medicine

Retinal Degeneration: Natural Solutions, Inc.

Homotoxicology

BHI/Heel Inc.

REFERENCES

Western medicine references

Aguirre G, Progressive Retinal Atrophy (PRA) in Bernese Mountain Dogs, PRA Task Force of the BMDCA.

Glaze MB, Gelatt KN. Feline Ophthalmology. In: Gelatt KN, ed. Veterinary Ophthalmology, 3rd ed., (Baltimore: Lippincott, Williams and Wilkins). 1999. 997–1052.

Narfström K, Ekesten B. Diseases of the canine ocular fundus. In: Gelatt KN, ed., Veterinary Ophthalmology 3rd ed. Philadelphia: Lippincott Williams and Wilkins 1999;869–933.

Smith PJ. In: Tilley L, Smith FWK. The 5-Minute Veterinary Consult, Lippincott Williams and Wilkins, 2003.

Nutrition references

Davidson MG, Feoli FJ, Gilger BC, McLellan GJ, Whitley W. Retinal degeneration associated with Vitamin E deficiency in hunting dogs: *JAVMA* 1998; 213:645–651.

Kramer GA, Kittleson MD, Fox PR, Lewis J, Pion PD. Plasma taurine concentrations in normal and in dogs with heart disease. *J Vet Intern Med* 1995;9(4):253–258.

Monson W. Taurine's Role in the Health of Cats. *Vet. Med.*, Oct. 1989; 84(10): 1013–105.

Pion PD, Kittleson MD, Rogers QR, et al. Myocardial failure in cats associated with low plasma taurine: a reversible cardiomyopathy. *Science* 1987;237:764–768.

Pawlosky RJ, et al. Retinal and brain accretion of long-chain polyunsaturated fatty acids in developing felines: the effects of corn-based maternal diets. *Am J Clin Nutr* 1997;65:465–72.

Dagnelie G, Zorge IS, McDonald TM. Lutein improves visual function in some retinal degeneration patients: a pilot study via Internet. *Optometry* 2000;71, 147–64.

Chinese herbal medicine/acupuncture references

Bao GY, et al. Treating 32 cases of retinal vein obstruction with Xue Fu Zhu Yu Tang. *Henan Journal of TCM.* 1999;19(5):48–49.

Cheng et al. Fasting Plasma Zeaxanthin Response to Fructus Barbarum L. (Wolfberry; Kei Tze) in a Food-based Human Supplementation Trial. *British Journal of Nutrition* 2005; 93, 123–130.

Ling B. The Treatment of Diabetic Retinal Bleeding with Integrated Chinese-Western Medicine, Bei Jing Zhong Yi (*Beijing Chinese Medicine*), 3; 1999, p. 17–18.

Nan Jiang Zhong Yi Xue Yuan Xue Bao (*Journal of Nan Jing University of Traditional Chinese Medicine*), 1989; 1:43.

Wang D. The Treatment of 161 Cases of Diabetic Retinal Bleeding with Dan Qi Di Huang Tang (Salvia, Pseudoginseng and Rehmannia Decoction), Bei Jing Zhong Yi (Beijing Chinese Medicine), 5, 1999, p. 25–26.

Yang H, Yang Jian-hua. Clinical and TCD Observations on Frequency Spectrum of Ophthalmic Arterial Blood Flow in 61 Eyes with Diabetic Retinopathy Treated with Yi Shen Huo Xue Fang (Boost the Kidneys and Quicken the Blood Formula), Zhe Jiang Zhong Yi Za Zhi (*Zhejiang Journal of Chinese Medicine*), #1, 2001, p. 30–31.

Yao Xue Za Zhi (*Journal of Medicinals*), 1971; (91):1098.

Yun Nan Zhong Yi Za Zhi (*Yun Nan Journal of Chinese Medicine*), 1980; 2: 28.

Zhong Gou Zhong Yao Za Zhi (*People's Republic of China Journal of Chinese Herbology*) 1992; 17 (1):21.

Zhong Guo Zhong Yao Za Zhi (*People's Republic of China Journal of Chinese Herbology*), 1989; 14(7):47.

Zhong Yao Tong Bao (*Journal of Chinese Herbology*), 1986; 11 (11):37.

Zhong Yao Xue (*Chinese Herbology*), 1998; 106:108.

Zhong Yao Yao Li Yu Ying Yong (*Pharmacology and Applications of Chinese Herbs*), 1983:400.

Zhong Yao Zhi (*Chinese Herbology Journal*), 1993:183.

Homotoxicology references

Bianchi I. Homeopathic Homotoxicological Repertory. Aurelia Publishers, 1995. p. 117.

Reckeweg H. Biotherapeutic Index: Ordinatio Antihomotoxica et Materia Medica, 5th ed. Baden-Baden, Germany: Biologische Heilmittel Heel GMBH, 2000. p. 108.

Reckeweg H. Biotherapeutic Index: Ordinatio Antihomotoxica et Materia Medica, 5th ed. Baden-Baden, Germany: Biologische Heilmittel Heel GMBH, 2000. p. 236.

Heel. Practitioner's Handbook of Homotoxicology, 1st U.S. edition, 2003. p. 255.

Sradj N. Retinopathy (Pigmentary). Heel Protocols, CD compilation.

EAR MITES

Definition and cause

Ear mites are cause by Otodectes cynotis, and they cause a severe inflammation and waxy accumulation in the external ear canal of both dogs and cats. Secondary to the self-trauma, the pinnae and face can become excoriated (Scott 1995).

Medical therapy rationale, drug(s) of choice, and nutritional recommendations

After a thorough cleansing to remove the accumulated waxy build-up, the treatment is instilling a preparation that contains a chemical insecticide such as Pyrethrin or Ivermectin, as well as medications to soothe the ear and dissolve the wax.

Anticipated prognosis

If detected early before self-trauma of the ear and the potential to damage the eardrum, the prognosis is excellent.

Integrative veterinary therapies

Ear mites colonize the ear canal of cats, dogs, and many other mammalian species. Secondary infections are common, and ear mites are commonly encountered in clinical practice. Medical therapy is usually curative; however, chronic ear infections may result and integrative therapies can be helpful in reducing inflammation, protecting local cells and tissues, and improving general immune function.

Nutrition
General considerations/rationale

Nutritional support should be in combination with medical management to help reduce inflammation, boost immune function, and prevent chronic secondary infections.

Appropriate nutrients

Nutrition/gland therapy: Supports the ear and glands of the immune system in combination with antioxidants such as vitamins E, A, and C, which help prevent chronic infections.

Chinese herbal medicine
General considerations/rationale

Practitioners of TCM recognize ear mites to be external parasites.

Appropriate Chinese herbs

Cnidium fruit (She chuang zi): An effective antipruritic (Lin Chuang Pi Fu Ke Za Zhi 1983).

Dictamnus (Bai xian pi): Used for dermatological conditions. In one trial it was used to treat 45 people with chronic eczema as part of a formula called Qu Feng Zhi Yang (dispelling wind-pathogen and relieving itching) decoction. In addition to dictamnus, this formula contains Qin jiao (gentian root), Huang bo (sophora), Di Fu Zi (Kochia), Sheng Di Huang (rehmannia root), Wei Ling Xian (clematis), Huai Hua (Flos sophorae), Cang Er Zi (Xanthium), Chen Pi (citrus peel), Gan Cao (licorice), and Ku Shen (sophora root).

Qing Dai San, which contains dioscoria (Shan yao), dragons bones (Long gu), oyster shell (Mu li), cuttlebone (Hai Piao xiao), and madder (Qian cao gen), was applied topically. Fifty-eight percent of the patients had complete recovery, while another 24% improved (Wang 2000).

Realgar (Xiong huang): Has been used in moist types of skin lesions as part of a patent formula called San Huang Lotion. In addition to realgar, san huang lotion contains Da Feng Zi (hydnocarpi), Fang Feng (siler), Bai Xuan Pi (dittany bark), Huang Bo (phellodendrom), Huang Qin (scutellaria), and Ku Shen (sophora root). Of 54 patients, 51% had complete resolution of lesions, and another 33% improved (Dong 1999).

Sophora root (Ku shen): Effective against rashes, itching, and eczema (Zhong Cao Yao Tong Xun 1976).

Sulfur (Liu huang): A commonly used substance in dermatology (Gupta 2004). There is anecdotal evidence that it may have activity against mites (Ayres 1986).

Homotoxicology
General considerations/rationale

Ear mite infestation initially constitutes an Excretion Phase disorder and the body's physiological response is to increase ceruminous and glandular secretion within the ear canal. Secondary infections may ensue as a result of accumulation of desquamated skin, mite waste, and bacteria. The bacterial species involved are not generally malignant and are attempting to reduce the quantities of Excretion Phase byproducts. Long-term infections resulting from untreated ear mite infestations can lead to Deposition Phase, Impregnation Phase, and Degeneration Phase disorders in extreme cases. Conventional treatment involves cleaning the debris from the ear canal, treating any infection present, and using an acaricidal product. Environmental controls may be needed.

There is no evidence-based antihomotoxic agent for specific treatment of ear mites. Homotoxicology can be used to manage other symptoms and help remove homotoxins from the affected tissue.

Appropriate homotoxicology formulas

Clean ears with appropriate solutions and apply an acaracidal agent. Formulas to consider:

Belladonna homaccord: Treats severely red ear canals with localized inflammation.

Echinacea compositum: Used in cases with secondary bacterial otitis and suppurative discharges.

Graphites homaccord: Used in greasy cases with pigmentation and slow healing.

Psorinoheel: An Excretion Phase remedy.

Traumeel S: Reduces irritation and inflammation and speeds healing.

Authors' suggested protocols

Nutrition

Ear and immune support formulas: 1 tablet for every 25 pounds of body weight BID.

Chinese herbal medicine

The authors use herbal ear mite solution. The powder is mixed with water and cooked; then the solution is used to clean ears BID for 1 week. In addition to the herbs cited above, ear mite contains alum (Ming fan), bunge prickly ash peel (Hua jiao), indigo (Qing dai), and phellodendron bark (Huang bai), which increase the efficacy of the formulation.

Homotoxicology

In addition to standard ear cleaning and acaracidal therapy:

Sulfur-Heel: May aid in the intense itching phase and improve healing.

Traumeel S: Use orally or in the ear directly (oral vial, 5 drops orally and 5 drops in the ear canal) BID for cases with extreme inflammation.

Product sources

Nutrition

Ear and immune support formulas: Animal Nutrition Technologies. **Alternatives**: Immune System Support—Standard Process Veterinary Formulas; Immuno Support—Rx Vitamins for Pets; Immugen—Thorne Veterinary Products.

Chinese herbal medicine

Herbal ear mite solution: Natural Solutions, Inc.

Homotoxicology
BHI/Heel Corporation

REFERENCES

Western medicine reference
Scott DW, Miller WH, Griffin CE. Muller and Kirk's small animal dermatology, 5th ed. Philadelphia: Saunders, 1995.

Chinese herbal medicine/acupuncture references
Ayres S Jr. Demodex folliculorum as a pathogen. *Cutis* 1986; 37:441.
Dong XT, et al. 54 cases of eczema treated with San Huang Lotion. *Journal of Changchun College of TCM.* 1999;15(3):43.
Gupta A, Nicol K. The Use of Sulfur in Dermatology. *J of Drugs in Dermatology* 2004;July-Aug.
Lin Chuang Pi Fu Ke Za Zhi (*Journal of Clinical Dermatology*), 1983; 1:15.
Wang YY. 45 cases of chronic eczema treated with Qu Feng Zhi Yang Tang. *Heilongiang Journal of Traditional Chinese Medicine and Pharmacology.* 2000;(2):27.
Zhong Cao Yao Tong Xun (*Journal of Chinese Herbal Medicine*), 1976; 1:35.

EXTERNAL OTITIS

Definition and cause

An inflammatory process of the external ear canal. Causes can be allergic, parasitic, auto-immune, mechanical, foreign bodies, and neoplasia. Secondary bacterial infections are common (Griffin 1993, Werner 2003).

A proper diagnostic approach is needed to best handle otitis externa. Otoscopic examination is vital to determine the extent of the disease. Otitis media should be identified and properly treated because it can lead to otitis externa. The state of the tympanic membrane should be noted because selection of topical agents is drastically affected by the presence of an open tympanum. Cytology of the ear canal exudates gives vital information as to the precise nature of the pathogens present. Thyroid and other endocrine testing may be needed in recurrent cases. Culture and sensitivity may be needed to properly evaluate the antimicrobial therapy selected.

Medical therapy rationale, drug(s) of choice, and nutritional recommendations

Systemic and topical antibiotics, anti-inflammatories, antifungal, and/or anti-parasitic medications are all recommended based upon proper diagnostics and a full determination of the underlying cause(s).

Anticipated prognosis

The prognosis depends upon the stage of diagnosis and phase of disease. The prognosis for both external otitis and otitis media is good so long as there are no underlying complications such as stenosis of the canal. Recurrences are common (Griffin 1993, Werner 2003).

Integrative veterinary therapies

Chronic otitis externa with severe scarring and polyp formation carries a poor prognosis for cure, and the client should be advised that chronic maintenance (and not cure) is the goal in such cases. However, some cases make remarkable improvement once they are allowed to activate inflammation and undergo exudative processes with proper nutritional and biological therapy, so integrative treatments are a good option.

In simple infections, cleaning the ear may be all that is required. While antibiotic, anti-inflammatory, and antifungal agents are frequently used, these do not cure the predisposing cause. Rather, they only serve to suppress the symptoms of inflammation and allow for the return of homeostasis. This type of otitis externa has been observed in the period following routine vaccinations and likely represents regressive vicariation and healing. Biological therapy assists these cases greatly on their path to wellness (see Homotoxicology, below).

Exudative discharges must be removed regularly because they contain proinflammatory and toxic material. Bacteria and yeast rapidly overpopulate such environments in response to the increased nutrients provided by these exudates.

Nutrition
General considerations/rationale

Nutritional support should occur in combination with medical management to help reduce inflammation, boost immune function, and prevent chronic secondary infections.

Appropriate nutrients

Nutrition/gland therapy: Gland therapy to support the ear and glands of the immune system in combination with antioxidants such as vitamins E, A, and C are beneficial in preventing chronic infections.

Chinese herbal medicine/acupuncture
General considerations/rationale

External otitis is due to Damp and Heat in the Liver with Blood deficiency, leading to internal Wind. Damp and Heat are the purulent debris and inflammation is seen in the ear canal. If there is an accompanying Blood deficiency, the Liver is not nourished. When the Liver is not nourished there is a fluid (Yin) deficiency. Because Yin and Yang are supposed to be in balance, a Yin deficiency means there is a relative Yang excess. Yang is Heat. One can envision this Heat rising up and causing Wind, just as a fire can cause wind gusts. One can liken the wind blowing trees to the gait of a swaying ataxic individual. Internal Wind or Wind generated inside the body can lead to dizziness. In Western terms, this is the dizziness, and ataxia is seen when otitis externa extends into the middle ear.

Treatment is aimed at eliminating the underlying cause of the otitis (bacteria, fungi, inhaled allergens, etc.), decreasing inflammation, and controlling pain.

Appropriate Chinese herbs

Angelica (Bai zi): Has anti-inflammatory properties (Zhong Guo Zhong Yao Za Zhi 1991).

Atractylodes (Cang zhu): Has activity against Staphylococcus auerus and dermatophytes (Zhong Yao Xue (Chinese Herbology 1998).

Bupleurum (Chai hu): Decreases the effect of histamine release (Zhong Yao Yao Li Yu Ying Yong 1983) and has antibiotic effects against streptococci (Zhong Yao Xue 1998).

Cicada slough (Chan tui): Has been used successfully in humans to treat chronic urticaria (Pi fu Bing Fang Zhi Yan Jiu Tong Xun 1972). It may be useful in decreasing the inflammation of the lining of the aural canal.

Honeysuckle (Jin yin hua): Has antibiotic effects against Staphylococcus aureus, E. coli, and Pseudomonas aeruginosa (Xin Yi Xue 1975), and is anti-inflammatory (Shan Xi Yi Kan 1960).

Licorice (Gan cao): Inhibits the growth of Staphylococcus aureus (Zhong Yao Zhi 1993). It contains glycyrrhizine and glycyrrhentinic acid, which have corticosteroid activity (Zhong Cao Yao 1991).

Mint (Bo he): Relieves itching (Zhong Cao Yao Xue 1980) and has anti-inflammatory effects (Zhong Yao Xue 1998).

Moutan (Mu dan pi): Demonstrates anti-inflammatory actions via inhibition of prostaglandin synthesis and decreases vascular permeability (Sheng Yao Xue Za Zhi 1979, Zhong Guo Yao Ke Da Xue Xue Bao 1990). It inhibits the growth of Staphylococcus aureus, streptococci, and dermatophytes (Zhong Yao Cai 1991).

Platycodon (Jie geng): Decreases allergic reactions (Zhong Yao Yao Li Yu Ying Yong 1983).

Poria (Fu ling): Has inhibitory effects on Staphylococcus aureus (Zhong Yao Cai 1985).

Rehmannia (Sheng di huang): Has shown anti-inflammatory activity in mice (Zhong Yao Yao Li Yu Ying Yong 1983).

Siegesbeckia (Xi xian cao): Inhibits the growth of Staphylococcus aureus (Kim 1979).

White peony (Bai shao): Contains paeoniflorin, which is a strong anti-inflammatory (Zhong Yao Zhi 1993). It also has antibiotic effects against Staphylococcus aureus, some streptococci, E. coli, Pseudomonas aeruginosa, and some dermatophytes (Xin Zhong Yi 1989).

There are few reports in the literature concerning the use of acupuncture to treat otitis. Yu (1990) used acupuncture to treat 81 people with suppurative otitis with some success.

Homotoxicology
General considerations/rationale

Eighty-five percent of otitis externa cases are allergic in origin (food, inhalant, contact, flea, etc.). Allergies and many adverse reactions to drugs are Impregnation Phase homotoxicoses. Mild ear infections can occur and are Inflammation Phase conditions. Careful history and physical evaluation are advised, and therapy for allergies should be discussed with the client (also see Allergy protocols).

In some homotoxicoses, particularly Deposition, Impregnation, and Degeneration phases, an inflammatory response may be required so that homotoxins—and tissue damaged by homotoxins—may be removed and repaired. This process involves redness, itching, and discharge.

The discharge ordinarily begins as a crusty, waxy, greasy-type material and progresses to lighter, oily material, and finally to pus or serous exudates. These stages can be seen in patients recovering biologically from Impregnation Phase diseases and must be gently handled with biological agents instead of suppressive drug therapy for optimum results to occur. In otitis in which pigmentation is noted, the client should be advised that inflammation will likely follow successful biological therapy, and if a client is unwilling to proceed, such therapy should be avoided.

Zymox is an effective agent in many of these cases, and does not interfere biologically with healing. Pavia wound care ointment is also extremely helpful in assisting patients that are undergoing regressive vicariation. It should be used in the ear for no more than 5 days and discontinued. After use of Pavia wound cream, a thick, waxy discharge will occur that requires gentle removal for approximately 5 days. In responsive cases rapid change occurs following this treatment. If the condition worsens, then use conventional medications to get it under control.

Appropriate homotoxicology formulas

Belladonna homaccord: Used for focal, intensely red areas of inflammation and for reactions following vaccinations.

BHI-Ear: Same remedy as *BHI-Chamomilla*, used for otitis media and externa. In mild cases this remedy alone may suffice. Contains Aconitum (also in *Aconitum homac-*cord, *Barijodeel, Echinacea compositum, Traumeel, BHI-Chamomilla Complex, BHI-FluPlus*, and others) for surges of blood toward various organs, with a tendency for the capillaries to rupture. This results in petechial hemorrhages in the nasal and respiratory mucosa, catarrhs, neuralgic symptoms with paraesthesia, hyperthermia, encephalitis with very high temperatures (e.g., post-vaccinial encephalitis), and chronic middle-ear infections. Capsicum (also contained in *Sulphur-Heel*, etc.) is indicated for ulcerative glossitis, aphthae, pharyngitis, mastoiditis, purulent acute otitis media, and other Reactive Phases. Chamomilla (contained in *Traumeel, Calcoheel, BHI-Calming, BHI-Ear*, etc.) is particularly suited to states of nervous agitation as a tranquillizing remedy and for painful states such as toothache, catarrhs of the middle ear, rheumatism, and others. The typical Chamomilla earaches are pressive and tearing, and the ears are especially sensitive to cold air. Thus, it is useful in inflammatory illness (Inflammation Phase), in this case, otitis media, with violent episodes of pain, and other painful conditions.

The ingredient Ferrum phosphoricum (also in *Ferrum homaccord, Tonsilla compositum*, etc.) is indicated for feverish states, otitis media, pneumonia, or other feverish, inflammatory diseases of the respiratory organs. Hepar sulphuris calcareum (also in *Belladonna homaccord, Cantharis compositum, Coenzyme compositum, Echinacea compositum, Euphorbium compositum, Mercurius-Heel, Traumeel, BHI-Enzyme, BHI-Infection, BHI-Inflammation*, and *BHI-Injury*) is indicated for the following symptoms: hypersensitivity to touch, pain and cold air, and the tendency to suppuration or inflammation which rapidly changes to suppuration. Hepar sulph is also a remedy for chronic catarrhs of the respiratory organs, inflammation and suppuration of the skin and mucosae such as furuncles and pyoderma, and chronic purulent offensive discharge from the ears (possibly along with Graphites and other remedies), otitis media, and abscess of the palatine tonsils.

Plantago major (also in *Viburcol*, etc.) is for treatment of a disposition to lymphatic disorders The main indications are: otitis media, mastoiditis and post-operative fistulae, and skin rashes. Pulsatilla (in *Abropernol, Causticum compositum, Coenzyme compositum, Cruroheel, Echinacea compositum, Euphorbium compositum, Mucosa compositum, Thyreoidia compositum, Tonsilla compositum, Viburcol, BHI-Enzyme, BHI-Inflammation, BHI-Sinus*, and many others) is indicated when eyelids are inflamed and there is itching with lacrimation. The external auditory canal may also be swollen and inflamed, as may the nasal mucosa. This is also indicated for otitis media with violent, stinging, pulsating pain; skin diseases; inflammations of the respiratory passages; and a tendency for the common cold (Reckeweg 2002).

BHI-Enzyme: Contains Malicum acidum, which is also in *Coenzyme compositum*, *Cor compositum*, *Hepar compositum*, and *Thyroidea compositum*. This is indicated in seborrhea; chronic dry, scaly eczemas; and eczema and fissures in the auditory canal. See also allergy protocols.

BHI-Skin: Contains several remedies that are useful in otitis externa and media, and is also of value in atopic/allergic cases. The remedies with indications for otitis include Petroleum (*BHI-Body Pure*, etc.), which can be of value in conditions that affect the mucosa of the eyes, with dacryocystitis, lacrimation, as well as otitis externa with chronic inflammatory discharge. These are associated with tinnitus and hearing impairment and fistulae.

Lycopodium (also in *Crurohoheel*, *Hepar compositum*, *Hepeel*, *BHI-Allergy*, *BHI-Hair and Skin*, and many others) is a specific liver remedy. It can bring significant relief in liver damage, liver dysfunctions, and even in serious degenerative symptoms. A wide variety of symptoms depend on liver function, or else provide an alternate outlet for the elimination of homotoxins if the liver function is disordered. These include skin diseases such as urticaria or ulcers; pityriasis with alopecia; and skin conditions with moist eczemas, otorrhoea, and other reaction phase conditions.

Kreosotum (also in *Lamioflur*, *Mucosa compositum*, and many others) has an excoriating action on the skin and causes white patches on the oral mucosa and the tongue, followed by deeper destruction of the tissue. Excoriating, fetid, and burning discharges are characteristic, as are hemorrhages and ulcers. There may be pustular eczema with scurf on the extensor sides of the limbs, and possibly also Meibomian cysts and styes, burning, itching, moist eczema of the ears, and maybe chronic otitis media and tinnitus (Reckeweg 2002). General support comes from sepia and Sulphur.

Cutis compositum: Opens the skin to drainage, detoxification, and repair in all phases.

Echinacea compositum: Provides immune support in the face of infection.

Graphites homaccord: Used for pigmented, greasy, oily dermatitis and otitis externa in overweight animals.

Hormeel: Normalizes endocrine responses.

Lamioflur: Used for discharges and inflammation near mucocutaneous junctions. Contains several useful remedies, including Hydrastis canadensis (also in *Mucosa compositum*, *NasoHeel*, *Ubichinon compositum*, *BHI Sinus*, etc.). It is used principally in serious disorders of the autonomic nervous system; protracted catarrhs; influenza with great secretion of mucus; liver conditions with jaundice; cystitis; eczematous skin eruptions; congestive coryza; nasal ulcers; cholesteatoma; otorrhoea; and in any other acrid, raw, excoriating discharges when a general

deterioration of energy is present It also contains Kali sulphuricum, which has main indications for yellow mucus or purulent discharges from the bronchi, conjunctivitis, pustular and vesicular eruptions, eustachian catarrh with deafness, and chronic otitis media with yellow discharge (Reckeweg 2002). Also contains Kreosotum (see *BHI-Skin*).

Psorinoheel: A constitutional remedy containing sulfur that is good for polypoid otitis and chronic cases of otitis externa.

Schwef-Heel: Sulfur-containing agent useful in allergic cases.

Sulphur-Heel: Used for red, dry, greasy, or bad-smelling cases.

Traumeel S: Has nonsteroidal anti-inflammatory actions. This remedy may serve as a helpful agent in all phases and all cases of otitis.

Authors' suggested protocols

Nutrition

Ear and immune support formulas: 1 tablet for every 25 pounds of body weight BID.

Chinese herbal medicine/acupuncture

H52 ImmunoDerm and H67 DermGuard: 1 capsule of each for every 10 to 20 pounds twice daily. In addition to the herbs discussed above, these preparations contain scutellaria (Huang Qin), fleece flower root (He shou wu), siler (Fang feng), tokoro (Bi xie), schizonepeta (Jing jie), dandelion (Pu gong ying), oldenlandia (Bai hua she cao), kochia (Di fu zi), xanthium fruit (Cang Er zi), bitter orange (Zhi ke), Angelica radix (Dang gui), buffalo horn shavings (Sui Niu jiao), earthworm (Di long), silkworm (Jiang can), and cnidium (Chuan xiong). The combination of these two formulas has anti-inflammatory, antipruritic, and antibacterial effects.

The underlying cause of recurrent otitis should also be determined. This formula works well on atopic otitis but is not effective for food allergies. The only effective therapy for food allergies seems to be avoidance, in the author's opinion.

Recommended acupuncture points include ST36, LI11, and GB2 (Handbook of TCM Practitioners 1987).

Homotoxicology

In addition to treatment of predisposing causes (see allergy, Autoimmune disease, Hypothyroidism, Cushing's disease):

Simple otitis externa: Traumeel, Belladonna homaccord, Echinacea compositum, combined and given orally BID. Broadfoot starts severe cases with Belladonna homaccord plus Echinacea compositum IV and as an autosanguis, and Belladonna compositum tablets BID to

TID. Traumeel vials can be opened and placed directly in the ear canal to reduce pain and swelling in acute cases, or use Pure Ear Drops, which are Traumeel in plastic vials for instilling into ear canals. Lamioflur, Abropernol, and Cruroheel may be considered in resistant cases.

Chronic otitis externa: Use Psorinoheel, added to the above.

Allergic cases: Give Schwef-Heel plus the Simple Otitis Externa combination. In allergies, consider repairing hepatic enzymes, covered in the allergic dermatitis section.

Chronic otitis externa with greasy discharge: Graphites homaccord combined with the above items as indicated BID PO.

Product sources

Nutrition
Ear and immune support formulas: Animal Nutrition Technologies. **Alternatives:** Immune System Support—Standard Process Veterinary Formulas; Immuno Support—Rx Vitamins for Pets; Immugen—Thorne Veterinary Products.

Chinese herbal medicine
Formulas H52 ImmunoDerm and H67 DermGuard: Natural Solutions, Inc.

Chinese herbal medicine
BHI/Heel Corporation

REFERENCES

Western medicine references

Griffin CE. Otitis externa and otitis media. In: Griffin CE, Kwochka KW, MacDonald JM, eds. Current veterinary dermatology: the science and art of therapy. 1993. St. Louis: Mosby.

Werner AH. Otitis Externa and Media. In: Tilley L, Smith F. The 5-Minute Veterinary Consult: Canine and Feline, Blackwell Publishing, 2003.

Chinese herbal medicine/acupuncture references

Handbook of TCM Practitioners, Hunan College of TCM, Shanghai Science and Technology Press, Oct 1987, p 780.

Kim JH, Han KD, Yamasaki K, Tanaka O. *Phytochemistry*, 1979; 18(5):894–895.

Pi fu Bing Fang Zhi Yan Jiu Tong Xun (*Research Journal on Prevention and Treatment of Dermatological Disorders*), 1972; 3: 215.

Shan Xi Yi Kan (*Shanxi Journal of Medicine*), 1960; (10):32.

Sheng Yao Xue Za Zhi (*Journal of Raw Herbology*), 1979; 33(3): 178.

Xin Yi Xue (*New Medicine*), 1975; 6(3): 155.

Xin Zhong Yi (*New Chinese Medicine*), 1989; 21(3):51.

Yu W. The clinical report on acupuncture treatment of 81 cases of suppurant otitis media by propagated meridianal far away points. *Chin J Acupunct Moxibustion* 1990;3(3):187–8.

Zhong Cao Yao (*Chinese Herbal Medicine*) 1991; 22 (10):452.

Zhong Cao Yao Xue (*Study of Chinese Herbal Medicine*), 1980;932.

Zhong Guo Yao Ke Da Xue Xue Bao (*Journal of University of Chinese Herbology*), 1990;21 (4):222.

Zhong Guo Zhong Yao Za Zhi (*People's Republic of China Journal of Chinese Herbology*), 1991; 16(9):560.

Zhong Yao Cai (*Study of Chinese Herbal Material*), 1985; (2): 36.

Zhong Yao Cai (*Study of Chinese Herbal Material*), 1991; 14(2):41.

Zhong Yao Xue (*Chinese Herbology*), 1998; 89:91.

Zhong Yao Xue (*Chinese Herbology*), 1998;103:106.

Zhong Yao Xue (*Chinese Herbology*), 1998; 318: 320.

Zhong Yao Yao Li Yu Ying Yong (*Pharmacology and Applications of Chinese Herbs*), 1983: 400.

Zhong Yao Yao Li Yu Ying Yong (*Pharmacology and Applications of Chinese Herbs*), 1983; 866.

Zhong Yao Yao Li Yu Ying Yong (*Pharmacology and Applications of Chinese Herbs*), 1983; 888.

Zhong Yao Zhi (*Chinese Herbology Journal*), 1993:183.

Zhong Yao Zhi (*Chinese Herbology Journal*), 1993; 358.

Homotoxicology reference

Reckeweg H. Homoeopathia Antihomotoxica Materia Medica, 4th ed. Baden-Baden, Germany: Aurelia-Verlag GMBH, 2002. pp. 120–1, 207, 223–5, 299, 340–2, 344–5, 372, 378, 394, 484–5, 493, 504–5.

Chapter Thirteen

Diseases of the Musculoskeletal System

ARTHRITIS

Definition and cause

Arthritis is a degenerative, progressive disease of the cartilage and synovial surface of the joint. Although arthritis is distinguished from immune-mediated arthritis because it is classified as non-inflammatory, inflammation is believed to be an important part of the initiation and ongoing breakdown of tissue in the joint. Arthritis in dogs and cats is assumed to be related to the aging process as well as secondary to other factors such as injury, physical deformity, overuse, and other diseases such as dental disease. Continual loss or breakdown of the joint surface often leads to pain, inflammation, and permanent deformity (Beale 1993, 2003; Cook 1927; Pederson 1978, 1989).

Medical therapy rationale, drug(s) of choice, and nutritional recommendations

More integrative options exist for arthritis than any other disease condition. The conventional approach is the use of anti-inflammatory and pain-suppressing drugs such as corticosteroids and NSAIDs. The potential side effects from the chronic use of these drugs have led to alternative approaches such as reconstructive surgical procedures and joint replacement. Dietary management is most commonly used for weight reduction. The newer trend in arthritis management is toward chondroprotective agents such as Adequan®, and nutraceuticals such as glycosaminoglycan (glucosamine), pain-relieving agents such as methyl sulfonyl methane (MSM), and free radical scavengers such as superoxide dismutase (SOD) (Beale 2003, Todhunter 1994).

Anticipated prognosis

Arthritis is a progressive degenerative disease. The approach of medically addressing the symptoms and sur-

gically correcting the problem simply corrects the associated symptoms. The addition of chondroprotective agents, nutraceuticals, and a weight loss program greatly increases the likelihood of control of the disease and offers a much improved prognosis. Arthritis offers a good example of the proven effects of the integrative approach to treating a disease condition.

Integrative veterinary therapies

The conventional medical approach to arthritis focuses upon the signs and symptoms of the disease. While the degenerative process is physically located in the joints, the underlying mechanism begins with an inflammatory process at the cellular level. This process initiates the pain and swelling, but also results in the decrease in synovial fluid production, leading to further friction, inflammation, and degeneration. Adding nutritional and alternative therapies helps to reduce free radical production, decrease inflammation, enhance synovial fluid production, and slow or prevent further degeneration. In addition, if started early, it can reduce the dependence upon or minimize the use of medications.

Nonsteroidal anti-inflammatory drugs frequently have adverse effects, now more commonly known by consumers. They are useful for short-term therapy and in cases of severely advanced osteoarthritis in which safer therapies no longer suffice.

Nutrition
General considerations/rationale
Nutritional and gland support are directed toward reducing inflammation and protecting cells and tissue. Medication, on the other hand, covers up the inflammation; however, it does not get to the underlying cause nor does it confer cellular protection. Nutritional therapies also focus upon improving nutrient flow to the cells and tissues of the joints and help to prevent a decrease in the production of synovial fluid.

Appropriate nutrients

Chondroprotective agents: The body uses glucosamine to make and repair joint tissue and cartilage. Glucosamine has been clinically proven to significantly reduce the pain, inflammation, and swelling associated with osteoarthritis in both people and animals (Crolle 1980, D'Ambrosio 1981, Tapadinhas 1982, Giordano 1996). Glucosamine has been shown to have none of the side effects of drugs, and can be as effective as prescribed medications (Pujalte 1980, Vaz 1982).

Several studies have demonstrated the effectiveness of glucosamine and chondroitin in the management of arthritis in dogs (Das 2000, Guastella 2005). Setnikar et al. (1986) has described how these compounds actually stimulate the body's own repair mechanism and help in the process of developing new cartilage. Numerous double-blind studies have compared the effectiveness of glucosamine against various NSAIDs, resulting in as good or, in many cases, even better pain control and removal of the clinical signs associated with osteoarthritis (Prudden 1974, Vaz 1982, DeAmbrosia 1982).

Chondroitin sulfate (CS) is found in the lining of the joints, and clinical evidence in double-blind studies shows that supplementation with CS reduces pain and inflammation and increases joint mobility (Leeb 1996, Morreale 1996, Pipitone 1992, Uebelhart 1998). In the veterinary field, Anderson (1999) and Canapp (1999) showed that there was significant reduction in pain and improved mobility as reported by survey veterinarians.

Fatty acids: In a double-blind study of people with rheumatoid arthritis, Joe (1993) showed that a number of people had significant benefits from the addition of evening primrose oil (EPO). Kremer (1995) has shown that fish oil helps to reduce inflammation in people with arthritis.

Botanical Cox2 inhibitors: Botanical Cox2 inhibitors have been shown to have anti-oxidative and anti-inflammatory effects (Bemis 2005). Botanical Cox 2 inhibitors reduce inflammation without the inherent side effects of Cox2 medications.

Vitamin C: Vitamin C has been studied clinically in animals. Brown (1994), Berg (1990), and Newman (1995) reported on the benefits of vitamin C in the treatment of degenerative joint disease and movement in dogs and horses. Belfield (1981, 1998) reported on the beneficial effects of vitamin C in treating and preventing hip dysplasia in dogs.

Chinese herbal medicine/acupuncture
General considerations/rationale

Practitioners of TCM consider arthritis to be a combination of Wind, Damp, and Cold. The Kidney, which has the function of controlling the bones, is the main organ that is involved. Wind is a traveling pathogen, according to TCM. It refers to the tendency of arthritis to manifest in various joints on different days. Wind also refers to motion. Some animals with arthritis may have twitching of the muscles, spasms, or trembling in the affected area. Cold causes stiffness, as many practitioners note. Animals tend to have more trouble getting up and mobilizing on colder days. Cold also causes pain. The animals often prefer warm areas on cold days. People know from experience that a heating pad helps decrease the pain associated with arthritis. Damp refers to swelling in the joint, i.e., the accumulation of fluids in the joint.

In addition to treating the signs of arthritis, it is important to address the underlying cause, such as rickettsial diseases, bacterial infections, and excess weight. Immune-mediated arthritis must be treated differently than degenerative arthritis.

Appropriate Chinese herbs

Aconite (Fu zi): Effectively decreases joint inflammation (Zhong Yao Tong Bao 1988) and has analgesic properties (Zhong Guo Zhong Yao Za Zhi 1992).

Angelica (Bai zhi): Has anti-inflammatory and analgesic properties (Zhong Guo Zhong Yao Za Zhi 1991). It contains scopoletin, an effective muscle relaxant (Zhi Wu Yao Yao Xiao Cheng Fen Shou Ce 1986).

Atractylodes (Bai zhu): Has been shown to decrease pain related to chronic back and leg arthritis in humans (Hu Bei Zhong Yi Za Zhi 1982).

Bupleurum (Chai hu): Contains saikosaponin, which has analgesic properties (Shen Yang Yi Xue Yuan Bao 1984).

Cinnamon twigs (Gui zhi): Have analgesic effects (Zhong Yao Xue 1998). Licorice contains two compounds, glycyrrhizin and glycrrhetinic acid, which have shown efficacy in treating arthritis (Zhong Cao Yao 1991).

Ginger (Sheng jiang): Has been shown to be effective in decreasing arthritis pain in several studies (He Bai Xin Yi Yao 1972, Chi Zhi Jiao Yi Shi Za).

Notopterygium (Qiang huo): Has been shown to relieve muscular pain in mice (Zhong Cao Yao 1991).

Pubescent angelica root (Du huo): Has demonstrated anti-inflammatory and analgesic effects (Zhong Yao Yao Li Yu Ying Yong 1983).

White peony (Bai shao): Contains paeoniflorin, which is a strong anti-inflammatory (Zhong Yao Zhi 1993). It is an effective pain reliever (Shang Hai Zhong Yi Yao Za Zhi 1983), and in combination with gan cao is excellent for muscle spasms (Hu Nan Zhong Yi 1989, Zhong Yao Zhi 1993).

Acupuncture

Musculoskeletal disease is one of the most common reasons for seeking acupuncture treatment in this country.

Acupuncture has been used extensively and effectively in all types of arthritic conditions. There are generalized points one can choose for acupuncture. For example, bai hua is a good choice for treating generalized weakness associated with muscle atrophy. In addition to being a good point to increase the body's energy, it also serves as a local point for the hip joint, lumbar spine, and hind legs (Schoen A 1994).

Local points also may be chosen. The following is a list of specific areas and possible point choices according to the author's experience:

Neck: SI16, LI18, BL10
Shoulders: SI9, SI10, TH14
Elbow: LI11, Qiang Feng (Yu 2000).
Carpus: PC6, TH5
Back: Hua tuo jia ji (points just lateral to each vertebrae chosen according to the location of the pain)
Hip: BL54, GB28, GB29
Stifle: GB34, ST35
Hock: BL60, KI3

Homotoxicology
General considerations/rationale
Osteoarthritis, a degenerative, nonautoimmune form of arthritis, represents homotoxicoses in the Inflammation, Deposition, and Degenerative phases, and is a common entity in veterinary medicine. Therapy is aimed at reducing homotoxin levels, improving circulation and lymphatic flows, reducing inflammatory pain, and improving mobility. Proper diet, adequate exercise, and weight management are critical to the success of any program designed to assist the osteoarthritis patient. Agents should be chosen initially that have minimal risk to the patient. An initial treatment period of 5 to 8 weeks is needed to properly assess response. Biological agents frequently require a longer window to demonstrate their effects, and clients should be advised of this fact at the initiation of therapy.

Homotoxicology has many biological agents that assist in managing arthritis with a minimum of harmful side effects, and consumers appreciate this immensely. Many clinicians take their first steps toward biological therapy in pursuit of better methods of pain management and rehabilitation for their patients, as well as for themselves. Some evidence for the effectiveness of antihomotoxic pain medications is discussed in the homotoxicology chapter of this text.

Appropriate homotoxicology formulas
Homeopathic strategies vary depending upon the anatomical location of the osteoarthritis as well as the presence or absence of other aggravating factors (cold, damp, skin rashes, etc (also see Autoimmune Arthritis in Chapter 6). The following remedies have proven themselves in hundreds of cases in the authors' clinics:

Aconitum homaccord: Treats polyarthrtis, particularly when combined with *Rhododendroneel S* and *Bryaconeel*.

Aesculus compositum: Is primarily a peripheral circulatory agent, but contains Rhus tox, Ruta graviolens, and Arnica, which are all excellent arthritis remedies.

Atropinum compositum: Treats painful muscle spasms associated with arthropathy (Heel 2003).

BHI-Arthritis: Used for swollen, painful joints and muscle stiffness. Particularly useful for patients that are more affected in cold, wet weather (Heel 2002).

BHI-Back: Treats back pain, muscle spasm, arthropathy (Heel 2002).

Bryaconeel: Treats polyarthritis, particularly when combined with *Rhododendroneel S* and *Aconitum homaccord*.

Calcoheel: Used for disordered calcium metabolism.

Cimicifuga homaccord: Treats neck pain and chronic luxations of pedal joints.

Colnadul: Used for arthritis that worsens with wet weather. It is particularly suited to knee problems, e.g. chronic dislocations. The authors use this in stifle issues (Broadfoot 2004).

Colocynthis homaccord: Used as an initial therapeutic agent, particularly for acutely painful conditions involving the lower back and hips. Initially use it every 15 to 30 minutes, until relief is noted (Reckeweg 2000).

Cruroheel: Used particularly for afflictions of the hind limbs.

Discus compositum: Treats spinal arthropathy (Broadfoot 2003).

Dulcamara homaccord: Used for arthritis worsened by wet weather.

Ferrum homaccord: Treats shoulder pain and shoulderhand syndromes.

Gelsemium homaccord: Treats head and neck pain and lower limb weakness (Demers 2005).

Graphites homaccord: Used for deforming arthropathies.

Lithiumeel: Treats osteoarthritis of the hip joints, and is useful in conjunction with *Graphites homaccord* in hip-dysplasia-induced osteoarthritis.

Osteoheel: Treats ankle pain.

Psorinoheel: Indicated in chronic polyarthritis. There is some evidence for microbial causes of arthritides, e.g., mycoplasmas, and this remedy may have applicability for therapy.

Rheuma-Heel: Treats left-sided arthritis of the shoulder or knee.

Rhododendroneel S: Treats polyarthritis, particularly when combined with *Bryaconeel* and *Aconitum homaccord*.

Traumeel S: Useful in the form of vials, drops, tablets, ointment, and gel in many applications in osteoarthritis cases, particularly in the early phases for control of acute pain. This formula has more scientific research than any other homeopathic remedy and is listed in the Physician's Desk Reference as a nonsteroidal anti-inflammatory agent (see the homotoxicology chapter for references).

Zeel: Useful in the form of ampules, tablets, ointment, and gel as the main long-term remedy for osteoarthritis. Revitalizes tissues through Catilago suis, Funiculus umbilicus, and Placenta suis. It includes a number of homeopathic botanicals that are useful in arthritis (Rhus tox, Arnica, Solanum dulcamara, Symphytum officinale, and Sanguinaria). It also has agents that assist in metabolism (Sulphur, Nicotinamide adenine dinucleotide [NAD], Coenzyme A, alpha-lipoic acid, and sodium oxalacetate) (Reckeweg 2002). It is useful for arthritic pathology in any location, but it is best for stifle arthritis. Combine with other agents to target specific anatomical areas (See the homotoxicology chapter references).

Authors' suggested protocols

Nutrition
Cartilage/ligament/muscle/skeletal support formula: 1 tablet for every 25 pounds of body weight BID.

Eskimo fish oil: One-half to 1 teaspoon per meal for cats. 1 teaspoon for every 35 pounds of body weight for dogs.

Evening primrose oil: 1 capsule (500 mgs) for every 25 pounds of body weight daily.

Zyflamend: One-half dropper for every 25 pounds of body weight BID.

Chinese herbal medicine/acupuncture
JointGuard: 1 capsule per 10 to 20 pounds twice daily. This supplement has analgesic, anti-inflammatory, and antipyretic effects. In addition to the herbs mentioned above, JointGuard also contains amenarrhena (Zhi mu), allium (Cong bai), siler (Fang feng), cnidium (Chuan xiong), platycodon (Jie geng), bitter orange (Zhi ke), peucedanum (Qian hu), poria (Fu ling), and jujube fruit (Da Zao).

Homotoxicology
Initial therapy: Traumeel S drops BID and Zeel tablets twice daily; recheck in 3 weeks. Injection therapy, biopuncture, or autosanguis with these agents can be very useful and can be repeated every 2 weeks to speed up response. Select other agents to target specific locations or symptoms.

Product sources

Nutrition
Cartilage/ligament/muscle/skeletal support formula: Animal Nutrition Technologies. **Alternatives:** Cosequin—Nutramax Labs; Glycoflex—Vetri Science; Musculoskeletal support—Standard Process Veterinary Formulas; Nutriflex—Vet Rx Vitamins for Pets; Arthragen—Thorne Veterinary Products.

    Evening primrose oil: Jarrow Formulas.

    Eskimo fish oil: Tyler Encapsulations.

    Zyflamend: New Chapter. **Alternative:** Botanical Treasures—Natura Health Products.

Chinese herbal medicine
H1 and H95: Natural Solutions, Inc.

Homotoxicology
BHI/Heel Corporation

REFERENCES

Western medicine references
Beale BS, Goring RL. Degenerative joint disease. In: Bojarab MJ, ed. Disease mechanisms in small animal surgery, Philadelphia: Lea and Febiger, 1993:727–736.

Beale BS. In: Tilley L, Smith F. The 5-Minute Veterinary Consult: Canine and Feline, 2003. Blackwell Publishing.

Cook TG, Hardenbergh JG. A case of recurrent synovitis and myositis in the dog associated with dental infection. *North Am Vet* 1927;8:30.

Pedersen NC, Pool R. Canine joint disease. *Vet Clin North Am* 1978.8:265.

Pedersen NC. Joint diseases of dogs and cats. In: Ettinger SJ, ed. Textbook of veterinary internal medicine. 3rd ed. Philadelphia: Saunders, 1989:2329–2377.

Todhunter RJ, Lust G. Polysulfated glycosaminoglycan in the treatment of osteoarthritis, *J Am Vet Med Assoc* 1994;204:1245–1251.

Nutrition references
Das AK, Hammad TA. Efficacy of a combination of FCH-G49TM glucosamine hydrochloride, TRH122TM low molecular weight sodium chondroitin sulfate and manganese ascorbate in the management of knee osteoarthritis. *Osteoarthritis Cart* 2000;8(5):343–350.

Guastella DB, Cook JL, Kuroki K, et al. Evaluation of chondroprotective nutriceuticals in an in vitro osteoarthritis model. In: Proceedings of the 32nd Annual Conference Veterinary Orthopedic Society 2005;5.

D'Ambrosio E, Casa B, Bompani G, et al. Glucosamine sulphate: a controlled clinical investigation in arthrosis. *Pharmatherapeutica* 1981;2(8):5048.

Giordano N, Nardi P, Senesi M, et al. The efficacy and safety of glucosamine sulfate in the treatment of gonarthritis. *Clin Ter* 1996;147:99–105.

Joe LA, Hart LL. Evening primrose oil in rheumatoid arthritis. *Ann Pharmacother* 1993;27:1475–7.

Kremer JM, Lawrence DA, Petrillow GF, et al. Effects of high-dose fish oil on rheumatoid arthritis after stopping nonsteroidal antiinflammatory drugs. *Arthritis Rheum* 1995;38:1107–14.

Leeb BF, Petera P, Neumann K. Results of a multicenter study of chondroitin sulfate (Condrosulf) use in arthroses of the finger, knee and hip joints. *Wien Med Wochenschr* 1996;146:609–14.

Morreale P, Manopulo R, Galati M, et al. Comparison of the antiinflammatory efficacy of chondroitin sulfate and diclofenac sodium in patients with knee osteoarthritis. *J Rheumatol* 1996;23:1385–91.

Pipitone V, Ambanelli U, Cervini C, et al. A multicenter, triple-blind study to evaluate galactosaminoglucuronoglycan sulfate versus placebo in patients with femorotibial gonarthritis. *Curr Ther Res* 1992;52:608–38.

Prudden JF, Balassa LL. The Biological Activity of Bovine Cartilage Preparations. *Semin. Arthrit. Rheum.*, 1974;4:287–321.

Pujalte JM, Llavore EP, Ylescupidez FR. Double-blind clinical evaluation of oral glucosamine sulphate in the basic treatment of osteoarthrosis. *Curr Med Res Opin* 1980;7(2):110–4.

Setnikar I, Giachetti C, Zanolo G. Pharmacokinetics of Glucosamine in the Dog and in Man. *Arzneimittelforschung*, 1986;36:729–735.

Tapadinhas MJ, Rivera IC, Bignamini AA. Oral glucosamine sulphate in the management of arthrosis: report on a multicentre open investigation in Portugal. *Pharmtherapeutica* 1982;3:157–68.

Uebelhart D, Thonar EJ, Delmas PD, et al. Effects of oral chondroitin sulfate on the progression of knee osteoarthritis: a pilot study. *Osteoarthritis Cartilage* 1998;6(Suppl A):39–46.

Vaz AL. Double-blind clinical evaluation of the relative efficacy of ibuprofen and glucosamine sulphate in the management of osteoarthritis of the knee in outpatients. *Curr Med Res Opin* 1982;8(3):145–9.

Chinese herbal medicine/acupuncture references

Chi Jiao Yi Shi Za Zhi (*Journal of the Barefoot Doctors*), 1077; 11:13.

He Bai Xin Yi Yao (*Hebei New Medicine and Herbology*), 1972; 3:31.

Hu Bei Zhong Yi Za Zhi (*Hubei Journal of Chinese Medicine*), 1982; 6: 57.

Hu Nan Zhong Yi (*Hunan Journal of Traditional Chinese Medicine*), 1989;2:7.

Schoen A. Veterinary Acupuncture, Ancient Art to Modern Medicine. 1994.California: American Veterinary Publications, Inc.

Shang Hai Zhong Yi Yao Za Zhi(*Shanghai Journal of Chinese Medicine and Herbology*), 1983; 4:14.

Shen Yang Yi Xue Yuan Bao (*Journal of Shenyang University of Medicine*), 1984; 1(3):214.

Yu C, Chen ZB. Xian Dai Zhong Shou Yi Da Quan (Modern Complete Works of Traditional Chinese Veterinary Medicine), March 2000. p 347.

Zhi Wu Yao Yao Xiao Cheng Fen Shou Ce (Manual of Plant Medicinals and Their Active Constituents), 1986: 624,603,197.

Zhong Cao Yao (*Chinese Herbal Medicine*), 1991; 22(1): 28.

Zhong Cao Yao (*Chinese Herbal Medicine*) 1991; 22 (10): 452.

Zhong Guo Zhong Yao Za Zhi (*People's Republic of China Journal of Chinese Herbology*), 1991; 16(9): 560.

Zhong Guo Zhong Yao Za Zhi (*People's Republic of China Journal of Chinese Herbology*), 1992; 17(2): 104.

Zhong Yao Tong Bao (*Journal of Chinese Herbology*), 1988; 13(6): 40.

Zhong Yao Xue (*Chinese Herbology*), 1998; 65: 67.

Zhong Yao Xue (*Chinese Herbology*), 1998; 759: 765.

Zhong Yao Yao Li Yu Ying Yong (*Pharmacology and Applications of Chinese Herbs*), 1983; 796.

Zhong Yao Zhi (*Chinese Herbology Journal*), 1993:183.

Zhong Yao Zhi (*Chinese Herbology Journal*), 1993; 358.

Homotoxicology references

Broadfoot P. Homotoxicology for Musculoskeletal Problems. Heel/AHVMA Homotoxicology Seminar. May, 2003. Denver, CO. CD.

Demers J. Inflammation, Lameness, Pain and Homotoxicology, Vol 20, Small Animal and Exotics Proceedings, North American Veterinary Conference, 2005. Orlando, FL, p 35.

Heel. BHI Homeopathic Therapy: Professional Reference. Albuquerque, NM: Heel Inc. 2002. p 31, 34.

Heel. Veterinary Guide, 3rd English edition. Baden-Baden, Germany: Biologische Heilmettel Heel GmbH. 2003. p 25.

Reckeweg H. Biotherapeutic Index: Ordinatio Antihomotoxica et Materia Medica, 5th ed. Baden-Baden, Germany: Biologische Heilmittel Heel GMBH, 2000. p 92.

Reckeweg H. 2002. Homeopathia Antihomotoxica Materia Medica, 4th ed. Baden-Baden, Germany: Aurelia-Verlag, pp. 246–9, 388, 446, 456–8, 555–9.

HIP AND ELBOW DYSPLASIA

Definition and cause

Hip and elbow dysplasia is a degenerative condition of the hip or elbow joints leading to a malaligned joint and secondary arthritic changes. Genetics, nutrition, and developmental changes affect the degenerative process in both conditions (Cook 1996; McLaughlin 2003; Rettenmaier 1991; Schwarz 2000, 2003; Tomlinson 1996; Wind 1986). For more information, please refer to Arthritis, above.

Medical therapy rationale, drug(s) of choice, and nutritional recommendations

Medical treatment involves anti-inflammatories, analgesics, and NSAIDs such as aspirin, carprofen, deracoxib, meloxicam, or piroxicam; however, none of the medical therapies address the physical malformation nor stop the degenerative process. Diet is directed toward weight control. Surgical correction or hip replacement often works. For elbows, surgical exploration of the joint and removal of any loose fragments often works well (Kapatkin 2002; Manley 1993; McLaughlin 1996, 2003, Schwarz 2003; Tomlinson 1996).

Anticipated prognosis

Prognosis for hips with surgery is good. Prognosis for elbows is more guarded based upon surgical intervention, medical therapy, and the status of degeneration of the elbow (McLaughlin 2003, Schwarz 2003).

Integrative veterinary therapies

See Arthritis, above.

Nutrition
General considerations/rationale
See Arthritis remarks and rationale, above.

Appropriate nutrients
See Arthritis recommended therapy, above.

Chinese herbal medicine/acupuncture
General considerations/rationale
Arthritis is considered to be Blood and Essence deficiency in the Liver and Kidney. There is also Blood and Qi stagnation. The Liver and Kidney control the ligaments and bones, respectively. These organs are not nourished when there is Blood deficiency, leading to disease in the parts they control. Essence is the potential for growth known as genetic potential in Western terminology. There is a genetic predisposition to developing hip and elbow dysplasia. When the Essence of the Liver and Kidney are deficient their associated structures degenerate. Blood and Qi stagnation lead to pain.

Appropriate Chinese herbs
Alisma (Ze xie): An anti-inflammatory herb. It was shown to ameliorate 2, 4-chloronitrobenzene-induced contact dermatitis in mice (Dai 1991). It may be able to reduce inflammation in the joints.

Angelica root (Dang gui): Is as strong as aspirin at decreasing inflammation and is 1.7 times as strong as aspirin for pain relief (Yao Xue Za Zhi 1971). Thirty-eight people with elbow arthritis were treated with modified Dang Gui Si Ni Tang (angelica root [Dang gui], white peony [Bai shao], astragalus [Huang qi], cinnamon [Gui zhi], white mustard seed [Bai jie zi], wild ginger [Xi xin], mulberry twig [Sang zhi], notopterygium [Qiang huo], aurantium [Zhi qiao], chaenomeles [Mu gua], eupolyphaga [Tu bie chong], licorice [Gan cao], and tetrapanax

[Tong cao]). Twenty-four percent of the participants had complete resolution, 68% improved, and 8% did not respond (Hu 1998).

Astragalus (Huang qi): A mild analgesic (Zhong Yao Tong Bao 1986).

Atractylodes (Bai zhu): Has been shown to decrease chronic leg pain (Hu Bei Zhong Yi Za Zhi 1982).

Corydalis (Yan hu suo): Has anti-inflammatory properties; works for both acute and chronic inflammation (Kubo 1994). It has analgesic activity. Corydalis has 1/100 the activity of morphine (Zhong Yao Yao Li Yu Ying Yong 1983). It works synergistically with acupuncture in providing analgesia (Chen Tzu Yen Chiu 1994).

Jujube (Da zao): Has anti-inflammatory effects. It can prevent egg-white-induced toe swelling in rats (Li 1997). This property may help prevent inflammation in the joints.

Lycopodium (Shen jin cao): Has analgesic and anti-inflammatory effects. It was shown experimentally to decrease heat-induced pain and inhibit formaldehyde-induced inflammation in rat hocks (Zeng 1999).

Peach kernel (Tao ren): Has anti-inflammatory properties. It was shown to prevent egg-white-induced arthritis in mice (Liu 1989).

Rehmannia (Sheng di huang): Reduces swelling and inflammation (Zhong Yao Yao Li Yu Ying Yong 1983). It has been shown to be effective for arthritis pain (Tian Jing Yi Xue Za Zhi 1966).

White peony (Bai shao): Contains Paeoniflorin, which is a strong anti-inflammatory (Zhong Yao Zhi 1993). It has analgesic effects. In one trial, 65% of people with painful conditions responded (Shang Hai Zhong Yi Yao Za Zhi 1983).

Acupuncture
Osteoarthritis and lateral epicondylitis (tennis elbow) are on the World Health Organization's list of disorders responsive to acupuncture (World Health Organization 2006). This suggests that hip and elbow dysplasia should also be responsive.

Homotoxicology
General considerations/rationale
See Arthritis remarks and rationale.

Appropriate homotoxicology formulas
See Arthritis.

Authors' suggested protocols

Nutrition
Cartilage/ligament/muscle/skeletal support formula: 1 tablet for every 25 pounds of body weight BID.

Eskimo fish oil: One-half to 1 teaspoon per meal for cats. 1 teaspoon for every 35 pounds of body weight for dogs.

Evening primrose oil: 1 capsule (500 mgs) per 25 pounds of body weight daily.

Chinese herbal medicine/acupuncture

Formula H20 Osteophyte: 1 capsule per 10 to 20 pounds twice daily. In addition to the herbs discussed above, H20 Osteophyte also contains burreed tuber (Shan leng), carthamus (Hong hua), codonopsis (Dang shen), cnidium (Chuan xiong), lycopus (Ze lan), poria (Fu ling), red peony (Chi shao), and zedoaria (E zhu).

The authors use the following acupuncture points: ST36, GB30, Baihui, GV4, LI11, PC6, SI9, BL20, and BL23.

Homotoxicology

Osteoarthritis of the hip or elbow: Graphites homaccord (and/or Calcoheel), Galium-Heel, and Zeel tablets, combined and given BID PO. BHI-Arthritis, Causticum compositum, and Sulfur-Heel all have components for chronic ailments, and some specific remedies for hip and elbow issues. Aesculus compositum can be useful as intermittent therapy, because it has rheumatic indications and several remedies with an affinity for hip problems. Coenzyme compositum can be given twice weekly PO. In cases with extreme pain, use Traumeel S by injection weekly, orally 2 to 4 times daily, or topically in the gel as needed for pain control. In cases with marked joint proliferation, consider Lithiumeel BID PO. Osteoheel can be alternated with Traumeel at intervals as needed to control signs. Discus compositum may be given EOD. Colocynthis is a useful remedy for lower back, hip, and sciatic problems.

Product sources

Nutrition

Cartilage/ligament/muscle/skeletal support formula: Animal Nutrition Technologies. **Alternatives**: Cosequin—Nutramax Labs; Glycoflex—Vetri Science; Musculoskeletal support—Standard Process Veterinary Formulas; Nutriflex—Vet Rx Vitamins for Pets; Arthragen—Thorne Veterinary Products.

Evening primrose oil: Jarrow Formulas.
Eskimo fish oil: Tyler Encapsulations.

Chinese herbal medicine

Formula H20 Osteophyte: Natural Solutions, Inc.

Homotoxicology

BHI/Heel Corporation

REFERENCES

Western medicine references

Cook JL, et al. Pathophysiology, diagnosis, and treatment of canine hip dysplasia. *Compendium on Cont Ed Pract Vet* 1996.18: 853–867.

Kapatkin AS, Mayhew PD, Smith GK. Canine Hip Dysplasia: Evidence-Based Treatment. *Compendium*. 2002.August.

Manley PA. The hip joint. In: Slatter D, ed. Textbook of small animal surgery, 2nd ed. Philadelphia: Saunders, 1993:1786–1804.

McLaughlin RM, Tomlinson J. Alternative surgical treatments for canine hip dysplasia, *Vet Med* 1996;91:137–143.

McLaughlin RM, Tomlinson J. Treating canine hip dysplasia with triple pelvic osteotomy. *Vet Med* 1996;91:126–136.

McLaughlin, RM. Hip Dysplasia. In: Tilley L, Smith F. The 5-Minute Veterinary Consult: Canine and Feline, 2003. Blackwell Publishing.

Rettenmaier JL, Constantinescu GM. Canine hip dysplasia. *Compend Contin Educ Pract Vet* 1991;13:643–653.

Schwarz PD. Elbow dysplasia. In: Bonagura JD, Kersey R, eds. Current veterinary therapy XIII: Small animal practice. Philadelphia: Saunders, 2000:1004–1014.

Schwarz, PD. Elbow Dysplasia. In: Tilley L, Smith F. The 5-Minute Veterinary Consult: Canine and Feline, 2003. Blackwell Publishing.

Tomlinson J, McLaughlin RM. Canine hip dysplasia: developmental factors, clinical signs and initial examination steps. *Vet Med* 1996;91:26–33.

Tomlinson J, McLaughlin RM. Total hip replacement. *Vet Med* 1996;91:118–124.

Tomlinson J. Symposium on Canine Hip Dysplasia. *Veterinary Medicine*. 1996.January.

Wind AP. Elbow incongruity and developmental elbow diseases in the dog: parts I and II. *J Am Anim Hosp Assoc* 1986;22:711–724.

Integrative veterinary medicine references
See Arthritis references, above.

Nutrition references
See Arthritis references, above.

CHM/acupuncture references

Chen Tzu Yen Chiu (*Acupuncture Research*), 1994; 19(1):55–8.

Dai Y, et al. *China Journal of Chinese Medicine*. 1991;16(10): 622.

Hu Bei Zhong Yi Za Zhi (*Hubei Journal of Chinese Medicine*), 1982; 6: 57.

Hu WW. Treating 38 cases of scapulohumeral periarthritis with modified Dang Gui Si Ni Tang. *Guangxi Journal of Traditional Chinese Medicine*. 1998;21(1):24.

Kubo M, Matsuda H, Toluoka K, Ma S, Shiomoto H. Antiinflammatory activities of methanolic extract and alkaloidal components from Corydalis tuber. *Biol Pharm Bull*, 1994: Feb; 17(2):262–5.

Li XM, et al. *Journal of Shizhen Medicinal Material Research.* 1997;8(4):373–374.

Liu CH, et al. The pharmacology of Tao Ren. *Journal of Pharmacology and Clinical Application of TCM.* 1989;(2):46–47.

Shang Hai Zhong Yi Yao Za Zhi (*Shanghai Journal of Chinese Medicine and Herbology*), 1983; 4:14.

Tian Jing Yi Xue Za Zhi (*Journal of Tianjing Medicine and Herbology*), 1966; 3:209.

World Health Organization list of common conditions treatable by Chinese Medicine and Acupuncture. Available at: http//tcm/health-info.org/WHO-treatment-list.htm. Accessed 10/20/2006.

Yao Xue Za Zhi (*Journal of Medicinals*), 1971;(91):1098.

Zeng YE, et al. *Journal of Shizhen Medicine.* 1999;10(9):641–642.

Zhong Yao Tong Bao (*Journal of Chinese Herbology*), 1986; 11(9):47.

Zhong Yao Yao Li Yu Ying Yong (*Pharmacology and Applications of Chinese Herbs*), 1983:400.

Zhong Yao Yao Li Yu Ying Yong (*Pharmacology and Applications of Chinese Herbs*), 1983;447.

Zhong Yao Zhi (*Chinese Herbology Journal*), 1993:183.

Homotoxicology references
See Arthritis references, above.

LIGAMENT CONDITIONS: ACL AND LUXATING PATELLA

Definition and cause

Patella luxation is a displacement of the patella from the trochlear groove. In most cases the condition is inherited and based upon conformation. Trauma can also be the cause. It is graded based upon the severity of the luxation and the resultant inflammatory process and clinical signs. Anterior cruciate conditions can range from a mild inflammation to a complete tear of the ligament. Causes are classified as traumatic, immune-mediated, or age-related degeneration of the ligament and conformational abnormalities (Brinker 1997, Johnson 1993, Moore 1996, Slocum 1998, Schwarz 2003).

Medical therapy rationale, drug(s) of choice, and nutritional recommendations

For patella luxation, treatment is dependent upon the amount of movement and secondary inflammation. Medical therapy includes anti-inflammatories such as corticosteroids or NSAIDs such as aspirin, caroprfen, metacam, or piroxicam. For more severe luxations, surgery is the treatment of choice. For anterior cruciate issues, ruptures require surgical repair. For strained or inflamed ligaments, the treatment of choice is rest along with anti-inflammatories or NSAIDs (Arnoczky 1998,

Johnson 1993, Kirby 1993, Moore 1996, Schwarz 2003, Willauer 1997).

Dietary recommendation of both patella luxation and anterior cruciate ligament issues is focused upon weight loss.

Anticipated prognosis

For both patella and cruciate ligament problems, surgical repair offers a good prognosis. However, the prognosis is more guarded if there is underlying degenerative or immune-mediated arthritis. For strained, stretched, and inflamed ligaments, often the prognosis is good for the episode if the patient is treated with rest and medication, but recurrences are likely (Johnson 1993, Kirby 1993, Schwarz 2003).

Integrative veterinary therapies

Surgery is the treatment of choice for most cases of cruciate rupture as well as chronically luxating patella. Disrupted or unstable ligaments create an unstable stifle joint and degenerative osteoarthritis is quick to develop. Pain-suppressing medications such as NSAIDs address the pain and inflammation; however, they do not address the healing of these areas. Additionally, animals that are not quieted or restricted by pain often continue to exacerbate the inflammation by using inflamed joints that should be rested.

Because other orthopedic abnormalities may increase the risk of ligamentous rupture or injury, these may be addressed and benefited by other therapeutic modalities including chiropractics, acupuncture, nutrition, weight management, physical therapy, exercise restriction, and prolotherapy (see Homotoxicology, below, for prolotherapy).

Nutrition
General considerations/rationale
Ligaments and tendons contain similar cellular structure as joints, and respond favorably to similar nutritional therapies. The key in any inflamed tendon, ligament, cartilage etc. is to reduce and not cover up the inflammation. Nutritional therapies focus upon reducing inflammation, improving nutrient flow to the cells and tissues, as well as balancing the immune system and minimizing an inherent mediated cellular attack.

Appropriate nutrients
See Arthritis, above, for a description of tissue support nutrients.

Plant sterols: Betasitosterol has anti-inflammatory effects (Gupta 1980).

Chinese herbal medicine/acupuncture
General considerations/rationale

Ligamentous lesions are a result of trauma, Kidney and Spleen deficiency, Blood and Qi stagnation, or Wind and Damp invading the body. Trauma is understood similarly in both medical views. In TCM theory, the organs involved are the Kidney and Spleen. The Kidneys control the bones so it makes sense that a deficiency in the Kidney could result in skeletal disease. The muscles are controlled by the Spleen. Muscle atrophy is commonly seen due to the animal's tendency not to use the painful limb. Blood and Qi stagnation refer to the pain and weakness observed in the condition. Wind is believed to blow pathogens into and around the body. Damp makes the joint "sticky" or stiff.

Appropriate Chinese herbs

Achyranthes (Niu xi): Has analgesic effects. This was demonstrated in body torsion and hot plate experiments in mice (Li 1999). It also has anti-inflammatory effects. It can prevent egg-white-induced foot swelling and formaldehyde-induced arthritis (Xong 1963).

Aconite/chuan (Chuan wu): Has a centrally mediated analgesic effect. In mice it was shown to be effective for decreasing inflammation and pain. It is stronger than aspirin at reducing inflammation (Xian Dai Zhong Yao Yao Li Xue 1997). It controlled the signs in 92% of 150 human patients with arthritis when given in combination with Cao wu, Qiang huo, Du hua, Fu zi, Mo yao, Ru xiang, Dang gui, Chuan niu xi, Ma huang, Gui zhi, Wu gong, Chuan xiong, and Ma qian zi (Nei Meng Gu Zhong Yi Yao 1986).

Angelica (Bai zhi): Has demonstrated anti-inflammatory effects in mice. It also decreases pain (Zhong Guo Zhong Yao Za Zhi 1991).

Angelica root (Dang gui): As strong as aspirin at decreasing inflammation and is 1.7 times as strong as aspirin for pain relief (Yao Xue Za Zhi 1971). Dang Gui plus ligusticus (Chuan xiong) was 97% effective in treating lower back and leg pain (Xin Zhong Yi 1980).

Atractylodes (Cang zhu): Has analgesic effects. This was demonstrated using body torsion and heat-induced pain tests (Zhang 1999, Zhang 1996). It also has anti-inflammatory effects. It has been shown to prevent xylene-induced ear swelling and carrageenin-induced foot swelling (Zhang 1998).

Cinnamon bark (Rou gui): Inhibits both acute and chronic inflammation. It has demonstrated the ability to inhibit carrageenin-induced foot swelling and prevent adjuvant-induced arthritis (Li 1989).

Corydalis (Yan hu suo): Has anti-inflammatory properties. It inhibits histamine release and formation of edema in rats and has been shown to be effective for both acute and chronic inflammation (Kubo 1994). It increases the efficacy of acupuncture in inducing analgesia (Chen Tzu Yen Chiu 1994).

Dipsacus (Xu duan): Has anti-inflammatory properties. It can inhibit feet swelling in hamsters and dimethyl benzene-induced ear inflammation (Wang 1996).

Dragon's blood (Xue jie): Has been used to treat arthritis. In one study involving 150 participants with arthritis, 84% reported marked reduction in symptoms and 10% more reported some pain relief (Shan Xi Zhong Yi 1985).

Drynaria (Gu sui bu): Was used to treat 160 mice with osteoarthritis with good results (Zhong Yao Tong Bao 1987).

Eucommia bark (Du Zhong): An effective analgesic (Zhu 1986).

Jujube (Da zao): Has anti-inflammatory effects. It has been shown to prevent dimethylbenzene-induced ear swelling in mice and egg-white-induced toe swelling in rats (Li 1997).

Lycopodium (Shen jin cao): Has anti-inflammatory and analgesic effects. It ameliorates heat-induced pain and reduces dimethylbenzene-induced ear swelling (Zeng 1999).

Mastic (Ru xiang): Contains boswellic acids, which have anti-inflammatory effects in vivo and in vitro (Roy 2006). Mastic decreases signs of arthritis in dogs (Reichling 2004).

Myrrh (Mo yao): A very good analgesic, especially when combined with Ru xiang (Zhong Yao Xue 1998).

Pubescent angelica root (Du hou): Has demonstrated analgesic and anti-inflammatory effects in mice (Zhong Yao Yao Li Yu Ying Yong 1983).

White atractylodes (Bai zhu): Has been used with some success in patients suffering from chronic leg pain (Hu Bei Zhong Yi Za Zhi 1982).

White peony (Bai shao): Contains paeoniflorin, which is a strong anti-inflammatory (Zhong Yao Zhi 1993). In one trial, 65% of people suffering from painful conditions experienced relief when given Bai shao (Shang Hai Zhong Yi Yao Za Zhi 1983).

Acupuncture

Many people seek acupuncture therapy for musculoskeletal pain. Clinical trials have shown that arthritis can be treated successfully using acupuncture (Brattberg 1983, Junnila 1982).

Homotoxicology
General considerations/rationale

Traumatic tears of the cruciate ligament result in swelling and pain, which represent Inflammation Phase changes, while the destruction of the ligament and damage to joint structures is a Degenerative Phase disorder. Surgery is advised in most cases.

Prolotherapy (proliferation therapy) involves injecting a sclerosing agent (such as hypertonic dextrose) into an area so that fibroplasia and resultant fibrosis develop as new collagen is laid down. Experienced prolotherapists can assist degenerating cruciate ligament patients, and the procedure has been used in fully torn ligaments as well. Traumeel is used by some prolotherapists but many prefer to avoid it, voicing the concern it may decrease fibroplasia, which is the desired effect of prolotherapy. This concern may not be warranted; one study demonstrated that Traumeel actually decreases pain by increasing the rate of healing (Lussignoli, et al. 1999). Zeel or Discus compositum may be superior choices for use in prolotherapy due to their proposed activation of stem cells. No controlled studies exist to compare these therapeutic variations; therefore, at this time no specific recommendations can be made in this regard, and choice is based upon the preference and experience of individual practitioners.

Luxating patella is caused by a developmental error. Mild cases have been addressed with prolotherapy, but more severe cases may need surgery. Clients should be advised about their options as soon as this condition is diagnosed because early surgery decreases the severity of osteoarthritis that develops from continued trauma in unrepaired joints.

Antihomotoxic drugs can be useful in managing pain and increasing healing, and they may be added to the mixture used in prolotherapy.

Appropriate homotoxicology formulas
See also Arthritis, Autoimmune Arthritis.

Aesculus compositum: Used to improve circulation in the extremities.

BHI-Arthritis: Treats swollen, painful joints and muscle stiffness. It is particularly useful for those patients that are more affected in cold, wet weather.

Causticum compositum: The primary ingredient, from which this remedy's name is derived, is Causticum. It is used in cases of a neuralgic-rheumatic nature with restlessness and pains in the nerves and muscles, especially at night and in the legs. It is possibly associated with paralytic conditions that are often brought on by dry cold. Its symptom picture includes a typical stiffness in the joints, the whole musculature, the back, and the sacrum, and is often associated with a high degree of weakness, trembling, and an unsteady gait.

Colnadul: Treats arthritis that worsens with wet weather. It is particularly suited to knee problems, e.g., chronic dislocations. The authors use this in stifle issues (Broadfoot 2004).

Cruroheel: Provides ligamentous support.

Discus compositum: Provides deep tissue support of connective tissue.

Placenta compositum: Improves the condition of peripheral circulation.

Sulphur-Heel: See Arthritis protocols, above, for a discussion of sulphur.

Traumeel: A nonsteroidal anti-inflammatory that is useful in controlling pain and swelling in acute incidents and in chronically painful areas (Wright-Carpenter, et al. 2004).

Zeel: Provides support of joints and control of joint pain, as well as activation of stem cells.

Authors' suggested protocols

Nutrition
Cartilage/ligament/muscle/skeletal support formula: 1 tablet for every 25 pounds of body weight BID.

Eskimo fish oil: One-half to 1 teaspoon per meal for cats. 1 teaspoon for every 35 pounds of body weight for dogs.

Evening primrose oil: 1 capsule (500 mgs) per 25 pounds of body weight daily.

Betathyme: 1 capsule for every 35 pounds of body weight BID (maximum, 2 capsules BID.)

Chinese herbal medicine
Formula H97 HipGuard: 1 capsule per 10 to 20 pounds twice daily. For ACL rupture and meniscus injury, the higher dose of 1 capsule per 10 pounds body weight twice daily is used. It may take up to 6 to 9 months to completely stabilize the joint. Obesity, hip dysplasia, and lack of exercise can affect the response. It is strongly recommended that overweight dogs be placed on an appropriate diet.

The author recommends the following acupuncture points to treat ligamentous injuries: ST36, GB30, Baihui, BL60, and BL23.

Homotoxicology
For pain in acute ligamentous tears and postoperatively: Traumeel S QID for 3 days, then BID PRN. Zeel, given BID long-term. Causticum compositum, given BID, Coenzyme compositum, given BID, and BHI-Inflammation, given BID to QID.

For swelling postoperatively: Galium-Heel, Lymphomyosot, and Arnica-Heel, mixed together and given BID. Long-term therapy: BHI-Arthritis and/or Colnadul. Discus compositum, given EOD. Sulphur-Heel, given as needed.

Following prolotherapy: Aesculus compositum BID PO, Cruroheel BID PO. Discus compositum once weekly. Placenta compositum once weekly.

Product sources

Nutrition

Cartilage/ligament/muscle/skeletal support formula: Animal Nutrition Technologies. **Alternatives:** Cosequin— Nutramax Labs; Glycoflex—Vetri Science; Musculoskeletal support—Standard Process Veterinary Formulas; Nutriflex—Vet Rx Vitamins for Pets; Arthragen—Thorne Veterinary Products.

Evening primrose oil: Jarrow Formulas.

Eskimo fish oil: Tyler Encapsulations.

Betathyme: Best for Your Pet. **Alternative:** Moducare— Thorne Veterinary Products.

Chinese herbal medicine
Formula H97 HipGuard: Natural Solutions, Inc.

Homotoxicology
BHI/Heel Corporation

REFERENCES

Western medicine references

Arnoczky S, Tarvin G. Surgical repair of patella luxations and fractures. In: Bojrab MJ, ed. Current techniques in small animal surgery. 4th ed. Philadelphia: Lea and Febiger, 1998;1237–1244.

Brinker WO, Piermattei DL, Flo GL. Patellar luxations. In: Brinker WO, Piermattei DL, Flo GL, eds. Handbook of small animal orthopedics and fracture repair. 3rd ed. Philadelphia, Saunders, 1997;516–534.

Brinker WO, Piermattei DL, Flo GL. Physical examination for lameness. In: Handbook of small animal orthopedics and fracture repair. 3rd ed. Philadelphia: Saunders, 1997:228–230.

Brinker WO, Piermattei DL, Flo GL. In: Handbook of small animal orthopedics and fracture repair. 3rd ed. Philadelphia: Saunders, 1997:393–394.

Johnson JM, Johnson AL. Cranial cruciate ligament rupture: pathogenesis, diagnosis, and postoperative rehabilitation. In: Roush JK, ed. Stifle Surgery, *Vet Clin North Am Small Anim Pract* 1993;23:717–733.

Kirby BM. Decision-making in cranial cruciate ligament ruptures. In: Roush JK, ed. Stifle Surgery. *Vet Clin North Am Small Anim Pract* 1993;23:797–819.

Moore KW, Read RA. Rupture of the cranial cruciate ligament in dogs. Part I. *Compend Contin Educ Pract Vet* 1996;18:223–234.

Moore KW, Read RA. Rupture of the cranial cruciate ligament in dogs. Part II. Diagnosis and management. *Compend Contin Educ Pract Vet* 1996;18:381–405.

Slocum B, Slocum TD. Patella luxation. In: Bojrab MJ, ed. Current techniques in small animal surgery. 4th ed. Philadelphia: Lea and Febiger, 1998;1222–1236.

Slocum B, Slocum TD. Treatment of the stifle for cranial cruciate ligament rupture. In: Bojrab MJ, ed. Current techniques in small animal surgery. 4th ed. Philadelphia: Lea and Febiger, 1998:1187–11215.

Schwarz, PD. Patellar Luxation. In: Tilley L, Smith F. The 5-Minute Veterinary Consult: Canine and Feline, 2003. Blackwell Publishing.

Schwarz, PD. Cruciate Disease—Cranial. In: Tilley L, Smith F. The 5-Minute Veterinary Consult: Canine and Feline, 200. 3Blackwell Publishing.

Willauer C, Vasseur P. Clinical results of surgical correction of medial luxation of the patella in dogs. *Vet Surg* 1987;16: 31–36.

Nutrition reference

Gupta MB, Nath R, Srivastava N, et al. Anti-inflammatory and antipyretic activities of Beta sitosterol. *Planta Medica* 1980; 39: 157–163.

Chinese herbal medicine/acupuncture references

Brattberg G. Acupuncture therapy for tennis elbow. *Pain* 1983, 16:285–288.

Chen Tzu Yen Chiu (*Acupuncture Research*), 1994; 19(1):55–8.

Hu Bei Zhong Yi Za Zhi (*Hubei Journal of Chinese Medicine*), 1982; 6:57.

Junnila SYT. Acupuncture superior to piroxicam in the treatment of osteoarthritis. *American Journal of Acupuncture*, 1982, 10:341–345.

Kubo M, Matsuda H, Toluoka K, Ma S, Shiomoto H. Antiinflammatory activities of methanolic extract and alkaloidal components from Corydalis tuber. *Biol Pharm Bull*, 1994: Feb; 17(2):262–5.

Li JD. *Journal of Foreign Medicine*, vol. of Traditional Chinese Medicine. 1989;11(1):1.

Li XCh, et al. *Shannxi Journal of Medicine*. 1999;28(12): 735–736.

Li XM, et al. *Journal of Shizhen Medicinal Material Research*. 1997;8(4):373–374.

Nei Meng Gu Zhong Yi Yao (*Traditional Chinese Medicine and Medicinals of Inner Magnolia*), 1986;(3):7.

Reichling J, Schmokel H, Fitzi J, et al. Dietary support with Boswellia resin in canine inflammatory joint and spinal disease. *Schweiz Arch Tierheilkd.* 2004;146(2):71–9.

Roy S Khanna S, Krishnaraju AV, et al. Regulation of vascular responses to inflammation: inducible matrix metalloproteinase-3 expression in human microvascular endothelial cells is sensitive to anti-inflammatory Boswellia. *Antioxidants and Redox Signaling.* 2006;8(3 and 4):653–660.

Shan Xi Zhong Yi (*Shanxi Chinese Medicine*), 1985; 6(4):162.

Shang Hai Zhong Yi Yao Za Zhi (*Shanghai Journal of Chinese Medicine and Herbology*), 1983; 4:14.

Wang YT, et al. *Journal of TCM Pharmacology and Clinical Research*. 1996;12(3):20–30.

Xian Dai Zhong Yao Yao Li Xue (*Contemporary Pharmacology of Chinese Herbs*), 1997;425.

Xin Zhong Yi (*New Chinese Medicine*), 1980;2:34.

Xong ZY, et al. *Journal of Pharmacology*. 1963;10(12):708.

Yao Xue Za Zhi (*Journal of Medicinals*), 1971;(91):1098.

Zeng YE, et al. *Journal of Shizhen Medicine*. 1999;10(9): 641–642.

Zhang MF, et al. *Journal of Pharmacology and Clinical Application of TCM*. 1996;12(4):1–4.

Zhang MF, et al. *Journal of Pharmacology and Clinical Application of TCM.* 1998;14(6):12–16.

Zhang MF, et al. *Journal of Shizhen Medicine.* 1999;10(1): 1–3.

Zhong Guo Zhong Yao Za Zhi (*People's Republic of China Journal of Chinese Herbology*), 1991; 16(9):560.

Zhong Yao Tong Bao (*Journal of Chinese Herbology*), 1987; 12(10):41.

Zhong Yao Yao Li Yu Ying Yong (*Pharmacology and Applications of Chinese Herbs*), 1983; 796.

Zhong Yao Zhi (*Chinese Herbology Journal*), 1993:183.

Zhu LQ, et al. *Journal of Chinese Materia Medica.* 1986; 17(12):15.

Homotoxicology references

Broadfoot P. Homotoxicology for Musculoskeletal Problems. Heel/AHVMA Homotoxicology Seminar. May, 2003. Denver, CO. CD.

Lussignoli S, Bertani S, Metelmann H, Bellavite P, Conforti A. Effect of Traumeel S, a homeopathic formulation, on blood-induced inflammation in rats. *Complement Ther Med.* 1999. Dec;7(4): pp 225–30.

Wright-Carpenter T, Klein P, Schaferhoff P, Appell HJ, Mir LM, Wehling P. Treatment of muscle injuries by local administration of autologous conditioned serum: a pilot study on sportsmen with muscle strains. *Int J Sports Med.* 2004. Nov;25(8): pp 588–93.

OSTEOCHONDROSIS

Definition and cause

Osteochondrosis is a growth disturbance, often leading to an overproduction of cartilage. This thickened cartilage leads to degeneration and necrosis. Coupled with improper nutrition and trauma, this excessive cartilage can lead to ostechondritis dessecans in the shoulder, elbow, or stifle joint (Fox 1993; Paatsama 1971; Olsen 1975, 1976; Schwartz 2003). In addition, it is believed that improper nutrition and trauma to the cartilage surface contributes to the disease, often leading to a degenerative joint (Birkeland 1967, Hedhammer 1974, Palmer 1970, Schwarz 2003).

Medical therapy rationale, drug(s) of choice, and nutritional recommendations

Anti-inflammatory medications are used to control symptoms. They do not address the underlying degeneration, nor do they help to promote healing. Surgery is often indicated, especially when a flap of cartilage has formed. While surgery is often beneficial, it also does not address the underlying process and continual degeneration of the joint (Birkeland 1967, Clayton Jones 1970, Denny 1980, Smith 1975, Schwarz 2003).

Anticipated prognosis

Shoulder disease responds well to surgery and often results in pain-free and full mobility. The prognosis for other joints such as the stifle and elbow is more guarded. This depends upon the progression of the lesion and the extent of the associated degenerative joint disease (Grondalen 1979, Denny 1980, Schwarz 2003).

Integrative veterinary therapies

The cause of osteochondrosis is linked to developmental and nutritional factors. Suggested remedies include weight loss to ease the stress on the joint as well as chondroprotective agents that protect and strengthen the cartilage surfaces. In addition, the use of nutrients, antioxidants, phytonutrients, and anti-inflammatories that nourish tissues and reduce free radical cellular reaction as compared to medical suppression of the inflammation are beneficial for short- and long-term prognosis. Medicinal herbal and homeopathic remedies also further improve the prognosis.

Nutrition
General considerations/rationale

The focus of nutritional support is on reducing inflammation, nourishing joint cells and tissues, improving circulation, and enhancing healthy cellular and tissue formation.

Chondroprotective agents: Several studies have demonstrated the effectiveness of glucosamine and chondriotin in the management of arthritis in dogs (Das 2000, Guastella 2005). Numerous double-blind studies have compared the effectiveness of glucosamine against various NSAIDs, resulting in as good or, in many cases, even better pain control and removal of the clinical signs associated with osteoarthritis (Prudden 1974, Brown 1981, Vaz 1982, DeAmbrosia 1982). Additionally, the newer trend in the management of arthritis is toward chondroprotective agents such as glycosaminoglycans, pain-relieving agents such as methyl sulfonyl methane (MSM), and free radical scavengers such as superoxide dismutase (SOD) (Beale 2003, Todhunter 1994).

Super oxide dismutase: Super oxide dismutase (SOD) is a potent destroyer of free radicals that can protect cells against oxidative damage (Petkau 1975, Fridovich 1972). McCord (1974) reported that SOD can protect hyaluronate from free-radical damage and that it may have an anti-inflammatory effect (Salin and McCord 1975).

Vitamin C: Vitamin C has been studied clinically in animals. Brown (1994), Berg (1990), and Newman (1995) reported on the benefits of vitamin C in the treatment of degenerative joint disease and movement in dogs and in horses. Belfield (1981, 1998) reported on the beneficial effects of using vitamin C in treatment and prevention of hip dysplasia in dogs.

Botanical Cox2 inhibitors: Botanical Cox2 inhibitors have been shown to have anti-oxidative and anti-inflammatory effects (Bemis 2005). Botanical Cox 2 inhibitors offer the benefit of inflammation reduction without the inherent side effects of Cox2 medications.

Chinese herbal medicine/acupuncture
General considerations/rationale
Osteochondrosis is the result of Kidney Qi and Yang Deficiency. Wind, Cold, and Damp invade the body, leading to Qi and Blood stagnation. The Kidneys control the bones in TCM theory. When the Kidney is deficient in energy (Qi) and heat (Yang), the bones can suffer. Wind can blow pathogens into the body and from one joint to the other. Cold and Damp make the joint stiff and painful. Application of warmth eases discomfort. When Qi and Blood cannot flow they accumulate and cause pain. Treatment involves decreasing inflammation and pain. TCM is different from Western medicine as different areas of the body are treated differently, even in the face of a single Western diagnosis. Therefore, separate formulas and acupuncture points are given for forelimb verses hindlimb disease.

Appropriate Chinese herbs for hindlimb osteochondrosis
Achyranthes (Niu xi): Has analgesic effects. This was demonstrated in body torsion and hot plate experiments in mice (Li 1999). It also has anti-inflammatory effects. It can prevent egg-white-induced foot swelling and formaldehyde-induced arthritis (Xong 1963).

Aconite/chuan (Chuan wu): Has a centrally mediated analgesic effect. In mice it was shown to be effective for decreasing inflammation and pain. It is stronger than aspirin at reducing inflammation (Xian Dai Zhong Yao Yao Li Xue 1997). It controlled the signs in 92% of 150 human patients with arthritis when given in combination with Cao wu, Qiang huo, Du hua, Fu zi, Mo yao, Ru xiang, Dang gui, Chuan niu xi, Ma huang, Gui zhi, Wu gong, Chuan xiong, and Ma qian zi (Nei Meng Gu Zhong Yi Yao 1986).

Angelica (Bai zhi): Has demonstrated anti-inflammatory effects in mice. It also decreases pain (Zhong Guo Zhong Yao Za Zhi 1991).

Angelica root (Dang gui): As strong as aspirin at decreasing inflammation and is 1.7 times as strong as aspirin for pain relief (Yao Xue Za Zhi 1971). Dang Gui plus ligusticus (Chuan xiong) was 97% effective in treating lower back and leg pain (Xin Zhong Yi 1980).

Atractylodes (Cang zhu): Has analgesic effects. This was demonstrated using body torsion and heat-induced

pain tests (Zhang 1999, Zhang 1996). It also has anti-inflammatory effects. It has been shown to prevent xylene-induced ear swelling and carrageenin-induced foot swelling (Zhang 1998).

Cinnamon bark (Rou gui): Inhibits both acute and chronic inflammation. It has demonstrated the ability to inhibit carrageenin-induced foot swelling and prevent adjuvant-induced arthritis (Li 1989).

Corydalis (Yan hu suo): Has anti-inflammatory properties. It inhibits histamine release and formation of edema in rats and has been shown to be effective for both acute and chronic inflammation (Kubo 1994). It increases the efficacy of acupuncture in inducing analgesia (Chen Tzu Yen Chiu 1994).

Dipsacus (Xu duan): Has anti-inflammatory properties. It can inhibit foot swelling in hamsters and dimethyl benzene-induced ear inflammation (Wang 1996).

Dragon's blood (Xue jie): Has been used to treat arthritis. In one study involving 150 participants with arthritis, 84% reported marked reduction in symptoms and 10% more reported some pain relief (Shan Xi Zhong Yi 1985).

Drynaria (Gu sui bu): Was used to treat 160 mice with osteoarthritis with good results (Zhong Yao Tong Bao 1987).

Eucommia bark (Du Zhong): An effective analgesic (Zhu 1986).

Jujube (Da zao): Has anti-inflammatory effects. It has been shown to prevent dimethylbenzene-induced ear swelling in mice and egg-white-induced toe swelling in rats (Li 1997).

Lycopodium (Shen jin cao): Has anti-inflammatory and analgesic effects. It ameliorates heat-induced pain and reduces dimethylbenzene-induced ear swelling (Zeng 1999).

Mastic (Ru xiang): Contains boswellic acids, which have anti-inflammatory effects in vivo and in vitro (Roy 2006). Mastic decreases signs of arthritis in dogs (Reichling 2004).

Myrrh (Mo yao): A very good analgesic, especially when combined with ru xiang (Zhong Yao Xue 1998).

Pubescent angelica root (Du hou): Has demonstrated analgesic and anti-inflammatory effects in mice (Zhong Yao Yao Li Yu Ying Yong 1983).

White atractylodes (Bai zhu): Has been used with some success in patients suffering from chronic leg pain (Hu Bei Zhong Yi Za Zhi 1982).

White peony (Bai shao): Contains paeoniflorin, which is a strong anti-inflammatory (Zhong Yao Zhi 1993). In one trial, 65% of people suffering from painful conditions experienced relief when given white peony (Shang Hai Zhong Yi Yao Za Zhi 1983).

Appropriate Chinese herbs for forelimb osteochondrosis

Aconite/chuan (Chuan wu): See above.

Angelica (Bai zhi): See above.

Cinnamon twigs (Gui zhi): Have analgesic properties (Zhong Yao Xue 1998). In one trial, 30 patients were treated with a formula containing cinnamon twigs and other herbs. There was complete recovery in 50%, marked improvement in 20%, and some improvement in 17%. Thirteen percent did not respond (Shi Zhen Gua Yao Yan Jiu 1991).

Ginger (Sheng jiang): Has anti-inflammatory effects. It decreases dimethylbenzene-induced ear swelling in mice and egg-white-induced toe swelling in rats (Zhang 1989). It has been used to treat patients with arthritis. In one trial 113 of 125 people with arthritis responded to injections of ginger into acupoints (He Bai Xin Yi Yao 1972, Chi Jiao Yi Shi Za Zhi 1977).

Jujube fruit (Da zao): See above.

Licorice (Gan cao): Has analgesic effects, especially when administered with white peony (Bai shao) (Zhong Yao Xue 1998).

Lycopodium (Shen jin cao): See above.

Mastic (Ru xiang): See above.

Myrrh (Mo yao): See above.

Notopterygium (Qiang huo): Has both anti-inflammatory and analgesic effects. It can inhibit xylol-induced ear lobe swelling and carrageenin-induced foot swelling in mice, and increase the thermal pain threshold (Xu Hui Bo 1991).

White peony (Bai shao): See above.

Acupuncture

Many people seek acupuncture therapy for musculoskeletal pain. Clinical trials have shown that arthritis can be treated successfully using acupuncture (Brattberg 1983, Junnila 1982).

Homotoxicology
General considerations/rationale

Osteochondrosis represents a Deposition or Degeneration phase homotoxicosis. Therapy is directed at improving the status of the mesenchymal tissues. In early cases, these lesions may heal without surgery, and early intervention with antihomotoxic medications may assist the body in its innate reparative processes. Early diagnosis through radiography, MRI, or bone scans may assist in determining the optimal therapy for each patient.

Appropriate homotoxicology formulas

See Arthritis and Autoimmune Arthritis for a more complete discussion of remedies.

No controlled studies exist at this time for use of antihomotoxic agents in osteochondrosis, but appropriate selections include:

Coenzyme compositum: Supports energy metabolism. Succinate is useful in retarded development, which this condition may represent.

Discus compositum: Treats inflammation and degeneration of mesenchyme.

Lymphomyosot: Reduces swelling and improves lymphatic drainage with a corresponding decrease in local homotoxin levels.

Osteoheel: Supports bony structures. Can be alternated with *Traumeel* for maximal effect.

Placenta compositum: Provides support of stem cells and vasculature.

Molybdan compositum: Provides trace elements in degenerative conditions.

Thyroidea compositum: Acts on the thymus and therefore may assist in growth irregularities and support a wide variety of endocrine tissues. It is also a powerful agent in drainage of the mesenchyme.

Traumeel S: Used for inflammation and to unblock inactivated enzymes.

Ubichinon compositum: Provides support of energy metabolism in deeper homotoxicoses.

Zeel: An anti-inflammatory agent with regenerative potential through activation of stem cells.

Authors' suggested protocols

Nutrition

Cartilage/ligament/muscle/skeletal support formula: 1 tablet for every 25 pounds of body weight BID.

Eskimo fish oil: One-half to 1 teaspoon per meal for cats. 1 teaspoon for every 35 pounds of body weight for dogs.

Evening primrose oil: 1 capsule (500 mgs) per 25 pounds of body weight, daily.

Zyflamend: One-half dropper for every 25 pounds of body weight BID.

SOD: Follow manufacturer's suggested dosage.

Chinese herbal medicine

The author recommends Formula H3 ElboPhlex for osteochondrosis of the front legs and H97 HipGuard for osteochondrosis of the hind legs at a dose of 1 capsule per 10 to 20 pounds, twice daily. They can be combined with NSAIDs and/or nutraceuticals as needed. Generally speaking, it takes up to 3 to 6 months for complete resolution of signs in most cases.

H97 HipGuard: Contains achyranthes (Niu xi), aconite/chuan (Chuan wu), angelica (Bai zhi), angelica root (Dang gui), astragalus (Huang qi), atractylodes (Cang zhu), cinnamon (Rou gui), citrus (Chen pi), corydalis (Yan hu suo), curcuma (Yu jin), dioscorea (Chuan shan long), dipsacus (Xu duan), dragon's blood (Xue jie), drynaria (Gu sui bu), eucommia bark (Du Zhong), eupolyphaga

(Tu bie chong), jujube (Da zao), lycopodium (Shen jin cao), mastic (Ru xiang), morinda (Ba ji tian), myrrh (Mo yao), pubescent angelica root (Du huo), white atracty-lodes (Bai zhu), and white peony (Bai shao). The herbs not mentioned above (under Appropriate Chinese Herbs) help increase the efficacy of the formula.

H3 ElboPhlex: Contains aconite/chuan (Chuan wu), angelica (Bai zhi), centipede (Wu gong), cinnamon twigs (Gui zhi), codonopsis (Dang shen), dioscorea (Chuan shan long), ginger (Sheng jiang), jujube fruit (Da zao), licorice (Gan cao), lycopodium (Shen jin cao), mastic (Ru xiang), mulberry twig (Sang zhi), myrrh (Mo yao), not-opterygium (Qiang huo), papaya (Mu gua), pueraria (Ge gen), and white peony (Bai shao). The additional herbs not discussed above (under Appropriate Chinese Herbs) increase the efficacy of the formula.

For the hindlimbs, the author recommends the following acupuncture points: ST36, ST37, Baihui, BL60, GV4, and BL23. For the forelimbs, the author recommends LI11, PC6, SI9, Baihui, and BL23.

Homotoxicology

Discus compositum: Give every 3 days PO or SQ, alternating with Thyroidea compositum. Give Ubichinon compositum twice weekly.

Aesculus compositum, Traumeel, and Lymphomyosot: Mix together and give orally BID.

Osteoheel, Calcoheel, and/or BHI-Bone: Give orally BID as indicated by the individual case.

Zeel: Give tablets BID, and/or Zeel P vials injected into acupoints for the affected joint every week.

Molybdan SID: Use for mineral donor support.

Product sources

Nutrition

Cartilage/ligament/muscle/skeletal support formula: Animal Nutrition Technologies. **Alternative:** Cosequin—Nutramax Labs; Glycoflex—Vetri Science; Musculoskeletal support—Standard Process Veterinary Formulas; Nutriflex—Vet Rx Vitamins for Pets; Arthragen—Thorne Veterinary Products.

Evening primrose oil: Jarrow Formulas.

Eskimo fish oil: Tyler Encapsulations.

Zyflamend: New Chapter. **Alternative:** Botanical Treasures—Natura Health Products.

SOD: Cell Advance—Vetri Science; NaturVet SOD; BioPet International; N-Zymes.com.

Chinese herbal medicine
Formulas H3 ElboPhlex, H97 HipGuard: Natural Solutions, Inc.

Homotoxicology
BHI/Heel Corporation

REFERENCES

Western medicine references
Birkeland R. Osteochondritis dissecans in the humeral head of the dog. *Nord Vet Med* 1967.19:294.

Clayton Jones DG, Vaughan LC. The surgical treatment of osteochondritis dissecans of the humeral head in dogs. *J Small Anim Pract* 1970.11:803.

Denny HR, Gibbs C. The surgical treatment of Osteochondritis dissecans and ununited coronoid process in the canine elbow joint. *J Small Anim Pract* 1980.21:323.

Fox SM, Walker AM. The etiopathogenesis of osteochondrosis. *Vet Med* 1993;88:116–122.

Griffiths RC. Osteochondritis dissecans of the canine shoulder. *J Am Vet Med Assoc* 1968.153:1733.

Grondalen J. Arthrosis with special reference to the elbow joint of young rapidly growing dogs: III. *Nord Vet Med* 1979.31:520.

Hedhammer A, Wu FM, Krook L et al. Overnutrition and skeletal disease: An experimental study in growing Great Dane dogs. *Cornell Vet* 1974.64: 1.

Paatsama S, Rokkanen P, Jussila J, et al. A study of osteochondritis dissecans of canine humeral head using histological, OTC bone labeling, microradiographic and microangiographic methods. *J Small Anim Pract* 1971.12:603.

Olsson SE. Lameness in the dog: a review of lesion causing osteoarthrosis of the shoulder, elbow, hip, stifle and hock joints. *Proceedings of the American Animal Hospital Association*, 1975;42:363–370.

Olsson SE. Osteochondritis dissecans in the dog. *Proceedings of the American Animal Hospital Association* 1975.42:362.

Olsson SE. Osteochondrosis: A growing problem to dog breeders. *Gaines Progress*, 1976.1–11.

Palmer CS. Osteochondritis dissecans in Great Danes. *Vet Med/Small Anim Clin* 1970.65:994.

Schwarz PD. Osteochondrosis. In: Tilley L, Smith F. The 5-Minute Veterinary Consult: Canine and Feline, 2003. Blackwell Publishing.

Smith CW, Stowater JL. Osteochondritis dissecans of the canine shoulder joint: A review of 35 cases. *J Am Anim Hosp Assoc* 1975.11 :658.

IVM/nutrition references
Belfield WO. Orthomolecular Medicine: A Practitioners Prospective, in Alternative and Complementary Veterinary Medicine, Schoen A, Wynn S, eds. Mosby, 1998.p 113.

Belfield WO, Zucker M. How to have a healthy dog; the benefits of vitamin and minerals for your dogs life cycle, 1981. New York: New American Library.

Bemis DL, Capodice JL, Anastasiadis AG, Katz AE, Buttyan R. Zyflamend©, a Unique Herbal Preparation With Nonselective COX Inhibitory Activity, Induces Apoptosis of Prostate Cancer Cells That Lack COX-2 Expression, *Nutr Cancer.* 2005;52(2):202–12.

Berg J. Polyscorbate (C-Flex): an interesting alternative for problems on the support and movement apparatus in dogs; clinical trial of ester-C ascorbate in dogs, *Norweg Vet J.*, 1990;102:579.

Brown LP. Ester-C for Joint Discomfort—A Study. *Natural Pet*, 1994.Nov.-Dec.,

Brown LP. Vitamin C (Ascorbic Acid)—New Forms and Uses in Dogs. In: Proceeding of the North American Veterinary Conference, 1994.Orlando, FL.

Brown RA, Weiss JB. Neovascularization and its Role in the Osteoarthritic Process. *Ann. Rheum. Dis.*, 1981.4.

D'Ambrosia E, Casa B, Bompani R, Scali G, Scali M. Glucosamine Sulphate: A Controlled Clinical Investigation in Arthrosis. *Pharmatherapeutica* 1982.2:504–508.

Das AK, Hammad TA. Efficacy of a combination of FCH-G49TM glucosamine hydrochloride, TRH122TM low molecular weight sodium chondroitin sulfate and manganese ascorbate in the management of knee osteoarthritis. *Osteoarthritis Cart* 2000;8(5):343–350.

Fridovich I. Superoxide Radical and Superoxide Dismutase, *Acc Chem Res* 1972.5, 321.

Guastella DB, Cook JL, Kuroki K, et al. Evaluation of chondroprotective nutriceuticals in an in vitro osteoarthritis model. In: Proceedings of the 32nd Annual Conference Veterinary Orthopedic Society 2005;5.

McCord J. Free Radicals and Inflammations: Protection of Synovial Fluid by Superoxide Dismutase, *Science* 1974.185, 529.

Newman NL. Equine Degenerative Joint Disease, *Natural Pet*, 1995. March, April, p. 56.

Petkau A, Chelack W, Pleskach S, Meeker B, Brady C. Radioprotection of Mice by Superoxide Dismutase, *Biochem Biophys Res Commun* 1975.65, 886.

Prudden JF, Balassa LL. The Biological Activity of Bovine Cartilage Preparations. *Semin. Arthrit. Rheum.*, 1974.4:287–321.

Salin M, McCord J. Free Radicals and Inflammation. Protection of Phagocytosing Leukocytes by Superoxide Dismutase, *J Clin Invest* 1975.56, 1319.

Todhunter RJ, Lust G. Polysulfated glycosaminoglycan in the treatment of osteoarthritis, *J Am Vet Med Assoc* 1994;204:1245–1251.

Vaz AL. Double-blind Clinical Evaluation of the Relative Efficacy of Ibuprofen and Glucosamine Sulfate in the Management of Osteoarthritis of the Knee in Outpatients. *Curr. Med. Res. Opin.*, 1982.8:145–149.

Chinese herbal medicine/acupuncture references

Brattberg G. Acupuncture therapy for tennis elbow. *Pain* 1983, 16:285–288.

Chen Tzu Yen Chiu (*Acupuncture Research*), 1994; 19(1):55–8.

Chi Jiao Yi Shi Za Zhi (*Journal of the Barefoot Doctors*), 1077; 11:13.

He Bai Xin Yi Yao (*Hebei New Medicine and Herbology*), 1972; 3:31.

Hu Bei Zhong Yi Za Zhi (*Hubei Journal of Chinese Medicine*), 1982; 6:57.

Junnila SYT. Acupuncture superior to piroxicam in the treatment of osteoarthritis. *American Journal of Acupuncture*, 1982, 10:341–345.

Kubo M, Matsuda H, Toluoka K, Ma S, Shiomoto H. Antiinflammatory activities of methanolic extract and alkaloidal components from Corydalis tuber. *Biol Pharm Bull*, 1994: Feb; 17(2):262–5.

Li JD. *Journal of Foreign Medicine*, vol. of Traditional Chinese Medicine. 1989;11(1):1.

Li XC, et al. *Shannxi Journal of Medicine*. 1999;28(12):735–736.

Li XM, et al. *Journal of Shizhen Medicinal Material Research*. 1997;8(4):373–374.

Nei Meng Gu Zhong Yi Yao (*Traditional Chinese Medicine and Medicinals of Inner Magnolia*), 1986;(3):7.

Reichling J, Schmokel H, Fitzi J, et al. Dietary support with Boswellia resin in canine inflammatory joint and spinal disease. *Schweiz Arch Tierheilkd*. 2004;146(2):71–9.

Roy S Khanna S, Krishnaraju AV et al. Regulation of vascular responses to inflammation: inducible matrix metalloproteinase-3 expression in human microvascular endothelial cells is sensitive to anti-inflammatory Boswellia. *Antioxidants and Redox Signaling*. 2006;8(3and4):653–660.

Shan Xi Zhong Yi (*Shanxi Chinese Medicine*), 1985; 6(4):162.

Shang Hai Zhong Yi Yao Za Zhi (*Shanghai Journal of Chinese Medicine and Herbology*), 1983; 4:14.

Shi Zhen Gua Yao Yan Jiu (*Research of Shizen Herbs*), 1991; 5(4):36.

Wang YT, et al. *Journal of TCM Pharmacology and Clinical Research*. 1996;12(3):20–30.

Xian Dai Zhong Yao Yao Li Xue (*Contemporary Pharmacology of Chinese Herbs*), 1997;425.

Xin Zhong Yi (*New Chinese Medicine*), 1980;2:34.

Xong ZY, et al. *Journal of Pharmacology*. 1963;10(12):708.

Xu HB, et al. Pharmacology of Qiang Huo volatile oil. *Journal of Chinese Materia Medica*. 1991;22(1):28–30.

Yao Xue Za Zhi (*Journal of Medicinals*), 1971;(91):1098.

Zeng YE, et al. *Journal of Shizhen Medicine*. 1999;10(9):641–642.

Zhang MF, et al. *Journal of Pharmacology and Clinical Application of TCM*. 1996;12(4):1–4.

Zhang MF, et al. *Journal of Pharmacology and Clinical Application of TCM*. 1998;14(6):12–16.

Zhang MF, et al. *Journal of Shizhen Medicine*. 1999;10(1):1–3.

Zhang ZX, et al. *Journal of Chinese Materia Medica*. 1989;20(12):544, 545–546.

Zhong Yao Xue (*Chinese Herbology*), 1998; 65:67.

Zhong Yao Xue (*Chinese Herbology*), 1998; 759:765.

Zhong Guo Zhong Yao Za Zhi (*People's Republic of China Journal of Chinese Herbology*), 1991; 16(9):560.

Zhong Yao Tong Bao (*Journal of Chinese Herbology*), 1987; 12(10):41.

Zhong Yao Yao Li Yu Ying Yong (*Pharmacology and Applications of Chinese Herbs*), 1983; 796.

Zhong Yao Zhi (*Chinese Herbology Journal*), 1993:183.

Zhu LQ, et al. *Journal of Chinese Materia Medica*. 1986;17(12):15.

Homotoxicology reference

Heel. Veterinary Guide, 3rd English edition. Baden-Baden, Germany: Biologische Heilmettel Heel GmbH, 2003. p 53.

SPINAL ARTHRITIS/SPONDYLOSIS

Definition and cause

Spinal arthritis/spondylosis is a degenerative condition of the bony spinal column with associated osteophytic activity between vertebrae. It occurs in both dogs and cats and is believed to have an inherited predisposition or be the result of continual localized trauma and secondary inflammation to the bony vertebrae (Glenney 1956, Read 1966)(see Arthritis). Spondylosis is often discovered radiographically with no associated clinical signs (Joseph 2003).

Medical therapy rationale, drug(s) of choice, and nutritional recommendations

Once clinical signs of pain, inflammation, and reduced mobility become evident, the treatment is corticosteroids or NSAIDs such as carpofen, deracoxib, meloxicam, or aspirin. Nothing has been reported to prevent progression of the condition (Romatowski 1986, Joseph 2003).

Anticipated prognosis

The prognosis depends upon the extent of the arthritis and the resultant pain and impact upon the spinal cord. Pain and inflammation control offer good control of the signs. When the disease is progressive and has impacted the spinal cord and is causing neurological symptoms, the prognosis is more guarded (Hoerlein 1965, Joseph 2003).

Integrative veterinary therapies

Spinal arthritis occurs at the articular surfaces and has the same underlying mechanism as degenerative arthritis of the limbs. Medical treatment is directed toward the pain and inflammation, while integrative therapies are directed at the underlying cause of the inflammation and the associated degeneration that leads to the osteophytic process and potential compression of spinal nerves. Conventional medications address the inflammation and pain; however, they do not correct the underlying initiating inflammatory process.

Nutrition
General considerations/rationale
Nutritional and gland support are directed at reducing inflammation, protecting cells and tissue, and slowing the degenerative process.

Appropriate nutrients
Nutrition/gland support: Several studies have demonstrated the effectiveness of glucosamine and chondroitin in the management of arthritis in dogs (Das 2000, Guastella 2005). Setnikar et al (1986) has described how these compounds actually stimulate the body's own repair mechanism and help in the process of developing new cartilage. Numerous double-blind studies have compared the effectiveness of glucosamine against various NSAIDs, resulting in as good or, in many cases, even better pain control and removal of the clinical signs associated with osteoarthritis (Prudden 1974, Vaz 1982, DeAmbrosia 1982).

Fatty acids: In a double-blind study of people with rheumatoid arthritis, Joe (1993) showed that a number of people had significant benefits from the addition of evening primrose oil (EPO). Kremer (1995) has shown that fish oil helps to reduce inflammation in people with arthritis.

Botanical cox2 inhibitors: Botanical Cox2 inhibitors have been shown to have anti-oxidative and anti-inflammatory effects (Bemis 2005). Botanical Cox2 inhibitors offer the benefit of inflammation reduction without the inherent side effects of Cox2 medications.

Vitamin C: Vitamin C has been studied clinically in animals. Brown (1994), Berg (1990), and Newman (1995) reported on the benefits of vitamin C in the treatment of degenerative joint disease and movement in dogs and horses. Belfield (1981, 1998) reported on the beneficial effects of using vitamin C in treating and preventing hip dysplasia in dogs.

Lecithin/phosphatidyl choline: Lecithin/phosphatidyl choline is a phospholipid that is integral to cellular membranes. Lecithin/PC is an essential nutrient for the membranes of nerve cells and is essential for the proper conduction of nervous impulses (Hanin 1987).

Chinese herbal medicine/acupuncture
General considerations/rationale
Spinal arthritis is due to Wind, Damp, and Cold invading the body. This causes Kidney Qi and Yang deficiency, and Qi and Blood stagnation. Wind both blows the pathogen into the body and blows it around the body so the pain may wander from joint to joint. Damp causes stiffness and Cold implies that the condition tends to respond well to heat. Most people with degenerative skeletal conditions report that heat soothes the pain. Qi and Blood stagnation cause pain. The Kidney is charged with controlling bones, so when the Kidney suffers deficiency, arthritis may result. Again, as Yang is heat, a Kidney Yang deficiency may result in a sore skeletal lesion that responds well to heat therapy. Older patients are more likely to have degenerative spinal conditions and they are also more likely to have Kidney Yang deficiency. The Yang of the Kidney is used over the life of the individual.

Treatment options are designed to increase mobility and decrease pain and inflammation.

Appropriate Chinese herbs

Atractylodes (Cang zu): Increases the pain threshold (Zhang 1999). In addition, it can counteract xylene-induced ear swelling and carrageenin-induced foot swelling (Zhang Ming Fa 1998), which indicates that it may be useful in decreasing inflammation at the site of degenerative changes.

Aconite root (Fu zi): Reduces swelling and inflammation in joints (Zhong Yao Tong Bao 1988). It has been shown to have analgesic properties (Zhong Guo Zhong Yao Za Zhi 1992).

Angelica (Bai zhi): Has been shown to have anti-inflammatory and analgesic effects in mice (Zhong Guo Zhong Yao Za Zhi 1991).

Angelica root (Dang gui): As strong as aspirin at decreasing inflammation and is 1.7 times as strong as aspirin for pain relief (Yao Xue Za 1971).

Astragalus (Huang qi): Has demonstrated mild analgesic effects in mice (Zhong Yao Tong Bao 1986).

Cinnamon twigs (Gui zhi): Have analgesic properties (Zhong Yao Xue 1998). Cinnamon twigs were part of a formula used in 30 patients with arthritis. There was complete recovery in 50% of those treated, marked improvement in 20%, and some improvement in 17%. Thirteen percent did not respond (Shi Zhen Gua Yao Yan Jiu 1991).

Coix (Yi yi ren): Has analgesic and anti-inflammatory effects. It suppresses dimethylbenzene-induced auricular swelling and carrageenin-induced foot swelling in mice (Zhang Ming Fa 1998). It was shown to help women with severe menstrual cramps (Zhang Yong Luo 1998), which may indicate that it would be useful in treating the pain associated with spinal arthritis and spondylosis.

Earthworm (Di long): Has a significant analgesic effect (Chen 1996).

Jujube fruit (Da zao): Decreases inflammation. It was shown to reduce dimethylbenzene-induced auricular inflammation in mice and egg-white-induced toe swelling in rats (Li 1997). This implies that it may be useful for decreasing the inflammation involved with degenerative vertebral conditions.

Licorice (Gan cao): Contains glycyrrhizin and glycyrrhetinic acid, which have anti-inflammatory effects. They have approximately 10% of the corticosteroid activity of cortisone. They decrease edema and have anti-arthritic effects (Zhong Cao Yao 1991). Licorice has demonstrated analgesic effects in mice, especially when combined with white peony (Bai shao) (Zhong Yao Xue 1998).

Notopterygium root (Qiang huo): Has anti-inflammatory and analgesic effects. In mice it was shown to decrease xylol-induced ear lobe swelling and carrageenin-induced foot pad edema, and increase the thermal pain threshold (Xu 1991).

Sichuan aconite (Chuan wu): Seems to have a centrally mediated analgesic effect. In mice it was shown to be effective at decreasing inflammation and pain. It is stronger than aspirin at reducing inflammation (Xian Dai Zhong Yao Yao Li Xue 1997). It controlled the signs in 92% of 150 human patients with arthritis when given in combination with Cao wu, Qiang huo, Du hua, Fu zi, Mo yao, Ru xiang, Dang gui, Chuan niu xi, Ma huang, Gui zhi, Wu gong, Chuan xiong, and Ma qian zi (Nei Meng Gu Zhong Yi Yao 1986).

White peony (Bai shao): Contains paeoniflorin, which is a strong anti-inflammatory (Zhong Yao Zhi 1993). It has demonstrated specific effects on pain in the lower back (Yun Nan Zhong Yi 1990).

Acupuncture

The World Health Organization (2006) lists lower back pain as one of the indications for acupuncture. One study looked at the use of abdominal acupuncture and electroacupuncture for treatment of prolapsed lumbar intervertebral discs. In this study there was complete relief from symptoms in 35% of the patients, significant improvement in 45% of the participants, slight improvement in 16%, and no response in 4% (Guo 2003).

Homotoxicology
General considerations/rationale

Arthritis is a Deposition Phase disorder wherein material accumulates and eventually impedes the function of the joint. True arthritis of the spine occurs on the articular surfaces of the vertebral facets and is potentially painful. Spondylosis indicates degeneration of the spinal anatomy and is classified as a Degeneration Phase homotoxicosis. Spondylosis must be differentiated from spondylitis, and appropriate diagnostics conducted to rule out infectious agents.

Appropriate homotoxicology formulas

Also See Arthritis protocols, above, for a more detailed discussion of these remedies.

Atropinum compositum: Used for muscle spasm and pain. Currently only available in the United States as a tablet, but is extremely useful for acute, severe back pain.

BHI-Back: An important and commonly used formula supportive of the spinal column, and particularly the lower back. The component Colocynthis is indicated for sharp, tearing pain in the back that improves with warmth and deep pressure. Anger may be involved in these cases, and colitis may be an associated sign as well. Gnaphalium polycephalum is included for pain and/or numbness of the back and pelvis. Gelsemium sempervirens is included for neurologic weakness and muscle stiffness. Rhus toxicodendron is an important classical remedy for pain in tendons, ligaments, and soreness of condyles. Arsenicum album and Chamomilla complete this formula, with indications for cramps and neuralgia (Heel 2002).

BHI-Sciatic Rx: Used for sciatica and neuralgia of the legs.

BHI-Spasm-Pain: Treats muscle spasm and back pain. Components of this formula help with sharp pains and spasms. This is a good alternative due to *Atropinum compositum*. Febrile conditions with back pain may respond due to Aconitum nepellus. Treats inflammation of other serosal membranes (joints and the abdomen) due to Bryonia alba. Colocynthis and Cuprum sulfuricum are included for sharp pains and menstrual-like cramps and other muscle spasms (Heel 2002).

Cimicifuga homaccord: Treats pain and spasm of the cervical spine.

Coenzyme compositum: Supports energy metabolism.

Colocynthis homaccord: Treats lower back pain.

Discus compositum: Supports connective tissue that is associated with the spine.

Neuralgo-Rheum-Injeel: Contains Silicea, which is a major remedy for vaccinosis. Silicea is also contained in *BHI-Alertness, BHI-Migraine, BHI-Neuralgia, Cruroheel, Discus compositum, Spigelon, Strumeel,* and *Zeel.*

Osteoheel: Stimulates bone healing.

Spascupreel: Indicated for muscle spasm and pain. Compare its use to that of *Atropinum compositum* and *BHI-Spasm-Pain*. Contains Agaricus, a toxic mushroom indicated in homeopathic dilution for seizures, excitable conditions, motor tics, and sensitivity to cool air, among many other signs. It is helpful for migraine headaches and a wide variety of muscular spasmodic issues (Reckeweg 2000).

Testes compositum: Used for strengthening and draining the matrix in male patients with weakness. Contains Conium maculatum, which is useful in ascending hindlimb ataxia, weakness, and hemiplegia. Conium is also possibly useful in an older dog, and is also found in *Cerebrum compositum, Cocculus compositum, Ginseng compositum, Rauwolfia compositum, Thyroidea compositum, Tonsilla compositum, Ubichinon compositum, Vertigoheel, BHI-Circulation, BHI-Dizziness, BHI-Lightheaded,* and *BHI-Stramonium complex*. This remedy may cause detoxification/vicariation reactions and should be given with good observation and client education. It is highly useful in geriatric, male patients (Reckeweg 2000).

Traumeel S: A critically important formula that activates blocked enzymes. It is a nonsteroidal anti-inflammatory agent (See the homotoxicology Chapter for more extensive citations) (Heel 2003).

Zeel: A commonly used anti-inflammatory that reduces pain and improves mobility (see the homotoxicology chapter for more extensive citations) (Heel 2003).

Authors' suggested protocols

Nutrition

Cartilage/ligament/muscle/skeletal support and brain/nerve support formulas: 1 tablet for every 25 pounds of body weight BID.

Eskimo fish oil: One-half to 1 teaspoon per meal for cats. 1 teaspoon for every 35 pounds of body weight for dogs.

Evening primrose oil: 1 capsule (500 mgs) per 25 pounds of body weight daily.

Zyflamend: One-half dropper for each 25 pounds of body weight BID.

Lecithin/phosphatidyl choline: One-fourth teaspoon for every 25 pounds of body weight BID.

Chinese herbal medicine

Formula H39 Backrelief: 1 capsule per 10 to 20 pounds twice daily. It can be combined with NSAIDs and nutraceuticals if desired. It generally takes 2 to 4 weeks to see a response. In addition to the herbs listed above, Backrelief also contains aconite/cao (Cao wu), allium (Cong bai), carthamus (Hong hua), papaya (Mu gua), poria (Fu ling), and siler (Fang feng). These herbs increase the efficacy of the formula.

Recommended acupuncture points include BL23, BL40, GV4, ST36, Baihui, and GV3 (Handbook of TCM Practitioners 1987).

Homotoxicology

Symptom cocktail: Traumeel, Aesculus compositum, Cimicifuga homaccord (neck) or Colocynthis homaccord (lower spine), and Zeel, and/or BHI-Back mixed together and given orally BID to TID. Discus compositum given initially by injection and then orally 1 to 3 times weekly. Spascupreel, as an initial injection, then Atropinum compositum PRN (if available). Consider Dulcamara homaccord and Causticum compositum, if indicated, and Rhododendroneel, particularly if condition is worse with weather changes. Give Atropinum compositum tablets PRN.

Deep detoxification formula: Galium-Heel, Lymphomyosot, Hepar compositum, Solidago compositum, Thyroidea compositum, Coenzyme compositum, and Ubichinon compositum mixed together and given orally twice weekly for 2 to 4 weeks and then every other day. Adjust dosing based upon detoxification reactions observed.

Product sources

Nutrition

Cartilage/ligament/muscle/skeletal and brain/nerve support formulas: Animal Nutrition Technologies.

Alternatives: Cosequin—Nutramax Labs; Glycoflex—Vetri Science; Musculoskeletal support—Standard Process Veterinary Formulas; Nutriflex—Vet Rx Vitamins for Pets; Arthragen—Thorne Veterinary Products.

Evening primrose oil: Jarrow Formulas.

Eskimo fish oil: Tyler Encapsulations.

Zyflamend: New Chapter. **Alternative:** Botanical Treasures—Natura Health Products.

Lecithin/phosphatidyl choline: Designs for Health.

Chinese herbal medicine
Formula H39 Backrelief: Natural Solutions, Inc.

Homotoxicology
BHI/Heel Corporation

REFERENCES

Western medicine references
Glenney WC. Canine and feline spinal osteoarthritis (spondylitis deformans). *J Am Vet Med Assoc* 1956.129:61.
Hoerlein BF. Canine Neurology: Diagnosis and Treatment. 1965.Philadelphia: WB Saunders.
Joseph RJ. Spondylosis deformans. In: Tilley L, Smith F. The 5-Minute Veterinary Consult: Canine and Feline, 2003. Blackwell Publishing.
Read RM. Spondylosis deformans in the cat. Thesis, 1966. Bristol.
Romatowski J. Spondylosis deformans in the dog. *Compend Contin Educ Pract Vet* 1986;8:531–536.

IVM/nutrition references
Belfield WO. Orthomolecular Medicine: A Practitioners Prospective. In: Alternative and Complementary Veterinary Medicine, Schoen A, Wynn S, eds. Mosby,1998. p 113.
Belfield WO, Zucker M. How to have a healthy dog; the benefits of vitamin and minerals for your dog's life cycle, 1981. New York: New American Library.
Bemis DL, Capodice JL, Anastasiadis AG, Katz AE, Buttyan R. Zyflamend©, a Unique Herbal Preparation With Nonselective COX Inhibitory Activity, Induces Apoptosis of Prostate Cancer Cells That Lack COX-2 Expression, *Nutr Cancer.* 2005;52(2):202–12.
Berg J. Polyscorbate (C-Flex): an interesting alternative for problems on the support and movement apparatus in dogs; clinical trial of ester-C ascorbate in dogs, *Norweg Vet J.*, 1990.102:579.
Brown LP. Ester-C for Joint Discomfort—A Study. *Natural Pet*, 1994.Nov.-Dec.
Brown LP. Vitamin C (Ascorbic Acid)—New Forms and Uses in Dogs. In: Proceeding of the North American Veterinary Conference, 1994.Orlando, FL.
Das AK, Hammad TA. Efficacy of a combination of FCH-G49TM glucosamine hydrochloride, TRH122TM low molecular weight sodium chondroitin sulfate and manganese ascorbate in the management of knee osteoarthritis. *Osteoarthritis Cart* 2000;8(5):343–350.

Guastella DB, Cook JL, Kuroki K, et al. Evaluation of chondroprotective nutriceuticals in an in vitro osteoarthritis model. In: Proceedings of the 32nd Annual Conference Veterinary Orthopedic Society 2005;5.
D'Ambrosio E, Casa B, Bompani G, et al. Glucosamine sulphate: a controlled clinical investigation in arthrosis. *Pharmatherapeutica* 1981;2(8):5048.
Hanin IG, Ansell B. Lecithin: Technological, Biological, and Therapeutic Aspects, NY: Plenum Press, 1987. 180, 181.
Joe LA, Hart LL. Evening primrose oil in rheumatoid arthritis. *Ann Pharmacother* 1993;27:1475–7.
Kremer JM, Lawrence DA, Petrillow GF, et al. Effects of highdose fish oil on rheumatoid arthritis after stopping nonsteroidal antiinflammatory drugs. *Arthritis Rheum* 1995;38:1107–14.
Newman NL. Equine Degenerative Joint Disease, *Natural Pet*, March, April 1995. p. 56.
Prudden JF, Balassa LL. The Biological Activity of Bovine Cartilage Preparations. *Semin. Arthrit. Rheum.*, 1974.4:287–321.
Setnikar I, Giachetti C, Zanolo G. Pharmacokinetics of Glucosamine in the Dog and in Man. *Arzneimittelforschung*, 1986.36:729–735.
Vaz AL. Double-blind clinical evaluation of the relative efficacy of ibuprofen and glucosamine sulphate in the management of osteoarthritis of the knee in outpatients. *Curr Med Res Opin* 1982;8(3):145–9.

Chinese herbal medicine/acupuncture references
Chen BY, et al. Analgesic and antipyretic effects of Di Long powder in mice, rats and rabbits. *Journal of Shanghai Medical University.* 1996;23(3):225–226,240.
Guo F, Ma L, Gong L, Zhang H. 50 cases of prolapsed lumbar intervertebral disc using abdominal acupuncture. *Journal of Chinese Acupuncture and Moxibustion*, 2003. 23, p145.
Handbook of TCM Practitioners, Hunan College of TCM, Oct 1987.Shanghai Science and Technology Press.
Li XM, et al. *Journal of Shizhen Medicinal Material Research.* 1997;8(4):373–374.
Nei Meng Gu Zhong Yi Yao (*Traditional Chinese Medicine and Medicinals of Inner Magnolia*), 1986;(3):7.
Shi Zhen Gua Yao Yan Jiu (*Research of Shizen Herbs*), 1991; 5(4):36.
World Health Organization list of common conditions treatable by Chinese Medicine and Acupuncture. Available at: http://tcm.health-info.org/WHO-treatment-list.htm. Accessed 10/20/2006.
Xian Dai Zhong Yao Yao Li Xue (*Contemporary Pharmacology of Chinese Herbs*), 1997;425.
Xu HB, et al. Pharmacology of Qiang Huo volatile oil. *Journal of Chinese Materia Medica.* 1991;22(1):28–30.
Yao Xue Za Zhi (*Journal of Medicinals*), 1971;(91):1098.
Yun Nan Zhong Yi (*Yunnan Journal of Traditional Chinese Medicine*), 1990; 4:15.
Zhang MF, et al. Yi Yi Ren's analgesic, anti-inflammatory, and antithrombotic effects. *Journal of Practical TCM.* 1998;12(2):36–38.
Zhang MF, et al. *Journal of Pharmacology and Clinical Application of TCM.* 1998;14(6):12–16.

Zhang MF, et al. *Journal of Shizhen Medicine.* 1999;10(1): 1–3.

Zhang YL, et al. Sequential experiments on Yi Yi Ren's analgesic effect in severe functional Dysmenorrhea. *Journal of TCM.* 1998;39(10):599–600.

Zhong Cao Yao (*Chinese Herbal Medicine*) 1991;22 (10):452.

Zhong Guo Zhong Yao Za Zhi (*People's Republic of China Journal of Chinese Herbology*), 1991; 16(9):560.

Zhong Guo Zhong Yao Za Zhi (*People's Republic of China Journal of Chinese Herbology*), 1992; 17(2):104.

Zhong Yao Tong Bao (*Journal of Chinese Herbology*), 1988; 13(6):40.

Zhong Yao Xue (*Chinese Herbology*), 1998; 65:67.

Zhong Yao Xue (*Chinese Herbology*), 1998; 759:765.

Zhong Yao Zhi (*Chinese Herbology Journal*), 1993:183.

Homotoxicology references

Heel. BHI Homeopathic Therapy: Professional Reference. Albuquerque, NM: Heel Inc: 2002. pp 34, 97.

Heel. Veterinary Guide, 3rd English ed. Baden-Baden, Germany: Biologische Heilmittel Heel GMBH, 2003. pp 110–2, 116–8.

Reckeweg H. Biotherapeutic Index: Ordinatio Antihomotoxica et Materia Medica, 5th ed. Baden-Baden, Germany: Biologische Heilmittel Heel GMBH, 2000. pp 403.

TRAUMA: SPRAINS, STRAINS, AND FRACTURES

Definition and cause

Simple sprains, strains, and fractures represent an inflammatory process at the cellular and tissue level. Addressing these conditions depends upon the location and extent of the damage.

Medical therapy rationale, drug(s) of choice, and nutritional recommendations

Medical therapy is based upon the condition. Surgery, splinting, or bandaging is often required for fractures. Sprains and strains often require rest in combination with topical or systemic anti-inflammatory medication such as corticosteroids or NSAIDs, but these may reduce healing while controlling pain.

Anticipated prognosis

The prognosis depends on the injury and/or the location. The prognosis is generally favorable for healing.

Integrative veterinary therapies

The focus of integrative therapy for sprains, strains, and fractures is on the status of the body's healing ability and state of degeneration, rather than entirely on the injury or its location. First, animals that are in a stage of degeneration are more prone to injury. Second, the injury in a degenerating animal may heal on the surface; however, the trauma may exacerbate the process of degeneration. Finally, medications may also contribute to the degeneration by causing untoward side effects. The selection of appropriate therapeutic nutrients and biological therapies can help minimize side effects of medication, reduce inflammation, and improve the immune status of the body. An improved immune status can assist healing and help to stabilize or reverse underlying degeneration (Goldstein 2005).

Nutrition
General considerations/rationale

The understanding of the concept listed above in Integrative Veterinary Therapies can expand clinicians' focus to include not only the injury and location, but also the status of the healing and immune systems. The selection of appropriate therapeutic nutrients helps to reduce inflammation and free radicals, and enhances immune system balance and function.

Appropriate nutrients

Nutrition/gland support: Cartilage, antioxidants, and essential fatty acids that contain omega-3 and -6 acids help reduce inflammation and free radicals and support and improve immune function.

Fatty acids: In a double-blind study of people with rheumatoid arthritis, Joe (1993) showed that a number of people significantly benefited from the addition of oil of evening primrose oil (EPO). Kremer (1995) has shown that fish oil helps to reduce inflammation in people with arthritis.

Plant sterols: Betasitosterol is a plant sterol and immune-modulating agent that has immune-enhancing and anti-inflammatory effects (Bouic 1996, 1999; Gupta 1980; Vanderhaeghe 1999).

Chinese herbal medicine/acupuncture
General considerations/rationale

Trauma leads to Blood and Qi stagnation, which can cause pain. Western practitioners state that trauma leads to inflammation.

Appropriate Chinese herb

Notoginseng (San qi): Has nonsteroidal anti-inflammatory action. It has been shown to be more COX-2 selective than ibuprofen and naproxen (Seaver 2004).

Acupuncture

Acupuncture has been accepted as an effective modality for the treatment of musculoskeletal disorders by the World Health Organization (2006). It decreases the pain associated with the injury. In one study, 9 of 12 volunteers reported that acupuncture increased the pain threshold (Stacher 1975).

Homotoxicology
General considerations/rationale

Simple sprains, strains, and fractures represent Inflammation Phase disorders. In cases where the patient is in the Impregnation Phase, the tissues are less elastic and more prone to injury. Fractures can also occur in Degeneration and Dedifferentiation phases; therefore, the clinician should examine the case and determine if simple therapy with Traumeel S is sufficient, or if deeper homotoxicoses exist. Clients need to be fully educated about the patient's current phase so they are not surprised when the desired regressive vicariation reactions occur.

Corticosteroids can decalcify bone and decrease healing. Using excessive levels of nonsteroidal drugs can actually decrease fibroplasia and prolong recovery, as well as injure other organ systems such as the liver, kidney, and intestinal lining (Busti, et al. 2005; Adebayo, Bjarnason 2006). Because the intestinal lining is critical to proper immune function, these drugs can theoretically impact the immune system in ways far greater than currently understood. Use of biological therapy may avoid such damage and is desirable, and it is well tolerated by patients.

Topical therapy with Traumeel gel or ointment and Zeel ointment have brought good control of pain in simple strains and sprains, and are widely used by human athletes and their trainers with no known major adverse effects.

Appropriate homotoxicology formulas

Aesculus compositum: Promotes circulation and healing.

Belladonna homaccord: Used in cases with intense inflammation and redness.

BHI-Arthritis: Used for joint pain.

BHI-Arnica ointment: Can relieve pain associated with trauma when applied topically.

BHI-Inflammation: Treats joint pain and inflammation.

Placenta compositum: Assists extremity vasculature in poorly healing injuries.

Cruroheel: Treats sprains and strains, and assists with ligamentous healing.

Discus compositum: Used for tendency toward strains, and improves healing function.

Osteoheel: Stimulates bone healing and is used in ankle injuries of all kinds.

Traumeel S: When given orally in drops or applied topically as gel or ointment, assists in reducing inflammation and stimulating and accelerating healing (Lussignoli, et al. 1999).

Zeel: Used for bone and joint pain. Stimulates healing and pain control over several weeks' duration. Traumeel is more clinically effective for acute pain.

Authors' suggested protocols
Nutrition

Cartilage/ligament/muscle/skeletal support formula: 1 tablet for every 25 pounds of body weight BID.

Eskimo fish oil: One-half to 1 teaspoon per meal for cats. 1 teaspoon for each 35 pounds of body weight for dogs.

Evening primrose oil: 1 capsule (500 mgs) per 25 pounds of body weight daily.

Betathyme: 1 capsule for every 35 pounds of body weight BID (maximum, 2 capsules BID.)

Chinese herbal medicine

The authors use a patent formula called Yun Nan Bai Yao (also known as Yunnan Bai Yao or Yunnan Paiyao) at the supplier's recommended dose. In addition to the herb cited above, Yun Nan Bai Yao may also contain Dioscorea nipponica (Chuan shan long), erodium (Lao guan cao), inula flowers (Xuan fu hua), and/or other herbs, depending upon the manufacturer.

Acupuncture points for trauma include GB20, LI11, TH5, GB34, BL37, BL60, GB30, and ST36. (Basic and Express Acupuncture therapy 1969). The practitioner may also consider local points.

Homotoxicology

In all cases: Topical Traumeel gel mixed with Lymphomyosot gel, as needed for control of pain and swelling. Traumeel drops given every 15 minutes for 4 to 5 dosages, then QID day 1, TID days 2 and 3, and BID day 4 and as needed. Discus compositum given at the dose of 1 tablet every other day. BHI-Inflammation is also a useful remedy selection, if available.

In all cases: Topical Zeel ointment BID mixed with Traumeel gel. Zeel tablets given twice daily.

For fractures and other injuries involving bone: Osteoheel for fractures PO QID day 1, TID day 2, BID days 3 and beyond. BHI-Injury given BID, possibly alternating with Bone BID, particularly for non-union fractures.

For sprains and strains: Cruroheel PO BID alternated with Traumeel and Osteoheel as needed.

In cases of severe swelling: Lymphomyosot and Apis given orally QID day 1 and as needed afterward.

Product sources
Nutrition

Cartilage/ligament/muscle/skeletal and immune support formulas: Animal Nutrition Technologies. **Alternatives:** Cosequin—Nutramax Labs; Glycoflex—Vetri Science; Musculoskeletal support—Standard Process Veterinary Formulas; Nutriflex—Vet Rx Vitamins for Pets; Arthragen—Thorne Veterinary Products.

Betathyme: Best for Your Pet. Alternative: Moducare—Thorne Veterinary Products.

Eskimo fish oil: Tyler Encapsulations.

Evening primrose oil: Jarrow Formulas.

Chinese herbal medicine

Yun Nan Bai Yao (also known as Yunnan Bai Yao or Yunnan Paiyao): China Direct.

Homotoxicology

BHI/Heel Corporation

REFERENCES

IVM/nutrition references

Goldstein R, Goldstein S. The Goldstein Wellness and Longevity Program, 2005. Neptune City, NJ: TFH Publication.

Gupta MB, Nath R, Srivastava N, et al. Antiinflammatory and antipyretic activities of Beta sitosterol. *Planta Medica* 1980; 39: 157–163.

Joe LA, Hart LL. Evening primrose oil in rheumatoid arthritis. *Ann Pharmacother* 1993;27:1475–7 [review].

Kremer JM, Lawrence DA, Petrillow GF, et al. Effects of highdose fish oil on rheumatoid arthritis after stopping non-steroidal antiinflammatory drugs. *Arthritis Rheum* 1995;38: 1107–14.

Vanderhaeghe LR, Bouic PJD. The Immune System Cure: Optimize Your Immune System in 30 Days—The Natural Way! New York City: Kensington Books, 1999, p. 205.

Chinese herbal medicine/acupuncture references

Basic and Express Acupuncture Therapy. Air Force Shenyang hospital, July 1969.People's Health Press.

Seaver B, Smith J. Inhibition of COX Isoforms by Nutra-ceuticals. *J of Herbal Pharmacotherapy*. 2004;4(2):11–18.

Stacher G, Wancura I, Bauer P, Lahoda R, Schulze D. Effect of acupuncture on pain threshold and pain tolerance determined by electrical stimulation of the skin: a controlled study. *Am J Chin Med* 1975; Apr;3(2):143–9.

World Health Organization list of common conditions treatable by Chinese Medicine and Acupuncture. Available at: http://tcm.health-info.org/WHO-treatment-list.htm   Accessed 10/20/2006.

Homotoxicology references

Adebayo D, Bjarnason I. Is non-steroidal anti-inflammatory drug (NSAID) enteropathy clinically more important than NSAID gastropathy? *Postgrad Med J.* Mar;82(965): 2006. pp 186–91.

Busti AJ, Hooper JS, Amaya CJ, Kazi S. Effects of perioperative antiinflammatory and immunomodulating therapy on surgical wound healing. *Pharmacotherapy.* 2005. Nov;25(11): pp 1566–91.

Lussignoli S, Bertani S, Metelmann H, Bellavite P, Conforti A. Effect of Traumeel S, a homeopathic formulation, on blood-induced inflammation in rats. *Complement Ther Med.* 1999. Dec;7(4): pp 225–30.

Chapter Fourteen

Diseases of the Respiratory System

BRONCHITIS: ACUTE, ALLERGIC, AND CHRONIC

Definition and cause

Inflammation is the underlying mechanism in bronchitis. Acute and allergic forms are caused by exposure to environmental irritants, mechanical (collapse), allergens, infections, and toxins. Chronic bronchitis results from ongoing airway irritation, inflammation, swelling, increased mucus production, smooth muscle spasms, narrowing, and chronic coughing. It is common in both dogs and cats (see Feline Bronchial Asthma, below) (Bonagura 1991, 1994; Dye 1996; Forrester 1997; Johnson 1997; McKiernan 2003; Padrid 1990; Schaer 1989).

Medical therapy rationale, drug(s) of choice, and nutritional recommendations

Therapy for bronchitis is directed at the inflammation and cough. However, it is important to first rule out other underlying causes such as heart disease, dental disease, infection, infestation, and cancer. Commonly recommended drugs include antitussives such hydrocodone, antibiotics, corticosteroids, and bronchodilators such as aminophylline and theophylline. No dietary or supplemental guidelines are recommended (Forrester 1997, McKiernan 2003, Padrid 1990).

Anticipated prognosis

The prognosis depends on finding and addressing the underlying cause. Bronchitis is a progressive disease in which the signs can be controlled; however, it is not considered to be a curable disease (Padrid 1990).

Integrative veterinary therapies

The integrative approach to bronchitis focuses on enhancing toxin elimination and reducing inflammation. Allergic bronchitis involves the immune system's reaction to allergens, with the bronchus as the target organ for the inflammatory response. Local bacterial populations often invade secondary to the chronic irritation, resulting in bronchial infection. The medical focus is upon the cough, irritation, and infection, and does not address the underlying cause; therefore, recurrences are common, often leading to chronic bronchitis.

When nutritional, herbal, and biological therapies are added to the prevention and treatment protocols, cellular elimination of wastes is encouraged, cellular inflammation is reduced, and secondary bacterial invasion is less likely.

Nutrition
General considerations/rationale

Therapeutic nutrition adds nutrient and gland support for the lungs and organs of the immune system. In addition, nutrients can help decrease local cellular inflammation while improving elimination of toxins.

Appropriate nutrients

Nutrition/gland therapy: Glandular adrenal, thymus, bronchus, and lung provide intrinsic nutrients that nourish the organ, help to neutralize cellular inflammation, and help to balance the immune system (see Gland Therapy, Chapter 2, for a more detailed explanation).

Vitamin B_6 (pyridoxine): Vitamin B_6 can be beneficial for animals with allergic bronchitis similar to those with asthma. Asthmatics have reduced levels of vitamin B_6, which has a natural antihistaminic effect. This can be a real deficiency or a side effect of brochodilating medications such as theophylline, which can cause a B_6 deficiency (Collipp 1975, Weir 1990). In clinical trials, vitamin B_6 supplementation has been found to help reduce the levels of required medication as well as decrease the frequency of allergic reactions such as asthmatic episodes (Collipp 1975, Reynolds 1895). Other studies found that some asthmatic patients still required corticosteroids to control the symptoms (Sur 1993).

Quercetin: Quercetin is a flavonoid that has potent antioxidant properties. Quercetin also has been proven to inhibit cells from releasing histamines (Middleton 1986, Ogasawara 1985). This antihistamine attribute is beneficial in the treatment of allergic conditions such as asthma and can improve breathing in compromised conditions such as pneumonia. Quercetin inhibits the enzyme lipoxygenase, which contributes to the clinical signs associated with asthma (Welton 1986).

Bromelain: Bromelain is a proteolytic enzyme that comes from pineapples. It has anti-inflammatory properties and is beneficial for the upper respiratory system (Taub 1966). Ryan (1967) showed an improvement in the treatment of sinusitis with bromelain in a double-blind study. Another characteristic of bromelain is its ability to reduce the thickness of mucus in the respiratory system, which is beneficial for allergic conditions such as asthma and all inflammatory and infectious respiratory diseases (Schaefer 1985). In addition, bromelain has been shown to positively affect white blood cells and the immune response, which is also beneficial for respiratory infections (Desser 1994, Kelly 1996, Munzig 1995).

N-acetyl cysteine (NAC): N-acetyl cysteine is an amino acid derivative of cysteine that helps break down mucous accumulations. In double-blind clinical trials, people with bronchitis showed improved symptoms and a decrease in recurrences when supplemented with NAC (Bowman 1983, Grandjean 2000). NAC is also a potent antioxidant that is protective of bronchial and pulmonary tissues (Van Schayck 1998). NAC has been shown to help break up mucus, and in a double-blind study, people with chronic bronchitis showed reduced coughing and an improved ability to expectorate. Another trial linked these benefits to the reduced viscosity of the sputum (Jackson 1984, Tattersall 1983).

Chinese herbal medicine/acupuncture
General considerations/rationale
Practitioners of TCM recognize different patterns of bronchitis. Patients with dry, unproductive coughs have a diagnosis of Qi and Yin deficiency. Yin refers to the fluids of the body. A Yin-deficient cough is therefore dry and non-productive. Patients with a productive cough have Qi and Yang deficiency. Yang and Yin balance each other according to TCM theory. Therefore, a Yang deficiency leads to a relative Yin excess. Yin is cold and moist. Cold discharges are white. Put together, the term Yang-deficient cough translates into a wet, productive cough with slight to copious, clear to white discharge. It is important to clear these discharges.

The Qi deficiency leads to immunosuppression because the immune system is a function of the energy of Qi. Therefore, the patient is susceptible to secondary bacterial, fungal, or viral pathogens. A clinician treating a patient with bronchitis, even if not initially caused by a pathogenic organism, must be prepared to recognize and treat secondary infections.

Appropriate Chinese herbs for dry nonproductive coughs
Adenophora (Sha shen): Suppresses coughs (Zhong Hua Yi Xue Za Zhi 1956) and has antifungal activity (Zhong Hua Pi Fu Ke Xue Za Zhi 1957).

Anemarrhena (Zhi mu): Has antibacterial properties (Yao Xue Qing Bao Tong Xun 1987).

Apricot seeds (Xing ren): Decrease coughing (Zhang 1991).

Aster (Zi wan): Demonstrates significant expectorant activity and is effective against several bacteria, viruses, and fungi (Chang Yong Zhong Yao Cheng Fen Yu Yao Li Shou Ce 1994).

Licorice (Gan cao): Contains glycyrrhizin. This compound has demonstrated antiviral effects against several classes of viruses and antibiotic effects against various bacteria (Zhu 1996, Zhong Yao Zhi 1993). It suppresses coughing and has expectorant activity (Zhong Yao Yao Li Yu Ying Yong 1983).

Mulberry leaf (Sang ye): Has demonstrated antibacterial activity against several types of bacteria (Zhong Yao Yao Li Yu Ying Yong 1983).

Ophiopogon (Mai dong): Has demonstrated antibacterial effects (Zhong Yao Xue 1998).

Platycodon (Jie geng): Has both expectorant and antitussive activity (Zhong Yao Yao Li Yu Ying Yong 1983).

Schisandra (Wu Wei zi): Has demonstrated activity against many bacteria (Zhong Yao Xue 1998).

Stemoma (Bai bu): Acts on the central nervous system to suppress coughs (Zhong Yao Yao Li Yu Ying Yong 1983).

Tangerine peel (Chen pi): Causes bronchial dilation (Shang Hai Yi Yao Za Zhi 1957).

Appropriate Chinese herbs for productive coughs
As above, the following herbs can be used for their antibacterial effects:

Coltsfoot flower (Kuan dong hua): Suppresses coughs, decreases respiratory tract secretions, and relieves wheezing (Zhong Yao Yao Li Yu Ying Yong 1983).

Dolichos seed (Bian dou): Has antibacterial and antiviral effects (Dictionary of Chinese Medicines 1997).

Poria (Fu ling): Inhibits Staphylococcus aureus, Bacillus coli, and Bacillus proteus (Nanjing College 1976).

Schisandra (Wu Wei zi), ophiopogon (Mai men dong), licorice (gan cao), and aster (zi wan): Ophiopogon (Mai men dong) also increases mucociliary transport velocity in quails and decreased respiratory tract mucus secretion (Tai 2002).

Acupuncture points

LU1, BL13, CV22, LI11, GV14, and Ding-chuan can be used to stop coughing (Zhong Yi Shi Xi Yi Shi Sou Ce 1987).

Homotoxicology
General considerations/rationale

Acute bronchitis is an Inflammation Phase condition, but acute flares of inflammation often occur with deeper phase homotoxicoses as they attempt to improve through regressive vicariation. Allergic bronchitis represents an Impregnation Phase disorder and quickly may deteriorate into a Degeneration Phase problem. Chronic bronchitis usually occurs in the Impregnation and Degeneration phases. The body deposits many homotoxins into the pulmonary connective tissue and the Deposition Phase is generally asymptomatic. Iatrogenic damage from antibiotics and prior infections (viral particles, endotoxins, etc.) may play a part in the genesis of chronic bronchial and pulmonary diseases. The clinician needs to look carefully at the patient and medical history to determine which phase is most represented in choosing the therapy. Diagnostic procedures are indicated as needed to separate diagnoses and determine therapy.

It is not expected that a rapid cure will occur in cases to the right of the Biological Divide. Autosanguis therapy is indicated in such cases (Broadfoot 2004). These patients can undergo sudden and dramatic increases in the secretory activity of the bronchial mucosa. Such sudden changes represent movement to the left of the Six-Phase Table of Homotoxicology and are desirable, although they can present the clinician and owner with difficult choices. Generally, supporting treatments, which move the patient toward inflammation and excretion, will lead to improved conditions over longer periods of time.

As an example, Palmquist treated an aged poodle suffering from chronic allergies and chronic obstructive pulmonary disease with great success. On presentation the dog was nonresponsive to standard drug therapy and had failed therapy at a boarded internist's practice. This dog was treated with autosanguis therapy and developed immediate copious mucus excretion and severe coughing and dyspnea. The patient was treated for 2 years and gradually improved until it was able to function with no pharmaceutical drugs. Chronic antihomotoxic therapy was needed for patient comfort for the remainder of its life.

Appropriate homotoxicology formulas

Respiratory disease is a complex issue and there are many possible combinations of remedies needed to obtain a clinical result. The following major remedies provide a starting place for the clinician interested in biological therapy.

Aconitum homaccord: Used for animals that are fearful; avoid touch; or experience aggravations following dry, cold weather or very hot weather. Other symptoms: sensitive to noises, feels like water trapped in left ear, red eyes, epiphora, dry-short or hacking cough that is especially worse late at night (Boericke 1927; Skaltsa, Philianos, and Papaphilippou 1997); red, flushed skin; tachycardia with pain in left shoulder; intermittent fever and chills; cough with nausea (Reckeweg 2000). A recent study of a Brazilian homeopathic combination including Aconitum indicates a possible mechanism of action affecting macrophage function directly (de Oliveira, et al. 2006). Useful as first prescription in inflammation and inflammatory fevers.

Atropinum compositum: Oral and injectable vials are not currently available in the United States, but tablets are and can be very useful for spasmodic bronchial coughing.

Belladonna homaccord: Used for acute onset conditions; dry nose; mucus catarrhal discharge, possibly with blood; tickling dry cough; whooping cough, possibly with pain in the left hip; may cry out in sleep; painful, high fever (Boericke 1927); delirium; aggression; sudden biting behavior. Canine distemper patients often benefit from this remedy (Heel 2003). Echinacea supports immune response. *Belladonna homaccord* is frequently indicated after *Aconitum homaccord*, when the flu-like, chill symptoms of Aconite have passed the critical point and localized symptoms such as pharyngitis and bronchitis have commenced (Reckeweg 2002). Belladonna is found in a variety of remedies.

BHI-Bronchitis: Treats wet and dry coughs and coughs worsened by smoke exposure (Heel 2002).

BHI-Chest: Treats cough with rib pain.

BHI-Cough: Treats mild coughs, wet and dry coughs, and smoke-induced coughs. Contains Quebracho for bronchial asthma and asthmatic bronchitis with dyspnea; also in emphysema (Reckeweg 2002). Also found in *Tartephedreel*.

Bronchalis: Treats acute and chronic bronchitis. The remedy Kreosotum, which is also common to *BHI-Bronchitis*, *Lamioflur*, and *Mucosa compositum*, is useful in chronic mucosal conditions with offensive, acrid, excoriating discharges; chronic bronchitis; bronchiectasis; and spasmodic cough (Reckeweg 2002).

Bryaconeel: Treats chronic bronchitis and pulmonary changes, particularly in aging animals.

Coenzyme compositum: Activates energy pathways and provides repair following mitochondrial damage by antibiotics and other drugs. Contains Baryta oxalsuccinica, which is indicated for chronic bronchitis (Reckeweg 2002). This remedy is also found in *BHI-Enzyme*.

Drosera homaccord: Treats cough aggravated by or originating following cold, wet weather; bronchial asthma; and spasmotic cough.

Echinacea compositum: Treats inflammation and provides immune support in viral and bacterial infections and febrile disorders. The ingredient Sanguinaria canadensis is particularly useful; it is indicated for patients with a history of violent pains in the mouth, chest, larynx, and trachea when coughing and breathing, which are aggravated at night. Eructation during or after coughing is also a typical symptom. Also treats bronchitis with tough, thick mucus; bronchiectasis with spastic cough; and right-sided pneumonia. This remedy contains Thuja for asthmatic bronchitis with copious expectoration at night (Reckeweg 2002).

Engystol N: Provides sulfur and matrix drainage in viral cases, and increases activity of the immune system.

Euphorbium compositum: An antiviral that is useful in clearing upper respiratory passages in sinusitis. Consider its use in viral bronchitis. May be helpful during regressive vicariation with signs compatible with viral homotoxins.

Galium-Heel: Used for chronic cases and allergy. Provides cellular detoxification and matrix drainage.

Husteel homaccord: Treats dry cough, chronic nasal discharge, sore neck, and catarrhal respiratory tract. The remedy Arsenicum iodatum, which is common to *Tartephedreel*, is particularly indicated for purulent respiratory diseases (Reckeweg 2002).

Lamioflur: Used for putrefied sputum and foul nasal discharges.

Lymphomyosot: Provides drainage of connective tissue and lymphatics. Used for mucocutaneous lesions.

Mercurius-Heel S: Used for catarrhal, suppurative conditions. It is antiviral and antibacterial.

Mucosa compositum: Used in Degeneration Phase homotoxicoses and during the recovery phase following initial infection and to repair damage from pharmaceutical agents.

Phosphor homaccord: Treats laryngitis, cough tending to develop pneumonia, and bloody sputum. Constitutionally, these patients tend to be tall/long and thin. They may be fearful of thunderstorms (Boericke 1927) and they may experience frequent swallowing from a sensation of a ball in the throat (Reckeweg 2000).

Psorinoheel: Contains Bacillinum, which is indicated for chronic bronchitis (Reckeweg 2002).

Schwef-Heel: Contains sulfur, and is used in allergic cases, particularly allergic dermatitis. Sulfur is also present in *Engystol*, which is used more frequently in respiratory cases. These cases have red skin, itchiness, and a bad odor. May be used intermittently as the case shifts.

Spascupreel: Treats spasmodic coughing and bronchospasm.

Tartephedreel: Treats cough with ropey mucus, pain in the region of the third rib (star anise), coughs with nausea (ipecacuanha); and there is a history of asthma (Reckeweg 2000). Also contains Blatta orientalis, which is suited to corpulent patients and those that are aggravated in rainy weather. The lower potencies are preferred in acute attacks, and in chronic cases the higher ones are preferred (Reckeweg 2002). This component is common to *BHI-Cough*, as well.

Tonsilla compositum: Provides support of the endocrine system and immunity, particularly in chronic disorders. It is a phase remedy for Degeneration cases.

Thyroidea compositum: Drains matrix and supports endocrine function. It is a deep detoxification formula component and a phase remedy in Impregnation Phases.

Traumeel S: Used intermittently in inflammatory conditions and regulation rigidity.

Ubichinon compositum: Used as a Degeneration Phase remedy and following antibiotic therapy.

Authors' suggested protocols

Nutrition

Bronchus/lung and immune support formulas: 1 tablet for every 25 pounds of body weight BID.

Vitamin B$_6$: 25 mgs for every 25 pounds of body weight SID.

Bromelain: 100 mgs for each 25 pounds of body weight, with food.

Quercetin: 50 mgs for each 10 pounds of body weight SID.

N-acetyl cysteine (600-mg tablets): One-quarter tablet for each 25 pounds of body weight SID.

Chinese herbal medicine

For dry, unproductive coughs, the authors recommend the herbal supplement H1 at a dose of 1 capsule per 10 to 20 pounds twice daily. This supplement increases tracheal and bronchial secretions to moisten the respiratory tract, suppresses coughing, and inhibits bacterial growth. In addition to the herbs listed above, this formula also contains codonopsis (Dang shen), poria (Fu ling), angelica root (Dang gui), donkey skin gelatin (E jiao), angelica (Bai zhi), siler (Fang feng), and allium (Cong bai).

For productive coughs, the authors recommend the herbal supplement H95, which inhibits the tracheal and bronchial secretions, has expectorant effects, and inhibits bacterial growth. The dose is 1 capsule per 10 to 20 pounds twice daily. In addition to the herbs listed above, this supplement also contains ginseng (Ren shen), atractylodes (Bai zhu), ginger (Sheng jiang), and jujube fruit (Da Zao).

Homotoxicology (Dose: 10 drops PO for 50-pound dog; 5 drops PO for small dog or cat)

These are highly individualized cases, and it is difficult to recommend a "one size fits all" protocol, but as a starting point, we can consider the remedies below. The authors often inject the initial remedies, both IV and subcutaneously, in the manner of an autosanguis. In chronic cases, it can be of immense value to nebulize the saline-based injectable or oral remedies (do not nebulize alcohol-based remedies or tablets), because it then gives us direct access to the afflicted tissues.

Acute bronchitis: Engystol, Traumeel, and Coenzyme compositum as a mixed injection. Belladonna homaccord or Aconitum homaccord (if febrile), Lymphomyosot, Echinacea compositum (bacterial), Spascupreel, and Bronchalis mixed together and given every 15 minutes for 3 to 5 doses and then BID to TID orally.

Allergic bronchitis: Galium-Heel, Engystol N, Lymphomyosot, Phosphor homaccord, Coenzyme compositum, Hepeel, BHI-Allergy, and Tartephedreel, mixed together and given TID to BID orally. Deep detoxification formula consisting of Galium-Heel, Thryoidea compositum, Hepar compositum, and Solidago compositum, given orally every 3 days for 120 days.

Chronic bronchitis: Tonsilla compositum, preferably as an autosanguis. Psorinoheel, Lymphomyosot, Galium-Heel, Bronchalis, Engystol, and Ubichinon compositum combined and given orally TID to BID. Add deep detoxification formula as above for allergic bronchitis with the addition of Mucosa compositum given orally every 3 days for 120 days or until response wanes.

Product sources

Nutrition

Bronchus/lung and immune support formulas: Animal Nutrition Technologies. **Alternatives:** Immune System Support—Standard Process Veterinary Formulas; Immuno Support—Rx Vitamins for Pets; Immugen—Thorne Veterinary Products.

Bromezyme (Bromelain): Progressive Labs.

Quercetin: Source Naturals; Quercitone—Thorne Veterinary Products.

N-Acetyl Cysteine: Pure Encapsulations.

Chinese herbal medicine
H1, H95: Natural Solutions, Inc.

Homotoxicology
BHI/Heel Corporation

REFERENCES

Western medicine references

Bonagura JD. Bronchopulmonary disorders. In: Birchard SJ, Sherding RG, eds. Saunders manual of small animal practice, Philadelphia: Saunders, 1994:561–573.

Bonagura JD, Berkwitt L. Cardiovascular and pulmonary disorders. Quick Reference to Veterinary Medicine, WR Fenner, ed. JB Lippincott, 1991:117–175.

Dye JA, McKiernan BC, Rozanski EA, et al. Bronchopulmonary disease in the cat. Historical, physical, radiographical, clinicopathologic and pulmonary functional evaluation of 24 diseased and 15 healthy cats. *J Vet Intern Med* 1996;10: 385–400.

Forrester SD, Moon ML. Diseases of the lower airways and lungs. Practical Small Animal Internal Medicine. WB Saunders 1997, pp 1153–1185.

Johnson L. Bronchial disease. In: August JR, ed. Consultations in feline internal medicine, 3rd ed., Philadelphia: Saunders, 1997:303–309.

McKiernan BC. In: Tilley L, Smith F. The 5-Minute Veterinary Consult: Canine and Feline, 2003. Blackwell Publishing.

Padrid PA, Hornoff WJ, Kurpershoek CJ, Cross CE. Canine chronic bronchitis, *J Vet Intern Med* 1990;4:172–180.

Schaer M, et al. Clinical approach to the patient with respiratory disease. Textbook of Veterinary Internal Medicine. SJ Ettinger (ed), WB Saunders, 1989:747–767.

IVM/Nutrition References

Boman G, Bäcker U, Larsson S, et al. Oral acetylcysteine reduces exacerbation rate in chronic bronchitis: a report of a trial organized by the Swedish Society for Pulmonary Diseases. *Eur J Respir Dis* 1983;64:405–15.

Collipp PJ, Chen SY, Sharma RK, et al. Tryptophane metabolism in bronchial asthma. *Ann Allergy* 1975;35:153–8.

Collipp PJ, Goldzier S III, Weiss N, et al. Pyridoxine treatment of childhood bronchial asthma. *Ann Allergy* 1975;35:93–7.

Desser L, Rehberger A, Paukovits W. Proteolytic enzymes and amylase induce cytokine production in peripheral blood mononuclear cells in vitro. *Cancer Biother* 1994;9:253–63.

Grandjean EM, Berthet P, Ruffmann R, Leuenberger P. Efficacy of oral long-term N-Acetylcysteine in chronic bronchopulmonary disease: A meta-analysis of published double-blind, placebo-controlled clinical trials. *Clin Ther* 2000;22:209–21.

Jackson IM, Barnes J, Cooksey P. Efficacy and tolerability of oral acetylcysteine (Fabrol) in chronic bronchitis: a double-blind placebo controlled study. *J Int Med Res* 1984;12: 198–206.

Kelly GS. Bromelain: a literature review and discussion of its therapeutic applications. *Altern Med Rev* 1996;1:243–57 [review].

Munzig E, Eckert K, Harrach T, et al. Bromelain protease F9 reduces the CD44 mediated adhesions of human peripheral blood lymphocytes to human umbilical vein endothelial cells. *FEBS Lett* 1995;351:215–8.

Middleton E Jr. Effect of flavonoids on basophil histamine release and other secretory systems. *Prog Clin Biol Res*. 1986;213:493–506.

Ogasawara H, Middleton E Jr. Effect of selected flavonoids on histamine release (HR) and hydrogen peroxide (H2O2) generation by human leukocytes [abstract]. *J Allergy Clin Immunol*. 1985;75(suppl):184.

Reynolds RD, Natta CL. Depressed plasma pyridoxal phosphate concentrations in adult asthmatics. *Am J Clin Nutr* 1985; 41:684–8.

Ryan RE. A double-blind clinical evaluation of bromelains in the treatment of acute sinusitis. *Headache* 1967;7:13–7.

Sur S, Camara M, Buchmeier A, et al. Double-blind trial of pyridoxine (vitamin B₆) in the treatment of steroid-dependent asthma. *Ann Allergy* 1993;70:141–52.

Weir MR, Keniston RC, Enriquez JI, McNamee GA. Depression of vitamin B₆ levels due to theophylline. *Ann Allergy* 1990;65:59–62.

Schafer A, Adelman B. Plasma inhibition of platelet function and of arachidonic acid metabolism. *J Clin Invest* 1985; 75:456–61.

Tattersall AB, Bridgman KM, Huitson A. Acetylcysteine (Fabrol) in chronic bronchitis—a study in general practice. *J Int Med Res* 1983;11:279–84.

Taub SJ. The use of Ananase in sinusitis. A study of 60 patients. *EENT Monthly* 1966;45:96–8.

Van Schayck CP, Dekhuijzen PNR, Gorgels WJMJ, et al. Are anti-oxidant and anti-inflammatory treatments effective in different subgroups of COPD? A hypothesis. *Respir Med* 1998;92:1259–64.

Welton AF, Tobias LD, Fiedler-Nagy C, et al. Effect of flavonoids on arachidonic acid metabolism. *Prog Clin Biol Res* 1986;213:231–42.

Chinese herbal medicine/acupuncture references

Chang Yong Zhong Yao Cheng Fen Yu Yao Li Shou Ce (A Handbook of the Composition and Pharmacology of Common Chinese Drugs), 1994; 1678: 1681.

Dictionary of Chinese Medicines. Shanghai Science and Technology Press, 1986:174.

Nanjing College of Pharmacy. Materia Medica, vol. 2. Jiangsu: People's Press; 1976.

Shang Hai Yi Yao Za Zhi (*Shanghai Journal of Medicine and Herbology*), 1957; (3): 148.

Tai S, Sun F, O'Brien D, Lee M, Zayaz J, King M. Evaluation of a mucoactive herbal drug, Radix Ophiopogonis, in a pathogenic quail model. *J of Herbal Pharmacotherapy* 2002.

Yao Xue Qing Bao Tong Xun (*Journal of Herbal Information*), 1987; 5(4): 62.

Zhang WJ, et al. Processed Xing Ren: Its potency and acute toxicity. *Journal of Traditional Chinese Medicine Material.* 1991;14(8):38–40.

Zheng JL. Pharmacology research and clinical application of Bian Dou. *Journal of Shizhen Medicine.* 1997;8(4):330–331.

Zhong Hua Pi Fu Ke Xue Za Zhi (*Chinese Journal of Dermatology*), 1957; 5(4): 286.

Zhong Hua Yi Xue Za Zhi (*Chinese Journal of Medicine*), 1956; 42(10): 959.

Zhong Yao Xue (*Chinese Herbology*), 1998; 845:848.

Zhong Yao Xue (*Chinese Herbology*), 1998; 878:890.

Zhong Yao Yao Li Yu Ying Yong (*Pharmacology and Applications of Chinese Herbs*), 1983: 246.

Zhong Yao Yao Li Yu Ying Yong (*Pharmacology and Applications of Chinese Herbs*), 1983.

Zhong Yao Yao Li Yu Ying Yong (*Pharmacology and Applications of Chinese Herbs*), 1983; 419.

Zhong Yao Yao Li Yu Ying Yong (*Pharmacology and Applications of Chinese Herbs*), 1983; 866.

Zhong Yao Yao Li Yu Ying Yong (*Pharmacology and Applications of Chinese Herbs*); 1983; 1132.

Zhong Yao Zhi (*Chinese Herbology Journal*), 1993; 358.

Zhong Yi Shi Xi Yi Shi Sou Ce (Traditional Chinese Medicine Practitioners Handbook) Hunan College of Traditional Medicine, 1987.

Zhu LH. *China Journal of TCM Information.* 1996;3(3): 17–20.

Homotoxicology references

Boericke W. Materia Medica with Repertory, 9th ed. Santa Rosa, CA: Boericke and Tafel, 1927.

Broadfoot P. Autosanguis Therapy. In: Proceedings of AHVMA/ Heel Homotoxicology Seminar. 2004. Denver, CO.

de Oliveira C, de Oliveira S, Godoy L, Gabardo J, Buchi DF. Canova, a Brazilian medical formulation, alters oxidative metabolism of mice macrophages. *J Infect.* 2006. Jun;52(6): pp 420–32.

Heel. BHI Homeopathic Therapy: Professional Reference. Albuquerque, NM: Heel Inc. 2002. p 39, 44, 48.

Heel. Veterinary Guide, 3rd English ed. Baden-Baden, Germany: Biologische Heilmittel Heel GMBH, 2003. pp 26–7,30,72.

Reckeweg H. Biotherapeutic Index: Ordinatio Antihomotoxica et Materia Medica, 5th ed. Baden-Baden, Germany: Biologische Heilmittel Heel GMBH, 2000. pp 285–6, 383–4, 411–12.

Reckeweg H. Homeopathia Antihomotoxica Materia Medica, 4th edition. Baden-Baden, Germany: Arelia-Verlag GMBH, 2002. pp. 153, 164, 169–70, 175, 184, 379, 507, 520–22, 572.

Skaltsa H, Philianos S, Papaphilippou G. The Aconit described by Nicander and today [article in French]. *Rev Hist Pharm* (Paris) 1997. 45(316): pp 405–10.

FELINE BRONCHIAL ASTHMA

Definition and cause

Feline bronchial asthma is an allergic and inflammatory reaction in the airway that is most often secondary to allergen exposure and results in bronchoconstriction. Symptoms include wheezing, coughing, dyspnea, and potentially death from severe bronchoconstriction.

Common suspected underlying causes are environmental contaminants such as secondary smoke, chemical and household cleaners, pollen, and dust. Although unproven, many clinicians believe that there is a hereditary and/or and autoimmune component to feline asthma (Corcoran 1995, Moise 1989, Noone 2003).

Medical therapy rationale, drug(s) of choice, and nutritional recommendations

Therapy for asthma is directed at the inflammatory process in the upper airways. Corticosteroids, antihistamines, bronchodilators, anti-serotonin medication such as cyproheptadine, and immunomodulators such as cyclosporine have all be used to treat asthma, with varying degrees of success (Dye 1996, Padrid 1996, Livingstone 1994).

Anticipated prognosis

Prognosis for management is generally good if caught early. Success is totally dependent upon client compliance and response to medication. Relapses are common when medication is stopped (Dye 1992, 1996; Livingstone 1994; Noone 2003).

Integrative veterinary therapies

Allergies to any substance can worsen asthmatic symptoms. Pollen allergy is a common cause of aggravation in these cases and should be suspected in cases presenting with a history of seasonality. Mold spores can aggravate allergies and cause direct trauma to the respiratory tissues. Mold reactions may be particularly hard to control. Careful evaluation of medications and supplements is advised in asthmatic patients because adverse reactions to many substances can aggravate asthma.

Any agent that traumatizes respiratory membranes can aggravate asthma as a primary homotoxin. Environmental pollution is common, and oxides of sulfur and nitrogen combine with water in the respiratory tree to yield acids (nitric acid, nitrous acid, and sulfuric acid). Ozone can cause major injury to cell membranes and is present in general air pollution. It is also generated by many popular air-deodorizing devices. Authorities have expressed concern over ozone-generating air purifiers because these may aggravate asthma in humans (Britigan, et al. 2006).

One author has identified a case of feline asthma that improved following removal of ozone-generating air filtration equipment, and specifically recommends removal of any such equipment from the home of cats suffering from asthma (Palmquist 2005).

Tobacco smoke is another common irritant, as is the out-gassing of noxious chemicals from building materials and new carpeting. Perfumes, scented candles, incense, room deodorizing sprays, laundry detergents, fabric softeners, and aromatic oils can all elicit respiratory pathology in sensitive individuals. Some animals may be congenitally missing detoxification systems or membrane receptors resulting from genetic alterations, making them more susceptible to such effects. Such issues are known to occur in collies and most certainly involve other species as well (Geyer, et al. 2005).

Routine vaccinations may play a part in this condition, and avoidance of unnecessary vaccination is desirable. Certainly we know that allergic patients are more prone to vaccination reactions and immune imbalances, and

it is logical to assume that this condition operates similarly.

Integrative therapies can work well with medications because recovery and cure are not always possible. The conventional medical symptom control through suppression of the immune system and bronchodilation are key elements for day-to-day quality of life. The use of therapeutic nutrients, herbs, and biological therapies can help to control symptoms and decrease asthmatic episodes, and in many cases result in reduced use of pharmacologic agents.

Nutrition
General considerations/rationale

While medical therapy is focused locally upon the breathing and suppression of the immune response, therapeutic nutrition adds nutrients, antioxidants, and gland support to help reduce local cellular inflammation, balance immune response, and encourage toxin elimination via the respiratory system.

Appropriate nutrients

Nutritional/gland therapy: Glandular adrenal, thymus, and lung provide intrinsic nutrients that nourish the organ, help to neutralize cellular inflammation, and balance the immune system response (see Gland Therapy, Chapter 2, for a more detailed explanation).

Thymus extract: The oral administration of thymus extract has been shown in early and double-blinded clinical trials to improve the symptoms and course of asthma in people. It is believed that this effect is related to the thymus gland extract's ability to balance immune function and reaction (Bagnato 1989, Cazzola 1987, Genova 1983, Kouttab 1989).

Vitamin B_6 (pyridoxine): Asthmatics have reduced levels of vitamin B_6, which is considered to have natural antihistaminic effects. This could be a real deficiency or a side effect of brochodilating medications such as theophylline, which can cause a B_6 deficiency (Collipp 1975, Weir 1990). In clinical trials B_6 supplementation helped reduce the levels of required medication and decreased the frequency of asthmatic episodes (Collipp 1975, Reynolds 1895). However, other studies found that asthmatic patients still required corticosteroids to control the symptoms (Sur 1993).

Fish oil: In a double-blind clinical trial in people with asthma it was shown that there was some reduction in symptoms when the diet was supplemented with fish oil. In other double-blind trials, asthmatic children showed a significant improvement in symptoms when taking fish oil (Arm 1988, Nagakura 2000).

Quercetin: Quercetin is a flavonoid that has potent antioxidant properties. Quercetin also has been proven to inhibit cells from releasing histamines (Middleton 1986,

Ogasawara 1985). This antihistamine attribute is beneficial in the treatment of allergic conditions such as asthma and can improve breathing in compromised conditions such as pneumonia. Quercetin inhibits the enzyme lipoxygenase, which contributes to the clinical signs associated with asthma (Welton 1986).

Chinese herbal medicine
General considerations/rationale
According the TCM theory, asthma is due to Lung and Kidney Qi deficiency. Lung Qi deficiency causes weakness and coughing. According to TCM, one function of the Kidney Qi or Kidney energy is to grasp the breath from the Lung and pull it downward. With Kidney Qi deficiency, the Kidney is not able to grasp the Lung breath. Because there is no energy pulling the air downward, the patient cannot take a full, deep breath. The breathing becomes shallow and rapid.

Appropriate Chinese herbs
Aster root (Zi wan): Can help clear the respiratory tract of irritants or pathogens. It can increase the excretion of phenol red from the respiratory tracts of mice. Two components seem to play a major role in the expectorant effect: shionone and episuberol (Lu 1999). It also has an antitussive effect (Zhao 1999).

Astragalus (Huang qi): Was used in 41 human patients with asthma. They were treated with an astragalus preparation via injection into ST36. The patients were treated twice weekly for 3 months, then rested for 2 weeks. This protocol was repeated 3 to 4 times as required according to symptoms. Eighty-five percent had a significant improvement in symptoms (Zhong Hua Er Ke Za Zhi 1978).

Cordyceps (Dong cong xia cao): Can relieve asthma by dilating the bronchi (Fu Jian Yi Yao Za Zhi 1983).

Fritillaria (Bei mu): Dilates bronchi at low concentrations Zhong Yao Xue 1998). It contains peimine and peiminine, which have been shown to decrease coughing in rats (Chang Yong Zhong Yao Cheng Fen Yu Yao Li Shou Ce 1994).

Gecko (Ge jie): Has an antiasthmatic effect via the relaxation of the bronchi (Chang Yong Zhong Yao Cheng Fen Yu Yao Li Shou Ce 1994).

Mulberry bark (Sang bai pi): Decreases coughing (Zhong Yao Xue 1998).

Schisandra (Wu wei zi): Was used in a study involving 50 human patients with severe asthma. The treatment period ranged from 7 months to 2 years. Of the 50 participants, 1 achieved complete remission while 47 became stable. Two patients did not respond (Zhong Yi Za Zhi 1988). Schisandra also increases the depth of respiration (Zhong Yao Yao Li Yu Ying Yong 1983).

Homotoxicology
General considerations/rationale
Reckeweg reported more than 5 decades ago the observation that human childhood asthma seemed to appear as an Impregnation Phase disease following allopathic treatment of childhood diseases such as streptococcal pharyngitis and otitis media. He particularly identified the use of antibiotics as a causative or associated factor in the progressive vicariation following such treatment. According to this line of reasoning, the homotoxicosis surfaces in an Inflammation Phase disorder, which becomes an asymptomatic Deposition Phase disorder when suppressed allopathically. This later deteriorates into an Impregnation Phase homotoxicosis and disease signs resurface as the injured tissue's function is compromised. Further suppression leads to progressive vicariation into the Degeneration Phase (chronic obstructive lung disease, chronic bronchitis, etc.). Upon continuing suppression or concurrent actions of other homotoxins, this can develop into neoplasia. A similar situation exists in feline medicine with the association of exposure to tobacco smoke with increased rates of lymphosarcoma (Bertone et al. 2002). To date, no one has examined this specific cycle of pathogenesis in cats, but it seems a theory well worth pursuing.

Biological therapy strives to create circumstances that favor regressive vicariation. In accordance with Hering's Law, cats treated biologically frequently demonstrate mild signs of upper respiratory disease, fevers, skin problems (pruritus, miliary dermatitis, alopecia, and seborrhea), otitis externa and interna, mild gastrointestinal reactions, and sinusitis as homotoxins are excreted from the system and tissues begin repair. The process of biological healing may require several years. The veterinarian should support this process and avoid allopathic drugs wherever possible, while at the same time preserving the patient's life and health with needed interventions.

Appropriate homotoxicology formulas
Apis homaccord: Treats a desire for fresh air and lung congestion.

BHI-Allergy: Treats generalized allergic reactions involving the respiratory tree (Heel 2002).

BHI-Asthma: Soothes bronchial asthma symptoms (Heel 2002).

BHI-Bronchitis: Supports bronchial tissues.

Bronchalis: Provides bronchial support.

Causticum compositum: Promotes regressive vicariation for burning sensations in the airways and promotes metabolic pathways.

Coenzyme compositum: Provides metabolic support.

Cor compositum: Supports cardiac tissues. Helpful in asthma occurring in cardiac cases.

Echinacea compositum: Provides immune support and normalization.

Engystol N: An antiviral that is supportive of allergic conditions through Sulfur; often treats skin rashes concurrently. Several mechanisms may be involved in its action (Enbergs 2006; Oberbaum, et al. 2005; Fimiani, et al. 2000).

Galium-Heel: Treats allergies and provides cellular detoxification.

Lymphomyosot: Provides lymph drainage and detoxification.

Mucosa compositum: Supports mucosal tissues throughout the body. A phase remedy in Degeneration Phases.

Solidago compositum: Supports the kidney and urinary tract, and is a phase remedy in Deposition Phase disorders.

Spascupreel: Treats spasms of smooth muscle; may function as an effective emergency drug during acute attacks. It can be given prior to steroids in milder attacks and where avoidance of corticosteroids is advisable (diabetics, etc.).

Tarthephedreel: Treats bronchial asthma and bronchial coughs.

Tonsilla compositum: Provides support and detoxification of reticuloendotelial tissues, immune modulation, and support of the hypothalamus and adrenal glands.

Traumeel S: An anti-inflammatory that activates blocked sulfur-containing enzymes that are needed for detoxification.

Ubichinon compositum: Provides metabolic support.

Zeel: Has anti-inflammatory effects through its inhibition of COX and LOX enzymes. Asthma is a LOX-5-mediated condition, and Zeel moderates LOX-5, as well as COX-1 and COX-2, without the side effects of conventional drugs (Jaggi, et al. 2004).

Authors' suggested protocols

Nutrition

Immune and bronchus/lung support formulas: 1 tablet for each 10 pounds of body weight BID.

Quercetin: 50 mgs for each 10 pounds of body weight SID.

Eskimo fish oil: One-half to 1 teaspoon per meal for cats. 1 teaspoon for each 35 pounds of body weight for dogs.

Vitamin B$_6$: 35 mgs daily.

Chinese herbal medicine

H91 Asthma: 1 capsule per 10 to 20 pounds twice daily as needed to control signs. In addition to the herbs cited above, H91 Asthma contains cooked rehmannia (Shu di huang), ginseng (Ren shen), and walnut (Hu tao ren).

Homotoxicology (Cat dose: 5 drops PO)

This condition responds best to a combination of autosanguis and oral therapies and requires long-term treatment and frequent follow-ups. The authors use the following protocols and make therapeutic adjustments as required:

Autosanguis therapy:

1. BHI-Allergy
2. Engystol N plus Galium-Heel
3. Mucosa compositum
4. Echinacea compositum
5. Coenzyme plus Ubichinon compositae

Oral cocktail: Traumeel S, Causticum compositum, Lymphomyosot, Galium-Heel, Tarthephedreel, and Bronchalis OR BHI-Bronchitis mixed together and given BID PO.

Zeel: TID PO.

Cor compositum: Once a week.

Solidago compositum: Once a week.

Spascupreel: May be used frequently during attacks and may prove successful as an emergency drug in these cases.

Product sources

Nutrition

Immune and bronchus/lung support formulas: Animal Nutrition Technologies. **Alternatives:** Immune System Support—Standard Process Veterinary Formulas; Immuno Support—Rx Vitamins for Pets; Immugen—Thorne Veterinary Products.

Quercetin: Source Naturals; Quercitone—Thorne Veterinary Products.

Eskimo fish oil: Tyler Encapsulations.

Chinese herbal medicine

Formula H91 Asthma: Natural Solutions, Inc.

Homotoxicology

BHI/Heel Corporation

REFERENCES

Western medicine references

Corcoran BM, Foster DJ, Fuentes VL. Feline asthma syndrome: a retrospective study of the clinical presentation in 29 cats. *J Small Anim Pract* 1995 Nov;36(11):481–488.

Dye JA, McKiernan B, Rozanski EA, et al. Bronchopulmonary disease in the cat. Historical, physical, radiographic, clinicopathologic and pulmonary function evaluation of 24 diseased and 15 healthy subjects. *J Vet Intern Med* 1996;10:385–400.

Dye J. Feline bronchopulmonary disease. *Bet Clin N Am Small Anim Pract* 1992, 22:1187–201.

Livingstone C. In: Sherding RG, ed. The Cat: Diseases and Clinical Management, Harcourt Publishers, 1994. January 15, 524.

Moise NS, Weidenkeller D, Yeager AE, Blue JT, Scarlett J. Clinical, radiographic, and bronchial cytologic features of cats with bronchial disease: 65 cases (1980–1986). *J Am Vet Med Assoc* 1989, 194:1476–1473.

Noone KE. Asthma Bronchitis, Cat. In: Tilley L, Smith F. The 5-Minute Veterinary Consult: Canine and Feline, 2003. Blackwell Publishing.

Padrid P. New Treatment Strategies for Cats with Exacerbation of Asthma. *NAV;* 1996.

IVM/nutrition references

Arm JP, Horton CE, Eiser NM, et al. The effects of dietary supplementation with fish oil on asthmatic responses to antigen. *J Allergy Clin Immunol* 1988;81:183 [abstract #57].

Bagnato A, Brovedani P, Comina P, et al. Long-term treatment with thymomodulin reduces airway hyperresponsiveness to methacholine. *Ann Allergy* 1989;62:425–8.

Cazzola P, Mazzanti P, Bossi G. In vivo modulating effect of a calf thymus acid lysate on human T lymphocyte subsets and CD4+/CD8+ ratio in the course of different diseases. *Curr Ther Res* 1987;42:1011–7.

Collipp PJ, Chen SY, Sharma RK, et al. Tryptophane metabolism in bronchial asthma. *Ann Allergy* 1975;35:153–8.

Collipp PJ, Goldzier S III, Weiss N, et al. Pyridoxine treatment of childhood bronchial asthma. *Ann Allergy* 1975;35:93–7.

Genova R, Guerra A. A thymus extract (thymomodulin) in the prevention of childhood asthma. *Pediatr Med Chir* 1983;5:395–402.

Kouttab NM, Prada M, Cazzola P. Thymomodulin: Biological properties and clinical applications. *Med Oncol Tumor Pharmacother* 1989;6:5–9 [review].

Middleton E Jr. Effect of flavonoids on basophil histamine release and other secretory systems. *Prog Clin Biol Res.* 1986;213:493–506.

Nagakura T, Matsuda S, Shichijyo K, et al. Dietary supplementation with fish oil rich in omega-3 polyunsaturated fatty acids in children with bronchial asthma. *Eur Respir J* 2000;16: 861–5.

Ogasawara H, Middleton E Jr. Effect of selected flavonoids on histamine release (HR) and hydrogen peroxide ($H2O2$) generation by human leukocytes [abstract]. *J Allergy Clin Immunol.* 1985;75(suppl):184.

Reynolds RD, Natta CL. Depressed plasma pyridoxal phosphate concentrations in adult asthmatics. *Am J Clin Nutr* 1985;41: 684–8.

Sur S, Camara M, Buchmeier A, et al. Double-blind trial of pyridoxine (vitamin B_6) in the treatment of steroid-dependent asthma. *Ann Allergy* 1993;70:141–52.

Weir MR, Keniston RC, Enriquez JI, McNamee GA. Depression of vitamin B_6 levels due to theophylline. *Ann Allergy* 1990;65:59–62.

Welton AF, Tobias LD, Fiedler-Nagy C, et al. Effect of flavonoids on arachidonic acid metabolism. *Prog Clin Biol Res* 1986;213:231–42.

Chinese herbal medicine/acupuncture references

Chang Yong Zhong Yao Cheng Fen Yu Yao Li Shou Ce (A Handbook of the Composition and Pharmacology of Common Chinese Drugs), 1994; 1523:1524.

Chang Yong Zhong Yao Cheng Fen Yu Yao Li Shou Ce (A Handbook of the Composition and Pharmacology of Common Chinese Drugs), 1994; 1682:1685.

Fu Jian Yi Yao Za Zhi (*Fujian Journal of Medicine and Herbology*); 1983;5:311.

Lu YH, et al. Zi Wan's effect in expelling phlegm and relieving cough: the effective parts and active components. 1999; 30(5):360–362.

Zhao XG, et al. Zi Wan (III): A comparison of the herb's expectorant and anti-tussive effects among different origins. *Journal of Chinese Materia Medica.* 1999;30(1):353–7.

Zhong Hua Er Ke Za Zhi (*Chinese Journal of Pediatrics*), 1978; 2:87.

Zhong Yao Xue, Chinese Herbology, 1998; 620:622.

Zhong Yao Xue, Chinese Herbology, 1998; 648:650.

Zhong Yao Yao Li Yu Ying Yong (*Pharmacology and Applications of Chinese Herbs*), 1983:177.

Zhong Yi Za Zhi (*Journal of Chinese Medicine*), 1988; 9:47.

Homotoxicology references

Bertone ER, Snyder LA, Moore AS. Environmental tobacco smoke and risk of malignant lymphoma in pet cats. *Am J Epidemiol.* 2002.Aug 1;156(3):pp 268–73.

Britigan N, Alshawa A, Nizkorodov SA. Quantification of ozone levels in indoor environments generated by ionization and ozonolysis air purifiers. *J Air Waste Manag Assoc.* 2006. May;56(5): pp 601–10.

Enbergs H. Effects of the homeopathic preparation Engystol on interferon-gamma production by human T-lymphocytes. *Immunol Invest.* 2006. 35(1):pp 19–27.

Fimiani V, Cavallaro A, Ainis O, Bottari C. Immunomodulatory effect of the homeopathic drug Engystol-N on some activities of isolated human leukocytes and in whole blood. *Immunopharmacol Immunotoxicol.* 2000.Feb;22(1):pp 103–15.

Geyer J, Doring B, Godoy JR, Leidolf R, Moritz A, Petzinger E. Frequency of the nt230 (del4) MDR1 mutation in collies and related dog breeds in Germany. *J Vet Pharmacol Ther.* 2005. Dec;28(6):pp 545–51.

Jaggi R, Wurgler U, Grandjean F, Weiser M. Dual inhibition of 5-lipoxygenase/cyclooxygenase by a reconstituted homeopathic remedy; possible explanation for clinical efficacy and favourable gastrointestinal tolerability. *Inflamm Res.* 2004. Apr;53(4):pp 150–7.

Heel. BHI Homeopathic Therapy: Professional Reference. Albuquerque, NM: Heel Inc. 2002. p 9.

Oberbaum M, Glatthaar-Saalmuller B, Stolt P, Weiser M. Antiviral activity of Engystol: an in vitro analysis. *J Altern Complement Med.* 2005. Oct;11(5): pp 855–62.

PLEURAL EFFUSION

Definition and cause

Pleural effusion is fluid in the pleural space caused by an abnormal accumulation of fluid, a decrease in the resorption of fluid, or a combination of both. Accumulation of fluid can occur secondary to heart disease such as valvular disease or congestive heart failure, trauma such as a diaphragmatic hernia, osmotic pressure imbalance such as secondary to hypoalbuminemia, viral or bacterial infections such as pyothorax, lymphatic dysfunction such as chylothorax, or neoplasia (Bauer 1995, Forrester 1988, Fossum 1994, Lehmkuhl 2003, Padrid 1997, Sherding 1994, Wolf 1997).

Medical therapy rationale, drug(s) of choice, and nutritional recommendations

Because respiratory distress is the primary symptom, the initial treatment is thoracocentesis followed by a cytological evaluation of the fluid. Once the diagnosis is established, the appropriate therapy is selected. Ongoing thoracocentesis and diuretics are generally recommended for heart disease. Antibiotics are recommended for infectious causes. Surgery is often recommended for trauma and diaphragmatic hernia, chylothorax, and neoplasia (Bauer 1995, Forrester 1988, Fossum 1994, Sherding 1994, Wolf 1997).

Anticipated prognosis

The prognosis is related to identification and correction of the underlying cause. Trauma, once corrected, often results in a good prognosis. Most other causes of pleural effusion carry a poor or guarded prognosis (Fossum 1994, Lehmkuhl 2003).

Integrative veterinary therapies

The integrative approach depends upon a definitive diagnosis and identifying the underlying cause. The therapy is directed toward the cause. (For neoplasia, please see Chapters 31 through 34 on cancer). The addition of therapeutic nutrients, herbs, and biological therapies are directed at both the fluid accumulation as well as the underlying cause such as cardiac, trauma, etc.

Nutrition
General considerations/rationale
Once the underlying cause has been established, therapeutic nutrients will be recommended based upon the organ condition or malfunction.

Appropriate nutrients
Nutritional/gland therapy: Glandular bronchus/lung and heart provide intrinsic nutrients required by these organs for proper function. They also help to reduce associated inflammation and cellular degeneration

(see Chapter 2, Gland Therapy, for more detailed information).

Bromelain: Bromelain is a proteolytic enzyme that comes from pineapples. It also has anti-inflammatory properties and is beneficial for the upper respiratory system (Taub 1966). In a double-blind study, Ryan (1967) showed an improvement in the treatment of upper respiratory inflammation and sinusitis with bromelain. Another characteristic of bromelain is its ability to reduce the thickness of mucus in the respiratory system, which is beneficial for all inflammatory and infectious respiratory diseases (Schaefer 1985). In addition, bromelain has been shown to positively affect white blood cells and the immune response, which is beneficial for preventing upper respiratory inflammation and infections (Desser 1994, Kelly 1996, Munzig 1995).

Vitamin E: Besides its antioxidant functions, vitamin E is involved in the proper functioning of the heart muscle. It particularly improves cardiac output and circulation, and helps to reduce platelet aggregation (Traber 1999, 2001). Vitamin E reduces inflammation and improves circulation by helping vessels to dilate and reduce the agglutination of blood platelets.

Coenzyme Q10 (CoQ10 or ubiquinone): Clinical research in people has shown that CoQ10 is beneficial in controlling cardiac disease. Results of clinical studies showed an improvement in the related symptoms of heart diseases such as a reduction in dyspnea and edema and well as improvements in blood pressure and helping to normalize heart rate (Gaby 1996, Giugliano 2000).

Chinese herbal medicine/acupuncture
General considerations/rationale
Pleural effusion is a result of Qi and Blood deficiency in the Spleen and Lung. The Spleen then loses the ability to transport water and fluids and the Lung loses its ability to distribute the water, so that it accumulates in the chest cavity.

The Spleen takes the water that is ingested and prepares it for action by the Lung. The Lung then distributes the water to the body. When the Spleen and Lung become deficient, they cannot perform these functions. Fluid builds up in abnormal spaces. Treatment objectives include treating the underlying cause of the Qi and Blood deficiency and draining the excess fluid from the chest, either by direct diuretic action or by improving circulation.

Appropriate Chinese herbs
Astragalus (Huang qi): Has been shown to have diuretic actions in dogs, rats, and humans (Modern TCM Pharmacology 1997). It also increases cardiac output while decreasing hypertension (Xu 1999, Luo 1999). This may help patients with pleural effusion secondary to heart failure. Astragalus may also help patients with neoplastic

causes. It has been shown to inhibit some solid tumors (Liu 1999, Shi 1999).

Codonopsis (Dang shen): Can lower blood pressure, increase cardiac output, and improve blood perfusion (Zhong Yao Xue 1998).

Dianthus (Qu mai): May have diuretic effects (Li 1996), which may make it useful in draining pleural fluid.

Fritillaria (Bei mu): Has anti-neoplastic effects. It has been shown to inhibit the growth of cancerous cells in vitro and cause apoptosis (Li 1998).

Ophiopogon root (Mai men dong): Improves cardiac function. It has a positive inotropic effect and can increase cardiac output (Hua Xi Yao Xue Za Zhi 1991).

Platycodon root (Jie geng): Can decrease blood pressure and tachycardia (Zhong Yao Yao).

Scutellaria (Huang qin): Lowers blood pressure (Tong 1995). It contains baicalein, which has been shown to cause apoptosis of human melanoma cells in vitro (Zi 2005). It is possible that it may have efficacy against other cancers.

Trichosanthes root (Tian hua feng): Has demonstrated anti-neoplastic activity. It was shown to inhibit hepatocarcinoma in mice (Modern TCM Pharmacology 1997). It also inhibited the growth of colon and gastric carcinomas in mice (Xu 1997, Bi Li Qi 1998, Xu 1998, Bi Li Qi 1998), which indicates that it may have efficacy against other solid tumors.

White peony (Bai shao): Causes vasodilation and mildly reduces blood pressure (Zhong Guo Yao Li Xue Tong Bao 1986).

Acupuncture

Acupuncture has been shown in several studies to decrease dyspnea secondary to pulmonary diseases (Jobst 1995). It has also shown efficacy in decreasing hypertension. Williams found that stimulation of Liv3, St36, LI11, and a point in the groove behind the ear used for blood pressure modification caused a decrease in diastolic blood pressure (Williams 1991). A study by Ballegaard (1993) indicated that acupuncture may have the ability to normalize cardiovascular function.

Homotoxicology
General considerations/rationale
Pleural effusions typically represent Inflammation, Impregnation, Degeneration, or Dedifferentiation phase homotoxicoses. Exudates usually are inflammatory in nature and represent the organism's attempt to remove homotoxins through inflammatory reactions. Transudates occur due to microvascular or lymphatic malfunction and are commonly seen with more severe pathologies, which often represent Degeneration or Dedifferentiation phase disorders. These can occur during both progressive and regressive vicariation.

Appropriate homotoxicology formulas
Apis homaccord: Treats pulmonary edema.

Bryaconeel: A very useful remedy containing Bryonia, which is indicated for inflammation of serous membranes, bronchial cough with chill, following acute inflammation of the respiratory organs, pleura, and peritoneum. There are often catarrhs of the larynx, of the trachea with hoarseness, accumulation of tough mucus with a dry cough, constriction of the chest, and pleuritic pains with deep inspiration. Often useful in pleurisy accompanied by pneumonia (Reckeweg 2002). Bryonia is common to *Bronchalis, BHI-Bronchitis, Echinacea compositum,* and *BHI-Inflammation.* Other ingredients are Aconitum (acute febrile diseases, influenza) and Phosphorus (bronchopneumonia, nighttime cough, bloody expectorate, and diseases of the lung and larynx) (Reckeweg 2000).

Coenzyme compositum: Used in chronic diseases to activate energy metabolism and after therapy with allopathic medications that damage mitochondrial function (antibiotics)(Ouedraogo, et al. 2000).

Echinacea compositum: An important Inflammation Phase remedy. Also indicated in Impregnation Phases marked by recurring infections. Used as a natural antibiotic in bacterial and viral conditions. Contains major remedies consisting of Echinacea, Aconitum, Sanguinaria, Sulfur, Baptista, Lachesis, Bryonia, Eupatorium, Pulsatilla, Mercurious submlimatus, Thuja, Influenzium nosode, Phosphorus, Cortisonum, Streptococcus nosode, Staphylococcus nosode, Phytolacca, Zincum, Gelsemium, Hepar sulfuris, Rhus tox, Arnica, Arsenicum, Argentum and Euphorbium (Reckeweg 2000).

Engystol N: Used for viral infections through the action of Vincetoxicum and Sulfur. Excellent for asthma in cats and pneumonia. This remedy directly stimulates immune function. (Ben-Yakir 2004; Oberbaum, et al. 2005; Enbergs 2006).

Galium-Heel: A phase remedy in all phases from Deposition through Degeneration due to its draining effects on the matrix as well as its ability to improve and activate the greater defenses. A main remedy for any chronic disease.

Glyoxal compositum: Treats chronic diseases in the Degeneration and Dedifferentiation phases. Decouples homotoxins from receptors and other proteins such as enzymes.

Hepar compositum: Provides support of the liver. Part of the deep detoxification formula for use in chronic diseases. Contains Lycopodium, which may be useful in cases of allergic rhinitis (Colin 2006).

Lymphomyosot: Provides lymph drainage and support.

Phosphor homaccord: Treats pulmonary parenchymal disorders, laryngitis, and bleeding tendencies. Phosphorus has proved its worth in pneumonia (orally or injected, in the potencies 10, 30, 200, and 1,000 times) (Reckeweg 2002). This component is also common to *Apis compositum, Bryaconeel, Echinacea compositum, Galium-Heel, Gripp-Heel, Mucosa compositum, NasoHeel,* and *BHI-Bleeding.*

Tonsilla compositum: An important phase remedy for Impregnation and Dedifferentiation conditions. Supports the endocrine and immune systems in chronic disease.

Traumeel S: Treats inflammatory conditions anywhere in the body as well as sinusitis and rhinitis. It is useful in regulation rigidity and important after regressive vicariation following use of *Pulsatilla compositum*. Used intermittently in many cases to reduce inflammation and improve patient comfort and healing.

Ubichinon compositum: Contains Anthrachinon, which has strong indications in afflictions of the lungs, pleurisy, pneumonia, and respiratory illness, where there is effusion in most cases. The remedy Ubiquinone (Coenzyme Q10) is useful in chronic mucosal inflammations and suppurations with excoriating secretions, in septic cold infections, descending bronchitis, febrile pneumonia, and asthmatic attacks and those with persistent nocturnal cough, particularly when provoked by movement (Reckeweg 2002).

Authors' suggested protocols

Nutrition

Cardiac and bronchus/lung support formulas: 1 tablet for every 25 pounds of body weight BID.

Bromelain: 100 mgs for each 25 pounds of body weight, with food.

Vitamin E: 50 IU for each 20 pounds of body weight SID.

Coenzyme Q10: 15 mg per 10 pounds of body weight SID.

Chinese herbal medicine/acupuncture

Formula H38 pleural effusion/cardiac: 1 capsule per 10 to 20 pounds twice daily as needed. It may be combined with Western drugs such as steroids, chemotherapeutics, and cardiac medications as needed. In addition to the herbs cited above, H38 pleural effusion/cardiac also contains angelica root (Dang gui), lily bulb (Bai he), pharbitis (Qian niu zi), and talc (Hua shi). These help to increase the efficacy of the formula.

Acupuncture points which may be used include those mentioned above.

Homotoxicology (Dose: 10 drops PO for 50-pound dog; 5 drops PO for small dog or cat)

For pleural effusion, in addition to proper medical care, consider Traumeel-S, Galium-Heel, Lymphomyosot, and Apis Homaccord combined and taken orally TID. Treat

other disorders as diagnosis demonstrates (neoplasia, cardiac, infectious, foreign body, vascular permeability issues, hypoproteinemia, etc.) (see notes for Chylothorax in Chapter 7).

Product sources

Nutrition

Cardiac and bronchus/lung support formulas: Animal Nutrition Technologies. **Alternatives**: Formula CV—Rx Vitamins for Pets; Cardiac Support Formula—Standard Process Veterinary Formulas; Cardio-Strength—Vetri Science Laboratories; Bio-Cardio—Thorne Veterinary Products.

Bromezyme: Progressive Labs.

Coenzyme Q10: Vetri Science—Rx Vitamins for Pets; Integrative Therapeutics—Thorne Veterinary Products.

Chinese herbal medicine

Formula H38 pleural effusion/cardiac: Natural Solutions, Inc.

Homotoxicology

BHI/Heel Corporation

REFERENCES

Western medicine references

Bauer T, Woodfield JA. Pleura and pleural space disorders. In: Ettinger SJ, Feldman EC, eds. Textbook of veterinary internal medicine, vol 1. 4th ed. Philadelphia: Saunders, 1995:817–829.

Forrester SD, Troy GC, Fossum TW. Pleural effusions: pathophysiology and diagnostic considerations. *Compend Contin Educ Pract Vet.* 1988;10:121–138.

Fossum TW. Pleural Effusion. In: Birchard SJ, Sherding RG, eds. Saunders manual of small animal practice, Philadelphia: Saunders, 1994:580–586.

Lehmkuhl LB, Smith WK. In: Tilley L, Smith F. The 5-Minute Veterinary Consult: Canine and Feline, 2003. Blackwell Publishing.

Padrid P. Pulmonary diagnostics. In: August JR, ed. Consultations in feline internal medicine 3. Philadelphia: Saunders, 1997:292–302.

Sherding RG. Disease of the pleural cavity. In: Sherding RG, ed. The cat: diseases and clinical management. 2nd ed. New York: Churchill Livingstone, 1994:1053–1083.

Wolf AM. Diseases of the pleural space and mediastinum. Practical Small Animal Internal Medicine. WB Saunders, 1997, pp 1129–1151.

IVM/nutrition references

Desser L, Rehberger A, Paukovits W. Proteolytic enzymes and amylase induce cytokine production in peripheral blood mononuclear cells in vitro. *Cancer Biother* 1994;9:253–63.

Kelly GS. Bromelain: a literature review and discussion of its therapeutic applications. *Altern Med Rev* 1996;1:243–57 [review].

Munzig E, Eckert K, Harrach T, et al. Bromelain protease F9 reduces the CD44 mediated adhesions of human peripheral blood lymphocytes to human umbilical vein endothelial cells. *FEBS Lett* 1995;351:215–8.

Ryan RE. A double-blind clinical evaluation of bromelains in the treatment of acute sinusitis. *Headache* 1967;7:13–7.

Schafer A, Adelman B. Plasma inhibition of platelet function and of arachidonic acid metabolism. *J Clin Invest* 1985; 75:456–61.

Taub SJ. The use of Ananase in sinusitis. A study of 60 patients. *EENT Monthly* 1966;45:96–8.

Traber MG. Does vitamin E decrease heart attack risk? Summary and implications with respect to dietary recommendations. *J Nutr.* 2001;131(2):395S–397S.

Traber MG. Vitamin E. In: Shils M, Olson JA, Shike M, Ross AC, eds. Nutrition in Health and Disease. 9th ed. Baltimore: Williams and Wilkins; 1999:347–362.

Chinese herbal medicine/acupuncture references

Ballegaard S, Muteki T, Harada H, Ueda N, Tayama F, Ohishi K. Modulatory effect of acupuncture on the cardiovascular system: a cross-over study. *Acupunct Electrother Res.* 1993 Apr–Jun;18(2):103–15.

Bi LQ, et al. *China Journal of Experimental Clinical Immunology.* 1998;10(1):59–61.

Bi LQ, et al. *China Journal of Integrated Medicine.* 1998;18(1):35–37.

Hua Xi Yao Xue Za Zhi (*Huaxi Herbal Journal*), 1991; 6(1):13.

Jobst KA. A critical analysis of acupuncture in pulmonary disease: efficacy and safety of the acupuncture needle. *J Altern Comple Med* 1995; 1 (1):57–85.

Li DG, et al. The diuretic effect of Qu Mai of Shandong origin. *Journal of Traditional Chinese Medicine Material.* 1996;19(10): 520–522.

Li XG, et al. *China Journal of Integrated External Medicine.* 1998;4(2):100–103.

Liu H. *Journal of Stomatology.* 1999;19(2):60–61.

Luo XP, et al. *China Journal of Pathology and Physiology.* 1999;15(7):639–643.

Modern TCM Pharmacology. 1997.Tianjin: Science and Technology Press.

Shi RB. *Journal of Beijing University of TCM.* 1999;22(2): 63–64.

Tong JM, et al. *Journal of Popular Medicine of Chinese Ethnic Minorities.* 1995;(2):24–28.

Williams T, Mueller K, Cornwall MW. Effect of acupuncture point stimulation on diastolic blood pressure in hypertensive subjects: a preliminary study. *Phys Ther* 1991 Jul;71(7): 523–9.

Xu SA, et al. *China Journal of Pharmacy.* 1999;34(10): 663–665.

Xu ZW, et al. *Zhejiang Journal of Oncology.* 1997;3(2): 110–111.

Xu ZW, et al. *Journal of Gastroenteropathy and Hepatology.* 1998;7(1):67–71.

Zhong Guo Yao Li Xue Tong Bao (*Journal of Chinese Herbal Pharmacology*), 1986; 2(5):26.

Zhong Yao Xue (*Chinese Herbology*), 1998; 739:741.

Zhong Yao Yao Li Yu Ying Yong (*Pharmacology and Applications of Chinese Herbs*); 1983;866.

Zi M, Otsuyama KI, Liu SQ, Abroun S, Ishikawa H, Tsuyama N, Obata M, Li FJ, Zheng X, Maki Y, Miyamoto K, and Kawano MM. Baicalein, a component of *Scutellaria* radix from Huang-Lian-Jie-Du-Tang (HLJDT), leads to suppression of proliferation and induction of apoptosis in human myeloma cells. *Blood.* 2005; 105:3312–3318.

Homotoxicology references

Ben-Yakir S. Primary evaluation of homeopathic remedies injected via acupuncture points to reduce chronic high somatic cell counts in modern dairy farms, *Veterinary Acupuncture Newsletter*, 2004.Feb;27(1):pp 19–21.

Colin P. Homeopathy and respiratory allergies: a series of 147 cases. *Homeopathy.* 2006. Apr;95(2): pp 68–72.

Enbergs H. Effects of the homeopathic preparation Engystol on interferon-gamma production by human T-lymphocytes. *Immunol Invest.* 2006. 35(1):pp 19–27.

Oberbaum M, Glatthaar-Saalmuller B, Stolt P, Weiser M. Antiviral activity of Engystol: an in vitro analysis. *J Altern Complement Med.* 2005. Oct;11(5):pp 855–62. Erratum in: *J Altern Complement Med.* 2005 Dec;11(6):pp 1122.

Ouedraogo G, Morliere P, Santus R, Miranda M, Castell JV. Damage to mitochondria of cultured human skin fibroblasts photosensitized by fluoroquinolones. *J Photochem Photobiol B.* 2000. Oct;58(1):pp 20–5.

Reckeweg H. Biotherapeutic Index: Ordinatio Antihomotoxica et Materia Medica, 5th ed. Baden-Baden, Germany: Biologische Heilmittel Heel GMBH, 2000. pp 292–3, 302, 330–3, 333–4, 531.

Reckeweg H. Homeopathia Antihomotoxica Materia Medica, 4th ed. Baden-Baden, Germany: Aurelia-Verlag GMBH, 2002. pp. 115–6, 136–9, 141–2, 152, 198, 250, 525, 583–4.

Sourdeval M, Lemaire C, Brenner C, Boisvieux-Ulrich E, Marano F. Mechanisms of doxycycline-induced cytotoxicity on human bronchial epithelial cells. *Front Biosci.* 2006. Sep 1;11:pp 3036–48.

Yu F, Yu F, Li R, Wang R. Toxic effect of chloromycetin on the ultrastructures of the motor neurons of the Chinese tree shrew (Tupaia belangeri). *Can J Physiol Pharmacol.* 2004. Apr;82(4): pp 276–81.

PNEUMONIA

Definition and cause

Pneumonia is an inflammatory reaction to a foreign material in the lungs. The underlying cause for pneumonia can be broadly categorized as allergic (antigenic-allergens, heartworms), infectious (bacterial or viral), or fungal, and also can be secondary to other conditions such as aspiration, heartworm disease, and neoplasia (Bauer 1989, Hawkins 1995, Kuehn 1991, Greene 1998, Roudebush 2003).

Medical therapy rationale, drug(s) of choice, and nutritional recommendations

Medical therapy for pneumonia is dependent upon the underlying causative agent(s). Antibiotics are given for bacterial infections, corticosteroids are given for allergic causes, and antifungal drugs are used for fungal infestation (Bauer 1989, Hawkins 1995, Kuehn 1991, Roudebush 2003, Wolf 1995).

Anticipated prognosis

Prognosis also depends upon the underlying cause. Allergic causes—including heartworm infestation—if identified and eliminated, often offer a good prognosis. Bacterial infections if diagnosed and treated early also offer a good prognosis. Chronic bacterial, fungal, and pneumonias secondary to other serious diseases such as neoplasia often offer a guarded prognosis. Recurrences are common (Bauer 1989, Roudebush 2003, Taboada 1997).

Integrative veterinary therapies

While the medical approach to respiratory problems is to look for the causative agent (bacteria, viral, fungal etc), alternatives take into consideration that the lungs and the upper respiratory system is an avenue of toxin elimination. The enhancement of toxin elimination and the reduction of inflammation are the focus of the integrative approach. When nutritional, herbal and biological therapies are added, elimination is encouraged, cellular inflammation is reduced, secondary invaders such as bacteria cannot take hold, grow and cause the disease.

Nutritional treatment of respiratory disorders involves reducing toxin levels (providing clean, properly humidified air), correcting dehydration when present so that secretory efforts are assisted and promoted. Also, assuring proper nutrition with attention to those nutrients which assist secretion and thin mucus as well as protect against and overly acid or oxidative environment. Therapy also provides the proper mix of exercise to stimulate lung motion and lymphatic movement and periods of rest in order that damage can be repaired.

Nutrition
General considerations/rationale

Therapeutic nutrition adds nutrient and gland support for the lungs and organs of the immune system. In addition, nutrients can help decrease local cellular inflammation while improving elimination of toxins.

Pneumonia can be a serious disease of a major organ of detoxification and can affect the body and organs systemically. It is therefore recommended that blood be analyzed medically and physiologically to determine organ involvement and disease. This allows clinicians to formulate therapeutic nutritional protocols that address the upper respiratory system as well as other organs of elimination and detoxification such as the liver and kidney (see Chapter 2, Nutritional Blood Testing, for additional information).

Appropriate nutrients

Nutritional/gland therapy: Glandular lung, adrenal, and thymus supply the intrinsic nutrients used to reduce inflammation and improve organ function as well as enhance the cellular elimination of toxins (see Gland Therapy, Chapter 2, for a more detailed explanation).

Quercetin: Quercetin is a flavonoid that has potent antioxidant properties. Quercetin also has been proven to inhibit cells from releasing histamines (Middleton 1986, Ogasawara 1985). This antihistamine attribute is beneficial in the treatment of allergic conditions such as asthma and can improve breathing in compromised conditions such as pneumonia. Quercetin inhibits the enzyme lipoxygenase, which contributes to the clinical signs associated with asthma (Welton 1986). Knekt (1997) has reported that Quercetin has proved beneficial in the inhibition of lung and other cancers.

Bromelain: Bromelain is a proteolytic enzyme derived from pineapples. Bromelain has anti-inflammatory properties and is beneficial for the upper respiratory system (Taub 1966). In a double-blind study, Ryan (1967) showed an improvement in the treatment of sinusitis with bromelain. Another characteristic of bromelain is its ability to reduce the thickness of mucus in the respiratory system, which is beneficial for asthma and all inflammatory and infectious respiratory disease (Schaefer 1985). In addition, bromelain has been shown to positively affect white blood cells and the immune response, which is beneficial for upper respiratory infections such as pneumonia (Desser 1994, Kelly 1996, Munzig 1995).

N,N-Dimethylglycine (DMG): N,N-Dimethylglycine has been widely research in both humans and animals. DMG has been found to increase energy and enhance immune function (Barnes 1979, Graber 1981, Kendall 2000, Reap 1990, Walker 1988). In a double-blind study, Graber (1981) showed that DMG has a protective and therapeutic effect in people with pneumonia. DMG also can help the body to eliminate toxins that may predispose and cause the upper respiratory infections (Kendall 2003).

Chinese herbal medicine/acupuncture
General considerations/rationale

Pneumonia results from Wind and Heat leading to Yin and Qi deficiency in the Lungs. Wind is thought to blow the pathogen into the body; the pathogen then attacks the Lung. This causes Heat or inflammation in the Lung. The

Lung Qi and Yin become damaged by the pathogen. Initially, the cough is strong, as the body's defenses are strong, but as the condition becomes chronic, the Lung Qi is depleted and the cough becomes weaker. As the Yin, or fluids, becomes damaged, the cough becomes dry and hacking and potentially chronic if the Yin is not replenished.

Appropriate Chinese herbs

Anemarrhena (Zhi mu): Has exhibited inhibitory effects against multiple strains of bacteria (Yao Xue Qing Bao Tong Xun 1987).

Apricot seed (Xin ren): Contains amygdalin. This compound increases phagocytic activity of Kupffer's cells in the respiratory tract of mice (Li 1991). This helps to clear pathogens from the trachea, bronchi, and alveoli. It also has expectorant and antitussive effects (Zhang 1991).

Citrus (Chen pi): Has expectorant effects (Huang 1999).

Fritillaria bulb (Chuan bei mu): Was shown in one experiment to decrease coughing in mice that were exposed to ammonia. It also has an expectorant effect (Zhu 1992).

Houttuynia (Yu xing cao): Possesses antimicrobial effects. It is useful against both bacteria and some viruses (Zhong Yao Xue 1998). It increases phagocytic activity of white blood cells (Xin Yi Yao Xue Za Zhi 1973), which can help to clear pathogens. In one trial it was used in human patients with pneumonia. Response to herbal therapy in this trial was considered excellent (Zhong Hua Nei Ke Za Zhi 1963).

Gypsum (Shi gao): Increases the phagocytic activity of macrophages (Zhong Yao Xue 1998), which helps to clear the pathogen from the respiratory tract.

Licorice (Gan cao): Contains glycyrrhizin, which has been shown to inhibit various viruses (Zhu 1996). Licorice also has antibacterial properties (Zhong Yao Zhi 1993). In addition, it has antitussive and expectorant effects, as was demonstrated in experiments involving guinea pigs. It is thought to act on the central nervous system to mediate the cough suppressant effects (Zhong Yao Yao Li Yu Ying Yong 1983).

Morus bark (Sang bai pi): Has antitussive actions (Zhong Yao Xue 1998).

Ophiopogon (Mai men dong): Has antibacterial properties (Zhong Yao Xue 1998). It also enhances mucociliary clearance rates and decreases the secretion of mucus in the respiratory tract (Tai 2002).

Perilla seeds (Su zi): Decrease coughing. In one trial 40 patients with persistent cough were treated with perilla seeds. Sixty-two percent had excellent results and 37% had some improvement (Zhong Yao Tong Bao 1986).

Poria (Fu ling): Enhances cellular immunity. In one experiment it increased the phagocytic efficacy of macrophages in mice (Lu 1990). It also has direct antibacterial effects (Nanjing College of Pharmacy 1976).

Rhubarb (Da huang): Contains emodin, rhein, and aloe-emodin, which have antibiotic effects (Zhong Yao Xue 1998). It inhibits both aerobic and anaerobic bacteria (Zhao 1999, Yang 1997). Furthermore, it has demonstrated antiviral effects (Xie 1996). In addition to the direct activity against pathogens, it also enhances immunity. Rhubarb has been shown to decrease endotoxin-induced secretion of interleukin 6 by pulmonary macrophages, which helps protect the lungs from damage (Miao 1998). It has been shown to increase phagocytic activity by macrophages (Zhang 1997).

Trichosanthes root (Tian hua fen): Shows antimicrobial effects against a variety of bacteria and viruses (Zhong Yao Yao Li Yu Ying Yong 1983).

Acupuncture

Acupuncture can be used to help stop coughing, clear phlegm, decrease inflammation, and stop wheezing. In one trial, 106 people with chronic cough and asthma were treated by acupoint injections at BL13, CV22, Lu 1, CV17, and St 36. Three to 4 acupoints were used per treatment. Forty-six percent experienced significant improvement and 44% had some improvement (Dai 1991).

Homotoxicology
General considerations/rationale

Pneumonia represents an Inflammation Phase disorder of the respiratory tract. It can occur as a progressive vicariation as homotoxins injure delicate pulmonary tissue. This can occur due to overwhelming of the organism's greater defenses, particularly the upper respiratory tree. Failure to trap homotoxins and expel them by the action of the mucosa and local immune barriers leads to the necessity for inflammatory actions. Inflammation localizes and destroys many homotoxins, but it can do further damage to the organism as well.

The clinician should not forget that pneumonia can also occur as a regressive vicariation. When homotoxins become trapped and alter the matrix, tissue, and cells, the body may require inflammation so that damaged tissues can be liquefied and removed for later repair. Bacteria may gain access to compromised tissues and set up bacterial infections. It is possible that such bacterial infections may actually assist the body in freeing homotoxins. Pneumonias resulting from Deposition, Impregnation and Degeneration phase diseases may be quite difficult to treat and may well require allopathic medications to preserve a patient's life. As with all biological therapy, the long-term approach to deeper cases involving Impregnation, Degeneration and Dedifferentiation phases is indicated.

Antihomotoxic medications are used to speed excretion and activate the body's greater defense mechanisms. In this phase the practitioner should select those remedies that are indicated based upon classical homeopathic prescribing. These consist of the symptom remedies and homaccords. Each of these is discussed below. Simple detoxification using Heel's Detox Kit, which consists of Nux vomica homaccord, Berberis homaccord, and Lymphomyosot, is helpful after removing the patient from the area of contamination. Such homotoxicoses usually respond fairly rapidly.

Inflammation Phase homotoxicoses, such as pneumonia, result when the offending homotoxin cannot be adequately excreted or inactivated, resulting in further damage to the mucosal elements. Inflammation can occur in cases of more chronic irritation from harsh chemicals and particulates, or in the instance of overwhelming damage from exposure to homotoxins. Disruption of the mucosal barrier leads to invasion and activation of cellular and humeral elements of the immune system. The inflammatory reaction is an important response that is necessary to properly remove debris and bacterial endotoxins; however, excessive inflammation sets the stage for deeper homotoxicoses and pathology.

Serious inflammation can quickly cause progressive vicariation to the Degeneration Phase. Fever often occurs in this phase and should not be interfered with unless it is life threatening. Fever activates the immune elements, makes tissue inhospitable to pathogens, and assists in removing trapped homotoxins from the area. When properly selecting antihomotoxic medications, the patient will often be found to develop a febrile response and this is generally a good prognostic sign. This happens frequently with agents such as Engystol-N, Echinacea compositum, and Tonsilla compositum.

Inflammation Phase diseases are treated by selecting the proper symptom remedy, supporting tissue repair and drainage, and providing adequate support to the patient's efforts at recovery. Antibiotics may be needed but may cause progressive vicariation by their action of releasing increasing amounts of endotoxins into the environment, as well as damaging mitochondria and other cellular organelles (Ouedraogo, et al. 2000; Yu, et al. 2004; Sourdeval, et al. 2006). If antibiotics are necessary, the practitioner should realize that an Impregnation or Degeneration phase disorder will often result and steps should be taken to support the patient by administering proper remedies to help reverse these states.

Deposition Phase homotoxicoses are generally subclinical and asymptomatic, and pneumonia may develop through the process of regressive vicariation into the Inflammation Phase. The body's defenses deposit homotoxins into the large connective tissue volume of the lungs and associated tissues. Two common clues to the presence of Deposition Phase disease are the presence of obesity or pigmentary skin lesions. In patients suspected of being in this phase, the use of Solidago compositum, Galium-Heel, Lymphomyosot, and Placenta compositum actually drains away and cleanses the deeper matrix, commonly resulting in regressive vicariation and the appearance of inflammatory conditions such as pruritus, cough, or oculonasal discharges. All of these results represent desirable healing on the part of the patient's immune system. It may be that intercepting homotoxicosis in this phase prevents or delays the onset of Impregnation disorders. Because Deposition Phase diseases are more easily treated than those of the Impregnation Phase—which lie on the other side of the biological divide—clinicians should strive to begin biological therapy before the patient's disease progresses. Research into this theory may yield several very valuable techniques for the veterinarian's wellness practice.

Impregnation Phase disorders frequently involve the respiratory system and represent difficult conditions, which often frustrate owners and veterinarians alike. Allergic pneumonia, such as pulmonary infiltrates of eosinophils, and viral infections are common examples of Impregnation Phase homotoxicoses. Because the homotoxins present in this phase have altered normal structures such as enzymes and receptor sites, the cell's ability to repair and change its condition are sorely affected. Conventional therapy involves avoiding allergens, suppressing immune response, and hyposensitization. Many patients gradually worsen as the condition becomes more degenerative and as damage accumulates from use of allopathic agents. Biological therapy in these conditions involves deep detoxification and matrix repair and drainage. When this is done properly, it can yield surprisingly good results as the body undergoes regressive vicariation in its attempt to repair chronic disease states. Organ-building therapy and energy metabolism are critical components as well. The compositae class of antihomotoxic drugs plays an important role here and in all phases that follow this one.

Pneumonia can result from degradation of the host defenses in Degeneration Phase conditions such as collapsing trachea, chronic obstructive disease, emphysema, bronchiectasis, and pulmonary fibrosis. Rapid patient demise may occur and aggressive therapy using an integrative approach is indicated. Allopathic drugs are needed to save the patient's life and produce adequate comfort for proper rest and rehabilitation. Biological therapies help the patient become stronger and repair damage from both disease and iatrogenic factors. Degeneration Phase cases may give surprisingly good responses in some conditions when approached over long periods of time with compositae class antihomotoxic medicines, good nutrition, and client education. Patients that respond will likely remain with abnormal function, but their conditions can be greatly improved.

Both authors find that autosanguis therapy is an essential component of biological therapy for many respiratory diseases, including pneumonia. New practitioners should read Chapter 34 in this text on autosanguis therapy and develop some comfort with this procedure. Many cases of chronic respiratory disease will not make any progress until autosanguis is performed. An oral version of autosanguis can be done, but in the hands of the authors does not appear to work as well as the injectable form.

Appropriate homotoxicology formulas

Obtaining an excellent working knowledge of classical homeopathic remedy selection greatly assists clinicians as they design treatment protocols for pneumonia. A detailed discussion of these protocols is beyond the scope of this text. In many cases, recovery is so rapid that both client and practitioner are happily surprised when the proper homeopathic remedy is chosen and applied. In other cases, the response is slower. The following are only superficial descriptions of antihomotoxic medicines; deeper study will clarify many of their roles as the biological therapist gains more experience (Bellavite, et al. 2006). Note that the areas of application for specific antihomotoxic medicines are included in their description.

Aconitum homaccord: An initial remedy used in Inflammation Phase conditions that is useful for fever, chills, hot skin, painful/hard coughs, and influenza-like conditions. It is indicated in fearful cases (Reckeweg 2000).

Abropernol: Contains Abrotanum, which can be useful in chronic pleurisy with effusion and other exudative processes, including the after-effects of chest surgery for hydrothorax or empyema. Difficult respiration and a dry, persistent cough, plus sensitivity to cold air, are characteristic of this remedy. Nitricum acidum is contained in this remedy for mucosal and respiratory conditions (Reckeweg 2002).

Apis homaccord: Treats pulmonary edema.

Arnica-Heel: Contains many agents that are active in respiratory conditions, such as Bryonia (inflammation and pleuritis), Mercurialis perennis (influenza and sepsis), Eupatorium (influenza with intermittent fever), and Solanum (worsening after wet weather) (Reckeweg 2000).

Belladonna homaccord: An Inflammation Phase remedy that is used for focal, intensely inflamed lesions and all septic conditions such as septic pneumonia. Also used for acute phases of canine distemper (pneumonia, seizures, and vocalization) and bloody sputum (Macloed 1983, Reckeweg 2000).

BHI-Cough: Useful in mild cases of viral respiratory infections (Heel 2002).

Bronchalis-Heel: A major symptom remedy that is useful in bronchitis and smoker's catarrh (secondhand smoke injury in pets living in smoking households). Contains many major homeopathic respiratory remedies including Belladonna, Lungwort, Kalium stibyltartaricum, Kreosotum, Ipecacuanha, Lobelia, Hyoscyamus, and Bryonia.

Bryaconeel: A very useful remedy containing Bryonia, which is indicated for inflammation of serous membranes, bronchial cough with chill following acute inflammation of the respiratory organs, pleura, and peritoneum. There are often catarrhs of the larynx and of the trachea with hoarseness, accumulation of tough mucus with a dry cough, constriction of the chest, and pleuritic pains with deep inspiration. Bryaconeel is often useful in pleurisy accompanied by pneumonia (Reckeweg 2002). Bryonia is common to *Bronchalis* and *BHI-Bronchitis*, *Echinacea compositum*, and *BHI-Inflammation*. Other ingredients are Aconitum (acute febrile diseases and influenza) and Phosphorus (bronchopneumonia, nighttime cough, bloody expectorate, and diseases of the lung and larynx) (Reckeweg 2000). This remedy is very useful in the authors' clinics in treatment of chronic obstructive and geriatric lung diseases involving chronic cough. May be used long term.

Chelidonium homaccord: Contains Lycopodium for serious inflammation of the respiratory organs. This is especially helpful in cases of pneumonia that reach a dangerous stage, when expectoration is difficult to expel, is possibly purulent and yellow or greenish-yellow and offensive, and in many cases is attributable to a liver dysfunction. The Chelidonium component is helpful in right-sided pneumonia, which may occur as a consequence of liver disturbance (Reckeweg 2002). This remedy also contains Belladonna.

Coenzyme compositum: Used in chronic diseases to activate energy metabolism and after therapy with allopathic medications that damage mitochondrial function (antibiotics).

Drosera homaccord: The main constituent, Cuprum aceticum, is indicated for whooping-cough-like conditions, bronchiolitis, bronchial asthma, spasmodic coughing fits, and smooth muscle cramping with or without seizures (Macloed 1983, Reckeweg 2000).

Dulcamara homaccord: Used for conditions that worsen after wet weather, rhinitis, neuralgia and fever, and tonsillitis.

Echinacea compositum: An important Inflammation Phase remedy. Also indicated in Impregnation Phases marked by recurring infections. Used as a natural antibiotic in bacterial and viral conditions such as tonsillitis, bronchitis, and pneumonia. Contains major remedies consisting of Echinacea, Aconitum, Sanguinaria, Sulfur, Baptista, Lachesis, Bryonia, Eupatorium, Pulsatilla, Mercurious submlimatus, Thuja, Influenzium nosode, Phosphorus, Cortisonum, Streptococcus nosode, Staphylococcus nosode, Phytolacca, Zincum, Gelsemium, Hepar sulfuris, Rhus tox, Arnica, Arsenicum, Argentum, and Euphorbium (Reckeweg 2000).

Engystol N: Used for viral infections through the action of Vincetoxicum and Sulfur. Excellent in asthma in cats and in pneumonia. This remedy is not antiviral, but it directly stimulates immune function (Ben-Yakir 2004; Oberbaum, et al. 2005; Enbergs 2006).

Euphorbium compositum and nasal spray: Has antiviral activity. A mainstay remedy that is extremely useful in chronic rhinitis and sinusitis in cats and dogs.

Galium-Heel: A phase remedy in all phases from Deposition through Degeneration due to its draining effects on the matrix as well as its ability to improve and activate the greater defenses. A main remedy for any chronic disease.

Glyoxal compositum: Used for chronic diseases in the Degeneration and Dedifferentiation phases. Decouples homotoxins from receptors and other proteins such as enzymes.

Gripp-Heel: Provides excellent support of immunity in viral infections such as influenza and influenza-like syndromes. Used frequently by the authors in feline upper respiratory cases, bronchopneumonia, and some viral tracheobronchitis cases.

Hepar compositum: Provides liver support. Part of the deep detoxification formula for chronic diseases. Contains Lycopodium, which may be useful in cases of allergic rhinitis (Colin 2006).

Husteel: Used for coughs, chills, colds, spasmodic bronchitis, bronchopneumonia, and pleurisy. The cough characterizing this formula is more dry and irritating. Husteel is often selected for cardiac coughs in older patients.

Lymphomyosot: Provides lymph drainage and support.

Mucosa compositum: Provides repair and drainage of the mucosal tissues. Useful as a phase remedy in Degeneration Phase diseases and following recovery from illness. Also may assist in returning mucosal elements to normal after iatrogenic damage to the gut lining following antibiotic therapy.

Naso-Heel: A main antihomotoxic medicine for rhinitis and sinusitis that is acute or chronic in nature.

Natrium homaccord: Treats chronic catarrhal rhinitis.

Phosphor homaccord: Treats pulmonary parenchymal disorders, laryngitis, and bleeding tendencies. Phosphorus has proved its worth in pneumonia (orally or injected, in the potencies 10, 30, 200 and 1,000 times) (Reckeweg 2002). This component is also common to *Apis compositum*, *Bryaconeel*, *Echinacea compositum*, *Galium-Heel*, *Gripp-Heel*, *Mucosa compositum*, *Naso-Heel*, and *BHI-Bleeding*.

Pulsatilla compositum: A remedy for regulation rigidity and nasal and mucosal catarrhal reactions. May assist in reversing damage from corticosteroids (Cortisonum aceticum). Contains Pulsatilla and Sulfur, which is commonly used in human homeopathy for allergic rhinitis (Colin 2006). Inflammation may suddenly appear following use of this formula, and support of patient functions through *Traumeel S*, *Echinacea compositum*, *Tonsilla compositum*, and *Engystol N* may prove helpful in completing the inflammatory reaction without doing further iatrogenic damage from allopathic drug administration.

Tartephedreel: Treats bronchial coughs, bronchial asthma, and prolonged coughing, especially when catarrhal respiratory conditions exist (Reckeweg 2000).

Tonsilla compositum: An important phase remedy for Impregnation and Dedifferentiation conditions. Supports the endocrine and immune systems in chronic disease.

Traumeel S: Treats inflammatory conditions anywhere in the body, as well as sinusitis and rhinitis. Useful in regulation rigidity. *Traumeel S* is important after regressive vicariation following use of *Pulsatilla compositum*. It is used intermittently in many cases to reduce inflammation and improve patient comfort and healing.

Spascupreel: May soothe coughs associated with bronchospasm by relaxing smooth muscles.

Ubichinon compositum: Contains Anthracinon, which has strong indications in affections of the lungs, pleurisy, and pneumonia and respiratory illness, where there is effusion in most cases. The ingredient Ubiquinone (Coenzyme Q10) is useful in chronic mucosal inflammations and suppurations with excoriating secretions, septic cold infections, descending bronchitis, febrile pneumonia, asthmatic attacks, and in patients with persistent nocturnal cough, particularly when provoked by movement (Reckeweg 2002).

Authors' suggested protocols

Nutrition

Bronchus/lung and immune support formulas: 1 tablet for every 25 pounds of body weight BID.

Quercetin: 50 mgs for every 10 pounds of body weight SID.

Bromelain: 100 mgs for each 25 pounds of body weight, with food.

DMG: Liquid—one-half ml per 25 pounds of body weight (maximum, 2 mls); tablets—125 mg–1 tablet for every 40 pounds of body weight (maximum, 3 tablets).

Chinese herbal medicine/acupuncture

H23 Pneumonia: 1 capsule per 10 to 20 pounds twice daily for 2 to 4 weeks after signs have resolved, depending upon the severity of the pneumonia. In chronic cases, therapy may be continued indefinitely. This formula is indicated for pneumonia of various etiologies (bacterial, viral, eosinophilic, allergic) as well as kennel cough and bronchiopneumonitis. It can be combined with antibiotics or steroids if needed.

In addition to the herbs cited above, H23 Pneumonia also contains glehnia root (Sha shen), lophatherum (Zhu ye), mulberry leaves (Sang ye), pseudotellaria (Tai zi shen), and trichosanthes seeds (Gua lou ren) to increase the efficacy of the formula.

Schoen (1994) has recommended the following acupuncture points for pneumonia in horses: BL13, BL14, BL15, BL17, GV11, GV12, GV14, GV16, SP20, SP 1, GB 1, and LI16.

Homotoxicology (Dose: 10 drops PO for 50-pound dog; 5 drops PO for small dog or cat)

Echinacea compositum as an initial injection: In acute viral pneumonias, Gripp-Heel plus Engystol N are indicated. Chronic cases may benefit from an autosanguis therapy with Tonsilla compositum. The following remedies can be considered for oral therapy: Abropernol, Arnica-Heel, Phosphor homaccord, BHI-Inflammation, Ubichinon compositum, and Chelidonium homaccord for liver support. The selections may be mixed in an oral cocktail, often with the remains of the syringe which was used for the autosanguis therapy, and given 2 to 4 times daily, or as needed to control the symptoms.

Deep detoxification formula: Used in refractory or recurrent cases. Contains Galium-Heel, Lymphomyosot, Hepar compositum, Solidago compositum, Thryoidea compositum, Coenzyme compositum, Ubichinon compositum, and Mucosa compositum; given orally every 3 days for long periods of time.

Product sources

Nutrition

Bronchus/lung and immune support formulas: Animal Nutrition Technologies. **Alternatives:** Immune System Support—Standard Process Veterinary Formulas; Immuno Support—Rx Vitamins for Pets; Immugen—Thorne Veterinary Products.

   Quercetin: Source Naturals; Quercitone—Thorne Veterinary Products.

   Bromezyme: Progressive Labs.

   DMG: Vetri Science.

Chinese herbal medicine

H23 Pneumonia: Natural Solutions, Inc.

Homotoxicology

BHI/Heel Corporation

REFERENCES

Western medicine references

Bauer T. Pulmonary hypersensitivity disorders. In: Kirk RW, ed. Current veterinary therapy X. Philadelphia: Saunders, 1989:369–376.

Hawkins EC. Aspiration pneumonia. In: Bonagura JD, Kirk RW, eds. Current veterinary therapy XII. Philadelphia: Saunders, 1995:915–919.

Kuehn NF, Roudebush P. Allergic lung disease. In: Allen DG, ed. Small animal medicine. Philadelphia: Lippincott, 1991: 423–432.

Greene CE. Infectious diseases of the dog and cat. 2nd ed. Philadelphia: Saunders, 1998.

Roudebush P. In: Tilley L, Smith F. The 5-Minute Veterinary Consult: Canine and Feline, Blackwell Publishing, 2003.

Taboada J. Systemic mycoses. In: Morgan RV, ed. Handbook of small animal practice. 3rd ed. Philadelphia: Saunders, 1997:1113–1126.

Wolf AM, Troy GC. Deep mycotic diseases. In: Ettinger SJ, Feldman EC, eds. Textbook of veterinary internal medicine. 4th ed. Philadelphia: Saunders, 1995:439–463.

IVM/nutrition references

Barnes L. B15: The politics of ergogenicity. *Physicians and Sports Medicine.* 1979;7(11):17.

Desser L, Rehberger A, Paukovits W. Proteolytic enzymes and amylase induce cytokine production in peripheral blood mononuclear cells in vitro. *Cancer Biother* 1994;9:253–63.

Graber G, Goust J, Glassman A, Kendall R, Loadholt C. Immunomodulating Properties of Dimethylglycine in Humans. *Journal of Infectious Disease*, 1981. 143:101.

Kelly GS. Bromelain: a literature review and discussion of its therapeutic applications. *Altern Med Rev* 1996;1:243–57 [review].

Kendall R, Lawson JW. Recent Findings on N,N-Dimethylglycine (DMG): A Nutrient for the New Millennium, *Townsend Letter for Doctors and Patients*, 2000 May.

Kendall RV. Building Wellness with DMG, Topanga, CA: Freedom Press, 2003.

Knekt P, Jarvinen R, Seppanen R, et al. Dietary flavonoids and the risk of lung cancer and other malignant neoplasms. *Am J Epidemiol* 1997;146:223–30.

Le Marchand L, Murphy SP, Hankin JH, et al. Intake of flavonoids and lung cancer. *J Natl Cancer Inst* 2000;92:154–60.

Middleton E Jr. Effect of flavonoids on basophil histamine release and other secretory systems. *Prog Clin Biol Res.* 1986;213:493–506.

Munzig E, Eckert K, Harrach T, et al. Bromelain protease F9 reduces the CD44 mediated adhesions of human peripheral blood lymphocytes to human umbilical vein endothelial cells. *FEBS Lett* 1995;351:215–8.

Ogasawara H, Middleton E Jr. Effect of selected flavonoids on histamine release (HR) and hydrogen peroxide (H2O2) generation by human leukocytes [abstract]. *J Allergy Clin Immunol.* 1985;75(suppl):184.

Reap E, Lawson J. Stimulation of the Immune Response by Dimethylglycine, a non-toxic metabolite. *Journal of Laboratory and Clinical Medicine.* 1990;115:481.

Ryan RE. A double-blind clinical evaluation of bromelains in the treatment of acute sinusitis. *Headache* 1967;7:13–7.

Schafer A, Adelman B. Plasma inhibition of platelet function and of arachidonic acid metabolism. *J Clin Invest* 1985; 75:456–61.

Taub SJ. The use of Ananase in sinusitis. A study of 60 patients. *EENT Monthly* 1966;45:96–8.

Walker M. Some Nutri-Clinical Applications of N,N-Dimethylglycine. *Townsend Letter for Doctors.* 1988 June.

Welton AF, Tobias LD, Fiedler-Nagy C, et al. Effect of flavonoids on arachidonic acid metabolism. *Prog Clin Biol Res* 1986;213:231–42.

Chinese herbal medicine/acupuncture references

Dai CL, et al. 106 cases of chronic cough and asthma treated with acupoint injection of He Lao. *Journal of Beijing College of TCM.* 1991;14(6):48.

Huang M, et al. *China Journal of Wild Botanic Resources.* 1999;18(1):36–37.

Li CH, et al. Amygdalin's effect on mononuclear macrophages' phagocytotic function. *Journal of Shanxi College of Medicine.* 1991;22(1):1–3,79.

Lu SC, et al. *Journal of No. 1 Military Academy.* 1990;10(3):267.

Miao R, et al. *Journal of Chinese Materia Medica.* 1998;29(6):395–397.

Nanjing College of Pharmacy. Materia Medica, vol. 2. Jiangsu: People's Press; 1976.

Schoen A. Veterinary Acupuncture; Ancient Art to Modern Medicine. California: American Veterinary Publications, Inc., 1994 p 554.

Tai S, Sun F, O'Brien D, Lee M, Zayaz J, King M. Evaluation of a Mucoactive Herbal Drug, Radix Ophiopogonis, in a Pathogenic Quail Model. *J of Herbal Pharmacotherapy* 2002;2(4):49–56.

Xie YY, et al. *Journal of Shandong Medical University.* 1996;34(2):166–169.

Xin Yi Yao Xue Za Zhi (*New Journal of Medicine and Herbology*), 1973; (7):25.

Yang SZ, et al. *Liaoning Journal of Traditional Chinese Medicine.* 1997;24(4):187.

Yao Xue Qing Bao Tong Xun (*Journal of Herbal Information*), 1987; 5(4):62.

Zhang BS, et al. *Journal of Traditional Chinese Medicine Material.* 1997;20(2):85–88.

Zhang WJ, et al. Processed Xing Ren: Its potency and acute toxicity. *Journal of Traditional Chinese Medicine Material.* 1991;14(8):38–40.

Zhao MJ, et al. *Zhejiang Journal of Traditional Chinese Medicine.* 1999;34(12):544.

Zhong Hua Nei Ke Za Zhi (*Chinese Journal of Internal Medicine*), 1963;3:250.

Zhong Yao Tong Bao (*Journal of Chinese Herbology*), 1986; 8:56.

Zhong Yao Xue (*Chinese Herbology*), 1998, 115: 119.

Zhong Yao Xue (*Chinese Herbology*), 1998; 187:189.

Zhong Yao Xue (*Chinese Herbology*), 1998; 251:256.

Zhong Yao Xue (*Chinese Herbology*), 1998;648:650.

Zhong Yao Xue (*Chinese Herbology*), 1998; 845:848.

Zhong Yao Yao Li Yu Ying Yong (*Pharmacology and Applications of Chinese Herbs*), 1983: 149.

Zhong Yao Yao Li Yu Ying Yong (*Pharmacology and Applications of Chinese Herbs*), 1983:246.

Zhong Yao Zhi (*Chinese Herbology Journal*), 1993;358

Zhu AN, et al. *Journal of University of Pharmacology of China.* 1992;23(2):118–121.

Zhu LH. *China Journal of TCM Information.* 1996;3(3):17–20.

Homotoxicology references

Bellavite P, Conforti A, Pontarollo F, Ortolani R. Immunology and homeopathy. 2. Cells of the immune system and inflammation. *Evid Based Complement Alternat Med.* 2006. Mar;3(1): pp 13–24.

Ben-Yakir S. Primary evaluation of homeopathic remedies injected via acupuncture points to reduce chronic high somatic cell counts in modern dairy farms. *Veterinary Acupuncture Newsletter,* 2004. Feb;27(1):pp 19–21.

Colin P. Homeopathy and respiratory allergies: a series of 147 cases. *Homeopathy.* 2006. Apr;95(2): pp 68–72.

Enbergs H. Effects of the homeopathic preparation Engystol on interferon-gamma production by human T-lymphocytes. *Immunol Invest.* 2006. 35(1):pp 19–27.

Heel. BHI Homeopathic Therapy: Professional Reference. Albuquerque, NM: Heel Inc. 2002. pp 21, 48.

Macleod G. A Veterinary Materia Medica and Clinical Repertory with a Materia Medica of the Nosodes. Safron, Walden: CW Daniel Company, LTD, 1983. pp 29–30.

Oberbaum M, Glatthaar-Saalmuller B, Stolt P, Weiser M. Antiviral activity of Engystol: an in vitro analysis. *J Altern Complement Med.* 2005. Oct;11(5):pp 855–62. Erratum in: *J Altern Complement Med.* 2005 Dec;11(6):pp 1122.

Ouedraogo G, Morliere P, Santus R, Miranda M, Castell JV. Damage to mitochondria of cultured human skin fibroblasts photosensitized by fluoroquinolones. *J Photochem Photobiol B.* 2000.Oct;58(1):pp 20–5.

Reckeweg H. Biotherapeutic Index: Ordinatio Antihomotoxica et Materia Medica, 5th ed. Baden-Baden, Germany: Biologische Heilmittel Heel GMBH, 2000. p 285–6, 293–4, 299–300, 302, 328, 329, 332–3, 333–4, 401.

Reckeweg H. Homeopathia Antihomotoxica Materia Medica, 4th ed., Baden-Baden, Germany: Aurelia-Verlag GMBH 2002. pp 115–6, 187–9, 226–7, 394–6, 489, 584.

Sourdeval M, Lemaire C, Brenner C, Boisvieux-Ulrich E, Marano F. Mechanisms of doxycycline-induced cytotoxicity on human bronchial epithelial cells. *Front Biosci.* 2006. Sep 1;11:pp 3036–48.

Yu F, Yu F, Li R, Wang R. Toxic effect of chloromycetin on the ultrastructures of the motor neurons of the Chinese tree shrew (Tupaia belangeri). *Can J Physiol Pharmacol.* 2004.Apr;82(4):pp 276–81.

SINUSITIS AND RHINITIS

Definition and cause

Sinusitis and rhinitis occur in both dogs and cats and can be acute or chronic. The most common underlying causes are infectious (bacterial, viral, and fungal) and are more often secondary. In cats, sinusitis is most commonly caused by viral infections (see FIV and FIP in Chapter 18, Infectious Diseases). Noninfectious causes are secondary to allergy, trauma, foreign body, parasites, and neoplasia. Common signs are sneezing, nasal discharge, and bleeding (Davidson 2000, Forrester 1997, Gaskell 1999, Wolf 1997).

Medical therapy rationale, drug(s) of choice, and nutritional recommendations

Antibiotics are the treatment of choice for primary and secondary infections. Corticosteroids and antihistamines are recommended when there is an underlying allergic component. Antifungal drugs, both systemic and local, are recommended for fungal infestations. Neoplasia requires radiation therapy, chemotherapy, and surgical interventions. Chronic and nonresponsive cases may also require surgical intervention (Gaskell 1999, Mason 2003).

Anticipated prognosis

The prognosis is related to the underlying cause. Trauma and foreign bodies carry a good prognosis, while chronic infection, infestation, and neoplasia carry a more guarded prognosis (Mason 2003).

Integrative veterinary therapies

The reduction of inflammation and the enhancement of toxin elimination is the focus of the integrative approach to sinusitis. Immune system organs also require support when there is an allergic component involving an immune reaction to allergens and the sinuses are the target tissue. With chronic irritation, local bacteria can invade, leading to a more chronic, moist form of sinusitis.

When nutritional, herbal, and biological therapies are added to the prevention and treatment protocols, cellular elimination of wastes is encouraged, cellular inflammation is reduced, and secondary invaders such as bacteria are more controlled by a healthier, more balanced immune mechanism.

Nutrition
General considerations/rationale

Therapeutic nutrition adds nutrient and immune gland support. In addition, nutrients can help decrease local cellular inflammation while improving elimination of toxins.

Appropriate nutrients

Nutritional/gland therapy: Glandular adrenal and thymus supply the intrinsic nutrients that reduce cellular inflammation, thereby helping to improve organ function. This helps to spare these organs from cascading inflammation and eventual degeneration (see Gland Therapy in Chapter 2 for a more detailed explanation).

Bromelain: Bromelain is a proteolytic enzyme that comes from pineapples. In addition to being an enzyme, it has anti-inflammatory properties and is beneficial for the upper respiratory system (Taub 1966). In a double-blind study, Ryan (1967) showed an improvement in the treatment of sinusitis with bromelain. Bromelain also can reduce the thickness of mucus in the respiratory system, which is beneficial for sinusitis (Schaefer 1985). In addition, bromelain has been shown to positively affect white blood cells and the immune response, which can help to prevent sinusitis from becoming secondarily infected and chronic (Desser 1994, Kelly 1996, Munzig 1995).

Quercetin: Quercetin is a flavonoid that has potent antioxidant properties. Quercetin also has been proven to inhibit cells from releasing histamines (Middleton 1986, Ogasawara 1985). This antihistamine attribute is beneficial in the treatment of allergic conditions and can improve breathing in more compromised conditions such as pneumonia. Quercetin inhibits the enzyme lipoxygenase, which contributes to the clinical signs associated with asthma (Welton 1986).

N,N-Dimethylglycine (DMG): N,N-Dimethylglycine has been widely researched in both humans and animals. DMG has been found to increase energy and enhance immune function (Barnes 1979, Graber 1981, Kendall 2000, Reap 1990, Walker 1988). In a double-blind study, Graber (1981) showed that DMG has a protective and therapeutic effect in people with pneumonia. DMG also can help the body to eliminate toxins that may predispose and cause the upper respiratory infections (Kendall 2003).

Chinese herbal medicine/acupuncture
General considerations/rationale

According to TCM, sinusitis and rhinitis are due to Damp and Heat in the Lung and Liver (Handbook of Traditional Chinese Medicine Practitioner 1987).

Although it is not intuitive to Western practitioners, the Liver controls the face. The meridians of the Liver channels cover the face so Liver pathology can affect the face and sinuses. The Lung opens to the Nose and Sinuses so Dampness in the Lung refers to the mucoid secretions that block the nasal passages and fill the Sinuses. Heat refers to the inflammation, which may be a result of the interaction between the immune system and secondary invaders i.e., bacteria, viruses and fungi, a reaction to foreign bodies or neoplastic cells, or a result of allergic reactions. Treatment goals include decreasing the signs associated with the condition as well as treating the underlying cause of the disease.

Appropriate Chinese herbs

Angelica (Bai zhi): Has been shown to have anti-inflammatory effects in mice. In addition, it has analgesic properties (Zhong Guo Zhong Yao Za Zhi 1991).

Atractodes (Cang zhu): Has shown efficacy against viruses, bacteria, and fungi (Zhong Yao Xue 1998).

Magnolia flower (Xin yi hua): Has been shown to be quite effective for rhinitis and sinusitis in several studies. It decreases mucous secretion, reduces inflammation, and is effective against several bacteria that may cause secondary infections, such as staphylococcus and streptococcus (Zhong Yao Cai 1990, Zhong Yao Xue 1998, Zhong Yao Tong Bao 1985).

Pinellia (Ban xia): Has demonstrated anti-inflammatory effects (Shen 1998).

Schizonepeta (Jing jie): Has analgesic properties (Zhong Yao Cai 1989). Humans with sinusitis report headaches so it is reasonable to assume animals suffer the same pain.

Scutellaria (Huang qin): Has demonstrated antibacterial effects against bacteria, viruses, and fungi (Zhong Yao Xue 1988, Wang 2000). It also decreases inflammation related to allergic reactions in mice (Kubo 1984).

Rhinitis has been recognized by the World Health Organization as being responsive to acupuncture (World Health Organization list of common conditions treatable by Chinese medicine and acupuncture). One trial studied 45 people with allergic rhinitis and found that acupuncture was better at controlling symptoms than antihistamine therapy (Chari 1988).

Homotoxicology
General considerations/rationale

The respiratory system is a common location of pathology in veterinary patients. Homotoxins gain access directly via the airways, through hematogenous spread via the systemic circulation, and through direct traumatic incidents. The Six-Phase Table of Homotoxicology is extremely helpful in the creation of treatment plans for respiratory patients, and both the development of disease, as well as its resolution, follows this table. Hering's Law is also seen in very clear fashion while managing many of these cases.

Excretion Phase diseases occur when homotoxins first contact the mucosal elements of the respiratory system. Veterinarians in clinical settings commonly see simple, acute rhinitis and sinusitis. Exposure to harsh chemicals

(bleach, ozone, disinfectants, tobacco smoke, scented products, air pollutants, etc.) or particulates leads to direct respiratory mucosal insult and resulting physiological efforts to dilute and excrete the material. Serous and mucous secretions assist in dilution and removal of homotoxins. The epithelial, mucosal elements provide the primary barrier to invasion and damage of this system. Intimately associated with the mucosa are rich lymphatic and neurological components used in monitoring and defense. Providing support of the flushing effects of this humeral phase treats Excretion Phase conditions of the nose and sinuses.

Rhinitis and sinusitis often present to veterinarians as Inflammation Phase disorders. If inflammation is effective, such homotoxicoses demonstrate regressive vicariation to Exudation Phase homotoxicoses. This is seen clinically as the production of serous drainage following the Inflammatory Phase. It is often mistaken for further symptoms of disease and is suppressively treated by antihistamines and decongestants, which act to stop or block the removal of homotoxins and thereby prevent the organism from complete healing. Such homotoxins may be deposited into tissues and lead to a clinically silent Deposition Phase conditions.

Allergic and viral rhinitis and sinusitis represent Impregnation Phase diseases and can rapidly deteriorate into Degeneration Phase diseases. This is often seen in bracheocephalic, longhaired feline patients that are persistently infected by the feline herpes virus.

Treatment of all phases of rhinitis and sinusitis involves reducing homotoxin levels (providing clean, properly humidified air), correcting dehydration when present so that secretory efforts are assisted and promoted, assuring proper nutrition with attention to those nutrients which assist secretion and thin mucus as well as protect against and overly acid or oxidative environment, and providing a proper mix of exercise to stimulate lung motion and lymphatic movement and periods of rest so that damage can be repaired. Antihomotoxic medications are used to speed excretion and activate the greater defense mechanisms of the body. In this phase the practitioner should select those remedies that are indicated based upon classical homeopathic prescribing. These consist of the symptom remedies and homaccords, each of which is discussed below. Simple detoxification using Heel's Detox Kit, which consists of Nux vomica homaccord, Berberis homaccord, and Lymphomyosot, is helpful after removing the patient from the area of contamination. Such homotoxicoses usually respond fairly rapidly.

Inflammation Phase rhinitis and sinusitis result when the offending homotoxin cannot be adequately excreted or inactivated, resulting in further damage to the mucosal elements. Bacterial rhinitis and sinusitis are typical Inflammation Phase diseases. Inflammation can occur in cases of more chronic irritation from harsh chemicals and particulates, or from overwhelming damage from exposure to homotoxins. Disruption of the mucosal barrier leads to invasion and activation of cellular and humeral elements of the immune system. The inflammatory reaction is an important response that is necessary to properly remove debris and bacterial endotoxins; however, excessive inflammation sets the stage for deeper homotoxicoses and pathology.

Serious inflammation can quickly cause progressive vicariation to the Degeneration Phase. This is common in fungal rhinitis and sinusitis. Fever often occurs in this phase and should not be interfered with unless it is life threatening. Fever activates the immune elements, makes tissue inhospitable to pathogens, and assists in removing trapped homotoxins from the area. When properly selecting antihomotoxic medications, the patient will often be found to develop a febrile response and this is generally a good prognostic sign. This happens frequently with agents such as Engystol N, Echinacea compositum, and Tonsilla compositum.

Inflammation Phase diseases are treated by selecting the proper symptom remedy, supporting tissue repair and drainage, and providing adequate support to the patient's recovery efforts. Antibiotics may be needed but may cause progressive vicariation by releasing increasing amounts of endotoxins into the environment and damaging mitochondria and other cellular organelles (Ouedraogo 2000, Yu 2004, Sourdeval 2006). If antibiotics are necessary, the practitioner should realize that an Impregnation or Degeneration phase disorder will often result, and steps should be taken to support the patient by administering proper remedies to aid in reversal of these states.

Deposition Phase homotoxicoses of the nasal cavity and sinuses are generally subclinical. The body's defenses deposit homotoxins into the large connective tissue volume of the lungs and associated tissues. Deposition Phase disorders are often subclinical and asymptomatic. Two common clues to the presence of Deposition Phase disease are obesity or pigmentary skin lesions. In patients suspected of being in this phase, Solidago compositum, Galium-Heel, Lymphomyosot, and Placenta compositum actually drain away and cleanse the deeper matrix, commonly resulting in regressive vicariation and the appearance of inflammatory conditions such as pruritus, cough, or oculonasal discharges, all of which represent desirable healing on the part of the patient's immune system. It may be that intercepting homotoxicoses in this phase prevent or delay the onset of Impregnation disorders. Because Deposition Phase diseases are more easily treated than Impregnation Phase diseases, which lie on the other side of the biological divide, clinicians should strive to begin biological therapy before the disease progresses. Research into this theory may yield several very valuable techniques for the veterinarian's wellness practice.

Impregnation Phase disorders are frequently seen involving the nasal cavity and sinuses, and represent difficult conditions that often frustrate owners and veterinarians alike. Chronic, recurring allergic issues and viral infections are common examples of Impregnation Phase homotoxicoses. Because the homotoxins present in this phase have altered normal structures such as enzymes and receptor sites, the cell's ability to repair and change its condition is sorely affected. Conventional therapy involves avoiding allergens, suppressing immune response, and hyposensitization. Many patients gradually worsen as the condition becomes more degenerative and as damage accumulates from use of allopathic agents. Biological therapy in these conditions involves deep detoxification and matrix repair and drainage, and when properly done, can yield surprisingly good results as the body undergoes regressive vicariation in its attempt to repair chronic disease states. Organ-building therapy and energy metabolism are critical components as well. The compositae class of antihomotoxic drugs plays an important role here and in all phases that follow this one.

Degeneration Phase conditions such as destruction of the nasal turbinates and loss of normal immune barriers, as well as destruction of cellular organelles (such as mitochondrial, Golgi apparatus, or genetic damage) represent more advanced and potentially irreversible conditions. However, some conditions may give surprisingly good responses when approached over long periods of time with compositae class antihomotoxic medicines, good nutrition, and client education. Patients that respond will likely remain with abnormal function, but their conditions can be greatly improved.

Cases that have progressed to the Dedifferentiation Phase are dealt with in the section on neoplasia in this text.

Both authors find that autosanguis therapy is an essential component of biological therapy for many respiratory diseases. New practitioners should read the autosanguis section in Chapter 34 and develop some comfort with this procedure. Many cases of chronic sinusitis and rhinitis will not make any progress until autosanguis is performed. An oral version of autosanguis can be done, but in the hands of the authors does not appear to work as well as the injectable form.

Appropriate homotoxicology formulas

Obtaining an excellent working knowledge of classical homeopathic remedy selection greatly assists clinicians as they design treatment protocols for rhinitis and sinusitis. A detailed discussion of these is beyond the scope of this text. In many cases, recovery is so rapid that both client and practitioner are happily surprised when the proper homeopathic remedy is chosen and applied. In other cases, the response is slower. The following are only superficial descriptions of antihomotoxic medicines, and deeper study will clarify many of their roles as the biological therapist gains more experience (Bellavite, et al. 2006). Note that the areas of application for specific antihomotoxic medicines are included in their description.

Belladonna homaccord: An Inflammation Phase remedy that treats focal, intensely inflamed lesions and all septic conditions such as septic pneumonia. It also treats acute phases of canine distemper (pneumonia, seizures, vocalization) and bloody sputum (Macloed 1983, Reckeweg 2000).

BHI-Sinus: Useful in sinusitis cases (Heel 2002).

Coenzyme compositum: Used in chronic diseases to activate energy metabolism and after therapy with allopathic medications that damage mitochondrial function (antibiotics).

Echinacea compositum: An important Inflammation Phase remedy that is also indicated in Impregnation Phases marked by recurring infections. Used as a natural antibiotic in bacterial and viral conditions such as tonsillitis, bronchitis, and pneumonia. Contains major remedies consisting of Echinacea, Aconitum, Sanguinaria, Sulfur, Baptista, Lachesis, Bryonia, Eupatorium, Pulsatilla, Mercurious submlimatus, Thuja, Influenzium nosode, Phosphorus, Cortisonum, Streptococcus nosode, Staphylococcus nosode, Phytolacca, Zincum, Gelsemium, Hepar sulfuris, Rhus tox, Arnica, Arsenicum, Argentum, and Euphorbium (Reckeweg 2000).

Engystol N: Used for viral infections through the action of *Vincetoxicum* and *Sulfur*. Excellent in asthma in cats and in pneumonia. This remedy directly stimulates immune function (Ben-Yakir 2004; Oberbaum, et al. 2005; Enbergs 2006).

Euphorbium compositum and nasal spray: Has antiviral activity. A mainstay remedy that is extremely useful in chronic rhinitis and sinusitis in cats and dogs.

Galium-Heel: A phase remedy in all phases from Deposition through Degeneration due to its draining effects on the matrix as well as its ability to improve and activate the greater defenses. A main remedy for any chronic disease.

Glyoxal compositum: Treats chronic diseases in the Degeneration and Dedifferentiation phases. Decouples homotoxins from receptors and other proteins such as enzymes.

Gripp-Heel: Provides excellent support of immunity in viral infections such as influenza and influenza-like syndromes. Used frequently by the authors in feline upper respiratory cases, bronchopneumonia, and some viral tracheobronchitis cases.

Hepar compositum: Provides liver support and is part of the deep detoxification formula for chronic diseases. Contains Lycopodium, which may be useful in cases of allergic rhinitis (Colin 2006).

Lymphomyosot: Provides lymph drainage and support.

Mucosa compositum: Used for repair and drainage of the mucosal tissues. Useful as a phase remedy in Degeneration Phase diseases and following recovery from illness. Also may assist in returning mucosal elements to normal after iatrogenic damage to the gut lining following antibiotic therapy.

Naso-Heel: A main antihomotoxic medicine for rhinitis and sinusitis that is acute or chronic in nature.

Natrium homaccord: Treats chronic catarrhal rhinitis.

Phosphor homaccord: Treats pulmonary parenchymal disorders, laryngitis, and bleeding tendencies. Phosphorus has proved its worth in pneumonia (orally or injected, in the potencies 10, 30, 200, and 1,000 times) (Reckeweg 2002). This component is also common to *Apis compositum, Bryaconeel, Echinacea compositum, Galium-Heel, Gripp-Heel, Mucosa compositum, Naso-Heel*, and *BHI-Bleeding*.

Pulsatilla compositum: A remedy for regulation rigidity and nasal and mucosal catarrhal reactions. May assist in reversing damage from corticosteroids (Cortisonum aceticum). Contains Pulsatilla and Sulfur, which are commonly used in human homeopathy for allergic rhinitis (Colin 2006). Inflammation may suddenly appear following use of this formula, and support of patient functions through *Traumeel S, Echinacea compositum, Tonsilla compositum*, and *Engystol N* may prove helpful in completing the inflammatory reaction without doing further iatrogenic damage from allopathic drug administration.

Tonsilla compositum: An important phase remedy for Impregnation and Dedifferentiation conditions. Supports the endocrine and immune systems in chronic disease.

Traumeel S: Treats inflammatory conditions anywhere in the body, as well as sinusitis and rhinitis. Useful in regulation rigidity. Also important after regressive vicariation following use of *Pulsatilla compositum*. Used intermittently in many cases to reduce inflammation and improve patient comfort and healing.

Ubichinon compositum: Contains Anthracinon, which has strong indications in affections of the lungs, pleurisy, pneumonia, and respiratory illness, where there is effusion in most cases. The remedy Ubiquinone (Coenzyme Q10) is useful in chronic mucosal inflammations and suppurations with excoriating secretions, in septic cold infections, descending bronchitis, febrile pneumonia, and asthmatic attacks, and in those with persistent nocturnal cough that is provoked by movement (Reckeweg 2002).

Authors' suggested protocols

Nutrition

Gingival/mouth and immune support formulas: 1 tablet for each 25 pounds of body weight BID.

Bromelain: 100 mgs for each 25 pounds of body weight, with food.

Quercetin: 50 mgs for each 10 pounds of body weight SID.

DMG: Liquid—one-half ml per 25 pounds of body weight (maximum, 2 mls); Tablets—125 mg–1 tablet for every 40 pounds of body weight (maximum, 3 tablets).

Chinese herbal medicine/acupuncture

For chronic sinusitis or rhinitis caused by allergies or bacterial, fungal, or viral infections, the authors recommend H57 Sinusitis at a dose of 1 capsule per 10 to 20 pounds twice daily. Based on our clinical observation, H57 Sinusitis helps to clear the infection in the nasal cavity and sinuses and controls secondary bacterial, fungal, and viral infections in the nasal passage.

Foreign bodies must be removed for treatment to be effective. Neoplasia must be addressed with herbs that are designed for cancerous conditions (see cancer/nasal cancer in Chapters 32 and 33).

In addition to the herbs mentioned above, H57 Sinusitis also contains, arisaema root (Dan nan xing) and leaven (Shen qu). These herbs help to enhance the functions of the herbs cited above.

Acupuncture points recommended by the authors include LI4, LI11, BL13, BL18, GV24, GV25, and GV26.

Homotoxicology (Dose: 10 drops PO for 50-pound dog; 5 drops PO for small dog or cat)

Rhinitis: Euphorbium compositum, Nasoheel, Belladonna compositum, Natrium homaccord, and BHI Allergy mixed together and given orally TID. In bacterial rhinitis add Echinacea compositum. In viral rhinitis add Engystol-N. In fungal rhinitis add Tonsilla compositum and Galium-Heel. Nebulizing or using Euphorbium nasal spray can be extremely helpful in rhinitis cases. In refractory or recurrent cases use Deep Detoxification Formula for long periods of time.

Sinusitis: Euphorbium compositum mixed with saline and used as a nose drop BID to TID. Mix a cocktail of Lymphomyosot, Belladonna homaccord, Echinacea compositum, and Engystol as orally BID to TID. In mild cases BHI-Sinus may be adequate; use TID. In refractory or recurrent cases use deep detoxification formula for long periods of time.

Product sources

Nutrition

Gingival/mouth and immune support formulas: Animal Nutrition Technologies. **Alternatives:** Immune System Support—Standard Process Veterinary Formulas; Immuno Support—Rx Vitamins for Pets; Immugen—Thorne Veterinary Products.

Bromezyme: Progressive Labs.
Quercetin: Source Naturals; Quercitone—Thorne Veterinary Products.
DMG: Vetri Science.

Chinese herbal medicine
Formula H57 Sinusitis: Natural Solutions, Inc.

Homotoxicology
BHI/Heel Corporation

REFERENCES

Western medicine references
Davidson AP, et al. Diseases of the nose and nasal sinuses. Textbook of Veterinary Internal Medicine, Vol 2, 5th edition, Ettinger, Feldman, eds, 2000, pp 1003–1025.
Forrester SD. Diseases of the nasopharynx, larynx, and trachea. Practical Small Animal Internal Medicine. WB Saunders 1997, pp 1113–1128.
Gaskell R, Dawson S. Feline respiratory diseases. Infectious Diseases of the Dog and Cat 2nd ed, WB Saunders, 1999, pp 346–357.
Mason RA. In: Tilley L, Smith F. The 5-Minute Veterinary Consult: Canine and Feline, Blackwell Publishing, 2003.
Wolf AM. Diseases of the nasal cavity. Practical Small Animal Internal Medicine, WB Saunders, 1997, pp 1093–1112.

IVM/nutrition references
Barnes L. B15: The politics of ergogenicity. *Physicians and Sports Medicine.* 1979.7(11):17.
Desser L, Rehberger A, Paukovits W. Proteolytic enzymes and amylase induce cytokine production in peripheral blood mononuclear cells in vitro. *Cancer Biother* 1994;9:253–63.
Graber G, Goust J, Glassman A, Kendall R, Loadholt C. Immunomodulating Properties of Dimethylglycine in Humans. *Journal of Infectious Disease.* 1981.143:101.
Kelly GS. Bromelain: a literature review and discussion of its therapeutic applications. *Altern Med Rev* 1996;1:243–57 [review].
Kendall R, Lawson JW. Recent Findings on N,N-Dimethylglycine (DMG): A Nutrient for the New Millennium, *Townsend Letter for Doctors and Patients,* 2000. May.
Kendall, RV. Building Wellness with DMG, Topanga, CA: Freedom Press, 2003.
Middleton E Jr. Effect of flavonoids on basophil histamine release and other secretory systems. *Prog Clin Biol Res.* 1986;213:493–506.
Munzig E, Eckert K, Harrach T, et al. Bromelain protease F9 reduces the CD44 mediated adhesions of human peripheral blood lymphocytes to human umbilical vein endothelial cells. *FEBS Lett* 1995;351:215–8.
Ogasawara H, Middleton E Jr. Effect of selected flavonoids on histamine release (HR) and hydrogen peroxide (H2O2) generation by human leukocytes [abstract]. *J Allergy Clin Immunol.* 1985;75(suppl):184.

Reap E, Lawson J. Stimulation of the Immune Response by Dimethylglycine, a Non-toxic Metabolite. *Journal of Laboratory and Clinical Medicine*. 1990.115:481.

Ryan RE. A double-blind clinical evaluation of bromelains in the treatment of acute sinusitis. *Headache* 1967;7: 13–7.

Schafer A, Adelman B. Plasma inhibition of platelet function and of arachidonic acid metabolism. *J Clin Invest* 1985;75: 456–61.

Taub SJ. The use of Ananase in sinusitis. A study of 60 patients. *EENT Monthly* 1966;45:96–8.

Walker M. Some Nutri-Clinical Applications of N,N-Dimethylglycine. *Townsend Letter for Doctors*. 1988. June.

Welton AF, Tobias LD, Fiedler-Nagy C, et al. Effect of flavonoids on arachidonic acid metabolism. *Prog Clin Biol Res* 1986;213:231–42.

Chinese herbal medicine/acupuncture references

Chari P, Biwas S, Mann SB, Sehgal S, Mehra YN. Acupuncture therapy in allergic rhinitis. *American Journal of Acupuncture* 1988;16:143–148.

Handbook of Traditional Chinese Medicine Practitioner. Hunan College of TCM, Shang Hai Science and Technology Press. 1987:752.

Kubo M, Matsuda H, Tanaka M, and Kumura Y. Studies on Scutellariae radix. VII Anti-arthritic and anti-inflammatory actions of methanolic extract and flavonoid components from Scutellariae radix. *Chem Pharm Bull*, 1984; 32(7):2724–2729.

Shen YQ, et al. *Journal of Pharmacology and Clinical Application of TCM*. 1998;14(2):29–31.

Wang J, Yu Y, Hashimoto F, et al. *J Pharm Pharmacol* 2000 Mar;52(3):361–6.

World Health Organization list of common conditions treatable by Chinese Medicine and Acupuncture. Available at: http//tcm/health-info.org/WHO-treatment-list.htm.

Zhong Guo Zhong Yao Za Zhi (*People's Republic of China Journal of Chinese Herbology*), 1991; 16(9):560.

Zhong Yao Cai (*Study of Chinese Herbal Material*), 1989; 12(6):37.

Zhong Yao Cai (*Study of Chinese Herbal Material*), 1990; 13(9): 33.

Zhong Yao Tong Bao (*Journal of Chinese Herbology*), 1985;5:45.

Zhong Yao Xue (*Chinese Herbology*), 1998;84:85.

Zhong Yao Xue (*Chinese Herbology*), 1988;137:140.

Zhong Yao Xue (*Chinese Herbology*), 1998;318:320.

Homotoxicology references

Bellavite P, Conforti A, Pontarollo F, Ortolani R. Immunology and homeopathy. 2. Cells of the immune system and inflammation. *Evid Based Complement Alternat Med*. 2006. Mar;3(1): pp 13–24.

Ben-Yakir S. Primary evaluation of homeopathic remedies injected via acupuncture points to reduce chronic high somatic cell counts in modern dairy farms. *Veterinary Acupuncture Newsletter*, 2004. Feb;27(1):pp 19–21.

Colin P. Homeopathy and respiratory allergies: a series of 147 cases. *Homeopathy*. 2006. Apr;95(2): pp 68–72.

Enbergs H. Effects of the homeopathic preparation Engystol on interferon-gamma production by human T-lymphocytes. 2006. *Immunol Invest*. 35(1):pp 19–27.

Heel. BHI Homeopathic Therapy: Professional Reference. Albuquerque, NM: Heel Inc. 2002. pp 22–23, 95.

Macleod G. A Veterinary Materia Medica and Clinical Repertory with a Materia Medica of the Nosodes. Safron, Walden: CW Daniel Company, LTD, 1983. pp 29–30.

Oberbaum M, Glatthaar-Saalmuller B, Stolt P, Weiser M. Antiviral activity of Engystol: an in vitro analysis. *J Altern Complement Med*. 2005. Oct;11(5):pp 855–62. Erratum in: *J Altern Complement Med*. 2005 Dec;11(6):pp 1122.

Ouedraogo G, Morliere P, Santus R, Miranda M, Castell JV. Damage to mitochondria of cultured human skin fibroblasts photosensitized by fluoroquinolones. *J Photochem Photobiol B*. 2000. Oct;58(1):pp 20–5.

Reckeweg H. Biotherapeutic Index: Ordinatio Antihomotoxica et Materia Medica, 5th ed. Baden-Baden, Germany: Biologische Heilmittel Heel GMBH, 2000. pp 299–300, 330–3, 333–4, 401.

Reckeweg H. Homeopathia Antihomotoxica Materia Medica, 4th ed. Baden-Baden, Germany: Aurelia-Verlag GMBH, 2002. pp 115–6, 187–9, 226–7, 394–6, 489, 584.

Sourdeval M, Lemaire C, Brenner C, Boisvieux-Ulrich E, Marano F. Mechanisms of doxycycline-induced cytotoxicity on human bronchial epithelial cells. *Front Biosci*. 2006. Sep 1;11:pp 3036–48.

Yu F, Yu F, Li R, Wang R. Toxic effect of chloromycetin on the ultrastructures of the motor neurons of the Chinese tree shrew (Tupaia belangeri). *Can J Physiol Pharmacol*. 2004. Apr;82(4): pp 276–81.

Chapter Fifteen

Diseases of the Urogenital System

ACUTE AND CHRONIC NEPHRITIS

Definition and cause

Acute nephritis is the sudden onset of kidney disease, usually secondary to decreased blood flow, toxins, infection, or serious inflammation of the renal tissues. Chronic renal disease is the result of a slow degeneration of the kidney and often becomes symptomatic when more than 75% of renal tissue is no longer functional. As a result, the well-known signs and symptoms of azotemia, dehydration, anemia, polydysia, and polyuria are present.

Underlying causes besides idiopathic include congenital; nephrotoxins; urinary obstruction; infectious bacterial; leptospirosis; fungal; viral; or secondary to other diseases such as cancer, kidney or bladder stones, diabetes, and Addison's disease (Adams 2003; Brown 1992; Cowgill 2003; Grauer 1995; DiBartola 1995; Krawiec 1989; Kruger 1995; Polzin 1992, 1995).

Medical therapy rationale, drug(s) of choice, and nutritional recommendations

Dietary recommendations include low-protein, phosphorus, and sodium diets with higher levels of omega-3 fatty acids. Medical therapy is directed at the loss of kidney function and minerals as well as the elevated level of blood urea nitrogen and creatinine. Water-soluble vitamins B and C are recommended due to poor appetite. Fat-soluble vitamins such as vitamin A are not recommended because of storage and elevated levels in the body.

Additional recommendations include ongoing fluid diuresis and anti-nausea drugs such as famotidine and cimetidine, potassium supplementation, phosphate binders, calcitrol to increase blood calcium levels and prevent further bone loss, erythropoeitin to address the secondary anemia, and ACE inhibitors such as benazapril or enalapril for hypertension and glomerular support. Some people may elect kidney transplant surgery (Adams 2003; Brown 2000, 2003; Cowgill 2003; Grauer 2000; Gregory 1993; Jacob 2002; Mathews 2000).

Anticipated prognosis

The prognosis depends upon the damage to kidney function; the involvement of other organ diseases; and the severity of the azotemia, elevated phosphorus levels, anemia, adherence to dietary programs and continuous supportive therapy. The disease is progressive, and therefore requires continual adherence to the medical and dietary treatment plans (Adams 2003, Cowgill 2003, Syme 2003).

Integrative veterinary therapies

The veterinary literature makes it clear that there is no medicine that can restore lost nephrons; and therefore, prevention should be the main course of action for the clinician.

In a prevention-oriented approach, it is therefore important for the clinician to view and improve the body's overall metabolism because the kidney is a main receptacle for metabolic and toxic wastes. In homotoxicology, this is called second-hand homotoxicosis (see Homotoxicolgy, below, for a more detailed explanation). In therapeutic nutrition this is referred to as reducing the metabolic load on the kidney (see Chapter 2, Glandular Therapy, for a more detailed discussion).

Toxic wastes can arrive at the kidney from all parts of the body and can be from environmental toxicity, medications or vaccinations, chemically preserved foods, household chemicals, or toxins, etc. It is important that the clinician focus upon reducing the toxic load, preventing cascading free radicals, and improving the elimination capability of other organs responsible for toxin elimination, such as the skin, lungs, and bowel.

Chinese medicine has long seen a relationship between the Liver and the Kidney. These 2 blood-filtering organs work together to eliminate many toxins. If the Liver is

475

unable to remove waste material, then they remain in the circulation and arrive at the Kidney, Lung, and Skin for handling. If toxin elimination is blocked or negatively affected, then this accumulation of material leads to disease in the organ. Kidney tissue is very susceptible to the deposition and subsequent development of pathology from such toxicoses, and since the kidney has limited reparative ability, we expect to see this organ more frequently affected by inflammatory problems. This fact is borne out in clinical practice.

Integrating therapeutic nutrition, medicinal herbs, and biological therapies that address the elimination of these toxins and the reduction of inflammation is therefore important to preventing the disease and slowing organ degeneration.

Nutrition
General considerations/rationale
The nutritional approach to kidney disease adds nutrients, antioxidants, and gland support for the metabolic organs involved in urea production and metabolic waste excretion (kidney, pituitary, liver, thyroid, and adrenal glands). See Chapter 2, Gland Therapy, for a more complete discussion.

Appropriate nutrients
Nutritional/gland therapy: Glandular adrenal, pituitary, liver, thyroid, and kidney provide intrinsic nutrients that nourish organ cells, help neutralize cellular immune inflammation, and improve waste elimination (see Gland Therapy in Chapter 2 for a more detailed explanation).

Note: Kidney disease often involves multiple organ dysfunction and it is recommended that blood be analyzed both medically and physiologically to determine related organ involvement and disease. This allows for a more specific gland and nutritional support protocol (see Nutritional Blood Testing in Chapter 2).

Arginine: Double-blind studies in people have confirmed that arginine is beneficial in the treatment of congestive heart failure and helping to improve kidney function in these patients (Rector 1996, Watanabe 2000).

Alpha-lipoic acid: ALA is involved in mitochondrial activity and is referred to as the universal antioxidant. As a potent antioxidant, it has been proven to reduce oxidative stress and inflammation. It has also been shown to increase the effectiveness of other antioxidants, such as vitamins C and E, Coenzyme Q10, and glutathione, making them more readily available for bodily function (Busse 1992, Scholich 1989).

Essential fatty acids: Studies have shown that dietary essential fatty acids increase intestinal calcium absorption and assist vitamin D in decreasing urinary calcium losses (Hertz-Picciotto 2000). It has also been shown that

calcium may reduce the absorption of oxalates and may indirectly reduce the formation of kidney stones in people. Perhaps this is an area for veterinary researchers to study the increasing incidence of calcium oxalate crystals and stones in dogs and cats (Barilla 1978, Curhan 1993).

Vitamin E: Vitamin E is involved in the formation of scar tissue, and helps to reduce it. Vitamin E also has organ- and tissue-sparing properties (Myers 1982; Shklar 1982, 1987).

Vitamin B$_{12}$: Studies showed that people who supplemented their diets with vitamin B$_{12}$ had significantly reduced neuropathy and pain associated with kidney disease (Yamane 1995, Kuwabara 1999). Deficiencies of vitamin B$_{12}$ are also associated with anemia and decreased function of the immune system (Kondo 1998) showed that vitamin B$_{12}$ supplementation treats anemia.

Quercetin: Quercetin, a flavonoid, is a potent antioxidant; one of its main health benefits is its ability to help reduce inflammation (Ames 1993). Research has proven that flavonoids increase the body's level of the antioxidant glutathione, thereby helping to control, reduce, and eliminate inflammation at the pre-disease level. Several studies have indicated that flavonoids can help regulate the immune response and have a controlling effect of overreactivity of immune-mediated cells such as T- and b-lymphocytes, mast cells, and neutrophils (Middleton 1986, 1992; Myhrstad 2002; Panthong 1994; Roger 1998).

Chinese herbal medicine
General considerations/rationale
Renal failure is considered to be Yin and Yang deficiency in the Kidney and Spleen, accompanied by internal toxin accumulation. Yin and Yang deficiency of the Kidney is easily translated into loss of Kidney function in Western terms. Yang is the energy of the Kidney to perform its functions, and the loss of Yin can be thought of as dehydration in modern terms. The Spleen functions to make Blood, so a deficiency in the Spleen explains the anemia seen in chronic renal failure. The Spleen also controls the muscles, so a deficiency in the Spleen can lead to muscle wasting and weakness. Toxin accumulation translates into uremia.

Treatment is aimed at treating the deficiency of the Kidney and strengthening the body.

Appropriate Chinese herbs
Astragalus (Huang qi): Useful in cases of renal deficiency. It decreases the amount of protein present in the urine (Zhong Guo Sheng Li Ke Xue Hui, Di Er Ci Hui 1963). It has been shown to decrease blood pressure in dogs, rabbits, and cats, and may be useful in cases of renal secondary hypertension (Guo Wai Yi Xue Can Kao Za Zhi 1977). It also improves renal function in humans with glomeronephritis (Zhong Xi Yi Jie He Za Zhi 1987).

Atractylodes (Bai zhu): Protects the kidneys. It prevents degenerative changes, including sclerosis of renal corpuscles and the widening of Bowman's space (Jing 1997). It counteracts anemia by stimulating the bone marrow. It stimulates both the erythroid-colony-forming unit (CFU-E) and the burst-forming unit (BFU-E). These units are responsible for enhancing differentiation of red blood cells (Hou 1999).

Codonopsis (Dang gui): Can help in renal patients with anemia because it can increase the packed cell volume (Zhong Yao Xue 1998). Hypertension is common in cases of renal failure. Codonopsis can lower blood pressure yet increase cardiac output, and thus improve tissue blood perfusion (Zhong Yao Xue 1998).

Ginger (Sheng jiang): Inhibits thrombus formation (Gao 1996). We now know that anti-thrombin III is lost in the urine in advanced cases of renal failure, which can lead to thromboembolic disease. The addition of ginger to the supplement may help prevent this complication.

Jujube (Da zao): Increases body weight muscle strength in mice (Guo Wai Yi Xue Zhong Yi Zhong Yao Fen Ce 1985).

Oyster shell (Mu li): Has been shown to have efficacy in preventing gastric ulcers (Nie 1994). Because uremia has been shown to cause ulceration of the stomach, addition of this herb to supplements may help prevent ulcers from developing.

Peach pit (Tao ren): Helps prevent thromboembolism by helping to dissolve thrombi (Shang Hai Zhong Yi Yao Za Zhi 1985).

Red peony (Chi shao): Has been shown to have a strong anti-thromboembolic action. Red peony was able to prolong the prothrombin time and thrombin time in experiments involving rabbits (Deng 1991). It has been shown to inhibit thrombin and both the intrinsic and extrinsic coagulation systems (Wang 1990). Red peony inhibits platelet clumping in humans and rats (Lui 1983, Ji 1999).

Rhubarb (Da huang): Rhubarb preparations have been shown to decrease BUN and creatinine levels in humans (Chang Yong Zhong Yao Cheng Fen Yu Yao Li Shou 1994). Rhubarb was shown to prevent progression of the condition in rats with hyperplastic glomerulonephritis (Li 1999).

White peony (Bai shao): Decreases the secretion of gastric acid (Zhong Yao Zhi 1993), which may help to reduce the incidence of uremic gastritis. It also has mild anti-thrombolic abilities. It decreases the aggregation of platelets (Zhong Yao Xue 1998).

Homotoxicology
General considerations/rationale
Acute nephritis is an Inflammation Phase disorder, while chronic nephritis is usually an Impregnation or Degeneration phase disorder. In acute nephritis the organism's defense mechanisms mobilize to destroy homotoxins present in the area. In chronic nephritis the binding of homotoxins and resulting deterioration of protein structures negatively impacts the organism's ability to repair tissues, metabolize homotoxins, and excrete them, thereby hindering the defense mechanisms. The blockage of enzyme function and production is particularly important in this phase.

The clinician is well advised to search out distant causes of the reactions noted because often the kidney is involved in "secondhand" homotoxicoses, since homotoxins arrive from other areas and damage the delicate renal tissues. Homotoxins may be ingested or absorbed through various epithelial surfaces (drugs, heavy metals, pathologic bacteria, viruses, fungi, etc.). They may also be generated within the organism at a distant site, such as in periapical dental abscesses, chronic periodontal disease, and tumors. Therefore, in considering the genesis of any homotoxicoses involving the kidney, one needs to tend to the health of the immune system, gastrointestinal tract, respiratory system, skin, and particularly the liver.

Appropriate homotoxicology formulas
Aesculus compositum: Improves renal blood flow (Reckeweg 2000).

Apis compositum: Treats acute and chronic glomerulonephritis and nephrosis. For readers who own the Biotherapeutic Index, *Apis compositum* is listed as *Albumoheel* (Reckeweg 2000).

Apis homaccord: Used for renal edema and proteinuria.

Atropinum compositum: Treats painful spasms, urolith passage, renal colic.

Belladonna homaccord: Treats hyperemic inflammations, congestion, and acute painful issues. It also supports the immune system through Echinacea (Heel 2003).

Berberis homaccord: Treats inflammation of bile ducts and urogenital tract (Heel 2003). Berberines contained in this formula have demonstrated anti-inflammatory effects (Ikram 1997; Ivanovska, Philipov 1996).

BHI-Inflammation: Formerly contained *Staph* and *Strep nosodes* as well as host-defense-supporting Echinacea. It reduces inflammation similar to *Traumeel*. Note that the new product on the U.S. market has omitted the nosodes and seems to be less effective than its predecessor. The authors frequently use a combination of *Traumeel* and *Echinacea compositum* in its place.

BHI-Kidney: Used for renal pain, dysfunction and renal colic, hematuria, and albuminuria.

BHI-Spasm-Pain: Treats painful spasms associated with renal or bladder pathology.

BHI-Uri-Control: Used for minor urinary pain, increased urgency, and mild incontinence.

Cantharsis homaccord: Treats irritation of the urinary tract with painful, burning urination and a frequent need to urinate.

Coenzyme compositum: Supports energy metabolism functions.

Echinacea compositum: Stimulates the defenses in infection.

Engystol N: Provides support of the immune system.

Galium-Heel: Treats proteinuria and Deposition, Impregnation, and Degeneration phase disorders. Provides cellular detoxification and drainage.

Lymphomyosot: Used for lymph drainage and tubular swelling.

Mucosa compositum: Supports renal epithelial tissues. Contains the E. coli nosode. It is useful in recovery phases, as well as Degeneration Phase homotoxicoses.

Phosphor comaccord: Provides support for the kidney.

Populus comaccord: Treats recurring painful urination and burning, as well as urine dribbling.

Rauwolfia compositum: Supports cardiac function. Contains Ren suis for kidney function (Reckeweg 2000).

Reneel: Treats urinary passage inflammation, particularly in acute phases, and is used to detoxify urinary tissues (Reckeweg 2000).

Schwef-Heel: Used in cats per the Veterinary Guide (Heel 2003).

Solidago compositum: Provides drainage and support or urogenital tissues, especially in the Deposition, Impregnation, Degeneration, and Dedifferentiation phases (Reckeweg 2000).

Spascupreel: Treats spasms and pain.

Tonsilla compositum: Stimulates the defenses and helps activate enzymes through catalyst activity. Used in chronic cases that may have immune challenges.

Traumeel S: Used for hematuria and bladder inflammation and in regulation rigidity cases that are stuck in the Inflammatory phase. The components of *Traumeel S* directly affect the immune system (Bellavite 2006).

Ubichinon compositum: Provides deep support of mitochondrial function.

Authors' suggested protocols

Nutrition

Kidney and pituitary support formulas: 1 tablet for every 25 pounds of body weight BID.

Liver and thyroid support formulas: One-half tablet for each 25 pounds of body weight SID.

Alpha-lipoic acid: 20 mg per 10 pounds of body weight daily.

Vitamin E: 100 IU for each 25 pounds of body weight.

Arginine: 50 mg per 10 pounds of body weight daily.

Omega-3,6,9: 1 capsule for each 25 pounds of body weight with food.

Quercetin: 50 mgs for each 10 pounds of body weight SID.

Chinese herbal medicine

Kidney Guard: 1 capsule per 10 to 20 pounds twice daily. In addition to the herbs mentioned above, this formula contains aconite (Fu zi), angelica radix (Dang gui), bamboo shavings (Zhu Lu), carthamus (Hong hua), coptis (Huang lian), eupatorium (Liu yue xue), fossil bones (Long gu), licorice (Gan cao), ligustrum (Nu zhen zi), ophiopogon (Mai men dong), perilla seed (Zhi Shu zi), and pseudotellaria (Tai zi shen). This combination of herbs helps improve renal blood circulation, regulate blood pressure, eliminate toxic byproducts, stimulate the appetite, and improve hydration.

There are no reported Western trials on the effect of acupuncture on serum BUN, phosphorus, or creatinine levels. Practitioners of TCM have used acupuncture for centuries and feel that it helps. Some recommended points include CV3, CV4, SP6, BL23, GV4, GV20, ST36, and Baihui (Handbook of TCM Practitioner 1987).

Homotoxicology

Acute nephritis: Berberis homaccord, Belladonna Homaccord, Lymphomyosot, mixed together and given BID PO. Solidago compositum given every 3 days.

Chronic nephritis: Solidago compositum, Coenzyme compositum, Ubichinon compositum every 3 days orally or by injection into relevant acupuncture points. Berberis homaccord and Galium-Heel given BID PO.

Product sources

Nutrition

Kidney, pituitary, liver, and thyroid support formulas: Animal Nutrition Technologies. **Alternatives**: Hepato support—Rx Vitamins for Pets; Hepagen—Thorne Veterinary Products; Hepatic, renal, and thyroid support: Standard Process Veterinary Formulas; Renal Essentials—Vetri Science Laboratories.

Alpha-lipoic acid: Source Naturals.

Quercetin: Source Naturals; Quercitone—Thorne Veterinary Products.

Omega-3,6,9: Vetri Science.

Chinese herbal medicine

Kidney Guard: Natural Solutions, Inc.

Homotoxicology

BHI/Heel Corporation

REFERENCES

Western medicine references

Adams LG. Renal Failure—Chronic. In: Tilley L, Smith F. The 5-Minute Veterinary Consult: Canine and Feline, Blackwell Publishing, 2003.

Brown SA, Barsanti JA, Finco DR. Medical management of canine chronic renal failure. In: Kirk RW, Bonagura JD, eds. Current veterinary therapy XI Philadelphia: WB Saunders, 1992:842–847.

Brown SA, Finco DR, Brown CA, et al. Evaluation of the effects of inhibition of angiotensin-converting enzyme with enalapril in dogs with induced chronic renal insufficiency. *Am J Vet Res* 2003;64:321–327.

Brown SA, Brown CA, Crowell WA, et al. Effects of dietary polyunsaturated fatty acid supplementation in early renal insufficiency in dogs. *J Lab Clin Med* 2000;135:275–286.

Cowgill LD. Renal Failure—Acute. In: Tilley L, Smith F. The 5-Minute Veterinary Consult: Canine and Feline, Blackwell Publishing, 2003.

DiBartola SP. Familial renal disease in dogs and cats. In: Ettinger SJ, Feldman EC, eds. Textbook of veterinary internal medicine. 4th ed. Philadelphia: WB Saunders, 1995:1796–1801.

Grauer G, Greco D, Gretzy D, et al. Effects of enalapril treatment versus placebo as a treatment for canine idiopathic glomerulonephritis. *J Vet Intern Med* 2000;14:526–533.

Grauer GF, Lane IF. Acute renal failure. In: Ettinger SJ, Feldman EC, eds. Textbook of veterinary internal medicine. 4th ed. Philadelphia: Saunders 1995:1720–1733.

Gregory CR. Renal transplantation in cats. *Compend Contin Educ Pract Vet* 1993;15:1325–1339.

Jacob F, Polzin DJ, Osborne CA, et al. Clinical evaluation of dietary modification for treatment of spontaneous chronic renal failure in dogs. *J Am Vet Med Assoc* 2002;220:1163–1170.

Krawiec D, Gelberg H. Chronic renal disease in cats. In: Kirk RW, ed. Current Veterinary Therapy X. Philadelphia: WB Saunders Co, 1989:1170–1173.

Kruger JM, Osborne CA, et al.: Congenital and Hereditary Disorders of the Kidney. Veterinary Pediatrics Dogs and Cats from Birth to Six Months, 2nd ed. Hoskins JD, ed. Philadelphia: WB Saunders 1995: pp 401–406.

Mathews KA, Holmberg DL, Miller CW. Kidney transplantation in dogs with naturally occurring endstage renal disease. *J Am Anim Hosp Assoc* 2000;36: 294–301.

Polzin DJ, Osborne CA, Adams LG, Lulich JP. Medical management of feline chronic renal failure. In: Kirk RW, Bonagura JD, eds. Current veterinary therapy XI Philadelphia: WB Saunders, 1992:848–853.

Polzin DJ, Osborne CA, Bartges JW, et al. Chronic renal failure. In: Ettinger SJ, Feldman EC, eds. Textbook of veterinary internal medicine. 4th ed. Philadelphia: WB Saunders, 1995: 1734–1760.

Syme HM, Elliott J. Relation of survival time and urinary protein excretion in cats with renal failure and/or hypertension. *J Vet Int Med* 2003;17:405A.

IVM/nutrition references

Ames BN, Shigenaga MK, Hagen TM. Oxidants, antioxidants and the degenerative diseases of aging. *Proc Natl Acad Sci USA.* 1993. 90:7915–7922.

Barilla DE, Notz C, Kennedy D, Pak CYC. Renal oxalate excretion following oral oxalate loads in patients with ileal disease and with renal and absorptive hypercalciurias: effect of calcium and magnesium. *Am J Med* 1978;64:579–85.

Busse E, Zimmer G, Schorpohl B, et al. Influence of alpha-lipoic acid on intracellular glutathione in vitro and in vivo. *Arzneimittelforschung* 1992;42:829–31.

Curhan GC, Willett WC, Rimm EB, Stampfer MJ. A prospective study of dietary calcium and other nutrients and the risk of symptomatic kidney stones. *N Engl J Med* 1993;328: 833–83.

Hertz-Picciotto I, Schramm M, Watt-Morse M, Chantala K, Anderson J, Osterloh J. Patterns and determinants of blood lead during pregnancy. *Am J Epidemiol.* 2000;152(9):829–837.

Kondo H. Haematological effects of oral cobalamin preparations on patients with megaloblastic anaemia. *Acta Haematol* 1998;9:200–5.

Kuwabara S, Nakazawa R, Azuma N, et al. Intravenous methylcobalamin treatment for uremic and diabetic neuropathy in chronic hemodialysis patients. *Intern Med* 1999;38:472–5.

Lederle FA. Oral cobalamin for pernicious anemia. Medicine's best kept secret? *JAMA* 1991;265(1):94–5.

Myers CE, et al. Effect of Tocopherol and Selenium on Defenses Against Reactive Oxygen Species and their Effect on Radiation Sensitivity. *Annals of the NY Acad of Sci*, 1982. 393: 419–425.

Myhrstad MC, Carlsen H, Nordstrom O et al. Flavonoids increase the intracellular glutathione level by transactivation of the gamma-glutamylcysteine synthetase catalytical subunit promoter. *Free Radic Biol Med* 2002 Mar 1;32(5):386–93.

Panthong A, Kanjanapothi D, Tuntiwachwuttikul P, et al. Anti-inflammatory activity of flavonoids. *Phytomedicine* 1994;1:141–144.

Rector TS, Bank A, Mullen KA, et al. Randomized, double-blind, placebo controlled study of supplemental oral L-arginine in patients with heart failure. *Circulation* 1996; 93:2135–41.

Roger CR. The nutritional incidence of flavonoids: some physiologic and metabolic considerations. *Experientia* 1988;44(9): 725–804.

Scholich H, Murphy ME, Sies H. Antioxidant activity of dihydrolipoate against microsomal lipid peroxidation and its dependence on alpha-tocopherol. *Biochem Biophys Acta.* 1989;1001:256–61.

Shklar G. Oral Mucosal Carcinogenesis in Hamsters: Inhibition by Vitamin E. *J Natl Cancer Inst*, 1982.68:791–797.

Shklar G, Schwartz J, Trickler D, Niukian K. Regression by Vitamin E of Experimental Oral Cancer. *J Natl Cancer Inst*, 1987.78:987–992.

Watanabe G, Tomiyama H, Doba N. Effects of oral administration of L-arginine on renal function in patients with heart failure. *J Hypertens* 2000;18:229–34.

Yamane K, Usui T, Yamamoto T, et al. Clinical efficacy of intravenous plus oral mecobalamin in patients with peripheral neuropathy using vibration perception thresholds as an indicator of improvement. *Curr Ther Res* 1995;56:656–70 [review].

Chinese herbal medicine/acupuncture references

Chang Yong Zhong Yao Cheng Fen Yu Yao Li Shou Ce (A Handbook of the Composition and Pharmacology of Common Chinese Drugs), 1994; 226:323.

Deng CQ, et al. *Journal of Pharmacology and Clinical Application of TCM.* 1991;7(1):20–23.

Gao BB, et al. *Chinese Pharmacology Bulletin.* 1996;12(3):53.

Guo Wai Yi Xue Can Kao Za Zhi (*Foreign Journal of Medicine*), 1977; 4: 231.

Guo Wai Yi Xue Zhong Yi Zhong Yao Fen Ce (*Monograph of Chinese Herbology from Foreign Medicine*), 1985; 7(4): 48.

Handbook of TCM Practitioner. Shanghai Sci and Tech Press. Hunan Sollege of TCM, Oct 1987 p.305.

Hou D, et al. *Journal of Jiangxi College of TCM.* 1999; 11(1):28.

Ji ZQ, et al. *Journal of Traditional Chinese Medicine Research.* 1999;15(5):47–49.

Jing WZ, et al. *China Journal of Geriatrics.* 1997;17(6):365–367.

Li XJ, et al. *China Journal of Modern Medicine.* 1999;9(7):32–34.

Lui J. Effect of Paeonia obovata 801 in metabolism of thromboxane B2 and arachidonic acid and on platelet aggregation in patients with coronary heart disease and cerebral thrombosis. Chung Hua I Hsueh Tsa Chih (*Chin Med J*) 1983; 63:477–81.

Nie SQ, et al. *China Journal of Chinese Medicine.* 1994;19(7):405–407.

Shang Hai Zhong Yi Yao Za Zhi (*Shanghai Journal of Chinese Medicine and Herbology*), 1985; 7:45.

Wang YQ, et al. *Journal of Integrated Medicine.* 1990;10(2):101–102.

Zhong Guo Sheng Li Ke Xue Hui, Di Er Ci Hui (Chinese Convention on Biophysiology, 2nd Annual Convention), 1963: 63.

Zhong Xi Yi Jie He Za Zhi (*Journal of Integrated Chinese and Western Medicine*), 1987; 7:403.

Zhong Yao Xue (*Chinese Herbology*), 1998; 739:741.

Zhong Yao Xue (*Chinese Herbology*), 1998; 831:836.

Zhong Yao Zhi (*Chinese Herbology Journal*), 1993:183.

Homotoxicology references

Bellavite P, Conforti A, Piasere V, Ortolani R. Immunology and Homeopathy. 2. Cells of the Immune System and Inflammation. *eCAM.* 2006. February;3(1): pp 13–24; doi:10.1093/ecam/nek018. Website. http://ecam.oxfordjournals.org/cgi/content/full/3/1/13#BIBL

Heel. BHI Homeopathic Therapy: Professional Reference. Albuquerque, NM: Heel Inc. 2002. p 22.

Ikram M. A review on the chemical and pharmacological aspects of genus Berberis. *Planta Med.* 1975. Dec;28(4): pp 353 Albuquerque, NM: Heel Inc.8.

Ivanovska N, Philipov S. Study on the anti-inflammatory action of Berberis vulgaris root extract, alkaloid fractions and pure alkaloids. *Int J Immunopharmacol.* 1996. Oct;18(10): pp 553 Albuquerque, NM: Heel Inc.61.

Heel. Veterinary Guide, 3rd English edition. Baden-Baden, Germany: Biologische Heilmettel Heel GmbH, 2003. pp 51, 72–73.

Reckeweg H. Biotherapeutic Index: Ordinatio Antihomotoxica et Materia Medica, 5th ed. Baden-Baden, Germany: Biologische Heilmittel Heel GMBH, 2000. pp 196,288,395,396, 401.

GLOMERULAR NEPHRITIS

Definition and cause

Glomerular nephritis is the presence of immune complexes that cause immune-mediated glomerular damage. Inciting causes can be genetic predisposition, infectious agents, toxins, neoplasia, any sustained inflammatory process, or secondary to other disease processes such as Lyme disease (Dambach 1997). In dogs, common causes are secondary to tick-borne disease, and in cats, secondary to FIP or FeLV. This immune-mediated inflammatory process sets off a cascade reaction that can result in a deposition of proteinaceous material, cellular infiltrative (lymphocytes, macrophages), or swelling and thickening of the glomeruli interfering with kidney function (Cook 1996; Finco 1995; Grauer 1992, 2000, 2003; Jergens 1987; Kruger 1995).

Medical therapy rationale, drug(s) of choice, and nutritional recommendations

Immunosuppressing drugs such as corticosteroids and cyclosporine are often used to block the immune response; however, there are no proven clinical results regarding this choice. Dietary recommendations include a high-quality, low-protein diet; however, in people, this is now being questioned because of problems with hypoalbuminemia. No proof of this exists in animal studies (Finco 1995, Grauer 2003, Polzin 1986). ACE inhibitors such as benazopril and enalapril are often recommended to help control hypertension and reduce urinary protein loss (Grauer 2000).

Anticipated prognosis

Prognosis is always guarded and often the disease progresses in spite of medical therapy and dietary adjustments (Cook 1996, Grauer 2003).

Integrative veterinary therapies

Genetic predisposition may be a strong factor in some cases of glomerular nephritis. The accumulation of toxins results in damage to the delicate glomerular structures, which leads to an inability of the nephron to function optimally. A wide variety of agents can lead to such injury, including chronic viral infections, repeated vaccination, chronic bacterial infection, parasites, chemical injury, radiation, drug therapy, aflatoxins, endotoxins, hypertension, genetic error, hormonal imbalances, and pesticide exposure (Newman 2002, Sobel 2005).

The causation and progression of inflammatory changes associated with glomerular disease are widely researched and an area of intense interest due to the frequency of this condition in both veterinary and human patients. Conventional medicine is actively researching anti-inflammatory agents as potential therapeutic modalities due to this pathogenesis (Sugaru 2005).

Many changes involving development and improvement of glomerulonephritis are linked to the presence of cytokines and other inflammatory mediators, as well as mast cells themselves, and the interrelationships of the immune responses associated with these compounds (Border 1990, Okudal 1990, Hochegger 2005).

The use of nutrients, nutraceuticals, medicinal herbs, and combination homeopathics may help protect against destructive autoaggressive reactions through their anti-inflammatory, immune-balancing, and tissue-sparing effects (Goldstein 2005).

Nutrition
General considerations/rationale
The therapeutic nutritional approach to glomerular nephritis focuses upon kidney cell protection and balancing the immune system's response against this target organ. Adding nutrients, antioxidants, and gland support can help control inflammation and slow degeneration.

Appropriate nutrients
Nutritional/gland therapy: Glandular kidney, adrenal, thymus, liver, and pituitary provide the intrinsic nutrients that nourish organ cells and help neutralize cellular auto-immune inflammation and resultant cellular degeneration (see Gland Therapy, Chapter 2, for a more detailed explanation).

Note: Because glomerular nephritis can involve all glands and have multiple underlying causes, a medical and physiological blood evaluation is recommended to assess glandular and immune health. This allows clinicians to formulate therapeutic nutritional protocols that address the kidney as well as an associated immune-mediated cellular process (see Chapter 2, Nutritional Blood Testing, for additional information).

Alpha-lipoic acid: Alpha lipoic acid is involved in mitochondrial activity and is referred to as the universal antioxidant. It has been proven to reduce oxidative stress and inflammation. It has also been shown to increase the effectiveness of other antioxidants, such as vitamins C and E, Coenzyme Q10, and glutathione, making them more readily available for bodily function (Busse 1992, Scholich 1989).

Sterols: Plant-derived sterols such as betasitosterol show anti-inflammatory properties that appear to be similar to corticosteriods (Gupta 1980). A cortisone-like effect without the associated immune-suppressing effects is beneficial in immune-mediated disease. Bouic (1996) reports on the immune-enhancing and balancing effect of plant sterols, which are beneficial to animals with immune-mediated conditions.

Essential fatty acids: Research has demonstrated the importance of essential fatty acids in the daily diet and on the clinical management of various degenerative diseases (Reinhart 1996, Holub 1995, Herman 1998).

Vitamin E: Vitamin E is involved in the formation of scar tissue, and also helps to reduce it. Vitamin E also has organ- and tissue-sparing properties (Myers 1982; Shklar 1982, 1987).

Chinese herbal medicine/acupuncture
General considerations/rationale
Glomerulonephritis is due to Heat and Damp accumulation in the Lower Burner, which invades the Kidneys and Bladder. This can be due to excess Heat and Damp or to Qi and Yin deficiency in the Kidney and Spleen.

Author's interpretation
This is how ancient physicians described the chronic phase: The Lower Burner is the lower Abdomen and Pelvis. It is used to discuss the Kidney and Bladder. Heat and Damp refer to inflammation and purulent debris. This can be due to excess causes such as pathogens, toxins, or immune mediators. Later on the Qi, or Energy, can become deficient from fighting the excess, and the Yin, or fluids, can become deficient from evaporation by the heat.

The patient is weakened at this point in the progression of the disease. The inflammation may be greatly reduced because the immune system is now depressed. However, the organs are damaged and the patient is more ill despite the decrease in inflammation. The Kidney deficiency results in polyuria and polydipsia. However, the Spleen is also deficient at this stage and therefore does not have the Qi (energy) to extract the nutrients from the food well enough to heal the body. This explains why this is an irreversible condition.

Treatment is aimed at reversing the underlying pathology; controlling the cause of the damage; normalizing blood chemistries; and controlling secondary effects such as renal hypertension, anemia, hyperlipidemia, and thromboembolism.

Appropriate Chinese herbs
Achyranthes (Niu xi): Has anti-inflammatory effects. It decreases egg-white-induced foot swelling in rats (Xong 1963).

Angelica root (Dang gui): As strong as aspirin at decreasing inflammation (Yao Xue Za Zhi 1971). It inhibits platelet aggregation as well as aspirin (Yao Xue Xue Bao 1980). Angelica root has been shown to inhibit thrombus formation (Zhong Guo Yao Li Xue Tong Bao 1981). It also has antibacterial properties (Hou Xue Hua Yu Yan Jia 1981), which may be useful in controlling bacterial causes of glomerulonephritis.

Astragalus (Huang qi): Can increase serum albumin and decrease proteinuria, which in turn helps to preserve amino acids, and improves the dysfunctional protein metabolism in glomerulopath (Zhou 1999). It has demonstrated the ability to lower the blood pressure of cats, dogs, and rats under anesthesia (Modern TCM Pharmacology 1997, Xu 1999, Luo 1999).

Cnidium (Chuan xiong): Dilates blood vessels and reduces blood pressure (Zhong Yao Yao Li Yu Ying Yong 1989). It also inhibits blood platelet aggregation induced by ADP, collagen, and thrombase (Pharmaceutical Industry Research Institute of Beijing 1977). One component, chuanxiongzine, has been shown to inhibit the formation of arterial thrombi (Wu 1992).

Codonopsis (Dang shen): Can increase the hematocrit and lower blood pressure (Zhong Yao Xue 1998). It can decrease serum cholesterol in rats with experimental hyperlipidemia (Hua 1994), which may help to control the hypercholesterolemia seen in some patients with glomerulonephritis.

Corn silk (Yu mi xu): Has been shown to lower blood pressure in dogs (Zhong Yao Da Chi Dien 1977). In a trial involving 9 people with chronic nephritis, 3 recovered completely and 2 improved after 2 weeks to 6 months. Kidney function improved, edema was reduced, and urinary production loss decreased (Zhong Hua Yi Xue Za Zhi 1956).

Eucommia bark (Du Zhong): Lowers blood pressure. In humans, the zinc:copper ratio in RBC is elevated in hypertensive people as compared to individuals with normal blood pressure. Eucommia can lower the zinc: copper ratio and blood pressure (Wang 1997). One component, chlorogenic acid, has antibacterial effects (Wang 1993).

Fleece flower root (He shou wu): Decreases cholesterol (Zhao 1984, Mei 1979). It also has antibacterial properties (Zhen 1986). It may be of use in bacterial causes of glomerulonephritis.

Giant knotweed root (Hu zhang): Lowers blood pressure (Xi An Yi Ke Da Xue Xue Bao 1982). It has anti-inflammatory properties (Zhong Guo Yi Yuan Yao Xue Za Zhi 1988). One component, resveratrol, lowers serum cholesterol levels in rats (Zhong Yao Yao Li Yu Ying Yong 1983).

Honeysuckle (Jin yin hua): Contains chlorogenic acid and isochlorogenic acid, which have antibacterial func-

tions (Xin Yi Xue 1975, Jiang Xi Xin Yi Yao 1960). It has demonstrated anti-inflammatory effects in mice and rabbits (Shan Xi Yi Kan 1960). In addition, it decreases blood lipid levels. In rats it decreases absorption of cholesterol from the intestines (Ke Xue Chu Ben She 1963).

Imperata (Bai mao gen): Has been used to treat renal inflammation. In a trial of 11 children with acute nephritis who were treated with imperata, 9 recovered completely and 2 showed moderate improvement. Edema and hypertension resolved and hematuria and proteinuria cleared (Guang Dong Yi Xue 1965).

Isatis root (Ban lan gen): Has demonstrated antiviral and antibacterial properties in numerous studies (Xu 1987, Cao 1999, Li 1994).

Leonurus (Yi mu cao): Has anticoagulant properties. It was shown to decrease fibrinogen levels in rabbits (Han 1992). In one experiment it was shown to decrease renal damage in gentamicin-induced acute renal failure in rats (Xia 1997), which indicates that it has protective influences on the kidney. It may also protect the kidney from damage from immune mediators.

Moutan (Mu dan pi): Inhibits bacterial proliferation (Zhong Yao Cai 1991). It may be efficacious in treating underlying bacterial infections. It also possesses anti-inflammatory properties. In mice, it can prevent dimethylbenzene-induced ear inflammation and carrageenin-, formaldehyde-, or egg-white-induced foot swelling (Wu 1990). Moutan can decrease blood pressure (Liao Ning Yi Xue Za Zhi 1960).

Ophiopogon (Mai dong): Has antibiotic properties (Zhong Yao Xue 1998).

Phellodendron (Huang bai): Has antibacterial effects. It inhibits leptospirosis, a disease known to affect the kidneys (Zhong Yao Xue 1998, Zhong Yao Da Ci Dien 1977, Zhong Cao Yao 1985). It also decreases blood pressure (Zhong Guo Yao Li Xue Tong Bao 1989).

Poria (Fu ling): Has antibacterial effects (Nanjing College of Pharmacy 1976).

Rehmannia (Sheng di huang): Lowers blood pressure (Zhong Yao Xue 1998).

Salvia (Dan shen): Controlled the signs in 70% of 48 patients with chronic nephritis in one study (Shang Hai Yi Yao Za Zhi 1981). It also reduces blood pressure (Guo Wai Yi Xue Zhong Yi Zhong Yao Fen Ce 1991).

Scrophularia (Xuan shen): Can lower blood pressure (Zhang 1959). It also inhibits bacteria (Chen 1986, Zheng 1960).

White atractylodes (Bai zhu): Decreases platelet aggregation (Chang Yong Zhong Yao Cheng Fen Yu Yao Li Shou Ce 1994). It can increase the proliferation rate of CFU-E and BFU-E colonies (Hou 1999), which may make it useful for treating the anemia associated with glomerulonephritis. It also decreases the degeneration rate of the kidney (Jing 1997), which may help protect the kidney from damage from the immune complex deposition.

Wolfberry (Gou qi zi): Has several functions in an herbal supplement designed for renal disease. It increases the production of red blood (Zhong Yao Xue 1998), lowers serum cholesterol and LDL levels (Wang 1998), and decreases blood pressure (Zhong Yao Zhi 1984). It also has antibacterial effects (Jin 1995) and may be useful in bacteria-induced glomerulonephritis.

Homotoxicology
General considerations/rationale
Glomerulonephritis constitutes a progressive condition beginning as an Inflammation Phase and progressing to the Impregnation and Degeneration phases (Reckeweg 2000).

Autosanguis and antihomotoxic agents have long been used to treat this condition, and further research into their effects on immune responses, including Th1 and Th2 modulation, may help explain how they might benefit patients receiving these antihomotoxic and physiologic regulation medicines (Khan, et al. 2005, Heine 2004). The reader is referred to the Acute and Chronic Nephritis protocol, above, for a more detailed discussion of factors involved in urinary system phase response and therapeutic options.

Aspects contributing to this disease likely continue silently through the Deposition Phase.

Appropriate homotoxicology formulas
Because managing glomerulonephritis depends upon finding and handling the primary cause of the inciting chronic inflammatory reaction, literally any other medical issue may be involved. Elimination of dental disease is a critical issue. The clinician should seek these primary homotoxicoses out and apply whatever other protocol information from this text that may be needed. Particularly see the Acute and Chronic Nephritis protocol, above.

Apis compositum: A major remedy for renal disease (especially albuminuria and edema), formerly known as *Albumoheel.* It is also used for glomerulonephritis (acute and chronic) and nephrosis, renal edema *(Apis mellifica),* parenchymal damage and degeneration (Phosphorus), acute nephritis and bladder spasm *(Mercurius sublimates corrosives),* and bleeding from the kidney and bladder (Nux moschata). It also treats renal pain on the right side (Reckeweg 2000). This agent may modify mast cell activity, which may be a theoretical explanation of its mechanism of action.

Berberis homaccord: A major remedy for urinary issues. Treats biliary and urogenital irritation, nephrolithiasis, nephritis, and colic and collapse. It also acts as a stimulant for the adrenal gland.

Lymphomyosot: Provides lymph drainage and immune and endocrine support. Specific urinary tract support may be found in the component Equisetum hiemale, which is used for diseases of the kidneys and urinary tract. Nasturtium aquaticum is included for irritation of the urinary tract collection system. Sarsaparilla is included for urinary gravel, dribbling of urine when sitting, and inflammations and irritations of the urinary organs (Reckeweg 2002).

Populus compositum: Although this remedy is not currently available, it has been used for recurring albuminuria, cystitis, disturbance of renal function, cystopyelitis, nephrolithiasis, prostatic hypertrophy, hydronephrosis, urethritis, and bladder spasm with burning (Reckeweg 2000). It contains Mercurius sublimatus corrosivus, which exhibits characteristic mercurial action in acute affections of the mucosa, acute glomerulonephritis with albuminuria, hematuria, and tenesmus. Mental notes include shivering, trembling of the limbs, brain symptoms, fear, restlessness, and unquenchable thirst. This component is also found in *Solidago compositum* (Reckeweg 2002).

Rauwolfia compositum: Contains Ren suis and is used most often for hypertension associated with renal disease. Though primarily a cardiac remedy, Ren suis has specific urinary tract indications, including nephrolithiasis, hydronephrosis, urinary-tract infections, albuminuria, hypertrophy of the prostate, and nephroses. It is also used for edema, oxaluria, and depressed renal function with oliguria and hyperhydrosis. Do not give in the acute stage of glomerulonephritis (Reckeweg 2002). Also contains Lycopodium, which is indicated in cystitis, nephrolithiasis, and red sediment in the urine. It is said to be valuable in uric acid diathesis and when there is a tendency toward gravel and renal colic (Reckeweg 2002). Contains Belladonna (see *Belladonna homaccord*), Conium (see *Cerebrum compositum*), and Sulphur (see *Klimakteel*).

Reneel: Provides drainage and detoxification of the renal system. Can be used in cases with or without stone formation. Treats inflammatory diseases of urinary passages (Reckeweg 2000).

Solidago compositum: An extremely useful agent for Deposition, Impregnation, Degeneration, and Dedifferentiation phase disorders. Treats nephrosis, nephritis, uroliths, hydronephrosis, pyelonephritis, prostatic hypertrophy, urinary incontinence, acute glomerulonephritis, oxaluria, and stimulation of diuresis. It contains Coxsackie virus nosode, which is indicated in pyelonephritis and acute and chronic cystitis. It also treats nephritis, orchitis, and oophoritis (Reckeweg 2002). It is part of the deep detox formula used so often by homotoxicologists.

Appropriate homotoxicology formulas
Nutrition
Kidney and pituitary support formulas: 1 tablet for each 25 pounds of body weight BID.

Immune and liver support formulas: One-half tablet for each 25 pounds of body weight SID.

Alpha-lipoic acid: 20 mg per 10 pounds of body weight daily.

Betathyme: 1 capsule for each 35 pounds of body weight BID. (maximum, 2 capsules BID)

Omega-3,6,9: 1 capsule for each 25 pounds of body weight with food.

Vitamin E: 100 IU for each 25 pounds of body weight.

Chinese herbal medicine

H87 Shar pei fever: 1 capsule per 10 to 20 pounds twice daily. This supplement is designed for renal disease with an immune component. In addition to the herbs above, H87 also contains areca peel (Da fu pi), ciborium (Gou ji), fossil bones (Long gu), oldenlandia (Bai hua she cao), oyster shell (Mu li), pyrola (Lu xian cao), and tortoise plastron (Gui ban) and carapace (Bie jia).

Recommended acupuncture points include PC6, CV12, ST36, SP9, BL23, SP6, and BL28 (Handbook of TCM practitioners 1987).

Homotoxicology

Berberis homaccord, Populus compositum, Reneel, Apis compositum, and Lymphomyosot: Mix together and give orally BID. Solidago compositum given daily for 2 weeks and then twice weekly orally. In chronic cases such as chronic nephritis add the Deep Detox formula. Rauwolfia compositum may be added in chronic cases, twice weekly, particularly in animals with concurrent cardiac disease, but avoid this agent in acute glomerular diseases.

Product sources

Nutrition
Kidney, pituitary, immune and liver support formulas: Animal Nutrition Technologies. **Alternatives:** Hepato support—Rx Vitamins for Pets; Hepagen—Thorne Veterinary Products; Hepatic, Renal, and Thyroid support—Standard Process Veterinary Formulas; Renal Essentials—Vetri Science Laboratories; Immune System Support—Standard Process Veterinary Formulas; Immuno Support—Rx Vitamins for Pets; Immugen—Thorne Veterinary Products.

Alpha-lipoic acid: Source Naturals.

Betathyme: Best for Your Pet. **Alternative:** Moducare—Thorne Veterinary Products.

Omega-3,6,9: Vetri Science.

Chinese herbal medicine
H87 Shar pei fever: Natural Solutions, Inc.

Homotoxicology
BHI/Heel Corporation

REFERENCES

Western medicine references
Cook AK, Cowgill LD. Clinical and pathologic features of protein-losing glomerular disease in the dog. A review of 137 cases (1985–1992). *J Am Anim Hosp Assoc* 1996;32:313–322.

Dambach DM, Smith CA, Lewis RM, Van Winkle TJ. Morphologic, immuno-histochemical, and ultrastructural characterization of a distinctive renal lesion in dogs putatively associated with Borrelia burgdorferi infection: 49 cases (1987–1992). *Vet Pathol* 1997;34:85–96.

Finco DR. Urinary protein loss. In: Osborne CA, Finco DA, eds. Canine and Feline Nephrology and Urology, Baltimore: Lea and Febiger, 1995, 211–215.

Grauer GF. Glomerulonephritis, *Semin Vet Med Surg (Small Animal)* 1992;7:187–197.

Grauer GF, Dibartola SP. Glomerular disease. In: Ettinger SJ, Feldman EC, eds. Textbook of Veterinary Internal Medicine. Philadelphia: WB Saunders, 2000, 1662–1677.

Grauer, GF. Glomerulonephritis, In: Tilley L, Smith F. The 5-Minute Veterinary Consult: Canine and Feline, Blackwell Publishing, 2003.

Grauer GF, Greco DS, Getzy DM, et al. Effects of enalapril vs. placebo as a treatment for canine idiopathic glomerulonephritis. *J Vet Intern Med* 2000;14:526–533.

Jergens AE. Glomerulonephritis in dogs and cats. *Compendium on Continuing Education for the Practising Veterinarian* 1987, 9: 903–912.

Kruger JM, Osborne CA, et al. Congenital and Hereditary Disorders of the Kidney. Veterinary Pediatrics Dogs and Cats from Birth to Six Months, 2nd ed. Hoskins, JD, ed. Philadelphia: WB Saunders, 1995: pp 401–406.

Polzin DJ, Osborne CA. Update—Conservative Medical Management of Chronic Renal Failure. Current Therapy IX. Kirk RW, ed. Philadelphia: WB Saunders, 1986 pp 1167–1173.

IVM references
Border W, Seiya Okuda S, Languino L, Sporn M, Ruoslahti E. Suppression of experimental glomerulonephritis by antiserum against transforming growth factor beta 1, *Nature*. 1990. July 26, 346:pp 371–374.

Goldstein R, Goldstein S. The Goldstein Wellness and Longevity Program, Neptune City, NJ: TFH Publication, 2005.

Hochegger K, Siebenhaar F, Vielhauer V, Heininger D, Mayer G, Maurer M, Rosenkranz A. Clinical immunology: Role of mast cells in experimental anti-glomerular basement membrane glomerulonephritis. *Eur J Immunology*, 2005. 35(10): pp 3072–3082.

Newman S, Johnson R, Sears W, Wilcock B. Investigation of repeated vaccination as a possible cause of glomerular disease in mink. *Can J Vet Res*. 2002. Jul;66(3):pp 158–64.

Okuda S, Languino L, Ruoslahti E, and Border W. Elevated expression of transforming growth factor-beta and proteoglycan production in experimental glomerulonephritis. Possible role in expansion of the mesangial extracellular matrix. *J Clin Invest*. August; 1990. 86(2):pp 453–462.

Sobel E, Gianini J, Butfiloski E, Croker B, Schiffenbauer J, Roberts S. Acceleration of autoimmunity by organochlorine pesticides in (NZB x NZW)F1 mice. *Environ Health Perspect*. 2005. Mar;113(3):pp 323–8.

Sugaru E, Sakai M, Horigome K, Tokunaga T, Kitoh M, Hume WE, Nagata R, Nakagawa T, Taiji M. SMP-534 inhibits TGF-beta-induced ECM production in fibroblast cells and reduces mesangial matrix accumulation in experimental glomerulonephritis. 2005. *Am J Physiol Renal Physiol*. Nov;289(5):pp F998–1004.

Nutrition references

Bouic PJD, et al. Beta-sitosterol and beta-sitosterol glucoside stimulate human peripheral blood lymphocyte proliferation: Implications for their use as an immunomodulatory vitamin combination. *International Journal of Immunopharmacology*, 1996. 18:693–700.

Busse E, Zimmer G, Schorpohl B, et al. Influence of alpha-lipoic acid on intracellular glutathione in vitro and in vivo. *Arzneimittelforschung* 1992;42:829–31.

Gupta MB, Nath R, Srivastava N, et al. Anti-inflammatory and antipyretic activities of β-sitosterol. *Planta Medica* 1980;39: 157–163.

Reinhart GA. A Controlled Dietary Omega-6:Omega-3 Ratio Reduces Pruritus in Nonfood Allergic Atopic Dogs, *Recent Advances in Canine and Feline Nutritional Research: Iams Proceedings*, 1996. p 277.

Myers CE, et al. Effect of Tocopherol and Selenium on Defenses Against Reactive Oxygen Species and their Effect on Radiation Sensitivity. *Annals of the NY. Acad of Sc.*, 1982. 393: 419–425.

Scholich H, Murphy ME, Sies H. Antioxidant activity of dihydrolipoate against microsomal lipid peroxidation and its dependence on alpha-tocopherol. *Biochem Biophys Acta* 1989;1001:256–61.

Shklar G. Oral Mucosal Carcinogenesis in Hamsters: Inhibition by Vitamin E. *J Natl Cancer Inst*, 1982. 68:791–797.

Shklar G, Schwartz J, Trickler D, Niukian K. Regression by Vitamin E of Experimental Oral Cancer. *J Natl Cancer Inst*, 1987.78:987–992.

Chinese herbal medicine/acupuncture references

Cao ZS, et al. Research on antibacterial effects against pyloric helicobacterium in 50 kinds of Chinese herbs. *Strait Journal of Pharmacy*. 1999;11(3):53–54.

Chang Yong Zhong Yao Cheng Fen Yu Yao Li Shou Ce (A Handbook of the Composition and Pharmacology of Common Chinese Drugs), 1994; 739:742.

Chen SY, et al. *Fujian Journal of Chinese Medicine*. 1986;17(4):57.

Guang Dong Yi Xue (–), 1965; 3:28.

Guo Wai Yi Xue Zhong Yi Zhong Yao Fen Ce (*Monograph of Chinese Herbology from Foreign Medicine*), 1991; 13(3):41.

Han ZX, et al. *Journal of Shengyang College of Pharmacology*. 1992;9(3):196–199.

Handbook of TCM practitioners, Hunan College of TCM, Shanghai Science and Technology Press, Oct 1987, page 308–315.

Hou D, et al. *Journal of Jiangxi College of TCM*. 1999;11(1):28.

Hou Xue Hua Yu Yan Jia (Research on Blood-Activating and Stasis-Eliminating Herbs), 1981:335.

Hua YL, et al. Experimental research on Ming Dang Shen's effect in lowering blood lipid level. *Journal of Nanjing College of TCM*. 1994;10(4):31–32.

Jiang Xi Xin Yi Yao (*Jiangxi New Medicine and Herbology*), 1960 (1):34.

Jin ZC, et al. Antibacterial effects of Gou Qi Zi extract. *Inner Mongolia Journal of Medicine*. 1995;15(4):203.

Jing WZ, et al. *China Journal of Geriatrics*. 1997;17(6): 365–367.

Ke Xue Chu Ben She (Scientific Press), 1963: 387.

Li WW. Experimental research on Ban Lan Gen and Xi Shu Guo's effect in counteracting HFRSV and HSV-2. *Journal of Hunan University of Medicine*. 1994;19(4):309–311.

Liao Ning Yi Xue Za Zhi (*Liaoning Journal of Medicine*), 1960;(7):48.

Luo XP, et al. *China Journal of Pathology and Physiology*. 1999;15(7):639–643.

Mei MZ, et al. *Journal of Pharmacy*. 1979;14(1):8.

Modern TCM Pharmacology. Tianjin: Science and Technology Press; 1997.

Nanjing College of Pharmacy. Materia Medica, vol.2. Jiangsu: People's Press; 1976.

Pharmaceutical Industry Research Institute of Beijing. *China Journal of Medicine*. 1977;57(8):464.

Shan Xi Yi Kan (*Shanxi Journal of Medicine*), 1960; (10):32.

Shang Hai Yi Yao Za Zhi (*Shanghai Journal of Medicine and Herbology*), 1981; 1:17.

Wang CL, et al. *Journal of Trace Elements and Health Research*. 1997;14(4):33–34.

Wang DS, et al. The dose-effect relation in Gou Qi Zi's effect of counteracting experimental hyperlipidemia and liver lipid peroxidation. *Journal of Applied Integrated Medicine*. 1998;11(3):199–200.

Wang JL, et al. *Journal of Chinese Materia Medica*. 1993; 24(12):655–656.

Wu GZ, et al. *Journal of University of Pharmacology of China*. 1990;21(4).

Wu GX, et al. *China Journal of Pharmacology*. 1992;13(4): 330.

Xong ZY, et al. *Journal of Pharmacology*. 1963;10(12):708.

Xi An Yi Ke Da Xue Xue Bao (*Journal of Xian University School of Medicine*), 1982; 3(4):941.

Xia XH, et al. *China Journal of Pathology and Physiology*. 1997;13(2):183–187.

Xin Yi Xue (*New Medicine*), 1975; 6(3): 155.

Xu SA, et al. *China Journal of Pharmacy*. 1999;34(10): 663–665.

Xu Zhen Can, et al. Assessment of antibacterial effects of the Chinese herb Ban Lan Gen. *Journal of Chinese Patented Medicine Research*. 1987;11(12):9–11.

Yao Xue Xue Bao (*Journal of Herbology*), 1980;15(6):321.

Yao Xue Za Zhi (*Journal of Medicinals*), 1971;(91):1098.

Zhang BH. *Journal of Beijing Medical College*. 1959;(1):59.

Zhao B, et al. *Journal of Chinese Patent Medicine Research*. 1984;(10):6.

Zhen HC, et al. *Chinese Medicine Bulletin*. 1986;(3):53.

Zheng QY, et al. *Pharmacy Bulletin*. 1960;8(2):57.

Zhong Cao Yao (*Chinese Herbal Medicine*), 1985;16(1):34.

Zhong Guo Yao Li Xue Tong Bao (*Journal of Chinese Herbal Pharmacology*), 1981;1(2):35.

Zhong Guo Yao Li Xue Tong Bao (*Journal of Chinese Herbal Pharmacology*), 1989; 10(5):385.

Zhong Guo Yi Yuan Yao Xue Za Zhi (*Chinese Hospital Journal of Herbology*), 1988; 8(5):214.

Zhong Hua Yi Xue Za Zhi (*Chinese Journal of Medicine*), 1956; 10:922.

Zhong Yao Cai (*Study of Chinese Herbal Material*), 1991; 14(2):41.

Zhong Yao Da Chi Dien (Dictionary of Chinese Herbs), 1977; 1037.

Zhong Yao Da Chi Dien (Dictionary of Chinese Herbs), 1977:2032.

Zhong Yao Xue (*Chinese Herbology*), 1998; 144:146.

Zhong Yao Xue (*Chinese Herbology*), 1998; 156:158.

Zhong Yao Xue (*Chinese Herbology*), 1998; 739:741.

Zhong Yao Xue (*Chinese Herbology*), 1998; 845:848.

Zhong Yao Xue (*Chinese Herbology*), 1998; 860:862.

Zhong Yao Yao Li Yu Ying Yong (*Pharmacology and Applications of Chinese Herbs*), 1983;653:654.

Zhong Yao Yao Li Yu Ying Yong (*Pharmacology and Applications of Chinese Herbs*), 1989; (2):40.

Zhong Yao Zhi (*Chinese Herbology Journal*), 1984:484.

Zhou Q. *Journal of Chinese Materia Medica*. 1999;30(5): 386–388.

Homotoxicology references

Casal M, Dambach D, Meister T, Jezyk P, Patterson D, Henthorn P. Familial glomerulonephropathy in the bullmastiff. *Vet Pathol*. 2004. 41:pp 319–325.

Khan S, Cook H, Bhangal G, Smith J, Tam F, Pusey C. Antibody blockade of TNF-alpha reduces inflammation and scarring in experimental crescentic glomerulonephritis. *Kidney Int*. 2005. May;67(5):pp 1812–20.

Heine H. Homotoxicology and basic regulation: Bystander reaction therapy. *La Medicina Biologica*. 2004.Jan 1:pp 3–6.

Reckeweg H. Biotherapeutic Index: Ordinatio Antihomotoxica et Materia Medica, 5th ed. Baden-Baden, Germany: Biologische Heilmittel Heel GMBH; 2000. pp 288–9, 337–8, 357,387–8, 396.

Reckeweg H. Homeopathia Antihomotoxica Materia Medica, 4th ed. Baden-Baden, Germany: Arelia-Verlag GMBH, 2002. pp. 169–70, 172–5, 191, 205–6, 249–252, 282–4, 290–1, 340–2, 344–5, 370–2, 390, 394–6, 402, 418–20, 424, 438, 441, 480, 504–5, 510, 524, 531–33, 555–60, 572–6.

RENAL DYSPLASIA

Definition and cause

Renal dysplasia is a non-inflammatory disease of the kidney tissue with inadequate or malformed nephrons. These changes are either acquired or genetic and involve many possible errors in growth and development. Many individual defects can occur. Both feline and canine breeds are involved. The list of affected breeds and disorders continues to expand (Greco 2001, Morita 2005). Renal dysplasia is also referred to as juvenile renal disease or hereditary nephropathy (Bovee 1984, Finco 1995, Greco 2001, Kruger 2003).

Medical therapy rationale, drug(s) of choice, and nutritional recommendations

Treatment for renal dysplasia usually takes a quality of life approach with supportive fluid replacement therapy and phosphate binders along with the typical low-protein and low-phosphorus diets (Finco 1983, Polzin 1986). Transfusion and erythropoetin are recommended for associated anemia.

Anticipated prognosis

The prognosis depends upon the extent of the kidney tissue dysfunction. The disease is irreversible, and often requires ongoing medical and dietary support. In most instances the prognosis for long-term survival is poor (Bovee 1984, Greco 2001.)

Integrative veterinary therapies

Because this is a non-inflammatory disease, the approach to renal dysplasia focuses on nourishing kidney cells, making dietary adjustments, and providing gland support to help reduce metabolic wastes and support of the organs of protein metabolism (liver, pituitary, thyroid, and adrenal).

Nutrition

General considerations/rationale
The nutritional approach to kidney disease adds nutrients, antioxidants, and gland support for the metabolic organs involved in the production of urea and excretion of metabolic wastes (kidney pituitary, liver, thyroid, and adrenal glands) (see Chapter 2, Gland Therapy, for a more complete discussion).

Appropriate nutrients
Nutritional/gland therapy: Glandular adrenal, pituitary, liver, thyroid, and kidney provide intrinsic nutrients that nourish organ cells and improve waste elimination (see Gland Therapy in Chapter 2 for a more detailed explanation).

Note: Because renal dysplasia can involve multiple organ systems, a medical and physiological blood evaluation is recommended to assess glandular and immune health. This allows clinicians to formulate therapeutic nutritional protocols that address the kidney as well as an associated immune-mediated cellular process (see Chapter 2, Nutritional Blood Testing, for additional information).

Arginine: Double-blind studies in people have confirmed that arginine is beneficial in the treatment of congestive heart failure and helping to improve kidney function in these patients (Rector 1996, Watanabe 2000).

Essential fatty acids: Studies have shown that dietary essential fatty acids increase intestinal calcium absorption and help vitamin D decrease urinary calcium losses. (Hertz-Picciotto 2000). It has also been shown that calcium may reduce the absorption of oxalates and may indirectly reduce the formation of kidney stones in people. Perhaps this is an area for veterinary researchers to study the increase incidence of calcium oxalate crystals and stones in dogs and cats (Barilla 1978, Curhan 1993).

Vitamin E: Vitamin E is involved in the formation of scar tissue, and also helps to reduce it. Vitamin E also has organ- and tissue-sparing properties (Myers 1982; Shklar 1982, 1987).

Vitamin B_{12}: Neuropathy and pain associated with diabetes or kidney disease were significantly reduced in studies with people who supplemented their diets with vitamin B_{12} (Yamane 1995, Kuwabara 1999). Deficiencies of vitamin B12 are associated with anemia and decreased function of the immune system (Kondo 1998); therefore, supplementation will treat the condition.

Chinese herbal medicine/acupuncture
General considerations/rationale

Renal dysplasia is due to Vital Essence deficiency with Qi and Yang deficiency in the Spleen and Kidney. This leads to Qi and Blood stagnation and internal toxin accumulation. Any congenital condition is considered to be a deficiency of the Vital Essence.

The Vital Essence is the basic genetic makeup of the individual. When deficient, the affected individual either has birth defects or does not mature properly. The Kidney and Spleen are considered to be the seat of genetic and environmental contributions, respectively, to the growth and development of the organism. The Kidney is what the parents of an organism contribute. In modern terms, this would translate into the genetic makeup of the individual. The Spleen is the environmental source of energy for growth because it is charged with the transformation of food into life energy. Yang is the warmth of life and Qi is the energy of life.

When the Kidney and Spleen lack energy there is no way for the affected individual to develop correctly. In the case of renal dysplasia this deficiency is expressed by the clinical signs of polyuria and polydipsia, which are easily attributed to the Kidneys. Other signs include

weight loss and anemia, which the practitioners of TCM assigned to the Spleen because it is responsible for turning food into Blood and the Spleen controls the muscles. Internal toxins are called uremic toxins by Western practitioners.

Blood and Qi stagnation are evidenced by lethargy and fatigue.

Appropriate Chinese herbs

Astragalus (Huang qi): Useful in cases of renal deficiency for several reasons. It decreases the amount of protein present in the urine (Zhong Guo Sheng Li Ke Xue Hui, Di Er Ci Hui 1963). It has been shown to decrease blood pressure in dogs, rabbits, and cats, and may be useful in cases of renal secondary hypertension (Guo Wai Yi Xue Can Kao Za Zhi 1977). It also improves renal function in humans with glomeronephritis (Zhong Xi Yi Jie He Za Zhi 1987).

Atractylodes (Bai zhu): Protects the kidneys. It prevents degenerative changes, including sclerosis of renal corpuscles and the widening of Bowman's space (Jing 1997). It counteracts anemia by stimulating the bone marrow and stimulates both the erythroid colony-forming unit (CFU-E) and the burst-forming unit (BFU-E). These units are responsible for enhancing differentiation of red blood cells (Hou 1999).

Codonopsis (Dang gui): Can help in renal patients with anemia because it can increase the PCV (Zhong Yao Xue 1998). Hypertension is common in cases of renal failure. Codonopsis can lower blood pressure yet increase cardiac output, and therefore improve tissue blood perfusion (Zhong Yao Xue 1998).

Ginger (Sheng jiang): Inhibits thrombus formation (Gao 1996). We now know that anti-thrombin III is lost in the urine in advanced cases of renal failure, which can lead to thrombo-embolic disease. The addition of ginger to the supplement may help prevent this complication.

Jujube (Da zao): Increases body weight and muscle strength in mice (Guo Wai Yi Xue Zhong Yi Zhong Yao Fen Ce 1985).

Oyster shell (Mu li): Has been shown to have efficacy in preventing gastric ulcers (Nie 1994). Since uremia has been shown to cause ulceration of the stomach, adding this herb to supplements may help prevent this development.

Peach pit (Tao ren): Helps prevent thromboembolism by helping to dissolve thrombi (Shang Hai Zhong Yi Yao Za Zhi 1985).

Red peony (Chi shao): Has been shown to have a strong anti-thromboembolic action. In experiments involving rabbits, red peony was able to prolong the prothrombin time and thrombin time (Deng 1991). It has been shown to inhibit thrombin and both the intrinsic and extrinsic coagulation systems (Wang 1990). It also inhibits platelet clumping in humans and rats (Lui 1983, Ji 1999).

Rhubarb (Da huang): Preparations have been shown to decrease BUN and creatinine levels in humans (Chang Yong Zhong Yao Cheng Fen Yu Yao Li Shou 1994). In rats with hyperplastic glomerulonephritis, rhubarb was shown to prevent progression of the condition (Li 1999).

White peony (Bai shao): Decreases the secretion of gastric acid (Zhong Yao Zhi 1993), which may help to reduce the incidence of uremic gastritis. In addition, it has mild anti-thrombolic abilities. It decreases the aggregation of platelets (Zhong Yao Xue 1998; 831:836).

Homotoxicology
General considerations/rationale
Diseases in this category represent the Degeneration Phase, and as such, they are not curable. However, support and proper care can extend the quality and quantity of life for individuals so affected. Palmquist has treated 3 exotic cats for polycystic kidney disease and all have done well clinically. The oldest of these cats is now 11 years old and still has normal renal parameters in spite of severe changes confirmed on ultrasound. The treatment strategy for these cats is to support the remaining kidney tissue and avoid factors that might further damage renal function.

Regular laboratory screening and physical examination is indicated in all such patients. Urine cultures and blood pressure monitoring are particularly important. Renal failure is treated according to standard approaches for chronic renal disease.

Appropriate homotoxicology formulas
Also see the Acute and Chronic Nephritis protocol, above.

Galium-Heel: Particularly applicable to all congenital and cellular phases. Affects renal tubular function through Apis. Used in feline polycystic kidney disease cases by the authors.

Psorinoheel: Used for its deep acting characteristics. Treats miasmic disorders.

Authors' suggested protocols

Nutrition
Kidney and pituitary support formulas: 1 tablet for each 25 pounds of body weight BID.

Liver support formula: One-half tablet for each 25 pounds of body weight BID.

Vitamin E: 100 IU for each 25 pounds of body weight.

Arginine: 50 mg per 10 pounds of body weight daily.

Omega-3,6,9: 1 capsule for each 25 pounds of body weight with food.

Chinese herbal medicine/acupuncture
Kidney Guard: 1 capsule per 10 to 20 pounds twice daily. In addition to the herbs mentioned above, this formula contains aconite (Fu zi), angelica radix (Dang gui), bamboo shavings (Zhu Lu), carthamus (Hong hua), coptis (Huang lian), eupatorium (Liu yue xue), fossil bones (Long gu), licorice (Gan cao), ligustrum (Nu zhen zi), ophiopogon (Mai men dong), perilla seed (Zhi Shu zi), and pseudotellaria (Tai zi shen). This combination of herbs helps improve renal blood circulation, regulate blood pressure, eliminate toxic byproducts from the body, stimulate the appetite, and improve hydration.

There are no reported Western trials on the effect of acupuncture on serum BUN, phosphorus, or creatinine levels. Practitioners of TCM have used acupuncture for centuries and feel that it helps. Some recommended points include CV3, CV4, SP6, BL23, GV4, GV20, ST36, and Baihui (Handbook of TCM Practitioner 1987).

Homotoxicology
The following is a theoretical discussion because with the exception of polycystic kidney disease, the authors are unable to document treatment results of any of the other diagnoses in this list through biological therapy.

Renal agenesis: As for acute and chronic nephritis.

Renal ectopia, tubulo-interstitial nephropathy: As for acute and chronic nephritis.

Polycystic kidney disease: Initially Galium-Heel, and as disease progresses as for acute and chronic nephritis.

Renal telangiectasis (vascular abnormalities in multiple organs): Consider experimental use of Aesculus compositum and/or Placenta compositum.

Renal amyloidosis: As for acute and chronic nephritis.

Nephroblastoma, renal cystadenocarcinoma: See cancer sections, chapters 31 through 34.)

Fanconi syndrome and primary renal glucosuria: As for acute and chronic nephritis.

Congenital nephrogenic diabetes insipidus: See Diabetes Insipidus, Chapter 16.

Product sources

Nutrition
Kidney, pituitary, and liver support formulas: Animal Nutrition Technologies. **Alternatives:** Hepagen—Thorne Veterinary Products; Renal Essentials:—Vetri Science; Hepato support—Rx Vitamins for Pets; Renal and Hepatic support—Standard Process Veterinary Formulas.

Omega-3,6,9: Vetri Science. **Alternative:** Ultra EFA—Rx Vitamins for Pets.

Chinese herbal medicine
Formula Kidney Guard: Natural Solutions, Inc.

Homotoxicology
BHI/Heel Corporation

REFERENCES

Western medicine references
Bovee KC. Inherited and Metabolic Renal Disease in Canine Nephrology, Harwal Pub. 1984.

Finco DR. Inherited and congenital renal disorders. In: Osborne CA, Finco DR, eds. Canine and feline nephrology and urology. 2nd ed. Baltimore: Williams and Wilkins, 1995:471–483.

Finco DR. The Role of Phosphorus Restriction in the Management of Chronic Renal Failure of the Dog and Cat; *Proc 7th Kal Kan Sypm, Veterinary Learning Systems.* Lawrenceville, NJ 1983; pp 131–133.

Greco DS. Congenital and inherited renal disease of small animals. *Vet Clin North Am Small Anim Pract.* 2001, Mar;31(2):pp 393–9.

Kruger, JM, Osborne, CA, Fitzgerald, SD. Renal Disease, Congenital and Developmental. In: Tilley L, Smith F. The 5-Minute Veterinary Consult: Canine and Feline, Blackwell Publishing, 2003.

Morita T, Michimae Y, Sawada M, Uemura T, Araki Y, Haruna A, Shimada A. Renal dysplasia with unilateral renal agenesis in a dog. *J Comp Pathol.* 2005. Jul;133(1):64–7.

Polzin DJ, Osborne CA. Update—Conservative Medical Management of Chronic Renal Failure. Current Therapy IX Kirk RW, ed. Philadelphia: WB Saunders. 1986. pp 1167–1173.

IVM/nutrition references
Kondo H. Haematological effects of oral cobalamin preparations on patients with megaloblastic anaemia. *Acta Haematol* 1998;9:200–5.

Kuwabara S, Nakazawa R, Azuma N, et al. Intravenous methylcobalamin treatment for uremic and diabetic neuropathy in chronic hemodialysis patients. *Intern Med* 1999;38:472–5.

Lederle FA. Oral cobalamin for pernicious anemia. Medicine's best kept secret? *JAMA* 1991;265(1):94–5.

Myers CE, et al. Effect of Tocopherol and Selenium on Defenses Against Reactive Oxygen Species and their Effect on Radiation Sensitivity. *Annals of the NY Acad of Sci.* 1982. 393: 419–425.

Rector TS, Bank A, Mullen KA, et al. Randomized, double-blind, placebo controlled study of supplemental oral L-arginine in patients with heart failure. *Circulation* 1996;93:2135–41.

Watanabe G, Tomiyama H, Doba N. Effects of oral administration of L-arginine on renal function in patients with heart failure. *J Hypertens* 2000;18:229–34.

Yamane K, Usui T, Yamamoto T, et al. Clinical efficacy of intravenous plus oral mecobalamin in patients with peripheral neuropathy using vibration perception thresholds as an indicator of improvement. *Curr Ther Res* 1995;56:656–70 [review].

Chinese herbal medicine/acupuncture references
Chang Yong Zhong Yao Cheng Fen Yu Yao Li Shou Ce (A Handbook of the Composition and Pharmacology of Common Chinese Drugs), 1994; 226:323.

Deng CQ, et al. *Journal of Pharmacology and Clinical Application of TCM.* 1991;7(1):20–23.

Gao BB, et al. *Chinese Pharmacology Bulletin.* 1996;12(3):53.

Guo Wai Yi Xue Can Kao Za Zhi (*Foreign Journal of Medicine*), 1977; 4: 231.

Guo Wai Yi Xue Zhong Yi Zhong Yao Fen Ce (*Monograph of Chinese Herbology from Foreign Medicine*), 1985; 7(4): 48.

Handbook of TCM Practitioner. Shanghai Science and Technology Press. Hunan College of TCM, Oct 1987 p.305.

Hou D, et al. *Journal of Jiangxi College of TCM.* 1999;11(1): 28.

Ji ZQ, et al. *Journal of Traditional Chinese Medicine Research.* 1999;15(5):47–49.

Jing WZ, et al. *China Journal of Geriatrics.* 1997; 17(6):365–367.

Li XJ, et al. *China Journal of Modern Medicine.* 1999; 9(7):32–34.

Lui J. Effect of Paeonia obovata 801 in metabolism of thromboxane B2 and arachidonic acid and on platelet aggregation in patients with coronary heart disease and cerebral thrombosis. Chung Hua I Hsueh Tsa Chih (*Chin Med J*) 1983; 63:477–81.

Nie SQ, et al. *China Journal of Chinese Medicine.* 1994;19(7): 405–407.

Shang Hai Zhong Yi Yao Za Zhi (*Shanghai Journal of Chinese Medicine and Herbology*), 1985; 7:45.

Wang YQ, et al. *Journal of Integrated Medicine.* 1990; 10(2):101–102.

Zhong Guo Sheng Li Ke Xue Hui, Di Er Ci Hui (Chinese Convention on Biophysiology, 2nd Annual Convention), 1963: 63.

Zhong Xi Yi Jie He Za Zhi (*Journal of Integrated Chinese and Western Medicine*), 1987; 7:403.

Zhong Yao Xue (*Chinese Herbology*), 1998; 739:741.

Zhong Yao Xue (*Chinese Herbology*), 1998; 831:836.

Zhong Yao Zhi (*Chinese Herbology Journal*), 1993:183.

Homotoxicology reference
Palmquist R. Treatment of three cases of polycystic kidney disease in cats (one Siamese and two Persian cats). 2004. Unpublished research data on file.

CYSTITIS

Definition and cause

Cystitis is an inflammatory process in the urinary bladder. Causes are most commonly idiopathic, infection, urolithiasis, or secondary to other diseases such as kidney disease or cancer. Signs are frequent urination, straining, blood in urine, and continual licking of the genitals. Chronic recurrences are labeled interstitial cystitis. Dietary causes related to high mineral or magnesium content as well as the feeding of dry foods are actively debated in feline lower urinary tract disease syndrome. In cats, cystitis is part of the lower urinary tract syndrome, and besides the above causes, also has a behavioral and litter box component (Bartges 2003; Buffington 1999; Grauer 1992; Lees 1986, 2003; Lulich 1995; McCall 1989; Osborne 1996, 2000, 2003).

Medical therapy rationale, drug(s) of choice, and nutritional recommendations

Treatment focuses on the clinical signs and the underlying cause. Antibiotics are generally recommended for infection. Additional common recommendations include giving urinary acidifiers and antispasmotics, increasing water consumption, and changing from dry-food diets to canned or fresh, low-mineral content foods (Buffington 1998, 1999; Lees 1986; Markwell 1999).

Anticipated prognosis

A good prognosis is expected when cystitis is treated early; however, recurrences are common when the underlying cause has not been identified and addressed (Grauer 1992, Lees 1986).

Integrative veterinary therapies

Antibiotics are the accepted therapy for urinary tract infections. Concerns regarding the relationship between continual use of antibiotics in urinary tract infections and the development of antibiotic-resistant strains of pathogens have been raised (Reid 1990, Lidifelt 1991). An integrative approach to urinary tract infection focuses on reducing inflammation and protecting the cells of the urogenital tract. The use of nutrients, nutraceuticals, medicinal herbs, and combination homeopathics that have anti-inflammatory, tissue-sparing, and regenerative effects on the bladder wall cells may reduce reliance on chronic medication.

Nutrition
General considerations/rationale
Therapeutic nutrition adds nutrients, antioxidants, and gland support for the tissues of the urogenital tract. These nutrients can help to reduce inflammation, are cellular protective, and help in the elimination of metabolic wastes and toxins.

Appropriate nutrients
Nutritional/gland therapy: Glandular adrenal, thymus, and kidney provide intrinsic nutrients that nourish and help neutralize cellular immune inflammation and degeneration (See Gland Therapy in Chapter 2 for a more detailed explanation).

Vitamin A: Vitamin A has been shown to help prevent and treat many types of infections, and is protective of the skin and mucous membrane linings of the body

(Halliwell 1994, Hussey 1990). People taking multivitamin combinations that are high in vitamins A and C showed an improved immune function and a significant reduction in infections, including those of the urinary tract (Chandra 1992).

Vitamin C: Vitamin C has been recommended for both acute and chronic urinary tract infections. It has been proven effective against E. coli, one of the main causes of UTI in people. Vitamin C (ascorbic acid) temporarily acidifies the urine, which provides a less unfriendly environment for bacterial growth (Axelrod 1985, Sirsi 1952).

Bromelain: The proteolytic enzyme bromelain has been shown to enhance the effectiveness of antibiotics in people with urinary tract infections. A double-blind study showed that 100% of the people taking the enzyme had complete resolution of the UTI as compared to 46% for those taking the placebo (Mori 1972).

Cranberry and blueberry: Research suggests that the use of cranberry or blueberry extract is beneficial in the treatment of cystitis. In double-blind trials, adding cranberry to the diet decreased the urine bacterial count and the frequency of urinary tract infections (Avorn 1994, Dignam 1997, Walker 1997). A study using blueberry showed prevention of bacterial adhesion to the wall of the bladder (Ofek 1991). The author suggests that the underlying mechanism of these fruit extracts may also be related to the phytonutrient and antioxidant levels (Goldstein 2006) (see Phytonutrients and Antioxidants in Chapter 2 for a more detailed explanation).

Chinese herbal medicine/acupuncture
General considerations/rationale
According to TCM theory, cystitis is due to Heat and Dampness in the Lower Burner affecting the Kidney and Bladder. There is associated Qi stagnation and water distribution disturbance. The Lower Burner is the lower one-third of the body. Heat refers to the inflammation, i.e., the pain and hematuria associated with urinary tract infections. Dampness refers to the cloudy appearance of the urine due to white blood cells and protein. Qi stagnation causes pain. Animals with cystitis may experience pain upon urination. Qi stagnation may also lead to insufficient energy to void properly, resulting in stranguria. The term water distribution disturbance refers to the inability to have normal urine flow.

To treat the cystitis, the practitioner must decrease inflammation by eliminating its cause. We now recognize bacteria and uroliths as common causes of the inflammation seen in cystitis. The ancient Chinese did not know about bacteria, yet many of the herbs used to treat cystitis were later shown to have significant antibacterial properties.

When faced with a patient with recurrent cystitis, modern veterinarians often recommend increasing water intake to induce diuresis to prevent subsequent episodes. The ancient Chinese used herbs with diuretic properties to drain the "Heat" from the urinary tract. Although the terminology used differs between the two forms of practice, it is clear that the objective is the same—flush the urinary tract and remove the cause of the condition.

Appropriate Chinese herbs

Angelica root (Dang gui): Has an immunostimulatory effect. It increases phagocytic activity of macrophages (Zhong Hua Yi Xue Za Zhi 1978).

Bupleurum (Chai hu): Stimulates both humoral and cellular immunity in mice (Shang Hai Yi Ke Da Xue Xue Bao 1986).

Dianthus (Qu mai): Causes diuresis (Li 1996).

Glechoma (Jin qian cao): Acts to dissolve urinary tract stones and prevent their reformation. In addition to the effect on uroliths, glechoma has a significant diuretic effect (Guang Xi Zhong Yi Yao 1990). Furthermore, glechoma has demonstrated efficacy against E. coli and Staphylococcus aureus (Zhong Yao Yao Li Yu Ying Yong 1983).

Scutellaria (Huang qin): Contains baicalin, which has antibiotic activity against E. coli, Stapylococcus aureus, b-hemolytic streptococcus, Pseudomonas aeruginosa, and leptospira. Furthermore, baicilin has shown synergistic effects with ampicillin, amoxicillin, methacillin, and cefotaxime. It can help overcome B-lactam resistance (Zhong Yao Xue 1988, Liu 2000). Additionally, scutellaria can help flush bacteria from the renal tract via its diuretic effects (Zhong Yao Xue 1988).

Sophora root (Ku shen): Has antibiotic efficacy against one of the most common causes of urinary tract infections, namely E. coli. E. coli is implicated in up to 50% of chronic urinary tract infections. Sophora root is also efficacious against several other bacteria such as Bacillus proteus, B hemotlyic strep, and Staph (Zhong Yao Xue 1988). Sophora root has immunostimulant effects. One experiment demonstrated its ability to stimulate the production of interferon in mice (Zhu Li 1998).

Wolfberry (Gou qi zi): Wolfberry extract has demonstrated significant antibacterial effects on multiple strains of bacteria, including Staphylococcus species, Bacillus species, and Pseudomonas aeruginosa (Jin Zhi Cui 1995). Experiments on the immunostimulatory effects of wolfberry have shown that it increases both the phagocytic activity of macrophages and the total T cell count (Geng 1988). It also has been shown to increase the production of white blood cells in mice (Zhong Yao Xue 1998).

Homotoxicology
General considerations/rationale

In the purest sense, cystitis is an inflammatory reaction of the bladder; however, many cases of cystitis represent deeper homotoxicoses and vicariation reactions, especially Impregnation and Deposition phase disorders.

The sudden appearance of cystitis may represent regressive or progressive vicariation. The clinician must carefully examine the health history to determine the direction in which the case is shifting on the Six-Phase Table of Homotoxicology. When simple remedies do not solve the problem, it is likely rooted in deeper pathology that has shifted in a beneficial manner toward the Inflammation Phase, because the homotoxins are eliminated from the urinary tract through the action of inflammatory cells and mucus secretion. Bacteria may well play a beneficial role by consuming such homotoxins as they are mobilized and eliminated. The presence of a deeper homotoxicosis should then be considered in any case that presents with a history of recurrent cystitis.

Appropriate homotoxicology formulas

Apis compositum: Used for acute nephritis, albuminuria, burning with scant urine, copius casts, and when the last drops burn. Patients may cry or run away on last bit of urination.

Belladonna homaccord: Treats localized inflammation, sudden and painful cystitis, urine retention and pain on passing urine, and dark urine with bloody casts. Echinacea agustifolia supports the immune system for inflammation of any kind (Reckeweg 2000).

Berberis homaccord: Drains the urinary tract and liver, and supports adrenal tissue. Treats mucus with red tinge and polyuria alternating with reduced urine production. It is useful in general detoxification of the urinary tract. The components Veratrum album and Citrullus colocynthis are useful for renal colic and spasmodic pain associated with cystitis. Also useful in cases of urolithiasis (Reckeweg 2000).

BHI-Bladder: Treats cystitis, urinary pain, urinary tract infection, peripheral edema, albuminuria, and hematuria.

BHI-Kidney Rx: Treats straining, stones, and bloody urination.

BHI-Uri-Cleanse: Indicated for strong urine, urine with bad odor, kidney pain, red urine, scanty urine, and urinary pain.

BHI-Uri-Control: Treats burning urination, the constant desire to urinate, and straining.

Cantharis compositum: Treats stranguria, straining, and urinary pain.

Echinacea compositum: Provides support during any bacterial infection, and is a phase remedy for Inflammation Phase conditions. Contains Aconitum, Gelsemium, Hepar sulphuris, Mercurius corrosivus, Pulsatilla, Streptococcus nosode, and Thuja, which all have bladder indications (Reckeweg 2002).

Mercurius homaccord: May be useful in cases of localized inflammation and sepsis due to its antibacterial and antiviral effects.

Mucosa compositum: Rehabilitates the body's mucosal elements, particularly the urinary tract. Used in Degeneration Phase disorders and following antibiotic therapy.

Populus homaccord: Used in obstructed male cats and prostatitis cases which suffer from intense burning and difficulty in urination.

Reneel: Provides drainage and detoxification of renal and urinary tissues. Treats cystitis, urolithiasis, and stranguria. Contains Causticum Hahnemanni for bladder atony and aluminum oxide for bladder paresis. Also treats albuminuria and nephrosclerosis (Heel 2003).

Solidago compositum: Stimulates the defense mechanisms of the urinary tract and treats bladder and kidney inflammation and infection. A phase remedy for Deposition Phase homotoxicoses and part of the deep detoxification formula.

Spascupreel: Used for spasmodic, cutting pain. A previous remedy, *Atropinum compositum*, which is only available in tablet form in the United States, is excellent for these patients, but in its absence *Spascupreel* is the next best choice.

Tonicoheel: Useful for the mental and emotional aspects that often characterize this problem. Contains several remedies that are valuable in bladder issues: Hypericum, Kali Phos, Helonias dioica, and Nux vomica (Reckeweg 2002).

Tonsilla compositum: Supports immune function in Impregnation and Dedifferentiation phases.

Traumeel S: Used as an intermittent agent in all inflammatory reactions.

Appropriate homotoxicology formulas

Nutrition
Urinary support formulas: 1 tablet for each 25 pounds of body weight BID.

Immune support formula: One-half tablet for each 25 pounds of body weight BID.

Bromelain: 250 mgs for each 25 pounds of body weight with food.

Cranberry extract: 100 mg for every 25 pounds of body weight.

Chinese herbal medicine/acupuncture
Formula H51 Chronic cystitis: 1 capsule per 10 to 20 pounds twice daily. In acute cases 2 weeks may be sufficient. In chronic cases long-term use is advised. If the animal develops recurrent problems upon discontinuation of the herbal supplement, it may be used continuously for years with no side effects.

In addition to the herbs cited above, H51 Chronic cystitis also contains amber (Hu po), fritillaria (Bei mu), licorice (Gan cao), lophatherum (Dan zhu ye), mantis egg case (Sang piao xiao), and rehmannia (Sheng di huang).

Because cystitis is a complicated condition, no single protocol can resolve every case.

Homotoxicology
Symptom formula: Populus homaccord, Cantharis compositum, BHI-Bladder mixed together and given 4 to 5 times daily for the first day or until symptoms improve, then given BID PO. Solidago compositum, Coenzyme compositum, and Ubichinon compositum as a mixed injection to start. Berberis homaccord can also help with the considerable spasm. For extremely painful cases, Cantharis compositum, Spascupreel, and Traumeel may also be considered as injections. Tonicoheel may be considered for the emotional strain on these pets, particularly in cats. If bacterial or viral issues are part of the pathology, Echinacea compositum may be tried as a regulating agent.

General detoxification: Detox Kit (Lymphomyosot, Nux vomica homaccord, Berberis homaccord) PO BID for 30 days in simple cases.

Deep detoxification: Galium-Heel, Lymphomyosot, Hepar compositum, Solidago compositum, Thyroidea compositum mixed together and given PO every 3 days for 120 days. Use this in chronic or recurring cases, particularly those in Impregnation, Degeneration, and Dedifferentiation phase cases.

Product sources

Nutrition
Urinary and immune support formulas: Animal Nutrition Technologies. Alternatives: UT Strength—Vetri Science; Immune System Support—Standard Process Veterinary Formulas; Immuno Support—Rx Vitamins for Pets; Immugen—Thorne Veterinary Products.

Bromezyme (bromelain): Progressive Labs.

CranberryPlus: Progressive Labs.

Chinese herbal medicine
Formula H51 Chronic cystitis: Natural Solutions, Inc.

Homotoxicology
BHI/Heel Corporation

REFERENCES

Western medicine references
Bartges J. Hematuria. In: Tilley L, Smith F. The 5-Minute Veterinary Consult: Canine and Feline, Blackwell Publishing, 2003.

Buffington CAT, Chew DJ. Effects of diets on cats with non-obstructive lower urinary tract diseases: a review. *J Anim Phsyiol and Anim Nutr.* 1998;80:120–127.

Buffington CAT, Chew DJ, Woodworth BE. Feline Interstitial Cystitis. *Journal of the American Veterinary Medical Association* 1999;215:682–687.

Buffington CAT, Chew DJ. Diet therapy in cats with lower urinary tract disorders. *Veterinary Medicine* 1999;94:625–630.

Grauer GF. Urinary tract infections. In: Nelson RW, Couto CG, eds. Essentials of small animal internal medicine. St. Louis: Mosby-Year Book, 1992:494–500.

Lees GE, Rogers KS. Treatment of urinary tract infections in dogs and cats, *J Am Vet Med Assoc* 1986;189:648–652.

Lees GE. Lower Urinary Tract Infection. In: Tilley L, Smith F. The 5-Minute Veterinary Consult: Canine and Feline, Blackwell Publishing, 2003.

Lulich JP, Osborne CA. Bacterial infections of the urinary tract. In: Ettinger SJ, Feldman EC, eds. Textbook of veterinary internal medicine. 4th ed. Philadelphia: Saunders, 1995:1775–1788.

Markwell PJ, Buffington CAT, Chew DJ, et al. Clinical evaluation of commercially available urinary acidification diets in the management of idiopathic cystitis in cats. *Journal of the American Veterinary Medical Association* 1999;214:361–365.

McCall Kaufman G. Hematuria—dysuria. In: Ettinger SJ, ed. Textbook of veterinary internal medicine. 3rd ed. Philadelphia: Saunders, 1989:160–164.

Osborne CA, Kruger JM, Lulich JP, eds. Disorders of the feline lower urinary tract I. Etiology and pathophysiology. *Vet Clin North Am* 1996;26:169–421.

Osborne CA, Kruger JM, Lulich JP, eds. Disorders of the feline lower urinary tract II. Etiology and pathophysiology. *Vet Clin North Am* 1996;26:423–665.

Osborne CA, Kruger JM, Lulich JP, et al. Feline lower urinary tract diseases. In: Ettinger SJ, Feldman EC, eds. Textbook of veterinary internal medicine. 5th ed. Philadelphia: Saunders, 2000:1710–1747.

Osborne C, Kruger JM, Lulich JP, Polzin DJ. Feline Idiopathic Lower Urinary Tract Diseases. In: Tilley L, Smith F. The 5-Minute Veterinary Consult: Canine and Feline, Blackwell Publishing, 2003.

Osborne CA, Lulich JP, Kruger JM. Disorders of feline lower urinary tract I Etiology and Pathophysiology. WB Saunders, 1996.

IVM/nutrition references

Avorn J, Monane M, Gurwitz JH, et al. Reduction of bacteriuria and pyuria after ingestion of cranberry juice. *JAMA* 1994;271:751–4.

Axelrod DR. Ascorbic acid and urinary pH. *JAMA* 1985;254:1310–1.

Chandra RK. Effect of vitamin and trace-element supplementation on immune responses and infection in elderly subjects. *Lancet* 1992;340:1124–7.

Dignam R, Ahmed M, Denman S, et al. The effect of cranberry juice on UTI rates in a long term care facility. *J Am Geriatr Soc* 1997;45:S53.

Goldstein R. Personal communication, 2006.

Halliwell B. Free Radicals and Antioxidants: a Personal View. *Nutr. Rev.*, 52:253, 1994.

Hussey GD, Klein M. A randomized, controlled trial of vitamin A in children with severe measles. *N Engl J Med* 1990;323:160–4.

Lidelfelt KG, Bollgren I, Nord CE. Changes in Periurethral Microflora after Antimicrobial Drugs, *Arch Dis Child* 66, 1991, p. 683–685.

Mori S, Ojima Y, Hirose T, et al. The clinical effect of proteolytic enzyme containing bromelain and trypsin on urinary tract infection evaluated by double blind method. *Acta Obstet Gynaecol Jpn* 1972;19:147–53.

Ofek I, Goldhar J, Zafriri D, et al. Anti-Escherichia coli adhesin activity of cranberry and blueberry juices. *New Engl J Med* 1991;324:1599 [letter].

Reid C, Bruce AW, Cook, RL. Effects on Urogenital Flora of Antibiotic Therapy of Urinary Tract Infection, *Scand J Infect Dis* 22, 1990, p43–47.

Sirsi M. Antimicrobial action of vitamin C on M. tuberculosis and some other pathogenic organisms. *Indian J Med Sci* 1952;6:252–5.

Sobota AE. Inhibition of bacterial adherence by cranberry juice: Potential use for the treatment of urinary tract infections. *J Urol* 1984;131:1013–6.

Walker EB, Barney DP, Mickelsen JN, et al. Cranberry concentrate: UTI prophylaxis. *J Family Pract* 1997;45:167–8.

Chinese herbal medicine/acupuncture references

Geng C, Wang G, Lin Y, et al. Effects on Mouse Lymphocyte and T Cells from Lycium Barbarum Polysaccharide (LBP). Zhong Cao Yao (*Chinese Herbs*). 1988,19(7):25.

Guang Xi Zhong Yi Yao (*Guangxi Chinese Medicine and Herbology*), 1990; 13(6):40.

Jin ZC, et al. Antibacterial effects of Gou Qi Zi extract. *Inner Mongolia Journal of Medicine.* 1995;15(4):203.

Li DG, et al. The diuretic effect of Qu Mai of Shandong origin. *Journal of Traditional Chinese Medicine Material.* 1996;19(10):520–522.

Liu IX, Durham DG, Richards RM. Baicalin synergy with beta-lactam antibiotics against methicillin-resistant Staphylococcus aureus and other beta-lactam-resistant strains of S. aureus. *J Pharm Pharmacol.* 2000 Mar;52(3):361–6.

Shang Hai Yi Ke Da Xue Xue Bao (*Journal of Shanghai University of Medicine*), 1986; 13(1):20.

Zhong Hua Yi Xue Za Zhi (*Chinese Journal of Medicine*), 1978;17(8):87.

Zhong Yao Xue (*Chinese Herbology*), 1988;137: 140.

Zhong Yao Xue (*Chinese Herbology*), 1988;148: 151.

Zhong Yao Yao Li Yu Ying Yong (Pharmacology and Applications of Chinese Herbs); 1983;696.

Zhu L, et al. Ku Shen total alkaloids' effect on mouse splenocytes' production of interferon. *Journal of Shanghai Second Medical University.* 1998;18(3):104–106.

Homotoxicology references

Reckeweg H. Biotherapeutic Index: Ordinatio Antihomotoxica et Materia Medica, 5th ed. Baden-Baden, Germany: Biologische Heilmittel Heel GMBH, 2000. pp 299–300, 300–1.

Reckeweg H. Homeopathia Antihomotoxica Materia Medica, 4th ed. Baden-Baden, Germany: Arelia-Verlag GMBH, 2002. pp.120–1, 315–6, 337, 340–2, 352, 370–2, 402, 420, 462, 504–5, 548–9, 572–6.

Heel. BHI Homeopathic Therapy: Professional Reference. Albuquerque, NM: Heel Inc. 2002. pp 35, 74, 102, 103.

Heel. Veterinary Guide, 3rd English edition. Baden-Baden, Germany: Biologische Heilmittel Heel GMBH, 2003. pp 106–7.

FELINE LOWER URINARY TRACT DISEASE SYNDROME (FLUTDS/FUS)

Definition and cause

Feline lower urinary tract disease syndrome is defined as a group of disorders of the urinary tract of cats that cause blood in the urine, straining, and increased frequency of urination that can be complicated with urolithiasis and blockages. Causes include bacterial or viral infection, dietary imbalances, drinking inadequate amounts of fluids, feeding dry food, feeding food that is too acid or alkaline, elevated ash and magnesium levels in the food, interstitial or recurrent cystitis, etc. The basic underlying process is inflammation of the lower urinary tract leading to the disease process (Osborne 1996, 2000, 2003).

Medical therapy rationale, drug(s) of choice, and nutritional recommendations

Dietary management should include increasing water consumption and feeding moist foods that are acidifying or alkalinizing if there is consistent urolithiasis (Buffington 1998, 1999). Depending on the underlying cause, medical therapy usually consists of antibiotics, antispasmotics, pain management, and urinary acidifiers in some cases. There is some evidence that suggests that some cats may benefit from the addition of glycoaminoglycans to the diet, which protects the membrane lining of the bladder (Buffington 1996) (see IVM below for more details). Some clinicians give cats suffering from FLUTDS corticosteroids with the idea that they may relieve swelling and reduce inflammation. A double-blind clinical study failed to demonstrate efficacy of this practice (Osborne 1996). Other rare issues, such as prostatic neoplasia, can be responsible for symptoms (Caney 1998). Surgery is indicated for blockages.

Anticipated prognosis

While most cases of FLUTDS respond well to medical therapy, recurrence and chronic infections are common and often require ongoing medical therapy, dietary restrictions, and urinary acidifiers or alkalinizers (Osborne 2003).

Integrative veterinary therapies

In FUS, cats fed a dry, high-vegetable/-cereal diet containing excess magnesium levels and reduced water intake become dehydrated. High magnesium levels in the diet can couple with high urine pH to favor the development of struvite crystals and calculi, and this combination of mucus and struvite can lead to blockage and urinary discomfort. When other diets are fed, the physiological scale tips and we see oxalate stones form. The cat's attempt to remove the material through inflammation results in clinical signs and presentation to the veterinarian for diagnosis and treatment.

The cause of FLUTDS is unclear at this time. Large population studies show definite differences in the incidence of differing types of diseases encountered in cats. Breed, age, sex, surgical alteration, and diet have all been associated with differing risk factors (Lekcharoensuk 2001). Surgically altered pets have higher risks in many categories (Lekcharoensuk 2001). Some evidence exists that affected cats may have problems with the protective layer of glycoaminoglycans in the mucous secretion of the bladder (Buffington 1996). These cases may benefit from supplementation of a product containing these agents, but this has not been proven in studies. Clinically, some cats with refractory disease improve suddenly following administration of glycoaminoglycan products, and because these agents are generally safe, it may be sensible to consider their use in difficult cases. Whether these defects are solely genetic or acquired is not known, but it is likely that genetic differences may predispose some individuals to these conditions. Because all proteins are produced through genetic encoding, a myriad of physiological errors can occur with genetic alterations.

As in all frustrating disease entities, there is a strong intention to assist these patients in their discomfort, and many medications are used in to attempt to manage this condition. It is important to assess the risk-to-benefit ratio of any agent given because pharmaceutical agents may do harm as well as assist. The practice of routinely administering antibiotics to these cats is questionable and controversial, because many have sterile urine. However, routine testing cannot identify all infected cats and antibiotic trials may be needed in difficult or recurring cases. Likewise, assuming that stress is the cause and automatically administering antidepressant medication makes little sense from a biological therapy view, because these drugs simply do further harm to the autoregulatory centers of the body and have not been shown to assist with symptoms of patients presenting with acute signs. In fact, they have actually worsened recovery by increasing risk of recurrence (Kruger 2003).

A theory exists regarding vaccination-strain live virus impregnating into the bladder of cats and later being expelled. This has not been supported by studies; however, wild viruses have been recovered (Kruger 1996). No studies have yet been designed to examine the rate of these conditions in cats vaccinated routinely, those with reduced exposure to vaccinations, or those that have received no vaccinations and have been raised on raw food diets. Whether these viruses recovered from FLUTDS cats constitute causative agents is not clear. Other unknown pathogens, such as impregnated viral particles, mycoplasma, or L-forms, may be involved. An attempt to identify Mycoplasma and Ureaplasma by PCR yielded negative results (Abou 2006). Fungi are also associated, and when present often indicate serious homotoxicoses and terrain imbalance.

Emotional and personality issues may be involved, and treatment steps to address these issues can be rewarding. Whether the response to stress is learned or genetic or a combination of the two, personality type seems to be associated with risk factors for this condition. A new study by Buffington (2006) observed, "Cats with clinical signs of lower urinary tract disease had significantly greater owner-observed gastrointestinal tract signs and scratching, fearful, nervous, and aggressive behaviors."

The aforementioned study is interesting to CAVM practitioners, because Traditional Chinese Medicine has postulated this for many years. Bach flower remedies for stress relief have long been used for this condition, and the connection between gastrointestinal complaints and disorders of the psychoneuroendocrine-immune system is tempting, to say the least, because factors which increase gastrointestinal permeability can cause widely divergent physical symptomology. These cats might be yet another manifestation of inflammatory bowel-like disease, a fact that makes dietary therapy very intriguing.

Finally, these data could reflect differences in owner psychological status because guardians who are more concerned with litter box contents might be found to be overly worried or anxious about their cat's health. The final word is still out, but this area provides fascinating opportunities for research and understanding. From the simplest standpoint, stress can reduce water consumption and the resulting dehydration by itself may predispose some of these cats to clinical breaks. On a positive note, use of chin pheromone diffusers has shown promise in cats thought to have emotional causations as well.

Water intake and dietary type are major factors in these cases. Dry commercial foods may place these cats in an abnormal situation wherein they fail to adequately excrete homotoxins, which accumulate and ultimately trigger the Inflammation Phase. Many cases respond to dietary changes involving feeding less dry food and more canned food, or use of a prescription diet designed for the cat's particular situation. FUS cats may respond to acidification

of urine and magnesium restriction, but this is not always needed for cats in the FLUTDS category of disease, and excess acidification may cause other metabolic problems that are also of concern.

The authors have seen many chronically affected cats respond to raw food diets, and while increased water intake may be the case, there may be other factors at work in these cats' recovery as well. Our present state of knowledge in this area is simply incomplete, but we know that cats are not small dogs in regard to dietary needs. Clients may present data to veterinarians that raw food diets completely prevent FLUTDS or FUS, but this is not the experience of Palmquist, who has seen several cats requiring strict prescription diets to control their problems after becoming obstructed on raw foods. Furthermore, raw diet formulation must be carefully supervised to prevent dietary nutritional drift, and guardians must be aware that their cats may shed fecal pathogens such as salmonella. However, many cats seem to do well on raw food diets, and perhaps these few cats which have problems on raw diets represent a genetic predisposition or another factor yet undiscovered, which explains their tendency for problems in this area.

An integrative approach to FLUTDS focuses upon reducing inflammation and protecting urogenital tract cells. FLUTDS is complex in its approach due to the numerous factors that have been researched and remain unresolved (diet, ash, acid, alkaline, antibiotics, urinary acidifiers). Therefore, the approach must be preceded by a complete workup, medical history, and understanding of the condition for that patient. At that point the appropriate nutrition, herbal, and biological program can be specifically designed (with medication or as a free-standing protocol) for the patient.

Nutrition
General considerations/rationale
Therapeutic nutrition consists of nutrients, antioxidants, and gland support for the tissues of the urogenital tract. These nutrients can help to reduce inflammation, are cellular protective, and enhance the elimination of metabolic wastes and toxins. The following nutrients are the basic nutritional support recommendations. Additional nutrients can be added after a complete evaluation of the patient. For example, an acid-forming supplement program should be recommended with struvite crystals, and an alkaline-forming supplement program should be chosen for calcium oxalate (see Cystitis, above, for additional protocol recommendations).

Appropriate nutrients
Nutritional/gland therapy: Glandular adrenal, thymus, kidney, and pituitary provide intrinsic nutrients that nourish and help neutralize cellular immune inflammation

and degeneration (see Gland Therapy, Chapter 2, for a more detailed explanation).

Bromelain: The proteolytic enzyme bromelain has been shown to enhance the effectiveness of antibiotics in people with urinary tract infections. A double-blind study showed that 100% of the people taking the enzyme had complete resolution of the UTI as compared to 46% for those taking the placebo (Mori 1972).

Glycoaminoglycans (glucosamine): There is some evidence that enhancing the protective layer of glycoaminoglycans in the bladder may be beneficial for cats, particularly those with refractory disease (Buffington 1996). Because these compounds are safe, they are indicated particularly in these nonresponsive cases.

Chinese herbal medicine/acupuncture
General considerations/rationale
Feline urological syndrome is a result of Heat and Damp accumulation in the Lower Burner. Qi stagnation is associated with the Lower Burner. Heat refers to the inflammation and hematuria. Damp may refer to proteinuria or the mucin plugs that may block the urethra. Stagnation leads to pain, so Qi stagnation refers to the pain associated with the condition. With Qi stagnation, the patient is unable to urinate because there is no energy to make the urine stream move.

Appropriate Chinese herbs
Glechoma (Jin qian cao), licorice (Gan cao), lygopodium (Hai jin sha), plantago (Che qian zi): 7 human patients with uroliths were treated with an herbal supplement containing these herbs in combination with dianthus (Qu mai), talc (Hua shi), clematis (Chuan mu tong), and cyathula (Chuan niu xi). 100% eliminated the stones within 10 days (Zhe Jiang Zhong Yi Za Zhi 1983).

Achyranthes (Niu xi): Has anti-inflammatory properties (Zhong Yao Tong Bao 1988). This may help to control the signs of FUS by decreasing inflammation in the lower urinary tract.

Alisma (Ze xie): Decreases calcium oxalate crystal formation in the renal tubule in hamsters, inhibiting the formation of kidney stones (Yi 1996, Yi 1997). It has been proven to have diuretic effects in people. It also increases sodium and urea output (Shi 1962, Xu 1963, Deng 1961).

Centipede (Wu gong): Has antibacterial effects (Chang Yong Zhong Yao Cheng Fen Yu Yao Li Shou Ce 1994).

Earthworms (Di long): Earthworms are potent analgesics (Chen 1996). They may help decrease the discomfort associated with bladder irritation.

Eupolyphaga (Tu bie cong): Has analgesic properties (Zhe Jiang Zhong Yi Za Zhi 1983). Humans have reported discomfort associated with urinary dysfunction, so it is reasonable to assume animals also suffer.

Glechoma (Jin qian cao): Helps to dissolve urinary tract stones and has been shown to prevent their reformation. It is more efficacious against renal uroliths than cystic calculi. It also has a significant diuretic action (Guang Xi Zhong Yi Yao 1990).

Phellodendron (Huang bai): Has demonstrated antibiotic efficacy against a variety of pathogens (Zhong Yao Xue 1998, Zhong Yao Da Ci Dian 1977). Therefore, it may be of use in bacterial causes of FUS.

Pyrrosia leaf (Shi wei): Has demonstrated antiviral activity (Zhong Guo Yao Li Xue Tong Bao 1989). Some researchers have hypothesized a viral etiology for FUS, so this herb may be useful for this condition.

Vaccaria seed (Wang bu liu xing): A component of a formula used to treat 95 patients with urinary tract stones with an 88% success rate (An Hui Zhong Yi Xue Yuan Xue Bao 1986).

Wolfberry (Gou qi zi): Has antibacterial effects against many strains of bacteria (Jin 1995). In addition, it has immunostimulant properties. It can increase the phagocytosis rate of macrophages (Geng 1988). These abilities may make it valuable for use in bacterial causes of FUS.

Acupuncture has been used successfully to treat urolithiasis. Most practitioners combine acupuncture with herbal therapy. In one study involving 127 human patients, 69% had complete resolution and 20% experienced improvement when treated with a combination of auricular acupuncture, body acupuncture, and herbal supplements (Cao 1989).

Homotoxicology
General considerations/rationale
In the purest sense, cystitis-urethritis is an inflammatory reaction, however, many cases represent deeper homotoxicoses and vicariation reactions, especially Impregnation and Deposition phase disorders. It is the author's belief that many cases of FLUTDS and FUS fall into this latter category. The general medical aspects have been summarized in conventional literature (Gerber 2005, Hostutler 2005).

The clinician needs to carefully examine the patient's health history to determine which way the case is shifting on the Six-Phase Table of Homotoxicology. All cats presenting with urinary signs should have a dietary and environmental history taken; receive a full physical examination; and have at minimum a urinalysis; and preferentially a urinalysis, urine culture and sensitivity, and full blood evaluation. Identifying the correct cause of FLUTDS is critical to successfully handling these cats, and the cause may not be apparent even with complete testing. The lack of growth on a routine culture may not rule out bacterial infection, either, because cat urine is antibacterial and may suppress bacterial growth in transit to the laboratory. Furthermore, some agents may not grow on routine media (i.e. *Mycoplasma*). Bacteria, although part of the pathogenesis of infectious causes, may appear and persist because of primary changes in the biological terrain and may well play a beneficial role by consuming such homotoxins as they are mobilized and eliminated.

A recent study showed that when *Corynebacterium urealyticum* was isolated, treated with appropriate antibiotic medication, and the affected bladder lining was surgically stripped, these patients improved and resolved the infection with *Corynebacterium* only to commonly recur with another bacterial agent, an indication of compromise of the basic immune functions in the area (Bailiff 2005). Thus, we see the theoretical application of antihomotoxic agents in accordance with the Six-Phase Theory of Reckeweg may decrease the risk of future infections by cleaning the terrain and improving immune function, while failing to damage further mucosal borders and permeability of gut and urinary mucosal elements.

The presence of a deeper homotoxicosis should then be considered in any case which presents with a history of recurrent cystitis.

As with all chronic and recurring conditions, treatment can be frustrating. No one protocol works for all patients. Some may respond very slowly while others respond remarkably fast, and clients need to be counseled to watch for signs of urinary obstruction during the 2 to 4 weeks after first presentation, so that more serious urinary blockage can be detected if it occurs. When simple symptom remedies and food changes do not solve the problem, it is likely rooted in deeper pathology that has shifted in a beneficial manner toward the Inflammation Phase as the homotoxins are eliminated from the urinary tract through the action of inflammatory cells and mucus secretion. Homotoxicology remedies alone are usually not sufficient in these cases and response rates seem to be best when these agents are combined with integrative methods such as proper diet, increased water intake, and stress reduction, along with herbal and nutritional support. This area is open for research and improved clinical approach.

Appropriate homotoxicology formulas

Apis compositum: Used for acute nephritis, albuminuria, burning with scant urine, copius casts, and when the last drops burn. Patients may cry or run away on last bit of urination.

Atropinum compositum: Incredibly effective for pain relief in cases of renal colic/spasm. Not currently available as a vial, but may still be obtained as a tablet in the United States. The company will do special runs if sufficient quantity is ordered (Reckeweg 2000). Contains several useful therapeutics, including Pareira brava (also in *Reneel, Solidago compositum, BHI-Kidney, BHI-Uri-Cleanse*) for unremitting strangury with overwhelming pain and urine with thick, viscous, white mucus or brick-

dust sediment. Also treats hypertrophy of the prostate and renal colic (Reckeweg 2002).

Belladonna homaccord: Used for localized inflammation, sudden and painful cystitis, urine retention and pain on passing urine, and dark urine with bloody casts. Echinacea agustifolia supports the immune system for inflammation of any kind (Reckeweg 2000).

Berberis homaccord: Drains the urinary tract and liver, and supports adrenal tissue. Treats mucus with red tinge and polyuria alternating with reduced urine production. Useful in general detoxification of the urinary tract. Veratrum album and Citrullus colocynthis are included for renal colic and spasmodic pain associated with cystitis. Also useful in cases of urolithiasis (Reckeweg 2000).

BHI-Bladder: Treats cystitis, urinary pain, urinary tract infection, peripheral edema, albuminuria, and hematuria.

BHI-Inflammation: Reduces inflammation and provides immune support.

BHI-Kidney Rx: Used for straining, stones, and bloody urination.

BHI-Uri-Cleanse: Used for strong urine, urine with bad odor, kidney pain, red urine, scanty urine, and urinary pain.

BHI-Uri-Control: Treats burning urination, a constant desire to urinate, and straining. Broadfoot reports some success with placing this agent in the food for patients that are difficult to medicate.

Cantharsis compositum: Used for stranguria, straining, and urinary pain.

Echinacea compositum: Provides support during any bacterial infection.

Mercurius homaccord: May be useful in cases of localized inflammation and sepsis due to the antibacterial and antiviral effects of this remedy. It is not intended for long-term use.

Mucosa compositum: Rehabilitates the mucosal elements of the body, particularly the urinary tract. Also used in Degeneration Phase disorders and following antibiotic therapy.

Populus homaccord: Used in obstructed male cats and prostatitis cases that suffer from intense burning and difficulty urination.

Reneel: Provides drainage and detoxification of renal and urinary tissues. Treats cystitis, urolithiasis, and stranguria. Treats bladder atony through Causticum Hahnemanni and bladder paresis through aluminum oxide. Also used for albuminuria and nephrosclerosis (Heel 2003).

Sabal homaccord: Treats cystalgia, as in prostatic diseases with straining and difficult urination, and urine leakage (Reckeweg 2000).

Solidago compositum: Stimulates the defense mechanisms of the urinary tract and treats bladder and kidney inflammation and infection. A phase remedy for Deposition Phase homotoxicoses and part of the Deep Detoxification formula.

Spascupreel: Treats painful spasm of the urinary tract.

Tonsilla compositum: Supports immune function in Impregnation and Dedifferentiation phases.

Traumeel S: An intermittent agent in all inflammatory reactions.

Authors' suggested protocols

Nutrition
Urinary support formulas: 1 tablet BID.
 Immune support formula: One-half to 1 tablet BID.
 Bromelain: One-fourth capsule with food.
 Glucosamine sulfate: 125 mgs BID.

Chinese herbal medicine/acupuncture
Formula H27 CrystaClair: 1 capsule per 10 to 20 pounds twice daily. This formula is indicated for a variety of crystals and stones as well as inflammatory diseases of the lower urinary tract. The lower dose is used for prevention and the higher dose for dissolution of the uroliths. In addition to the herbs mentioned above, CrystaClair also contains centipede (Wu gong), eupolyphaga (Tu bie cong), lindera (Wu yao), malva (Dong kui zi), scorpion (Quan xie), and wolfberry (Gou qi zi). These additional herbs help increase the efficacy of the formula. In general, no diet change or drugs are needed.

The authors use the following acupuncture points: BL28, SP6, CV3 and SP9 (Handbook of TCM Practitioners 1987).

Homotoxicology
Symptom formula per Broadfoot and Palmquist: Populus homaccord, Cantharsis compositum, and BHI-Bladder mixed together and given 4 to 5 times daily for the first day or until symptoms improve, then given BID PO. If Populus homaccord is not available, substitute Berberis homaccord and Sabal homaccord. If spasm is bad, consider Atropinum compositum or Spascupreel.

Alternative protocol per Martin Goldstein: Combine 4 BHI-Inflammation and 4 BHI-Bladder with 1 ounce of spring water and succuss. Give orally BID to QID depending upon symptoms. Keep mixture refrigerated (Goldstein 1999).

General detoxification: Detox Kit (Lymphomyosot, Nux vomica homaccord, and Berberis homaccord) PO BID for 30 days in simple cases.

Deep detoxification: Galium-Heel, Lymphomyosot, Hepar compositum, Solidago compositum, Thyroidea compositum, Coenzyme compositum, Ubichinon compositum, and Mucosa compositum mixed together and given PO every 3 days for 120 days in cases that recur or do not respond.

Product sources

Nutrition
Urinary and immune support formulas: Animal Nutrition Techologies. **Alternatives**: UT Strength—Vetri Science; Immune System Support—Standard Process Veterinary Formulas; Immuno Support—Rx Vitamins for Pets; Immugen—Thorne Veterinary Products.
 Bromezyme (Bromelain): Progressive Labs.
 Glucosamine: Progressive Labs.

Chinese herbal medicine
Formula H27 CrystaClair: Natural Solutions Inc.

Homotoxicology
BHI/Heel Corporation

REFERENCES

Western medicine references
Buffington CAT, Chew DJ. Calcium oxalate urolithiasis in cats. *Endourology* 1999;13:659–663.
Buffington CAT, Chew DJ. Effects of diets on cats with non-obstructive lower urinary tract diseases: a review. *J Anim Phsyiol and Anim Nutr.* 1998;80:120–127.
Buffington CAT, Chew DJ. Diet therapy in cats with lower urinary tract disorders. *Veterinary Medicine* 1999;94:625–630.
Markwell PJ, Buffington CAT, Chew DJ, et al. Clinical evaluation of commercially available urinary acidification diets in the management of idiopathic cystitis in cats. *Journal of the American Veterinary Medical Association* 1999;214:361–365.
Osborne CA, Kruger JM, Lulich JP. Disorders of the feline lower urinary tract I. Etiology and pathophysiology. *Vet Clin North Am* 1996;26:169–421.
Osborne CA, Kruger JM, Lulich JP, et al. Feline lower urinary tract diseases. In: Ettinger SJ, Feldman EC, eds. Textbook of veterinary internal medicine. 5th ed. Philadelphia: Saunders, 2000:1710–1747.
Osborne CA, Kruger JM, Lulich PP, Polzin DJ. Feline Idiopathic Lower Urinary Tract Diseases. In: Tilley L, Smith F. The 5-Minute Veterinary Consult: Canine and Feline, Blackwell Publishing, 2003.
Osborne CA, Lulich JP, Kruger JM. Disorders of feline lower urinary tract I Etiology and Pathophysiology: WB Saunders, 1996.

IVM references
Abou N, Houwers D, van Dongen A. PCR-based detection reveals no causative role for Mycoplasma and Ureaplasma in feline lower urinary tract disease. *Vet Microbiol.* 2006. Aug 25;116(1–3):pp 246–7.

Buffington C, Blaisdell J, Binns SP Jr, Woodworth B. Decreased urine glycosaminoglycan excretion in cats with interstitial cystitis. *J Urol.* 1996. May;155(5):pp 1801–4.

Buffington CA, Westropp JL, Chew DJ, Bolus RR. Risk factors associated with clinical signs of lower urinary tract disease in indoor-housed cats. *J Am Vet Med Assoc.* 2006 Mar 1;228(5): pp 722–5.

Lekcharoensuk C, Osborne C, Lulich J. Epidemiologic study of risk factors for lower urinary tract diseases in cats. *J Am Vet Med Assoc.* 2001. May 1;218(9):pp1429–35.

Lekcharoensuk C, Osborne C, Lulich J, Pusoonthornthum R, Kirk C, Ulrich L, Koehler L, Carpenter K, Swanson L. Association between dietary factors and calcium oxalate and magnesium ammonium phosphate urolithiasis in cats. *J Am Vet Med Assoc.* 2001.Nov 1;219(9):pp 1228–37.

Kruger J, Conway T, Kaneene J, Perry RL, Hagenlocker E, Golombek A, Stuhler J. Randomized controlled trial of the efficacy of short-term amitriptyline administration for treatment of acute, nonobstructive, idiopathic lower urinary tract disease in cats. *J Am Vet Med Assoc.* 2003. Mar 15;222(6): pp 749–58.

Kruger J, Osborne C, Venta P, Sussman M. Viral infections of the feline urinary tract. *Vet Clin North Am Small Anim Pract.* 1996. Mar;26(2):pp 281–96.

Nutrition reference

Mori S, Ojima Y, Hirose T, et al. The clinical effect of proteolytic enzyme containing bromelain and trypsin on urinary tract infection evaluated by double blind method. *Acta Obstet Gynaecol Jpn* 1972;19:147–53.

Chinese herbal medicine/acupuncture references

An Hui Zhong Yi Xue Yuan Xue Bao (*Journal of Anhui University School of Medicine*), 1986;5(3):33.

Cao GF, Lin HQ, Yu Y. Urinary calculi treated by electric stimulation at ear and body acupoints combined with Chinese herbal drugs: Report of 127 cases. *Liaoning JTCM* 1989 13(6):37–38.

Chang Yong Zhong Yao Cheng Fen Yu Yao Li Shou Ce (A Handbook of the Composition and Pharmacology of Common Chinese Drugs), 1994; 1725:1728.

Chen BY, et al. Analgesic and antipyretic effects of Di Long powder in mice, rats and rabbits. *Journal of Shanghai Medical University.* 1996;23(3):225–226,240.

Deng ZP, et al. *China Journal of Medicine.* 1961;47(1):7–11.

Geng C, Wang G, Lin Y, et al. Effects on Mouse Lymphocyte and T Cells from Lycium Barbarum Polysaccharide (LBP). Zhong Cao Yao (*Chinese Herbs*). 1988,19(7):25.

Guang Xi Zhong Yi Yao (*Guangxi Chinese Medicine and Herbology*), 1990; 13(6):40.

Jin ZC, et al. Antibacterial effects of Gou Qi Zi extract. *Inner Mongolia Journal of Medicine.* 1995;15(4):203.

Shi JL, et al. *Haerbin Journal of Traditional Chinese Medicine.* 1962;(1):60–6.

Xu WF. *Fujian Journal of Chinese Medicine.* 1963;8(1):42–44.

Yi CP, et al. *Journal of Tongji Medical University.* 1996;25(4): 321–322.

Yi CP, et al. *Journal of Tongji Medical University.* 1997; 26(2):99–101.

Zhe Jiang Zhong Yi Za Zhi (*Zhe Jiang Journal of Chinese Medicine*), 1983; 4:177.

Zhe Jiang Zhong Yi Za Zhi (*Zhejiang Journal of Chinese Medicine*), 1983; 11:493.

Zhong Guo Yao Li Xue Tong Bao (*Journal of Chinese Herbal Pharmacology*), 1989; 10(1):85.

Zhong Yao Da Ci Dien (Dictionary of Chinese Herbs), 1977:2032.

Zhong Yao Tong Bao (*Journal of Chinese Herbology*), 1988; 13(7):43.

Zhong Yao Xue (*Chinese Herbology*), 1998; 144: 146.

Homotoxicology references

Caney SM, Holt PE, Day MJ, Rudorf H, Gruffydd-Jones TJ. Prostatic carcinoma in two cats. *J Small Anim Pract.* 1998. Mar;39(3):pp 140–3.

Gerber B, Boretti F, Kley S, Laluha P, Muller C, Sieber N, Unterer S, Wenger M, Fluckiger M, Glaus T, Reusch C. Evaluation of clinical signs and causes of lower urinary tract disease in European cats. *J Small Anim Pract.* 2005. Dec;46(12):pp 571–7.

Goldstein M. 1999. Personal communication.

Heel. BHI Homeopathic Therapy: Professional Reference. Albuquerque, NM: Heel Inc. 2002. pp 35, 74, 102, 103.

Heel. Veterinary Guide, 3rd English edition. Baden-Baden, Germany: Biologische Heilmittel Heel GMBH, 2003. pp 106–7.

Hostutler R, Chew D, DiBartola S. Recent concepts in feline lower urinary tract disease. *Vet Clin North Am Small Anim Pract.* 2005. Jan;35(1):pp 147–70, vii.

Osborne C, Kruger J, Lulich J, Johnston G, Polzin D, Ulrich L, Sanna J. Prednisolone therapy of idiopathic feline lower urinary tract disease: a double-blind clinical study. *Vet Clin North Am Small Anim Pract.* 1996. May;26(3):pp 563–9.

Reckeweg H. Biotherapeutic Index: Ordinatio Antihomotoxica et Materia Medica, 5th ed. Baden-Baden, Germany: Biologische Heilmittel Heel GMBH, 2000. pp 299–300, 300–1, 398.

URINARY INCONTINENCE

Definition and cause

Urinary incontinence is the inability to store urine and the loss of control of urination. The underlying cause is most commonly post spaying or neutering and decrease in hormonal control of the sphincter. Neurological deficits (spinal cord, central nervous system), bladder storage deficits, chronic inflammation or infection, urolithiasis, and anatomical abnormalities are the other common underlying causes (Arnold 1992; Goodkin 1996; Labato 1994; Lane 1994, 2003).

Medical therapy rationale, drug(s) of choice, and nutritional recommendations

The underlying cause should be determined and addressed before initiating therapy if possible. The treatment of choice for hormonal imbalances is hormone replacement therapy (diethylstilbesterol and testosterone). Alternatively, adrenergic agonists such as phenyl-propanolamine are also effective. Surgery may be recommended in refractory cases (Holt 1992; Moreau 1989; Richter 1985, 1989).

Anticipated prognosis

Many animals respond well to medical therapy and are controlled; however, the potential for medication side effects increases because the therapy is lifelong. The prognosis is more guarded when the incontinence is secondary to other diseases, blockages, chronic urinary infections, and urolithiasis.

Integrative veterinary therapies

The integrative approach to urinary incontinence is multifaceted, focusing upon the nervous and muscular control of the bladder and urethra, the reduction of inflammation in the lower urogenital system, and general nutrient support for the endocrine (hormonal) glands. In some cases the reliance on drugs to control the incontinence may be reduced or eliminated.

Nutrition
General considerations/rationale

Therapeutic nutrition focuses upon nutrients that can help to improve organ function and hormonal control.

Appropriate nutrients

Nutritional/gland therapy: Glandular pituitary, hypothalamus, brain, and ovary/uterus or prostate/testicular supply the intrinsic nutrients that help reduce cellular inflammation and improve organ function. These glandular materials are hormone free and support general gland function even when the animal has been spayed or neutered. In these animals the pituitary and adrenal glands, which are responsible for picking up the "hormonal slack," receive nutrient support (see Gland Therapy in Chapter 2 for a more detailed explanation).

Magnesium: Magnesium has been associated with neuromuscular function and conditions such as muscle cramping, weakness, and neuromuscular dysfunction. Magnesium is recommended for weakening muscle function (Bibley 1996, Levin 2002).

Lecithin/phosphatidyl choline: Phosphatidyl choline is a phospholipid that is integral to cellular membranes particularly those of nerve and brain cells. It helps to move fats into the cells and is involved in acetylcholine uptake, neurotransmission, and cellular integrity. As part of the cell membranes, lecithin is an essential nutrient that is required by the nerves and all of the body's cells for general health and wellness (Hanin 1987).

Phosphatidyl serine: Phosphatidyl serine is a phospholipid and an essential ingredient in cellular membranes, particularly those of brain cells. It has been studied in people with altered mental functioning and degeneration with positive results (Crook 1991, Cenacchi 1993). The addition of PS in people with Alzheimer's disease resulted in a mild to significant clinical improvement (Delewaide 1986, Engel 1992, Funfgeld 1989).

Chinese herbal medicine/acupuncture
General considerations/rationale

Urinary incontinence is due to Qi and Yang deficiency in the Lung, Spleen, and Kidney. There is associated Blood stagnation and Phlegm accumulation. The Blood stagnation and Phlegm block the meridians to the Brain. With Kidney Qi and Yang deficiency there is not enough energy to hold the urine. The Lung and Spleen help to properly distribute water. Incontinence can result when either one lacks energy. Quite often, patients with incontinence are older. These patients sleep deeper and may be senile. They may not sense that the urine is coming, which leads to incontinence. This confusion is attributed to Phlegm because it is thought that Phlegm can fog the mind.

Appropriate Chinese herbs

Mantis egg case (Sang piao xiao): Has been used to treat bedwetting in adults and children. In one study 45 of 50 patients had complete resolution using an herbal supplement containing sang piao xiao (Xin Yi Xue 1974). Another study of 11 patients who experienced bedwetting were given a different herbal supplement containing mantis egg case. All experienced improvement (Zhong Yi Za Zhi 1965). Three patients with frequent urination were treated with Ma Zi Ren Wan (Ma zi ren, Da huang, Shan yao, Zhi zi, Hou po and Xing ren) modified by the addition of Fu pen zi and Sang piao xiao. All reported improvement in signs (Wu 1985).

Rubus (Fu pen zi): Has been shown to have estrogen-like activity on the vaginal mucosa (Chang Yong Zhong Yao Xian Dai Yan Jiu Yu Lin Chuan 1995). Many spayed female dogs experience urinary incontinence that is responsive to estrogenic hormones, indicating that rubus may help improve urinary retention ability.

Acupuncture

Studies have shown that acupuncture is an efficacious modality for treating incontinence. In one study 15 elderly women who had not responded sufficiently to standard pharmacological therapy for incontinence were treated with acupuncture. Most responded well, with 80% still reporting improvement 3 months after acupuncture therapy ended (Bergstrom 2000). In another study of 76 men, electroacupuncture at 200 hz was delivered to CV3, St28, BL23, BL28, SP6, SP9, KI3, and scalp points. Half were cured and 26% more reported improvement (Zhang 1999).

Homotoxicology
General considerations/rationale

Urinary incontinence represents an Impregnation/Degeneration Phase homotoxicosis. Such urinary incontinence can be common in bitches following routine ovariohysterectomy. There are obviously many different causes for this condition, but if the body is damaged to the point of incontinence one can be sure that the patient has crossed the biological divide. Incontinence can be frustrating to treat for this reason, and pharmaceutical therapy may be needed. Careful evaluation of the musculoskeletal, neurological, endocrine, and urinary systems are advised in all such cases. Neoplasia can cause incontinence; this represents Dedifferentiation Phase disease.

Appropriate homotoxicology formulas

BHI-Uri-Control (**Also known as** *BHI-Bladder*): Treats burning urination, a constant desire to urinate, straining, minor urinary pain, increased urgency, and mild incontinence. Indicated for urinary gravel, dribbling of urine when sitting, and pain on micturition (strangury) (Reckeweg 2002).

Berberis homaccord: Supports adrenal functions and urinary drainage. Treats pain from renal calculi, especially renal colic, as well as other diseases of the genitourinary system, such as cystitis with pyelitis and urinary tenesmus with cloudy, mealy, red, or flaky urine. Also treats adrenal exhaustion (Reckeweg 2002). Contains Colocynthis, which is helpful in cases of weakened lower back and even straining to pass stool, especially if colitis-type signs are present.

Cerebrum compositum (**behavioral**): Supports cerebral tissue and detoxification, and improves mentation. Contains Conium for inability to finish mating, along with involuntary interruption of the flow of urine. Conium-containing formulas may be useful, particularly in hypertrophy of the prostate. Such cases may be accompanied by cystitis with purulent urine. Also consider Conium in the neoplastic and preneoplastic phases (Reckeweg 2002). Embryo suis is included for burning pain in the bladder and urethra with urine that is strong and offensive. Gelsemium is quite particularly indicated in states of paralysis, e.g., after apoplexy, in weakness of the bladder and urinary incontinence, and in spastic states. Hyoscyamus is included for paralysis of the sphincters of the bladder and anus. Kali phosphoricum, considered to be the universal nerve remedy, can be invaluable in cases of urine incontinence and in bladder irritation, and is a supporting remedy in albuminuria. Manganum phosphoricum is indicated for spinal paralysis, frequent urination with pressure in kidneys, and incontinence when walking (must urinate frequently to prevent this). Medorrhinum is well indicated in nocturnal enuresis, renal colic, cystitis, and urethritis along with general itching and leucorrhea.

Phosphoricum acidum is included for irritable conditions of the bladder, prostatorrhoea before urination, frequent urination at night, burning or cutting pains during urination, retention of urine, or when urine has red sediment and a greasy layer on the surface. Selenium is included for catarrh of the bladder, with dribbling of urine after urination and involuntary passage of urine while walking. In the past, selenium was often used as a chief remedy in chronic, post-gonorrheal urethritis, along with Sepia, Kali iodatum, and Sulphur. Thuja has some additional urinary indications, such as sharp pains in the kidneys (possibly associated with inflammatory symptoms); burning-hot urine; and nonspecific inflammations such as cystitis or urethritis, pyelitis, and paralysis of the bladder. Thuja also may be valuable in prostatitis with a constant urging to urinate and yet the patient must wait a long time before being able to pass urine (Reckeweg 2002).

Discus compositum: Used in cases originating from neurological disease involving the back.

Gelsemium homaccord: Used in classical homeopathy for rear leg weakness and urinary incontinence. Treats bladder paralysis, dilute urine, dizziness or lethargy, cases with fearful history, and weakness and trembling of limbs. Gelsemium is particularly indicated in states of paralysis, e.g., after apoplexy, and in weakness of the bladder and urinary incontinence. It can be useful in spastic conditions and urinary incontinence (Reckeweg 2002).

Hormeel: Supports endocrine functions (Heel 2003). Sepia is included for hyperactivity; nervous disorders with a sensation of bearing-down and fullness in the urinary organs, pressure on the bladder, and frequent passing of urine with flatulence in the lower abdomen; and inflammations of the urinary organs. The urine contains a sediment like clay, and may also have an offensive odor; this is also useful in cases manifesting disorders in voiding from the urinary bladder. In enuresis, the incontinence usually takes place during first sleep. Mentals include conditions of exhaustion; disorders of emotional or otherwise psychological nature; and depressive emotional discord or upset. This remedy also contains Pulsatilla, which has as an indication for disorders of voiding from the bladder (Reckeweg 2002).

Ovarium compositum: May help to improve connective tissue function when the ovaries have been removed.

Plantago homaccord: Treats urine leakage and burning, cystalgia, and urinary incontinence (Reckeweg 2002). Many dogs have been successfully treated using this remedy. It can take several weeks before any change is noted, so patience is recommended. A 60-day trial is not inappropriate.

Populus homaccord: Used for urine dribbling and in obstructed male cats and prostatitis cases that suffer from recurring painful intense burning and difficulty urination. Contains Populus compositum with Kreosotum for incontinence at night as well as profuse pale urine and a violent urging to urinate. Also contains Mercurius sublimatus corrosivus for affections of the mucosa, acute glomerulonephritis with albuminuria, hematuria, and tenesmus. Mental notes include shivering, trembling of the limbs, brain symptoms, fear, restlessness, and unquenchable thirst. Populus homaccord is also found in *Solidago compositum* (Reckeweg 2002). Uva ursi is included for cystitis, pyelitis, urethritis, and urinary incontinence (Reckeweg 2002). Other remedies in this combination include: Equisetum, Solidago, Berberis, and a number of other well-indicated components.

Reneel: Contains Causticum. Low potencies are indicated for urinary incontinence following ovariohysterectomy (Day 1990). This single component is used in disorders of the respiratory passages, disorders of the urinary tract, chronic eczema, chronic disorders in the field of rheumatic diseases, spasmodic contractions, paralysis, emotional discord or upset, itching of the urethral orifice, tenesmus of urine, tenesmus at stool, fruitless attempts at urination, raw pain in the bladder, and enuresis day or night. Treats stress incontinence of urine, especially on coughing, blowing the nose, or sneezing (Reckeweg 2002). Provides drainage and detoxification of the urinary system and treats urinary passage inflammation, particularly in acute phases (Reckeweg 2000). Also treats cystitis, urolithiasis, and stranguria. Causticum Hahnemanni is included for bladder atony and aluminum oxide is included for bladder paresis. Treats nephrosclerosis (Heel 2003) and albuminuria.

Sabal homaccord: Treats difficult urination and dribbling urine. Particularly well suited in prostatic issues. Also used for paralysis of the urinary sphincter (Boericke 1927).

Solidago compositum: Phase remedy for Deposition Phases and in detoxification and drainage of the urinary tract.

Spascupreel: Well suited for spasms, pain, and cutting pain. A previous remedy, Atropinum compositum, is excellent for these patients, but is now only available as tablets. The Gelsemium component of *Spascupreel* is particularly indicated in states of paralysis, or weakness of the bladder and urinary incontinence (Reckeweg 2002).

Authors' suggested protocols

Nutrition

Female or male, pituitary/hypothalamus/pineal support formulas: 1 tablet for each 25 pounds of body weight BID.

Brain nerve support formula: One-half tablet for each 25 pounds of body weight BID.

Magnesium: 10 mgs for every 10 pounds of body weight SID.

Lecithin/phosphatidyl choline: One-fourth teaspoon for each 25 pounds of body weight BID.

Phosphatidyl serine: 20 mgs for each 15 pounds of body weight SID.

Chinese herbal medicine/acupuncture

Formula H37 Incontinence Support: 1 capsule per 10 to 20 pounds twice daily. In addition to the herbs discussed above, H37 Incontinence Support also contains alpinia fruit (Yi zhi ren), astragalus (Huang qi), cinnamon bark (Rou gui), codonopsis (Dang shen), cornus (Shan zhu yu), dioscorea (Shan yao), fossil bones (Long gu), lindera (Wu yao), oyster shell (Mu li), psoralea (Bu gu zhi), rehmannia (Shu di huang), and schizandra (Wu wei zi). These additional herbs increase the efficacy of the formula.

Acupuncture points commonly employed include SP6, ST36, CV3, and CV4 (Basic and Express Acupuncture Therapy 1969).

Homotoxicology

Proper diagnosis is important to long-term treatment plans. Conventional medication may be necessary.

Palmquist starts most cases on Plantago homaccord and Reneel orally BID, then reassesses the case and responds as is appropriate. For refractory cases, continue the protocol below.

Ovarium compositum: Inject weekly for 4 to 6 weeks.

Gelsemium homaccord, Plantago homaccord, Sabal homaccord, Reneel, and Hormeel: Combine and give orally twice daily for several weeks. Continue as needed for ongoing control.

Broadfoot begins with Cerebrum compositum as an injection, and continues 2 to 3 times weekly. Give Gelsemium homaccord BID. Consider Hormeel, Testis compositum, and Tonico-Heel.

Product sources

Nutrition

Female or male, pituitary/hypothalmaus/pineal, and brain/nerve support formulas: Animal Nutrition Technologies.

Lecithin/phosphatidyl choline: Designs for Health.

Phosphatidyl serine: Integrative Therapeutics.

Chinese herbal medicine

H37 Incontinence Support: Natural Solutions, Inc.

Homotoxicology

BHI/Heel Corporation

REFERENCES

Western medicine references

Arnold S. Relationship of incontinence to neutering. In: Kirk RW, Bonagura J, eds. Current veterinary therapy XI. Philadelphia: Saunders, 1992:875–877.

Gookin JL, Stone EA, Sharp NJ. Urinary incontinence in dogs and cats. Part 1. Urethral Pressure Profilometry. *Comp Cont Ed Pract Vet* 1996.18:407–418.

Holt PE. Pathophysiology and treatment of urethral sphincter mechanism incompetence in the incontinent bitch. *Vet Int* 1992;3:15.

Labato MA. Micturition Disorders. In: Birchard SJ, Sherding RG. Manual of Small Animal Practice, Philadelphia: WB Saunders Co, 1994, pp 857–864.

Lane IF, Barsanti JA. Urinary incontinence. In: August J, ed. Consultations in feline internal medicine. 2nd ed. Philadelphia: Saunders, 1994:373–382.

Lane IF. Urinary Incontinence. In: Tilley L, Smith F. The 5-Minute Veterinary Consult: Canine and Feline, Blackwell Publishing, 2003.

Moreau PM, Lappin MR. Pharmacologic manipulation of micturition. In: Kirk RW, ed. Current veterinary therapy X. Philadelphia: Saunders, 1989:1214–1222.

Richter K. Use of urodynamics in micturition disorders in dogs and cats. In: Kirk RW, ed. Current veterinary therapy X. Philadelphia: Saunders, 1989:1145–1150.

Richter KP, Ling GV. Clinical response and urethral pressure profile changes after phenylpropanolamine in dogs with primary sphincter incompetence. *J Am Vet Med Assoc* 1985;187:605–11.

IVM/nutrition references

Bilbey Douglas LJ. Prabhakaran, VM. Muscle cramps and magnesium deficiency: case reports. *Canadian Family Physician*, 1996;Vol. 42, July, pp. 1348–51.

Cenacchi T, Bertoldin T, Farina C, et al. Cognitive decline in the elderly: a double-blind, placebo-controlled multicenter study on efficacy of phosphatidylserine administration. *Aging (Milano)* 1993;5:123–33.

Crook TH, Tinklenberg J, Yesavage J, et al. Effects of phosphatidylserine in age-associated memory impairment. *Neurology* 1991;41:644–9.

Delwaide PJ, Gyselynck-Mambourg AM, Hurlet A, et al. Double-blind randomized controlled study of phosphatidylserine in senile demented patients. *Acta Neurol Scand* 1986;73:136–40.

Engel RR, Satzger W, Gunther W, et al. Double-blind cross-over study of phosphatidylserine vs. placebo in patients with early dementia of the Alzheimer type. *Eur Neuropsychopharmacol* 1992;2:149–55.

Fünfgeld EW, Baggen M, Nedwidek P, et al. Double-blind study with phosphatidylserine (PS) in Parkinsonian patients with senile dementia of Alzheimer's type (SDAT). *Prog Clin Biol Res* 1989;317:1235–46.

Hanin IG, Ansell B. Lecithin: Technological, Biological, and Therapeutic Aspects, 1987, NY: Plenum Press, 180, 181.

Horrocks LA, et al. Phosphatidyl Research and the Nervous System, Berlin: Springer Verlach. 1986.

Levin C. Canine Epilepsy. Oregon City, OR: Lantern Publication, 2002 P 18–19.

Chinese herbal medicine/acupuncture references

Basic and Express Acupuncture Therapy. PRC Air Force Shenyang hospital, People's Health Press, July 1969.

Bergstrom MK, Carlsson CPO, Lindholm C, Widengren R. Improvement of urge- and mixed-type incontinence after acupuncture treatment among elderly women: a pilot study. *Journal of the Autonomic Nervous System* 2000, vol 2–3 p 173–180.

Chang Yong Zhong Yao Xian Dai Yan Jiu Yu Lin Chuan (Recent Study and Clinical Application of Common Traditional Chinese Medicine), 1995; 691:692.

Wu XB. Treating micturition with Ma Zi Ren Wan. *Shanghai Journal of Traditional Chinese Medicine and Herbs.* 1985;3(4):19.

Xin Yi Xue (*New Medicine*), 1974;3:139.

Zhang H. Scalp acupuncture plus body acupuncture for senile urinary incontinence. *Int J Clin Acupuncture.* 1999; 10:101–104.

Zhong Yi Za Zhi (*Journal of Chinese Medicine*), 1965; 11:30.

Homotoxicology references

Boericke W. Materia Medica with Repertory, 9th ed. Santa Rosa, CA: Boericke and Tafel. 1927. p 451.

Day C. The Homeopathic Treatment of Small Animals: Principles and Practice. Saffron Walden, Essex: CW Daniel Company, LTD. 1990. p 86.

Heel. Veterinary Guide, 3rd English edition. Baden-Baden, Germany: Biologische Heilmettel Heel GmbH, 2003. p 66.

Reckeweg H. Homeopathia Antihomotoxica Materia Medica, 4th ed. Baden-Baden, Germany: Arelia-Verlag GMBH, 2002. pp. 180–2, 217–220, 254–6, 315–6, 337, 404, 408–10, 462, 370–2, 379, 420, 486–8, 504–5, 524, 528–529, 531–3, 572–6, 588.

UROLITHIASIS: CALCIUM OXALATE, STRUVITE, URATE

Definition and cause

Urolithiasis is one of the most researched conditions of dogs and cats. Volumes of well-researched clinical and scientific studies have been conducted, and diets have been designed to prevent and treat urolithiasis. It is beyond the scope of this book to present an in-depth discussion of the cause and medical, dietary, and surgical approaches to this condition. A number of references that thoroughly discuss the cause, prevention, and treatment of urolithiasis in domestic animals appear below. The causes of urolithiasis include infection, diet (including dry foods), elevated ash and magnesium content, acidifying and alkalinizing diets, supersaturated urine, and genetic predisposition (Lulich 2000, 2003; Osborne 1995, 1996, 1999, 2000, 2003).

Medical therapy rationale, drug(s) of choice, and nutritional recommendations

Treatment of urolithiasis in dogs and cats is multifaceted and depends on the animal, underlying cause, behavior, and diet. Common treatment methods include restricted and specially formulated diets such as Hills C/D, U/D, and S/D; antibiotics; urinary acidifiers or alkalinizers; surgery; retrograde urohydropropulsion; and behavior modification techniques (Abdullahi 1984; Bartges 1996, 1999, 2003; Collins 1998; Lulich 1992, 1993, 2001; Osborne 1981, 1990; Sorenson 1993).

Anticipated prognosis

Medical therapy, surgery, dietary adjustments, and behavior techniques can produce good results and prognosis; however, recurrences are often likely and client compliance is mandatory (Lulich 2000; Osborne 2000, 2003).

Integrative veterinary therapies

An integrative approach to urolithiasis considers reducing inflammation, enhancing elimination of toxins and metabolic wastes, tissue sparing of the cells of the urogenital tract, and supporting the organs of the immune system (see Cystitis, above, for more detailed information). Nutrients, nutraceuticals, medicinal herbs, and combination homeopathics that have anti-inflammatory, tissue-sparing, and regenerative effects on the glands of the urogenital and immune systems can be used with or independent from required medication are beneficial.

Struvite stones may be dissolved once normal urinary terrain is established, but oxalate and urate stones present a challenge. Homotoxicology and other alternative modalities, especially Traditional Chinese Medicine, may result in reduction of stone size and the breaking apart of larger stones, and integrate nicely into treatment plans for patients suffering from nonemergency urolithiasis. Surgery and chronic antibiotic therapy may be needed. In many cases, this is a recurrent problem and continued diet management along with long-term detoxification strategies are needed to obtain control of the situation.

Nutrition
General considerations/rationale

Therapeutic nutrition adds nutrients, antioxidants, and gland support for the tissues of the urogenital tract. These nutrients can help to reduce inflammation, are cellular protective, and can enhance the elimination of metabolic wastes and toxins.

Appropriate nutrients

Nutritional/gland therapy: Glandular adrenal, thymus, kidney, and pituitary provide intrinsic nutrients that nourish, reduce cellular inflammation, and improve elimination of metabolic wastes (see Gland Therapy in Chapter 2 for a more detailed explanation).

Bromelain: The proteolytic enzyme bromelain has been shown to enhance the effectiveness of antibiotics in people with urinary tract infections. A double-blind study showed that 100% of the people taking the enzyme had complete resolution of the UTI as compared to 46% for those taking the placebo (Mori 1972).

Essential fatty acids: Studies have shown that dietary essential fatty acids increase intestinal calcium absorption, thus assisting vitamin D in decreasing urinary calcium losses (Hertz-Picciotto 2000). Calcium may reduce the absorption of oxalates and may indirectly reduce the formation of kidney stones in people. Perhaps veterinary researchers will study the increased incidence of calcium oxalate crystals and stones in dogs and cats (Barilla 1978, Curhan 1993).

Vitamin E: Vitamin E is involved in the formation of scar tissue, and also helps to reduce it. Vitamin E also has organ- and tissue-sparing properties (Myers 1982; Shklar 1982, 1987).

Chinese herbal medicine/acupuncture
General considerations/rationale

In traditional Chinese Medicine, urolithiasis is due to Qi and Blood stagnation with Heat and Damp accumulation in the Lower Burner. Heat refers to the inflammation and hematuria. Damp refers to proteinuria. Stagnation leads to pain, so Qi and Blood stagnation refer to the pain associated with the condition. With Qi stagnation, the patient is unable to urinate because there is no energy to make the urine stream move.

Appropriate Chinese herbs

Glechoma (Jin qian cao), licorice (Gan cao), lygopodium (Hai jin sha), and plantago (Che qian zi): Seven human patients with uroliths were treated with an herbal supplement containing these herbs in combination with dianthus (Qu mai), talc (Hua shi), clematis (Chuan mu tong), and cyathula (Chuan niu xi). There was a 100% success rate in eliminating the stones within 10 days (Zhe Jiang Zhong Yi Za Zhi 1983).

Alisma (Ze xie): Decreases calcium oxalate crystal formation in the renal tubule in hamsters, inhibiting the formation of kidney stones (Yi 1996, Yi 1997). It has been proven to have diuretic effects in people. It increases sodium and urea output (Shi 1962, Xu 1963, Deng 1961).

Glechoma (Jin qian cao): Helps to dissolve urinary tract stones and has been shown to prevent their reformation.

It is more efficacious against renal uroliths than cystic calculi. It also has a significant diuretic action (Guang Xi Zhong Yi Yao 1990).

Vaccaria seed (Wang bu liu xing): A component of a formula used to treat 95 patients with urinary tract stones with an 88% success rate (An Hui Zhong Yi Xue Yuan Xue Bao 1986).

Homotoxicology
General considerations/rationale
Uroliths represent Deposition Phase disease. Stones can form for a wide variety of reasons, but homotoxicology views this issue as stemming from homotoxins that have accumulated in the area. Inflammatory Phase disease can progress to stone formation (Deposition Phase) and symptomatic Impregnation Phase disease (former toxin ingestion, vaccination impregnation, iatrogenic damage from drugs, etc.), which can begin to improve through regressive vicariation leading to the development of stones. Dietary imbalances can contribute to urolith formation. Primary organ failure or serious disease (hepatic shunt, hypercalcemia, and neoplasia) can lead to stone formation. Infection by bacteria, viruses, and fungi can also contribute, but biological therapists view such infections as predispositioned by the presence of homotoxins.

Therapy is aimed at eliminating the homotoxins, repairing damaged tissues, controlling infection, removing stones, and exercising preventative maintenance.

Appropriate homotoxicology formulas
Arsuraneel: Used in cases involving the right kidney.

Atropinum compositum: Very effective for painful urethral spasm but only available in the United State in tablet form. The authors hope that the oral or injectable vials are brought back due to their high efficacy in relieving pain.

Berberis homaccord: Antihomotoxic medication of choice for nephrolithiasis. Often combined with other remedies. Berberis drains the urinary tract and hepatobiliary tract, and supports adrenal function (Reckeweg 2000).

BHI-Uri-Cleanse: Treats pain and burning on urination, urinary urgency, strong smelling or scanty urine, pain in the kidney region, and renal colic with dribbling after urination (Heel 2002). The component Pareira brava is a classical remedy for pain from urinary calculi (Day 1994).

Cantharis compositum: Treats burning urination.

Coenzyme compositum: Used for cytosol energy production.

Engystol N: Helpful in cases involving the left kidney when used in combination with *Veratrum homaccord*. Consider *Engystol* when allergy or viral disease may be involved.

Galium-Heel: Deposition phase remedy.

Lithiumeel: Indicated for articular deposition of uric acid. Possibly consider its use in urate uroliths as an experimental application (Reckeweg 2000).

Lymphomyosot: Phase remedy that is useful for lymph drainage and immune/endocrine support.

Sabal homaccord: Treats prostatic disease and urethral narrowing that results in difficult urination.

Mucosa compositum: Rehabilitates the mucosal elements of multiple organs, including the urinary tract. Useful after antibiotic therapy or infection.

Plantago compositum: Used for hypersensitivity to sounds, localized inflammation phases, nocturnal enuresis, increased urine flow, popular dermatitis, and itching.

Populus compositum: Used in cases with prostatic disease, urethral burning, and narrowed urine stream.

Solidago compositum: A urinary Deposition Phase remedy. It is an E. coli nosode.

Spascupreel: Used for renal colic and spasmodic pain associated with uroliths (Heel 2003).

Reneel: Supports and detoxifies the urinary tract. Useful in cases of renal colic (Reckeweg 2000).

Ubichinon compositum: Used after antibiotics and in cases that have shifted to the Degeneration Phase.

Veratrum homaccord: Used when there is left kidney involvement, nausea, collapse, shock, or psychosis.

Authors' suggested protocols

Nutrition
Urinary support formula: 1 tablet for each 25 pounds of body weight BID.

Immune and pituitary support formulas: One-half tablet per 25 pounds of body weight SID.

Bromelain: 250 mgs for each 25 pounds of body weight with food.

Vitamin E: 100 IU for each 25 pounds of body weight SID.

Omega-3,6,9: 1 capsule for each 25 pounds of body weight with food.

Chinese herbal medicine/acupuncture
CrystalClair: Use for both prevention of urolithiasis and to dissolve stones. For dissolution, use 1 capsule per 5 to 10 pounds twice daily. For prevention, use 1 capsule per 20 pounds twice daily. In addition to the herbs mentioned above, CrystalClair also contains achyranthes (Niu xie), centipede (Wu gong), earthworm (Di long), eupolyphaga (Tu bie cong), lindera (Wu yao), malva (Dong kui zi), phellodendron (Huang bai), pyrrisia (Shi wei), scorpion (Quan xie), and wolfberry (Gou qi zi). In general, no diet change or drugs are needed to control the condition when using this herbal supplement.

Homotoxicology

Symptom Formula: Berberis homaccord, Reneel, and Spascupreel (if painful) mixed together and given orally BID to TID.

Detoxification: Lymphomyosot, Galium-Heel, Solidago compositum, Coenzyme compositum, and Mucosa compositum mixed together and given twice weekly for 10 to 12 weeks minimum.

Product sources

Nutrition
Urinary, immune, and pituitary support formulas: Animal Nutrition Technologies. **Alternatives:** Immune System Support—Standard Process Veterinary Formulas;, Immuno Support—Rx Vitamins for Pets; Immugen—Thorne Veterinary Products.

Bromezyme: Progressive Labs.
Omega-3,6,9: Vetri Science.

Chinese herbal medicine
CrystalClair: Natural Solutions, Inc.

Homotoxicology remedies
BHI/Heel Corporation

REFERENCES

Western medicine references

Abdullahi SU, Osborne CA, Leininger JR, et al. Evaluation of a calculolytic diet in female dogs with induced struvite urolithiasis. *Am J Vet Res*, 1984.45:1508–1519.

Bartges JW, Osborne CA, Lulich JP, et al. Canine urate urolithiasis: Etiopathogenesis, diagnosis, and management. *Vet Clin No Amer* 1999.29:161–191.

Bartges JW, Osborne CA, et al. Influence of four diets on uric acid metabolism and endogenous acid production in healthy beagles. *Am J Vet Res* 1996.57: 324–328.

Bartges, JW. Urate Urolithiasis. In: Tilley L, Smith F. The 5-Minute Veterinary Consult: Canine and Feline, Blackwell Publishing, 2003.

Collins RL, Birchard SJ, Chew DJ, et al. Surgical treatment of urate calculi in Dalmatians: 38 cases (1980–1995). *J Am Vet Med Assoc* 1998;213: 833–838.

Lulich JP, Osborne CA, Lekcharoensuk C, et al. Effects of hydrochlorothiazide and diet in dogs with calcium oxalate urolithiasis. *J Am Vet Med Assoc* 2001.218:1583–1586.

Lulich JP, Osborne CA, Bartges JW, et al. Canine lower urinary tract disorders. In: Ettinger SJ, Feldman EC: Textbook of Veterinary Internal Medicine, 5th ed. Philadelphia: WB Saunders Co, 2000 pp 1747–1781.

Lulich JP, Osborne CA, Carlson M, et. al. Nonsurgical removal of uroliths in dogs and cats by voiding urohydropropulsion. *J Am Vet Med Assoc* 1993. 203: 660–663.

Lulich JP, Osborne CA. Catheter-assisted retrieval of urocystoliths from dogs and cats. *J Am Vet Med Assoc* 1992.210: 111–113.

Lulich JP, Osborne CA. Urolithiasis, Calcium Oxalate. In: Tilley L, Smith F. The 5-Minute Veterinary Consult: Canine and Feline, Blackwell Publishing, 2003.

Osborne CA, Kruger JM, Lulich JP, et al. Feline lower urinary tract diseases. In: Ettinger SJ, Feldman EC. Textbook of Veterinary Internal Medicine, 5th edition, Philadelphia: WB Saunders Co., 2000. pp 1710–1747.

Osborne CA, Klausner JS, Krawiec DR. Canine struvite urolithiasis: Problems and their dissolution. *J Am Vet Med Assoc* 1981179:239–244.

Osborne CA, Lulich JP, Kruger JM et al. Medical dissolution of feline struvite uroliths. *J Am Vet Med Assoc* 1990.196: 1053–1063.

Osborne CA, Lulich JP, Thumchai R, et al. Feline Urolithiasis: Etiology and Pathophysiology. *Vet Clin North Am* 1996; 26:217–232.

Osborne CA, Lulich JP, Thumchai R, et al. Diagnosis, Medical Treatment and Prognosis of Feline Urolithiasis, *Vet Clin North Am* 1996;26:589–628.

Osborne CA, Kruger JM, Lulich JP, et al. Feline lower urinary tract diseases. In: Ettinger SJ, Feldman EC, eds. Textbook of veterinary internal medicine. 5th ed, Philadelphia: Saunders, 1999.

Osborne CA, Kruger JM, Lulich JP. Urolithiasis, Struvite—Cats. In: Tilley L, Smith F. The 5-Minute Veterinary Consult: Canine and Feline, Blackwell Publishing, 2003.

Osborne CA, Lulich JP, Bartges JW, et al. Canine and feline urolithiasis: relationship of etiopathogenesis to treatment and prevention. In: Osborne CA, Finco DR, eds. Canine and feline nephrology and urology. Baltimore: Williams and Wilkins, 1995:798–888.

Osborne CA, Lulich JP, Polzin DJ, et al. Medical dissolution and prevention of canine struvite urolithiasis: twenty years of experience. *Vet Clin North Am* 1999;29:73–111.

Osborne CA, Lulich JP, Polzin PJ. Urolithiasis, Struvite—Dogs. In: Tilley L, Smith F. The 5-Minute Veterinary Consult: Canine and Feline, Blackwell Publishing, 2003.

Sorenson JL, Ling GV. Diagnosis, prevention, and treatment of urate urolithiasis in Dalmatians. *J Am Vet Med Assoc*, 1993.203:863–869.

Sorenson JL, Ling GV. Metabolic and genetic aspects of urate urolithiasis in Dalmatians. *J Am Vet Med Assoc* 1993;203: 857–862.

IVM/nutrition references

Barilla DE, Notz C, Kennedy D, Pak CYC. Renal oxalate excretion following oral oxalate loads in patients with ileal disease and with renal and absorptive hypercalciurias: effect of calcium and magnesium. *Am J Med* 1978;64: 579–85.

Curhan GC, Willett WC, Rimm EB, Stampfer MJ. A prospective study of dietary calcium and other nutrients and the risk of symptomatic kidney stones. *N Engl J Med* 1993;328: 833–83.

Hertz-Picciotto I, Schramm M, Watt-Morse M, Chantala K, Anderson J, Osterloh J. Patterns and determinants of blood lead during pregnancy. *Am J Epidemiol.* 2000;152(9):829–837.

Mori S, Ojima Y, Hirose T, et al. The clinical effect of proteolytic enzyme containing bromelain and trypsin on urinary tract infection evaluated by double blind method. *Acta Obstet Gynaecol Jpn* 1972;19:147–53.

Myers CE, et al. Effect of Tocopherol and Selenium on Defenses Against Reactive Oxygen Species and their Effect on Radiation Sensitivity. *Annals of the NY Aca. of Sci*, 1982.393: 419–425.

Shklar G. Oral Mucosal Carcinogenesis in Hamsters: Inhibition by Vitamin E. *J Natl Cancer Inst* 1982.68:791–797.

Shklar G, Schwartz J, Trickler D, Niukian K. Regression by Vitamin E of Experimental Oral Cancer. *J Natl Cancer Inst* 1987.78:987–992.

Chinese herbal medicine/acupuncture references

An Hui Zhong Yi Xue Yuan Xue Bao (*Journal of Anhui University School of Medicine*), 1986;5(3):33.

Deng ZP, et al. *China Journal of Medicine*. 1961;47(1):7–11

Guang Xi Zhong Yi Yao (*Guangxi Chinese Medicine and Herbology*), 1990; 13(6):40.

Shi JL, et al. *Haerbin Journal of Traditional Chinese Medicine*. 1962;(1):60–6.

Xu WF. *Fujian Journal of Chinese Medicine*. 1963;8(1):42–44.

Yi CP, et al. *Journal of Tongji Medical University*. 1996; 25(4):321–322.

Yi CP, et al. *Journal of Tongji Medical University*. 1997; 26(2):99–101.

Zhe Jiang Zhong Yi Za Zhi (*Zhejiang Journal of Chinese Medicine*), 1983;(11):493.

Homotoxicology references

Day C. The Homeopathic Treatment of Small Animals: Principle and Practice. Walden: CW Daniel, 1992. p 77.

Heel. BHI Homeopathic Therapy: Professional Reference. Albuquerque, NM: Heel Inc. 2002. p 102.

Heel. Veterinary Guide, 3rd English edition. Baden-Baden, Germany: Biologische Heilmittel Heel GMBH, 2003. p 66.

Reckeweg H. Biotherapeutic Index: Ordinatio Antihomotoxica et Materia Medica, 5th ed. Baden-Baden, Germany: Biologische Heilmittel Heel GMBH, 2000. pp 195–6, 359.

Chapter Sixteen

Metabolic and Endocrine Diseases

ADDISON'S DISEASE

Definition and cause

Addison's disease may be defined as a pathological reduction in the production of glucocorticoid and/or mineralocorticoid hormones by the adrenal glands. The most common cause of this reduced production is an autoimmune process. Other causes include pituitary gland underproduction, histoplasmosis, trauma, reaction to medications such as o,p-DDD, granulomatous disease, and cancer (Bonagura 2000, Ettinger 1989, Feldman 1996, Kintzer 2003, Verge 1995, Volpe 1977). Because of the central role of the adrenal glands in metabolism and immune function, multiple organs are often affected, leading to multiple, simultaneous diseases (Bowen 1986, Greco 2001, Nuefeld 1981).

Medical therapy rationale, drug(s) of choice, and nutritional recommendations

The recommended treatment for Addison's disease is lifelong replacement therapy with prednisone, fluorocortisone, or DOCP (Kintzer 2003).

Anticipated prognosis

The prognosis is generally favorable with lifelong replacement therapy, except when there are multiple associated organ diseases (Bonagura 2000, Greco 2001, Kintzer 2003).

Integrative veterinary therapies

The adrenal glands are exhausted and function is low in Addison's disease, and stabilization is required with medical therapy. Nutrients, nutraceuticals, medicinal herbs, and combination homeopathics that have tissue-sparing and regenerative effects on cells can help the adrenals and all of the body's other interrelated glands such as the pituitary gland.

If animals with Addison's disease are diagnosed early and medicated properly, the integration of alternative therapies may help with stability and a return of normal adrenal function. In certain animals it may be possible to reduce medication to lower levels along with appropriate organ systems management.

Nutrition
General considerations/rationale

While medical therapy is focused upon adrenal stability, the nutritional approach adds nutrients, antioxidants, and gland support for the adrenal glands and other related organ systems.

Because Addison's disease is serious and affects multiple organ systems, a medical and physiological evaluation of the blood is recommended to assess total glandular health. This information helps clinicians formulate therapeutic nutritional protocols that address adrenal support as well as underlying organ conditions that may be or have been affected by the compromised adrenal function (see Chapter 2, Nutritional Blood Testing, for additional information).

Appropriate nutrients

Nutritional/gland therapy: Glandular adrenal, thymus, kidney, liver, pituitary, and hypothalamus provide the intrinsic nutrients that nourish and help improve overall organ function and help to slow degeneration (see Gland Therapy in Chapter 2 for a more detailed explanation).

N,N-Dimethylglycine (DMG): N,N-Dimethylglycine (DMG) has been widely researched in both humans and animals. DMG has been found to increase energy and enhance immune function (Barnes 1979, Graber 1981, Kendall 2000, Reap 1990, Walker 1988).

Vitamin C (ascorbic acid): Studies have shown that vitamin C can help balance, attenuate, and balance circulating cortisol levels (Brody 2002, Peters 2001).

Chinese herbal medicine
General considerations/rationale
According to TCM, Addison's disease is due to a Yang deficiency in the Spleen and Kidney. Yang can be thought of as energy or heat. The lack of Yang causes the hypometabolic state that is seen in patients with hypoadrenocorticism. The Spleen controls the muscles so a deficiency in Spleen Yang causes the weakness that is exhibited by patients. Kidney Yang warms the body so a deficiency could lead to the hypothermia that is often seen. In some cases there may be melena and or hematemsis. The Spleen is responsible for digestion and holding the blood in the vessels according to TCM, so a deficiency in Spleen Yang explains these signs. Treatment involves treating the slow metabolism (bradycardia) and weakness. When possible, TCM aims to restore the body to normal levels. Therefore, herbs that increase the adrenocortical hormones to normal levels are indicated.

Appropriate Chinese herbs
Astragalus (Huang qi): Increases the basal metabolic rate in mice (Zhong Yao Yao Li Yu Lin Chuang 1985).

Cinnamon (Rou gui): Contains cinnamaldehyde, which has positive inotropic and chronotropic effects on the heart (Yuan 1981).

Cornus (Shan zhu yu): Has demonstrated positive inotropic effects in cats. This lead to increased blood pressure and better peripheral perfusion (Hu 1988).

Deer horn gelatin (Lu jiao jiao): Strengthens muscles. When given to mice, there was a significant increase in the length of time they were able to swim (Wang 1992).

Dioscorea (Shan yao): Decreases muscular fatigue (Zhang 1996).

Epimedium (Yin yang huo): Increases the secretion of corticosterone and cortisol (Zhong Yao Da Ci Dian 1977).

Licorice (Gan cao): Possesses glucocorticoid and mineralocorticoid effects due to the glycyrrhizin and glycyrrhetinic acid components. These compounds cause reabsorption of sodium and water and potassium excretion and they prolong the effect of cortisones in the body either by decreasing its metabolism in the liver or by increasing the plasma concentration by decreasing protein binding (Zhong Yao Zhi 1993). Licorice was shown to be very effective in treating Addison's disease in a group human patients (Bai Qui En Yi Ke Da Xue Xue Bao 1978).

Rehmannia (Shu di huang): Has been shown to increase the plasma levels of adrenocortical hormone (Zhong Yao Xue 1998).

Homotoxicology
General considerations/rationale
Addison's disease is a Degeneration Phase disorder. Endocrine function of the adrenal gland is so depressed that sudden collapse and even death can occur. If patients are caught in earlier phases, improvement may be achieved through rest and support of the adrenal functions. Therapy with pharmaceutical agents is indicated, and after some time the practitioner may attempt to decrease the dosage of drugs but should monitor the patient's biochemical and physical status carefully.

Some cases will be found to require markedly lower doses of hormonal replacement after biological therapy (Palmquist 2003).

Appropriate homotoxicology formulas
The first 3 antihomotoxic medicines are the most important in this protocol, but combination with other formulas is needed to individualize therapy.

Berberis homaccord: A mainstay of therapy in adrenal gland disease (Heel 2003). It provide drainage and detoxification of the adrenal gland, kidney, and liver. A wide range of bioactive compounds are present in Berberis vulgaris extracts. Research is ongoing in this area (Food Consortium 2005, Fatei, et al. 2005).

China homaccord: Used for generalized weakness, collapse and shock, and hypotension (Reckeweg 2000).

Coenzyme compositum: A catalyst that supports cytoplasmic energy production.

Galium-Heel: A cellular and matrix detoxification and drainage formula with support for kidney. It is a phase remedy for diseases involving the Deposition, Impregnation, Degeneration, and Dedifferentiation phases.

Ginseng compositum: Used for exhaustion and weakness.

Glyoxal compositum: Depolymerizes homotoxins from cell membrane systems that block receptor recognition and function as well as other enzyme actions.

Hormeel: Normalizes hormonal functions.

Ovarium compositum: Provides drainage of the matrix and support of endocrine function in females.

Phosphor homaccord: Provides antihomotoxic benefits in all parenchymal organ diseases.

Testes compositum: Provides drainage of the matrix and support of endocrine function in males.

Thalamus compositum: Supports the central nervous components and endocrine system from a top-down approach. Provides glandular support for the pineal gland, optic thalamus, and adrenal gland. Cyclic AMP in dilution stimulates regulatory enzyme activity in cellular phases of the disease (Broadfoot, Demers, Palmquist 2006).

Thyroidea compositum: Provides normalization of hormonal function and matrix drainage in deep cases.

Tonsilla compositum: Offers immune support and deep support for the endocrine system. Alternate with *Thyroidea compositum* in endocrine dysfunction cases.

Ubichinon compositum: A catalyst that supports mitochondrial function and deblocking of enzyme function.

Authors' suggested protocols

Nutrition

Adrenal and kidney support formulas: 1 tablet for each 25 pounds of body weight BID.

Pituitary/hypothalamus/pineal and liver support formulas: One-half tablet for each 25 pounds of body weight BID.

DMG: Liquid—One-half ml per 25 pounds of body weight (maximum, 2 mls); tablets—125 mg–1 tablet for every 40 pounds of body weight (maximum, 3 tablets).

Vitamin C: 100 mgs for each 15 pounds of body weight BID.

Chinese herbal medicine/acupuncture

Formula H101 Addison's disease: 1 capsule per 10 to 20 pounds to effect twice daily. This supplement also contains alisma (Ze xie), codonopsis (Dang shen), ligustrum (Nu zhen zi), loranthus (Sang ji sheng), mouton (Mu dan pi), poria (Fu ling), psoralea (Bu gu zhi), and wolfberry (Gou qi zi). These herbs help increase the efficacy in patients with hypoadrenocorticism. The herbal combination helps to regulate pituitary-adrenal functions and helps the body to produce more natural cortisol. It may be used alone or with low doses of corticosteroids if necessary.

Homotoxicology (Dose: 10 drops PO for 50-pound dog; 5 drops PO for small dog or cat)

Symptom formula: Berberis homaccord, Galium-Heel, China homaccord, and Phosphor homaccord mixed together and given orally BID to TID. After initial crisis is over alternate Hormeel BID with China homaccord. Give Ginseng compositum if there is weakness or infirmity, particularly in geriatric animals.

Deep detoxification formula: Lymphomyosot, Hepar compositum, Solidago compositum, Thyroidea compositum, Tonsilla compositum, Coenzyme compositum, and Ubichinon compositum mixed together and given twice weekly for 12 weeks. Glyoxal compositum given by injection initially and at intervals when improvement has waned. Thalamus compositum as an initial injection and repeated intermittently.

Testes compositum or Ovarium compositum: Base on patient gender; give weekly by injection, especially in neutered pets.

Product sources

Nutrition

Adrenal, kidney, liver, and pituitary/hypothalamus/pineal support formulas: Animal Nutrition Technologies. Alternatives: Renal and Adrenal Support—Standard Process Veterinary Formulas; Renal Essentials—Vetri Science Laboratories.

DMG: Vetri Science Laboratories.

Chinese herbal medicine

Formula H101 Addison's disease: Natural Solutions Inc.

Homotoxicology

BHI/Heel Corporation

REFERENCES

Western medicine references

Bonagura J. Kirk's Current Veterinary Therapy XII. Philadelphia: WB Saunders Co.; 2000.

Bowen D, Schaer M, Riley W. Autoimmune polyglandular syndrome in a dog: A case report. *J Am Anim Hosp Assoc* 1986; 22:649–654.

Bruyette DS, Feldman EC. Primary hypoparathyroidism in the dog. *J Vet Intern Med* 1988; 2:7–14.

Ettinger S. Textbook of Veterinary Internal Medicine. Philadelphia: WB Saunders Co. 1989.

Feldman EC, Nelson RW. Canine and Feline Endocrinology and Reproduction. 2nd ed. Philadelphia: WB Saunders, 1996:55–57.

Greco D. Endocrinology: Addison's Disease and ACTH Testing Procedures, Lecture at the DCVMA, 2001.

Kintzer PP, Peterson ME. Treatment and long-term follow-up of 205 dogs with hypoadrenocorticism. *J Vet Int Med* 1997;11(2):43–49.

Kintzer P. Hypoadrenocorticism In: Tilley L, Smith F. The 5-Minute Veterinary Consult: Canine and Feline, Blackwell Publishing, 2003.

Nuefeld M, Maclaren NK, Blizzard RM. Two types of autoimmune Addison's disease associated with different polyglandular autoimmune syndromes. *Medicine* 1981; 60:355–362. 4.

Peterson ME, Greco DS, Orth DR. Hypoadrenocorticism in ten cats. *J Vet Int Med* 1989:3:55–58.

Schaer M, Riley W, Buergelt C, et al. Autoimmunity and Addison's disease in the dog. *J Amer Anim Hosp Assoc* 1986; 22:789–794.

Verge CF. Immunoendocrinopathy syndromes. In: Williams Textbook of Endocrinology, 7th ed. Wilson JD, Foster DW, Kronenberg HM, Larsen PR, eds. Philadelphia: WB Saunders, 1995:1651–1662.

Volpe R. The role of autoimmunity in hypoendocrine and hyperendocrine function. *Annals Int Med* 1977; 87:86–99.

Willard MD, Schall WD, McCaw DE, Nachreiner RF. Canine hypoadrenocorticism: Report of 37 cases and review of 39 previously reported cases. *J Amer Vet Med Assoc* 1986; 180(1):59–62.

IVM/nutrition references

Barnes L. B15: The politics of ergogenicity. *Physicians and Sports Medicine.* 1979;7(#11):17.

Brody S, Preut R, Schommer K, et al. A randomized controlled trial of high dose ascorbic acid for reduction of blood pressure, cortisol, and subjective responses to psychological stress. *Psychopharmacology* (Berl). 2002 Jan;159(3):319–24.

Kendall R, Lawson JW. Recent Findings on N,N-Dimethylglycine (DMG): A Nutrient for the New Millennium, *Townsend Letter for Doctors and Patients*, 2000; May.

Peters EM, Anderson R, Nieman DC, et al. Vitamin C supplementation attenuates the increases in circulating cortisol, adrenaline and anti-inflammatory polypeptides following ultramarathon running. *Int J Sports Med.* 2001 Oct;22(7):537–43.

Reap E, Lawson J. Stimulation of the Immune Response by Dimethylglycine, a non-toxic metabolite. *Journal of Laboratory and Clinical Medicine.* 1990.115:481.

Walker M. Some Nutri-Clinical Applications of N,N-Dimethylglycine. *Townsend Letter for Doctors.* 1988.June.

Chinese herbal medicine/acupuncture references

Bai Qui En Yi Ke Da Xue Xue Bao (*Journal of Baiqiuen University of Medicine*), 1978;4:54.

Hu XY, et al. *Journal of Nanjing College of TCM.* 1988;(3):28–29.

Wang L, et al. A comparative study of six different kinds of gelatins. *Chinese Journal of Chinese Medicine.* 1992;17(1):48–50.

Yuan-Tian-Zheng-Min. *Journal of Foreign Medicine*, vol. of *Traditional Chinese Medicine.* 1981;3(4):227.

Zhang N, et al. *China Journal of Sports Medicine.* 1996;15(2):114–117.

Zhong Yao Da Ci Dian (Dictionary of Chinese Herbs), 1977:2251.

Zhong Yao Xue (Chinese Herbology), 1998, 156:158.

Zhong Yao Yao Li Yu Lin Chuang (Pharmacology and Clinical Applications of Chinese Herbs), 1985.

Zhong Yao Zhi (*Chinese Herbology Journal*), 1993;358.

Homotoxicolgy references

Broadfoot P, Demers J, Palmquist R. Endocrine cases, on taped proceedings of AHVMA/Heel Annual Homotoxicology Seminar, 2006. Denver, CO.

Fatehi M, Saleh TM, Fatehi-Hassanabad Z, Farrokhfal K, Jafarzadeh M, Davodi S. A pharmacological study on Berberis vulgaris fruit extract. *J Ethnopharmacol.* 2005. Oct 31;102(1):46–52.

Heel. Veterinary Guide, 3rd English edition. Biologische Baden-Baden, Germany: Heilmettel Heel GmbH, 2003. p 23.

The Local Food Consortium. Understanding local Mediterranean diets: a multidisciplinary pharmacological and ethnobotanical approach. *Pharmacol Res.* 2005. Oct;52(4):353–66.

Palmquist RE. Canine Hypoadrenocorticism: Reduced oral corticosteroids utilized in successful management following biological therapy. Unpublished case material. 2003.

Reckeweg HH. Biotherapeutic Index: Ordinatio Antihomotoxica et Materia Medica, 5th ed. Baden-Baden, Germany: Biologische Heilmittel Heel GMBH, 2000. p 311.

HYPERADRENALCORTICISM (CUSHING'S DISEASE)/ PITUITARY-DEPENDANT HYPERADRENOCORTICISM (PDH)

Definition and cause

Hyperadrenocorticism (Cushing's disease) is defined as an excessive production or presence of cortisol, which has indirect and pronounced effects on multiple organ systems. The cause is most commonly due to oversecretion of ACTH by the pituitary gland, and is caused by hyperplasia or a tumor. It is less commonly caused by an adrenal tumor (or hyperplasia) or the excessive administration of glucocorticoids. In all cases the pituitary can no longer recognize, respond to, or control the elevated blood cortisol levels. The literature reports an increased incidence of Cushing's disease in Golden and Labrador Retrievers; Poodles; Boston, Scottish, and Yorkshire Terriers; Boxers; Dachshunds; and German Shepherds (Feldman 2004, Kemppainen 1997, Kintzer 2003, Peterson 1984, Witt 2004). The disease is rare in cats (Duesberg 1997).

Medical therapy rationale, drug(s) of choice, and nutritional recommendations

Therapy focuses on the affected gland and ultimately reduces the production of circulating cortisol. The most commonly used drugs for cortisol reduction are o,p-DDD (Mitotane, Lysodren), Ketaconazole, Deprenyl, and Vetoryl (Trilostane). Other options include surgery and/or radiation therapy (Barker 2005; Braddock 2004; Bruyette 1997; Kintzer 1994, 1995, 2003; Peterson 1997; Witt 2004). Nutritional recommendations address secondary complications such as diabetes, kidney disease, or polyarthritis. Vitamin C may be indicated to help reduce cortisol levels (Brody 2002).

Anticipated prognosis

Untreated Cushing's disease carries a poor prognosis. Due to the excessive circulating cortisol and the associated immunosuppressing effects, numerous secondary diseases can worsen the prognosis. Short-term response for 4 to 6 months is quite favorable. Average survival time is about 2 years, considerably less with a malignancy of the adrenal gland. The goal of therapy is to reduce the hormonal load, thereby improving the day-to-day quality of life and minimizing secondary organ system disease (Barker 2005; Braddock 2004; Bruyette 1997; Duesbery 1997; Feldman 2004; Kintzer 1994, 1995, 2003; Peterson 1997; Ramsey 2004; Sannello 2004; Witt 2004).

Integrative veterinary therapies

The pituitary and adrenal glands have major metabolic and control responsibilities in the body, and therefore are often overworked and prone to degeneration. At the cellular level, stress, exposure to chemicals and toxins, improper nutrition, and lack of antioxidants can lead to local inflammation, excessive production of free radicals, and the production of auto-antibodies. This process can result in degeneration or inflammation of the pituitary or adrenal gland. Progression of this free-radical-based inflammatory process can lead to hyperplasia and set the stage for a malignancy. The appropriate use of antioxidants, vital nutrients, herbs, and homeopathic remedies can address this inflammatory/degenerative process by either quieting or slowing the process and thereby reducing the dependent need for medication and improving quality of life. For a more in-depth discussion of causes of cancer, toxicity, and loss of control over cellular division, refer to Chapters 31 through 34.

While chemotherapeutics are the drugs of choice for Cushing's disease, these medications are directed at the destruction of the hormone-secreting cells, thereby reducing the secondary effects of excessive levels. Medical therapy for Cushing's disease does not reduce the cellular inflammation that leads to the hyperplasia, nor does it ameliorate the degenerative process that sets the stage for formation of adenoma or carcinoma. It is in these areas that integrative veterinary therapies are beneficial. They improve the response to medication and reduce cellular inflammation, which protects and spares cells from the side effects of the drugs, helps to balance the gland response of the immune system, and improves the animal's day-to-day quality of life. In addition, certain nutrients and herbs reduce cortisol levels and therefore can be used as a freestanding therapy (Craveri 1971, Kosaka 1966).

Nutrition
General considerations/rationale

Besides the many metabolic processes and the production of cortisol, the adrenal glands play a central role in the immune system. The cells of the adrenal glands can begin to overfunction during periods of chronic inflammation related to excess free radicals and depleted antioxidant reserves. As the inflammation spreads to surrounding glands, a cascade effect can occur, leading to glandular hyperactivity. While this is a Degenerative Phase disease at the cellular level, there is either hyperactivity or even tumor formation, and the use of antioxidants and anti-inflammatory nutrients can often help to reduce the inflammatory response and lessen the hyperproduction of cortisol.

Appropriate nutrients

Glandular therapy: Glandular adrenal, pituitary, pineal, and liver have been shown to have an anti-inflammatory and regenerative effects on the adrenal gland and can improve general function (Craveri 1971). See Gland Therapy in Chapter 2 for a complete description and mechanism of action.

Dehydroepiandrosterone (DHEA): DHEA has been shown to lower the plasma levels of cortisol such as those produced by hyperactive adrenal glands (Kroboth 2003). In addition, it has also been shown that a lack or decrease in the amounts of available DHEA may have an overall suppressing effect on the immune system in general (Kroboth 2003, Wisniewski 1993, Morio, et al. 1996).

Vitamin C (ascorbic acid): Studies have shown that vitamin C can help balance, attenuate, and reduce circulating cortisol levels (Brody 2002, Peters 2001). In addition, vitamin C can help offset the high alkalinity often associated with Cushing's disease and the secondary increase in the levels of alkaline phosphatase in the blood.

Vitamin B_6 (pantothenic acid): Vitamin B_6 has an overall anti-inflammatory effect in the body and also has been shown to help decrease circulating cortisol levels (Kosaka 1966, Tahiliani 1991, Tarasov 1985).

Phosphatidylserine: Phosphatidylserine is a phospholipid that is a structural component of the biological membranes in animals and plants. In studies, supplemental PS has been shown to improve mood and blunt the release of cortisol in response to physical stress (Monteleone, et al. 1990, Kelly 1999, Benton, et al. 2001).

Melatonin: Melatonin is produced by the pineal gland and has been proven to affect the sleep-awake cycles and the circadian rhythm and help induce normal sleep. It has been proven that in both adrenal and pituitary Cushing's disease patients, the levels of melatonin in the blood are significantly reduced and that the addition of melatonin increases the actual ratio of DHEA to cortisol (Soszynski, et al. 1989, Pawlikowski, et al. 2002).

Chinese herbal medicine
General considerations/rationale

Many herbs can be combined to treat pituitary hyperadrenocorticism, which is a complex condition that affects the body in a multitude of ways. The authors primarily approach this disease as a pituitary tumor condition and also address the associated physical abnormalities such as hypertension and hyperglycemia. If the diagnosis is confirmed as an adrenal tumor, then the CHM program is adjusted as listed below.

Appropriate Chinese herbs

Some herbs can be combined to treat hyperadrenocorticism because it is a complex condition affecting the body in a multitude of ways.

Some herbs, such as scrophularia (xuan shen) (Zhong Yao Yao Li Du Li Yu Lin Chuan 1992) and atractylodes (cang zhu) (Zhong Hua Yi Xue Za Zhi 1985), decrease blood glucose levels.

The following herbs help lower blood pressure, a common sequelum of Cushing's disease: astragalus root (Huang qi) (Gou Wai Yi Xue Can Kao Za Zhi 1977), rehmannia (Sheng di huang) (Zhong Yao Xue 1998), milettia (Ji xue teng) (Zhong Cao Yao Yao Li Xue 1983), ginseng (ren shen) (Ji Lin Yi Xue, 1983), and apricot seed (xing ren) (Chinese Medical Herbology and Pharmacology 2001).

Some herbs have hepatoprotective effects such as astragalus root (Huang qi) (Shang Hai Yi Yao Za Zhi 1998) and rehmannia (sheng di huang) (Zhong Yao Xue 1998).

Other herbs have been shown to decrease blood cholesterol or triglyceride levels. Myrrh (Mo yao) (Zhong Yi Za Zhi 1988) and sargassum (hai zao) (Shi Yong Nei Ke Za Zhi 1987) are included in this category.

Because some animals with Cushing's disease have a neoplastic etiology, herbs that inhibit neoplastic cell proliferation may be helpful. Cremastra (shan ci gu) (Chang Yong Zhong Yao Xian Dai Yan Jiu Yu Lin 1995) and barbat skullcap (ban zhi lian) (Wong 1996) have this action.

Note: If the diagnosis is an adrenal mass, the following herbs can be used: achyranthes (Niu xi), agrimony (Xian he cao), amber (Hu po), angelica radix (Dang gui), astragalus (Huang qi), atractylodes (Bai zhu), barbat skullcap (Ban zhi lian), burreed tuber (San leng), centipede (Wu gong), Chinese sage (Shi jian chuan), cinnamon bark (Rou gui), cnidium (Chuan xiong), codonopsis (Dang shen), corydalis tuber (Yan hu suo), kelp (Kun bu), licorice (Gan cao), mastic (Ru xiang), myrrh (Mo yao), notoginseng (San qi), oldenlandia (Bai hua she cao), oyster shell (Mu li), peach kernel (Tao ren), poria (Fu ling), pteropus (Wu ling zi), red peony (Chi shao), rehmannia (Sheng di huang), rhubarb (Da huang), scorpion (Quan xie), and zedoaria (E zhu). Please see Chapters 34 through 35 on cancer for more details on the treatment of tumors.

Homotoxicology
General considerations/rationale
Both functionally hypersecreting hypophyseal and adrenal tumors represent Dedifferentiation Phase disorders. Because these conditions are right of the biological division, therapy is generally palliative. However, spontaneous regression of hypophyseal masses may occur (Reckeweg 2000). These conditions represent end-stage homotoxicoses involving deep cellular damage and neoplastic transformation with subsequent loss of inherent autocontrol mechanisms. While no evidence-based veterinary protocols using antihomotoxic medica-

tions exist for this condition, therapy is commonly directed at reconditioning cellular organelles, especially energy production systems, draining toxic materials away from the diseased area, improving the microenvironment of the matrix, and improving detoxification and repair capabilities. Antihomotoxic medicines in the compositae category are especially helpful (Reckeweg 2000, Smit 2004).

Appropriate homotoxicology remedies
Berberis homaccord: Provides support of diseased adrenal gland, liver, and renal tissue.

Coenzyme compositum: Activates cellular energy production pathways.

Cutis compositum: Provides support and drainage for the skin. Useful in all phases of cutaneous disorders, especially in cases of pruritus (Heel 2003).

Galium-Heel: Activates the host's greater defense mechanisms in cellular phases.

Glyoxal compositum: Provides decoupling and activation of metabolism in enzyme blocked systems.

Graphites compositum: Provides constitutional support.

Hormeel: Normalizes hormonal pathways (Reckeweg 2000).

Hypothalamus compositum: Supports pituitary and hypothalamic tissue.

Lymphomyosot: Provides lymph drainage and immunoendocrine support.

Ovarium compositum or *Testis compositum*: Supports gender-based hormonal axis.

Placenta compositum: Provides vascular and stem cell support.

Pulsatilla compositum: Provides support in cases of damage from corticosteroids and in cases of regulation rigidity.

Solidago compositum: Used for drainage, detoxification, and support of urinary organs.

Thyroidea compositum: Provides deep tissue drainage and hormonal support. Phase remedy in Impregnation Phase disorders. Used as a deep detoxification remedy and in cases of regressive vicariation. Patients taking this medication frequently discharge material from body orifices. This generally is a beneficial sign of the excretion of homotoxins, and as such, should not be interfered with by suppressive medicants. Pigmentary lesions often regress into inflammatory lesions and may cause pruritus as homotoxins deposits are mobilized (Reckeweg 2000).

Tonsilla compositum: Supports the immune system in Dedifferentiation Phase disorders.

Traumeel S: Activates sulfur-containing enzymes and supports inflammatory processes.

Ubichinon compositum: Used for mitochondrial rehabilitation and support of aerobic metabolism.

Authors' suggested protocols

Nutrition

Adrenal and pituitary/hypothalamus/pineal support formulas: 1 tablet for each 25 pounds of body weight BID.

Liver support formula: One-half tablet for each 25 pounds of body weight BID.

Melatonin: 1 mg for each 20 pounds of body weight SID (maximum, 5 mgs).

Phosphatidyl serine: 25 mgs for each 25 pounds of body weight BID.

Dehydroepiandrosterone (DHEA): 5 mgs for each 20 pounds of body weight SID.

Vitamin C (ascorbic acid): 100 mgs per 10 pounds of body weight BID.

Vitamin B_6 (pantothenic acid): 25 mgs for each 25 pounds of body weight SID (maximum, 100 mgs).

Chinese herbal medicine

Uro-G-Plus: 1 capsule for each 10 pounds of body weight BID. Decrease to 1 capsule for every 20 pounds of body weight twice daily if indicated based upon results of an ACTH response test.

IMPORTANT NOTE: The authors use the Uro-G-Plus formula, which also contains prunella (Xia ku cao), scrophularia (xuan shen), subprostrata sophora root (shan dou gen), and codonopsis (dang shen). These additional herbs help balance the formula. Do not combine Uro-G-Plus with lysodren or ketoconazole to avoid a potential Addisonian crisis. For adrenal tumors, the authors recommend Adrenal Tumor (H83) at a dose of 1 capsule per 5 to 8 pounds twice daily along with dietary restrictions appropriate for patients with neoplasia.

Homotoxicology (Please refer to the Dosage Schedule, Table 4.6 in Chapter 4, for homotoxicology remedies)

In pituitary tumors:

Deep detoxification—Lymphomyosot, Solidago compositum, Hepar compositum, Thyroidea compositum, Coenzyme compositum, Ubichinon compositum, Hypothalamus compositum, Placenta compositum, Testis compositum OR Ovarium compositum PO every 3 days.
Hormeel, Galium-Heel, Berberis homaccord: PO BID.
Tonsilla compositum: 1 tablet PO EOD.
Glyoxal: 1 tablet weekly.

In adrenal tumors (surgery if possible):

Deep detoxification—Lymphomyosot, Solidago compositum, Hepar compositum, Thyroidea compositum, Tonsilla compositum, Coenzyme compositum, Ubichinon compositum, Cutis compositum. PO every 3 days.
Galium-Heel, Traumeel, Graphites homaccord, Berberis homaccord: PO BID.
Glyoxal compositum: 1 tablet weekly.

Product sources

Nutrition

Adrenal, pituitary/hypothalamus/pineal, and liver support formulas: Animal Nutrition Technologies. Alternatives: Hepatic and Adrenal Support—Standard Process Veterinary Formulas; Hepato Support—Rx Vitamins for Pets; Hepagen—Thorne Veterinary Products.

Phosphatidyl serine: Integrative Therapuetics.
Melatonin: Thorne Veterinary Products.
Dehyrone (DHEA): Thorne Veterinary Products.
Vitamins C and B_6: Over the counter.

Chinese herbal medicine

Uro-G-Plus, Adrenal Tumor (H83): Natural Solutions, Inc.

Homotoxicology

BHI/Heel Corporation

REFERENCES

Western medicine references

Barker EN, et al. A comparison of the survival times of dogs treated with Mitotane or Trilostane for pituitary-dependent hyperadrenocorticism. *J Vet Intern Med* 2005;19:810–815.

Braddock JA, et al. Inefficacy of Selegiline in treatment of canine pituitary-dependent hyperadrenocorticism. *Aust Vet J* 2004; 82:272–277.

Bruyette DS, Ruehl WW, Entrikent TL, et al. Management of canine hyperadrenocorticism with l-deprenyl (Anipryl). *Vet Clin North Am* 1997;27(2):273–286.

Duesberg C, Peterson ME. Adrenal disorders in cats. *Vet Clin North Am* 1997;27(2):321–348.

Feldman EC. In: Ettinger SJ, Feldman EC, editors. Hyperadrenocorticism, Textbook of Veterinary Internal Medicine, 2004. WB Saunders.

Kemppainen R, Behrend E. Adrenal Physiology. *Vet Clin N Am: Sm Anim Pract* 1997;27:173–186.

Kintzer PP, Peterson ME. Mitotane treatment of cortisol secreting adrenocortical neoplasia: 32 cases (1980–1992). *J Am Vet Med Assoc* 1994;205:54–61.

Kintzer PP, Peterson ME. Mitotane therapy of canine hyperadrenocorticism. In: Kirk RW, Bonagura JD, eds. Current veterinary therapy XII. Philadelphia: Saunders, 1995.

Kintzer PP. In: Tilley L, Smith F. The 5-Minute Veterinary Consult: Canine and Feline, Blackwell Publishing, 2003.

Peterson ME, Kintzer PP. Medical therapy of pituitary-dependent hyperadrenocorticism: mitotane. *Vet Clin North Am* 1997;27(2):255–272.

Peterson M. Hyperadrenocorticism. *Vet Clin N Am: Small Animal Pract* 1984;14:731–749.

Ramsey IK, et al. Hyperparathyroidism in dogs with hyperadrenocorticism. *J Small Anim Pract* 2004;46:531–536.

Witt AL, Neiger R. Adrenocorticotropic hormone levels in dogs with pituitary-dependent hyperadrenocorticism following trilostane therapy. *Vet Rec* 2004;154:399–400.

Nutrition references

Brody S, Preut R, Schommer K, et al. A randomized controlled trial of high dose ascorbic acid for reduction of blood pressure, cortisol, and subjective responses to psychological stress. *Psychopharmacology* (Berl). 2002 Jan;159(3):319–24.

Craveri F, De Pascale V. Activity of orally administered adrenocortical extract. I. Effect on the survival test. *Boll Chim Farm* 1971;110:457–62.

Craveri F, De Pascale V. Activity of orally administered adrenocortical extract. II. Effect on liver glycogenesis and sodium retention. *Boll Chim Farm* 1971;110:457–62.

Craveri F, De Pascale V. Activity of orally administered adrenocortical extract. III. Effect in tests based on muscular work. *Boll Chim Farm* 1971;110:457–62.

Kosaka M, Kikui S, Fujiwara T, Kimoto T. Action of pantetheine on the adrenal cortex. *Horumon To Rinsho* 1966 Oct;14(10):843–847.

Kroboth PD, Amico JA, Stone RA, Folan M, Frye RF, Kroboth FJ, Bigos KL, Fabian TJ, Linares AM, Pollock BG, Hakala C. Influence of DHEA administration on 24-hour cortisol concentrations, *J Clin Psychopharmacol.* 2003; 23(1):96–9 (ISSN: 0271-0749) Pharmacodynamic Research Center, University of Pittsburgh, Pittsburgh, Pennsylvania 15261, USA. krobothpd@msx.upmc.edu.)

Monteleone P, Beinat L, Tanzillo C, et al. Effects of phosphatidylserine on the neuroendocrine response to physical stress in humans. *Neuroendocrinology.* 1990 Sep;52(3):243–8.

Morio H, Terano T, Yamamoto K, et al. Serum levels of dehydroepiandrosterone sulfate in patients with asymptomatic cortisol producing adrenal adenoma: comparison with adrenal Cushing's syndrome and non-functional adrenal tumor. *Endocr J.* 1996 Aug;43(4):387–96.

Pawlikowski M, Kolomecka M, Wojtczak A, et al. Effects of six months melatonin treatment on sleep quality and serum concentrations of estradiol, cortisol, dehydroepiandrosterone sulfate, and somatomedin C in elderly women. *Neuroendocrinol Lett.* 2002 Apr;23 Suppl 1:17–9.

Peters EM, Anderson R, Nieman DC, et al. Vitamin C supplementation attenuates the increases in circulating cortisol, adrenaline and anti-inflammatory polypeptides following ultramarathon running. *Int J Sports Med.* 2001 Oct;22(7):537–43.

Peters EM, Anderson R, Theron AJ. Attenuation of increase in circulating cortisol and enhancement of the acute phase protein response in vitamin C-supplemented ultramarathoners. *Int J Sports Med.* 2001 Feb;22(2):120–6.

Soszynski P, Stowinska-Srzednicka J, Kasperlik-Zatuska A, et al. Decreased melatonin concentration in Cushing's syndrome. *Horm Metab Res.* 1989 Dec;21(12):673–4.

Sennello KA et al. Treating adrenal neoplasia in dogs and cats. *Vet Med* 2004;99:172–185.

Tahiliani AG, Beinlich CJ. Pantothenic acid in health and disease. *Vit Horm* 1991;46:165–227.

Tarasov I, Sheibak VM, Moiseenok AG. Adrenal cortex functional activity in pantothenate deficiency and the administration of the vitamin or its derivatives. *Vopr Pitan.* 1985 Jul;(4):51–4.

Wisniewski TL, Hilton CW, Morse EV, et al. The relationship of serum DHEA-S and cortisol levels to measures of immune function in human immunodeficiency virus-related illness. *Am J Med Sci.* 1993 Feb;305(2):79–83.

Chinese herbal medicine/acupuncture references

Chang Yong Zhong Yao Xian Dai Yan Jiu Yu Lin (Recent Study and Clinical Application of Common Traditional Chinese Medicine), 1995;165:166.

Chinese Medical Herbology and Pharmacology, Art of Medicine Press, Inc. 2001;220.

Gou Wai Yi Xue Can Kao Za Zhi (*Foreign Journal of Medicine*) 1977;4:231.

Ji Lin Yi Xue (*Jilin Medicine*), 1983;3:51.

Shang Hai Yi Yao Za Zhi (*Shanghai Journal of Medicine and Herbology*) 1998;(4):4.

Shi Yong Nei Ke Za Zhi (*Practical Journal of Internal Medicine*), 1987;11:580.

Wong BY, Lau BH, Jia TY, Wan CP. Oldenlandia diffusa and Scutellaria barbata augment macrophage oxidative burst and inhibit tumor growth. *Cancer Biother Radiopharm* 1996 Feb; 11(1);51–6.

Zhong Cao Yao Yao Li Xue (Herbology of Chinese Medicinals) 1983;200.

Zhong Hua Yi Xue Za Zhi (*Chinese Journal of Medicine*) 1985;44(2):150.

Zhong Yao Xue (Chinese Herbology) 1998;156:158 REHMANNIA.

Zhong Yao Yao Li Du Li Yu Lin Chuan (Pharmacology, Toxicology and Clinical Applications of Chinese Herbs), 1992;50.

Homotoxicology references

Bianchi I. Homeopathic Homotoxicological Repertory. Aurelia Publishers 1995. pp. 135, 138, 144, 197, 200.

Heel. Practitioner's Handbook of Homotoxicology, 1st US edition, 2003. p. 32.

Reckeweg H. Biotherapeutic Index: Ordinatio Antihomotoxica et Materia Medica, 5th ed. Baden-Baden, Germany: Biologische Heilmittel Heel GMBH, 2000. p 50.

Reckeweg H. Biotherapeutic Index: Ordinatio Antihomotoxica et Materia Medica, 5th ed. Baden-Baden, Germany: Biologische Heilmittel Heel GMBH, 2000. pp. 22–3.

Reckeweg H. Biotherapeutic Index: Ordinatio Antihomotoxica et Materia Medica, 5th ed. Baden-Baden, Germany: Biologische Heilmittel Heel GMBH, 2000. p 114.

Reckeweg H. Biotherapeutic Index: Ordinatio Antihomotoxica et Materia Medica, 5th ed. Baden-Baden, Germany: Biologische Heilmittel Heel GMBH, 2000. p 416.

Smit A. Cancer and Chronic Disease, on lecture proceedings CD. 2004. Heel.

DIABETES MELLITUS (TYPES 1 AND 2)

Definition and cause

Diabetes mellitus is categorized as the inability to remove and use sugar from the blood; however, metabolically, the disease affects all body systems, organs, and tissues. Pancreatic metabolism dysfunction, secondary kidney disease, neuropathy, and retinal changes occur with the disease. Causes include genetic predisposition, immune-mediated, pancreatic infections, adverse drug reactions, or are secondary to other diseases that lead to insulin deficiency, inadequacy, or inability to properly use insulin.

Long-standing insulin deficiency leads to ketoacidosis, an emergency situation that requires intensive medical therapy (Crenshaw 2003; Nelson 1995; Nichols 1995; Norsworthy 1995; Wallace 1990, 2003).

A recent study has revealed that early changes in intestinal permeability precede the development of type 1 diabetes in human patients (Bosi 2006). Dietary and environmental factors (high-carbohydrate diets, obesity, reduced exercise, etc.) are contributors. Insulin-dependent or type 1 diabetes mellitus is most commonly diagnosed in cats and dogs, but a metabolic-like syndrome exists in overweight cats that can manifest as persistently elevated blood glucose levels. In older reports this is referred to as type 2 diabetes.

Medical therapy rationale, drug(s) of choice, and nutritional recommendations

Dietary therapy focuses upon weight reduction and increasing fiber content. Increased dietary fiber has been shown to help with obesity and improve control of blood glucose levels. The diet should also contain complex vs. simple carbohydrates (Nelson 1995; Plotnick 1995; Wallace 1990, 2003). A high-fiber, low-fat diet may benefit some cats, and most diabetic cats do better on higher protein, moderate-fat diets such as those produced by prescription diet companies. Homemade or commercial raw food diets may be well accepted by many patients as well. Glargine insulin has been associated with improved remission rates in cats, as have high protein diets (Weaver, et al. 2006).

The drug of choice for both dogs and cats is insulin (Greco 1995). Oral hypoglycemic agents such as Glipizide may be helpful in type 2 diabetes (Ford 1995; Garcia 1998; Miller 1995; Nelson 1994, 1995; Norsworthy 1995).

Anticipated prognosis

The prognosis is generally good for both dogs and cats with proper dietary and medical therapies. The disease is considered permanent in dogs. Complications such as ketoacidosis carry a much more guarded prognosis (Crenshaw 2003; Wallace 1990, 2003).

Integrative veterinary therapies

Causes of diabetes include genetic predisposition, immune-mediated, pancreatic infections, adverse drug reactions, or

are secondary to other disease, and result in insulin deficiency, inadequacy, or inability to properly use insulin.

The underlying mechanism of the insulin deficiency or improper utilization is most commonly inflammatory (auto-immune, infection, drug reaction, etc.). The integrative approach therefore is aimed at reducing the inflammatory process and protecting pancreatic cells. In addition, it is important to include multi-glandular support because diabetes and sugar metabolism affect all cells.

The addition of nutrients, nutraceuticals, medicinal herbs, and combination homeopathics that have anti-inflammatory, protective, and regenerative effects is indicated. If instituted early, integrative therapies can help slow progressive inflammation and improve overall organ function.

Nutrition
General considerations/rationale

Medical therapy is focused upon the regulation of blood glucose levels. Therapeutic nutrients, antioxidants, and gland support should focus upon multiple organ systems. Sugar metabolism affects all cells and organs, and therefore it is important to support overall bodily function. A medical and physiological blood evaluation is recommended to assess glandular health. This helps clinicians to formulate therapeutic nutritional protocols that address not only blood sugar regulation but also other organs that are affected by or contribute to the condition (see Chapter 2, Nutritional Blood Testing, for a more detailed discussion).

Appropriate nutrients

Nutritional/gland therapy: Glandular adrenal, thymus, spleen, pancreas, pituitary, thyroid, and liver provide intrinsic nutrients that nourish and help neutralize cellular immune inflammation and degeneration and can help improve organ function (See Gland Therapy in Chapter 2 for a more detailed explanation).

Vitamin E: It has been shown that people with lower blood levels of vitamin E are more prone to the development of both type 1 and 2 diabetes (Knekt 1999, Salonen 1995). In addition, it has been shown that vitamin E supplementation has improved glucose tolerance (Paolisso 1993). Vitamin E has also been shown to be beneficial in diabetic side effects such as retinopathy and nephropathy (Bursell 1999, Ross 1982).

Magnesium: It has been shown that diabetic people are traditionally low in magnesium, which is corrected with supplementation (Eibl 1995, Paolisso 1990). In addition, magnesium supplementation has been shown to improve the production of insulin in people with type 2 diabetes (Paolisso 1989). Studies also have shown that the requirements for insulin in people with type 1 diabetes are lower when supplemented with magnesium and that retinopathy is more likely to occur when magnesium is deficient in the diet (McNair 1978). The American Diabetes Association suggests that there is a "strong association . . . between magnesium deficiency and insulin resistance;" however, the association will not confirm that this is a connection between a deficiency and the risk of developing diabetes (American Diabetes Association 1992).

Zinc: Type 1 diabetes in people has been linked to zinc deficiencies, which also may adversely affect general immune function (Nakamura 1991, Mocchegiani 1989). It has also been shown that supplementing the diet with zinc can help to lower blood glucose levels (Rao 1987).

Alpha-lipoic acid (ALA): ALA, which is involved metabolically in sugar and fat metabolism, has been clinically shown to be beneficial in the management and treatment of diabetes and diabetic neuropathy often found in people (Konrad 1999, Nickander 1996, Packer, 1997). Estrada has shown that ALA has improved glucose uptake in animals. The American Diabetes Association recommends ALA along with vitamin E for helping to prevent diabetic complications such as neuropathy, atherosclerosis, and cataract formation (Ou 1996, Yi 2006).

Coenzyme Q10: Coenzyme Q10 (CoQ10) is required for the normal metabolism of sugar. Studies have shown that animals with diabetes are reported to be deficient in CoQ10. People with type 2 diabetes have been shown to have significantly lower levels of coenzyme Q10 than healthy subjects (Miyake 1999). In another study it was shown that diabetics' blood sugar levels declined more than 30% when supplemented (Shigeta 1966).

Chromium: Chromium helps release sugar from the blood to the muscles and other tissues, and is indicated in the treatment of diabetes mellitus. Early reports in the literature show that brewer's yeast, which is rich in chromium, can be helpful in the treatment of diabetes and the improvement of glucose tolerance (Anderson 1998, 2000; Offenbacher 1980). Improvement has been reported in people with both type 1 and 2 diabetes, which is believed to be due to improved sensitivity to insulin (Gaby 1996, Evans 1989).

Chinese herbal medicine/acupuncture
General considerations/rationale
Diabetes is a result of Yin deficiency in the Lung, Stomach, and Kidney. This may be secondary to improper diet, stress, lack of exercise, and/or excess Dry and Heat.

Yin deficiency in the Lung allows the heat resulting from the relative Yang excess to dry up the body fluids, leading to thirst. The Yin deficiency in the Stomach makes the patient polyphagic in an attempt to cool the fire in the Stomach. The deficiency in the Kidneys leads to polyuria.

Stress, diet, and lack of exercise are all risk factors for diabetes in Western medicine. A tendency to suffer from

Dry or Heat is a term used in TCM to indicate a constitutional characteristic. It can be translated into a genetic tendency toward development of diabetes in Western terminology.

Appropriate Chinese herbs
Achyranthes (Niu xi): Contains ecdysterone and inokosterone. Experimentally, these compounds have been shown to inhibit hyperglycemia induced by glucagon, alloxan, and anti-insulin serum (Song 1970, Ogawa 1974, Ye 1986).

Anemarrhena (Zhi mu): Contains anemarns A, B, C, and D, which all lower blood glucose (Ri Ben Yao Wu Xue Za Zhi 1971).

Ophiopogon (Mai men dong): Has been shown to decrease blood glucose in mice with alloxan-induced diabetes (Wan 1998).

Acupuncture
Some practitioners use acupuncture to treat type 2 diabetes. One study found that BL18, 20; ST25; SP8; LI11; and GB9 increased pancreatic output. Some physicians use BL13, 20, 21, 23; RN4; SP6; and ST36 to control the symptoms of diabetes (Li 2000).

Homotoxicology
General considerations/rationale
Diabetes mellitus represents a Degeneration Phase homotoxicosis. This disease probably represents a continuum of progressive vicariation and may have genetic causation in some patients. In some cases, it may result as a consequence of chronic pancreatitis.

Insulin-dependent diabetes mellitus must be treated appropriately with insulin replacement therapy. Homotoxicology can assist these patients generally because it provides support for the Impregnation and Degeneration phases that affect the patient. Type 2 patients can greatly benefit from biological therapies and can even reverse their disease in some instances. This can happen with dietary therapy alone or when combined with proper homeopathic and herbal support.

Appropriate homotoxicology formulas
In addition to the remedies below, also see the protocols for pancreatitis, obesity, and cardiac disease.

Aesculus compositum: Provides vascular support. Contains a wide array of remedies for peripheral circulatory support. Should be combined with *Placenta compositum* for maximum efficacy.

Arsuraneel: Indicated for emaciation, dystrophy, diabetes mellitus, and anemia. The primary ingredient, Arsenicum album, is included for exhaustion, restlessness, anxiety, insatiable thirst, and emaciation. Contains Aceticum acidum for edematous swellings, waxy appearance, diabetes mellitus, anemia, and excessive thirst. Has Curare (see *Syzygium compositum*) and Secale (see *Placenta compositum*).

BHI-Pancreas: Contains Podophyllum. Also found in *Leptandra homaccord, Momordica compositum,* and *Ubichinon compositum*, which may be used in a wide range of potencies in the treatment of pancreatic problems, including acute and chronic pancreatitis. Momordica (also in *Momordica compositum,* and *Mucosa compositum*) is indicated in pancreatitis (Reckeweg 2002). The herb Momordica charantia has been shown to help regenerate the beta cells in type I diabetes by providing the insulin-like substance P-insulin (polypeptide-P) that lowers blood sugar (Broadfoot 2006). Contains Leptandra, Pancreatinum, and other pancreatic support remedies.

Coenzyme compositum: Provides metabolic support. One of the most effective injections for diabetes mellitus is *Coenzyme compositum*, which is useful for diabetic gangrene along with *Circulo-Injeel*. It contains alpha-Ketoglutaricum acidum (common to *Causticum compositum, Cor compositum, Hepar compositum, Syzygium compositum, Thyroidea compositum, BHI-Enzyme,* and others). It is an active factor in the citric acid cycle and redox systems, and in Impregnation Phase pathologies helps to improve cell respiration. Natrum pyruvicum (see *Placenta compositum*) and Sulphur, a critical component in the makeup of the mesenchymal support system, are included. Defined in physiological, chemical, or enzymological terms, its function is the reactivation of enzyme-based detoxifying procedures which have been altered biochemically (Reckeweg 2002).

Galium-Heel: Provides cellular detoxification and supports kidney function.

Lymphomyosot: Provides lymphatic drainage. Has been shown to benefit human diabetics in reducing lymphoedema and distal extremity pathology and in improving wound healing.

Chelidonium homaccord: Supports liver excretion and gallbladder function. Bitter melon has been shown to assist diabetics.

Glyoxal compositum: Has catalytic and unblocking action on damaged respiratory enzymes and toxins, and is indicated in all cellular phase and viral diseases. It is given in infrequent doses.

Hepeel: Used intermittently to support liver detoxification and repair.

Hepar compositum: Deep detoxification formula that supports liver, gastrointestinal, and pancreatic function. The ingredient Molybdan compositum is a tremendously useful mineral donor for enzymatic function. Kali asparaginicum (Potassium asparate), one of the potassium salts, is one of its components; it serves as a coupling factor to potassium through salt formation and shows a particular affinity for important intermediate conversions. Aspartic acid is known to be a sugar former, a so-called glucoplastic amino acid. Because potassium salts perform an important function of the so-called "sodium pump" in the cell membrane, the combination with aspartic acid appears especially noteworthy for influencing intracellular enzyme mechanisms, and thus, is generally used in preparations aimed at stabilizing or regenerating the enzyme functions. Manganum gluconicum (also in *BHI-Enzyme*) contains manganese salts which have a strong enzyme action (e.g., in the citric acid cycle), in which energy in the mitochondria is obtained from glucose. Manganese salts in the form of an organic compound (with gluconic acid) afford the opportunity for rapid entry into the cell.

Gluconic acid occupies a key position in the oxidation of glucose via the pentose-phosphate cycle (Warburg-Dickens-Horecker schema). Manganese gluconate is usually given in combination with other enzyme-activating factors. Zincum gluconicum, which is gluconic acid coupled with zinc, allows for enhancement of various enzyme functions. Zinc has many trace element functions to fulfill in the body, and is the second most abundant trace element, after iron. Zinc forms complexes with insulin when the peptide chains in the insulin crystal are attached to the imidazole groups because of a chelation. The insulin-producing cells of the islets of Langerhans are particularly rich in zinc, so they are probably attached to zinc complexes. Pancreatic carboxypeptidase also contains zinc. Thus, by administering zinc compounds, it is possible to influence important enzyme functions (e.g., in anemia, diabetes mellitus, liver damage, kidney diseases, and Degeneration Phases) (Reckeweg 2002). Sulphur is also contained in this remedy, along with a host of other critical components.

Mucosa compositum: Can be thought of as a cellular "washing agent" which helps to normalize the mucosal surfaces throughout the body. Based on the individual homeopathic constituents of Mucosa compositum, there are therapeutical possibilities for the affections of the mucosa, as well as of the digestive glands. This is also a possible auxiliary remedy for pancreatitis, cholecystitis, and cholangitis. Furthermore, it is possible that it can be used to purify the homotoxic terrain in neoplasm phases. Mucosa compositum contains numerous mucous membranes and anti-inflammatory agents (Argentum nitricum, Belladonna, etc.), as well as preparations intended specifically for the treatment of the epigastrium, pylorus, pancreas, and small and large intestines (Veratrum).

Mucosa compositum also exerts a prophylactic action against progressive vicariation (in the sphere of the cellular phases). It contains Momordica balsamina for gripping, colicky pains in the epigastrium, gastrocardiac syndrome, and pancreopathy. It treats ceanothus—a "tangled" sensation on the left side—diabetes, and splenic disorders. Pancreas suis (see *Syzygium compositum*, below) is included for pancreopathy, chronic enteritis, marasmus, and cachexia (Reckeweg 2000). Kreosotum is included for neuralgias, particularly of the sciatic nerve and primarily accompanying diabetes or albuminuria. A sickness of a wide variety of mucosa runs throughout the whole symptom picture of Kreosotum, so that profuse and loathsome discharges with ulceration and severely depleted vital energy are typical (Reckeweg 2002). Sulphur (see *Coenzyme compositum*) is also contained in this remedy.

Placenta compositum: Stimulates the peripheral circulation of the blood in arteriosclerosis, gangrenous conditions of the distal limbs caused by diabetes mellitus, gangrenous ulcers, and decubitus. *Placenta compositum* is the parenteral equivalent of *Aesculus compositum* drops, and should be administered in combination for arteriosclerotic deficiency phenomena to relieve the connective tissues more rapidly from Deposition Phase homotoxins. It contains numerous revitalizing factors, such as Arteria suis (Artery). The attenuations of this sarcode are prepared from the fresh arteries of a healthy pig, and are indicated for disturbances of circulation, periarteritis, and venous spasm. Useful in diabetes mellitus, gangrene, and cramps in the calf muscles. A catalytic remedy, l(+)-Lacticum acidum (sarcolactic acid), is useful for disturbed cell respiration, with specific indications for diabetes mellitus. Natrum pyruvicum is a remedy that should be considered in disorders of glucose metabolism, especially when there is a circulatory disturbance (diabetic gangrene). Secale is included for blood circulatory disorders associated with arterial diseases (Reckeweg 2002).

Solidago compositum: Deep detoxification formula that supports urogenital tissues.

Syzygium compositum: Supports the pancreas and a wide variety of tissues that are negatively affected by diabetic pathology. Contains Hepar suis for liver repair. This is a broad reaching, diabetes-mellitus-specific remedy (Reckeweg, 2000). *Syzygium compositum* represents an important preparation for long-term medication. Syzygium jambolanum, whose main indication is diabetes mellitus, is included. Pancreas suis (also found in *Hepar compositum* and *Mucosa compositum*) is useful in diabetes mellitus (of pancreatic origin), cachexia, enteritis, enterocolitis, metabolic support, pancreatic repair, and malabsorption. Small quantities of Phlorizine, injected subcutaneously, precipitate a severe glycosuria, which occurs without any preceding hyperglycaemia and continues even when the blood-sugar level becomes low because the kidney has become permeable to lower levels of blood glucose. Glycosuria occurs late, or minimally in kidney disease. Thus, it seems obvious and consistent with the Law of Similars and the reversal effect (Arndt-Schulz) to use Phlorizine in the treatment of diabetes mellitus.

However, in most cases of diabetes mellitus we are dealing with Degeneration Phases or genetically determined phases on the right of the Biological Divide that are difficult to cure with single homeopathic remedies.

A number of curative possibilities can be realized through E. Bürgi's synergistic principle, such as combination remedies. These are especially effective if they are used parenterally, and thus come into close contact with the body's greater defensive system, and possibly undiluted. Curare has some specific indications for diabetes mellitus and muscular debility.

This remedy also contains alpha-ketoglutaricum (see *Coenzyme compositum*) and Secale (also found in *Aesculus compositum*, *Arsuraneel*, *Circuloheel*, *Placenta compositum*, *Arteria-Heel*, *Syzygium compositum*, *BHI-Varicose*, and others), which are useful when there is a sensation of numbness, cramps and paralysis of the extremities, gangrene (especially in diabetics with excess fat tissue), venous spasms, and varicose ulcers (Reckeweg 2002). Arsenicum album (see *Arsuraneel*) and Plumbum metallicum (for arteriosclerosis, nephrosclerosis, paresis with emaciation, muscular atrophy) are included. Acidum phosphoricum is indicated for physical and mental exhaustion and emaciation. Acidum sulfuricum treats chronic gastritis and diabetes. Acidum L (+)-lacticum (sarcolactic acid) is used for acid-base regulation in the connective tissues. Kreosotum (beech tar creosote) treats catarrh of the mucosa with acrid secretions and secondary conditions from diabetes such as pruritus, cataract, gangrene, and disorders of the peripheral circulation. Kalium picrinicum is included for symptoms of exhaustion (Reckeweg 2000).

Thyroidea compositum: Provides deep detoxification and support of endocrine functions.

Tonsilla compositum: Supports the immune system and endocrine system; used in alteration with *Thyroidea compositum*.

Ubichinon compositum: Provides metabolic support. Has many enzyme activators, including Naphthaquinone with indications for patients that either gradually lose more and more weight in spite of eating well, or is used for obese patients with pale, yellowish, sallow skin. Para-benzoquinone is useful in degenerative diseases of the eyes (retina) and diabetes mellitus. Alpha-lipoic acid (see *Syzygium compositum*), Podophyllum (see *BHI-Pancreas*), and Sulphur (see *Coenzyme compositum*) are also included.

Authors' suggested protocols

Nutrition

Immune, pancreas, endocrine/exocrine, and liver support formulas: 1 tablet for each 25 pounds of body weight BID.

Magnesium: 10 mgs for every 10 pounds of body weight SID.

Zinc: 15 mg for each 25 pounds of body weight SID.

Vitamin E: 100 IU for each 25 pounds of body weight.

Alpha-lipoic acid: 20 mg per 10 pounds of body weight daily.

Coenzyme Q10: 25 mgs for every 10 pounds of body weight daily.

Pan chelate (chromium GTF): 1 capsule for each 35 pounds of body weight SID.

Chinese herbal medicine

Ketoacidotic crises require emergency Western medication for stabilization. The recommended patent formula is Yu Nu Jian, which contains achyranthes (Niu xi), anemarrhena (Zhi mu), gypsum (Shi gao), ophiopogon (Mai men dong), and rehmannia (Shu di huang). In the author's experience, this formula may decrease the amount of insulin required for the patient, but rarely is sufficient on its own. It is given at the supplier's recommended rate.

Some acupuncture points to consider include ST36, KI3, BL13, BL20, LI11, CV4, and BL23 (Handbook of TCM practitioners 1987).

Homotoxicology (Dose: 10 drops PO for 50-pound dog; 5 drops PO for small dog or cat)

Symptom remedy: Syzygium compositum, Lymphomyosot, Aesculus compositum mixed together and given BID long-term. The dosage is adjusted according to the disease, the clinical picture, and the stage of the illness. In the first stage of therapy give this combination 6 times daily orally, and as time passes use it BID to QID orally. Give Placenta compositum, Mucosa compositum, and Coenzyme compositum as intercurrent injections, possibly as an autosanguis.

Deep detoxification: Galium-Heel, Hepar compositum, Solidago compositum, Thyroidea compositum, Coenzyme compositum, Ubichinon compositum mixed together and given every 3 days for 3 to 6 months or until phase shift occurs. Give Glyoxal compositum once a week. BHI-Pancreas, Leptandra, and/or Momordica compositum can be given BID for long-term pancreatic support.

Product sources

Nutrition

Immune, pancreas endocrine/exocrine, and liver support formulas: Animal Nutrition Technologies. **Alternatives:** Hepatic and Immune System Support—Standard Process Veterinary Formulas; Hepato Support—Rx Vitamins for Pets; Hepagen—Thorne Veterinary Products; Immuno Support—Rx Vitamins for Pets; Immugen–Thorne Veterinary Products.

Alpha-lipoic acid: Source Naturals.

Coenzyme Q10: Vetri Science; Rx Vitamins for Pets; Integrative Therapeutics; Thorne Veterinary Products.

Pan chelate: Progressive Labs.

Chinese herbal medicine

Yu Nu Jian: Blue Light, Inc.

Homotoxicology

BHI/Heel Corporation

REFERENCES

Western medicine references

Crenshaw KL. Diabetes Mellitus, Ketoacidotic. In: Tilley L, Smith F. The 5-Minute Veterinary Consult: Canine and Feline, Blackwell Publishing, 2003.

Ford SL. NIDDM in the cat: Treatment with the oral hypo-glycemic medication, glipizide. In Greco DS, Peterson ME, eds. The Veterinary Clinics of North America Small Animal Practice: Diabetes Mellitus. Philadelphia: WB Saunders Co. 1995; 599–616.

Garcia JL, Bruyette DS. Using oral hypoglycemic agents to treat diabetes mellitus in cats. *Veterinary Medicine.* 1998 (August); 736–742.

Greco DS, Broussard JD, Peterson ME. Insulin therapy. In Greco DS, Peterson ME, eds. The Veterinary Clinics of North America Small Animal Practice: Diabetes Mellitus. Philadelphia: W.B. Saunders Co. 1995;677–690.

Miller E. Long-term monitoring of the diabetic dog and cat: Clinical signs, serial blood glucose determinations, urine glucose, and glycated blood proteins. In Greco DS, Peterson ME, eds. The Veterinary Clinics of North America Small Animal Practice: Diabetes Mellitus. Philadelphia: W.B. Saunders Co. 1995;571–584.

Nelson RW. Diabetes mellitus. In: Ettinger SJ, Feldman EC, eds. Textbook of veterinary internal medicine. Philadelphia: Saunders, 1995;1510–1537.

Nelson RW. Diabetes mellitus. In: Birchard SJ, Sherding RG, eds. Saunders Manual of Small Animal Practice. Philadelphia: W.B. Saunders Co. 1994;249–256.

Nichols R, Crenshaw KL. Complications and concurrent disease associated with diabetic ketoacidosis and other severe forms of diabetes mellitus. In: Bonagura JB, ed. Small animal practice current veterinary therapy XII. Philadelphia: Saunders, 1995;384–386.

Norsworthy G. Performing a blood glucose curve in a diabetic cat. *Veterinary Medicine.* 1998 (May);425–428.

Peterson ME. Diagnosis and management of insulin resistance in dogs and cats with diabetes mellitus. In Greco DS, Peterson ME, eds. The Veterinary Clinics of North America Small Animal Practice: Diabetes Mellitus. Philadelphia: W.B. Saunders Co. 1995;691–714.

Plotnick AN, Greco DS. Home management of cats and dogs with diabetes mellitus: common questions asked by veterinarians and clients. In Greco DS, Peterson ME, eds. The Veterinary Clinics of North America Small Animal Practice:

Diabetes Mellitus. Philadelphia: W.B. Saunders Co. 1995; 753–759.

Wallace MS, Kirk CA. The diagnosis and treatment of insulin-dependent and non-insulin-dependent DM in the dog and the cat. *Probl Vet Med* 1990;2:573–590.

Wallace MS. Diabetes Mellitus—Uncomplicated. In: Tilley L, Smith F. The 5-Minute Veterinary Consult: Canine and Feline, Blackwell Publishing, 2003.

IVM/nutrition references

American Diabetes Association. Magnesium supplementation in the treatment of diabetes. *Diabetes Care* 1992;15:1065–7.

Bursell SE, Schlossman DK, Clermont AC, et al. High-dose vitamin E supplementation normalizes retinal blood flow and creatinine clearance in patients with type I diabetes. *Diabetes Care* 1999;22:1245–51.

Eibl NL, Schnack CJ, Kopp H-P, et al. Hypomagnesemia in type II diabetes: effect of a 3-month replacement therapy. *Diabetes Care* 1995;18:188.

Estrada DE, Ewart HS, Tsakiridis T, et al. Stimulation of glucose uptake by the natural coenzyme alpha-lipoic acid/thioctic acid: participation of elements of the insulin signaling pathway. *Diabetes.* 1996;45(12):1798–1804.

Anderson RA. Chromium in the prevention and control of diabetes. *Diabetes Metab* 2000;26:22–7 [review].

Anderson RA. Chromium, glucose intolerance and diabetes. *J Am Coll Nutr* 1998;17:548–55 [review].

Evans GW. The effect of chromium picolinate on insulin controlled parameters in humans. *Int J Biosocial Med Res* 1989;11:163–80.

Gaby AR, Wright JV. Diabetes. In: Nutritional Therapy in Medical Practice: Reference Manual and Study Guide. Kent WA, ed. 1996, 54–64 [review].

Gaby AR, Wright JV. Nutritional protocols: diabetes mellitus. In: Nutritional Therapy in Medical Practice: Protocols and Supporting Information. Kent WA, ed. 1996, 10.

Konrad T, Vicini P, Kusterer K, Hoflich A, Assadkhani A, Bohles HJ, Sewell A, Tritschler HJ, Cobelli C, Usadel KH. alpha-Lipoic acid treatment decreases serum lactate and pyruvate concentrations and improves glucose effectiveness in lean and obese patients with type 2 diabetes. *Diabetes Care.* 1999 Feb;22(2):280–7.

Knekt P, Reunanen A, Marniumi J, et al. Low vitamin E status is a potential risk factor for insulin-dependent diabetes mellitus. *J Intern Med* 1999;245:99–102.

Miyake Y, Shouzu A, Nishikawa M, et al. Effect of treatment of 3-hydroxy-3-methylglutaryl coenzyme I reductase inhibitors on serum coenzyme Q10 in diabetic patients. *Arzneimittelforschung* 1999;49:324–9.

McNair P, Christiansen C, Madsbad S, et al. Hypomagnesemia, a risk factor in diabetic retinopathy. *Diabetes* 1978;27:1075–7.

Mocchegiani E, Muzzioli M. Therapeutic application of zinc in human immunodeficiency virus against opportunistic infections. *J Nutr.* 2000;130(5S Suppl):1424S–1431S.

Mocchegiani E, Boemi M, Fumelli P, Fabris N. Zinc-dependent low thymic hormone level in type I diabetes. *Diabetes* 1989;12:932–7.

Muller GH, Kirk RW, Scott DW. Small Animal Dermatology, 4th ed. Philadelphia: W.B. Saunders. 1989;1–48.

Nakamura T, Higashi A, Nishiyama S, et al. Kinetics of zinc status in children with IDDM. *Diabetes Care* 1991;14:553–7.

Nickander KK, McPhee BR, Low PA, Tritschler H. Alpha-lipoic acid: antioxidant potency against lipid peroxidation of neural tissues in vitro and implications for diabetic neuropathy. *Free Radic Biol Med.* 1996;21(5):631–9.

Offenbacher EG, Pi-Sunyer FX. Beneficial effect of chromium-rich yeast on glucose tolerance and blood lipids in elderly subjects. *Diabetes* 1980;29:919–25.

Ou P, Nourooz-Zadeh J, Tritschler HJ, Wolff SP. Activation of aldose reductase in rat lens and metal-ion chelation by aldose reductase inhibitors and lipoic acid. *Free Radic Res* 1996;25:337–346.

Packer L, Tritschler HJ, Wessel K. Neuroprotection by the metabolic antioxidant alpha-lipoic acid. *Free Radic Biol Med.* 1997;22(1–2):359–78.

Paolisso G, Sgambato S, Pizza G, et al. Improved insulin response and action by chronic magnesium administration in aged NIDDM subjects. *Diabetes Care* 1989;12:265–9.

Paolisso G, D'Amore A, Giugliano D, et al. Pharmacologic doses of vitamin E improve insulin action in healthy subjects and non-insulin dependent diabetic patients. *Am J Clin Nutr* 1993;57:650–6.

Paolisso G, Scheen A, D'Onofrio FD, Lefebvre P. Magnesium and glucose homeostasis. *Diabetologia* 1990;33:511–4.

Rao KVR, Seshiah V, Kumar TV. Effect of zinc sulfate therapy on control and lipids in type I diabetes. *J Assoc Physicians India* 1987;35:52.

Salonen JT, Nyssonen K, Tuomainen T-P, et al. Increased risk of non-insulin dependent diabetes mellitus at low plasma vitamin E concentrations: a four year follow up study in men. *BMJ* 1995;311:1124–7.

Shigeta Y, Izumi K, Abe H. Effect of coenzyme Q7 treatment on blood sugar and ketone bodies of diabetics. *J Vitaminol (Kyoto)* 1966;12:293–8.

Yi X, Maeda N. Alpha-Lipoic Acid Prevents the Increase in Atherosclerosis Induced by Diabetes in Apolipoprotein E-Deficient Mice Fed High-Fat/Low-Cholesterol Diet, *Diabetes,* 2006; 55(8): 2238–44.

Chinese herbal medicine/acupuncture references

Handbook of TCM Practitioners, Hunan College of TCM, Shanghai Science and Technology Press, Oct 1987, p 317–319.

Li-ping W, Yu-xin J. Diabetes [Teaching Rounds]. *Int J Clin Acupuncture.* 2000;11:115–120.

Ogawa S, et al. Investeg Endocrinol Horm Heterophylly. 1974:341.

Ri Ben Yao Wu Xue Za Zhi (*Japan Journal of Pharmacology*), 1971;67(6):223

Song THX, et al. *Japanese Journal of Pharmacology.* 1970;66:551.

Wan HJ, et al. *China Journal of TCM Science and Technology.* 1998;5(4):218–219.

Ye Ye Hong. Foreign Medicine Volume of TCM. 1986;8(1):42.

Homotoxicology references

Broadfoot P. Diabetes. In: Proceedings of AHVMA/Heel Homotoxicology Veterinary Conference, 2006. Denver CO.

Bosi E, Molteni L, Radaelli MG, Folini L, Fermo I, Bazzigaluppi E, Piemonti L, Pastore MR, Paroni R. Increased intestinal permeability precedes clinical onset of type 1 diabetes. *Diabetologia*. 2006. Oct 7; [Epub ahead of print]

Reckeweg H. 2000. Homeopathia Antihomotoxica Materia Medica, 5th ed. Baden-Baden, Germany: Aurelia-Verlag GMBH, pp 384–5, 408–10.

Reckeweg H. Homeopathia Antihomotoxica Materia Medica, 4th ed. Baden-Baden, Germany: Aurelia-Verlag GMBH, 2002. pp 117, 154, 176, 268, 365, 373, 377–8, 383, 404, 450–1, 476, 486, 495–7, 525–8, 555–60, 564, 608–10.

Weaver K, Rozanski E, Mahony O, Chan D, Freeman L. Use of glargine and lente insulins in cats with diabetes mellitus. *J Vet Intern Med*. 2006. Mar-Apr;20(2):pp 234–8.

DIABETES INSIPIDUS

Definition and cause

Diabetes insipidus (DI) is an uncommon entity in veterinary medicine, and little is known about the physiopathology involved in its development. Two basic syndromes exist: (1) Central diabetes insipidus, in which there is a deficiency in secretion of antidiuretic hormone (ADH); and (2) Nephrogenic diabetes insipidus, whereby toxins affect the kidney and block the physiologic action of ADH. As an example, drugs like alcohol bind to receptor sites for ADH and block its action, leading to diuresis and loss of fluids and electrolytes. It is defined as an imbalance in water metabolism, which leads to polydypsia, polyuria, and low urine specific gravity. Central DI commonly involves genetic inheritance. Nephrogenic DI may be inherited or secondary to kidney disease or metabolic/endocrine diseases such as hyperadrenocorticism (Feldman 1997; Gunn-Moore 2005; Nichols 2001, 2003).

Medical Therapy Rationale, Drug(S) of Choice, and Nutritional Recommendations

Once diagnosed, the therapy of choice for CDI is Desmopressin (DDAVP) and for NDI is chlorothiazide (Nichols 2003).

Anticipated prognosis

The prognosis for medical control is generally good. Underlying causes such as trauma and neoplasia carry a more guarded prognosis. In all instances, continual medical therapy is often required; otherwise death will occur. Current genetic research is focusing on identifying the underlying genetic cause with the goal of correcting the genetic malformation (Nichols 2003).

Integrative veterinary therapies

Because DI is most commonly inherited, the IVM approach is to support pituitary health. In other causes, such as nephrogenic, see the appropriate disease protocol. The recommended protocols include nutraceuticals, medicinal herbs, and combination homeopathics that have anti-inflammatory, tissue-sparing, and regenerative effects on the cells.

Nutrition
General considerations/rationale

Nutritional and glandular support focuses upon the posterior pituitary gland and kidney and their function.

Appropriate nutrients

Nutritional/gland therapy: Glandular pituitary, hypothalamus, and kidney supply intrinsic nutrients that are used to improve organ function and reduce cellular inflammation. This helps to spare these organs from continued degeneration (Cima 2000, Goldstein 2000) (see Gland Therapy in Chapter 2 for a more detailed explanation).

Chinese herbal medicine/acupuncture
General considerations/rationale

In TCM, diabetes insipidus is due to Spleen and Kidney Yang deficiency with Cold accumulation. The Spleen and Kidney are responsible for water metabolism in the body. When there is a Yang deficiency in these organs, one result may be an inability to maintain normal water homeostasis. One sign of Cold in the body, according to TCM, is copious clear urination.

Appropriate Chinese herbs

Because diabetes insipidus is a rare condition, there is little Western research into the use of herbs. The following herbs have actions that may, in the author's opinion, be the mechanism behind their efficacy. Similarly, no Western studies have addressed diabetes insipidus.

Astragalus (Huang qi): Can help promote kidney function. It increases plasma proteins and helps decrease the output of urinary protein (Zhou 1999). Astragalus helped to protect the kidneys of mice with experimental diabetes mellitus (Shi 1999). It may have a similar effect of protecting kidneys in other disease processes.

Rubus (Fu pen zi): Has been shown to increase hormone secretion from the hypothalamus and pituitary (Chen 1996). It also may be able to increase the secretion of vasopressin, although no studies have yet been published.

Gypsum (Shi gao): Was shown to decrease spontaneous water consumption in mice (Zhong Yao Xue 1998).

Homotoxicology
General considerations/rationale
Reckeweg considers DI an Impregnation or Degeneration phase disorder, but there is absolutely nothing published in any homotoxicology literature regarding this condition, so the following is simply theoretical discussion from the author. Tumors can result in diabetes insipidus and represent Dedifferentiation Phase disease. Because all of these phases lie on the right of the Six-Phase Table of Homotoxicology, it is thought that many cases that are so involved would not resolve and would require hormone replacement therapy, aggressive medical management, and careful evaluation of drugs used in the case (Gunn-Moore 2005, Nichols 2001). The emphasis is on management and not cure. Attention to hydration is critical because dehydration can lead to renal compromise and death. Recovery may occur in the event of nephrogenic cases resulting from toxin exposure because diuresis is an Excretion Phase physiologic response that leads to removal of the offending homotoxin. The prognosis for traumatic cases may be better and management of trauma may lead to recovery.

The theoretical approach to such a case involves phase remedies to approach the chronic Impregnation Phase or Degeneration Phase conditions. Clinicians treating such cases biologically must inform owners of the experimental nature of antihomotoxic agents in this condition, and they should carefully record their treatment plans and results and share these with others interested in forwarding biological therapy.

Appropriate homotoxicology formulas
No veterinary studies exist on the use of antihomotoxic agents in diabetes insipidus. Neither author has treated a case biologically. Theoretical possibilities include:

Arteria-Heel: This remedy, renamed *Secale*, addresses peripheral vasculature.

Berberis homaccord: Supports the renal tubular excretion phase and adrenal cortical function (Reckeweg 2000).

Bryaconeel: Indicated in neuralgias and commonly used in geriatric medicine. Acts on serous membranes and meninges.

Coenzyme compositum: Supports energy production through enzyme induction and repair, and is useful in repairing damage to enzyme systems of metabolism and following administration of drugs injurious to metabolism. Phase remedy in Degeneration and Dedifferentiation phases.

Galium-Heel: Phase remedy in matrix and cellular phases. Provides powerful support of the immune system (Echinacea augustifolia). Assists in drainage of cell and matrix, is supportive of renal tubular function, and decreases swelling and edema (Apis mellifica, Galium aparine, and Galium mollugo). It is a critical component in the deep detoxification formula. Dosing should consider clinical condition and response, with the dose reduced if strong reactions are noted (Reckeweg 2000).

Glyoxal compositum: Provides mitochondrial repair of damaged enzyme systems in Degeneration and Dedifferentiation phase disorders.

Hepeel: Provides liver drainage and detoxification.

Lymphomyosot: Used after cortisone therapy and mesenchymal purging in chronic disease states.

Nervoheel: Ignatia and Sepia officinalis are well known remedies for depression and anxiety. These and other ingredients have affinity for neurological tissues.

Ovarium compositum: Provides organ support and drainage of ovaries in females.

Placenta compositum: Supportive of hypophysis after cortisone therapy. Contains sulfur to support enzyme and metabolic repair and repairs vascular structures. Regenerative of hypophyseal-adrenal axis. Used intermittently in endocrine disorders.

Pulsatilla compositum: Used in regulation rigidity cases. Contains Pulsatilla pratensis, Sulfur, and Cortisonum aceticum, and is useful for repairing damage following steroid administration. Often a case will rapidly activate following administration of this agent, and in cases of strong regressive vicariation the administration of *Traumeel S* moves the patient toward healing and resolution. Used in conjunction with catalyst therapy.

Solidago compositum: Deposition Phase remedy that is needed to remove debris from the matrix after regressive vicariation begins.

Syzygium compositum: Reckeweg lists this as a component of basic therapy for diabetes insipidus, but no explanation is presented in any of his writings (Reckeweg 2000).

Testes compositum: Provides organ support and drainage in males.

Thalamus compositum: Supports thalamus, pineal gland, adrenal gland, and cellular regulation through glandular content and homeopathically diluted cyclic adenonsine monophosphate (cAMP). Assists in establishing autoregulation of pyschoneuro-endocrine immune functions (Reckeweg 2000).

Thyroidea compositum: Provides matrix drainage and repair of autoregulation. Contains low levels of thyroid, pineal, spleen, bone marrow, umbilical cord, and liver to support glandular function and repair. Galium aparine drains matrix and cellular components. Cortisonum aceticum, in low potency, assists in repairing damage from excess levels of cortisone. Precursors and Krebs cycle constituents promote energy metabolism through the Michaelis-Menten law of enzyme activity. Pulsatilla and Sulfur assist in regulation rigidity-type situations. Part of the deep detoxification formula (Reckeweg 2000).

Tonsilla compositum: The main antihomotoxic drug for repairing chronic diseases involving endocrine disorders. Supports a wide number of tissues including tonsil, lymph node, bone marrow, umbilical cord (stem cell precursors), spleen, hypothalamus, liver, embryo, and adrenal cortex (Heine 2004). Contains Cortisonum aceticum and thyroid hormone in nanodilutions. Also contains Psorinum for deep constitutional, lack-of-reaction cases. Degeneration phase agent (Reckeweg 2000).

Traumeel S: Provides anti-inflammatory action that is useful in trauma cases and possibly other forms of disease.

Ubichinon compositum: Provides mitochondrial repair of energy production mechanisms. Used in chronic diseases and iatrogenic injury to mitochondria from antibiotic therapy, and is part of the deep detoxification formula.

Authors' suggested protocols

Nutrition
Pituitary/hypothalmus/pineal and kidney support formulas: 1 tablet for each 25 pounds of body weight BID.

Chinese herbal medicine/acupuncture
Formula CDI: 1 capsule per 10 to 20 pounds twice daily according to response. In addition to the herbs mentioned above, CDI contains aconite (Fu zi), albizzia flower (He huan hua), anemarrhena (Zhi mu), cimicifuga (Sheng ma), cinnamon bark (Rou gui), cornus (Shan zhu yu), crataegus (Shan zha), dendrobium (Shi hu), dioscorea (Shan yao), licorice (Gan cao), polygonum stem (Ye jiao teng), poria (Fu ling), rehmannia (Sheng di huang), and wolfberry (Gou qi zi). These additional herbs help increase efficacy.

Monitor urine production and specific gravity. If necessary, combine the herbal supplement with Western therapy. About 50% to 60% of animals need concurrent Western therapy.

Some acupoints that may be of use include ST36, BL20, BL23, and BL13 (Handbook of TCM practitioners 1987).

Homotoxicology (Dose: 10 drops PO for 50-pound dog; 5 drops PO for small dog or cat)
All homotoxicology is done in conjunction with conventional therapy, including hormonal supplementation. Some cases may be able to reduce supportive drug therapy levels after a period of time, but most require lifetime pharmaceutical support.

Reckeweg's oral protocol for humans: Arteria-Heel TID, Nervoheel TID, and Bryaconeel TID as primary therapy. Possibly give those 2 to 6 times daily. Give Syzygium compositum and Traumeel intermittently (Reckeweg 2000).

Reckeweg's injection therapy for humans: Autosanguis therapy with Hypophysis-Suis Injeel, Arsenicum album-Injeel, Bryaconeel Injeel S, and Galium-Heel. Give Hepeel, Acidum phosphoricum-InjeelS, and Acidum lacticum-Injeel for thirst. Give coenzyme compositum and Ubichinon compositum at intervals. Use the collective catalyst pack with Testes compositum for males and Ovarium compositum for females (Reckeweg 2000).

Product sources

Nutrition
Pituitary/hypothalmus/pineal and kidney support formulas: Animal Nutrition Technologies. **Alternatives:** Renal support—Standard Process Veterinary Formulas; Renal Essentials—Vetri Science Laboratories.

Chinese herbal medicine
Formula CDI: Natural Solutions, Inc.

Homotoxicology
BHI/Heel Corporation

REFERENCES

Western medicine references
Feldman EC, Nelson RW. Canine and feline endocrinology and reproduction, Philadelphia: Saunders, 1997.
Gunn-Moore D. Feline endocrinopathies. *Vet Clin North Am Small Anim Pract.* 2005 Jan;35(1):pp 171–210.
Nichols R. Polyuria and polydipsia. Diagnostic approach and problems associated with patient evaluation. *Vet Clin North Am Small Anim Pract.* 2001, Sep;31(5):pp 833–44.
Nichols R. Diabetes Insipidus, In: Tilley L, Smith F. The 5-Minute Veterinary Consult: Canine and Feline, Blackwell Publishing, 2003.

IVM/nutrition references
Cima J. Biochemical Blood Chemistry Evaluation, Palm Beach Gardens, FL., March 2000.
Goldstein R, et al. The BNA Handbook: A Working Manual for Veterinarians, Westport, CT: Animal Nutrition Technologies, 2000. p 47.

Chinese herbal medicine/acupuncture references
Chen SH, et al. Fu Pen Zi water soluble extract solution's effect on hypothalamus-pituitary-gonad axis in rats. *China Journal of Chinese Medicine.* 1996;21(9):560–562.
Handbook of TCM practitioners. Hunan College of TCM, Shanghai Sci and Tech Press, Oct 1987.

Shi JH, et al. *China Journal of TCM Science and Technology.* 1999;15(4):32–34.

Zhong Yao Xue (Chinese Herbology), 1998, 115:119.

Zhou Q. *Journal of Chinese Materia Medica.* 1999;30(5):386–388.

Homotoxicology references

Broadfoot P. The Neuroendocrine System. In: Proceedings of 2006 Homotoxicology Seminar, AHVMA/Heel, Denver, CO, 2006. May 19–21; pp 33–53.

Feldman E, Peterson M. Hypoadrenocorticism. *Vet Clin N Am*; 1984. 14: pp 751–766.

Gunn-Moore D. Feline endocrinopathies. Vet Clin North Am Small Anim Pract. 2005 Jan;35(1):pp 171–210.

Heel. Veterinary Guide, 3rd English edition. Biologische Baden-Baden, Germany: Heilmettel Heel GmbH. 2003. p 23.

Heine H. Homotoxicology and basic regulation: Bystander reaction. *La Medicina Biologica.* 2004.January (1): p 5. Available at http://www.gunainc.com/AllLanguages/ElencoScheda/Elenco_Scheda.asp?SelectionMenu=-1096&xid=9BEB85D787A84914AEED43918A937DBB&id_BoxContent=1077.

Nichols R. Polyuria and polydipsia. Diagnostic approach and problems associated with patient evaluation. Vet Clin North Am Small Anim Pract. 2001. Sep;31(5):pp 833–44.

Reckeweg H. Biotherapeutic Index: Ordinatio Antihomotoxica et Materia Medica, 5th ed. Baden-Baden, Germany: Biologische Heilmittel Heel GMBH, 2000. pp 120, 300–1, 337–8, 414, 415–6, 418–20.

HYPOTHYROIDISM

Definition and cause

True hypothyroidism is a common endocrinopathy in dogs, but is not a significant clinical entity in cats unless their thyroid glands have been damaged directly (i.e., in surgery or radiation). The most common diagnosis in dogs is an immune-mediated autoimmune thyroiditis, wherein lymphocytes attack and destroy vital thyroid tissue, resulting in an inability to produce adequate thyroid hormone. Less common causes include neoplasia, dietary deficiency of iodine, and are secondary to pituitary disease (Chastain 1995; Panciera 1994, 1998; Tyler 2003; Reed 1998).

The basic underlying result is a direct decrease in the production of thyroid hormone and a corresponding decrease in metabolic activity. Congenital hypothyroidism is an infrequent cause (Tyler 2003).

Medical therapy rationale, drug(s) of choice, and nutritional recommendations

Treatment is thyroid hormone replacement, and response to therapy is generally good unless there are additional causes or there is secondary disease (Dixon 2002, Ferguson 2002, Greco 2000, Panciera 1997, Tyler 2003).

Anticipated prognosis

The prognosis for control of hypothyroidism is generally good; however, continual thyroid replacement medication is required to control disease signs. Hypothyrodism that is secondary, or other diseases such as neoplasia or pituitary disease, often have a more guarded prognosis (Tyler 2003, Reed 1998).

Integrative veterinary therapies

The most common underlying cause of hypothyroidism is an autoimmune process. Environmental agents can aggravate this condition, and a link between rabies vaccination and an increase in antithyroid antibody has been reported (Scott-Moncrieff, et al. 2002). Dodds has noticed a connection between vaccination and the appearance of hypothyroidism in purebred dogs and has recommended prudent use of vaccinations in dogs that are at risk (Dodds 1995, 2001, 2002, 2003). Sick euthyroid syndrome is a common entity in small animal practice. In this situation, the thyroid levels are found to be low in association with the presence of other pathologies. Thyroid levels return to normal if these pathologies are successfully addressed. Pharmaceutical agents such as general anesthesia, glucocorticoids, potentiated sulfas, radio-contrast dyes, phenobarbital, iodine, furosemide, aspirin, and phenylbutazone can cause artificially lowered serum thyroid levels and a careful drug history should be taken in cases in which hypothyroidism is encountered (Nelson 1995).

Conventional medical therapy focuses on replacing deficient thyroid hormone, rather than upon the autoimmune process. Hypothyroidism is a classic example of a cellular autoimmune reaction, whereby the target organ begins to weaken from multiple causes such as a vaccine reaction or free radical inflammation. Thyroid cells die and the cellular debris evokes autoantibody production, resulting in an immune attack, cascading inflammation, further cell death, and finally a hypofunctioning gland. The introduction of therapeutic nutrients, medicinal herbs, and biological therapies can often help quiet the autoimmune process and slow ongoing organ degeneration, and may even help reduce the dose of or the reliance upon medication.

There are additional medical options. In clinical studies, the use of desiccated thyroid, which contains both T3 and T4, used in conjunction with thyroxine was more effective than L-thyroxine alone (Bunevicius 1999). Dessicated thyroid (Armour) is a good option to maintain thyroid hormone levels along with alternative therapies. Another study showed that iodine deficiencies can also lead to hypothyroidism, and therefore dietary sources are important (Thilly 1993).

Nutrition
General considerations/rationale
While medical therapy is focused upon thyroid hormone replacement, the nutritional approach adds nutrients, iodine, antioxidants, and gland support for the pituitary/thyroid axis. These nutrients nourish organ cells and help control ongoing inflammation.

Appropriate nutrients
Nutritional/gland therapy: Glandular thyroid, pituitary, and hypothalamus supply the intrinsic nutrients that are used to reduce cellular inflammation and improve organ function. This helps to spare these organs from further immune attack, cascading inflammation, and eventual degeneration (see Gland Therapy in Chapter 2 for a more detailed explanation).

Note: Because hypothyroidism can affect multiple organ systems such as the skin, gastrointestinal, cardiovascular, and central nervous, a medical and physiological blood evaluation is recommended to assess general glandular health. This allows clinicians to formulate therapeutic nutritional protocols that address the pituitary and thyroid glands as well as other organ disease that may be present (Cima 2000, Goldstein 2000)(see Chapter 2, Nutritional Blood Testing, for additional information).

Alpha-lipoic acid (ALA): ALA is involved in mitochondrial activity and is referred to as the universal antioxidant. A potent antioxidant, it has been proven to reduce oxidative stress and inflammation. It has also been shown to increase the effectiveness of other antioxidants, such as vitamins C and E, Coenzyme Q10, and glutathione, making them more readily available for bodily function (Busse 1992, Scholich 1989). This is important in autoimmune reactions such as thyroiditis.

Marracci (2002) and Morini (2004) found that ALA slowed progression of the autoimmune response and the disease process. Free radical inflammation is implicated as the initiator of many disease processes that are discussed in this book. ALA and other antioxidants have the proven function of reducing this initiating inflammation, and therefore are indicated in the prevention of many of these disease conditions.

Coenzyme Q10: CoenzymeQ10 is a strong antioxidant that helps reduce the associated inflammation that is the predecessor to many chronic diseases. CoQ10 has indications in the prevention and treatment of common diseases such as gingivitis and periodontal disease, heart disease, arthritis, diabetes, and many types of cancer (Gaby 1998, Shigeta 1966).

Chinese herbal medicine/acupuncture
General considerations/rationale
Hypothyroidism is a result of Spleen and Kidney Qi and Yang deficiency. The Spleen controls the muscles; therefore, Qi and Yang deficiency in the Spleen can lead to muscle weakness. The patient usually feels cold, with poor blood circulation, and fatigue, which is due to Kidney Qi and Yang deficiency.

Treatment is aimed at increasing the thyroid hormone levels and reversing the secondary signs such as high cholesterol and muscle weakness.

Appropriate Chinese herbs
Alisma (Ze xie): Lowers the serum cholesterol and LDL levels (Institute of Pharmacy 1976).

Dioscorea (Shan yao): Contains diosgenin, a compound which decreases intestinal cholesterol absorption and therefore blood cholesterol levels (Cayen 1979, Zagoya 1971). It also increases muscular endurance and improves muscle contractility (Zhang 1996).

Rehmannia (Shu di huang): Can increase serum T4 levels (Qu 1998, Zhang 1999, Hou 1992).

Sage tangle (Kun bu): Can reverse hypothyroidism due to iodine deficiency (Jiangsu New Medical College 1998). In addition, it treats the sequela of hypothyroidism. It can decrease total serum cholesterol, b-lipoprotein, and triglyceride, and can raise the levels of HDL-C and HDL2-C (Tang 1989). It promotes the elimination of cholesterol (Huang 1998).

Sargassum (Hai zao): Contains high levels of iodine (Zhong Yao Xue 1998).

Wolfberry (Gou qi zi): Lowers the total serum cholesterol, triglyceride level and the LDL-C fraction (Wang 1998).

Acupuncture has successfully treated hypothyroidism. In one study, acupuncture was used to treat hypothyroidism in patients recovering from serious brain injuries. Thyroid function improved in all 14 patients and the T4 and T3 values returned to normal (Yu 1996).

Homotoxicology
General considerations/rationale
Autoimmune thyroiditis represents an Impregnation Phase disorder in the early stages, which may progress rapidly to a Degeneration Phase homotoxicosis. Patients with genetic defects may be properly classified as Degeneration Phase cases and handled appropriately. Sick euthyroid syndrome cases can be assisted by organ support, detoxification, drainage, and excretion of homotoxins through various antihomotoxic agents. Proper diagnosis, treatment, and monitoring are required to assure maximum success, and the clinician should recognize that in many cases hormone replacement therapy is vital to long-term health and well being.

Autoimmune thyroiditis can be attenuated by the use of antihomotoxic drugs (particularly Thyroidea compositum). Early screening with the purpose of identifying at-risk dogs may assist breeders in reducing the incidence of this condition, and may have the further benefit of identifying dogs with a predisposition to thyroid dysfunction. Such dogs may benefit from early treatment with antihomotoxic drugs. Supplementation with thyroid hormone is needed in cases with low levels and thyroid hormone replacement therapy is compatible with antihomotoxic drugs.

Appropriate homotoxicology formulas

As with all homotoxicoses, therapy should begin in the earlier phases of the disorder. Common remedies that may prove useful in hypothyroidism include:

BHI-Enzyme: Contains Baryta (also found in *Coenzyme compositum*) for goiter (Reckeweg 2002).

Coenzyme compositum: Provides metabolic support of cytoplasmic energy production. Degeneration Phase remedy.

Echinacea compositum: The components Influenzinum and Staphylococcus nosodes both have indications in cases of thyroid dysfunction. Staph nosode can be used to good effect in connective tissue lesions (possibly also in obesity) and in thyroid illnesses. It is especially effective in combination with Streptococcus haemolyticus nosode, which is also contained in *Echinacea compositum*. Influenzinum is used in patients with a tendency to corpulence and adiposity—even in children—arising from thyroid hypofunction. It has tonic action in exhaustion, tiredness, and chronic hoarseness (Reckeweg 2002).

Galium-Heel: Provides cellular drainage and detoxification. Important phase remedy in Deposition, Degeneration, and Dedifferentiation phase homotoxicoses.

Hepar compositum: Assists in detoxification, drainage, and organ support of the liver. Used as part of the deep detoxification formula that is commonly applied to patients in deeper phases (Deposition, Impregnation, Degeneration, and Dedifferentiation).

Lymphomyosot: Provides lymph drainage and support. Contains Levothyroidinum (Thyroxine) in homeopathic dilution, which can stimulate endocrine function per the Arndt-Schulz Principle. This formula should be used with caution in patients that are sensitive to compounds that contain iodine. It is an important drainage and detoxifying agent in all Impregnation, Degeneration, and Dedifferentiation phase disorders.

Molybdan compositum: Supplements trace minerals and regulates mineral metabolism. Use 1 tablet for trace mineral supplementation daily for 3 to 4 days and then every second or third day. If undesirable symptoms occur, discontinue for several days and restart as needed at a longer dose frequency such as once weekly. No adverse side effects are expected at normal dosing, but use caution with this preparation if combining therapy with other trace mineral supplements (Reckeweg 2000). Keep out of the reach of children or pets. The authors have experienced no undesirable effects from this product when properly dosed.

Mucosa compositum: Supports mucosal elements and helps with repair and detoxification. Phase remedy in Degeneration Phase disorders.

Placenta compositum: Provides repair and detoxification of vascular structures in chronic disease. Useful for patients with cold extremities. May assist stem cell function in repair.

Psorinoheel: Constitutional remedy that is useful in Excretion Phase and Degeneration Phase disorders. Consider in suspect genetic cases, especially those with dermal issues and/or seizure disorders.

Solidago compositum: Assists in detoxification, drainage, and organ support of the kidney and urogenital systems. Used as part of the deep detoxification formula that is commonly applied to patients in deeper phases (Deposition, Impregnation, Degeneration, and Dedifferentiation).

Strumeel: Contains Calcium iodatum for chronic glandular indurations, goiter, and tonsillar hypertrophy. The iodine component of this remedy activates metabolic processes and connective tissue function (Reckeweg 2002). This remedy also contains Fucus vesiculosis and Spongia tosta, as found in *Thyroidea compositum*.

Thyroidea compositum: The main formula for hypothyroidism; it is also indicated in Impregnation Phase cases. It is particularly useful in deep matrix drainage and detoxification. Contains glandular therapy elements of thyroid, thymus, pineal gland, spleen, bone marrow, umbilical cord (stem cell elements), and liver, which gives it a far reaching organotrophic effect. Early use may delay onset of clinical disease; some patients have thyroid hormone levels improve some weeks to months after initial therapy (Palmquist 2005). Also contains Cortisonum aceticum (cortisone acetate) for adrenal cortex damage and iatrogenic damage from prior steroid therapy, and numerous metabolic precursors of the citric acid cycle that benefit metabolism. Galium (goose grass) drains cellular elements. It is helpful in a wide variety of preneoplastic and neoplastic conditions (Reckeweg 2000).

This agent may bring on desirable regressive vicariation and should be assisted with proper biological support. Areas of depigmentation and alopecia may become inflamed as homotoxins are metabolized and excreted. It is not uncommon for patients undergoing regressive vicariation to have discharge from the eyes, ears, and other mucous membranes. These are not adverse reactions, but rather helpful biological responses. If they are excessive, reduce the dosage frequency and continue forward gently. Long-term therapy is often needed. This is an ingredient in the deep detoxification formula that is so commonly used in deeper homotoxicoses. It also has components with specific affinity for thyroid disorders: Calcium fluoratum, Fucus vesiculosis, and Spongia tosta (Reckeweg 2002).

Tonsilla compositum: Contains Thyroxine. If the thyroid gland is absent, either in thyroid aplasia or thyroidectomy, a typical deficiency disease known as myxoedema develops. The metabolism of food and energy is reduced by up to 50% in degeneration of the thyroid gland, and possibly in cases of goiter with colloid atrophy, but it can be normalized again by the administration of thyroid hormone. The thyroid hormone has particular importance for the functioning of the interstitial mesenchyme, which is generally accelerated and activated by thyroxine, thyroidinum, or the thyroid hormones. Thus, doses of the hormone are given not in substitutive, but in excitative dosage (higher potencies), and are included in combination remedies that are aimed at activating the mesenchyme and removing the homotoxic deposits in the connective tissue.

Ubichinon compositum: Provides metabolic support of mitochondrial elements. Degeneration phase remedy that is useful in reversing damage from antibiotics to the mitochondrial membrane and enzyme system.

Authors' suggested protocols

Nutrition
Thyroid and pituitary support formulas: 1 tablet for each 25 pounds of body weight BID.

Alpha-lipoic acid: 10 mgs per 15 pounds of body weight daily (maximum, 100 mgs).

Coenzyme Q10: 25 mgs for every 10 pounds of body weight daily.

Chinese herbal medicine/acupuncture
Formula H81 Hypothyroidism: 1 capsule per 10 to 20 pounds twice daily to effect. In addition to the herbs described above, H81 Hypothyroidism also contains aconite (Hei fu zi), angelica root (Dang gui), antler (Lu jiao), cinnamon bark (Rou gui), cistanche (Rou cong rong), cnidium (Chuan xiong), cornus (Shan zhu yu), cuscata (Tu si zi), eucommia bark (Du zhong), ginger (Gan jiang), and laminaria (Hai dai). These herbs increase the efficacy of the formula.

The authors recommend the following acupuncture points: BL20, BL23, and GV4 (Lei 1996).

Homotoxicology (Dose: 10 drops PO for 50-pound dog; 5 drops PO for small dog or cat)
Symptom remedy: Thyroidea compositum, as a single remedy by injection (SQ, IV, IM) or 1 tablet 1 to 3 times weekly PO, or as part of the deep detoxification formula listed below. Abropernol and Strumeel given BID. All these can be combined and then administered BID orally.

Deep detoxification formula: Galium-Heel, Lymphomyosot, Hepar compositum, Solidago compositum, Thyroidea compositum, Coenzyme compositum, Ubichinon compositum mixed together and given 1 to 3 times weekly PO.

Product sources

Nutrition
Thyroid and pituitary/hypothalamus/pineal support formulas: Animal Nutrition Technologies. **Alternative**: Canine Thyroid Support—Standard Process Veterinary Formulas.

Alpha-lipioic acid: Source Naturals.

Coenzyme Q10: Vetri Science; Rx Vitamins for Pets for Pets; Integrative Therapeutics; Thorne Veterinary Products.

Chinese herbal medicine
Formula H81 Hypothyroidism: Natural Solutions, Inc.

Homotoxicology
BHI/Heel Corporation

REFERENCES

Western medicine references

Chastain CB, Panciera DL. Hypothyroid diseases. In: Ettinger SJ, Feldman EC, eds. Textbook of veterinary internal medicine. 4th ed. Philadelphia: WB Saunders, 1995:1487–1501.

Dixon RM, Reid SWJ, Mooney CT. Treatment and therapeutic monitoring of canine hypothyroidism. *Journal of Small Animal Practice* 2002;43, 334–340.

Ferguson DC. Thyroid hormone replacement therapy—the numbers game. A physiological perspective. Proceedings of the 20th Annual ACVIM Forum, Dallas, TX, 2002. 681–682.

Greco DS. Use of endogenous thyrotropin and free thyroxine determinations for monitoring thyroid replacement treatment in dogs with hypothyroidism. In: Bonagura JD, ed. Kirk's Current Veterinary Therapy XIII. Small Animal Practice. Philadelphia: WB Saunders Company, 2000. 330–333.

Panciera DL. Hypothyroidism in dogs: 66 cases (1987–1992). *J Am Vet Med Assoc* 1994;204:761–767.

Panciera DL. Treatment of hypothyroidism: consequences and complications. *Canine Practice* 1997;22(1):57–58.

Panciera DL. Canine hypothyroidism. In: Mooney CT, Torrance A, eds. BSAVA Manual of Small Animal Endocrinology, 2nd ed. Cheltenham BSAVA Publications, 1998; pp 103–113.

Tyler W. Hypothyroidism. In: Tilley L, Smith F. The 5-Minute Veterinary Consult: Canine and Feline, Blackwell Publishing, 2003.

Reed Larsen P, Davies TF, Hay ID. The thyroid gland. In: Wilson JD, Foster DW, Kronenberg HM, Reed Larsen P, eds. Williams Textbook of Endocrinology, 9th ed. Philadelphia: WB Saunders Company, 1998. pp 389–515.

IVM references

Bunevicius R, Kazanavicius G, Zalinkevicius R, Prange AJ Jr. Effects of thyroxine as compared with thyroxine plus triiodothyronine in patients with hypothyroidism. *N Engl J Med* 1999;340:424–9.

Dodds WJ. Estimating disease prevalence with health surveys and genetic screening. *Adv Vet Sc Comp Med.* 1995. 39:pp 29–96.

Dodds WJ. Vaccination protocols for dogs predisposed to vaccine reactions. *J Am An Hosp Assoc.* 2001. 38:pp 1–4.

Dodds WJ. Complementary and alternative veterinary medicine: the immune system. *Clin Tech Sm An Pract,* 2002. 17:pp 58–63.

Dodds WJ. Advocate for serologic testing after vaccination. *J Am Vet Med Assoc.* 2003. 222:pp 149–150.

Scott-Moncrieff JC, Azcona-Olivera J, Glickman NW, Glickman LT, Hogen, Esch H. Evaluation of antithyroglobulin antibodies after routine vaccination in pet and research dogs. *J Am Vet Med Assoc.* 2002. Aug 15;221(4):pp 515–21.

Thilly CH, Swennen B, Bourdoux P, et al. The epidemiology of iodine-deficiency disorders in relation to goitrogenic factors and thyroid-stimulating-hormone regulation. *Am J Clin Nutr* l 1993;57(2 Suppl):267S–70S.

Nutrition references

Busse E, Zimmer G, Schorpohl B, et al. Influence of alpha-lipoic acid on intracellular glutathione in vitro and in vivo. *Arzneimittelforschung* 1992;42:829–31.

Cima J. Biochemical Blood Chemistry Evaluation, Palm Beach Gardens, FL., March 2000.

Gaby AR. Coenzyme Q10. In: A Textbook of Natural Medicine, by Pizzorno JE, Murray MT. Seattle: Bastyr University Press, 1998, V:CoQ10-1-8.

Goldstein R, et al. The BNA Handbook: A Working Manual for Veterinarians, Westport, CT: Animal Nutrition Technologies 2000.

Marracci GH, Jones RE, McKeon GP, Bourdette DN. Alpha lipoic acid inhibits T cell migration into the spinal cord and suppresses and treats experimental autoimmune encephalomyelitis. *J Neuroimmunol.* 2002;131(1–2):104–114.

Morini M, Roccatagliata L, Dell'Eva R, et al. Alpha-lipoic acid is effective in prevention and treatment of experimental autoimmune encephalomyelitis. *J Neuroimmunol.* 2004; 148(1–2):146–153.

Scholich H, Murphy ME, Sies H. Antioxidant activity of dihydrolipoate against microsomal lipid peroxidation and its dependence on alpha-tocopherol. *Biochem Biophys Acta* 1989;1001:256–61.

Shigeta Y, Izumi K, Abe H. Effect of coenzyme Q7 treatment on blood sugar and ketone bodies of diabetics. *J Vitaminol* 1966;12:293–8.

Chinese herbal medicine/acupuncture references

Cayen MN, Dvornik D. Effect of diosgenin on lipid metabolism in rats. *J Lipid Res* 1979;20(2):162–174.

Hou SL, et al. *China Journal of Materia Medica.* 1992;17(5):301.

Huang ZS, et al. *China Journal of Ocean Medicinal Products.* 1998;17(1):35–37.

Lei YM, et al. Chinese famous TCM doctors formulas for terminal illness. Guang Xi Sci and Tech Press, Dec 1996.

Institute of Pharmacy. People's Experiment Hospital of Zhejiang. Chinese Materia Medica Bulletin. 1976;(7):26–30.

Jiangsu New Medical College (ed). Dictionary of Chinese Medicines. Shanghai Science and Techonology Press; 1998.

Qu FY, et al. *Heilongjiang Journal of TCM.* 1998;21(5):6.

Tang ZL, et al. *Journal of Integrated Medicine.* 1989;9(4): 223–225.

Wang DS, et al. The dose-effect relation in Gou Qi Zi's effect of counteracting experimental hyperlipidemia and liver lipid peroxidation. *Journal of Applied Integrated Medicine.* 1998;11(3): 199–200.

Yu Q, et al. Acupuncture use to treat hypothyroidism in patients recovering from severe brain injuries. *China Journal of Acupuncture.* 1996;16(8):1–3.

Zagoya JCD, Lagun J, Guzman-Garcia J. Studies on the regulation of cholesterol metabolism by the use of structural analogue, diosgenin. *Biochemical Pharmacologiy* 1971;20: 3471–3480.

Zhang N, et al. *China Journal of Sports Medicine.* 1996;15(2):114–117.

Zhang PX, et al. *China Journal of Gerontology.* 1999;19(3):174–175.

Zhong Yao Xue (Chinese Herbology), 1998; 629:631.

Homotoxicology references

Broadfoot PJ, Demers J, Palmquist R. Proceedings of 2006 AHVMA and Heel Homotoxicology Seminar: Endocrinology. 2006. May 19–21, pp 38, 61, 86–90, 103–5.

Nelson R, Feldman E. The endocrine system and metabolic disorders. In: Siegal M, ed. University of California-Davis School of Veterinary Medicine. Books of dogs: a complete medical reference for dogs and puppies. New York: HarperCollins, 1995;pp 313–314.

Reckeweg H. Biotherapeutic Index: Ordinatio Antihomotoxica et Materia Medica, 5th ed. Baden-Baden, Germany: Biologische Heilmittel Heel GMBH, 2000. pp 366–7, 415–6.

Reckeweg H. Homeopathia Antihomotoxica Materia Medica, 4th ed. Baden-Baden, Germany: Arelia-Verlag GMBH, 2002. pp. 169, 197–8, 305, 358, 543, 544, 576.

HYPERTHYROIDISM

Definition and cause

Hyperthyroidism, defined as an excessive production of thyroid hormone by the thyroid gland, is one of the most common endocrine diseases of senior cats. It is less frequently seen in dogs, and is usually associated with malignancy of the thyroid gland.

In cats, the underlying pathology is a hyperplastic, overactive gland or a nodular or adenomatous mass that is usually benign. Because of the thyroid gland's central role in metabolism, many organ systems are affected by the overactivity of the gland and the resultant increased levels of thyroid hormone (Feldman 1996; Graves 1992, 1997, 2003; Mooney 2002; Peterson 1994).

Medical therapy rationale, drug(s) of choice, and nutritional recommendations

After the positive diagnosis of hyperthyroidism, medical therapy is directed at the hyperactivity and the resultant elevation in circulating thyroid hormone levels. Treatment may involve surgical removal of the overactive gland, radioactive iodine, or anti-thyroid medication such as methimazole or ipodate (Oragraffin). Because hyperthyroidism can affect multiple organ systems, therapy must take into consideration damage from elevated blood pressure and other affected organs such as the heart and kidney (Graves 1995, 2003; Hoffman 2003; Mooney 1997; Murray 1997).

Because of the elevated rates of metabolism, a highly bioavailable and absorbable diet that is rich in protein is recommended (Martin 2002, Graves 2003).

Anticipated prognosis

The prognosis is dramatically improved if there are no secondary organ system problems such as heart or kidney damage. Medical management is based upon client compliance and potential side effects from the drugs, and therefore a better prognosis is seen with either surgical removal or radioactive iodine treatments (Graves 2003).

Integrative veterinary therapies

Proper handling of hyperthyroid patients is important to preserve their health because of the toxic effects of excessive thyroid hormone on the heart, kidney, and liver. Hypertension and cardiac and renal disease frequently result from hyperthyroidism.

Recent studies have shown a significant difference in the survival of cats depending upon their treatment. The use of methimazole followed by I_{131} isotope therapy gave excellent results (Milner 2006). It is recommended that red blood cell and white blood cell levels be monitored while the patient is on pharmaceutical agents to detect toxic reactions to medications. Careful supervision of renal function is strongly recommended.

IVM offers viable alternatives to clients that resist surgery, radioactive iodine treatment, or methimazole because of side effects such as vomiting, anorexia, and weight loss. The use of lower doses of methimazole in combination with alternative therapies, nutraceuticals, medicinal herbs, and antihomotoxic agents offers these clients a good alternative along with proper monitoring of thyroxine levels.

Nutrition
General considerations/rationale

The cause of thyroid gland enlargement or overproduction of hormones remains unclear. The authors' opinion is that a possible mechanism can be a process similar to goiter in people, which can be caused by an autoimmune process or exposure to environmental toxins or medication (Gaitan 1988, 1990; Goldstein 2005).

This cellular immune attack of the thyroid can result in gland hyperactivity in cats and similarly gland hypofunctioning in dogs. The therapeutic nutritional approach therefore is directed at quieting the underlying free-radical-induced inflammatory process (from exposure to environmental chemicals, overvaccination, other diseases, etc.), ultimately leading to the overactive thyroid gland.

Appropriate nutrients

Nutritional/gland therapy: Glandular thyroid, pituitary, and hypothalamus as well as kidney and heart supply the intrinsic nutrients that are used to reduce cellular inflammation and improve organ function. This helps to protect and spare the thyroid (and other organs) from ongoing immune attack, cascading inflammation, and eventual degeneration (see Gland Therapy in Chapter 2 for a more detailed explanation).

Alpha-lipoic acid: ALA is involved in mitochondrial activity and is referred to as the universal antioxidant. A potent antioxidant, it has been proven to reduce oxidative stress and inflammation. It has been shown to increase the effectiveness of other antioxidants such as vitamins C and E, Coenzyme Q10, and glutathione, making them more readily available for bodily function (Busse 1992, Scholich 1989).

Marracci (2002) and Morini (2004) found that ALA slowed progression of the autoimmune response and the disease process. Free radical inflammation is implicated as the initiator of many diseases discussed in this book. ALA and other antioxidants have the proven function of reducing this initiating inflammation, and therefore are indicated in the prevention of many cellular autoimmune disease conditions.

Coenzyme Q10 (CoQ10 or ubiquinone): Coenzyme Q10 is a strong antioxidant that helps reduce the associated inflammation that is the predecessor to many chronic diseases. CoQ10 has indications in the prevention and treatment of common diseases (Gaby 1998, Shigeta 1966).

Chinese herbal medicine
General considerations/rationale

In TCM, hyperthyroidism is a combination of Qi and Phlegm stagnation, Yang excess in the Liver, and Yin deficiency in the Liver and Heart.

Excess Yang energy causes nervousness, tachycardia, and hypertension. This increased blood pressure in turn causes the elevated liver enzymes or renal damage often associated with a hyperthyroid state. Yin deficiency can lead to a relative Yang excess. In Western terms this can be manifested as panting to cool the body. The Shen (Mind) resides in the Heart. The Yin is the fluid aspect of the body. It nourishes the body. Yin deficiency in the Heart means that the Shen is not nourished. Behavioral changes occur when the Mind is not nourished. This refers to crying at night, aggressive behaviors, nervousness, etc. Because the Liver is responsible for the smooth flow of Qi, it causes irritability when there is Qi stagnation in the Liver. Phlegm stagnation is a mass, i.e., the hypertrophied thyroid gland.

Appropriate Chinese herbs

Dioscorea bulb (Huang yao zi): Was used to treat 25 patients with thyroid tumors with a 80% efficacy rate (Fu Jian Yi Xue Yuan Xue Bao, 1964). There was no effect on normal thyroid glands in rats, but it markedly reduced the size of the gland in rats with experimentally induced thyroid gland hypertrophy (Chang Yong Zhong Yao Xian Dai Yan Jiu Yu Lin Chuan 1995).

Figwort root (Xuan shen): Has been shown to cause vasodilation in rabbits and mice. In addition to lowering blood pressure, it can also decrease the heart rate (Zhong Yao Yao Li Yu Ying Yong 1983).

Fritillaria (Bei mu): Has antihypertensive effects (Zhong Yao Xue 1998).

Gentiana (Long dan cao): Demonstrates hepatoprotective effects from a variety of insults and increases the content of hepatic glycogen. Two of the components, gentiopicroside and sweroside, counteract CCl4- or GALN-induced liver damage. Gentiopicroside also reduces liver lipid peroxidation in hungry mice (Zhang 1991, Zhong Guo Yao Li Xue Tong Bao, 1986, Hu 1989). In addition, it decreased liver enzymes in humans with chronic infectious hepatitis (Shang Hai Zhong Yi Yao Za Zhi 1965). Another component, gentianine, has sedative effects (Lei 1982).

Prunella (Xia ku cao): Helps to normalize blood pressure in patients with hypertension (Zhong Yao Yao Li Yu Ying Yong 1983).

Rehmannia (Sheng di huang): In an experiment in which rehmannia was given to hyperthyroid mice, it lowered the concentration level of T3 and increased the level of T4. This resulted in a decrease in polydipsia and polyuria and prevented the weight loss associated with hyperthyoridism (Hou 1992). In addition, it also decreases blood pressure (Zhong Yao Xue 1998).

Sage tangle (Kun bu): Contains laminine, which reduces blood pressure (Yao Xue Za Zhi 1983). In one study, sage tangle was capable of slowing the metabolic rate and relieving the signs in people with hyperthyroidism (Jiangsu New Medical College). Another study in 110 humans showed a 76.4% efficacy in treating hypertension (Zhong Cao Yao Tong Xun 1974).

Salvia (Dan shen): Decreases blood pressure (Guo Wai Yi Xue Zhong Yi Zhong Yao Fen Ce 1991). It has hepatoprotective effects. Salvia promotes the regeneration of liver cells and has been used in mice with cirrhosis (Zhong Xi Yi Jie He Za Zhi 1988).

Scorpion (Quan xie): Decreases the heart rate and causes prolonged decreases in blood pressure (Shen Yang Yi Xue Yuan Xue Bao 1987).

Tortoise shell (Bie jia): Has been shown to decrease the size of nodules and masses and may help to decrease the size of the thyroid gland (Zhong Cao Yao Xue 1980).

White peony (Bai shao): Can cause mild vasodilation and thereby reduce blood pressure (Zhong Guo Yao Li Xue Tong Bao 1986). It also has sedative effects to help with the anxiety or irritability hyperthyroid patients experience (Zhong Yao Tong Bao 1985).

Homotoxicology
General considerations/rationale

Hyperthyroidism most commonly occurs in small animal veterinary medicine due to a benign tumor in the thyroid of cats or a malignant tumor in dogs. This represents a Dedifferentiation Phase disorder. Short-term elevation of serum thyroid hormone can occur during recovery from illness and is a natural and desirable response that does not require specific treatment.

Dobias (2006) has reported limited success in treating hyperthyroid cats using homeopathy, particularly with a remedy known as *Natrum muraticum* (Nat mur), which consists of homeopathically prepared sodium chloride. Patients that fit this symptom picture may respond, and this response could suggest toxicity from excessive levels of sodium chloride in pet diets or some other imbalance in halogen metabolism that later negatively impacts the thyroid gland, leading to disease. This is an interesting area for further investigation (Dobias 2006).

Appropriate homotoxicology formulas

Surgery or radiation therapy is recommended in cases of likely malignant neoplasia. Antihomotoxic drugs can be given according to the patient's condition (see Cardiac Arryhthmias, Cardiomyopathies, and Congestive Heart Failure in Chapter 9; Acute and Chronic Nephritis in Chapter 15; and cancer in chapters 31 and 32). Other hyperthyroid patients may benefit from the following:

Aletris-Heel: Treats exhaustion, anemia, weakness, and thyrotoxicosis.

China homaccord: Treats weakness and exhaustion.

Coenzyme compositum: Provides metabolic support.

Engystol N: May help to clear the matrix in cases of viral impregnation.

Gelsemium homaccord: Used for affectations of the head, headache, and weakness of the head and posterior.

Glyoxal compositum: Used in all Dedifferentiation Phase disorders as a phase remedy.

Glonoin homaccord: Nitroglycerin, the active agent, supports heart function and is effective for the sensation of palpitations that originate in the chest and extend up the neck (which causes cats to vocalize loudly at night). Glonoin is also useful for a sensation of imminent death. It contains Lycopus for tachyarrythmias and Crataegus for cardiac muscle support (Reckeweg 2000).

Natrum homaccord: Contains Natrum muraticum, which may prove useful according to work in classical homeopathy by Dobias. Its effectiveness is unproven at this time. Palmquist has attempted two feline cases with no measurable benefit.

Strumeel: Supports thyroid tissues following initial therapy for thyrotoxicosis.

Thalamus compositum: Used for central control, particularly in neoplastic phases.

Thyroidea compositum: Supports hormonal axes, and the thyroid in particular. Viscum is indicated in Dedifferentiation Phases. Also provides central support of the hypothalamus and pituitary.

Tonico-Injeel: Used for hypertension, exhaustion, depression, neural injury, neuroasthenia, and gastric and hepatic upsets.

Traumeel: Used for inflammatory phases, which may contribute to the progression of this disease.

Ubichinon compositum: Provides metabolic support.

Veratrum homaccord: Treats vomiting, diarrhea, and personality changes that tend toward psychosis.

Authors' suggested protocols

Nutrition

Kidney and cardiac support formulas: One-half capsule BID.

Thyro complex: One-half capsule SID.

Alpha-lipoic acid: 35 mgs daily.

Coenzyme Q10: 30 mgs for daily.

Chinese herbal medicine

Formula H55 Hyperthyroidism: 1 capsule per 10 to 20 pounds twice daily. The dose is adjusted based upon clinical and laboratory findings. Clinical observation found this formula helps to reduce T3 and T4 levels, the size of thyroid glands in most the cases, and the heart rate, and improves the liver functions.

In addition to the herbs mentioned above, Hyperthyroidism contains anemarrhena (Zhi mu), cremastra (Shan ci gu), gentiana root (Long dan cao), gypsum (Shi gao), oyster shell (Mu li), sargassum (Hai zao), tortoise plastron (Gui ban), vaccaria (Wang bu liu xing), and zedoaria (E zhu).

Homotoxicology (Dose: 10 drops PO for 50-pound dog; 5 drops PO for small dog or cat)

Symptom formula: Glonoin homaccord, Gelsemium homaccord, Aletris-Heel (thyrotoxicosis), or Tonico-Injeel (thyrotoxicosis and hypertension) mixed together and given PO TID.

Deep detoxification formula: Galium-Heel, Thyroidea compositum, Hepar compositum, Coenzyme compositum, Ubichinon compositum mixed together and given every 3 days.

Product sources

Nutrition

Kidney and cardiac support formulas: Animal Nutrition Technologies. **Alternatives:** Formula CV—Rx Vitamins for Pets; Cardiac Support Formula—Standard Process Veterinary Formulas; Cardio-Strength—Vetri Science Laboratories; Bio-Cardio—Thorne Veterinary Products; Renal Support—Standard Process Veterinary Formulas; Renal Essentials—Vetri Science Laboratories.

Thyro complex: Professional Complementary Health Products.

Alpha-lipioic acid: Source Naturals.

Coenzyme Q10: Vetri Science; Rx Vitamins for Pets; Integrative Therapeutics; Thorne Veterinary Products.

Chinese herbal medicine

Formula H55 Hyperthyroidism: Natural Solutions, Inc.

Homotoxicology

BHI/Heel Corporation

REFERENCES

Western medicine references

Feldman EC, Nelson RW. (Feline Hyperthyroidism. In: Canine and Feline Endocrinology and Reproduction, 2nd ed. Philadelphia: Oxford University Press, 1996.pp.1447–1479.

Graves TK, Peterson ME. Occult hyperthyroidism in cats. In: Kirk RW, Bonagura JD, eds. Current veterinary therapy XI. Philadelphia: Saunders, 1992:334–337.

Graves TK. Complications of treatment and concurrent illness associated with feline hyperthyroidism. In: Kirk RW, Bonagura JD, eds. Current veterinary therapy XII. Philadelphia: Saunders, 1995.

Graves TK. Hyperthyroidism and the kidney. In: August JR, ed. Consultations in feline internal medicine 3, Philadelphia: Saunders, 1997.

Graves TK. Feline hyperthyroidism: an update. Proceedings of the 9th annual Fred Scott Feline Symposium, Cornell University, 1997.

Graves TK. In: Tilley L, Smith F. The 5-Minute Veterinary Consult: Canine and Feline, Blackwell Publishing, 2003.

Hoffman G, Marks SL, Taboada J, et al. Transdermal methimazole treatment in cats with hyperthyroidism. *J Feline Med Surg;* 2003;5: 77–82.

Martin K, Rossing M, et al. Evaluation of dietary and environmental risk factors for hyperthyroidism in cats. *J Amer Vet Med Assoc* 2000.217(6):853.

Mooney C. Update on the medical management of hyperthyroidism. In: August JR, ed. Consultations in Feline Internal Medicine 3, Philadelphia: WB Saunders. , p. 155, 1997.

Mooney CT. Pathogenesis of feline hyperthyroidism. *J Feline Med Surg.* 2002;4:167–169.

Murray LAS, Peterson ME. Ipodate treatment of hyperthyroidism in cats. *J Amer Vet Med Assoc* 1997;211:63.

Peterson ME. Hyperthyroid diseases. In: Ettinger SJ, Feldman EC, eds. Textbook of veterinary internal medicine. 4th ed. Philadelphia: Saunders, 1994.

IVM reference

Milner R, Channell C, Levy J, Schaer M. Survival times for cats with hyperthyroidism treated with iodine 131, methimazole, or both. *JAVMA,* 2006. Feb 15;228(4): pp 559–563.

Nutrition references

Busse E, Zimmer G, Schorpohl B, et al. Influence of alpha-lipoic acid on intracellular glutathione in vitro and in vivo. *Arzneimittelforschung* 1992;42:829–31.

Gaby AR. Coenzyme Q10. In: A Textbook of Natural Medicine, by Pizzorno JE, Murray MT. Seattle: Bastyr University Press, 1998, V:CoQ10-1-8.

Gaitan E. Goitrogens. *Baillieres Clin Endocrinol Metab* 1988;2:683–702.

Gaitan E. Goitrogens in food and water. *Annu Rev Nutr* 1990;10:21–39.

Marracci GH, Jones RE, McKeon GP, Bourdette DN. Alpha lipoic acid inhibits T cell migration into the spinal cord and

suppresses and treats experimental autoimmune encephalomyelitis. *J Neuroimmunol.* 2002;131(1–2):104–114.

Morini M, Roccatagliata L, Dell'Eva R, et al. Alpha-lipoic acid is effective in prevention and treatment of experimental autoimmune encephalomyelitis. *J Neuroimmunol.* 2004; 148(1–2):146–153.

Scholich H, Murphy ME, Sies H. Antioxidant activity of dihydrolipoate against microsomal lipid peroxidation and its dependence on alpha-tocopherol. *Biochem Biophys Acta* 1989;1001:256–61.

Shigeta Y, Izumi K, Abe H. Effect of coenzyme Q7 treatment on blood sugar and ketone bodies of diabetics. *J Vitaminol* 1966;12:293–8.

Chinese herbal medicine/acupuncture references

Chang Yong Zhong Yao Xian Dai Yan Jiu Yu Lin Chuan (Recent Study and Clinical Applications of Common Traditional Chinese Medicine), 1995;464:465.

Fu Jian Yi Xue Yuan Xue Bao (*Journal of Fujian University of Medicine*), 1964;2:21.

Guo Wai Yi Xue Zhong Yi Zhong Yao Fen Ce (Monograph of Chinese Herbology from Foreign Medicine), 1991; 13(3):41.

Hou SL, et al. *China Journal of Materia Medica.* 1992;17(5):301.

Hu RQ, et al. The effect of sweroside on the spleen volume of mice with GALN-induced acute liver damages. *Journal of Yunan College of TCM.* 1989;12(2):8.

Jiangsu New Medical College (ed). Dictionary of Chinese Medicines. Shanghai Science and Technology Press; 1998.

Lei WY, et al. Swertiamarin's central inhibitory effects. *Journal of Chinese Materia Medica.* 1982;13(8):368.

Shang Hai Zhong Yi Yao Za Zhi (*Shanghai Journal of Chinese Medicine and Herbology*), 1965;4:4.

Shen Yang Yi Xue Yuan Xue Bao (*Journal of Shenyang University of Medicine*), 1987;4(2):109.

Yao Xue Za Zhi (*Journal of Medicinals*), 1983;103(6): 683.

Zhang Y. Advances in pharmacological research on gentiopicroside. *Yunan Journal of Medicine.* 1991;12(5): 304.

Zhong Cao Yao Tong Xun (*Journal of Chinese Herbal Medicine*), 1974;3:39.

Zhong Cao Yao Xue (Study of Chinese Herbal Medicine), 1980; 1445.

Zhong Guo Yao Li Xue Tong Bao (*Journal of Chinese Herbal Pharmacology*), 1986;2(5):26.

Zhong Xi Yi Jie He Za Zhi (*Journal of Integrated Chinese and Western Medicine*), 1988;8(3):161.

Zhong Yao Tong Bao (*Journal of Chinese Herbology*), 1985; 10(6):43.

Zhong Yao Xue (Chinese Herbology), 1998; 156:158.

Zhong Yao Xue (Chinese Herbology), 1998; 620:622.

Zhong Yao Yao Li Yu Ying Yong (Pharmacology and Applications of Chinese Herbs), 1983;370.

Zhong Yao Yao Li Yu Ying Yong (Pharmacology and Applications of Chinese Herbs), 1983:883.

Homotoxicology references

Dobias P. Principles of Using Periodic Table of Elements in Animal Prescribing. In: Proceedings of the 2006 Annual Conference, AHVMA, Louisville, KY, 2006. pp 129–141.

Reckeweg H. Biotherapeutic Index: Ordinatio Antihomotoxica et Materia Medica, 5th ed. Baden-Baden, Germany: Biologische Heilmittel Heel GMBH, 2000. p 342.

Chapter Seventeen

Neurological Disorders

COGNITIVE DYSFUNCTION

Definition and cause

Cognitive dysfunction (CD) is broadly defined as the onset of age-related behavioral changes that are not associated with any physical or medical causes. CD can occur in both dogs and cats. Some of the common symptoms are lethargy, apathy, loss of house training, confusion, restless sleep, pacing, staring into walls or corners, howling, or other abnormal vocalization. Ruehl (1996) surveyed companions who lived with elderly dogs and found that more than 60% had at least 1 symptom of CD. One of the common findings in people with Alzheimer's disease and dogs and cats with CD is the deposition of amyloid plaques (Cummings 1996, Landsberg 1997).

Medical therapy rationale, drug(s) of choice, and nutritional recommendations

Selegiline (Anipryl) is the recognized treatment for CD. It appears to be able to slow the progressive degeneration of cognition. Treatment is generally recommended for the life of the animal (Landgsberg 1997).

Anticipated prognosis

When CD is diagnosed early, before multiple clinical symptoms appear and are medically treated, the prognosis is good. The prognosis is more guarded with longstanding CD and when there are underlying complicating diseases.

Integrative veterinary therapies

An integrative approach to cognitive dysfunction takes into consideration not only the brain and nerves, but all of the organ systems. The focus is upon the initiating inflammation that precedes the degenerative process, the deposit of amyloid, and the resulting behavior changes.

The use of nutrients, antioxidants, phytonutrients, medicinal herbs, and combination homeopathics that have anti-inflammatory, tissue-sparing, and regenerative effects on brain and nerve cells can help improve the clinical picture and slow the degenerative process. Numerous studies and references show the benefits of alternative therapies in people with age-related cognitive decline and dementia (Brayne 1995, Craik 1992, Hanninen 1996, Levy 1994, Smith 1996).

Nutrition
General considerations/rationale

Cotman (2002) and Milgram (2002) documented the benefits of improved, antioxidant-rich diets for the clinical picture of dogs with cognitive dysfunction. Joseph (1998) showed that diets that are rich in antioxidants and phyto-nutrients help slow the progression of a cognitive decline. Nutritional supplements that improve circulation, reduce free radical load and inflammation, protect brain and nerve cells, and supply the necessary nutrients for proper function have a positive effect on the animal's quality of life and help to control or eliminate symptoms of CD.

Appropriate nutrients

Nutritional/gland therapies: Glandular brain supplies intrinsic nutrients and can help improve circulation and reduce inflammation in the brain and central nervous system (Goldstein 2000) (see Gland Therapy in Chapter 2). Phospholipids found in glandular brain are a source of unsaturated omega-3 fatty acids, which are now thought to play a vital role in the development and maintenance of the central nervous system. High concentrations of phosphatidyl choline and serine are found in brain tissue. Horrocks (1986) reported on the potential clinical use of these nutrients in chronic neurological conditions.

Phosphatidyl serine (PS): Phosphatidyl serine is a phospholipid that is essential for cellular membranes, particularly those of brain cells. It has been studied and shown positive results in people with impaired mental functioning and degeneration (Crook 1991). In people with

Alzheimer's disease the addition of PS led to a mild to significant clinical improvement (Delewaide 1986, Engel 1992, Funfgeld 1989).

PS was found to improve cognition in another human study (Maggioni 1990). In a double-blind study of 494 geriatric people, PS showed significant improvement in both cognition and behavior. (Cennachi 1993).

Lecithin/phosphatidyl choline: Phosphatidyl choline is a phospholipid that is integral to cellular membranes, particularly those of nerve and brain cells. It helps to move fats into the cells and is involved in acetylcholine uptake, neurotransmission, and cellular integrity. Lecithin, as part of the cell membranes, is an essential nutrient that is required by all of the cells of the body for general health and wellness (Hanin 1987).

Acetyl-L-carnitine: Acetyl-L-carnitine is a derivative of the amino acid L-carnitine, which is involved in the production of acetylcholine and the proper function of the brain and the transmission of nerve impulses. Studies have indicated that acetyl-L-carnitine can slow the development of Alzheimer's disease and improve cognition in people. People taking acetyl-L-carnitine showed an improvement in memory and their day-to-day demeanor and mood (Cipoli 1990, Genazzani 1990, Garzya 1990).

Blue-green algae: Blue-green algae has been observed to create a generalized feeling of well being in humans, and it may prove helpful in veterinary patients. Its effects are usually observed to be slower in onset; the benefits take 3 to 4 weeks to appear. This may be due in part to their content of natural antihistaminic compounds or their levels of omega-3 fatty acids (Bruno 2001).

Many recent studies have confirmed the beneficial results from these critical fatty acids. Aphanizomenon flos aquae, a blue-green algae, has been shown in clinical settings to have positive effects on brain function. In addition to the aforementioned omega-3 fatty acids, it contains a full spectrum of essential amino acids, a broad-based mineral content, a rapidly assimilable glyolipoprotein cell wall, and a wide variety of vitamins. It has mild chelating properties, and thus may be valuable in heavy metal toxicoses such as Thimerosol reactions. It is a tremendous asset as a micronutrient resource and figures prominently in many treatment programs (Broadfoot 1997).

Chinese herbal medicine/acupuncture
General considerations/rationale
Cognitive dysfunction is a result of Liver and Kidney Qi and Blood deficiency, Yin and Yang deficiency, Phlegm accumulation, and blockage of the meridians.

Author's interpretation
Cognitive dysfunction is seen in the elderly. These patients are deficient in Blood, Yang, Yin, and Qi because they have used these substances up during life. The Liver nourishes the Kidney, and it cannot perform this function when it becomes deficient. The Kidney houses the Essence, or life potential, so when it becomes deficient in all substances, the individual suffers the ravages of old age, including senility.

Phlegm can be thought of as sticky substances that "gum up" the mind, to use a colloquial expression. If it blocks the meridians' flow of thought, the result is forgetfulness.

Appropriate Chinese herbs
Curcuma root (Yu jin): May be able to prevent free radical tissue damage (Cui 1990). Free radical damage has been implicated in degenerative changes.

Fleece-flower root (He shou wu): Has been shown to increase life expectancy and slow aging in laboratory animals (Zhong Yao Yao Li Yu Lin Chuang 1989).

Gastrodia (Tian ma): Causes proliferation of large gliocytes in rats, indicating that it may improve the patient's memory (Liu 1997). It can increase SOD levels in the blood (Bai Xiu Rong 1996). Gastrodia also was shown to improve the learning and memory of mice that have suffered from cerebral ischemia (Du 1999).

Grassleaved sweetflag rhizome (Shi chang pu): May improve the ability to learn. One study compared the ability of mice to navigate a maze with and without grassleaved sweetflag root treatment. The mice were placed in the same maze for 6 days. Mice that received grassleaved sweetflag root made fewer mistakes and finished the maze faster than those given saline (Zhong Cao Yao 1992). This suggests that the herb improved the mice's memory of the maze.

Scorpion (Quan xie): May protect the brain. One study examined people suffering from a cerebral embolism. Most of the patients treated with scorpion seemed to respond positively (Ji Lin Zhong Yi Yao 1989).

White peony (Bai shao): Improves memory. It contains paeoniflorin, which can help scopolamine-damaged rats improve maze performance (Ohta 1993).

Zizyphus (Suan zao ren): Increases the activity of superoxide dismutase, creatine phosphatase, and lactic dehydrogenase in the brain, and can decrease the content of lactic acid (Bai 1996). These actions may prevent nerve cell damage and may help improve memory.

Acupuncture
Acupuncture may help improve the condition of the central nervous system. One study found that comatose patients recovered better if acupuncture was added to the customary Western treatments (Frost 1976). Another study found that patients who suffered from vascular dementia experienced quicker and more complete recovery when treated with acupuncture (Zhuang 1998).

Homotoxicology
General considerations/rationale
This condition generally represents Degeneration Phase changes in the neurological system. Oxidative damage is indicated as a contributory factor (Rofina et al. 2006). Therapy is aimed at removing homotoxins, rehabilitating organelles and cellular function, and improving circulation in the area. Interest in complementary and integrative approaches has recently increased (Kline 2002). Of particular interest to homotoxicologists and other physiological regulation medicine practitioners is the use of mitochondrial enzyme cofactors (Milgram 2002). The authors are unaware of any controlled, evidence-based studies on homeopathic agents in this condition, although a nonrefereed publication dealing with dementia in human patients has recently appeared (Smit 2006).

Application of the Six-Phase Table of Homotoxicology can be helpful in such cases. Often cognitive dysfunction represents congestion and clogging of the matrix followed by decreasing efficacy of cellular function and elimination of wastes. Typically this process is silent in the Deposition and early Impregnation phases and becomes more evident in the late Impregnation and Degeneration phases of pathogenesis. Most patients in this category benefit from the deep detoxification formula because it supports elimination organs and provides drainage of the cells and matrix. Further judicious use of catalyst therapy can greatly assist geriatric patients by providing adequate cellular energy metabolism to perform the requested tasks involved in homotoxin removal and excretion. Such cleansing is a fundamental requirement for cellular healing to occur.

Regressive vicariation of the central nervous system can be a startling experience for client and clinician alike. Patients suffering from subclinical Impregnation disease that undergo regressive vicariation can experience depression, headache, photophobia, sleep disorder, muscle twitching, and both petit mal and grand mal seizures. The client needs to be fully informed before such steps are taken in elderly pets, and while such signs usually represent healing and are beneficial, in the acute phases they can be alarming and require medical attention. The key to minimizing such events is the slow progression of both organ support and drainage. If a patient is affected by strong neurological signs, the biological therapist will know to reduce the frequency and dose of the detoxification and drainage remedies, thus allowing the body time to remove and process homotoxins that have been liberated through healing.

Impregnation and Degeneration phase disorders are usually not curable, but can be managed with long-term therapy and an integrative approach. Clients will often report improved conditions in 2 to 4 weeks of therapy. Brighter eyes and more interest in play and other activities are most often reported. An initial period of deep rest and reduced activity may occur, especially with the use of catalysts such as Glyoxal compositum, and this is believed to be due to initial movement of homotoxins out of organelles and into the matrix. Palmquist recommends using the deep detoxification formula only twice per week for 3 to 4 weeks prior to raising the dosage or beginning other therapies on such patients. Nutritional therapy during this period seems very helpful (Milgram, et al. 2002).

The importance of rehabilitative exercise and play cannot be overstated. Numerous studies have shown that proper mental stimulation, challenge and play, and exercise directly assists in drainage through improved circulation and lymph milking by skeletal muscles during exercise (Goldstein 2005). Once again the clinician must be aware of homotoxins moving into connective tissue and the resultant discomfort that can occur. Such patients frequently have an initial exacerbation of musculoskeletal discomfort and this can be greatly helped by use of biological therapeutic agents which assist the patient in moving toxins. Lymphomyosot (lymph motion and drainage), Byaconeel (pain in small joints of the hand and feet resulting from regressive vicariation), Cruroheel (connective tissue drainage and support in regressive vicariation), and Arsuraneel (serious vicariations) are commonly required in these stages (Reckeweg 2000). The use of compositae class remedies provides support for connective tissue and stem cell elements and seems to diminish such negative symptoms as well (Reckeweg 2000).

Appropriate homotoxicology formulas
Aesculus compositum: Useful in improving circulation following stroke or reduced cerebral circulation (Aesculus hippocastanum and Secale cornutum). Contains Arteria suis for support of arteries. Solanum nigrum further supports cerebral function, particularly in cases with confusion, epileptic seizures, or disorientation. Several other agents support removal of homotoxins and improve vessel stability (Reckeweg 2000). Baryta iodata (also in *Circuloheel*, *BHI-Circulation*, and *BHI-Stramonium Complex*) is included for arteriosclerosis, coronary ischemia, and heart problems in aged pets. Dulcamara is used for certain states of confusion and dull headache coupled with hardness of hearing, and is also very useful for the rheumatic afflictions that occur with damp weather. Plumbum metallicum (also in *Placenta compositum* and others) is included.

This remedy treats arteriosclerosis with fatty heart and ventricular hypertrophy; bleak, despondent mood; emaciation in paretic syndromes and other diseases of the nervous system; hepatic disorders; and states of confusion. Rhus toxicodendron treats a multiplicity of symptoms that suggest a rheumatic origin and include mental confused, difficulty in understanding, and absent-mindedness.

Secale cornutum treats the emotional and intellectual functions that are particularly disordered. Predominant symptoms include difficulty in thinking, deficient understanding and comprehension, a certain dullness of intellect, great forgetfulness and sensory delusions, and sometimes vertigo and staggering and an inability to stand upright. Secale also treats the impairment of the central emotional control by the brain or the impairment of the autonomic central control, with spastic symptoms developing in the whole abdomen. Viscum album (also in *Ginseng compositum, Rauwolfia compositum, Secale, Thalamus compositum, Thyroidea compositum,* and *Viscum compositum*) is included for melancholia, hypotension and hypertension, sensations of vertigo, coronary stenosis, arrhythmia, and articular diseases of attrition (Reckeweg 2002).

Apis homaccord: Generally useful in edema, but also in cerebral sensitivity. May assist cardiac-induced cerebral weakness through Scilla, Apisinum, and Apis mellifica.

Barijodeel: Useful in senile dementia, cerebral sclerosis, memory failure, anxiety, arteriosclerosis, and depression. Very useful agent in geriatric patients (Reckeweg 2000). The primary component is Baryta carbonica (also in Placenta compositum, Tonsilla comp, and Ginkgo), which is suited to anxious patients who shun the company of others and exhibit weakness and slowness of mental activity. It is also helpful for hypertension and angiosclerosis (Reckeweg 2002). The remaining remedies are also very strongly suited to the mental and emotional issues that accompany aging pets and the attendant behavior and physical changes, and are common components of therapies used in older animals (Broadfoot 2006).

BHI-Alertness: Used for depressed, dull, geriatric patients.

BHI-Ginkgo complex: Supports cerebral blood flow and improves awareness. Contains the remedy Ginkgo for symptoms of senility disorders: forgetfulness, mental exhaustion, lack of concentration, numbness, vagueness, dull mental state, avoidance of company, confusion, apathy, and irrational fears. The physical symptoms include vertigo, insomnia, and vision impairment. This remedy strongly affects the kidney and lung channels, according to Traditional Chinese Medicine, and is used in cases with phlegm; wheezing, asthma, and leukorrheal discharge; frequent urination; incontinence; dysphagia; and dry mouth. The abdomen is tense and swollen and the patient may experience cough, dyspnea, etc. The urogenital area and respiratory symptoms, as well as the mentals, all relate to TCM's connection to the kidney channel. This remedy also contains Baryta carbonica (see Barijodeel).

BHI-Recovery: Used for post-stroke recovery.

Cactus compositum: Supports cardiac function in senile dementia that originates from a weakening cardiac status.

Causticum compositum: The remedy picture of Causticum, the primary remedy, embraces complaints of a neuralgic-rheumatic nature that are possibly associated with paralytic conditions. They include a high degree of weakness, frequent association with trembling and an unsteady gait, and nocturnal enuresis. On the emotional side, Causticum corresponds to sadness and depression. Causticum complements Rhus tox and Sulphur well, especially in the treatment of rheumatism. Embryo suis (also found in *Cerebrum compositum, Placenta compositum, Testis compositum,* and others) is useful for anxiety, impaired concentration, confusion, mental dullness, and fatigue. Fumaricum acidum (also in *Coenzyme compositum, Thyroidea compositum,* and *BHI-Enzyme,* to name a few) is used for disturbances of lipids and steroids in the metabolism and with premature arteriosclerosis. It works in combination with malic acid to treat hypertension. And also treats and prevents embolism and is used for a feeling of weakness or relaxation that leads to sleep or excessive physical irritability. The component alpha-Ketoglutaricum (also in *Coenzyme compositum, Thyroidea compositum,* and *BHI-Enzyme*) may be used for paralysis following a stroke, as well as total exhaustion, restlessness at day and night, and poor appetite. Fatigue and daytime sleepiness are prominent symptoms with mental dullness, forgetfulness, irritability, concentration issues, anxiety, and mental confusion (Reckeweg 2002). This remedy also contains Natrum oxalaceticum (see *Ginseng compositum*).

Cerebrum compositum: Supports cerebral tissue, stem cells, and vessels (Cerebrum suis, Placenta suis, Placenta suis, Arnica montana). It helps to improve memory (Selenium, Thuja occidentalis, Acidum phosphoricum, Manganum phospohoricum, Semecarpus anacardium, Ambra grisea, Conium maculatum, and Medorrhinum-Nosode). This remedy also supports cerebral function and vascular structures (Kalium phophoricum). It treats vertigo, stupor, and headache (Gelsemium sempervirens, Kalium bichromicum, and Ruta graveolens) and supports capillary and other circulation as well as lymph (Aesculus hippocastanum). Further indications include anxiety (Aconitum napellus) and exhaustion (China, Amarita cocculus).

Cerebrum compositum supports enzyme systems and helps with difficulty sleeping (Hyoscyamus niger) (Reckeweg 2000). It contains Ambra grisea (also found in *Cocculus compositum, Vertigoheel, BHI-Dizziness, BHI-Lightheaded,* and *BHI-PMS-Mulimen*) and is used for nervous excitement, hearing impairment, and difficulty in concentration. Predominant in its symptom picture we find nervous symptoms of a primarily chronic nature such as nervous weakness of vision and hearing, vertigo, weakness of memory, deterioration of brain function and senility with general mental prostration, nervous hyperexcitability and nervous exhaustion, insomnia, autonomic dysregulation, angiosclerosis, and premature aging (Reckeweg 2002).

A case study in a *Biological Therapy Journal* article profiles adjuvant therapy of Alzheimer's patients with age-related dementias, and extrapolation to canine patients may prove interesting. Regular, intensive memory training is important in human patients, and antihomotoxic medicine offers an interesting therapeutic option for detoxification and metabolism activation using catalyst preparations and suis organ preparations. This study used *Cerebrum compositum*, *Coenzyme compositum*, and *Ubichinon compositum* to good effect (Shperling 1996). *Cerebrum compositum* was studied in a large group of patients, and showed very good therapeutic efficacy and was well tolerated. The preparation's broad spectrum of efficacy is the result of its variety of botanical and mineral components; as well as Cerebrum suis, Embryo suis, Hepar suis, and Placenta suis, which specifically stimulate organic function; and the nosodes Luesinum and Medorrhinum, two constitutional remedies for exerting a positive influence on the organism's general responsive status. The overall action of *Cerebrum compositum* is directed not only toward improving brain function, but also toward alleviation and prevention of arteriosclerotic circulatory disturbances with attendant deterioration in cerebral performance, a factor particularly valuable in the treatment of aged patients (Weiser 1995).

Coenzyme compositum: Provides metabolic support and energy. Used in cases of exhaustion.

Galium-Heel: Used for support of chronic disease states; is a cellular phase remedy.

Gelsemium homaccord: Treats neuralgia and nerve pain, headache, and posterior weakness. Commonly required in aging large breed dogs.

Ginseng compositum: Increases energy and awareness in geriatric pets. Primarily named for the Ginseng component Aralia quinquefolia (also in *Testis compositum*). The principal indications are: states of nervous exhaustion, weakness of intellect, confusion, and dulled senses. There may be vertigo, and a tendency to sleep, or weakness of vision with hypersensitivity to light. ATP (Adenosine Triphosphate, which is also found in *Coenzyme compositum*, *Thyroidea compositum*, *Ubichinon compositum*, and *BHI-Enzyme*) is useful for damage to the energy-utilizing systems (e.g., citric acid cycle and others), especially iatrogenic damage. Patients may be angry, excitable, or irritable, and demonstrate restlessness with difficult concentration. The Conium component (common to *Cerebrum compositum*, *Cocculus compositum*, *Testis compositum*, et al.) can be considered when there is a history of paralysis which ascends from below.

Rotatory vertigo is one of the main indications for Conium. Other symptoms include old age, arteriosclerosis and progressive cachexia, and symptoms of sensory irritation. In the area of brain function, Conium can treat weakness of memory, reduced mental ability, and possibly also tremors, tinnitus and sleeplessness. In the mucosa we may see irritation with dryness, and ulcers with offensive discharge.

Natrum oxalaceticum (also in *Causticum compositum*, *Coenzyme compositum*, *Thyroidea compositum*, *Ubichinon compositum*, and others) is indicated for vertigo that does not respond to other remedies; vertigo and cerebral ischemia; anxiety; mental confusion; depression and sadness; and nerve pain with hypersensitivity to noise, light, and touch. Viscum album (also in *Aesculus compositum*, *Thalamus compositum*, *Thyroidea compositum*, *Viscum compositum*, and others) is mainly indicated for hypotension and hypertension, sensations of vertigo, coronary stenosis, arrhythmia, and articular diseases of attrition (Reckeweg 2002).

Glyoxal compositum: Supports metabolism and unblocks receptors and enzymes.

Lymphomyosot: Provides lymph drainage.

Ovarium compositum: Supports ovarian tissue and drainage.

Placenta compositum: Used for vascular support and headache.

Selenium homaccord: Treats diminished mental activity and cerebral function, especially as it relates to atherosclerosis (Reckeweg 2000).

Testis compositum: Supports testicular function and provides drainage. Primary remedy is Testis suis with premature senility as the main indication. States of exhaustion are another indication. This remedy, which also contains Ginseng and Conium (see *Ginseng compositum*), raises the level of vitality (Reckeweg 2002).

Ubichinon compositum: Supports deep metabolism and the cytochrome oxidase system.

Vertigoheel: Possibly increases cerebral circulation (Klopp, Niemer, Weiser 2005).

Authors' suggested protocols

Nutrition

Brain/nerve and behavior emotional support formulas: 1 tablet for each 25 pounds of body weight BID.

Phosphatidyl serine: 25 mgs for each 25 pounds of body weight BID.

Lecithin/phosphatidyl choline: One-fourth teaspoon for each 25 pounds of body weight BID.

Acetyl-L-carnitine (500 mgs): One-half capsule per 25 pounds of body weight daily.

Blue-green algae: One-fourth teaspoon for each 25 pounds of body weight daily.

Chinese herbal medicine/acupuncture

Senility B: 1 capsule per 10 to 20 pounds twice daily. In addition to the herbs discussed above, Senility B contains angelica root (Dan gui), antler powder (Lu jiao jiao), arisaema/bile (Dan nan xing), black sesame seeds (Hei zhi ma), bulrush (Pu huang), fossil teeth (Long chi), licorice (Gan cao), longan fruit (Long yan rou), mulberry (Sang shen zi), polygala (Yuan zhi), poria (Fu ling), pseudotellaria root (Tai zhi shen), red peony (Chi shao), rehmannia (Shu di huang), salvia (Dan shen), silkworm fungus (Jiang can), and trichosanthes (Quan gua lou). These herbs help improve the function of the formula.

The classically recommended acupuncture points are KI1 and KI4 (Lei 1999). In addition, the author also recommends ST36, PC6, Baihui, SP6, BL18, BL20, and BL23.

Homotoxicology (Dose: 10 drops PO for 50-pound dog; 5 drops PO for small dog or cat)

Symptom remedy: Cerebrum compositum given by injection and then orally 1 to 3 times weekly. Can be added to the following detoxification formula and used long term.

Detoxification therapy: Galium-Heel, Lymphomyosot, Hepar compositum, Solidago compositum, Thyroidea compositum Coenzyme compositum, Ubichinon compositum, and Placenta compositum mixed together and given twice weekly for 3 to 4 months. Add Mucosa compositum if diarrhea or other gastrointestinal issues arise.

Product sources

Nutrition

Brain/nerve and behavior support formulas: Animal Nutrition Technologies.

Phosphatidyl serine: Integrative Therapuetics.
Lecithin/phosphatidyl choline: Designs for Health.
Acetyl-L-carnitine: Thorne Research.
Blue-green algae: Cell Tech (Simplexity) or BlueGreen Foods, Inc.

Chinese herbal medicine

Formula Senility B: Natural Solutions Inc.

Homotoxicology

BHI/Heel Corporation

REFERENCES

Western medicine references
Cummings BJ, Satou T, Head E, et al. Diffuse Plaques Contain c-terminal AB42 and not AB40: Evidence from Cats and Dogs, *Neurobiol Aging* 1996 Jul–Aug;17(4):653–9.

Milgram NW, Ivy GO, Head E, et al: The effect of l-deprenyl on behavior, cognitive function and biogenic amines in the dog. *Neurochemical Research* 18:1211, 1993.
Cotman CW, Head E, Muggenburg BA, Zicker S, Milgram NW. Brain aging in the canine: a diet enriched in antioxidants reduces cognitive dysfunction, *Neurobiol Aging.* 2002 Sep–Oct;23(5):809–18.
Landsberg G, Hunthausen W, Ackerman L. Handbook of Behaviour Problems of the Dog and Cat, Butterworth-Heinemann, 1997.
Landsberg GM, Ruehl WR, Geriatric Behavioural Problems, *Veterinary Clinics of North America*, 1997, pp. 1537–1559.
Milgram NW, Zicker SC, Head E, Muggenburg BA, Murphey H, Ikeda-Douglas CJ, Cotman CW. Dietary enrichment counteracts age-associated cognitive dysfunction in canines. *Neurobiol Aging.* 2002 Sep–Oct;23(5):737–45.
Ruehl WW, Hart BL. Canine cognitive dysfunction. In: Dodman NH, Shuster L, eds. Psychopharmacology of Animal Behavior Disorders. Boston: Blackwell Science Inc., (in press).

IVM references
Brayne C, Gill C, Paykel ES, et al. Cognitive decline in an elderly population—a two wave study of change. *Psychological Study of Medicine* 1995;25:673–83.
Craik FIM, Salthouse TA. Handbook of Aging and Cognition. Hillsdale, NJ: Erlbaum, 1992.
Hänninen T. Age-associated memory impairment: A neuropsychological and epidemiological study. *Neurologian klinikan julkaisusarja* 1996;39 [abstract].
Levy R. Aging-associated cognitive decline. *Int Psychogeriatr* 1994;6:63–8.
Smith GE, Petersen RC, Parisi JE, et al. Definition, course, and outcome of mild cognitive impairment. *Aging Neuropsychol Cogn* 1996;3:141–7.

Nutrition references
Broadfoot P. Personal communication. 1997.
Bruno J. Edible Microalgae: A Review of the Health Research. Center for Nutritional Psychology, 2001. p 23.
Cenacchi T, Bertoldin T, Farina C, et al. Cognitive decline in the elderly: a double-blind, placebo-controlled multicenter study on efficacy of phosphatidylserine administration. *Aging (Milano)* 1993;5:123–33.
Cipolli C, Chiari G. Effects of L-acetylcarnitine on mental deterioration in the aged: initial results. *Clin Ter* 1990;132(6 Suppl):479–510 [in Italian].
Fünfgeld EW, Baggen M, Nedwidek P, et al. Double-blind study with phosphatidylserine (PS) in Parkinsonian patients with senile dementia of Alzheimer's type (SDAT). *Prog Clin Biol Res* 1989;317:1235–46.
Garzya G, Corallo D, Fiore A, et al. Evaluation of the effects of L-acetylcarnitine on senile patients suffering from depression. *Drugs Exp Clin Res* 1990;16(2):101–6.
Genazzani E. A controlled clinical study on the efficacy of L-acetylcarnitine in the treatment of mild to moderate mental deterioration in the aged. Conclusions. *Clin Ter* 1990;132(6 Suppl):511–2.
Hanin IG, Ansell B. Lecithin: Technological, Biological, and Therapeutic Aspects, 1987, NY: Plenum Press, 180, 181.

Joseph JA, Shukitt-Hale B, Denisova NA, et al. Long-term dietary strawberry, spinach, or vitamin E supplementation retards the onset of age-related neuronal signal-transduction and cognitive behavioral deficits. *J Neurosci* 1998;18(19): 8047–55.

Maggioni M, Picotti GB, Bondiolotti GP, et al. Effects of phosphatidylserine therapy in geriatric patients with depressive disorders. *Acta Psychiatr Scand* 1990;81(3):265–70.

Salvioli G, Neri M. L-acetylcarnitine treatment of mental decline in the elderly. *Drugs Exp Clin Res* 1994;20(4):169–76.

Chinese herbal medicine/acupuncture references

Bai XL, et al. Suan Zao Ren total saponin's effect on ischemic brain damages and cerebral biochemical indicators in rats. *China Journal of Chinese Medicine.* 1996;20(6):369–370.

Bai XR, et al. *Journal of Mathematical Medicine.* 1996;9(2): 180–182.

China Journal of Chinese Medicine. 1996;20(6):369–370.

Cui XL, et al. *China Bulletin of Pharmacology.* 1990;7(2):20.

Du GY, et al. *China Journal of Chinese Medicine.* 1999;24(10): 626–628.

Frost EAM. Acupuncture for the comatose patient. *American Journal of Acupuncture,* 1976 4(1):45–48.

Ji Lin Zhong Yi Yao (*Jilin Chinese Medicine and Herbology*), 1989;(4):15.

Lei YM, et al. Chinese Famous Doctors Secret Formulas for Chronic Terminal Ill Patients. Guangxi Science and Technology Press, July 1999. p 944.

Liu JX, et al. *China Journal of TCM Theories.* 1997; 3(6):23–25.

Ohta H, Ni JW, Matsumoto K, et al. Paeony and its major constituent, paeoniflorin, improve radial maze performance impaired by scopolamine in rats. *Pharmacol Biochem Behav* 1993;45:719–23.

Zhong Cao Yao (*Chinese Herbal Medicine*), 1992;23(8):417.

Zhong Yao Yao Li Yu Lin Chuang (*Pharmacology and Clinical Applications of Chinese Herbs*), 1989;5(3):19.

Zhuang L, Li Y, Zheng L, Yang W. Clinical observation on combined treatment of vascular dementia with acupuncture, moxibustion and Chinese medicinal herbs. *World J Acupuncture Moxibustion.* 1998;8:7–11.

Homotoxicology references

Dalpé R. A Homeopathic Analysis of Ginkgo biloba. URL: http://www.onlinehomeopath.com/ginkgo.shtml.

Goldstein R, Goldstein S. The Goldstein's Wellness and Longevity Program. Neptune City, NJ: TFH Publications, 2005. pp 190–4.

Kline K. Complementary and alternative medicine for neurologic disorders. *Clin Tech Small Anim Pract.* 2002. Feb;17(1):pp 25–33.

Klopp R, Niemer W, Weiser M. Microcirculatory effects of a homeopathic preparation in patients with mild vertigo: an intravital microscopic study. *Microvascular Res.* 2005. 69(2): pp 10–16.

Milgram N, Zicker SC, Head E, Muggenburg B, Murphey H, Ikeda-Douglas CJ, Cotman C. Dietary enrichment counteracts age-associated cognitive dysfunction in canines. *Neurobiol Aging.* 2002.Sep–Oct;23(5):pp 737–45.

Reckeweg H. Biotherapeutic Index: Ordinatio Antihomotoxica et Materia Medica, 5th ed. Baden-Baden, Germany: Biologische Heilmittel Heel GMBH, 2000. p 22–3, 286–9, 295–6, 299, 302, 308–9, 400–401.

Reckeweg H. Homeopathia Antihomotoxica Materia Medica, 4th ed. Baden-Baden, Germany: Arelia-Verlag GMBH, 2002. pp. 131, 159–160, 168–9, 170, 217–20, 254–6, 282–4, 286–8, 307–8, 320, 373–6, 446–8, 495, 512–3, 525–8, 598–9.

Rofina J, Van Ederen A, Toussaint M, Secreve M, Van der Spek A, Van der Meer I, Van Eerdenburg F, Gruys E. Cognitive disturbances in old dogs suffering from the canine counterpart of Alzheimer's disease. *Brain Res.* 2006. Jan 19, 1069(1):pp 216–26.

Shperling M, Chabanov D. Alzheimer's disease: A case study. Reprinted from *Biblogische Medizin*; 1996. August; 180–81. *Biol Ther.* 14(319): p 263.

Smit A. Central nervous system disorders and homotoxicology. *J Biomed Therapy.* 2006. Summer, pp 6–7.

Weiser M, Zenner S. Cerebral function disorders and biological therapy: An application study with 731 patients. Reprinted from *Biologische Medizin* 5:pp. 277–283, in *Biol Ther.* 1994. 134(31995): pp 85–90.

DEGENERATIVE MYELOPATHY

Definition and cause

Degenerative myelopathy (DM) is a slow, progressive degeneration of the spinal cord, which often leads to loss of motor control of the hind legs. While no proven cause is known, it is believed that an autoaggressive process may be involved with the observed degeneration of the spinal cord. Although it is most commonly found in German Shepherds, DM has also been seen in other breeds such as old English Sheepdogs, Belgium Shepherds, and Weimaraners (LeCouteur 1989, Sisson 2003).

Medical therapy rationale, drug(s) of choice, and nutritional recommendations

Once diagnosed, there is no proven therapy for DM. Clemmons (1989) states that "the current treatment of DM is designed to suppress the immune disease, but does nothing to correct the immune alterations which led to the disease state." Clemmons has proposed an immune-mediated cause in German Shepherds, and as such recommends a combination of controlled exercise to improve tone and circulation, vitamins and other supplements, n-acetyl-cysteine, and aminocaproic acid (EACA), which have shown an improvement or stabilization of the condition in more than 50% of the animals with DM. No controlled trials have been reported, however (Clemmons 1989, Sisson 2003).

Anticipated prognosis

Most animals diagnosed with degenerative myelopathy slowly lose nervous control and become non-ambulatory within 1 to 2 years of diagnosis. Late-stage DM is often complicated with both fecal and urinary incontinence (Sisson 2003). Clemmons (1989) offers a better prognosis (see medical therapy above).

Integrative veterinary therapies

The authors recommend an augmented version of Dr. Roger Clemmons' protocol for the treatment of DM in dogs (Clemmons 2002). The enhancements to Dr. Clemmons' program include adding the authors' specific glandular, Chinese herbal, acupuncture, and homotoxicology remedies to his published protocol.

Nutrition

Gland therapy: Glandular brain, adrenal, thymus, and spleen supply the intrinsic nutrients that help reduce autoimmune cellular inflammation, neutralize free radicals, and improve organ and nerve function. This helps to slow and spare the nerves from progressive degeneration (see Gland Therapy in Chapter 2 for a more detailed explanation).

Phospholipids found in glandular brain are a source of unsaturated omega-3 fatty acids, which are now believed to play a vital role in the development and maintenance of the central nervous system. High concentrations of phosphatidyl choline and serine are found in brain tissue. Horrocks (1986) reported on the potential clinical use of these nutrients in chronic neurological conditions.

General considerations/rationale

Many of the following considerations and recommendations are taken from the web site of Clemmons (2002): http://neuro.vetmed.ufl.edu/neuro/DM_Web/DMofGS. htm. Updated August 27, 2002.

"Diet may have a powerful influence on the development of chronic degenerative diseases. New information suggests a significant connection between dietary regulation and the progression and development of diseases such as multiple sclerosis. Eliminating toxins from processed food may help prevent a number of immune-related disorders. The current treatment of DM is designed to suppress the immune disease, but does nothing to correct the immune alterations which led to the disease state.

Diet might help to correct this defect and allow the immune system in DM dogs to stabilize. The principles of dietary therapy, including a homemade diet, are outlined here. For those who cannot cook for their dog, the basic diet should be supplemented with the additional ingredients listed below. It is best to choose a dog food that is close in protein content and is as natural as possible. Wild dogs were not meat eaters. They ate bodies, including intestinal contents that were often laden with plants and plant materials. Dogs have evolved so that eating animal fats and protein do not cause them to suffer the same problems as humans when eating these sources of saturated fats. Even so, dogs probably suffer from the same causes of dietary and environmental intoxication that affect humans.

Basic diet (1 serving for 30 to 50 pounds body weight)

2 oz. boneless pork center loin chop (boiled, baked, or fried in olive oil)

4 oz. tofu

8 oz. long grain brown rice (3 oz. cooked in 6 oz. water)

2 teaspoons extra virgin olive oil

1/4 cup molasses

2 carrots (boiled and then chopped)

1 cup spinach (cooked)

4 tablespoons green bell pepper (chopped and steamed)

4 broccoli spears (boiled and chopped)

This diet provides approximately 1,160 to 1,460 calories per serving. Poultry meat, beef, and lamb can be substituted for the pork chop. This alters the composition slightly, mainly by adding fat. The weight of the meat is based upon boneless weight. Most of the items can be prepared in a microwave.

Based upon the dog's body weight, more or less will need to be prepared. For example, multiply all the ingredients by 1.5 times to 2.5 times for dogs weighing 80 pounds (daily caloric requirements may vary by dog).

This recipe can be made in advance, divided into appropriate quantities, and frozen. Just before feeding, thaw in hot or boiling water or defrost in the microwave.

To complete the diet, add the following combination before serving (recipe makes 1 serving; multiply or divide as needed):

1 teaspoon dry ground ginger

2 raw garlic cloves (crushed)

1/2 teaspoon dry mustard

1 teaspoon bone meal

Approximately 1 serving of the above diet equals 1 can of commercial dog food. The exact requirements for a dog can be approximated by substituting the diet on that basis. The dog should be weighed each week, and the amount of the diet increased if it is losing weight (or decreased if the dog is gaining weight). Eventually, the correct amount will be clear.

Many German Shepherds have sensitive stomachs; therefore, it may be wise to phase in the new diet by mixing it with existing food until the dog adapts. Start by mixing the diet with existing food in equal amounts. After 1 week increase the diet to replace 75% of the original food. After another week, switch completely to the new diet. This diet is balanced and high in most of the vitamins and minerals that dogs need. Any shortcomings can be corrected with the supplements given below."

Appropriate nutrients

B-complex: B vitamins are water-soluble, and any excess amount is eliminated through the urine. They may help in neural regeneration and should be given to dogs. No dog should die while having cheap urine. There is altered absorption of some B vitamins in DM, and supplementation can correct this.

Vitamin E: Vitamin E is an important nutrient that has been shown to have a number of physiologic and pharmacologic effects. It is a potent antioxidant that reduces fat oxidation and increases the production of HDL cholesterol. At higher doses it also reduces cyclooxygenase and lipooxygenases activities, decreasing production of prostaglandins and leukotreines. As such, it is a potent anti-inflammatory drug. It reduces platelet function and prolongs the bleeding time slightly in healthy individuals. There are no known side effects to vitamin E at levels less than 4,000 to 6,000 IU per day (except in cats, where levels over 400 IU/day might create hepatolipidosis). This drug slows the progression of DM and corrects for low serum and tissue levels. In DM, there appears to be a deficient absorption and tissue-binding protein which accounts for the low serum and tissue concentrations of vitamin E.

Vitamin C: Vitamin C works with vitamin E and helps with its regeneration, potentiating its antioxidant effect. Vitamin C supplementation does no harm, because the excess is excreted through the kidney. While dogs produce vitamin C in their bodies (unlike humans, pigs, and guinea pigs, who must obtain it from their diet), they may need vitamin C in excess of their manufacturing capacity when they are suffering from stress or disease.

Selenium: Selenium is an important mineral that has antioxidant properties similar to vitamin E. Vitamin E can replace the requirement for selenium in the body, but selenium cannot substitute for vitamin E. In addition, selenium does not cross the blood-brain barrier like vitamin E. On the other hand, selenium may help vitamin E to be more effective. Many plant sources are low in selenium and supplementation may be important.

Omega-3 fatty acids: Omega-3 fatty acids such as EPA (eicosapentaenoic acid) and DHA (docosahexaenoic acid) are the constituents of fish oils that act as anti-inflammatory agents. They may be worth trying in dogs with autoimmune disorders or arthritis.

Gammalinolenic acid: Borage oil, evening primrose oil, and black currant oil are natural sources of gammalinolenic acid, a fatty acid that is hard to get in the diet. GLA is an effective anti-inflammatory agent with none of the side effects of anti-inflammatory drugs. It also promotes healthy growth of skin, hair, and nails. It may be good for skin conditions, arthritis, and autoimmune disorders. It takes 6 to 8 weeks to see changes after adding GLA to the diet.

Soybean lecithin: Lecithin is a fat-like substance found in the cells of the body. It may combat atherosclerosis, improve memory, and fight Alzheimer's disease in people. However, there is no scientific evidence to support these claims. On the other hand, lecithin is harmless. It is not necessary as a supplement unless a dog has DM and the client elects not to use the diet outlined above (tofu contains plenty of soybean lecithin).

Coenzyme Q: Coenzyme Q, also called CoQ10, is a natural substance that assists in oxidative metabolism. It may improve the use of oxygen at the cellular level, and patients with heart, muscle, and nerve problems may find it worth trying in doses of 30 to 100 mg per day. Some people report that it increases their aerobic endurance.

Medication: The following medications are recommended by Clemmons:

Over the last 2 decades, we have found 2 medications which appear to prevent progression or result in clinical remission of DM in many (up to 80%) of patients: aminocaproic acid (EACA) and n-acetylcysteine (NAC). Clemmons recommends giving EACA as a solution, using the generic product. This product, while designed for injection, can be mixed with chicken broth to provide a palatable solution for oral usage. Clemmons recommends mixing 2 parts of aminocaproic acid solution (250 mg/ml) with 1 part chicken broth and giving 3 ml of this mixture orally every 8 hours. In his experience, this mixture has been equally, if not more, effective to the tablet form of EACA. Furthermore, the solution is much less expensive than the tablets. The generic form of EACA solution can be obtained from American Regent, 1-(800) 645-1706 (outside of New York). The generic drug from American Regent may be obtained through prescription with the help from a local pharmacy.

An alternative source for EACA is to have a compounding pharmacy make the solution from chemical grade EACA. WestLab Pharmacy in Gainesville, Florida, can be reached at 1-800-4WESTLA (1-352-373-8111) and can mail the medication and bill the client directly. Occasional gastrointestinal irritation is the only side effect that has been attributed to EACA. This only presents a problem in a few patients, usually those who have pre-existing GI problems that the medication might exaggerate. A local pharmacist can help determine whether any additional drugs might be contraindicated or lead to possible drug interactions with the recommended therapy. The only known interaction is with estrogen compounds, and only in high doses.

Acetylcysteine is a potent antioxidant that has powerful neuroprotective effects. Clemmons gives 75 mg/kg divided in 3 doses a day for 2 weeks. After that, give the 3 doses every other day. The N-acetylcysteine comes as a 20% solution and must be diluted with chicken broth (or other compatible substitute) to 5% to prevent stomach upset. This new treatment is expensive unless purchased through compounding pharmacies. Again, WestLab Pharmacy has this product and can send it to clients upon veterinary prescription. Using N-acetylcysteine at the above dose does not appear to have side effects. It can produce vomiting and may increase the bleeding time. The GI upset is likely due to the sodium content of the pharmaceutical product, which requires high concentration of base to buffer to pH 7.4. WestLab's product does not have as many side effects because the pH is reduced during preparation. Giving fresh ginger 30 minutes before and giving the NAC with food (or on a full stomach) often reduces this effect.

The combination of aminocaproic acid, N-acetylcysteine, dietary supplements, and exercise is the best treatment we have discovered. It corrects those aspects of the immune dysfunction, which we can treat, based upon our belief that DM is an immune-mediated inflammatory disease. We always hope that all patients will respond to our treatment protocol. Although it does not work in all cases, this combined treatment has been up to 80% effective in patients diagnosed at the University of Florida. The chances of successful treatment are improved if the therapy is begun early in the course of DM rather than later. A response to the drugs should be evident within the first 7 to 10 days. There are no other medications that Clemmons has found to provide any real benefits in the longterm treatment of DM. For further information about treatments for DM, Clemmons recommends Current Therapy X, pages 830–833, and *Vet. Clin. Nor. Am.* 22:965–971, 1992.

Chinese herbal medicine/acupuncture
General considerations/rationale
Degenerative myelopathy is due to Qi, Blood, Yin, and Essence deficiency in the Kidney, Liver, Spleen, and Stomach. The Spleen and Stomach produce the nutrients that in turn nourish the Muscles and Nerves and support the Kidney. Therefore, deficiencies in these organs lead to deficiencies it those structures. The Liver controls ligaments and the Spleen controls Muscles, so Blood and Yin deficiency in these organs leads to weakness and atrophy. The Kidneys control the Marrow or interior of Bones. The Spinal Cord is inside the Vertebrae, so this structure falls under the auspices of the Kidney. Qi deficiency in these organs defines the weakness seen in the condition. The Stomach also suffers from deficiency of Qi, preventing it from extracting enough Blood and fluids from food to reverse the pathology. There seems to be a genetic predisposition to development of degenerative myelopathy. It is

most often seen in German shepherds. This suggests a deficiency of Essence, or genetic predisposition in Western terms.

Appropriate Chinese herbs
Achyranthes (Niu xi): Has anti-inflammatory effects. It can ameliorate egg white-induced foot swelling in rats (Xong 1963), which may make it efficacious in decreasing inflammation in the spinal cord.

Licorice (Gan cao): Contains glycyrrhizin and glycyrrhetinic acid. These compounds have 10% of the corticosteroid activity of cortisone (Zhong Cao Yao 1991). If an autoimmune etiology is truly the cause, this property could be quite beneficial.

Milletia (Ji xue teng): May modify the immune system. It has an inhibitory effect on cellular immunity (Yang 1997, Xu 1993). It may decrease immune-mediated destruction of the nervous system.

Rehmannia/cooked (Shu di huang): Has anti-inflammatory properties (Zhong Yao Yao Li Yu Ying Yong 1983) and has been used for nervous system inflammation. It was one component of a supplement that also contained Rou cong rong, Lu han cao, Gu sui bu, Yin yang huo, Ji xue teng, and Lai fu zi that was used in 1,100 patients with myelitis. Seventy-three percent had significant improvement in clinical signs, and another 13% had moderate improvement (Liao Ning Zhong Yi Za Zhi 1982).

Sichuan aconite (Chuan wu): Decreases inflammation (Xian Dai Zhong Yao Yao Li Xue 1997).

Acupuncture
Degenerative myelopathy is similar to multiple sclerosis in people. Acupuncture has been shown to help decrease symptoms in affected humans. Naeser (1996) reviewed studies in human medicine related to spinal cord disorders and multiple sclerosis. A total of 42 people participated in the various studies. Acupuncture was shown to improve incontinence and muscle spasms. One woman who had been unable to walk without assistance was able to walk short distances after 1 year of treatment. Clemmons (2006) has found that acupuncture therapy slows the rate of progression of the degenerative myelopathy in dogs.

Homotoxicology
General considerations/rationale
Degenerative myelopathy is a progressive Degeneration Phase disease with no known cure. Practitioners are unable to address such homotoxicoses until too late in the pathophysiology for cure. This condition may represent a genetic deterioration involving only a few breeds. Autoimmune disease is another possible cause. Theoretical approaches to such conditions involve draining the matrix, supporting organelle repair, and supporting energy metabolism.

The authors have not used homotoxicology as a sole agent to treat any patients with confirmed diagnosis of degenerative myelopathy, and are unaware of any published cases that have responded favorably in a measurable way. Success in assisting these patients has been reported by Wynn and Marsden using acupuncture, herbs, and nutriceuticals (Wynn, Marsden 2003).

Clemmons feels there may be similarities to multiple sclerosis in humans, a homotoxicosis that has some history of therapy in homotoxicology. Unfortunately, many of the constituents of this experience are not available in the United States (Reckeweg 2000).

Classical homeopathic doctors have reported success in individual cases. While no controlled studies on homeopathy for degenerative myelopathy exist, further research may reveal useful information based upon known data on the use of aminocaproic acid and n-acetylcysteine (NAC) in conjunction with antioxidant therapy, Chinese herbs, and acupuncture as the desired foundational therapy.

Appropriate homotoxicology formulas

Aesculus compositum: Supports vascular tissues.

Arsuraneel: Useful when the patient feels there is no hope. Symptoms include weakness, exhaustion, disability, and polyneuritis. Contains Curare (also contained in *Circulo-Injeel*, *Syzygium compositum*, and *Testis compositum*).

BHI-Recuperation: Contains Causticum, Gelsemium sempervirens, and Plumbum metalicum, which are commonly indicated for weakness and paralysis.

Causticum compositum: Usually indicated for burns, radiation injuries, and other sharp burning pains, Causticum is useful for weakness of the rear legs and paralysis of single parts. Unsteady walking is a symptom. It is also contained in *Barijodeel*, *Husteel*, *Neuralgo-Rheum-Injeel*, *Reneel*, *Rheuma-Heel*, *BHI-Arthritis*, *BHI-Bladder*, *BHI-Recuperation*, *BHI-Throat*, and *BHI-Uricontrol*. The ingredient Embryo suis has been used for muscular dystrophy. Other ingredients support chronic degenerative conditions.

Circulo-Injeel: Contains Curare for weakness and paralysis, as well as polyneuritis.

Coenzyme compositum: Supports metabolism.

Discus compositum: Combination remedy that supports connective tissue.

Echinacea compositum: May normalize inflammatory reactions.

Galium-Heel: Treats cellular diseases and provides matrix drainage. Contains Galium mollugo for detoxification (Reckeweg 2000). Also treats precancerous conditions. Echinacea augustifolia strengthens immunity and is used in inflammatory conditions. Useful in autoimmune conditions.

Gelsemium homaccord: Main remedy for rear leg weakness; trembling is common. Gelsemium is also contained in *BHI-Back*, *BHI-Headache*, *BHI-Heart RX*, *BHI-Neuralgia*, *BHI-Recovery*, *BHI-Recuperation*, *BHI-Sciatic*, *Cerebrum compositum*, *Echinacea compositum*, *Spascupreel*, and *Spigelon*.

Ginseng compositum: Treats weakness and exhaustion.

Glyoxal compositum: Depolymerizes homotoxins from receptors and enzymes and assists in energy production and receptor activation.

Graphites homaccord: Treats weakness in the lower back in overweight patients with history of skin affectations and constipation. Patients are easily chilled.

Lymphomyosot: Provides lymph drainage and immune support.

Lyssin-Injeel: Not available in the United States, but is included because this is homeopathically prepared rabies virus. Due to the possibility of progressive vicariation reactions resulting from vaccination, this remedy may prove helpful in some cases.

Medulla spinalis suis-Injeel: Nosode therapy for the spinal cord.

Neuralgo-Rheum-Injeel: Contains Silicea, and is a major remedy for vaccinosis. Also contained in *BHI-Alertness*, *BHI-Migraine*, *BHI-Neuralgia*, *Cruroheel*, *Discus compositum*, *Spigelon*, *Strumeel*, and *Zeel*.

Phosphor homaccord: Supports spinal weakness in thin animals that are prone to hemorrhage. Constitutional remedy.

Psorinoheel: Miasmic medicine that reaches deep homotoxicoses for all chronic diseases. Also act as an Excretion Phase remedy.

Schwef-Heel: Contains homeopathic dilutions of Sulfur, which activate blocked enzyme systems, assist in construction of structural substances of the matrix, activate blocked or stalled cases, and treat heaviness or paretic limbs (Boercke 1927).

Selenium homaccord: Treats weakness and exhaustion.

Testes compositum: Provides strengthening and drainage of the matrix in male patients with weakness. Contains Conium maculatum for ascending hindlimb ataxia, weakness, and hemiplegia. This also may be helpful for older dogs. Also found in *Cerebrum compositum*, *Cocculus compositum*, *Ginseng compositum*, *Rauwolfia compositum*, *Thyreoidea compositum*, *Tonsilla compositum*, *Ubichinon compositum*, *Vertigoheel*, *BHI-Circulation*, *BHI-Dizziness*, *BHI-Lightheaded*, and *BHI-Stramonium Complex*.

Traumeel S: Anti-inflammatory agent which activates blocked enzyme systems. Treats regulation rigidity.

Ubichinon compositum: Supportive of metabolism in cellular diseases and Degeneration Phase diseases.

Authors' suggested protocols

Nutrition

Brain/nerve and immune support formulas: 1 tablet for each 25 pounds of body weight BID. These formulations contain glandular brain, adrenal, lymph, thymus, spleen, alpha-lipoic acid, L-carnitine, N-acetyl cysteine, phosphatidyl choline, and phosphatidyl serine.

The combination of these brain/nerve and immune support formulas contains the following nutrients per serving for a 75-pound dog:

Vitamin A—3,750 IU
Vitamin E—525 IU
Vitamin C—750 mg
N-Acetyl Cysteine—75 mg
Selenium—105 mcg
Lecithin—300 mg
Phosphatidyl serine—75 mg

In addition to the above 2 formulations which add multiple glandular support, Clemmons recommends adding the following nutrients and additional vitamins and minerals to those listed above to achieve his recommended, target dosage schedule of:

Vitamin C—1,000 mg BID
Vitamin E—2000 IU daily
Selenium—200 mcg daily

Vitamin B complex: Give high potency B-complex (with approximately 50 mg of most of the B components) to healthy dogs. Dogs with DM should receive stress formula B-complex with 100 mg of most of the B components.

Coenzyme Q10: 100 mgs daily.

Fatty acids: Many versions of these substances are on the shelves of health food stores, from salmon oil to capsules of concentrated EPA. However, eating some cooked salmon or sardines may have benefits over capsular forms of the fish oils. Alternatively, dogs can be given ground flax seeds, flax oil, or hemp oil as a dietary supplement instead of fish oils. These materials reduce platelet function for a brief period in dogs, but it seems that dogs compensate for this within about 8 weeks. Omega-3 fatty acids replace the 2-series fatty acids over time. As such, cellular stimulation produces 3-series prostaglandins and thromboxanes. The latter does not cause inflammation nor does it reduce blood flow like the 2-series thromboxanes do. All dogs should receive 1,000 mg of fish oil capsule, 1 tablespoon ground flax seeds, or 2 sardines every day.

Gamma-linolenic acid: 500 mgs BID.

Lecithin/phosphatidyl choline: One-fourth teaspoon for each 25 pounds of body weight BID.

Oil of evening primrose: 1 capsule for every 25 pounds of body weight SID.

Blue-green algae: One-fourth teaspoon for each 25 pounds of body weight daily.

Chinese herbal medicine/acupuncture

The authors use a formula called Degenerative Myelopathy at a dose of 1 capsule per 10–20 pounds twice daily to effect. In addition to the herbs discussed above, Degenerative Myelopathy also contains Antler gelatin (Lu jiao shuang), arisaema/bile (Dan nan xing), astragalus (Huang qi), bamboo silicea (Tian zhu huang), centipede (Wu gong), citrus (Chen pi), dragon's blood (Xue jie), earthworm (Di long), ginger (Ren shen), salvia (Dan shen), silkworm (Jiang can), and uncaria (Gou teng). These herbs help increase the efficacy of the formula.

The authors recommend the following acupuncture points: Bl18, BL23, BL30, BL60, ST36, Baihui, and GV4.

Homotoxicology (Dose:10 drops PO for 50-pound dog; 5 drops PO for small dog or cat)

The two protocols below are strictly experimental. The first is based upon current protocols used by Broadfoot; the second is based upon Reckeweg's protocol for multiple sclerosis. Results, positive or negative, should be reported for further evaluation.

Broadfoot's protocol for neurological degeneration:
Autosanguis Therapy (for the full procedure, see Advanced Homotoxicology: Autosanguis Therapy, chapter 33): (give half of each injection subcutaneously to patient and place the remainder in the symptom cocktail formula which follows below): Traumeel S, Galium-Heel plus Neuralgo Rheum, Circulo Injeel plus Engystol N, Discus Compositum, and Coenzyme compositum plus.

Ubichinon compositum. Give half of each injection subcutaneously to the patient and place the remainder in the following symptom cocktail:

Symptom cocktail: Phosphor homaccord, Gelsemium homaccord, Aesculus compositum, Ginseng compositum, and autosanguis (above) mixed together and given orally BID. Arsuraneel at 1 tablet BID orally.

Glyoxal compositum: 1 vial weekly. Circulo-Heel at 1 vial weekly.

Multiple sclerosis per Reckeweg:
Psorinoheel, Galium-Heel, Schwef-Heel, Graphites homaccord, Lymphomyosot mixed together and given 2 to 6 times daily. Injection therapy using Echinacea compositum (forte) and Cerebrum compositum every 2 to 4 days. Ubichinon compositum and Coenzyme compositum at intervals. Glyoxal compositum given once and repeated once change ceases. Medulla spinalis-Injeel (if available) given once weekly IM. Autosanguis therapy using the above-mentioned injections are recommended.

Product sources

Nutrition

Brain/nerve and immune support formulas: Animal Nutrition Technologies. *Alternatives:* Immune System Support—Standard Process Veterinary Formulas; Immuno Support—Rx Vitamins for Pets; Immugen—Thorne Veterinary Products.

Coenzyme Q10: Vetri Science; Rx Vitamins for Pets; Integrative Therapeutics.

Lecithin/phosphatidyl choline: Designs for Health.

N-acetyl cysteine: Pure Encapsulations.

Blue-green algae: Simplexity.

Beyond essential fats: Natura Health Products. **Alternatives:** Hemp oil—Nature's Perfect Oil; Flax oil—Barlean's Organic Oils; Eskimo fish oil—Tyler Encapsulations; Ultra EFA—Rx Vitamins for Pets; Omega-3,6,9—Vetri Science; Evening primrose oil—Jarrows Formulas.

Chinese herbal medicine
Natural Solutions, Inc.

Homotoxicology
BHI/Heel Corporation

REFERENCES

Western medicine references
Clemmons RM. Degenerative myelopathy. In: Kirk RW, ed. Current veterinary therapy X. Philadelphia: Saunders, 1989:830–833.
LeCouteur RA, Child G. Diseases of the spinal cord: degenerative myelopathy of dogs. In: Ettinger SJ, ed. Textbook of veterinary internal medicine. 3rd ed. Philadelphia: Saunders, 1989:648–649.
Sisson A. Myelopathy, Degenerative. In: Tilley L, Smith F. The 5-Minute Veterinary Consult: Canine and Feline, Blackwell Publishing, 2003.

IVM/nutrition references
Clemmons R. Degenerative Myelopathy German Shepherd Dogs. http://neuro.vetmed.ufl.edu/neuro/DM_Web/DMofGS.htm.
Horrocks LA, et al. Phosphatidyl Research and the Nervous System, Berlin: Springer Verlach, 1986.

Chinese herbal medicine/acupuncture references
Clemmons. http://neuro.vetmed.ufl.edu/neuro/DM_Web/DMofGS.htm. Accessed 10/20/06.
Liao Ning Zhong Yi Za Zhi (*Liaoning Journal of Chinese Medicine*), 1982;3:40.
Naeser (*Journal of Alternative and Complementary Medicine*) Vol. 2, 1996, pp. 211–248.
Xian Dai Zhong Yao Yao Li Xue (Contemporary Pharmacology of Chinese Herbs), 1997;425.
Xong ZY, et al. *Journal of Pharmacology.* 1963;10(12):708.

Xu Q, et al. *Journal of Pharmacology and Clinical Application of TCM.* 1993;9(4):30–33.
Yang F, et al. *China Journal of Experimental Clinical Immunology.* 1997;9(1):49–52.
Zhong Cao Yao (*Chinese Herbal Medicine*) 1991;22 (10):452.
Zhong Yao Yao Li Yu Ying Yong (Pharmacology and Applications of Chinese Herbs), 1983: 400.

Homotoxicolgy references
Boericke W. Materia Medica with Repertory, 9th ed. Santa Rosa, CA: Boericke and Tafel, 1927. pp 497–500.
Clemmons R. Degenerative Myelopathy: German Shepherd Dogs. http://neuro.vetmed.ufl.edu/neuro/DM_Web/DmofGS.htm
Reckeweg H. *Biotherapeutic Index: Ordinatio Antihomotoxica et Materia Medica*, 5th ed. Baden-Baden, Germany: Biologische Heilmittel Heel GMBH, 2000. pp 189, 337–338,
Wynn S, Marsden S. Manual of Natural Veterinary Medicine: Science and Tradition. St Louis: Mosby. 2003. pp 452–458.

EPILEPSY

Definition and cause

Epilepsy is defined as a seizuring condition in which there are no physical conditions or lesion in the brain. While the mechanism that incites epilepsy and convulsions is not known, it is believed that there is an underlying biochemical imbalance. Epilepsy is more common in Golden and Labrador retrievers, St. Bernards, Springer spaniels, Shetland sheepdogs, and Corgis. It is rare in cats.

Seizures can originate from a wide variety of causes. Anything that interferes with the complex and delicate neurophysiological, autoregulatory system may trigger seizure activity, and a partial list of precipitating causes includes acute trauma, hypoxia, infectious agents, parasites, brain swelling, scar tissue, impregnation of viral particles or toxins, metabolic disturbances, adverse reactions to medications, allergies, psychosomatic stressors, organ diseases (cardiovascular, hepatic, endocrine), electromagnetic disturbances, radiation damage, genetic factors, enzyme deficiencies or damage, and neoplasia (Dayrell-Hart 1991; Ettinger 1989; Lane 1990; Podell 1994, 1996; Trepanier 1995). The presence of seizures alone is not sufficient to diagnose epilepsy (Bagley 2005).

Medical therapy rationale, drug(s) of choice, and nutritional recommendations

The most popular therapy is a combination of phenobarbital and potassium bromide. Other therapies that are often recommended include dilantin, diazepam, and primadone (Ettinger 1989). There is little evidence to support diet in the control of seizures; however, several reports point to food allergies as the source of the seizures via an immune-mediated process. These studies indicate that a restricted diet was responsible for the resolution of the seizures. In people, studies have indicated that seizures can be controlled with a hypoallergenic type of diet; they showed that the seizures began again when other foods were reintroduced (Collins 1994, Crayton 1981). Despite the little amount of evidence, many veterinarians recommend a hypoallergenic type of diet when managing dogs and cats with epilepsy, often with surprisingly good results.

Anticipated prognosis

While control of seizures is possible with combinations of drugs such as phenobarbital and potassium bromide, complete control is often difficult. Side effects of medications that are refractory to chronic medications and the potential for status epilepticus lessen the course and prognosis.

Integrative veterinary therapies

Epilepsy is a chemical and electrical imbalance in the brain. Medical therapies are prescribed to stop seizures; however, they do not address the underlying cause or inciting factors leading to this imbalance. When approaching epilepsy from an integrative viewpoint, a double phase approach must be taken. First, the diagnosis must be confirmed and the proper medical or alternative therapies that control the convulsions implemented. Second, if possible, the approach should include a determination of the cause and the necessary steps to eliminate inciting factors. Assessing the animal's internal and external environments is important. In addition, the diet should be thoroughly examined; all chemical additives, preservatives, environmental toxins, and other potential seizure-causing substances should be eliminated; side effects of medications should be considered; and prior and future vaccinations should be evaluated for the long-term control of seizures (Gorham 1996, Levin 2002).

General considerations/rationale

Epilepsy has been linked to allergic food reactions. One report showed that there was significantly more biological evidence to an allergy component to epileptic people than non-epileptic people (Campbell 1973, Crayton 1981, Stevens 1965).

Appropriate nutrients

Nutritional/gland therapy: Glandular brain, pituitary, hypothalamus, pineal, liver, and adrenal glands supply the intrinsic nutrients that help to reduce cellular inflammation and improve the function of the brain and nerves, liver, and adrenal glands (see Gland Therapy in Chapter 2 for a more detailed explanation).

Note: Epilepsy can have multiple causes, and therefore a medical and physiological blood evaluation is recommended to assess general glandular health. This helps clinicians to formulate therapeutic nutritional protocols that address the central nervous system as well as other organ weaknesses (Cima 2000, Goldstein 2000) (see Chapter 2, Nutritional Blood Testing, for additional information).

Vitamin E: Research has found that adding vitamin E to medical therapy reduced the frequency of seizures (Horn 1991, Ogunmekan 1989, Sullivan 1990, Tupeev 1993).

Fatty acids: In preliminary studies it was found that omega-3 fatty acids significantly reduced the frequency of seizures in human patients (Schlanger 2002).

Phosphatidyl serine (PS): Phosphatidyl serine is a phospholipid that is essential in cellular membranes, particularly those of brain cells. It has been studied in people with mental functioning and degeneration with positive results (Crook 1991, Cenacchi 1993).

Lecithin/phosphatidyl choline: Phosphatidyl choline is a phospholipid that is integral to cellular membranes, particularly those of nerve and brain cells. It helps to move fats into the cells and is involved in acetylcholine uptake, neurotransmission, and cellular integrity. As part of the cell membranes, lecithin is an essential nutrient required by all the cells of the body for general health and wellness (Hanin 1987).

Magnesium: Physiologically, magnesium activates adenosine triphosphatase, which is required for the proper functioning of the nerve cell membranes and fuels the sodium potassium pump. Magnesium has also been associated with neuromuscular function and conditions such as muscle cramping, weakness, and neuromuscular dysfunction. Magnesium is recommended for therapy for epilepsy and weakening muscle function (Bibley 1996, Levin 2002).

Chinese herbal medicine
General considerations/rationale

According to Traditional Chinese Medicine, epilepsy is caused by Wind and Phlegm obstructing the Mind. There is also Liver Qi stagnation.

Author's interpretation

In Western terms, wind is motion. Epilepsy is a form of motion (wind) that is manifested by tonic/clonic muscular activity. Wind also refers to a condition that comes and goes suddenly, just as a gust of wind may do. Seizures tend to have this pattern. The patient is normal between episodes.

According to TCM, the Liver controls the Tendons and Ligaments. Therefore, smooth flow of Liver Qi is needed to keep the Limbs supple. When the suppleness is lost, movement becomes spastic.

The loss of consciousness experienced during a seizure is defined as interference with the functioning of the Mind (phlegm obscuring the Mind). When the Mind does not function properly, the patient is unable to interact normally with the environment (in other words, the patient loses consciousness).

The central nervous system must be sedated to prevent wind from creating the excess nerve activity that leads to seizures.

Appropriate Chinese herbs

In cases of active seizing, valium, barbiturates or inhalant anesthetics should be administered as required. Herbal therapy is helpful in decreasing the frequency, severity, or duration of seizures. The following herbs have demonstrated anti-epileptic effects:

Scorpion (Quan xie): Decreased the severity, duration, and frequency of seizures when administered to rats with induced epilepsy (Shen Yang Yi Xue Yuan Xue Bao 1988).

Silkworm (Jiang can): Reduces the frequency of seizures in humans (Jiang Su Yi Yao 1976).

Grass-leaf sweet-flag (Shi chang pu): Decreases seizure activity in humans (Yao Xue Tong Bao 1982).

Polygala root (Yuan zhi): Can help decrease seizure frequency (Zhong Yao Yao Li Yu Ying Yong 1983).

Uncaria (Gou teng): Contains rhynchophilline, a chemical that has been shown to decrease spontaneous activity and strengthen phenobarbital-induced sedation in mice (Shi 1993). It has been proven to prevent seizures in animals (Hsieh 1999).

In addition to herbal therapy, acupuncture may be considered to decrease the duration or frequency of the seizures. The efficacy of acupuncture reported in the literature varies greatly. Some researchers find that it has no effect, while others are more positive. In one study, 5 dogs with intractable epilepsy were treated with gold bead implants in acupuncture points. Three dogs responded but 2 dogs relapsed after 5 months. Reports of 2 other dogs treated with acupuncture in the ear (Shen-men point) demonstrated that acupuncture was able to decrease seizure episodes by 80% (Joseph 1992, van Niekerk 1988).

Homotoxicology
General considerations/rationale

Seizuring cases may represent Inflammation to Dedifferentiation phase homotoxicoses. For that reason, and because selection of correct antihomotoxic medicines depends upon proper identification of phase, the clinician must properly diagnose the condition and identify any extrinsic factors associated with the onset of seizures.

Typically, idiopathic epilepsy is thought to represent a Degeneration Phase disorder (Reckeweg 2000).

In cases in which other causes of seizure activity have been eliminated and the signs and history indicate idiopathic epilepsy, homotoxicology therapy can decrease seizure activity and reduce dependency upon pharmaceutical agents, and may help improve other pathological processes in a patient's condition. Antihomotoxic medicants are appropriate and can be used in conjunction with a wide variety of other supportive and pharmaceutical agents to manage seizures. Drugs are necessary and recommended for patients that have severe, life-threatening seizures, or when seizure intervals are too short.

Patients so treated often undergo regressive vicariation and it should be noted that in some instances, the seizure activity might worsen as neurological tissues become inflamed, swell, and discharge homotoxins. Many of these patients recover from their disease signs following such responses. Canine distemper virus signs, including mentation changes (with or without misemotional states), fever, tonic-clonic tics, oculonasal mucoid discharge, and coughing, can occur (Palmquist 2003). Such biological responses are predicted by Hering's Law and are necessary for healing; however, clients may not accept them readily, and they should be well informed before beginning such treatment.

Appropriate homotoxicology formulas

Autosanguis therapy may be needed to shift the organism's position to the left on the Six-Phase Table. A large number of homeopathic remedies are indicated for seizures, and a complete listing is not practical in such a text. The following list covers major antihomotoxic formulas; others may be indicated depending upon the entire case's manifestations:

Aconitum homaccord: Treats seizures aggravated by or associated with fear, fever, or red skin. Use early in the history because this is an Inflammation Phase remedy.

Apis homaccord: Reduces swelling.

Atropinum compositum: Treats convulsions and muscle spasms. Argentum nitricum is indicated in epilepsy when the pupils are enlarged for hours or days before the attack. It seldom produces a full and final cure; however, distinct improvements can often be achieved, e.g. in the frequency and violence of the attacks. Also note that it is absolutely necessary (for humans) to maintain a diet that is strictly free of pork toxins. The remedy also contains Atropinum sulphuricum, which acts like Belladonna but is to be preferred in neuralgias, painful states, biliary colic, and epilepsy. It should be used if Belladonna fails. This remedy is also found in Spascupreel. Cuprum aceticum is considered in diseases accompanied by a tendency to spasmodic conditions, such as cerebral seizure disorders (Reckeweg 2002).

Belladonna homaccord: Used in Inflammation Phase disorders and in acute seizures to reduce severity and length. It is the agent of first choice for acute seizure.

BHI-Body-Pure: Treats environmental toxicity issues, especially petroleum products, tobacco, drug exposure, and emotional upset.

BHI-Calming: Used for stress-induced issues.

Cerebrum compositum: Supports cerebral tissues with the help of Hyoscyamus. The indications include states of excitement with great restlessness, mobility, depression to the point of melancholia, dull apathy, delirium, weakness of thinking and memory, and a dulling of the powers of comprehension. Attacks of epileptic spasms with tetany, convulsions, trismus, congestion of blood in the head, and headaches are also typical. The eyes have a glazed stare and an unusual sheen, and there may be protrusion, distortion, and spasms of the eye muscles. Further indications are conjunctival discharge, marked pupil enlargement, dullness of vision, weakness of vision, and myopia (these are also indications for Belladonna).

A summary of the main Hyoscyamus symptoms presents the following remedy picture: symptoms of cerebral irritation with convulsions, muscle twitching, catalepsy, and epileptiform spasms. Another contributing note comes from Ignatia, which should also be borne in mind in numerous retoxic phases. The irritability of the nervous system may provide a clue (effects of strychnine and brucine), because this is characteristic of Ignatia and constitutes the organic foundation for the changing symptoms that occur in Impregnation Phases. It is a nerve remedy above all, suited to hypersensitivity of the sensory organs, including the skin, nasal organs, and taste. This remedy also treats trembling and twitching. It is used for Sydenham's chorea and epileptiform attacks (Reckeweg 2002).

Coenzyme compositum: Provides catalyst support of the metabolism. Important in nearly all cases.

Galium-Heel: Use in most epilepsy cases. It is a Deposition, Impregnation, Degeneration, and Dedifferentiation phase remedy that is very important in cellular detoxification and matrix drainage and cellular repair. It contains a wide variety of agents, especially Apis, which reduces swelling.

Hepar compositum: Provides liver detoxification and support.

Solidago compositum: Provides kidney support and detoxification.

Hepeel: Detoxifies and supports the liver.

Lymphomyosot: Used for lymph drainage and swelling reduction, especially when combined with *Apis homaccord* and/or *Traumeel*.

Lyssinum-Injeel: Not available in the United States but can be useful in cases of seizures associated with rabies vaccination reactions (Reckeweg 2000).

Molybdan compositum: Treats trace mineral disorders and chronic diseases.

Nux vomica homaccord: Treats gastrointestinal issues, food allergy, adverse reactions to food or food additives, emotional upsets, and anger.

Psorinoheel: Deep acting remedy that contain Bufo (toad venom), which is useful in Inflammation and Degeneration phase homotoxicoses. Signs may include alternating torpor and convulsions, and epileptiform attacks occur. A peculiar state of agitation is noticed before these symptoms appear, and deep sleep may be seen after the convulsions (Reckeweg 2002).

Also found is Cicuta virosa. The main indications include pica appetite, convulsions with worm infestation, epileptiform attacks, and meningitis with hypersensitivity and attacks. It is a complementary remedy in tubercular meningitis, and is indicated in a wide variety of psychoses and conditions of the brain and spinal cord that include cramps that may be caused by worms. There also may be stomach cramps with hematemesis, paralysis of the bladder, and skin diseases with simultaneous disturbances of the peripheral nervous system.

Spascupreel: Treats convulsions and muscle spasm. Agaricus muscarius is included for Sydenham's chorea, tics, states of agitation, epileptiform attacks, itching, crawling sensations, burning pains, sensations of numbness, general restlessness of the muscles with a compulsion to move in unusual ways (cf. Stramonium). The symptoms may change to tetany, stupor, conditions of excessive excitement, reduction of excitability of the nervous system, sequelae of drug and medication abuse, state of confusion, and cerebral seizure disorders (Reckeweg 2002).

Schwef-Heel: Sulfur-containing enzyme that is used for reactivation and detoxification. Dosing is intermediate (Heel 2003).

Strophanthus compositum: Contains Aesthusa cynapium for convulsions associated with vomiting (Reckeweg 2000). The tincture of Fool's Parsley produces considerable toxic effects that are particularly noticeable in disturbances of the nervous system: various kinds of spasms, dulling of faculties, loss of consciousness, oppressed mood with anxiety, restlessness, irritability, possibly hallucinations, delirium, and sleepiness, sometimes to the point of unconsciousness. Epileptiform spasms also may occur, along with dilated pupils and particularly great weakness of the lower limbs (Reckeweg 2002).

Thyroidea compositum: Provides hormonal support and matrix drainage. Corpus Pineale Suis exhibits certain counterpoint actions to the pituitary. May be tried experimentally as a supporting or intercurrent remedy in epilepsy, Sydenham's chorea, and Degeneration Phases generally (Reckeweg 2002).

Traumeel: Reduces inflammation in traumatic or inflammatory issues.

Ubichinon compositum: Provides catalyst support of the metabolism in later cases. Naphthoquinone is also indicated in epilepsy with a brief aura, traumatic epilepsy, shock following serious head injury, and threatened vaccinial encephalitis from which seizures may result (Reckeweg 2002).

Valerianaheel: Mildly neurotonic and tranquilizing for stress-induced issues or difficulty sleeping. Contains Kali Bromatum (potassium bromide). The main indications are: restlessness, always busy and occupied, trembling hands, nervousness, conditions of excessive excitement associated with the central nervous system, cerebral seizure disorders, nightmares, sleepwalking, insomnia, reduced cerebral emotivity as with paralysis, and sequelae of cerebrovascular accidents (Reckeweg 2002). This component is also found in *Nervoheel*.

Viscum compositum: Used in Dedifferentiation Phase cases.

Authors' suggested protocols

Nutrition

Brain/nerve support formula: 1 tablet for each 25 pounds of body weight BID.

Pituitary/hypothalamus/pineal and immune support formulas: One-half tablet for each 25 pounds of body weight SID.

Lecithin/phosphatidyl choline: One-fourth teaspoon for each 25 pounds of body weight BID.

Phosphatidyl serine: 25 mgs for each 25 pounds of body weight BID.

Omega-3 fatty acids: Eskimo fish oil—one-half to 1 teaspoon per meal for cats, 1 teaspoon for each 35 pounds of body weight for dogs; hemp or flax oil—1 teaspoon for every 25 pounds of body weight with food.

Additional vitamin E: 50 IU for each 25 pounds of body weight.

Magnesium: 10 mgs for every 10 pounds of body weight SID.

Chinese herbal medicine

Epitrol (White Crane Herbs): 1 capsule per 10 to 20 pounds BID to effect.

Important note: The Epitrol formulation also contains the following herbs: Abalone shell (Shi jue ming), snake skin slough (She tui), typhonium gigantium rhizome (Bai fu zi), arisaema pulvis (Dan nan xing), bamboo shavings (Zhu ru), red tangerine peel (Ju hong), gentiana root (Long dan cao), scutellaria (Huang qin), forsythia (Lian qiao), gypsum/raw (Shi gao), and hoelen spirit (Fu shen). These herbs help to balance the formula and increase the efficacy of the herbs mentioned above. They also help to increase the antiseizure activity of the formula.

The authors occasionally use the following acupuncture points for treatment of active seizing or to prevent future seizures; they are generally used in conjunction with herbal or Western therapy: GB20, Bai hui, PC6, St36, Bl15, and Bl18.

Homotoxicology (Dose: 10 drops PO for 50-pound dog; 5 drops PO for small dog or cat)

Symptom formula: Start cases on the following mixture for 8 to 12 weeks: Galium-Heel, Spascupreel, Belladonna homaccord, Atropinum compositum BID to TID PO as needed. In acute seizures this mixture can be given several times in close succession. Adjust this mixture as the case dictates. In cases in which constitutional seizures are suspected, consider Psorinoheel if no or poor response is obtained.

Deep detoxification formula: Thyroidea compositum, Hepar compositum, Solidago compositum, Coenzyme compositum every 3 days for several months. Handle regressive vicariation as needed during this process.

Note: After several months attempt to reduce anticonvulsant dosage slowly.

Product sources

Nutrition

Brain/nerve, pituitary/hypothalmus/pineal, and immune support formulas: Animal Nutrition Technologies. **Alternatives**: Immune System Support—Standard Process Veterinary Formulas; Immuno Support—Rx Vitamins for Pets; Immugen—Thorne Veterinary Products.

Lecithin/phosphatidyl choline: Designs for Health.

Phosphatidyl serine: Integrative Therapuetics.

Eskimo fish oil: Tyler Encapsulations. **Alternatives**: Flax oil—Barlean's Organic Oils; Hemp oil—Nature's Perfect Oil; Ultra EFA—Rx Vitamins for Pets; Omega-3,6,9—Vetri Science.

Chinese herbal medicine

Epitrol: White Crane Herbs.

Homotoxicology

BHI/Heel Corporation

REFERENCES

Western medicine references

Collins JR. Seizures and other neurologic manifestations of allergy. *Veterinary Clinics of North America: Small Animal Practice* 1994; 24: 735–48.

Conrack CN, Gerard VA. Identifying the cause of an early onset of seizures in puppies with epileptic parents. *Veterinary Medicine*, 1991; 1060–1061.

Crayton JW. Epilepsy precipitated by food sensitivity: Report of a case with double-blind placebo controlled assessment. *Clinical Electroencephalography*1981; 12:192–198.

Dayrell-Hart B, Steinberg SA, Van Winkle TI. Hepatoxicity of phenobarbital in dogs: 18 cases (1985–1989). *Journal of the American Veterinary Medical Association* 1991; 199:1060.

Ettinger SJ. Seizures. In: Textbook of Veterinary Medicine, Diseases of the Dog and Cat, Anonymous. Philadelphia: WB Saunders Company 1989, p. 66–69.

Lane S, Bunch SE. Medical management of recurrent seizures in dogs and cats. *Journal of Veterinary Internal Medicine* 1990; 4:26.

Podell M. Seizures in the dog. *Veterinary Clinics of North America: Small Animal Practice* 1996;26(4):779–809.

Podell M, Fenner WR. Use of bromide as an antiepileptic drug in dogs. *Compendium Continuing Education Practicing Veterinary* 1994;16:767–773.

Trepanier LA. Use of bromide as an anticonvulsant for dogs with epilepsy. *Journal of the American Veterinary Medical Association* 1995207:163.

IVM/nutrition references

Bilbey DLJ, Prabhakaran, VM. Muscle cramps and magnesium deficiency: case reports. *Canadian Family Physician*, 1996;Vol. 42, July, pp. 1348–51.

Campbell M. Neurologic manifestations of allergic disease. *Ann Allergy* 1973;31:485–98 [review].

Cenacchi T, Bertoldin T, Farina C, et al. Cognitive decline in the elderly: a double-blind, placebo-controlled multicenter study on efficacy of phosphatidylserine administration. *Aging (Milano)* 1993;5:123–33.

Cima J. Biochemical Blood Chemistry Evaluation, Palm Beach Gardens, FL., March 2000.

Crayton JW, Stone T, Stein G. Epilepsy precipitated by food sensitivity: report of a case with double-blind placebo-controlled assessment. *Clin Electroencephalogr* 1981;12:192–8.

Crook TH, Tinklenberg J, Yesavage J, et al. Effects of phosphatidylserine in age-associated memory impairment. *Neurology* 1991;41:644–9.

Goldstein R, et al. The BNA Handbook: A Working Manual for Veterinarians, Westport, CT: Animal Nutrition Technologies, 2000.

Gorham ME. Epilepsy significant clinical problem in canines; logical evaluation of patients imperative. *DVM Newsmagazine*: 1S, 1996.

Levin DL. Canine Epilepsy—An Owner's Guide to Living With or Without Seizures, Oregon City, OR: Lantern Publications, 2002.

Hanin IG, Ansell B. Lecithin: Technological, Biological, and Therapeutic Aspects, 1987, NY: Plenum Press, 180, 181.

Hom AC, Weaver RC, Aldersen JJ. Efficacy of D-alpha tocopherol acetate as adjunctive antiepileptic agent in patients with refractory epilepsy and profound developmental disability. A prospective, randomized, double-blind, placebo-controlled trial. *Epilepsia* 1991;32(suppl 3):63.

Levin C. Canine Epilepsy, Oregon City, OR: Lantern Publications, 2002 P 18–19.

Ogunmekan AO, Hwang PA. A randomized, double-blind, placebo-controlled, clinical trial of D-alpha tocopheryl acetate (vitamin E), as add-on therapy, for epilepsy in children. *Epilepsia* 1989;30:84–9.

Schlanger S, Shinitzky M, Yam D. Diet enriched with omega-3 fatty acids alleviates convulsion symptoms in epilepsy patients. *Epilepsia* 2002;43:103–104.

Stevens H. Allergy and epilepsy. *Epilepsia* 1965;6:205–16.

Sullivan C, Capaldi N, Mack G, Buchanan N. Seizures and natural vitamin E. *Med J Aust* 1990;152:613–4 [letter].

Tupeev IR, Kryzhanovskii GN, Nikushkin EV, et al. The antioxidant system in the dynamic combined treatment of epilepsy patients with traditional anticonvulsant preparations and an antioxidant—alpha-tocopherol. *Bull Eksp Biol Med* 1993;116:362–4.

Chinese herbal medicine/acupuncture references

Hsieh C-L, Tang N-Y, Chiang S-Y, et al. Anticonvulsive and free radical scavenging actions of two herbs, Uncaria Rhynchophylla (MIQ) jack and Gastrodia Elata BL., in kainic acid-treated rats. *Life Sci* 1999;65:2071–82.

Jiang Su Yi Yao (*Jiangsu Journal of Medicine and Herbology*), 1976;2:33.

Joseph R. Neurologic Evaluation and its Relation to Acupuncture. *Problems in Veterinary Medicine*, 1992;4:1, 98–206.

Life Sci 1999; 65(20): 2071–82.

Shen Yang Yi Xue Yuan Xue Bao (*Journal of Shenyang University of Medicine*), 1988;5(2):110.

Shi JS, et al. *China Journal of Pharmacology*. 1993;14(2): 114–117.

van Niekerk J, Eckersley GN. The Use of Acupuncture in Canine Epilepsy. *Journal of the South African Vet Association*, 1988.59:1, 5.

Yao Xue Tong Bao (Report of Herbology) 1982; 9:50.

Zhong Yao Yao Li Yu Ying Yong (Pharmacology and Applications of Chinese Herbs) 1983; 477.

Homotoxicology references

Bagley R. Fundamentals of Veterinary Clinical Neurology. Ames, IA: Blackwell. 2005. pp 363, 365.

Heel. Veterinary Guide, 3rd English edition. Baden-Baden, Germany: Biologische Heilmittel Heel GMBH, 2003. p 37.

Palmquist R. Distemper-like symptoms seen during regressive vicariation and seizure onset in a dog under treatment for dedifferentiation phase disorders: Hering's law illustrated. Unpublished case report. 2003.

Reckeweg H. Biotherapeutic Index: Ordinatio Antihomotoxica et Materia Medica, 5th ed. Baden-Baden, Germany: Biologische Heilmittel Heel GMBH, 2000. p. 136–7, 529.

Reckeweg H. Homeopathia Antihomotoxica Materia Medica, 4th ed. Baden-Baden, Germany: Aurelia-Verlag, 2002. pp 125–6, 127, 147, 161, 235, 257–8, 267, 350–1, 367, 437.

ENCEPHALITIS

Definition and cause

Encephalitis is an inflammatory process of the brain that may or may not involve the meninges and/or the spinal cord. It is often caused by infections and immune-mediated processes, especially in pugs and Maltese dogs. Encephalitis occurs in both dogs and cats, and is commonly associated with the following causes: viral (canine distemper or feline viral diseases), bacterial, rickettsial, protozoan, and mycotic (Appel 1969, Braund 1994, Greene 1990, Sisson 2003, Summers 1995, Vandevelde 1980). There is some evidence of post-vaccinal encephalitis (Bestetti 1978, Cornwell 1988, Hartley 1974).

Medical therapy rationale, drug(s) of choice, and nutritional recommendations

Therapy is directed to the underlying causes along with symptomatic treatment such as the control of seizuring. Specific therapies are directed to the causative agent or process once the diagnosis is made. Common medical therapies include corticosteroids, antibiotics, antifungal agents, and mannitol to reduce edema (Braund 1994, Sisson 2003, Summers 1995).

Anticipated prognosis

The prognosis depends upon the underlying cause and the extent of the inflammatory process. The prognosis for infectious agents is generally fair if treated promptly. Viral and immune-mediated processes carry a more cautious prognosis. Post-vaccinal encephalitis can be mild but often causes permanent damage to the brain (Braund 1994, Sisson 2003). Pug encephalitis is difficult to manage and is often fatal (Hasegawa 2000).

Integrative veterinary therapies

The underlying process is inflammatory and more commonly immune-mediated. The integrative approach, therefore, is to use nutrients, medicinal herbs, and combination homeopathics that have anti-inflammatory properties and that can help balance the immune system and quiet the exaggerated response. Clinicians should use any appropriate therapy in these cases. Integrative therapy using conventional medicine, nutrition, and biological agents may speed recovery, as well as improve patient comfort (Kline 2002).

Nutrition
General considerations/rationale
After the cause of the encephalitis is identified, the clinician should include nutritional support for the brain and nervous system, as well as the immune glands and the liver along with indicated medical therapy.

Appropriate nutrients
Nutritional/gland therapies: Glandular brain, adrenal, thymus, spleen, and liver supply intrinsic nutrients, help protect the organs' cells, reduce inflammation, and improve circulation to the brain (see Gland Therapy in Chapter 2).

Phospholipids found in glandular brain are a source of unsaturated omega-3 fatty acids, which are now thought to play a vital role in the development and maintenance of the central nervous system. High concentrations of phosphatidyl choline and serine are found in brain tissue. Horrocks (1986) reported on the potential clinical use of these nutrients in chronic neurological conditions.

Betasitosterol: Betasitosterol is a plant-derived sterol that has anti-inflammatory properties similar to those of corticosteroids and aspirin (Gupta 1980). Sterols also have been proven to enhance immune function (Bouic 1996). They have been found to be able to enhance T-lymphocyte production and moderate B cell activity, thereby helping to balance the immune response and indirectly reducing the risk of an auto-immune reaction (Bouic 1996).

N,N-Dimethylglycine (DMG): DMG has been widely researched in both humans and animals. It has been found to increase energy and enhance immune function (Barnes 1979, Graber 1981, Kendall 2000, Reap 1990, Walker 1988).

Chinese herbal medicine/acupuncture
General considerations/rationale
Encephalitis is caused by Heat and Wind accumulation in the Heart and Lung, which dries the body fluid into Phlegm. The Phlegm in turn moves upward to brain and blocks the meridians. The Heart houses the Shen, or Mind. Heat in the Heart can upset the Mind. The term "Phlegm blocking the meridians" translates into a clouding of the mind. In other words, in this condition the patient cannot interact properly with its environment. It also refers to the decrease of consciousness. Heat can also refer to the fevers seen in some cases. The term Wind refers to seizure activity.

Appropriate Chinese herbs
Centipede (Wu gong): Has antiseizure effects (Zhong Yao Xue 1998). It also inhibits various bacteria (Chang Yong Zhong Yao Cheng Fen Yu Yao Li Shou Ce 1994).

Curcuma (Yu jin): Contains curdione, which has sedative effects on the central nervous system (Hao 1994).

Forsythia (Lian qiao): Decreases inflammation by decreasing capillary permeability, which contributes to its inhibitory effect on edema. It also decreases fever (Ke Yan Tong Xun 1982, Ma 1982) and pain (Rui 1999). Forsythia has antiviral and antibacterial effects (Zhang 2002, 1982).

Grass-leaf sweet-flag root (Shi chang pu): Contains alpha-asarone, which has demonstrated an efficacy of approximately 85% in treating seizures in 90 people (Yao Xue Tong Bao 1982).

Gypsum (Shi gao): Has antipyretic effects. In one study of 200 patients with fevers, 90% experienced a significant reduction of temperature (Xin Zhong Yi 1980). It stimulates the phagocytic activity of macrophages (Zhong Yao Xue 1998) and concurrently decreases inflammation (Zhong Hua Wai Ke Za Zhi 1960).

Honeysuckle (Jin yin hua): Contains multiple compounds with antibacterial effects. The strongest among these are chlorogenic acid and isochlorogenic acid (Xin Yi Xue 1975, Jiang Xi Xin Yi Yao 1960). In addition, honeysuckle has demonstrated anti-inflammatory and antipyretic effects in rabbits and mice (Shan Xi Yi Kan 1960).

Isatis leaves (Da qing ye): Has antibacterial and antiviral activity (Health and Epidemic Prevention Station of Lingling 1975, Wang 1983). In addition to direct antipathogen effects, it enhances the immune system by increasing the phagocytic activity of macrophages and increasing serum lysozyme (Li 1996). Finally, isatis leaves have an anti-inflammatory action (Li 1996).

Licorice (Gan cao): Has glycyrrhizin and glycyrrhetic acid, which have significant anti-inflammatory effects. They have approximately 10% of the corticosteroid activity of cortisol and can help prevent the formation of granulomas (Zhong Cao Yao 1991). Licorice has an analgesic effect (Zhong Yao Xue 1998). It also has demonstrated both antibacterial and antiviral effects (Zhong Yao Zhi 1993, 1996).

Lophatherum (Zhu ye): Decreases fevers. It is as effective as phenacetin. It also has diuretic effects (Zhong Yao Yao Li Yu Ying Yong 1977), which may help decrease cerebral edema.

Red peony (Chi shao): Contains paeoniflorin, a compound that has demonstrated antiseizure and sedative effects in animals (Zhong Yao Xue 1998).

Saussurea (Mu xiang): Has demonstrated antibacterial effects against several strains of bacteria (Zhong Yao Yao Li Yu Ying Yong 1983).

Scorpion (Quan xie): Has been shown experimentally to control caffeine- or megimide-induced seizures in mice (Shen Yang Yi Xue Yuan Xue Bao 1988). A similar study of induced seizures in rats showed a decrease in severity, duration, and recurrence rates (Shen Yang Yi Xue Yuan Xue Bao 1989).

Silkworm (Jiang can): Has been proven effective at decreasing seizure activity in mice with experimentally induced seizures (Zhong Cao Yao Xue 1980). In one trial, 77% of humans with epilepsy who were treated with Jiang can responded well (Jiang Su Yi Yao 1976). It was shown to have synergistic activity with phenobarbitol in mice (Chang Yong Zhong Yao Cheng Fen Yu Yao Li Shou Ce 1994). It is especially efficacious in cases of pyrexia-induced seizures (Zhong Guo Nong Cun Yi Xue 1984). As an added benefit, it has been shown to inhibit several strains of bacteria (Zhong Yao Xue 1998).

Uncaria (Gou teng): Has been shown to prevent seizures in animals (Hsieh 1999).

Acupuncture

There are few studies involving the use of acupuncture for encephalitis per se. Schoen (1991) postulated that it would be helpful in cases of encephalitis by decreasing inflammation and preventing muscle spasms. It helps alleviate seizures, possibly by causing the release of serotonin and GABA (Wu 1988).

Homotoxicology
General considerations/rationale

Acute bacterial encephalitis represents an Inflammation Phase condition. Parasitic encephalitides are found in the Deposition Phase, while viral conditions are categorized as Impregnation Phase homotoxicoses. Most other inflammatory conditions are Impregnation or Degeneration phase disease manifestations. Such conditions can undergo rapid progressive vicariation to the Degeneration Phase.

Treatment involves supporting the immune system in its efforts to eliminate pathogens and associated homotoxins, as well as controlling swelling and pain to minimize damage to the delicate central nervous system. Moderate fevers help to remove homotoxins. The overuse of nonsteroidal antipyretics is undesirable from a biological therapy viewpoint.

Appropriate homotoxicology formulas

No veterinary studies exist on the use of antihomotoxic agents in encephalitis and meningitis, but Reckeweg developed protocols for human patients that can be applied to veterinary patients when biological therapy is desired. Appropriate remedies for consideration include:

Aconitum homaccord: Aconitum (also common to *Barijodeel, Bryaconeel, Cerebrum compositum, Echinacea compositum, Gripp-Heel, Pectus-Heel, Rhododendroneel, Spascupreel, Strophanthus compositum, Traumeel, BHI-Chamomilla Complex, BHI-FluPlus, BHI-Injury,* and *BHI-Spasm-Pain*) is the main remedy. It is one of the most important homeopathic fever remedies, especially when the skin is hot, there is alternating fever and chills, and there is possible hyperthermia and paresthesia. Often, the patient exhibits great anxiety and a rapid, tense pulse that is strong and possibly dysrhythmia. Low potencies are normally given in pyrexia and organic complaints, catarrhs, neuralgic symptoms with paresthesia, hyper-thermia, and encephalitis with very high temperatures (e.g., post-vaccinal encephalitis or meningoencephalitis (Reckeweg 2002).

Aesculus compositum: Helps to improve circulation following stroke or reduced cerebral circulation (Aesculus hippocastanum and Secale cornutum). Areteria suis supports the arteries. Solanum nigrum further supports cerebral function, particularly in cases with confusion, epileptic seizures, or disorientation. Several other agents support homotoxin removal and improve vessel stability (Reckeweg 2000). This remedy also contains Baptisia, which is also found in *Arnica-Heel*, *Atropinum compositum*, *Echinacea compositum*, *Populus homaccord*, and *Solidago compositum*. It has indications in typhoid fevers, sepsis, and septic sore throat, as well as encephalitis and meningitis with states of confusion. It should be given intercurrently in all septic fevers (Reckeweg 2002).

Apis mellifica, a central component of several other remedies such as *Apis compositum*, *Belladonna homaccord*, *Apis homaccord*, *Arnica-Heel*, *Cruroheel*, *Galium-Heel*, and *Populus compositum,* is also included. There is also a certain oversensitivity to touch and frequently to any jarring, so that the patient yells out at the slightest bump. This may occur in meningeal irritation. In the latter, regarding human patients, such a typical penetrating scream (known as the "cri encephalique") may begin with no apparent cause. Thus, Apis is a remedy that is frequently indicated in inflammatory conditions of the serous membranes, the meninges, the synovial membranes, or the mucous membranes (Reckeweg 2002).

Apis homaccord: Generally useful in edema, but also in cerebral sensitivity. May assist cardiac-induced cerebral weakness through Scilla, Apisinum, and Apis mellifica. See *Aesculus compositum*, above.

Arsuraneel: Used for patients that do not respond to initial therapy. This formula may move them into a recovery phase through stimulation of the general defenses. It is useful in cases with seizures, anxiety feeling worse at night, paresis, and muscular disability (Reckeweg 2000).

Belladonna homaccord: With an affinity for the central nervous system, Belladonna is useful in patients who manifest seizures and scream out at night. Violent delirium is characteristic of Belladonna, above all in fever. Belladonna's typical action on the eyes is also well known, It is used for cramps in the muscles of the eyes and eyelids, and enlargement of the pupils, particularly in an inflammatory or irritative condition of the conjunctiva with great photophobia, epiphora, and pain. Belladonna is indicated in incipient boils; tonsillitis; surface inflammations such as erysipelas, conjunctivitis, and scarlet fever; otitis; cholangitis; meningitis; and other inflammatory affections. A delirious state occurs with a violent rise in temperature with considerably raised sensitivity of all the senses and a disproportionate sensitivity to touch, noises, light, cold air (especially draughts and jarring) as can be the case in meningitis. Along with nasal catarrhs, there

may be catarrhs of the larynx and trachea, with slight mucus, accompanied a typical cough that is dry, rough, and barking, with hoarseness. In the digestive organs, Belladonna affects acute gastric catarrhs (Reckeweg 2002).

Bryaconeel: Treats neuralgia, serous membrane inflammation such as meningitis *(Bryonia cretica)*, acute feverish conditions, and influenza-like signs. Contains Phosphorus to support parenchymatous organs such as the lung and liver. Moderates severe or overaggressive vicariations. Used in meningitis in cases that do not respond to primary therapy (Reckeweg 2000).

Cerebrum compositum: Supports cerebral tissue, stem cells, and vessels (Cerebrum suis, Placenta suis, and Arnica montana). Cerebrum suis is indicated in states of mental exhaustion and disturbances in development. Symptoms include functional weakness, circulatory disturbances of the brain, progressive paralysis (retrospective treatment), paraplegia, arteriosclerotic dementia, encephalomalacia (Reckeweg 2002), memory loss, and forgetfulness (Selenium, Thuja occidentalis, Acidum phosphoricum, Manganum phospohoricum, Semecarpus anacardium, Ambra grisea, Conium maculatum, Medorrhinum-Nosode). Supports cerebral function and vascular structures (Kalium phophoricum). Treats vertigo, stupor, and headache (Gelsemium sempervirens, Kalium bichromicum, Ruta graveolens), anxiety (Aconitum napellus), and exhaustion (China, Amarita cocculus). Supports capillary and other circulation, as well as lymph (Aesculus hippocastanum) and enzyme systems and difficulty sleeping (Hyoscyamus niger) (Reckeweg 2000).

Coenzyme compositum: Supports energy production through enzyme induction and repair, and is useful in repairing damage to enzyme systems of metabolism and following administration of drugs injurious to metabolism. Phase remedy in Degeneration and Dedifferentiation phases.

Cruroheel: Has strong connective tissue effects and is useful in difficult cases or those with strong vicariation signs.

Echinacea compositum: Contains Zincum metallicum (also in *Discus compositum*, *BHI-FluPlus*, etc.) Zincum metallicum is a great nerve remedy, exerting a fundamental action on the brain and the autonomic centers and the sympathetic and the parasympathetic nervous systems. Symptoms of cerebral irritation occur after vaccination and when there is a threat of viral encephalitis. In these cases, Zincum metallicum, together with other medicaments which provoke a regressive vicariation, is able to release the homotoxins from the nervous system and break them down by way of the vaccination pustules, which once more become inflamed. Similar action has been known in Sulphur and Cuprum. In particular, these effects of reactivating blocked enzyme systems have often been described with reference to Sulphur. Chronic nerve pains and muscular twitching, as well as a general nervousness and hypersensitivity and high degree of excitability with emaciation, exhaustion, and paralytic weakness, may also indicated a need for Zincum. These conditions may proceed to the point of complete paralysis or hemiparesis with twitching, tremors, and weakness, as well as spasmodic conditions, neuralgia, and diseases that afflict the spine, brain, and spinal cord (Reckeweg 2002).

Engystol N: Has antiviral effects through immunostimulation.

Galium-Heel: Phase remedy in matrix and cellular phases. Provides powerful support of the immune system (Echinacea augustifolia). Assists in drainage of cell and matrix, is supportive of renal tubular function, and decreases swelling and edema (Apis mellifica, Galium aparine, and Galium mollugo). It is a critical component in the deep detoxification formula. Doses should be administered with regard to clinical condition and response, with the dose reduced if strong reactions are noted (Reckeweg 2000).

Gelsemium homaccord: Treats neuralgia and nerve pain, headache, and posterior weakness. Commonly required in aging, large-breed dogs.

Glyoxal compositum: Provides mitochondrial repair of damaged enzyme systems in Degeneration and Dedifferentiation phase disorders.

Lymphomyosot: Used after cortisone therapy and mesenchymal purging in chronic disease states.

Placenta compositum: Supports hypophysis after cortisone therapy. Contains sulfur to support enzyme and metabolic repair. Regenerative of hypophyseal-adrenal axis. Repairs vascular structures and is used intermittently in endocrine disorders.

Secale compositum: The principle remedy (also found in *Aesculus compositum, Arsuraneel, Circulo-heel, Discus compositum, Placenta compositum, Secale* [also known as *Arteria-Heel*], *Syzygium compositum, BHI-Headache II, BHI-Migraine,* and *BHI-Varicose*). Symptoms of meningitis may occur, with stiffness of the neck, muscular weakness, and periodic muscular pain with spasm and heaviness of the limbs and drawing and jerking pains. There also may be cramps, twitching and trembling of the limbs, or rigidity and stiffness of the limbs and joints (Reckeweg 2002).

Solidago compositum: Deposition Phase remedy needed to remove debris from the matrix after regressive vicariation begins. Contains Coxsackie Virus Nosode with indications that include abacterial meningitis and headache, possibly including pareses (Reckeweg 2002).

Spigelon: Helpful for symptoms of headache, cerebral conditions with inflammation, and weakness of connective tissues (Reckeweg 2000).

Thyroidea compositum: Provides matrix drainage and repair of autoregulation. Contains low levels of thyroid, pineal, spleen, bone marrow, umbilical cord, and liver to support glandular function and repair. Galium aparine drains matrix and cellular components. Cortisonum aceticum, in low potency, assists in repairing damage from excess levels of cortisone. Precursors and Krebs cycle constituents promote energy metabolism through the Michaelis-Menten law of enzyme activity. Pulsatilla and Sulfur assist in regulation rigidity-type situations. Part of the deep detoxification formula (Reckeweg 2000).

Tonsilla compositum: Main antihomotoxic drug for repairing chronic diseases involving endocrine disorders. Supports a wide number of tissues including tonsil, lymph node, bone marrow, umbilical cord (stem cell precursors), spleen, hypothalamus, liver, embryo, and adrenal cortex (Heine 2004). Contains Cortisonum aceticum and thyroid hormone in nanodilutions. Also contains Psorinum for deep constitutional, lack of reaction cases. Degeneration phase agent (Reckeweg 2000).

Ubichinon compositum: Provides mitochondrial repair of energy production mechanisms. Used in chronic diseases and iatrogenic injury to mitochondria from antibiotic therapy. Part of deep detoxification formula.

Authors' suggested protocols

Nutrition

Brain/nerve support: 1 tablet for 25 pounds of body weight BID.

Immune support formula: One-half tablet for each 25 pounds of body weight BID.

Liver support formula: One-half tablet for each 25 pounds of body weight SID.

Betathyme: 1 capsule for each 35 pounds of body weight BID (maximum, 2 capsules BID).

DMG: Liquid—One-half ml per 25 pounds of body weight (maximum, 2 mls); tablets—125 mg to 1 tablet for every 40 pounds of body weight (maximum, 3 tablets).

Chinese herbal medicine

Formula H90 Encephalitis: 1 capsule per 10 to 20 pounds twice daily. It can be used in both acute and chronic encephalitis and is especially effective in cases with seizures. In addition to the herbs discussed above, H90 Encephalitis also contains arisaema/bile (Dan nan xing), orange peel (Ju hong), pinellia (Ban xia), and salvia (Dan shen), which increase the efficacy of the formula.

This formula can be combined with any Western therapy as needed (i.e., anticonvulsants, antibiotics, anti-inflammatories). Some acupuncture points to consider include PC6, SP6, PC7, ST40, CV26, GV14, and KI3 (Handbook of TCM Practitioners 1987).

Homotoxicology (Dose: 10 drops PO for 50-pound dog; 5 drops PO for small dog or cat)
According to Reckeweg, the following protocol is useful. Note that it has not been tested in animals.

Initial therapy: Belladonna homaccord and Apis homaccord mixed together and used orally TID. In viral issues, give Engystol N by injection or orally daily. In bacterial infections, consider Echinacea compositum given daily by injection (the initial dose is often given I.V., followed by sub-q dosing, often in the manner of an autosanguis injection). Spigelon given daily by injection or orally if there are signs of headache. Aesculus compositum and Echinacea comp forte, BID to TID orally.

In refractory cases that do not respond to initial therapy after 1 to 2 days: Cruroheel-S, Arsuraneel, and Bryaconeel mixed together and taken orally every 15 to 30 minutes. Aesculus compositum given in massive initial doses every 5 to 10 minutes and then TID orally as an aid to circulatory issues.

Following improvement: Cerebrum compositum, Placenta compositum, and Tonsilla compositum to improve cerebral, vascular, and lymphatic/immune status. Initially given by injection, then followed by oral dosing either together or on alternate days in succession twice weekly.

Product sources

Nutrition
Brain/nerve, immune, and liver support formulas: Animal Nutrition Technologies. **Alternatives:** Immune system and Hepatic support—Standard Process Veterinary Formulas; Hepagen—Thorne Veterinary Products; Immuno and Hepato Support—Rx Vitamins for Pets.

Betathyme: Best for Your Pets; Moducare; Thorne Veterinary Products.

DMG: Vetri Science.

Chinese herbal medicine
Formula H90 Encephalitis: Natural Solutions, Inc.

Homotoxicology
BHI/Heel Corporation

REFERENCES

Western medicine references
Appel MJ. Pathogenesis of canine distemper. *Am J Vet Res* 1969; 30:1167–1182.
Bestetti G, Fatzer R, Frankhauser R. Encephalitis following vaccination against distemper and infectious hepatitis in the dog. An optical and ultrastructural study. *Acta Neuropathol* (Berl) 1978; 43:69–75.
Braund KG. Clinical syndromes in veterinary neurology. 2nd ed. St. Louis: Mosby, 1994.
Braund KG. Encephalitis and meningitis. *Vet Clin North Am Small Anim Pract* 1980; 10:31–56.
Cornwell HJ, Thompson H, McCandlish IA, et al. Encephalitis in dogs associated with a batch of canine distemper (Rockborn) vaccine. *Vet Rec* 1988; 122:54–59.
Greene CE. Infectious diseases of the dog and cat. Philadelphia: Saunders, 1990.
Hartley WJ. A post-vaccinal inclusion body encephalitis in dogs. *Vet Pathol* 1974; 11:301–312.
Hasegawa T, Uchida K, Sugimoto M, et al. Long-term management of necrotizing meningoencephalitis in a pug dog. *Canine Practice* 2000; 25:20–22.
Sisson A. Encephalitis. In: Tilley L, Smith F. The 5-Minute Veterinary Consult: Canine and Feline, Blackwell Publishing, 2003.
Summers BA, Cummings JF, de Lahunta A. Veterinary neuropathology. Baltimore: Mosby, 1995.
Vandevelde M, Kristensen B, Braund KG, et al. Chronic canine distemper virus encephalitis in mature dogs. *Vet Pathol* 1980; 17:17–28.

IVM reference
Kline K. Complementary and alternative medicine for neurologic disorders. *Clin Tech Small Anim Pract*. 2002. Feb;17(1):pp 25–33.

Nutrition references
Barnes L. B15: The politics of ergogenicity. *Physicians and Sports Medicine*. 1979.7(#11):17.
Kendall R, Lawson JW. Recent Findings on N,N-Dimethylglycine (DMG): A Nutrient for the New Millennium, *Townsend Letter for Doctors and Patients*, 2000 May.
Bouic PJD, et al. Beta-sitosterol and beta-sitosterol glucoside stimulate human peripheral blood lymphocyte proliferation: Implications for their use as an immunomodulatory vitamin combination. *International Journal of Immunopharmacology* 1996;18:693–700.
Gupta MB, Nath R, Srivastava N, et al. Anti-inflammatory and antipyretic activities of β-sitosterol. *Planta Medica* 1980;39: 157–163.
Horrocks LA, et al. Phosphatidyl Research and the Nervous System, Berlin: Springer Verlach, 1986.
Reap E, Lawson J. Stimulation of the immune response by Dimethylglycine, a non-toxic metabolite. *Journal of Laboratory and Clinical Medicine*. 1990;115:481.
Walker M. Some Nutri-Clinical Applications of N,N-Dimethylglycine. *Townsend Letter for Doctors*. June 1988.

Chinese herbal medicine/acupuncture references
Chang Yong Zhong Yao Cheng Fen Yu Yao Li Shou Ce (A Handbook of the Composition and Pharmacology of Common Chinese Drugs), 1994; 1725:1728.
Chang Yong Zhong Yao Cheng Fen Yu Yao Li Shou Ce (A Handbook of the Composition and Pharmacology of Common Chinese Drugs), 1994; 1810:1812.
Handbook of TCM practitioners. Hunan College of TCM. Shanghai Science and Technology Press, Oct 1987; 249.

Hao HQ, et al. Curdione's regulatory effect on cats' sleeping rhythmic electric activity. *Journal of Chinese Materia Medica.* 1994;25(8):423–424.

Health and Epidemic Prevention Station of Lingling. 287 herbs' antibacterial effects. *Hunan Journal of Medicine and Herbs.* 1975;2(1):46.

Hsieh CL, Tang NY, Chiang SV, Hsieh CT, Lin JG. Anticonvulsive and free radical scavenging actions of two herbs, Uncaria rhynchophylla (MIQ) Jack and Gastrodia elata Bl., in kainic acid-treated rats. *Life Sci* 1999; 65(20):2071–82.

Jiang Su Yi Yao (*Jiangsu Journal of Medicine and Herbology*), 1976;2:33.

Jiang Xi Xin Yi Yao (*Jiangxi New Medicine and Herbology*), 1960 (1):34.

Ke Yan Tong Xun (*Journal of Science and Research*), 1982;(3):35.

Li MZ, et al. The pharmadynamics of Re Du Qing Injection. *China Journal of Experimental Recipes.* 1996;2(6):24–30.

Ma ZY. *Shannxi Journal of Traditional Chinese Medicine and Herbs.* 1982;(4):58.

Rui J. *Journal of Chinese Materia Medica.* 1999;30(1):43–45.

Schoen A. Acupuncture therapy for Chronic Lyme disease in the canine and equine. Proc 17th Ann Mtg IVAS, 1991. pp 52–55.

Shan Xi Yi Kan (*Shanxi Journal of Medicine*), 1960; (10):32.

Shen Yang Yi Xue Yuan Xue Bao (*Journal of Shenyang University of Medicine*), 1988; 5(2):110.

Shen Yang Yi Xue Yuan Xue Bao (*Journal of Shenyang University of Medicine*), 1989; 6(2):95.

Wang YS, et al. TCM Pharmacology and Application, 1st ed. Beijing: People's Health Press; 1983.

Wu D: Suppression of epileptic seizures with acupuncture. *Am J Acupuncture* 1988;16:113–118.

Xin Yi Xue (*New Medicine*), 1975; 6(3):155.

Xin Zhong Yi (*New Chinese Medicine*), 1980;6:28.

Yao Xue Tong Bao (*Report of Herbology*), 1982;9:50.

Zhang G, Song S, Ren J, Xu S. A New Compound from Forsythia suspense (Thunb.) Vahl with Antiviral Effect on RSV. *J of Herbal Pharmacotherapy.* 2002;2(3):35–39.

Zhong Cao Yao (*Chinese Herbal Medicine*) 1991;22(10):452.

Zhong Cao Yao Xue (Study of Chinese Herbal Medicine), 1980;1423.

Zhong Guo Nong Cun Yi Xue (*Chinese Agricultural Medicine*), 1984;(2):20.

Zhong Hua Wai Ke Za ZHi (*Chinese Journal of External Medicine*), 1960;4:366.

Zhong Yao Xue (Chinese Herbology), 1998, 115:119.

Zhong Yao Xue (Chinese Herbology), 1998; 162:164.

Zhong Yao Xue (Chinese Herbology), 1998, 704:706.

Zhong Yao Xue (Chinese Herbology), 1998, 706:708.

Zhong Yao Xue (Chinese Herbology), 1998; 759:765.

Zhong Yao Yao Li Yu Ying Yong (Pharmacology and Applications of Chinese Herbs), 1977:2253.

Zhong Yao Yao Li Yu Ying Yong (Pharmacology and Applications of Chinese Herbs), 1983;169.

Zhong Yao Zhi (*Chinese Herbology Journal*), 1993;358.

Zhu LH. *China Journal of TCM Information.* 1996;3(3):17–20.

Homotoxicology references

Heine H. Homotoxicology and basic regulation: Bystander reaction. *La Medicina Biologica.* 2004. January (1): p 5. http://www.gunainc.com/AllLanguages/ElencoScheda/Elenco_Scheda.asp?SelectionMenu=1096andxid=9BEB85D787A849 14AEED43918A937DBBandid_BoxContent=1077.

Reckeweg H. Biotherapeutic Index: Ordinatio Antihomotoxica et Materia Medica, 5th ed. Baden-Baden, Germany: Biologische Heilmittel Heel GMBH, 2000.p 22–3, 286–9, 295, 299–300, 302, 308–9, 337–8, 404, 415–6, 418–19.

Reckeweg H. Homeopathia Antihomotoxica Materia Medica, 4th ed. Baden-Baden, Germany: Arelia-Verlag GMBH, 2002. pp. 120, 167–8, 172–5, 222, 259, 525–8, 610–11.

GRANULAMATOUS MENINGOENCEPHALITIS(GME)/ PERIPHERAL NEUROPATHIES

Definition and cause

Peripheral neuropathies may represent numerous specific diagnoses. Many are inherited and have no successful treatment. When diagnosing such conditions it is helpful to divide them into categories of disease, including degenerative, genetic, idiopathic, inflammatory-noninfectious, inflammatory-infectious, metabolic, neoplasia, trauma, and vascular. Each particular case has a pathophysiology responsible for neurological dysfunction, and this identification may be immensely helpful in selecting proper biological therapy.

Often, the pathophysiology of many of these cases is never fully elucidated and clinicians may be forced to select therapy without a full understanding of the true condition. Common causes are immune-mediated, infectious, secondary to degenerative diseases such as diabetes or cancer, or secondary to a toxic reaction to chemotherapeutics or chemical toxins.

Establishing a complete diagnosis is well worth the effort. It may be very helpful to cooperate with internists and neurologists to determine successful treatment plans for patients suffering from neuropathies. Clients need to be counseled early on that these conditions may not respond and may even continue to deteriorate, even if the correct causation is determined (Braund 1980, 1982, 1988, 1995; Cuddon 1997; Cumming 1982, 1991; Griffiths 1985; Towell 1994).

Medical therapy rationale, drug(s) of choice, and nutritional recommendations

Medical therapy depends upon the underlying cause. If properly diagnosed and treated, the hope is that the neuropathy will resolve. Immune-mediated neoplasia most often require ongoing immunosuppressing therapies such as corticosteroids and chemotherapeutics (Braund 1995, Cuddon 1997, Cummings 1992).

Anticipated prognosis

The prognosis depends upon determining the underlying cause. Generally, a response is seen 1 to 3 months after initiating the therapy. The prognosis is poor to guarded if there is no response to the initial medical therapy (Cuddon 1997).

Integrated veterinary medicine

The underlying process is inflammation of the central nervous system. While the specific cause is not reported, inflammation and immune-mediated processes most often necessitate the selection of corticosteroids as the primary therapy. The integrative approach, therefore, is to use nutrients, nutraceuticals, medicinal herbs, and combination homeopathics that have anti-inflammatory properties and can help to balance the immune system and reduce an exaggerated response. Clinicians should use any appropriate therapy in these cases; integrative therapy using conventional medicine, nutrition, and biological agents may speed recovery and improve patient comfort (Kline 2002).

Nutrition
General considerations/rationale

While medical therapy is focused locally upon inflammation, the nutritional approach adds glandular support for the organs of the immune system as well as nutrients to help improve brain and nerve function.

Note: Because GME and its symptoms can range from local to systemic, it is recommended that blood be analyzed both medically and physiologically to determine concurrent disease. This helps clinicians to formulate therapeutic nutritional protocols that address the central nervous system as well as other organ systems (Cima 2000, Goldstein 2000) (see Chapter 2, Nutritional Blood Testing, for additional information).

Appropriate nutrients

Nutritional/gland therapy: Glandular brain, nerve, adrenal, and thymus supply the intrinsic nutrients that help to reduce cellular inflammation and improve nerve and immune function. This helps to spare the brain and nerve from ongoing immune attack and helps slow degeneration and loss of function (see Gland Therapy in Chapter 2 for a more detailed explanation).

Phospholipids found in glandular brain are a source of unsaturated omega-3 fatty acids, which are now thought to play a vital role in the development and maintenance of the central nervous system. High concentrations of phosphatidyl choline and serine are found in brain tissue. Horrocks (1986) reported on the potential clinical use of these nutrients in chronic neurological conditions.

Phosphatidyl serine: Phosphatidyl serine is a phospholipid that is essential for the integrity of cell membranes, particularly those of nerve and brain cells. It has been studied extensively in people with impaired mental functioning and degeneration with positive results (Cenacchi 1993).

Lecithin/phosphatidyl choline: Phosphatidyl choline is a phospholipid that is integral to cellular membranes, particularly those of nerve and brain cells. It helps to move fats into the cells and is involved in acetylcholine uptake, neurotransmission, and cellular integrity. As part of the cell membranes, lecithin is an essential nutrient required by all of the body's cells for general health and wellness (Hanin 1987).

Magnesium: Physiologically, magnesium activates adenosine triphosphatase, which is required for the proper functioning of the nerve cell membranes and fuels the sodium potassium pump. Magnesium is associated with neuromuscular function and conditions such as muscle cramping, weakness, and neuromuscular dysfunction. Magnesium is recommended for therapy for epilepsy and weakening muscle function. (Bibley 1996, Levin, 2002).

Sterols: Plant-derived sterols such as betasitosterol show anti-inflammatory properties that appear to be similar to corticosteroids (Gupta 1980). A cortisone-like effect without the associated immune suppressing effects is beneficial in any inflammatory process in the central nervous system. (Bouic 1996) reports on the immune enhancing and balancing effect of plant sterols that are also beneficial to animals with immune-mediated diseases.

Essential fatty acids: Research also confirms the benefits of essential fatty acids' calming effect on the central nervous system (Erasmus 1993).

Chinese herbal medicine/acupuncture
General considerations/rationale

GME is a combination of External Wind, Heat, and Toxin invading the Ying and Blood, which affects Wei and Qi at the same time. This leads to Heart and Pericardium disturbances.

Peripheral neuropathy may be a result of trauma or it may be due to Cold and Wind invasion, leading to Qi and Blood stagnation in the Meridians.

In GME, the Wind blows the pathogenic influence into the body. Heat and Toxins then invade the Ying and Blood layers of the body. The Heat refers to fever and inflammation. Toxins are the substances that cause the inflammation. Wei is the immune system, so there is a disruption of immunoregulation, which is in agreement with the Western understanding of an immune basis to this disease. Neurological signs appear when the Ying level is affected. At the Xue level, the Heart and Pericardium, which house and protect the mind, are disturbed. When this occurs, the patient does not react properly to the environment. This can explain the seizures with the attendant loss of consciousness.

Treatment is aimed at decreasing the inflammation, fever, and pain, and normalizing the neurological function.

In peripheral neuropathy the ancient Chinese physicians were well aware of the ability of trauma to damage nerves. When they could not point to trauma as a cause, they theorized that Wind blew Cold into the body. Cold was able to slow the transit of Blood and Qi in the Meridians. Without a normal flow of Blood and Qi, the limbs could not function properly. Treatment is aimed at normalizing limb function.

Appropriate Chinese herbs for GME

Achyranthes (Niu xi): Has shown analgesic effects. In mice it was shown to decrease pain reactions to body torsion and hot plates (Li 1999). It also demonstrated anti-inflammatory effects (Xong 1963).

Arctium Niu bang zi: Has anti-inflammatory and antipyretic effects (Zhong Yao Xue 1998).

Buffalo horn shaving (Niu jiao): A strong pain reliever that also decreases edema (Mao 1997).

Coix (Yi yi ren): Can help control pain and inflammation. It helps prevent carrageenin-induced foot swelling and dimethylbenzene-induced ear swelling in mice (Zhang Ming Fa 1998). A study involving 26 women with severe dysmenorrhea found that coix significantly decreased pain by more than 90% (Zhang Yong Luo 1998).

Forsythia (Lian qiao): Has anti-inflammatory, analgesic, and anti-pyretic effects and can prevent edema (Ma 1982, Rui 1999).

Gastrodia (Tian ma): Can help decrease pain. It decreases the level of dopamine in the brain, and this may be responsible for the analgesic effect (Huang 1993). It was shown to decrease agar-induced swelling in mice and carrageenin- and 5-HT-induced swelling in the feet of rats (Yu 1989). This anti-inflammatory action may be useful in treating GME.

Grass-leaf sweet-flag root (Shi chang pu): Contains alpha-asarone, which demonstrated an efficacy of approximately 85% in treating seizures in a group of 90 people (Yao Xue Tong Bao 1982). It may help decrease seizures in patients with GME.

Honeysuckle (Jin yin hua): An anti-inflammatory and antipyretic herb (Shan Xi Yi Kan 1960).

Isatis (Da qing ye): Has anti-inflammatory effects (Li 1996).

Licorice (Gan cao): Contains glycyrrhizin and glycyrrhetinic acid, which have anti-inflammatory effects. They have approximately 10% of the corticosteroid activity of cortisone. They decrease edema and decrease the formulation of granulomas (Zhong Cao Yao 1991).

Lophatherum (Dan zhu ye): An antipyretic herb (Zhong Yao Yao Li Yu Ying Yong 1977).

Mint (Bo he): Decreases fever and inflammation (Zhong Yao Xue 1998).

Platycodon (Jie geng): Contains platycodin, which has antipyretic effects (Li 1984, Zhang 1984). It also has anti-inflammatory effects via its ability to increase corticosterone secretion (Li 1984, Zhang 1984, Zhou 1979).

Pueraria (Ge gen): Reduces fevers (Modern TCM Pharmacology 1997).

Schizonepeta (Jing jie): Has analgesic properties (Zhong Yao Cai 1989).

Scutellaria (Huang qin): Contains baicalin and biacalein, which have been shown to suppress inflammation in mice (Kubo 1984). It also can lower fever (Xu 1999).

Silkworm (Jiang can): Has been shown to be effective in stopping experimentally induced seizures in mice (Zhong Cao Yao Xue 1980). In one trial, 77% of humans with epilepsy who were treated with Jiang responded well (Jiang Su Yi Yao 1976). This suggests that it may help reduce seizure activity in patients with GME.

Uncaria (Gou teng): Has been proven to prevent seizures in animals (Hsieh 1999).

Acupuncture for GME

The World Health Organization recognizes the efficacy of acupuncture for the treatment of headache (World Health Organization 2006). In addition, acupuncture has been shown to be better than phenobarbital at stopping fever-induced seizures in children (He 1997). This may have a dual effect of addressing both the seizure and fever aspects of GME.

Appropriate Chinese herbs for forelimb neuropathies

Angelica root (Dang gui): Increases phagocytic activity of macrophages (Zhong Hua Yi Xue Za Zhi 1978), which may help patients with infectious peripheral neuropathies. It also decreases inflammation (Yao Xue Za Zhi 1971), which may make it beneficial in inflammatory etiologies.

Astragalus (Huang qi): Can improve humoral and cellular immune functions (Jiao 1999), which may help in the case of bacterial or viral neuropathies.

Centipede (Wu gong): Has antibiotic properties. It inhibits cancer cells in vitro (Chang Yong Zhong Yao Cheng Fen Yu Yao Li Shou Ce 1994), which indicates that it may be useful for neuropathies secondary to these causes.

Cinnamon twig (Gui zhi): Inhibits some bacteria and viruses (Zhong Yao Xue 1998).

Earthworm (Di long): Has anti-neoplastic effects. The mechanism is not yet elucidated, but it may be due to enhanced immunity and scavenging of free radicals (Wang 1991). This may help in some forms of neoplastic neuropathy.

Jujube fruit (Da zao): Can inhibit dimethylbenzene-induced ear swelling in mice, and egg white-induced toe swelling in rats (Li 1997). It may also ameliorate inflammatory neuritis.

Licorice (Gan cao): Inhibits bacteria (Zhong Yao Zhi 1993) and viruses (Zhu 1996). It may be efficacious in viral and bacteria-mediated neuropathies.

Milettia (Ji xue teng): Has antiviral effects. It has been shown to inhibit herpes virus I (simplex), a virus known to be neurotropic (Meng 1995). In addition, it has demonstrated activity against cancers via increased NK activity in mice (Hu 1997, Xu 1996).

Rehmannia/cooked (Shu di huang): May help improve the conditions of nerves. One trial examined the results of an herbal supplement containing rehmannia with Rou cong rong, Lu han cao, Gu sui bu, Yin yang huo, Ji xue teng, and Lai fu zi in 1,100 patients with myelitis. 73% had significant improvement, and another 13% had moderate improvement in clinical signs (Liaoning Journal of Chinese Medicine 1982).

Tumeric (Jiang huang): May decrease neuronal inflammation. It inhibits MIP-2 (macrophage inflammatory protein-2) production. This chemical has been implicated in traumatic brain injury (Singh 2006), which strongly suggests applicability in patients with neuropathy.

White peony (Bai shao): Contains paeoniflorin, which is a strong anti-inflammatory (Zhong Yao Zhi 1993). In addition, it seems to have a neurotropic effect. It contains gallotannin, which prevents neuron damage in mice with cobalt-induced seizures (Sunaga 2004). This may make it a powerful herb for decreasing neuronal inflammation.

Wild ginger (Xi xin): Inhibits carrageenin-induced foot swelling (Xie 1995). It may prevent inflammation in the nervous system, thereby treating inflammatory neuropathies.

Appropriate Chinese herbs for hindlimb neuropathies

Achyranthes (Niu xi): Decreases egg-white-induced foot swelling in rats (Xong 1963). It may help decrease inflammation in the nervous system.

Alpinia (Yi zhi ren): Has demonstrated some anti-neoplastic activity (Zhong Guo Zhong Yao Za Zhi 1990).

Antler powder (Lu jiao jiao): Enhances the phagocytic function of macrophages and can be used as an adjuvant in cancer treatment (Du 1981).

Astragalus (Huang qi): See forelimb paralysis, above.

Cornus (Shan zhu yu): Can inhibit carrageenin-induced toe swelling in rats and mice (Zhao 1996). This suggests

that it may be useful in cases of inflammatory etiologies.

Dioscorea (Shan yao): Stimulates both the humoral and cellular immune system (Miao 1996). It may help with infectious causes of neuropathy.

Eucommia (Du zhong): Contains chlorogenic acid, which has antibacterial effects (Wang 1993). It stimulates cellular immunity (Liu 1998), which may make it useful when the neuropathy is due to infectious etiologies.

Ophiopogon (Mai men dong): Effective against Staphylococcus albus, Bacillus subtilis, E. coli, and Salmonella typhi (Zhong Yao Xue 1998).

Papaya (Mu gua): Has inhibitory effects on tumors (Zhong Cao Yao Tong Xun 1975).

Poria (Fu ling): Has antibiotic effects (Zhong Yao Cai 1985). It also stimulates cellular immunity (Lu 1990). Finally, it has demonstrated anti-neoplastic activity (Chen 1986).

Rehmannia/cooked (Shu di huang): See forelimb paralysis, above.

White atractylodes (Bai zhu): Has demonstrated anti-neoplastic efficacy (Zhong Liu Yu Zhi Tong Xun 1976).

Appropriate Chinese herbs for facial neuropathies

Angelica root (Dang gui): See forelimb neuropathies, above.

Centipede (Wu gong): See forelimb neuropathies, above.

Cnidium (Chuang xiong): Increases the phagocytic function of macrophages (Lang 1991). It may be helpful in infectious neuropathies.

Gastrodia (Tian ma): Decreases nerve pain from toxins and vascular causes (Ji Lin Yi Xue Yuan Xue Bao 1982).

Ginseng (Ren shen): Prevents the decrease in plasma T3 and T4 levels as laboratory animals age (Shi 1998). It may be useful in hypothyroid-induced neuropathies.

Siler (Fang feng): Has antibiotic properties (Zhong Yao Tong Bao 1988). It is also anti-neoplastic (Li 1999).

Silkworm (Jiang can): Can inhibit some bacteria (Zhong Yao Xue 1998).

White aconite (Bai fu zi): May help with facial nerve disorders. In one study, 90% of 418 people with facial numbness recovered completely when an herbal formula containing typhonium (Bai fu zi), angelica root (Dang gui), scorpion (Quan xie), sick silkworm (Jiang can), and centipede(Wu gong) was injected into acupoints (Hu Bei Zhong Yi Yao Za Zhi 1982).

Homotoxicology
General considerations/rationale
GME is an intracranial proliferative inflammatory process involving mesenchymal cells, which may present in a

generalized inflammatory form or a mass form. The cause is unknown. Lymphocytes and macrophages are the primary inflammatory cells that are present (Bagley 2005).

There is no published material on this condition in any homotoxicology references, which makes the material that follows an academic discussion. Goldstein (2006) has successfully used the protocol below in combination with other integrative modalities discussed in this section.

Because connective tissue elements function in an abnormal and deleterious manner, this condition represents a disease to the right of the Biological Divide, most likely the Impregnation and Degeneration phases. There may be Dedifferentiation Phase factors involved. Examination of such cases for chemical or viral agents may prove interesting in researching the cause. Antihomotoxic agents discussed in the encephalitis/meningitis section are applicable. Phase remedies and deep detoxification with support of energy-producing enzyme systems represent a logical clinical approach to this condition. The expected prognosis is guarded. The use of drugs such as corticosteroids and immunosuppressants are warranted to preserve patient comfort and ability. As with all neurological problems, use of a qualified neurologist may be helpful in establishing the correct diagnosis and most current treatment options.

Selecting symptom remedies and detoxification protocols is extremely important in neurology cases. Many homeopathic and herbal agents have affinity for neural tissue in specific body regions (neck, face, lumbar spine, extremities), and the integrative clinician should always be sure to consider the anatomical region is designing proper treatment programs. In traumatic cases, the use of simple single antihomotoxic formulas such as Traumeel S may give immediate improvement. Most cases of peripheral neuropathies presented to veterinarians represent deeper homotoxicoses and require combinations of therapy and careful monitoring of progress. Always remember that the goal of therapy is regressive vicariation and that signs of inflammation and discharge may well represent the beginning of healing in a patient. Inherited conditions generally carry a guarded prognosis, but may improve or stabilize with biological therapies integrated with conventional medical handlings, and it is beneficial to have a basic understanding of these approaches when faced with a nonresponsive or difficult case.

The development of acutely painful conditions similar to shingles in humans may represent the movement of homotoxins from chronic Impregnation and Degeneration phases to the Inflammation Phase, and should be welcomed as a potentially good sign. Other neurological signs may occur during these regressive vicariations (i.e., altered awareness, personality changes, tics, and seizures) and may require experienced handling as the patient

moves from right to left of the Six-Phase Table of Homotoxicology.

Appropriate homotoxicology formulas

Aesculus compositum: Useful in improving circulation following stroke or reduced cerebral circulation (Aesculus hippocastanum and Secale cornutum). Areteria suis supports the arteries. Solanum nigrum further supports cerebral function, particularly in cases with confusion, epileptic seizures, or disorientation. Several other agents support homotoxin removal and improve vessel stability (Reckeweg 2000).

Apis homaccord: Generally useful in edema, but also in cerebral sensitivity. May assist cardiac-induced cerebral weakness through Scilla, Apisinum, and Apis mellifica. The main symptoms of Apis may be summed up as follows for quick reference: sensitivity to touch and jarring; irritation of the meninges, especially from suppressed eruptions; diseases of the serosa, joints, and meninges; infiltration of the cellular tissues; and serous meningitis (Reckeweg 2002). Apis is also found in *Aesculus compositum*, *Cerebrum compositum*, *Placenta compositum*, and *Tonsilla compositum*.

Arsuraneel: Used for patients not responding to initial therapy; this formula may move them into a recovery phase through stimulation of the general defenses. Useful in cases with seizures, anxiety, feeling worse at night, paresis, and muscular disability (Reckeweg 2000).

Belladonna homaccord: Belladonna, which has an affinity for the central nervous system, is useful in patients manifesting seizures and who scream out at night. Violent delirium is characteristic of Belladonna, above all in fever. Belladonna's typical action on the eyes is also well-known, with cramps in the muscles of the eyes and eyelids, enlargement of the pupils and, in particular, an inflammatory or irritative condition of the conjunctiva with marked photophobia, lachrymation, and pain. Belladonna is indicated in incipient boils, tonsillitis, and surface inflammations such as erysipelas, conjunctivitis, scarlet fever, otitis, cholangitis, meningitis, and other inflammatory affections. A delirious state occurs with a violent rise in temperature with considerably raised sensitivity of all the senses and a disproportionate sensitivity to touch, noises, light, cold air—especially draughts and jarring—as can be the case in meningitis. Along with nasal catarrhs, there may be catarrhs of the larynx and trachea, with slight mucus, accompanied a typical cough, which is dry, rough, and barking, with hoarseness. In the digestive organs, Belladonna affects acute gastric catarrhs (Reckeweg 2002). Belladonna is also common to *Traumeel*, *Spigelon*, *Viburcol*, *BHI-Inflammation*, *BHI-Neuralgia*, and *BHI-Recovery* formulas.

BHI-Inflammation: Contains Rhus toxicodendron for cases of weakness and paresis. Cases may be aggravated after lying in wet grass. Patients that benefit may have pustular, pruritic skin conditions; joint pain; myelitis; vertigo/dizziness; intercostal pain; and other types of neuralgia. Commonly used in combination with other antihomotoxic agents.

Bryaconeel: Used for neuralgia, serous membrane inflammation such as meningitis (Bryonia cretica), acute feverish conditions, and influenza-like signs. Contains Phosphorus to support parenchymatous organs such as the lung and liver. Moderates severe or overaggressive vicariations. Used in meningitis in cases not responsive to primary therapy (Reckeweg 2000).

Cerebrum compositum: Supports cerebral tissue, stem cells, and vessels (Cerebrum suis, Placenta suis, Arnica montana). Treats memory loss and forgetfulness and improving memory (Selenium, Thuja occidentalis, Acidum phosphoricum, Manganum phospohoricum, Semecarpus anacardium, Ambra grisea, Conium maculatum, Medorrhinum-Nosode). Supports cerebral function and vascular structures (Kalium phophoricum). Treats vertigo, stupor, headache, and weakness (Gelsemium sempervirens, Kalium bichromicum, Ruta graveolens) anxiety (Aconitum napellus), and exhaustion (China, Amarita cocculus). Supports capillary and other circulation, as well as lymph (Aesculus hippocastanum) and enzyme systems and difficulty sleeping (Hyoscyamus niger) (Reckeweg 2000).

Coenzyme compositum: Supports energy production through enzyme induction and repair, and is useful in repairing damage to enzyme systems of metabolism and following administration of drugs injurious to metabolism. Sulfhydral groups in Cysteinum assist in repairing therapeutic damage and in cases of forelimb weakness. Phase remedy in Degeneration and Dedifferentiation phases.

Cruroheel: Has strong connective tissue effects and is useful in difficult cases or those with strong vicariations.

Discus compositum: Clears the deep matrix and supports connective tissue repair, and treats irritation originating in the spinal column. Contain a number of useful remedies that particularly benefit musculoskeletal function, including Funiculus umbicalis suis (also contained in *Cutis compositum, Placenta compositum, Thyroidea compositum, Tonsilla compositum,* and *Zeel*) for debility. Treats arteriosclerosis, cervical spondylosis, collagen diseases, scleroderma, fibromas, vascular pathology, geriatric indications of all kinds, dystonia of the autonomic nervous system, autoimmune diseases, damage from antibiotics and other drugs, general iatrogenic damage, multiple sclerosis, and muscular atrophy. Also contains Niconitamidum, which is used to activate the energy metabolism in insufficiencies of the respiratory chain. The substance, which occurs naturally in the body, is an important component of NAD and NADP. Treats deficiencies of Nicotinamidum that lead to mental and neurological disturbances (Reckeweg 2002). It is common to the remedies *Coenzyme compositum, Discus compositum, Ginseng compositum, Ubichinon compositum, Zeel,* and *BHI-Enzyme.*

Echinacea compositum: Contains Aconitum, which is indicated for catarrhs, neuralgic symptoms with paresthesia, hyperthermia, and encephalitis with very high temperatures (e.g. post-vaccinial encephalitis or meningo-encephalitis, which may be activated by the implantation of living cells). Low potencies are normally given in pyrexia and organic complaints (Reckeweg 2002). The component Aconitum is common to several useful remedies, including *Barijodeel, Bryanconeel, Cerebrum compositum, Gripp-Heel,* and *Traumeel.* Baptisia is included for meningitis and encephalitis, serious feverish infections, general blood poisoning, and states of confusion (Reckeweg 2002). *Aesculus compositum, Arnica-Heel,* and other complexes are also included.

Engystol N: Has antiviral effects through immunostimulation.

Galium-Heel: Phase remedy in the matrix and cellular phases. Provides powerful support of the immune system (Echinacea augustifolia). Assists in drainage of cell and matrix, supports renal tubular function, and decreases swelling and edema (Apis mellifica, Galium aparine, and Galium mollugo). It is a critical component in the deep detoxification formula. Doses should be administered with regard to clinical condition and response, with the dose reduced if strong reactions are noted (Reckeweg 2000).

Gelsemium homaccord: Treats neuralgia and nerve pain, headache, and posterior weakness. Commonly required in aging large-breed dogs. This is a major antihomotoxic agent used in many neuropathy cases. Think of this agent in trembling pets because Gelsemium is known as the "trembling" remedy.

Ginseng compositum: Treats eyelid weakness and exhaustion.

Glyoxal compositum: Provides mitochondrial repair of damaged enzyme systems in Degeneration and Dedifferentiation phase disorders.

Listeriosis nosode: This remedy is not available in any of the homotoxicology combinations, but could be useful as a single remedy. The zoonotic organism Listeria monocytogenes causes a disease characterized by granulomatous meningoencephalitis in small animals (Reckeweg 2002).

Lymphomyosot: Used after cortisone therapy and for mesenchymal purging in chronic disease states.

Neuralgo-Rheum-Injeel: The components Causticum Hahnemanni and Rhus toxicodenron are powerful neurological remedies that cover a wide variety of chronic rheumatic-arthritic complaints, skin conditions, and intercostal-sciatic neuralgias.

Placenta compositum: Supports hypophysis after cortisone therapy. Contains sulfur to support enzyme and metabolic repair. Regenerative of hypophyseal-adrenal axis, and repairs vascular structures. Used intermittently in endocrine disorders.

Psorinonheel: Useful in deep, constitutional/genetic homotoxicoses. Consider in experimental application in inherited conditions. This remedy contains Cicuta, which is indicated for meningitis with hypersensitivity. It is a complementary remedy in tuberculous meningitis (Reckeweg 2002).

Solidago compositum: Deposition Phase remedy needed to remove debris from the matrix after regressive vicariation begins. In Traditional Chinese Medicine, the Kidney Chi governs the Brain, and as such, neurological issues may benefit from support of the Kidney and related tissues. Part of the deep detoxification formula. An interesting indication in this remedy is for Coxsackie virus nosode, which is used for abacterial meningitis and encephalitis (Reckeweg 2002).

Spigelon: Helpful for symptoms of headache, cerebral conditions with inflammation, and weakness of connective tissues (Reckeweg 2000).

Thyroidea compositum: Used for matrix drainage and autoregulation repair. Contains low levels of thyroid, pineal, spleen, bone marrow, umbilical cord, and liver to support glandular function and repair. Galium aparine drains the matrix and cellular components. Cortisonum aceticum in low potency assists in repairing damage from excess levels of cortisone. Precursors and Krebs cycle constituents promote energy metabolism through the Michaelis-Menten law of enzyme activity. Pulsatilla and Sulfur assist in regulation rigidity-type situations. Part of the deep detoxification formula (Reckeweg 2000).

Tonsilla compositum: Main antihomotoxic drug for chronic diseases involving endocrine disorders. Supports a wide number of tissues including tonsil, lymph node, bone marrow, umbilical cord (stem cell precursors), spleen, hypothalamus, liver, embryo, and adrenal cortex (Heine 2004). Contains Cortisonum aceticum and thyroid hormone in nanodilutions. Also contains Psorinum for deep constitutional, lack of reaction cases. Degeneration Phase agent (Reckeweg 2000).

Ubichinon compositum: Provides mitochondrial repair of energy production mechanisms. Used in chronic diseases and iatrogenic injury to mitochondria from antibiotic therapy, and is part of the deep detoxification formula. Parabenzochinon, a critical component in this regard, is indicated for autoimmune issues, and has been recommended for a state of paresis occurring after poliomyelitis, encephalitis or vaccinations, disturbance in neuromuscular coordination, conditions such as multiple sclerosis and tumors in the spinal area with pains and paresis, and brain tumors. In many cases of meningeal irritation, parabenzoquinone deals with the terrible pains better than an opiate.

Authors' suggested protocols

Nutrition

Brain/nerve and immune support formulas: 1 tablet for each 25 pounds of body weight BID.

Phosphatidyl serine: 25 mgs for each 25 pounds of body weight BID.

Lecithin/phosphatidyl choline: One-fourth teaspoon for each 25 pounds of body weight BID.

Betathyme: 1 capsule for each 35 pounds of body weight BID (maximum, 2 capsules BID).

Essential fats: One-half teaspoon for every 35 pounds of body weight with food.

Magnesium: 10 mgs for every 10 pounds of body weight SID.

Chinese herbal medicine/acupuncture

For GME, the patent formula is Yin Qiao San. It contains arctium (Niu bang zi), forsythia (Lian qiao), honeysuckle (Jin yin hua), licorice (Gan cao), lophatherum (Dan zhu ye), mint (Bo he), phragmites root (Lu gen), platycodon (Jie geng), schizonepeta (Jing jie), and soybean (Dan dou chi). It is dosed according to the manufacturer's recommendation. Yin Qiao San has been shown experimentally to decrease inflammation. It inhibited dimethlybenzine-induced increase in skin capillary permeability (Fu 1993). It also has antipyretic effects similar to aspirin (Xu 1986, Shen 1987). In addition it has been shown to have antibacterial and antiviral efficacy (Zhang 1981, Wang 1958, Shanghai Health and Epidemic Prevention Station 1960). Finally, it has analgesic properties as demonstrated using hot plate and acetic torsion experiments in mice (Zhou 1990). It was used to treat encephalitis B in 37 people with good response (Liu 1958). In another study on people with encephalitis (nonspecified origin), 74 of 81 people recovered completely, 2 did not respond completely and 5 people died (Wu 1965).

An alternative herbal supplement is H25 GME Disorder at a dose of 1 capsule per 10 to 20 pounds twice daily. In addition to the herbs in Yin Qiao San, H25 GME also contains achyranthes (Niu xi), buffalo horn shavings (Niu jiao), chrysanthemum (ju hua), coix (Yi yi ren), gastrodia (Tian ma), grass-leaf sweet-flag root (Shi chang pu), hoelen spirit (Fu shen), isatis leaf (Da qing ye), isatis root (Ban lan gen), papaya (Mu gua), phellodendron (Huang bai), pueraria (Ge gen), scutellaria (Huang qin), silkworm (Jiang can), and uncaria (Gou teng).

These formulas can be combined with conventional drugs, but often are only needed for a short period of time.

The author uses the following acupuncture points for GME: ST36, GV14, CV17 and GB20.

For forelimb neuropathies, the authors recommend H41 Forelimb Paralysis at a dose of 1 capsule per 10 to 20 pounds twice daily. In addition to the herbs discussed above, H41 Forelimb Paralysis contains codonopsis (Dang shen) and scorpion (Quan xie), which increase the efficacy of the formula.

The author recommends the following acupuncture points: LI11, SI9, TH6, LI10, ST36, and Bai Hui.

For hindlimb neuropathies the authors recommend H 72 Hindlimb Paralysis/Incontinence at a dose of 1 capsule per 10 to 20 pounds twice daily. In addition to the herbs mentioned above, H72 Hindlimb Paralysis/Incontinence contains American ginseng (Xi yang shen), ciborium (Gou ji), cynomorium (Suo yang), fossil bones/raw (Long gu), lindera (Wu yao), mantis egg case (Sang piao xiao), polygonatum (Yu zhu), and tortoise plastron (Gui ban). These herbs enhance the function of the herbal supplement.

The author uses the following acupuncture points: ST36, UB60, BL30, and Bai Hui.

For facial neuropathies the authors use H 73 Facial Nerve Paralysis at a dose of 1 capsule per 10 to 20 pounds twice daily. In addition to the herbs listed above, H 73 Facial Nerve Paralysis contains scorpion (Quan xie) to improve the efficacy of the formula.

The author recommends the following acupuncture points: ST4, ST6, ST7, and SI9.

Homotoxicology

Deep detoxification may assist noninherited conditions, and support of energy metabolism through the use of catalysts should be considered. Use of antihomotoxic agents that match the patient's symptoms may be helpful. Treatment must be individualized to the specific patient's needs. Any clinician successfully treating either inherited or acquired polyneuropathies should report their findings for publication.

Granulomatous meningoencephalitis (GME)
Symptom formula: Two protocols exist.

1. Administer Echinacea compositum IV and Solidago compositum and Galium-Heel as an autosanguis, and dispense anoral cocktail consisting of Traumeel, Psorinoheel, and Aesculus compositum BID to TID. Use Ubichinon compositum orally BID. Administer Spigelon for pain and inflammation associated with the illness, and consider Listeria nosode, obtained from a single remedy company, or Heel-Germany.
2. Administer Gelsemium homaccord, BHI-Inflammation, Spigelon, and Traumeel S mixed together and given PO BID for 3 weeks, then alternate with Pulsatilla compositum in an attempt to shift regulation rigidity. Give Cerebrum compositum 1 to 3 times weekly. Consider autosanguis therapy.

Deep detoxification formula: Galium-Heel, Lymphomyosot, Hepar compositum, Solidago compositum, Thyroidea compositum (alternated with Tonsilla compositum in inflammatory conditions), Coenzyme compositum, and Ubichinon compositum combined and given orally twice weekly. Consider giving these and the above symptom formula agents as autosanguis therapy.

Acquired peripheral neuropathies
In nearly all cases it would be appropriate to administer Neuralgo-Rheum and Discus compositum 2 to 3 times weekly by injection.

Deep detoxification formula: Galium-Heel, Lymphomyosot, Hepar compositum, Solidago compositum, Thyroidea compositum (alternated with Tonsilla compositum in inflammatory conditions), Coenzyme compositum, and Ubichinon compositum combined and given orally twice weekly. Consider giving these agents as autosanguis therapy.

Diabetic polyneuropathy
Lymphomyosot, Syzygium compositum, and Mucosa compositum given orally in conjunction with alpha-lipoic acid. (See also Diabetes mellitus protocol).

Hypothyroid polyneuropathy
Administer in addition to proper thyroid hormone replacement therapy. Thyroidea compositum given twice weekly alone or as part of the deep detoxification formula if the condition is stable.

Iatrogenic pharmaceutical injury (vincristine, vinblastine, and colchicines)
Deep detoxification formula, IV fluid support, and avoidance of the offending drug until it can be cleared.

Idiopathic
Deep detoxification formula, and also consider BHI-Body Pure for 1 to 3 months.

Immune-mediated (autoimmune such as systemic lupis erythmatosis)
See autoimmune protocols.

Infectious (Neospora caninum and FeLV)
Use clindimycin for Neospora. See the FeLV protocol section. Tonsilla compositum given twice weekly and Echinacea compositum daily by injection during acute involvement. Engystol may improve immune function given daily. Traumeel S if acute inflammation or swelling is involved.

Toxic injury (metals, solvents such ascarbon tetracycline, organophosphate, insecticides)
Deep detoxification formula in conjunction with appropriate antidote, plus supportive and chelation therapy.

Product sources

Nutrition

Brain/nerve and immune support formulas: Animal Nutrition Technologies. **Alternatives:** Immune System Support—Standard Process Veterinary Formulas; Immuno Support—Rx Vitamins for Pets; Immugen—Thorne Veterinary Products.

Phosphatidyl serine: Integrative Therapuetics.

Lecithin/phosphatidyl choline: Designs for Health.

Betathyme: Best for Your Pet. **Alternative:** Moducare Thorne Veterinary Products.

Beyond essential fats: Natura Health Products. **Alternatives:** Flax oil—Barlean's Organic Oils; Hemp oil—Nature's Perfect Oil; Ultra EFA—Rx Vitamins; Omega- 3,6,9—Vetri Science.

Magnesium: Over the counter.

Chinese herbal medicine

Yin Qiao San: Mayway Corp.

Formulas H25 GME, H41 Forelimb Paralysis, H72 Hindlimb Paralysis/Incontinence, and H73 Facial Nerve Paralysis: Natural Solutions, Inc.

Homotoxicology

BHI/Heel Corporation

REFERENCES

Western medicine references

Braund KG. Peripheral nerve disorders. In: Ettinger SJ, Feldman EC, eds. Textbook of Veterinary Internal Medicine, 4th ed. Philadelphia: WB Saunders, 1995:701–728.

Braund KG, Mehta JR, Toivio-Kinnucan M, et al. Congenital hypomyelinating polyneuropathy in two Golden Retriever littermates. *Vet Pathol* 1989;26:202–208.

Braund KG, Luttgen PJ, Redding RW, et al. Distal symmetrical polyneuropathy in a dog. *Vet Pathol* 1980;17:422–435.

Braund KG, Steiss JE. Distal neuropathy in spontaneous diabetes mellitus in dogs. *Acta Neuropathol* 1982;57:263–269.

Cuddon P. Peripheral Neuropathies (Polyneuropathies). In: Tilley L, Smith F. The 5-Minute Veterinary Consult: Canine and Feline. Baltimore: William and Wilkins, 1997. pp 930–1.

Cummings JF. Canine inflammatory polyneuropathies. In: Kirk RW, Bonagura JD, eds. Current veterinary therapy XI. Small animal practice. Philadelphia: Saunders, 1992:1034–1037.

Cummings JF, Cooper BJ, de Lahunta A, et al. Canine inherited hypertrophic neuropathy. *Acta Neuropathol* 1981;53:137–143.

Griffiths IR. Progressive axonopathy: An inherited neuropathy of Boxer dogs: 1. Further studies of the clinical and electrophysiological features. *J Small Anim Pract* 1985;26:381–392.

Towell TL, Shell LC. Endocrinopathies that affect peripheral nerves of cats and dogs. *Compend Contin Educ Pract Vet* 1994;16:157–161.

IVM reference

Kline K. Complementary and alternative medicine for neurologic disorders. *Clin Tech Small Anim Pract.* 2002. Feb;17(1):pp 25–33.

Nutrition references

Bilbey Douglas LJ, Prabhakaran VM. Muscle cramps and magnesium deficiency: case reports, *Canadian Family Physician*, Vol. 42, July 1996, pp. 1348–51.

Bouic PJD, et al. Beta-sitosterol and beta-sitosterol glucoside stimulate human peripheral blood lymphocyte proliferation: Implications for their use as an immunomodulatory vitamin combination. *International Journal of Immunopharmacology* 1996;18:693–700.

Cenacchi T, Bertoldin T, Farina C, et al. Cognitive decline in the elderly: a double-blind, placebo-controlled multicenter study on efficacy of phosphatidylserine administration. *Aging (Milano)* 1993;5:123–33.

Cima J. Biochemical Blood Chemistry Evaluation, Palm Beach Gardens, FL., March 2000.

Erasmus U. Fats That Heal Fats That Kill. Alive Books; Revised and updated edition (January 1, 1993). The Complete Lecture, www.udoerasmus.com.

Goldstein R, et al. The BNA Handbook: A Working Manual for Veterinarians, Westport, CT: Animal Nutrition Technologies, 2000.

Gupta MB, Nath R, Srivastava N, et al. Anti-inflammatory and antipyretic activities of β-sitosterol. *Planta Medica* 1980;39:157–163.

Hanin IG, Ansell B. Lecithin: Technological, Biological, and Therapeutic Aspects, 1987, NY: Plenum Press, 180, 181.

Horrocks LA, et al. Phosphatidyl Research and the Nervous System, Berlin: Springer Verlach, 1986.

Levin C. Caninie Epilepsy. Oregon City, OR: Lantern Publications, 2002 P 18–19.

Chinese herbal medicine/acupuncture references

Chang Yong Zhong Yao Cheng Fen Yu Yao Li Shou Ce (A Handbook of the Composition and Pharmacology of Common Chinese Drugs), 1994;1725:1728.

Chen CX. *Journal of Chinese Materia Medica.* 1986;16(4):40.

Du YT. Lu Jiao Jiao injection's effect on the phagocytosis of macrophagocytes in patients of mammary cancer. *Journal of Traditional Chinese Medicine.* 1981;(3):36.

Fu HY, et al. *Journal of Pharmacology and Clinical Application.* 1993;(1):1.

He JX, et al. Therapeutic effect of acupuncture at LI4 in the treatment of infantile convulsion due to high fever.

Hsieh CL, Tang NY, Chiang SV, Hsieh CT, Lin JG. Anticonvulsive and free radical scavenging actions of two herbs, Uncaria rhynchophylla (MIQ) Jack and Gastrodia elata Bl., in kainic acid-treated rats. *Life Sci* 1999; 65(20):2071–82.

Hu Bei Zhong Yi Yao Za Zhi (*Hubei Journal of Chinese Medicine*), 1982; 1: 33.

Hu LP, et al. *Journal of Zhejiang College of TCM.* 1997;21(6): 29–30.

Huang S, et al. *Guizhou Journal of Medicine.* 1993;17(1): 14–15.

Ji Lin Yi Xue Yuan Xue Bao (*Journal of Jilin University of Medicine*), 1982; 1:28.

Jiang Su Yi Yao (*Jiangsu Journal of Medicine and Herbology*), 1976;2:33.

Jiao Y, et al. *China Journal of Integrated Medicine.* 1999;19(6):356–358.

Kubo M, Matsuda H, Tanaka M, Kimura Y, Okuda H, Higashino M, Tani T, Namba K, Arichi S. Studies on Scutellariae radix. VII. Anti-arthritic and anti-inflammatory actions of methanolic extract and flavonoid components from Scutellariae radix. *Chem Pharm Bull*, 1984; 32(7):2724–9.

Lang XC, et al. *Journal of Hebei Medical College.* 1991;12(3):140.

Li L, et al. *Journal of Beijing Medical University.* 1999;22(3):38–40.

Li MZ, et al. The pharmadynamics of Re Du Qing Injection. *China Journal of Experimental Recipes.* 1996;2(6):24–30.

Li XC, et al. *Shannxi Journal of Medicine.* 1999; 28(12):735–736.

Li XM, et al. *Journal of Shizhen Medicinal Material Research.* 1997;8(4):373–374.

Li Yin Fang (translator). *Foreign Medicine*, vol. of TCM. 1984;6(1):15–18.

Liaoning Journal of Chinese Medicine, 1982; 3:40.

Liu H. *Journal of Wannan Medical College.* 1998;17(3):238–240.

Liu ZM, et al. *Journal of Traditional Chinese Medicine.* 1958;(4):251.

Lu SC, et al. *Journal of No. 1 Military Academy.* 1990;10(3): 267.

Ma Zhen Ya. *Shannxi Journal of Traditional Chinese Medicine and Herbs.* 1982;(4):58.

Mao XJ, et al. Experimental research on mixture of Cao Wu and Shui Niu Jiao. *Journal of Yunnan College of TCM.* 1997; 19(7):33–34.

Meng ZM, et al. *Journal of University of Pharmacology of China.* 1995;26(1):33–36.

Miao MS. *Henan Journal of TCM.* 1996;16(6):349–50.

Modern TCM Pharmacology. Tianjin: Science and Technology Press; 1997.

Rui J. *Journal of Chinese Materia Medica.* 1999;30(1):43–45.

Shan Xi Yi Kan (*Shanxi Journal of Medicine*), 1960;(10):32.

Shanghai Health and Epidemic Prevention Station. *Shanghai Journal of Chinese Medicine.* 1960;(2):68.

Shen YJ, et al. *Journal of Pharmacology and Clinical Application.* 1987;(Suppl):14.

Shi RR, et al. *Journal of Traditional Chinese Medicine.* 1998;26(3):56–57.

Singh S, Khar A. Biological effects of curcumin and its role in cancer chemoprevention and therapy. *Anticancer Agents in Medicinal Chemistry*, 2006; 6(3):259–70.

Sunaga K, Sugaya E, Kajiwara K, Tsuda T, Sugaya A, Kimura M. Molecular Mechanism of Preventive Effect of Peony Root Extract on Neuron Damage. *J of Herbal Pharmacotherapy* 2004;4(1):9–20.

Wang JL, et al. *Journal of Chinese Materia Medica.* 1993;24(12):655–656.

Wang KW. Forecast of research on anti-cancer effects of Di Long capsules (912). *China Journal of Clinical Research on Tumor.* 1991;18(3):131–132.

Wang SL, et al. *Journal of Medical Science of China.* 1958;(3):275.

World Health Organization list of common conditions treatable by Chinese Medicine and Acupuncture. http://tcm.health-info. org/WHO-treatment-list.htm Accessed 10/20/2006.

Wu HR, et al. *Zhejiang Journal of Traditional Chinese Medicine.* 1965;(8):4.

Xie W, et al. *Ninxia Journal of Medicine.* 1995;17(2): 121–124.

Xong ZY, et al. *Journal of Pharmacology.* 1963;10(12):708.

Xu G, et al. *China Journal of TCM Science and Technology.* 1999;6(4):254–255.

Xu JJ, et al. *Chinese Medicine Bulletin.* 1986;(1):51.

Xu QL, et al. *Shanghai Journal of Immunology.* 1996;16(3): 141.

Yao Xue Tong Bao (Report of Herbology), 1982; 9:50.

Yao Xue Za Zhi (*Journal of Medicinals*), 1971;(91):1098.

Yu LS, et al. *Journal of Chinese Materia Medica.* 1989;20(5): 221–213.

Zhang JK. *Journal of Chinese Patent Medicine.* 1981;(9):22.

Zhang MF, et al. Yi Yi Ren's analgesic, anti-inflammatory, and antithrombotic effects. *Journal of Practical TCM.* 1998; 12(2):36–38.

Zhang SC, et al. *Journal of Chinese Patent Medicine Research.* 1984;(2):37.

Zhang YL, et al. Sequential experiments on Yi Yi Ren's analgesic effect in severe functional dysmenorrhea. *Journal of TCM.* 1998;39(10):599–600.

Zhao SP, et al. Journal of Sino-Japanese Friendship Hospital. 1996;10(4):295–298.

Zhong Cao Yao (*Chinese Herbal Medicine*) 1991;22 (10):452.

Zhong Cao Yao Tong Xun (*Journal of Chinese Herbal Medicine*), 1975; (6) 18.

Zhong Cao Yao Xue (Study of Chinese Herbal Medicine), 1980; 1423.

Zhong Guo Zhong Yao Za Zhi (*People's Republic of China Journal of Chinese Herbology*), 1990; 15(8):492.

Zhong Hua Yi Xue Za Zhi (*Chinese Journal of Medicine*),1978; 17(8):87.

Zhong Liu Yu Zhi Tong Xun (*Journal of Prevention and Treatment of Cancer*), 1976; 2:40.

Zhong Xi Yi Jiehe Shiyong Linchuang Jujiu (*Clinical Emergency by Integrated Chinese and Western Medicine*). 1997, 4(8):360–360 [in Chinese].

Zhong Liu Yu Zhi Tong Xun (*Journal of Prevention and Treatment of Cancer*), 1976; 2:40.

Zhong Yao Cai (*Study of Chinese Herbal Material*), 1985; (2):36.

Zhong Yao Cai (*Study of Chinese Herbal Material*), 1989; 12(6):37.

Zhong Yao Tong Bao (*Journal of Chinese Herbology*), 1988:13(6):364.

Zhong Yao Xue (Chinese Herbology), 1998; 89:91.

Zhong Yao Xue (Chinese Herbology), 1998; 65:67.

Zhong Yao Xue (Chinese Herbology), 1998; 91:92.

Zhong Yao Xue (Chinese Herbology), 1998; 706:708.

Zhong Yao Xue (Chinese Herbology), 1998; 845:848.

Zhong Yao Yao Li Yu Ying Yong (Pharmacology and Applications of Chinese Herbs), 1977:2253.

Zhong Yao Zhi (*Chinese Herbology Journal*), 1993:183.

Zhong Yao Zhi (*Chinese Herbology Journal*), 1993;358.

Zhou WZ, et al. *Pharmacy Bulletin.* 1979;14(5):202–203.

Zhou YP, et al. Chinese Patent Medicine. 1990;(1):22.

Zhu LH. *China Journal of TCM Information.* 1996;3(3): 17–20.

Homotoxicology references

Bagley R. Fundamentals of Veterinary Clinical Neurology. Blackwell Publishing Asia: Australia 2005, p 249.

Goldstein R. 2006. Personal communication.

Heine H. Homotoxicology and basic regulation: Bystander reaction. *La Medicina Biologica.* 2004. January (1): p 5. http://www.gunainc.com/AllLanguages/ElencoScheda/Elenco_Scheda.asp?SelectionMenu=-1096andxid=9BEB85D787A849 14AEED43918A937DBBandid_BoxContent=1077

Reckeweg H. Biotherapeutic Index: Ordinatio Antihomotoxica et Materia Medica, 5th ed. Baden-Baden, Germany: Biologische Heilmittel Heel GMBH, 2000. p 22–3, 286–9, 295, 299–300, 302, 308–9, 337–8, 404, 415–6, 418–19.

Reckeweg H. Homeopathia Antihomotoxica Materia Medica, 4th ed. Baden-Baden, Germany: Arelia-Verlag GMBH, 2002. pp. 120–1, 141–2,167–8, 172–5, 176–8, 235, 259, 310–12, 389, 456, 540.

LARYNGEAL PARALYSIS

Definition and cause

Laryngeal paralysis is a degenerative process that affects the normal functioning of the larynx, leading to an interference with the normal flow of air to the lungs. Secondarily, there may be gagging, excessive salivation, vomiting, and aspiration pneumonia. Underlying causes are believed to be genetic inheritance, trauma to the nervous ennervation of the larynx, neuropathy, chronic larynx disease, immune-mediated inflammation, or secondary to other diseases such as neoplasia (Braund 1995, Bjorling 1995, Harpster 2003, Harvey 1981, Venker-van Haagen 1992).

Medical therapy rationale, drug(s) of choice, and nutritional recommendations

The treatment of choice for laryngeal paralysis is a laryngeal tie-back surgery. This procedure is reported to produce good success rates. If the client declines surgery, medical therapy with tranquilizers or anti-inflammatory drugs may be used with varying degrees of success.

Surgery can offer patients tremendous relief but may be associated with high complication rates, particularly

death from pneumonia, and may require repeated procedures (Hammel, Hottinger, Novo 2006). A new procedure involving injection of autogenous cartilage shows some promise (Lee, et al. 2006).

In cases of trauma, temporary tracheostomies can be life saving. Neoplastic cases require appropriate therapy depending upon the type, location, and size of the tumor. Many cases of neoplasia in cats involve squamous cell carcinoma or lymphosarcoma. A larger complement of neoplastic types are involved in dogs. Patients suffering from laryngeal paralysis are prone to hypoxia, overheating, and difficulty swallowing; as a result, they have an increased chance of aspiration of resultant pneumonia and a more guarded prognosis (Braund 1995, Harvey 1981, Harpster 2003).

Anticipated prognosis

Surgical correction often improves the condition and results in a good prognosis. Multiple surgeries may be necessary in some animals. Paralysis secondary to neoplasia offers a guarded prognosis (Harpster 2003, Venker-van Haagen 1992).

Integrative veterinary therapies

Causes secondary to trauma and genetic inheritance require alternative therapy support. In chronic inflammatory and immune-mediated cases, the nerves, larynx, and glandular immune system should be taken into account. Reducing inflammation, protecting cells, and preventing ongoing degeneration and cell death will help improve the clinical picture, as will surgery if it is required. The use of nutrients, nutraceuticals, medicinal herbs, and combination homeopathics that have anti-inflammatory, tissue-sparing, and regenerative effects can often control the clinical signs and improve the day-to-day level of comfort for the animal.

Nutrition
General considerations/rationale

While surgery can often help with day-to-day comfort and function, nutritional therapies can help improve nerve control and gland support can help the immune system. This can help reduce inciting inflammation and slow degeneration.

Appropriate nutrients

Nutritional/gland therapy: Glandular brain, adrenal, thymus, pituitary, and hypothalamus supply the intrinsic nutrients that help to improve nervous system and organ function and reduce cellular inflammation. This helps to spare these organs from expanding inflammation and can slow degeneration (see Gland Therapy in Chapter 2 for a more detailed explanation).

Phospholipids found in glandular brain are a source of unsaturated omega-3 fatty acids, which are now thought to play a vital role in the development and maintenance of the central nervous system. High concentrations of phosphatidyl choline and serine are found in brain tissue. Horrocks (1986) reported on the potential clinical use of these nutrients in chronic neurological conditions.

Lecithin/phosphatidyl choline: Phosphatidyl choline is a phospholipid that is integral to cellular membranes, particularly those of nerve and brain cells. It helps to move fats into the cells and is involved in acetylcholine uptake, neurotransmission, and cellular integrity. As part of the cell membranes, lecithin is an essential nutrient that is required by nerves for general health and wellness (Hanin 1987).

Phosphatidyl serine (PS): Phosphatidyl serine is a phospholipid that is an essential ingredient in cellular membranes, particularly those of brain cells. It has been studied in people with altered mental functioning and degeneration with positive results (Crook 1991, Cenacchi 1993). When people with Alzheimer's disease were given PS, they showed a mild to significant clinical improvement (Delewaide 1986, Engel 1992, Funfgeld 1989).

Coenzyme Q10: Coenzyme Q10 (ubiquinone) is found in the mitochondria and is involved in the cells' energy production that is required for the daily functioning of the body. It is essential in the manufacture of ATP, the energy source for all the body's cells and tissues. CoQ10 is also a potent antioxidant and helps to neutralize free radicals and protect cells (Thomas 1997, Weber 1994).

Blue-green algae: Blue-green algae has been observed to create a generalized feeling of well being in humans, and may prove helpful in veterinary patients. Its effects are usually observed to be slower in onset, with the resultant benefits taking 3 to 4 weeks to appear. This may be due in part to their content of natural antihistaminic compounds or their levels of omega-3 fatty acids (Bruno 2001).

Many studies in recent years have confirmed the beneficial results from these critical fatty acids. Aphanizomenon flos aquae, a blue-green algae, has been shown in clinical settings to have positive effects on brain function. In addition to the aforementioned omega-3 fatty acids, it also contains a full scope of essential amino acids, a broad-based mineral content, a rapidly assimilable glyolipoprotein cell wall, and a wide variety of vitamins. It has mild chelating properties, and thus, can be valuable in heavy metal toxicoses such as Thimerosol reactions. It is a tremendous asset as a micronutrient resource and figures prominently in many treatment programs (Broadfoot 1997).

Chinese herbal medicine/acupuncture
General considerations/rationale
According to TCM, laryngeal paralysis is caused by Yin deficiency in the Lung and Kidney. The Lung controls the Throat. The Kidney is responsible for misting fluid up to the upper part of the body. If the Kidney has a Yin deficiency it cannot send fluids up to the Lungs. The Yin deficiency leads to a relative excessive Yang because Yin and Yang balance each other. Yang is warm, and the resulting heat, or inflammation, rises up, burning and paralyzing in the throat.

Treatment involves correcting the underlying etiology if possible and decreasing inflammation.

Appropriate Chinese herbs
NOTE: This section seems to overemphasize neoplastic etiologies. This reflects the lack of well-controlled studies concerning the use of herbs to treat laryngeal paralysis.

Astragalus (Huang qi): Has been shown to inhibit the growth of tumors (Liu 1999, Shi 1999). It may help control underlying neoplastic causes of laryngeal paralysis.

Belamcanda (She gan): Has demonstrated antiviral activity (Zhong Yao Yao Li Yu Ying Yong 1990). It may help control viral neuropathies.

Centipede (Wu gong): Has antineoplastic properties (Chang Yong Zhong Yao Cheng Fen Yu Yao Li Shou Ce 1994). It may help if the laryngeal paralysis is secondary to cancer.

Forsythia (Lian qiao): Has an anti-inflammatory effect (Ma 1982). Methanol-based extract of Lian qiao has anti-inflammatory and analgesic effects(Rui 1999).

Honeysuckle (Jin yin hua): Has anti-inflammatory effects (Shan Xi Yi Kan 1960).

Prunella (Xia ku cao): Has anti-inflammatory actions (Zhong Yao Xue 1998). It can increase serum cortisol levels (Jiang 1988), which may help decrease swelling.

Red peony (Chi shao): Has anticancer properties (Hu 1990).

Rehmannia (Sheng di): Reduces swelling and inflammation (Zhong Yao Yao Li Yu Ying Yong 1983). This may be useful in cases in which laryngeal paralysis is secondary to inflammatory conditions.

Salvia (Dan shen): Has anti-neoplastic effects (Li 1999). It may help treat neoplastic causes of laryngeal paralysis.

Subprostrata sophora (Shan dou gen): Has anticancer properties, most likely due to the matrine, oxymatrine, and sophocarpine components (Zhong Guo Yi Xue Ke Xue Xue Bao 1988). It may help control neoplastic etiologies.

Scorpion (Quan xie): Has antineoplastic properties (Jiang Su Yi Yao 1990).

Acupuncture
Many studies have been performed on stroke victims. EEG maps and somatosensory evoked potentials reveal

that patients treated with acupuncture improve faster than those who are not (Chen 1990). A review by Ionescu-Tirgoviste (1981) showed that some forms of peripheral neuritis respond to acupuncture. These studies show that the nervous system is amenable to treatment with acupuncture.

Homotoxicology
General considerations/rationale
Laryngeal paralysis is a significant disease in dogs, and is more rarely seen in cats. Trauma is a rare cause in both dogs and cats, and can represent the Inflammation Phase, or the Degenerative Phase in more severe injuries. Inherited conditions affect several breeds of dogs and represent Dedifferentiation Phase disease, because the genetic complement is no longer intact. Inherited cases generally present between 4 and 8 months of age. Tumors can also result in this condition; this is rare in dogs and more common in cats. Vagal neuropathies (cranial nerve X) in conjunction with abnormalities of the spinal accessory nerve (cranial nerve XI and its branch, the recurrent laryngeal nerve) result in this condition (Bagley 2005).

Many cases commonly seen in veterinary clinics represent idiopathic disease (Impregnation or Degeneration phase), and these most often present in dogs from 2 to 12 years of age. Many cases are beyond reversal by the time they are presented to the veterinarian for diagnosis (Harpster 1997). Other polyneuropathies can present with laryngeal signs (hypothyroidism, etc).

Appropriate homotoxicology formulas
Barijodeel: Contains Causticum Hahnemanni, which is indicated for intractable paralytic conditions such as Bell's palsy and laryngeal paralysis. Arnica, Ignatia, and Kali phos are other remedies with nerve damage or dysfunction indications that are included in this formula. All of these remedies have a particular affinity for neck, laryngeal, or pharyngeal dysfunctions (Reckeweg 2002). Causticum is also contained in *Causticum compositum, Neuralgo-Rheum-Injeel, Reneel,* and *Rheuma-Heel.*

BHI-Allergy: Though not an obvious first choice for laryngeal paralysis, this remedy nonetheless contains a number of useful components for this condition, among them the aforementioned Arnica and Ignatia. In addition, it contains Selenium for neurasthenia, laryngitis, hoarseness, and inflammation of the upper respiratory passages. *Sulphuricum acidum* in this remedy also has some laryngitis, coughing attacks with regurgitations, dyspnea, and shortness of breath as indications (Reckeweg 2002).

BHI-Inflammation: Used as an immune supportive agent. It combines effects similar to *Traumeel* along with Echinacea.

Coenzyme compositum: Supports energy production through enzyme induction and repair. It is useful in repairing damage to enzyme systems of metabolism and following administration of drugs injurious to metabolism. It is a phase remedy in Degeneration and Dedifferentiation phases.

Discus compositum: Useful in cleansing deep matrix and supports connective tissues.

Galium-Heel: Phase remedy in matrix and cellular phases. Provides powerful support of the immune system (Echinacea augustifolia). Assists in drainage of cells and matrix, supports renal tubular function, and decreases swelling and edema (Apis mellifica, Galium aparine, and Galium mollugo). It is a critical component in the deep detoxification formula. Dosing should be done with regard to clinical condition and response, with the dose reduced if strong reactions are noted (Reckeweg 2000).

Gelsemium homaccord: A generally useful remedy in neurological weakness and paralysis.

Glyoxal compositum: Provides mitochondrial repair of damaged enzyme systems in Degeneration and Dedifferentiation phase disorders.

Ignatia homaccord: Usually used in cases of depression and anxiety, this formula is also used for the sensation of a lump in the throat (globus hystericus) and might have usefulness in cases associated with shock or sadness from loss occurring prior to the onset of difficulties. Kent (1921) lists this remedy for use in difficulty breathing as well.

Lymphomyosot: Used after cortisone therapy and mesenchymal purging in chronic disease states.

Phosphor homaccord: Provides parenchymal organ support. Treats laryngitis and disorders of nutritive organs (Heel 2003).

Pulsatilla compositum: Used in regulation rigidity cases. Contains Pulsatilla pratensis, Sulfur, and Cortisonum aceticum for repairing damage following steroid administration. Often a case will rapidly activate following administration of this agent, and in cases of strong regressive vicariation the administration of Traumeel S moves the patient toward healing and resolution. It is used in conjunction with catalyst therapy.

Solidago compositum: Deposition Phase remedy needed to remove debris from the matrix after regressive vicariation begins.

Thyroidea compositum: Used for matrix drainage and repair of autoregulation. Contains low levels of thyroid, pineal, spleen, bone marrow, umbilical cord, and liver to support glandular function and repair. Galium aparine drains matrix and cellular components. Cortisonum aceticum in low potency assists in repairing damage from excess levels of cortisone. Precursors and Krebs cycle constituents promote energy metabolism. Pulsatilla and Sulfur assist in regulation rigidity-type situations. Part of Deep Detoxification Formula (Reckeweg 2000).

Traumeel S: Treats Inflammation Phase disorders, particularly in cases of trauma. May prove useful in reducing inflammation from laryngeal fluttering. It is an alternative to corticosteroids that is worthy of consideration and examination.

Ypsiloheel: Assists in central autoregulation. Contains Lachesis, which is indicated in laryngeal paralysis and globus hystericus (sensation of a ball in the throat, which may manifest in veterinary patients as extending the neck and swallowing frequently) (Kent 1927). Because Ypsiloheel can also assist in cases of centrally mediated vomiting, clinicians should be alert to these signs in selecting remedies.

Authors' suggested protocols

Nutrition
Brain/nerve and pituitary/hypothalmus/pineal support formulas: 1 tablet for each 25 pounds of body weight BID.

Immune support formula: One-half tablet for each 25 pounds of body weight BID.

Lecithin/phosphatidyl choline: One-fourth teaspoon for each 25 pounds of body weight BID.

Phosphatidyl serine: 25 mgs for each 25 pounds of body weight BID.

Coenzyme Q10: 25 mgs for every 10 pounds of body weight daily.

Blue-green algae: One-fourth teaspoon for each 25 pounds of body weight daily.

Other fatty acid sources: Beyond Essential Fats—one-half teaspoon for every 35 pounds of body weight with food (maximum, 100 pounds); oil of evening primrose, hemp oil, flax oil, and fish oil—follow manufacturer's dose recommendations.

Chinese herbal medicine
Formula H53 Laryngeal Paralysis at a dose of 1 capsule per 10 to 20 pounds twice daily. In addition to the herbs discussed above, H53 Laryngeal Paralysis contains adenophora (Sha shen), codonopsis (Dang shen), ophiopogon (Mai men dong), phragmites (Lu gen), and scrophularia (Xuan shen) to help improve the efficacy of the formula.

The author uses the following acupuncture points: LI11, CV22, CV23, BL13, and BL23.

Homotoxicology
Proper treatment depends upon the causation involved.

Traumatic cases: Tracheostomy as needed. Traumeel S given orally or by injection TID for 3 days and then BID for 2 days.

Idiopathic cases: Surgery is likely needed. Barijodeel and BHI-Allergy, given TID orally. Also consider Traumeel-S and Phosphorus homaccord if laryngitis is present. Possibly also give Gelsemium homaccord BID orally. Deep detoxification formula consisting of Galium-Heel, Lymphomyosot, Hepar compositum, Solidago composi-

tum, Thyroidea compositum, Coenzyme compositum, and Ubichinon compositum mixed together and given orally twice weekly.

Neoplasia: See chapters 31 and 32, cancer and IVM Cancer Treatment Protocols.

Product sources

Nutrition
Brain/nerve, pituitary/hypothalmus/pineal, and immune support formulas: Animal Nutrition Technologies. **Alternatives:** Immune System Support—Standard Process Veterinary Formulas; Immuno Support—Rx Vitamins for Pets; Immugen—Thorne Veterinary Products.

Lecithin/phosphatidyl choline: Designs for Health.

Phosphatidyl serine: Integrative Therapuetics.

Coenzyme Q10: Vetri Science; Thorne Veterinary Products.

Blue-green algae: Cell Tech (Simplexity); BlueGreen Foods, Inc.

Beyond essential fats: Natural Health Products. **Alternatives:** Hemp oil—Nature's Perfect Oil; Flax oil—Barlean's Organic Oils; Eskimo fish oil—Tyler Encapsulations; Ultra EFA—Rx Vitamins for Pets; Omega- 3, 6, 9—Vetri Science; Evening primrose oil—Jarrows Formulas.

Chinese herbal medicine
Formula H53 Laryngeal Paralysis: Natural Solutions, Inc.

Homotoxicology
BHI/Heel Corporation

REFERENCES

Western medicine references
Braund KG. Peripheral nerve disorders. In: Ettinger EJ, Feldman EC, eds. Textbook of Veterinary Internal Medicine Toronto: WB Saunders Co. 1995, p. 701–726.
Bjorling DE. Laryngeal paralysis. In: Bonagura JD and Kirk RW, eds. Kirk's Current Veterinary Therapy XII Small Animal Practice. Toronto: WB Saunders Co. 1995, p. 901–901.
Harpster NK. Laryngeal Disease. In: Tilley L, Smith F. The 5-Minute Veterinary Consult: Canine and Feline, Blackwell Publishing, 2003.
Harvey CE. The larynx. In: Bojrab MJ, ed. Pathophysiology in small animal surgery. Philadelphia: Lea and Febiger, 1981:350–358.
Venker-van Haagen AJ. Diseases of the larynx. *Vet Clin North Am Small Anim Pract* 1992;22:1155–1172.

IVM/nutrition references
Broadfoot P. 1997. Personal communication.
Bruno J. Edible Microalgae: A Review of the Health Research. Center for Nutritional Psychology, 2001. p 23.

Hanin IG, Ansell B. Lecithin: Technological, Biological, and Therapeutic Aspects, 1987, NY: Plenum Press, , 180, 181.

Horrocks LA, et al. Phosphatidyl Research and the Nervous System. Berlin: Springer Verlach, 1986.

Cenacchi T, Bertoldin T, Farina C, et al. Cognitive decline in the elderly: a double-blind, placebo-controlled multicenter study on efficacy of phosphatidylserine administration. *Aging (Milano)* 1993;5:123–33.

Crook TH, Tinklenberg J, Yesavage J, et al. Effects of phosphatidylserine in age-associated memory impairment. *Neurology* 1991;41:644–9.

Fünfgeld EW, Baggen M, Nedwidek P, et al. Double-blind study with phosphatidylserine (PS) in Parkinsonian patients with senile dementia of Alzheimer's type (SDAT). *Prog Clin Biol Res* 1989;317:1235–46.

Thomas SR, Neuzil J, Stocker R. Inhibition of LDL oxidation by ubiquinol-10. A protective mechanism for coenzyme Q in atherogenesis? *Mol Aspects Med* 1997;18:S85–103.

Weber C, Jakobsen TS, Mortensen SA, et al. Antioxidative effect of dietary coenzyme Q10 in human blood plasma. *Int J Vitam Nutr Res* 1994;64:311–5.

Chinese herbal medicine/acupuncture references

Chang Yong Zhong Yao Cheng Fen Yu Yao Li Shou Ce (A Handbook of the Composition and Pharmacology of Common Chinese Drugs), 1994; 1725:1728.

Chen DZ, et al. Evaluation of therapeutic effects of acupuncture in treating ischemic cerebrovascular disease. *Chinese Journal of Integrated Traditional and Western Medicine*, 1990, 10(9):526–528 (in Chinese).

Hu SK, et al. *China Journal of Medicine.* 1990;5(3):22–23.

Ionescu-Tirgoviste C, Phleck-Khhayan, Danciu A, Bigu V, Cheta D. The treatment of peripheral polyneuritis by electroacupuncture. *Am J Acupunct* 1981;9(4):303–9.

Jiang Su Yi Yao (*Jiang Su Journal of Medicine and Herbology*), 1990;16(9):513.

Jiang Y, et al. *Gansu Journal of TCM.* 1988;7(4):4–7.

Li XF, et al. In vitro anti-tumor effects of Dan Shen and Dan Shen compound injection. *Zhejiang Journal of Integrated Medicine.* 1999;9(5):291–292.

Liu H. *Journal of Stomatology.* 1999;19(2):60–61.

Ma ZY. *Shannxi Journal of Traditional Chinese Medicine and Herbs.* 1982;(4):58.

Rui J. *Journal of Chinese Materia Medica.* 1999;30(1):43–45.

Shan Xi Yi Kan (*Shanxi Journal of Medicine*), 1960; (10):32.

Shi RB. *Journal of Beijing University of TCM.* 1999;22(2):63–64.

Zhong Guo Yi Xue Ke Xue Xue Bao (*Journal of Chinese Medical Science University*), 1988; 10(1): 39.

Zhong Yao Xue (Chinese Herbology), 1998; 128:130.

Zhong Yao Yao Li Yu Ying Yong (Pharmacology and Applications of Chinese Herbs), 1983:400.

Zhong Yao Yao Li Yu Ying Yong (Pharmacology and Applications of Chinese Herbs), 1990; 6(6): 28.

Homotoxicology references

Bagley R. Fundamentals of Veterinary Clinical Neurology. Blackwell Publishing Asia: Australia, 2005. p 103.

Hammel S, Hottinger H, Novo R. Postoperative results of unilateral arytenoid lateralization for treatment of idiopathic laryngeal paralysis in dogs: 39 cases (1996–2002). *J Am Vet Med Assoc.* 2006. Apr 15;228(8):pp 1215–20.

Harpster N. Laryngeal Paralysis. In: Tilly L, Smith F. The 5-Minute Consult: Canine and Feline, 3rd ed. Baltimore: Williams and Wilkins, 1997. pp 758–9.

Heel. Veterinary Guide, 3rd English edition. Baden-Baden, Germany: Biologische Heilmettel Heel GmbH. 2003. p 23.

Kent J. Repertory of the Homeopathic Materia Medica and a Word Index. Paharganj, New Delhi: B. Jain, LTD 1921. p 755.

Lee B, Wang S, Goh E, Chon K, Lee C, Lorenz R. Histologic evaluation of intracordal autologous cartilage injection in the paralyzed canine vocal fold at two and three years. *Otolaryngol Head Neck Surg.* 2006. Apr;134(4):pp 627–30.

Reckeweg H. Biotherapeutic Index: Ordinatio Antihomotoxica et Materia Medica, 5th ed. Baden-Baden, Germany: Biologische Heilmittel Heel GMBH, 2000. pp 300–1, 3337–8, 414, 415–6, 418–20.

Reckeweg H. Homeopathia Antihomotoxica Materia Medica, 4th ed. Baden-Baden, Germany: Arelia-Verlag GMBH, 2002. pp. 148–9, 217–9, 355–6, 370–1, 528–9, 561–2.

INTERVERTEBRAL DISC DISEASE—PARESIS/PARALYSIS

Definition and cause

Intervertrebal (IV) disc disease is a degeneration of the intervertebral disc, which is characterized by leakage of the disc material, leading to spinal cord compression and neurological deficits. While no proven genetic link has been determined, certain breeds such as dachshunds, beagles, and corgis are more predisposed to the condition. The literature links the cause to aging and degeneration of the disc tissue. The neurological deficits are secondary to compression (Braund 1993, Gage 1975, Hoerlein 1987, Smith 2003, Toombs 1993).

Medical therapy rationale, drug(s) of choice, and nutritional recommendations

The medical or surgical approach to IV disc disease, pain, paresis, and paralysis depends upon the severity of the inflammation and the compression of the cord. Restricted activity or cage rest is recommended in most cases. Corticosteroids are often recommended for their anti-inflammatory effects. Surgical intervention (hemilaminectomy or fenestration) is often necessary because pain or neurological deficits are common. The dietary recommendation focuses on weight reduction in obese animals. Vitamin E is beneficial for cats but has no proven indications for dogs (Braund 1993, Smith 2003).

Anticipated prognosis

The prognosis depends upon the damage to the cord. Patients with painful episodes generally carry a better prognosis than animals with neurological deficits, paralysis, paresis, and incontinence. The prognosis with surgery is good if the surgery occurs within 48 hours of the rupture (Gage 1975, Toombs 1993, Smith 2003).

Integrative veterinary therapies

Paresis refers to weakness of motor function without total paralysis. Paralysis is a lack of motor function. Anything that negatively impacts function of the motor unit can result in signs of paresis or paralysis. Damage to the upper motor neuron or central nervous system can result in paresis due to loss of conscious proprioceptive functions. Nervous tissue is extremely susceptible to a wide variety of injurious processes, and determining the cause of paresis can be challenging. Paresis in this section of text refers to neurological deficits, but the reader should remember that musculoskeletal problems can also lead to gait weaknesses, and that all paresis is not necessarily neurological in origin.

An integrative approach to IV disc-related paresis focuses upon the integrity of the disc itself as well as the secondary compression, inflammation, and resultant cell death. The addition of nutrients, nutraceuticals, medicinal herbs, and combination homeopathics that have anti-inflammatory and potentially regenerative effects on the nerves and IV disc cells can often help improve the clinical signs and the day-to-day level of comfort, and can enhance the healing process. In addition, complementary and alternative veterinary modalities (CAVM) can also strengthen surrounding discs and help prevent recurrences in adjacent locations.

Nutrition
General considerations/rationale
While surgery can help relieve the compression and improve clinical function, nutritional therapies can help improve nerve regeneration and return of function.

Appropriate nutrients
Nutritional/gland therapy: Glandular brain and cartilage supply intrinsic nutrients that help to improve nervous and organ function, reduce cellular inflammation, and strengthen connective tissue (see Gland Therapy in Chapter 2 for a more detailed explanation).

Phospholipids found in glandular brain are a source of unsaturated omega-3 fatty acids, which are now thought to play a vital role in the development and maintenance of the central nervous system. High concentrations of phosphatidyl choline and serine are found in brain tissue. Horrocks (1986) reported on the potential clinical use of these nutrients in chronic neurological conditions.

Lecithin/phosphatidyl choline: Phosphatidyl choline is a phospholipid that is integral to cellular membranes, particularly those of nerve and brain cells. It helps to move fats into the cells and is involved in acetylcholine uptake, neurotransmission, and cellular integrity. As part of the cell membranes, lecithin is an essential nutrient that is required by cells for general health and wellness (Hanin 1987).

Coenzyme Q10: Coenzyme Q10 (ubiquinone) is found in the mitochondria and is involved in the cells' energy production that is required for the daily functioning of the body. It is essential in the manufacture of ATP, the energy source for all of the body's cells and tissues. CoQ10 is also a potent antioxidant that helps to neutralize free radicals and protect cells (Thomas 1997, Weber 1994).

Chinese herbal medicine/acupuncture
General considerations/rationale
Intervertebral disc disease may be a result of trauma, as in Western theory. It may also result from Wind, Damp, and Cold invading the Kidneys, which leads to Qi and Yang deficiency.

Trauma is self-explanatory. It was also thought that Wind could blow Cold into the body, where it could attack the Joints. Application of Heat often relieves the signs in these patients. Damp tends to make things tight and sticky, which explains the stiffness many patients feel in damaged Joints. The Kidneys control the Bones, so Kidney pathology can cause Osseous and Joint lesions. When there is Qi and Yang deficiency, the patient has little energy to move and too little warmth to warm his body and Joints.

Treatment is aimed at decreasing the inflammation associated with injuries, increasing mobility, and decreasing pain.

Appropriate Chinese herbs
Atractylodes (Cang zu): Increases the pain threshold (Zhang 1999). In addition, it can counteract xylene-induced ear swelling and carrageenin-induced foot swelling (Zhang Ming Fa 1998). This indicates that it may be useful in decreasing inflammation at the site of disc disease.

Aconite root (Fu zi): Reduces swelling and inflammation in joints (Zhong Yao Tong Bao 1988). It has been shown to have analgesic properties (Zhong Guo Zhong Yao Za Zhi 1992).

Angelica (Bai zhi): Has been shown to have anti-inflammatory and analgesic effects in mice (Zhong Guo Zhong Yao Za Zhi 1991).

Angelica root (Dang gui): Is as strong as aspirin at decreasing inflammation and is 1.7 times as strong as aspirin for pain relief (Yao Xue Za 1971).

Astragalus (Huang qi): Has demonstrated mild analgesic effects in mice (Zhong Yao Tong Bao 1986).

Cinnamon twig (Gui zhi): Has analgesic properties (Zhong Yao Xue 1998). It was part of a formula used in 30 patients with arthritis; 50% recovered completely, 20% showed marked improvement, 17% showed some improvement, and 13% did not respond (Shi Zhen Gua Yao Yan Jiu 1991).

Coix (Yi yi ren): Has analgesic and anti-inflammatory effects. It suppresses dimethylbenzene-induced auricular swelling and carrageenin-induced foot swelling in mice (Zhang Ming Fa 1998). It was shown to help women with severe menstrual cramps (Zhang Yong Luo 1998), which may indicate that it would be useful in treating the pain associated with intervertebral disc disease.

Earthworm (Di long): Has a significant analgesic effect (Chen 1996).

Jujube fruit (Da zao): Decreases inflammation. Jujube fruit was shown to reduce dimethylbenzene-induced auricular inflammation in mice and egg-white-induced toe swelling in rats (Li 1997), which implies that it may be useful for decreasing the inflammation involved with intervertebral disc disease.

Licorice (Gan cao): Contains glycyrrhizin and glycyrrhetinic acid, which have anti-inflammatory effects. They have approximately 10% of the corticosteroid activity of cortisone. They decrease edema and have anti-arthritic effects (Zhong Cao Yao 1991). Licorice has demonstrated analgesic effects in mice, especially when combined with white peony (Bai shao) (Zhong Yao Xue 1998).

Notopterygium root (Qiang huo): Has anti-inflammatory and analgesic effects. In mice, it was shown to decrease xylol-induced ear lobe swelling and carrageenin-induced foot pad edema, and increase the thermal pain threshold (Xu 1991).

Sichuan aconite (Chuan wu): Seems to have a centrally mediated analgesic effect. In mice, it was shown to be effective for decreasing inflammation and pain. It is stronger than aspirin at reducing inflammation (Xian Dai Zhong Yao Yao Li Xue 1997). It controlled the signs in 92% of 150 human patients with arthritis when given in combination with Cao wu, Qiang huo, Du hua, Fu zi, Mo yao, Ru xiang, Dang gui, Chuan niu xi, Ma huang, Gui zhi, Wu gong, Chuan xiong, and Ma qian zi (Nei Meng Gu Zhong Yi Yao 1986).

White peony (Bai shao): Contains paeoniflorin, which is a strong anti-inflammatory (Zhong Yao Zhi 1993). It has demonstrated specific effects on pain in the lower back (Yun Nan Zhong Yi 1990).

Acupuncture

The World Health Organization lists lower back pain as one of the indications for acupuncture (World Health Organization 2006). One study looked at the use of abdominal acupuncture and electroacupuncture for treatment of prolapsed lumber intervertebral discs. In this study there was complete relief from symptoms in 35% of the patients, significant improvement in 45% of the participants, slight improvement in 16%, and no response in 4% (Guo 2003).

Homotoxicology
General considerations/rationale

It is beyond the scope of this text to fully deal with all causes of paralysis and paresis. This section primarily addresses fibrocartilagenous embolic and intervertebral disease, which represents Impregnation or Degeneration phase homotoxicoses.

Appropriate homotoxicology formulas

Aesculus compositum: Treats post-embolic circulatory disorders such as infarct and stroke. It is worthy of evaluation in fibrocartilagenous embolic disease, but no studies exist. Supportive of circulation (Aesculus hippocastanum, Secale cornutum, Tabacum, Solanum nigrum, Arnica Montana, Barium iodatum, Hamamelis virginiana, Arteria suis, and Rhuta graveolens). Cuprum assists with spasm. Aesculus has specific antiCOX-1 and COX-2 inhibitory effects; other agents also affect vascular structures (Sato, et al. 2005; Suter, Bommer, Rechner 2006; Fujimura, et al. 2006). It is supportive of joints and muscles and is useful for sharp pains and counteracting the effects of cold, wet weather (Solanum dulcamara). *Apis* helps reduce swelling and pain (Reckeweg 2000).

Atropinum compositum: The oral and injectable vials are currently off the market in the United States, but oral tablets are available. This agent is highly effective for spasm and pain associated with diseases of the spine and back. If this remedy is not available consider *Spascupreel* in its place.

Barijodeel: Treats paresis post stroke.

BHI-Inflammation: Rhus toxicodendron assists in cases of paresis. Cases may be aggravated after lying in wet grass. Patients may have pustular, pruritic skin conditions, joint pain, myelitis, vertigo/dizziness, intercostal pain, and other types of neuralgia. Commonly used in combination with other antihomotoxic agents.

Cerebrum compositum: Used in the recovery phase. Placenta suis assists in peripheral circulation while improving vitality and awareness, particularly in aged patients.

Cimcifuga homaccord: Has regional affinity for cervical spine neuralgia and pain originating in the sacral area and passing cranially. Treats cervical spine spasm.

Coenzyme compositum: Supports energy production through enzyme induction and repair. Useful in repairing damage to enzyme systems of metabolism and following administration of drugs injurious to metabolism. Phase remedy in the Degeneration and Dedifferentiation phases.

Colocynthis homaccord: Regional remedy for pain in the sacral and lumbar region. Useful in colitis cases and for sciatica (Reckeweg 2000).

Discus compositum: The principal antihomotoxic medication for intervertebral disc disease. *Discus compositum* contains 37 ingredients, making it a balanced agent that helps a wide variety of spinal and matrix-clearing issues. Signs of homotoxin off-load is common following use of *Discus compositum* (Reckeweg 2000, 2002).

This compositae class agent combines animal, mineral, and plant agents to assist in healing, drainage, and detoxification. Tissue receives direct support through Discus intervertebralis suis (intervertebral disc), Funiculus umbilicus suis (umbilical cord, which supports vascular and stem cell tissues), Cartilago suis (cartilage), Medulla ossis suis (bone marrow), Embryo suis (embryo), and Glandula suprarenalis suis (adrenal gland). It is useful in all cases of intervertebral or degenerative spinal disease. This remedy treats sciatica and sciatic neuralgia (Citrullus colocynthis, Cimcifiga racemosa, Picric acid, Ammonium chloride). It also supports energy metabolism and tissue repair (vitamin C, vitamin B$_1$, vitamin B$_2$, vitamin B$_6$, Nicotinamide, Coenzyme A, Nicotinamide Adenine Dinucleatide, Sodium osalacetate, Thioctic acid, Calcium phosphate, Silicic acid, and Sulphur). Zincum metallicum is a strong nerve remedy that is included for peripheral symptoms in the nervous system, with numbness of the soles of the feet and cutting pains in the heel, which may proceed to the point of complete paralysis or hemiparesis with twitching, tremors and weakness.

Engystol N: Creates a "channeling effect" in the mesenchymal tissues and lymphatic system (Reckeweg 2000).

Galium-Heel: This phase remedy in matrix and cellular phases provides powerful support of the immune system (Echinacea augustifolia). Assists in drainage of cell and matrix, supports renal tubular function, and decreases swelling and edema (Apis mellifica, Galium aparine, and Galium mollugo). It is a critical component in the deep detoxification formula. Dosing should be done with regard to clinical condition and response, with the dose reduced if strong reactions are noted (Reckeweg 2000).

Gastricumeel: Useful in supporting gastric and duodenal function following spinal pathology (Heel 2003).

Gelsemium homaccord: Used for headache, depression, posterior weakness, and fear of open spaces (Reckeweg 2000). Main formula for paresis. Gelsemium semperervirens has long been used in herbal medicine because it has an affinity for nervous tissues. Strong neuroprotection results from low-dose use of Gelsemium (Bousta 2001).

Glyoxal compositum: Used to unblock cellular receptors and provides mitochondrial repair of damaged enzyme systems in Degeneration and Dedifferentiation phase disorders.

Lymphomyosot: Used after cortisone therapy and mesenchymal purging in chronic disease states. Reduces swelling and pressure. Contains Aranea diadema for periodic neuralgia, spinal nerve irritation, paralgesia, and painful articular disease. Calcium phosphoricum is indicated for calcium deficiency and spinal affections. Fumaria officinalis has indications for tightness in the back over the right kidney. Treats back pain and cutting pain on the right side, along with lumbar pain or sudden weakness in the lumbar region and cervical tension on the right side. Myosotis arvensis is used for conditions that include left-sided cervical pain or constriction in the cervical region. This also treats pressing pain in the lumbar region and right-side scapular pain that is stabbing (Reckeweg 2002).

Nux vomica homaccord: Provides enteric protection following spinal injury (Heel 2003).

Ovarium compositum: Supports gonadal tissue in geriatric patients.

Placenta compositum: Supports hypophysis after cortisone therapy. Contains sulfur to support enzyme and metabolic repair. Regenerative of hypophyseal-adrenal axis and vascular stem cells. Repairs vascular structures and is used intermittently in endocrine disorders.

Rhododendroneel S: Treats paresis of the radial nerve (Reckeweg 2000).

Solidago compositum: Deposition Phase remedy needed to remove debris from the matrix after regressive vicariation begins.

Spascupreel: Treats stabbing pains, muscle spasm, and neuralgia. Very useful in managing spasmodic pain. It is an alternative for *Atropinum compositum*.

Testes compositum: Supports connective tissue.

Thalamus compositum: Supports thalamus, pineal gland, adrenal gland, and cellular regulation through glandular content and homeopathically diluted cyclic adenonsine monophosphate (*cAMP*). Assists in establishing autoregulation of pyschoneuroendocrine-immune functions (Reckeweg 2000). Assists in resetting pain thresholds.

Thyroidea compositum: Used for matrix drainage and repair of autoregulation. Contains low levels of thyroid, pineal, spleen, bone marrow, umbilical cord, and liver to support glandular function and repair. Galium aparine drains matrix and cellular components. Cortisonum aceticum in low potency assists in repairing damage from excess levels of cortisone. Precursors and Krebs cycle constituents promote energy metabolism through the Michaelis-Menten law of enzyme activity. Pulsatilla and Sulfur assist in regulation rigidity-type situations. Part of the deep detoxification formula (Reckeweg 2000).

Traumeel S: Has nonsteroidal anti-inflammatory effects. Useful in acute intervertebral disc herniation to reduce swelling (Apis) and pain, and activates blocked enzymes. Listed in the Physician's Desk Reference.

Ubichinon compositum: Provides mitochondrial repair of energy production mechanisms. Used in chronic diseases, iatrogenic injury to mitochondria from antibiotic therapy, and is part of the deep detoxification formula.

Zeel: Useful for its anti-inflammatory effects and supportive qualities for chronic arthritis.

Authors' suggested protocols

Nutrition
Brain/nerve and cartilage/ligament/muscle/skeletal support formulas: 1 tablet for each 25 pounds of body weight BID.

Coenzyme Q10: 25 mgs for every 10 pounds of body weight daily.

Lecithin/phosphatidyl choline: One-fourth teaspoon for each 25 pounds of body weight BID.

Chinese herbal medicine/acupuncture
Formula H39 BackRelief: 1 capsule per 10 to 20 pounds twice daily. If necessary it can be combined with steroids, nonsteroidal anti-inflammatory drugs, and nutraceuticals. (**NOTE:** it is never recommended to combine NSAIDS and steroids). In addition to the herbs listed above, BackRelief also contains aconite/cao (Cao wu), allium (Cong bai), carthamus (Hong hua), papaya (Mu gua), poria (Fu ling), and siler (Fang feng). These herbs increase the efficacy of the formula.

Recommended acupuncture points are "AShi" points, BL23,BL25, BL57, BL40, Baihui, ST36, and GB30 (Handbook of TCM Practitioner 1987).

Homotoxicology (dose: 10 drops PO for 50-pound dog; 5 drops PO for small dog or cat)
Symptom formula: Traumeel S and Discus compositum given initially by injection, preferably into applicable acupoints. Traumeel Gel and Lymphomyosot Gel mixed together and massaged into the affected areas BID to TID. Spascupreel, Aesculus compositum, Lymphomyosot, and Traumeel S combined and given orally BID to TID. Add Cimicifuga homaccord (cervical disc or pain), Gelsemium homaccord (posterior weakness), Colocynthis homaccord

(lumbosacral disease or sciatica). Zeel and Discus compositum orally twice per week and Cerebrum compositum weekly.

Deep detoxification formula: Galium-Heel, Hepar compositum, Solidago compositum, Thyroidea compositum, Coenzyme compositum, Ubichinon compositum mixed together and given orally twice weekly to every other day.

Product sources

Nutrition
Brain/nerve and cartilage/ligament/muscle/skeletal formulas: Animal Nutrition Technologies. **Alternatives:** Cosequin—Nutramax Labs; Glycoflex—Vetri Science; Musculoskeletal Support—Standard Process Veterinary Formulas; Nutriflex—Vet Rx Vitamins for Pets; Arthragen—Thorne Veterinary Products.

Coenzyme Q10: Vetri Science, Thorne Veterinary Products.

Lecithin/phosphatidyl choline: Designs for Health.

Chinese herbal medicine
Formula H39 BackRelief: Natural Solutions, Inc.

Homotoxicology
BHI/Heel Corporation

REFERENCES

Western medicine references
Braund KG. Canine intervertebral disc disease. In: Bojrab MJ, ed. Disease mechanisms in small dog surgery. Philadelphia: Lea and Febiger, 1993:960–969.

Gage ED. Modifications in Dorsolateral Hemilaminectomy and Disc Fenestration in the Dog. *J. Am. Anim. Hosp. Assoc.* 1975, 11: 407–411.

Hoerlein BF. Intervertebral disc disease. In: Oliver JE, Hoerlein BF, Mayhew, IG, Veterinary neurology. Philadelphia: WB Saunders, 1987, pp. 321–340.

Toombs JT, Bauer MB. Intervertebral disk disease. In: Slatter DH, ed. Textbook of small dog surgery. 2nd ed. Philadelphia: Saunders, 1993:1070–1086.

Smith MO. In: Tilley L, Smith F. The 5-Minute Veterinary Consult: Canine and Feline, Blackwell Publishing, 2003.

IVM/nutrition references
Hanin IG, Ansell B. Lecithin: Technological, Biological, and Therapeutic Aspects, 1987, NY: Plenum Press, 180, 181.

Horrocks LA, et al. Phosphatidyl Research and the Nervous System, Berlin: Springer Verlach, 1986.

Thomas SR, Neuzil J, Stocker R. Inhibition of LDL oxidation by ubiquinol-10. A protective mechanism for coenzyme Q in atherogenesis? *Mol Aspects Med* 1997;18:S85–103.

Weber C, Jakobsen TS, Mortensen SA, et al. Antioxidative effect of dietary coenzyme Q10 in human blood plasma. *Int J Vitam Nutr* Res 1994;64:311–5.

Chinese herbal medicine/acupuncture references
Chen BY, et al. Analgesic and antipyretic effects of Di Long powder in mice, rats and rabbits. *Journal of Shanghai Medical University*. 1996;23(3):225–226,240.
Guo F, Ma L, Gong L, Zhang H. 50 cases of prolapsed lumbar intervertebral disc using abdominal acupuncture. *Journal of Chinese Acupuncture and Moxibustion*, 2003; 23, p145.
Handbook of TCM Practitioner. Hunan College of TCM, Oct 1987, P671–672.
Li XM, et al. *Journal of Shizhen Medicinal Material Research*. 1997;8(4):373–374.
Nei Meng Gu Zhong Yi Yao (*Traditional Chinese Medicine and Medicinals of Inner Magnolia*), 1986;(3):7.
Shi Zhen Gua Yao Yan Jiu (Research of Shizen Herbs), 1991; 5(4):36.
World Health Organization list of common conditions treatable by Chinese Medicine and Acupuncture. http://tcm.health-info.org/WHO-treatment -list.htm. Accessed 10/20/2006.
Xian Dai Zhong Yao Yao Li Xue (Contemporary Pharmacology of Chinese Herbs), 1997;425.
Xu HB, et al. Pharmacology of Qiang Huo volatile oil. *Journal of Chinese Materia Medica*. 1991;22(1):28–30.
Yao Xue Za Zhi (*Journal of Medicinals*), 1971;(91):1098.
Zhang MF, et al. Yi Yi Ren's analgesic, anti-inflammatory, and antithrombotic effects. *Journal of Practical TCM*. 1998; 12(2):36–38.
Yun Nan Zhong Yi (*Yunnan Journal of Traditional Chinese Medicine*), 1990; 4:15.
Zhang MF, et al. Yi Yi Ren's analgesic, anti-inflammatory, and antithrombotic effects. *Journal of Practical TCM*. 1998;12(2):36–38.
Zhang MF, et al. *Journal of Pharmacology and Clinical Application of TCM*. 1998;14(6):12–16.
Zhang MF, et al. *Journal of Shizhen Medicine*. 1999;10(1):1–3.
Zhang YL, et al. Sequential experiments on Yi Yi Ren's analgesic effect in severe functional dysmenorrhea. *Journal of TCM*. 1998;39(10):599–600.
Zhong Cao Yao (*Chinese Herbal Medicine*) 1991;22 (10):452.
Zhong Guo Zhong Yao Za Zhi (*People's Republic of China Journal of Chinese Herbology*), 1991; 16(9):560.
Zhong Guo Zhong Yao Za Zhi (*People's Republic of China Journal of Chinese Herbology*), 1992; 17(2):104.
Zhong Yao Tong Bao (*Journal of Chinese Herbology*), 1988; 13(6):40.
Zhong Yao Xue (Chinese Herbology), 1998; 65:67.
Zhong Yao Xue (Chinese Herbology), 1998; 759:765.
Zhong Yao Zhi (*Chinese Herbology Journal*), 1993:183.

Homotoxicology references
Bousta D, Soulimani R, Jarmouni I, Belon P, Falla J, Froment N, Younos C. Neurotropic, immunological and gastric effects of low doses of Atropa belladonna L., Gelsemium sempervirens L. and Poumon histamine in stressed mice. *J Ethnopharmacol*. 2001.Mar 3;74(3):pp 205–15.

Broadfoot P. The Neuroendocrine System. In: Proceedings of 2006 Homotoxicology Seminar, AHVMA/Heel, 2006. Denver, CO, May 19–21; pp 33–53.
Feldman E, Peterson M. Hypoadrenocorticism. *Vet Clin N Am*; 1984;14: pp 751–766.
Fujimura T, Moriwaki S, Hotta M, Kitahara T, Takema Y. Horse Chestnut Extract Induces Contraction Force Generation in Fibroblasts through Activation of Rho/Rho Kinase. *Biol Pharm Bull*. 2006;Jun;29(6):pp 1075–81.
Heel. Veterinary Guide, 3rd English edition. Baden-Baden, Germany: Biologische Heilmettel Heel GmbH. 2003. p 45.
Reckeweg H. Biotherapeutic Index: Ordinatio Antihomotoxica et Materia Medica, 5th ed. Baden-Baden, Germany: Biologische Heilmittel Heel GMBH, 2000. pp 213–14, 286–7, 318, 326–27, 333–4, 339–40, 414, 415.
Reckeweg, H. Homeopathia Antihomotoxica Materia Medica, 4th ed. Baden-Baden, Germany: Arelia-Verlag GMBH, 2002. pp. 145, 198–9, 213–5, 236–7, 247–8, 279, 281–2,305–7, 310–2, 322–3, 432, 449, 457–8, 610.
Sato I, Suzuki T, Kobayashi H, Tsuda S. Antioxidative and antigenotoxic effects of Japanese horse chestnut (Aesculus turbinata) seeds. *J Vet Med Sci*. 2005. Jul;67(7):pp 731–4.
Suter A, Bommer S, Rechner J. Treatment of patients with venous insufficiency with fresh plant horse chestnut seed extract: a review of 5 clinical studies. *Adv Ther*. 2006. Jan-Feb;23(1):pp 179–90.

RADIAL NERVE PARALYSIS

Definition and cause

Radial paralysis is most commonly associated with trauma, and more specifically with a fracture of the humerus (Browne 1960, Hoerlein 1978, Knecht 1974). More often, however, the trauma involves multiple nerves of the brachial plexus. Radial nerve damage also can ensue from space-occupying lesions involving the brachial plexus of dogs and cats (Knecht 1974, 1985).

Medical therapy rationale, drug(s) of choice, and nutritional recommendations

Surgical exploration of the brachial plexus is recommended in compression and space-taking lesions, as well as neoplasia. Other treatments include a splint, fusing the joint, and amputation (Knecht 1977, Swaim 1978).

Anticipated prognosis

If the trauma results in stretching as compared to rupture, the prognosis is much improved. Surgical removal of a space-occupying lesion improves the prognosis; however, the tumor type also affects prognosis (Knecht 1985).

Integrative veterinary therapies

Cases with no deep pain perception and no reflexes carry a grave prognosis. If deep pain is present, then long-term therapy may yield results. Regular evaluation is recommended at 24 hours, 1 week, 2 weeks, 1 month, and 2 months post injury. Some lesions may slowly improve, and final decisions should not be made before allowing sufficient time for healing to manifest. Neuritis and accompanying neurodermatitis may result during healing and must be managed to avoid further injury. During recovery it is vital to protect the foot from further trauma. Boots, bandages, and reduced exercise with physical therapy are all important steps for long-term care.

An integrative approach to radial paralysis focuses upon the damaged nerve, local inflammation, regenerating nerve cells, and improving nervous function. Nutrients, medicinal herbs, and combination homeopathics that have anti-inflammatory and potentially regenerative effects on the nerves can help improve healing.

Nutrition
General considerations/rationale
Nutritional therapies can often help improve nerve function and speed up regeneration of nerves and surrounding tissues.

Appropriate nutrients
Nutritional/gland therapy: Glandular brain supplies intrinsic nutrients that help to reduce associated inflammation and improve nerve cell metabolism and healing (see Gland Therapy in Chapter 2 for a more detailed explanation).

Phospholipids found in glandular brain are a source of unsaturated omega-3 fatty acids, which are now thought to play a vital role in the development and maintenance of the central nervous system. High concentrations of phosphatidyl choline and serine are found in brain tissue. Horrocks (1986) reported on the potential clinical use of these nutrients in chronic neurological conditions.

Lecithin/phosphatidyl choline: Phosphatidyl choline is a phospholipid that is integral to cellular membranes, particularly those of nerve and brain cells. It helps to move fats into the cells and is involved in acetylcholine uptake, neurotransmission, and cellular integrity. As part of the cell membranes, lecithin is an essential nutrient required by all of the cells of the body for general health and wellness (Hanin 1987).

Coenzyme Q10: Coenzyme Q10 (ubiquinone) is found in the mitochondria and is involved in the cells' energy production that is required for the daily functioning of the body. It is essential in the manufacture of ATP, the energy source for all the body's cells and tissues. CoQ10 is also a potent antioxidant that helps to neutralize free

radicals and protect cells (Thomas 1997, Weber 1994).

Acetyl-L-carnitine: Acetyl-L-carnitine is a derivative of the amino acid L-carnitine, which is involved in the production of acetylcholine and the proper function of the brain and the transmission of nerve impulses. Studies have indicated that acetyl-L-carnitine can slow the development of Alzheimer's disease and improve cognition in people. People taking acetyl-l-carnitine showed an improvement in memory and their day-to-day demeanor and mood (Cipoli 1990, Genazzani 1990, Garzya 1990).

Chinese herbal medicine/acupuncture
General considerations/rationale
Peripheral neuropathy may be due to trauma, as in Western medicine, or it may be due to Cold and Wind invasion leading to Qi and Blood stagnation in the Meridians.

Wind has the ability to blow a pathogen into the body. In physics, we were shown how cold can thicken fluids, making them flow more slowly. In the TCM concept of peripheral neuropathy, Cold can slow the flow of Qi and Blood in the Meridians. When Blood does not flow to a limb, the limb is not nourished and will atrophy, and it will have no energy to move.

Appropriate Chinese herbs
Disclaimer: Few Western studies use herbs for radial paralysis, so the authors were unable to find well-controlled clinical trials. The following herbs have shown effects on the nervous system, which may indicate that they are useful for radial nerve paralysis. Controlled studies must be conducted to further evaluate their efficacy.

Rehmannia (Shu di): Has an effect on the central nervous system. It was used as part of a supplement along with Rou cong rong, Lu han cao, Gu sui bu, Yin yang huo, Ji xue teng, and Lai fu zi in 1,100 patients with myelitis. Seventy-three percent had significant improvement, and another 13% had moderate improvement in clinical signs (Liaoning Journal of Chinese Medicine 1982). It also may be able to affect peripheral nerves, although this must be further investigated.

Scorpion (Quan xie) and centipede (Wu gong): May have a positive effect on nerves. In one trial, 47 people experiencing a first-time episode of cerebral embolism were treated with scorpion (Qian xie), bungarus (Bai hua she), and centipede (Wu gong). Twenty-four patients recovered completely and 17 showed some response. Six did not respond (Ji Lin Zhong Yi Yao 1989). This suggests that these herbs may be useful in other neuropathies.

White peony (Bai shao) and licorice (Gan cao): These herbs were used in a study of 10 patients with congenital myotonia. One participant had marked improvement and 4 more showed moderate improvement when treated with a decoction containing white peony (Bai shao), licorice (Gan cao), achyranthes (Niu xi), cicada (Chan tui), coix (Yi yi ren), silkworm (Jiang can), and chaenomeles (Mu gua)(Zhong Xi Yi Jie He Za Zhi 1984). While its use for radial paralysis has not been studied specifically, these other findings suggest that it may be useful in a variety of neurological diseases. White peony (Bai shao) has also been shown to stop the pain of trigeminal neuralgia (Zhong Yi Za Zhi 1983), which is further evidence that it may have an effect on nerves.

Acupuncture

The World Health Organization has listed peripheral neuropathies as an indication for acupuncture (World Health Organization Accessed 2006). Acupuncture may help nerves repair themselves. Neurological function was improved as a result of acupuncture therapy in studies on hemiplegic patients who suffered as a result of cerebral infarctions (Hu 1993, Bai 1993).

Homotoxicology
General considerations/rationale

Mild traumatic lesions are Inflammation Phase disorders, while more severe traumatic lesions can be Impregnation Phase (partial damage) or Degeneration Phase (more severe damage with nerve fiber death) disorders. In rare cases radial paralysis can result from neoplasia, and this represents a Dedifferentiation Phase disease. For a discussion of neoplasia see Chapters 31 through 34. The following discussion relates to less severe injuries in which nerve fibers still exist and there is some hope of regeneration.

Appropriate homotoxicology formulas

Aesculus compositum: Provides vessel repair. More specifically, *Aesculus* has indications for paraesthesia and a paralytic sensation in the left hand and left arm (Reckeweg 2002).

Apis homaccord: For use if edema is marked.

Arnica-Heel: Used in acute trauma.

BHI-Neuralgia: Contains Spigelia, Gelsemium, Silicea, and other connective tissue and nerve-related remedies (Reckeweg 2002).

Coenzyme compositum: Assists energy metabolism in deeper homotoxicoses.

Discus compositum: Provides deep matrix clearing of connective tissue, and stem cell activation.

Galium-Heel: Used in cellular and matrix phases, this remedy assists with swelling and drainage of homotoxins.

Glyoxal compositum: Used in Degeneration and Dedifferentiation phase disorders to reduce homotoxin polymerization and enzyme blockage.

Lymphomyosot: Provides lymph drainage.

Placenta compositum: Provides stem cell activation and vessel repair in peripheral vasculature.

Spigelia: Contains Castoreum as a nerve remedy for rheumatic and neuralgic conditions with spasmodic tension in the intercostal region and the musculature of the neck, shoulders, and back; and neuralgias of the arm (Reckeweg 2002).

Spigelon: Treats neuralgia, stabbing pains, headache, neuropathy, neuritis, and general weakness of connective tissue (Reckeweg 2000).

Traumeel S: Given systemically by injection or orally by liquid or tablet; has nonsteroidal anti-inflammatory mechanisms.

Ubichinon compositum: Assists with energy metabolism in deeper homotoxicoses.

Authors' suggested protocols

Nutrition

Brain/nerve support formula: 1 tablet for each 25 pounds of body weight BID.

Acetyl-L-carnitine (500 mgs): One-half capsule per 25 pounds of body weight daily.

Coenzyme Q10: 25 mgs for every 10 pounds of body weight daily.

Lecithin/phosphatidyl choline: One-fourth teaspoon for each 25 pounds of body weight BID.

Chinese herbal medicine/acupuncture

Formula H41 Forelimb Paralysis: 1 capsule per 10 to 20 pounds twice daily. In addition to the herbs mentioned above, H41 Forelimb Paralysis contains angelica root (Dang gui), astragalus (Huang qi), cinnamon twig (Gui zhi), codonopsis (Dang shen), earthworm (Di long), jujube fruit (Da zao), milettia (Ji xue teng), tumeric (Jiang huang), and wild ginger (Xi xin). These herbs increase the efficacy of the formula.

The authors use the following acupuncture points: LI11, SI9, TH6, LI10, ST36, and Bai Hui.

Homotoxicology (dose: 10 drops PO for 50-pound dog; 5 drops PO for small dog or cat)

Traumeel S: Given IV and then QID for 2 days, then TID for 3 days.

Lymphomyosot and Aesculus compositum: Given orally BID for 2 to 4 weeks. BHI-Neuralgia given BID.

Discus compositum and Placenta compositum: Alternated and given with Spigelon twice weekly.

Product sources

Nutrition

Brain/nerve support formula: Animal Nutrition Technologies.

Acetyl-L-carnitine: Thorne Research.
Coenzyme Q10: Vetri Science; Thorne Veterinary Products.
Lecithin/phosphatidyl choline: Designs for Health.

Chinese herbal medicine
Formula H41 Forelimb: Natural Solutions, Inc.

Homotoxicology
BHI/Heel Corporation

REFERENCES

Western medicine references
Bowne JG. Radial paralysis syndrome in the dog. *Iowa State Univ Vet* 1960; 22:73.
Hoerlein BF, Bowen JM. Clinical disorders of nerves and muscles. In: Hoerlein BF, ed. Canine Neurology, Philadelphia: WB Saunders, 1978. pp 280–296.
Knecht CD. Radial-brachial paralysis. In: Kirk RW, ed. Current Veterinary Therapy V, Philadelphia: WB Saunders, 1974. pp 658–662.
Knecht CD, Greene JA. Surgical approach to the brachial plexus in small animals. *J Am Anim Hosp Assoc* 1977;13:592.
Knecht CD, Raffe MR. In: Textbook of Small Animal Orthopaedics, Newton CD, Nunamaker DM, eds. Lippincott Company, 1985.
Swaim SF. Peripheral nerve surgery. In: Hoerlein BF, ed. Canine Neurology, Philadelphia: WB Saunders, 1978. pp 296–315.

IVM/nutrition references
Cipolli C, Chiari G. Effects of L-acetylcarnitine on mental deterioration in the aged: initial results. *Clin Ter* 1990;132(6 Suppl):479–510 [in Italian].
Garzya G, Corallo D, Fiore A, et al. Evaluation of the effects of L-acetylcarnitine on senile patients suffering from depression. *Drugs Exp Clin Res* 1990;16(2):101–6.
Genazzani E. A controlled clinical study on the efficacy of L-acetylcarnitine in the treatment of mild to moderate mental deterioration in the aged. Conclusions. *Clin Ter* 1990;132(6 Suppl):511–2.
Hanin IG, Ansell B. Lecithin: Technological, Biological, and Therapeutic Aspects, 1987, NY: Plenum Press, 180, 181.
Horrocks LA, et al. Ed. Phosphatidyl Research and the Nervous System, Berlin: Springer Verlagh, 1986.
Thomas SR, Neuzil J, Stocker R. Inhibition of LDL oxidation by ubiquinol-10. A protective mechanism for coenzyme Q in atherogenesis? *Mol Aspects Med* 1997;18:S85–103.
Weber C, Jakobsen TS, Mortensen SA, et al. Antioxidative effect of dietary coenzyme Q10 in human blood plasma. *Int J Vitam Nutr Res* 1994;64:311–5.

Chinese herbal medicine/acupuncture references
Bai XY et al. [A comparative study of acupuncture and Western medicine in the treatment of stroke]. *Chinese Acupuncture and Moxibustion*, 1993, 13(1):1–4 [in Chinese].
Hu HH, et al. A randomized controlled trial on the treatment for acute partial ischemic stroke with acupuncture. *Neuroepidemiology*, 1993, 12:106–113.
Ji Lin Zhong Yi Yao (*Jilin Chinese Medicine and Herbology*), 1989; (4):15.
Liaoning Journal of Chinese Medicine, 1982; 3:40.
World Health Organization list of common conditions treatable by Chinese Medicine and Acupuncture. http://tcm.health-info.org/WHO-treatment-list.htm. Accessed 10/20/2006.
Zhong Yi Za Zhi (*Journal of Chinese Medicine*), 1983; 11;9.

Homotoxicology reference
Reckeweg H. Homeopathia Antihomotoxica Materia Medica, 4th ed. Baden-Baden, Germany: Arelia-Verlag GMBH, 2002 pp. 124, 216, 534–536, 541–2.

VESTIBULAR SYNDROMES

Definition and cause

Vestibular syndromes are defined as a head tilt along with other signs associated with a dysfunction of the vestibular apparatus: ataxia, loss of balance, falling toward the head tilt, nystagmus, etc. The cause of the vestibular imbalance is most often an inflammatory reaction secondary to bacterial/viral infection; exposure to toxins or drugs such as metronidazole; immune-mediated such as a polyneuropathy; or secondary to other conditions such as trauma, otitis involving the inner ear, polyneuropathy, or neoplasia. The literature also reports vestibular ataxia secondary to a thiamine deficiency (Bagley 2005, Cochrane 2003, de Lahunta 1993, Thomas 2000).

Medical therapy rationale, drug(s) of choice, and nutritional recommendations

Medical therapy depends upon the severity of the clinical signs. Topical and systemic antibiotics are recommended when the cause is confirmed secondary to inner ear problems. Corticosteroids are often recommended to reduce inflammation as well as suppress the immune reactions. Thiamine is recommended with those animals that have confirmed vitamin B_1 deficiencies. When the vestibular disease is secondary to other conditions such as hypothyroidism or cancer, the primary therapy must include the primary disease (Bagley 2005, Clemmons 1997).

Anticipated prognosis

Primary vestibular disease often responds well to medical therapy consisting of reducing inflammation and giving antimicrobials. The prognosis is less favorable if the vestibular disease is secondary to other conditions such as GME or cancer.

Integrative veterinary therapies

Vestibular syndrome covers a wide variety of neurological disorders, including anomalous, metabolic, neoplastic, idiopathic, infectious inflammatory, noninfectious-inflammatory, traumatic, toxic, vascular, and metabolic categories (Bagley 2005). The term "idiopathic vestibular syndrome" is not a comprehensive diagnosis and can consist of a myriad of actual abnormalities that lead the patient to manifest disturbances in the functioning of the vestibular system. Patients with infections, parasites, allergies, masses, or vascular lesions all require different selections of appropriate conventional and complementary veterinary medical therapies. The contribution of iatrogenic vestibular conditions is very important.

Evaluation of a patient in this category should include careful assessment of drug history, because ototoxic medications such as aminoglycoside antibiotics, furosemide, chlorhexidine, and cisplatin, as well as metronidazole, can cause adverse effects that result in vestibular signs. In some instances, removal of the drug leads to rapid improvement as the patient undergoes regressive vicariation (Deposition and Impregnation phases), while in other instances such changes may be permanent (Degeneration Phase iatrogenic homotoxicoses) (Paquette and Sammut 2006)(see Chapter 4, Homotoxicology). Clinicians need accurate diagnoses to properly select and implement maximally effective treatment plans. An in-depth history (including diet, travel, and drug history; physical and neurological examination (including otoscopic examination); blood work consisting of CBC, biochemistries, and thyroid testing; and any necessary medical imaging should be considered. Otitis media and otitis interna cases can sometimes be difficult to diagnose, and can mislead clinicians during the diagnostic process. MRI and CT scans may offer critical data to properly understand and treat many patients afflicted by vestibular syndrome.

Because vestibular syndrome is an inflammatory process, often with an immune component, the use of nutrients, medicinal herbs, and combination homeopathics that have anti-inflammatory effects are beneficial for the restoration of equilibrium and healing.

Nutrition
General considerations/rationale

While medical therapy is focused locally upon the reduction of inflammation and control of infections, nutritional therapies including antioxidants and glands help to reduce inflammation and support the immune system organs.

Appropriate nutrients

Nutritional/gland therapy: Glandular adrenal, thymus, and brain supply the intrinsic nutrients that reduce cellular inflammation and improve organ function (see Gland Therapy in Chapter 2 for a more detailed explanation).

Lecithin/phosphatidyl choline: Phosphatidyl choline is a phospholipid that is integral to cellular membranes, particularly those of the nerve and brain cells. It helps to move fats into the cells and is involved in acetylcholine uptake, neurotransmission, and cellular integrity. As part of the cell membranes, lecithin is an essential nutrient required by the cells of the body for general health and wellness (Hanin 1987).

Phosphatidyl serine (PS): Phosphatidyl serine is a phospholipid that is essential for cellular membranes, particularly those of brain cells. It has been studied in people with impaired mental functioning and degeneration with positive results (Crook 1991, Cenacchi 1993). People with Alzheimer's disease who were treated with PS showed a mild to significant clinical improvement (Delewaide 1986, Engel 1992, Funfgeld 1989).

Betasitosterol: Betasitosterol is a plant-derived sterol that has anti-inflammatory properties similar to corticosteroids and aspirin (Gupta 1980). In addition, sterols have been proven to enhance immune function (Bouic 1996). Sterols have been found to be able to enhance T-lymphocyte production and moderate B cell activity, thereby helping to balance the immune response and indirectly reducing the risk of an autoimmune reaction (Bouic 1996).

Chinese herbal medicine/acupuncture
General considerations/rationale

Vestibular disease is due to Wind in the Liver with rising Yang. There may be Yin, Yang, Qi, and/or Blood deficiency.

Wind can be a description of ataxia. The swaying of an ataxic individual is similar to the swaying of trees in the wind. It can also be responsible for blowing a pathogen into the body, i.e., a bacterium for otitis media. The Liver is given the responsibility for ensuring the smooth flow of energy in the body. When there is Liver pathology, energy becomes affected and function may become jerky. When the Heat or Yang of the Liver rises there may be dizziness, irritability, and headaches.

This condition is seen quite often in elderly patients. They may be dehydrated (deficient in fluids or Yin), weak (deficient in energy or Q), coolness and heat seeking (deficient in Heat or Yang), and/or anemic (deficient in Blood). If these conditions exist they must also be addressed. Basic therapy is aimed at treating the dizziness, any underlying cause of the disorder, and the inflammation that the etiologic agent incites.

Appropriate Chinese herbs

Angelica root (Dang gui): Has antibiotic activity against both gram-positive and gram-negative bacteria (Hou Xue Hua Yu Yan Jia 1981).

Astragalus (Huang qi): Has demonstrated efficacy against various strains of bacteria (Zhong Yao Zhi 1949).

Bupleurum (Chai hu): Contains an anti-inflammatory chemical called saikosaponin (Shen Yang Yi Xue Yuan Bao 1984). It is one component of Fu Yuan Hou Xue Tang. This patent formula also contains trichosanthes (Gua lou), angelica root (Dang gui), licorice (Gan cao), pangolin scales (Pao shan jia), peach pit (Tao ren), carthamus (Hong hua), pueraria (Ge gen), and clematis (Wei ling xian). When it was used to treat 38 people with vertigo, 68% of the participants had complete resolution of signs and another 18% improved (Tang 1997).

Citrus (Chen pi): An anti-inflammatory. It decreases the permeability of blood vessels and reduces inflammation (Zhong Yao Yao Li Yu Ying Yong 1983). It also seems to have a dual effect on the immune system. It increases serum lysozyme levels but decreases the T-lymphocyte transformation rate (Jin 1992).

Fleece flower root (He sou wu): Has demonstrated antibacterial action against a variety of bacteria (Zhen 1986).

Ginger (Sheng jiang): Has anti-inflammatory effects. It can decrease capillary permeability (Zhang 1989). In addition, it is a strong anti-emetic (Xi 1990), which is helpful when the vestibular disease causes vomiting.

Haematite (Dai zhe shi): Has been used to treat people with vertigo. It was part of a supplement that also contained Ban xia, Che qian cao, and Xia ku cao. It was 94% effective in a trial involving 86 patients (Zhong Cao Yao Tong Xun 1972).

Jujube (Da zao): Can decrease inflammation and swelling (Li 1997).

Licorice (Gan cao): Contains glycyrrhizin and glycyrrhetinic acid, which have anti-inflammatory effects. They have approximately 10% of the corticosteroid activity of cortisone (Zhong Cao Yao 1991). But while licorice is anti-inflammatory, it is also an immunomodulant. It can either stimulate or inhibit the phagocytic activity of macrophages (Zhong Yao Xue 1998). This indicates that it may be able to normalize the immune system. It may improve the immunodeficient patient but also decrease immunoreactivity in immune-mediated disease.

Poria (Fu ling): Inhibits various bacteria (Nanjing College of Pharmacy 1976).

Scutellaria (Huang qin): Contains baicalin, which has antibiotic activity against a wide variety of viruses and bacteria, and also has a synergistic effect with ampicillin, amoxicillin, methacillin, and cefotaxime (Zhong Yao Xue 1988, Liu 2000). In addition, baicalin and another component, baicalein, are anti-inflammatory (Kubo 1984).

Acupuncture

Several studies have shown that vertigo is quite responsive to acupuncture therapy. Zhou treated 63 patients with acupuncture at GV20, PC6, and ST36, along with additional points as required based upon the TCM pattern. Sixty-five percent of the patients recovered fully while another 29% improved (Zhou 1998).

Meniere's disease is a condition seen in humans that seems to be related to increased pressure in the inner ear due to increased amounts of endolymphatic fluid. This condition can cause severe, even debilitating, vertigo. Yan then treated 189 patients with Meniere's syndrome with acupuncture at SP6, Kid3, GV20, GB20, GB34, PC6, HT7, ST40, and CV4. Ninety-two percent had complete resolution of symptoms while another 6% improved (Yan 1999).

Homotoxicology
General considerations/rationale

As in all conditions, it is useful to determine the relative position on the Six-Phase Table of Homotoxicology. Many of these patients are found to the left of the biological divide. Impregnation Phase diseases (chronic inflammation, allergy, viral, and some hemorrhages), Degeneration Phase diseases (embolic stroke and hemorrhage), and Dedifferentiation Phase homotoxicoses (congenital anomalies and neoplasia) are common causes, but Inflammation Phase cases (meningitis, abscess, infection, and trauma) may also occur. It is important to realize that earlier homotoxicoses may ultimately lead to a vestibular syndrome and it is desirable to treat these as earlier, less irreversible conditions. Proper use of biological therapies may resolve a condition before progressive vicariation occurs. Deposition Phase signs such as obesity and inactivity should warn the practitioner of ongoing disease and steps should be taken as early as possible to prevent the patient's crossing over the biological divide.

Appropriate homotoxicology formulas

Also see the allergy protocols located in Chapter 10, Diseases of the Dermatological System.

BHI-Recovery: Used as a reparative agent following stroke. Contains Gelsemium sempervirens (vertigo and difficulty swallowing) and Melilotus officinalis (hypertension and blood congestion of the cranium) (Heel 2002).

Aesculus compositum: Although it is considered to be in the realm of a primary peripheral circulatory remedy, this combination includes a large group of remedies with some specific indications for vertiginous syndromes: Aesculus hippocastanum (for headaches, especially above the eyes, accompanied by flickering vision, with a heavy sensation, as if numbed, with vertigo, and especially with occipital pain), Aethusa (see Strophanthus, below), Secale (for a subcutaneous sensation of crawling; there may be a preponderance of nervous symptoms such as lassitude, vertigo, and convulsive twitching alternating with spasmodic contractions of individual areas of muscle; there may be symptoms similar to those indicated for Strophanthus), Tabacum, and Viscum album (hypotension and hypertension, sensations of vertigo, coronary stenosis, and arrhythmia) (Reckeweg 2002).

Cactus compositum: Used in cases resulting from cardiac causes.

Carbo compositum: Used for cerebral hemorrhage, collapse, circulatory failure, and brain congestion (Reckeweg 2000).

Cerebrum compositum: Useful in many cases of vestibular syndrome, especially stroke (Morawiec-Bajda, Wasilewski 2000; Kuznetsova, Lukach 2004).

Cocculus homaccord: A classical remedy for dizziness and motion sickness.

Coenzyme compositum: Supports cytosol energy mechanics.

Cralonin: Used in circulatory disturbances stemming from cardiac disease (See Chapter 9, Diseases of the Cardiovascular System, for more details).

Galium-Heel: Provides matrix and cellular drainage and support. Part of the deep detoxification formula.

Gelsemium homaccord: Used for headache, depression, and posterior weakness, as well as fear of open spaces (Reckeweg 2000). Gelsemium sempererviens has long been used in herbal medicine because of its affinity for nervous tissues. It has been shown to have antiseizure activity in rats that have undergone experimental neurological damage (Peredery, Persinger 2004). Also provides strong neuroprotection from low doses of Gelsemium (Bousta 2001).

Ginseng compositum: At first glance, this remedy may seem less likely as a first line of therapy. Nonetheless, it contains some very useful vertigo remedies: ATP and Nadidum have general indications for vertigo. Natrum oxalaceticum can be used in cases that are unresponsive to other remedies. This combination also contains Conium (see *Vertigoheel*) and Pulsatilla for consideration in cases in which there may be vertigo with a tendency to vomit and aggravation when lying down. Viscum album (see *Aesculus compositum*) is also included. Finally, the ingredient for which it takes its name, Ginseng (Aralia quinquefolia), is used for vertigo, hemicrania with ptosis of the eyelids, heat in the head, and tendency to sleep, characteristic paralytic ptosis, difficulty in opening the upper lids, a certain weakness of vision with hypersensitivity to light, visual distortion, and double vision (Reckeweg 2002).

Glyoxal compositum: Used for unblocking receptors and activating blocked enzymes in cellular phase homotoxicoses.

Hamamelis homaccord: A hemorrhage remedy that also treats venous congestion and thromboembolic diseases. If seizures are present, also consider *Belladonna homaccord*, *Traumeel S*, and *Cruroheel* (Reckeweg 2000).

Hepar compositum: Provides liver support and drainage. Part of the deep detoxification strategy.

Lymphomyosot: Provides lymphatic drainage and immune support.

Phosphor compositum: Useful in bleeding issues, it also contains Argentum nitricum for vertigo that is accompanied by general weakness, trembling, and tinnitus, such as one finds in Meniere's syndrome.

Solidago compositum: Used for support and drainage of the kidney, which is involved in the function and degeneration of the brain in Traditional Chinese Medicine. It is a component in the deep detoxification formula.

Spigelon: Useful for headache.

Strophanthus compositum: Used primarily as a cardioactive remedy, it contains Aethusa for disturbances of the nervous system, with various kinds of spasms, dulling of faculties, or loss of consciousness. It is also used for reflex vomiting, gastrointestinal symptoms, and great exhaustion with a sensation of coldness and a tendency to develop vertigo, as well as loss of consciousness. Tabacum is another useful component; it is useful in collapse with pallor and cold sweat, trembling, coldness of the limbs, neuralgia, vertigo and Meniere's syndrome. Tormentilla is indicated for lightheadedness, vertigo that is better while lying down and worse on rising or standing or walking, and intermittent nausea (Reckeweg 2002). Also contains Carbo veg for bleeding, collapse, and shock, and Latrodectus mactans for lowered coagulability (thus, it is potentially valuable in cases of stroke).

Thyroidea compositum: Provides matrix drainage and endocrine support, and is part of the deep detoxification formula.

Traumeel S: A nonsteroidal anti-inflammatory agent that is useful in stroke, trauma, Inflammation Phases, and hemorrhage cases.

Ubichinon compositum: Provides mitochondrial support and detoxification, and supports improved energy mechanics.

Vertigoheel: Highly effective agent that is useful for vertigo of many differing causations. Major remedy for vertigo/dizziness that apparently treats microvascular circulation (Klopp, Niemer, Weiser 2005). Commonly used in human medicine for senile vertigo (Issing, Klein, Weiser 2005). Contains an array of vertigo-specific therapeutics, most notably Ambra grisea, a remedy for nervous symptoms of a predominantly chronic nature such as nervous weakness of vision and hearing, vertigo, weakness of memory, deterioration of brain function, and senility with general mental prostration. Cocculus is for vertigo, which occurs on traveling, and Meniere's syndrome with migraine-like symptoms and nausea and vomiting. Conium treats rotary vertigo, and petroleum treats vertigo, often with nausea, heaviness, swimming in the head, and tinnitus associated with dull, drawing headaches (Reckeweg 2002).

Viscum compositum: Useful for sudden attacks of vertigo and precancerous and Dedifferentiation Phase diseases. Supports intracellular regulation via *cAMP*. It is also a useful geriatric medication (Reckeweg 2000).

Ypsiloheel: Thuja occidentalis is a constitutional remedy used for many purposes, including proliferative processes and hemorrhagic stroke of the left frontal lobe. Used to assist in regaining cranial autoregulation. Also useful in many centrally mediated conditions as an intermittent remedy (Reckeweg 2000).

Authors' suggested protocols

Nutrition

Ear support formula: 1 tablet for each 25 pounds of body weight BID.

Immune support formula: One-half tablet for each 25 pounds of body weight BID.

Lecithin/phosphatidyl choline: One-fourth teaspoon for each 25 pounds of body weight BID.

Phosphatidyl serine: 25 mgs for each 25 pounds of body weight BID.

Betathyme: 1 capsule for each 35 pounds of body weight BID (maximum, 2 capsules BID.) **Alternative:** Moducare—follow manufacturer's directions.

Vitamin B$_1$ (thiamine): Cats—25 mgs SID; dogs—25 mgs for each 35 pounds of body weight SID.

Chinese herbal medicine/acupuncture

Formula Vestibular Disease: 1 capsule per 10 to 20 pounds twice daily as needed. In addition to the herbs cited above, Vestibular Disease contains alisma (Ze xie), bamboo shavings (Zhu ru), codonopsis (Dang shen), haliotis (Shi jue ming), pinellia (Ban xia), and uncaria (Gou teng). These herbs increase the efficacy of the formula.

Recommended acupuncture points include GV20, PC6, ST36, SP6, and SI9 (Handbook of TCM practitioners 1987).

Homotoxicology (dose: 10 drops PO for 50-pound dog; 5 drops PO for small dog or cat)

Also see protocols for individual diseases such as otitis, neoplasia, meningitis/encephalitis, GME, etc.

Embolic stroke: Vertigoheel orally TID. Carbo compositum, a wonderful remedy that is no longer available, given initially by injection or orally. Consider Strophanthus compositum as an alternative, especially if known cardiac issues exist. Arnica-Heel alternated with Traumeel, given orally every 30 to 60 minutes for 5 hours, then TID for 3 days and BID for 2 days. Cerebrum compositum alternated with Cor compositum every week.

Hemorrhagic stroke: Vertigoheel, Cinnamomum homaccord (if available; as an alternative consider BHI-Bleeding and/or Strophanthus compositum), and Phosphor homaccord mixed together and given orally TID. Hamamelis homaccord is an intermediate remedy given during early phases of hemorrhage. Cerebrum compositum given twice weekly in recovery phases.

Idiopathic vestibular syndrome: Vertigoheel TID orally. Aesculus compositum twice daily. Barijodeel and/or Ginseng compositum, twice daily, may be useful in refractory cases, particularly in aged animals with circulatory deficits.

Deep detoxification in cases that are right of the biological divide: Galium-Heel, Lymphomyosot, Hepar compositum, Solidago compositum, Thyroidea compositum, Coenzyme compositum, and Ubichinon compositum mixed together and given orally twice per week, alternating with Cerebrum compositum and Placenta compositum twice weekly.

Product sources

Nutrition

Ear and immune support formulas: Animal Nutrition Technologies. **Alternatives:** Immune System Support—Standard Process Veterinary Formulas; Immuno Support—Rx Vitamins for Pets; Immugen—Thorne Veterinary Products.

Lecithin/phosphatidyl choline: Designs for Health.

Betathyme: Best for Your Pets; Moducare; Thorne Veterinary Products.

Phosphatidyl serine: Integrative Therapuetics.

Vitamin B$_1$ (thiamine): Over the counter.

Chinese herbal medicine

Formula Vestibular Disease: Natural Solutions, Inc.

Homotoxicology

BHI/Heel Corporation

REFERENCES

Western medicine references

Clemmons, RM. Vestibular Disease. In: Tilley L, Smith F. The 5-Minute Veterinary Consult: Canine and Feline, Blackwell Publishing, 2003.

de Lahunta A. Veterinary neuroanatomy and clinical neurology. 2nd ed. Philadelphia: Saunders, 1983.

Oliver JE, Lorenz MD. Handbook of veterinary neurologic diagnosis. 2nd ed. Philadelphia: Saunders, 1993.

Thomas WB. Vestibular dysfunction. *Vet Clin Small Anim Pract* 2000;30:227–249.

IVM reference
Bagley R. Fundamentals of Veterinary Clinical Neurology. Blackwell Publishing Asia: Australia, 2005. p 198.

Nutrition references
Bouic PJD, et al. Beta-sitosterol and beta-sitosterol glucoside stimulate human peripheral blood lymphocyte proliferation: Implications for their use as an *International Journal of Immunopharmacology* 1996;18:693–700.

Gupta MB, Nath R, Srivastava N, et al. Anti-inflammatory and antipyretic activities of β-sitosterol. *Planta Medica* 1980; 39:157–163.

Cenacchi T, Bertoldin T, Farina C, et al. Cognitive decline in the elderly: a double-blind, placebo-controlled multicenter study on efficacy of phosphatidylserine administration. *Aging* (Milano) 1993;5:123–33.

Crook TH, Tinklenberg J, Yesavage J, et al. Effects of phosphatidylserine in age-associated memory impairment. *Neurology* 1991;41:644–9.

Fünfgeld EW, Baggen M, Nedwidek P, et al. Double-blind study with phosphatidylserine (PS) in Parkinsonian patients with senile dementia of Alzheimer's type (SDAT). *Prog Clin Biol Res* 1989;317:1235–46.

Hanin IG, Ansell B. Lecithin: Technological, Biological, and Therapeutic Aspects, 1987, NY: Plenum Press, 180, 181.

Chinese herbal medicine/acupuncture references
Handbook of TCM practitioners, Hunan College of TCM, Shanghai Science and Technology Press, Oct 1987, p 785–786.

Hou Xue Hua Yu Yan Jia (Research on Blood-Activating and Stasis-Eliminating Herbs), 1981:335.

Jin ZC, et al. *Journal of Chinese Materia Medica.* 1992;23(11):612.

Kubo M, Matsuda H, Tanaka M, Kimura Y, Okuda H, Higashino M, Tani T, Namba K, Arichi S. Studies on Scutellariae radix. VII. Anti-arthritic and anti-inflammatory actions of methanolic extract and flavonoid components from Scutellariae radix. *Chem Pharm Bull*, 1984; 32(7):2724–9.

Li XM, et al. *Journal of Shizhen Medicinal Material Research.* 1997;8(4):373–374.

Liu IX, Durham DG, Richards RM. Baicalin synergy with beta-lactam antibiotics against methicillin-resistant Staphylococcus aureus and other beta-lactam-resistant strains of S. aureus. *J Pharm Pharmacol.* 2000 Mar;52(3):361–6.

Nanjing College of Pharmacy. Materia Medica, vol 2. Jiangsu: People's Press; 1976.

Shen Yang Yi Xue Yuan Bao (*Journal of Shenyang University of Medicine*), 1984; 1(3):214.

Tang SQ. Treating 38 cases of vertigo with modified Fu Yuan Huo Xue Tang. *Xinjiang Journal of Traditional Chinese Medicine.* 1997;15(2):20.

Xi Ye Shi Lang. *Journal of Nanjing College of TCM.* 1990; 6(2):60.

Yan S-M. Acupuncture for Meniere's syndrome: short and long term observation of 189 cases. *Int J Clin Acupuncture.* 1999;10(3):303–304.

Zhang ZX, et al. *Journal of Chinese Materia Medica.* 1989;20(12):544, 545–546.

Zhen HC, et al. *Chinese Medicine Bulletin.* 1986;(3):53.

Zhong Cao Yao (*Chinese Herbal Medicine*) 1991;22 (10): 452.

Zhong Cao Yao Tong Xun (*Journal of Chinese Herbal Medicine*), 1972; 4:57.

Zhong Yao Xue (Chinese Herbology), 1988; 137:140.

Zhong Yao Xue (Chinese Herbology), 1998; 759:766.

Zhong Yao Yao Li Yu Ying Yong (Pharmacology and Applications of Chinese Herbs), 1983;567.

Zhong Yao Zhi (*Chinese Herbology Journal*), 1949;(12):648.

Zhou Y. Vertigo treated by acupuncture: an analysis of 63 cases. *Shanghai J Acupuncture Moxibustion.* 1998:19–21.

Homotoxicology references
Bousta D, Soulimani R, Jarmouni I, Belon P, Falla J, Froment N, Younos C. Neurotropic, immunological and gastric effects of low doses of Atropa belladonna L., Gelsemium sempervirens L. and Poumon histamine in stressed mice. *J Ethnopharmacol.* 2001. Mar 3;74(3):pp 205–15.

Heel. BHI Homeopathic Therapy: Professional Reference. Albuquerque, NM: Heel Inc. 2002. p 90.

Issing W, Klein P, Weiser M. The homeopathic preparation Vertigoheel versus Ginkgo biloba in the treatment of vertigo in an elderly population: a double-blinded, randomized, controlled clinical trial. *J Altern Complement Med.* 2005;Feb;11(1): pp 155–60.

Klopp R, Niemer W, Weiser M. Microcirculatory effects of a homeopathic preparation in patients with mild vertigo: an intravital microscopic study. *Microvasc Res.* 2005; Jan;69(1–2):pp 10–6.

Kuznetsova S, Lukach O. Effect of cerebrum compositum preparation on functional state of the central nervous system in elderly patients with ischemic stroke. *Lik Sprava.* 2004. Jul-Sep;(5–6):pp 88–93.

Morawiec-Bajda A, Wasilewski B. Myogenic vestibular evoked potentials used to objective estimation of effectiveness of central action drugs. *Otolaryngol Pol.* 2000; 54(3):pp 327–36.

Paquette D, Sammut V. A case of metronidazole toxicity. *Pulse,* 2006; August 48(8):pp 6–19.

Peredery O, Persinger MA. Herbal treatment following post-seizure induction in rat by lithium pilocarpine: Scutellaria lateriflora (Skullcap), Gelsemium sempervirens (Gelsemium) and Datura stramonium (Jimson Weed) may prevent development of spontaneous seizures. *Phytother Res.* 2004; Sep;18(9):pp 700–5.

Reckeweg H. Biotherapeutic Index: Ordinatio Antihomotoxica et Materia Medica, 5th ed. Baden-Baden, Germany: Biologische Heilmittel Heel GMBH, 2000. pp 305–6, 340, 347, 429–32, 433.

Reckeweg H. Homeopathia Antihomotoxica Materia Medica, 4th ed. Baden-Baden, Germany: Aurelia-Verlag GMBH, 2002. pp 124, 125–126, 131, 146–7, 156, 159, 244–5, 254–5, 320, 434–5, 446–7, 471, 484–5, 504, 525–6, 578–9.

SECTION 3

Integrative Therapy Protocols for Infectious Diseases

Chapter Eighteen

Integrative Therapy Protocols for Infectious Diseases

CANINE CORONAVIRUS DIARRHEA

Definition and cause

Coronavirus diarrhea in puppies is similar to parvovirus; however, death from the disease is not as prevalent. The disease is characterized by severe inflammation in the intestines, leading to persistent diarrhea and dehydration. Vomiting is generally not associated with coronavirus enteritis. The disease is passed from infected animals by contact with the stool. Vaccination for coronavirus generally prevents the disease (Carmichael 2005; Decaro 2004; Ettinger 1995; Pratelli 2001, 2005).

Medical therapy rationale, drug(s) of choice, and nutritional recommendations

There is no specific treatment for the virus. Supportive care of antibiotics, antidiarrheal medication, and fluid therapy is indicated. The diarrhea generally lasts 2 to 3 weeks, unless the puppy has other complicating diseases such as parvovirus.

Anticipated prognosis

If the virus is detected early and is not complicated by other disease, the chance of complete resolution is above 90%.

Integrative veterinary therapies

Although the intestines are the target tissue of coronavirus infection, the organs of the immune system are also compromised, allowing the virus to propagate. An integrative approach takes into consideration the intestines and control of diarrhea as well as general immune system support. The use of nutrients, nutriceuticals, medicinal herbs, and combination homeopathics that have anti-inflammatory, tissue-protective and regenerative effects on the intestines and immune system organs helps to control symptoms as well as speed recovery.

Nutrition
General considerations/rationale

Therapeutic nutrition takes into consideration support and protection of the gastrointestinal tract, the immune system, and the viral-induced inflammation and tissue destruction. The nutritional approach is multifaceted and consists of reducing intestinal inflammation, supporting the intestines and immune system organs (thymus, adrenal, bone marrow) with nutrients, and enhancing the elimination of metabolic wastes and toxins.

Appropriate nutrients

Nutrition/gland therapy: Glandular adrenal, thymus, bone marrow, and intestines help to neutralize viral-induced inflammation and protect the intestines and organs of the immune system (see Gland Therapy in Chapter 2).

Note: Because coronavirus disease and the associated diarrhea can be serious in puppies, it is recommended that blood be analyzed both medically and physiologically to determine organ involvement and disease. This can help the clinician specifically formulate nutritional support based upon the animal's individual needs (Cima 2000, Goldstein 2000) (see Chapter 2, Nutritional Blood Testing, for additional information).

Sterols and sterolins: Animal studies have demonstrated that phytosterols have anti-inflammatory and antipyretic effects (Gupta 1980). Pegel (1997) feels that sterols are essential for a properly functioning immune system. In studies on cats with FIV, sterols are believed to have an immune-modulating effect and help to maintain proper lymphocyte levels (Bouic 1997). While the sterols have no direct antiviral properties, the balancing and stimulation of the immune system is enough to control the spread and effects of the virus.

N,N-Dimethylglycine (DMG): DMG has been shown to support immune function and improve toxin removal (Verdova 1965). DMG has immune modulating ability and has been clinically proven to increase both tumor necrosis factor (TNF) and interferon production (Graber 1986, Kendall 2003, Reap 1990, Wang 1988).

Vitamin C: Vitamin C has been clinically proven to be a potent antioxidant and immune-enhancing agent specifically against infectious agents (Pauling 1976). Vitamin C in large doses may help puppies with coronavirus, but no controlled studies exist. Preservative-free vitamin C should be used if this is part of the treatment plan.

Glutamine: Glutamine can enhance immune function, is beneficial for the intestinal tract, and can help improve cellular integrity as well as permeability (Souba 1985, Windmueller 1982, Yoshimura 1993).

Chinese herbal medicine
General considerations/rationale
According to TCM, this type of diarrhea is caused by Heat, Dampness, and toxins in the Blood.

Author's interpretation
Heat refers to Blood in the diarrhea and Dampness refers to any pus. The toxins translate into the viral or secondary bacterial particles in modern terminology.

Appropriate Chinese herbs
Ash bark (Qin pi): Had an 80% success rate in treating people with bacterial dysentery (Zhong Yao Xue 1998).

Coptis root (Huang lian): Caused marked improvement in all participants in a study of 100 people with acute gastroenteritis (Si Chuan Yi Xue Yuan Xue Bao 1995).

Phellodendron bark (Huang bai): Has been used for chronic bacterial diarrhea (Zhong Yi Za Zhi 1959).

Homotoxicology
General considerations/rationale
Canine coronavirus, like all viral infections, initially constitutes an Impregnation Phase disorder that can rapidly lead to a Degeneration Phase condition. Young puppies without proper maternal or vaccinal protection are most likely to be infected with coronavirus. Most infections are minor and, therefore, coronavirus is not included in the recommended core vaccinations for canine patients.

Standard medical therapy consists of supportive aggressive fluid and electrolyte therapy, antibiotics, and antiemetics when needed for patient comfort. Antiemetics have been associated with prolonged hospitalizations in canine parvovirus enteritis and their use should be carefully considered before they are administered (Mantione 2005). Biological therapeutic theory considers vomiting and diarrhea as effective methods for the elimination of excess viral particles and other homotoxins.

Use of antihomotoxic medications can assist these patients in recovering and can help handle signs which may occur from latent healing, which manifests as regressive vicariation.

Appropriate homotoxicology formulas
See also Canine Parvovirus.

BHI-Bleeding: Treats severe intestinal hemorrhage.

Cactus compositum: Used for coronary insufficiency, endocarditis, and myocarditis, and for improved circulation in febrile or septic conditions.

Coenzyme compositum: Provides metabolic assistance.

Cor compositum: Provides cardiac support after injury.

Cralonin: Supports cardiac function.

Diarrheel: Used as a symptomatic agent for profound diarrhea. Not used in most cases.

Duodenoheel: Treats vomiting later in the course as the virus damages the duodenum and lower gastrointestinal tract. Use when the patient does not respond to *Gastricumheel*.

Echinacea compositum: Effective against bacterial invasion.

Engystol N: Stimulates white blood cell activity through Vincetoxicum. This remedy is commonly used in viral infections to activate the host immune response. It is not specifically antiviral.

Gastricumheel: Used in cases of vomiting early in infection, especially when *Veratrum homaccord* has not been successful.

Mercurius Heel: Has antiviral and antibacterial effects in diarrhea.

Mucosa compositum: Helps the bowel to heal following trauma and Degeneration Phase disorders. Helps with leaky gut and may reduce sensitization to food items that can occur following parvovirus infection.

Nux vomica homaccord: Used for intestinal complaints.

Podophyllum compositum: Treats gushing diarrhea with jelly-like mucus, colicky pain, and vomiting.

Tanacet-Heel: Used for concurrent worm infestations and collateral damage to the GI system.

Tonsilla compositum: Provides immune support in Impregnation and Degeneration phase conditions. Supports the spleen and bone marrow.

Ubichinon compositum: Provides mitochondrial resuscitation following antibiotics, and is used as a phase remedy in Degeneration Phase homotoxicoses.

Veratrum homaccord: Indicated for bloody vomitus, rapid depression, collapse, and shock.

Vomitusheel: Treats vomiting.

Authors' suggested protocols

Nutrition
Immune and intestinal/IBD support formulas: 1 tablet for each 25 pounds of body weight BID.

Betathyme: 1 capsule for each 35 pounds of body weight BID (maximum, 2 capsules BID).

Maitake DMG: 1 ml per 25 pounds of body weight BID.

Glutimmune: One-fourth scoop per 25 pounds of body weight daily.

Vitamin C: 100 mgs per 10 pounds of body weight BID. Care should be taken because oral vitamin C may cause diarrhea in some animals and a lower dose adjustment may be required.

Chinese herbal medicine

The patent formula, Bai Tou Weng Tang, contains pulsatilla (Bai tou weng), phellodenron bark (Huang bai), coptis root (Huang lian), and ash bark (Qin pi). This formula has strong antibacterial, antiviral, and antiparasitic effects. It also helps to control diarrhea and abdominal pain. It is dosed according to the label on the bottle.

Homotoxicology (Dose: 10 drops PO for 50-pound dog, 5 drops PO for small dog)

Broadfoot routinely uses the following approach on initial presentation: Nux vomica homaccord as an IV, then Engystol N, Coenzyme compositum, and Gripp-Heel, plus Aconitum homaccord or Traumeel as an autosanguis on presentation (especially for desperately ill puppies).

Symptom formula: Veratrum homaccord, Engystol N, Echinacea homaccord, Mercurius-Heel, Cactus compositum, Cralonin 6 to 8 times daily as needed, then tapered to TID.

Detoxification and repair following improvement: Galium-Heel, Mucosa compositum, Coenzyme compositum, Ubichinon compositum every 3 days for 2 to 3 weeks.

Product sources

Nutrition

Immune and intestinal support formulas: Animal Nutrition Technologies. Alternatives: Immune System and Enteric Support—Standard Process Veterinary Formulas; Immuno Support and NutriGest—Rx Vitamins for Pets; Immugen—Thorne Veterinary Products.

Betathyme: Best for Your Pet. Alternative: Moducare—Thorne Veterinary Products.

Glutimmune: Well Wisdom. Alternatives: L-Glutamine powder—Thorne Veterinary Products.

Maitake DMG: Vetri Science.

Vitamin C: Over the counter.

Chinese herbal medicine

Bai Tou Weng Tang: CHM Treasure of the East/Bluelight, Inc.

Homotoxicology
BHI/Heel Corporation

REFERENCES

Western medicine references

Carmichael L. In: Recent Advances in Canine Infectious Diseases, International Veterinary Information Service, Ithaca NY (www.ivis.org), Last updated: 29-Apr-2005; A0105.0405.

Decaro N, Pratelli A, Tinelli A, et al. Fecal immunoglobulin A antibodies in dogs infected or vaccinated with canine coronavirus. *Clin Diagn Lab Immunol* 2004 Jan; 11:102–5.

Ettinger SJ, Feldman EC. Textbook of Veterinary Internal Medicine, 4th ed., WB Saunders Company. 1995.

Pratelli A. Canine Coronavirus Infection. In: Recent Advances in Canine Infectious Diseases, Carmichael L, ed. International Veterinary Information Service, Ithaca NY (www.ivis.org), Last updated: 29-Apr-2005.

Pratelli A, Martella V, Elia G, et al. Severe enteric disease in an animal shelter associated with dual infections by canine adenovirus type 1 and canine coronavirus. *J Vet Med B Infect Dis Vet Public Health* 2001; 48:385–392.

IVM/nutrition references

Bouic PJD. Immunomodulation in HIV/AIDS: The Tygerberg Stellenbosch University experience. AIDS Bulletin published by the Medical Research Council of South Africa Sept. 1997.6(3):18–20.

Cima J. Biochemical Blood Chemistry Evaluation, Palm Beach Gardens, FL., March 2000.

Goldstein R, et al. The BNA Handbook: A Working Manual for Veterinarians, Westport, CT: Animal Nutrition Technologies, 2000.

Graber G, Kendall R. N,N-Dimethylglycine and Use in Immune Response, US Patent 4,631,189, Dec 1986.

Gupta MB, Nath R, Srivastava N, et al. Anti-inflammatory and antipyretic activities of β-sitosterol. *Planta Medica* 1980; 39:157–163.

Kendall RV. Building Wellness with DMG, Topanga, CA: Freedom Press, 2003.

Pauling L. Vitamin C: The common cold and the flu, San Francisco: WH Freeman, 1976.

Pegel KH. The importance of sitosterol and sitosterolin in human and animal nutrition. *South African Journal of Science* June 1997;93:263–268.

Souba W et al. Glutamine metabolism in the intestinal tract: invited review, *JPEN* 1985;9:608–617.

Verdova I, Chamaganova A. Use of vitamin B₁₅ for the treatment of certain skin conditions, Vitamin B₁₅ (Pangamic Acid) Properties, Functions and Use, Naooka, Moscow: Science Publishing, 1965.

Windmueller HG. Glutamine utilization by the small intestine, *Adv. Enzymol* 1982.53:201–237.

Yoshimura K, et al. Effects of enteral glutamine administration on experimental inflammatory bowel disease, *JPEN* 1993; 17:235.

Chinese herbal medicine/acupuncture references

Si Chuan Yi Xue Yuan Xue Bao (*Journal of Sichuan School of Medicine*), 1959;1:102.

Zhong Yao Xue (*Chinese Herbology*), 1998;197:199.

Zhong Yi Za Zhi (*Journal of Chinese Medicine*), 1959;8:23.

Homotoxicology reference

Mantione N, Otto C. Characterization of the use of antiemetic agents in dogs with parvovirus enteritis treated at the veterinary teaching hospital. *JAVMA*, 2005. Dec 1, 227(11): pp 1787–93.

CANINE DISTEMPER

Definition and cause

Canine distemper (CDV), which is caused by a morbilli-virus, is a contagious disease that affects the GI, respiratory, and central nervous systems. Canine distemper often causes signs such as fever, anorexia, weakness, and debilitation. While vaccination can cause high antibody titers, the vaccine can sometimes incite the disease (Durchfeld 1990, Montali 1983, Spencer 1992).

Often distemper begins as an upper respiratory infection resulting in sneezing, coughing, a thick yellowish ocular and nasal discharge, high fever, and intractable diarrhea. Left untreated, the disease can progress to encephalitis, head-tilt, circling, paralysis, convulsions, and finally, death. Most veterinarians recommend euthanasia when distemper manifests in the nervous system, but recovery is sometimes possible. Animals with a strong immune system often remain subclinical and survive (Appel 1987, 1999; Greene 1998; Spencer 1882).

Medical therapy rationale, drug(s) of choice, and nutritional recommendations

Medical therapy is symptom-oriented, such as antibiotics for secondary infections, fluid therapy, ocular ointments, anti-diarrheal, and anti-convulsive medications such as phenobarbital. Dietary recommendations are usually to feed whatever the dog will eat, and bland diets to address the diarrhea. Antiviral drugs have been reported to be ineffective (Appel 1999; Green 1987, 1998).

Anticipated prognosis

With good support medical care, the prognosis for an animal with an active, noncompromised immune system is generally 50%. Because this disease is so severe, vaccination is recommended for all dogs at least once after 12 weeks of age. Yearly boosters are not indicated for most dogs, and continuing immunity can be monitored by blood titers (Palmquist 2003). Many dogs obtain lifelong protection from one such vaccination (Durchfield 1990, Montali 1983, Spencer 1992, van Heerden 1980).

Dogs infected with this virus depend on their own immunocompetence and require intense clinical support to survive the disease cycle. Many survivors have marked physical damage resulting from cellular damage. With proper therapy a large number of such dogs may survive, but clients need to be advised of the possibility of death, and more importantly of the frequency of other issues (seizures, visual disturbances, dermatological syndromes, tonic tics, possible mentation changes, and general debility). Recovery is a protracted, labor-intensive process that not all clients or veterinarians are willing to undertake (Appel 1999, Green 1998).

Integrative veterinary therapies

Because conventional treatment offers few options except for supportive care, the addition of integrative modalities often improves the treatment success. This is primarily due to the nourishment of the body as well as the help in maintaining immune competence. In many instances the addition of therapeutic nutritional support as well as appropriate selected herbal and biological remedies help control the symptoms and the spread of the viral infection.

Nutrition
General considerations/rationale

The addition of therapeutic nutrition takes into consideration the immune system, the viral-induced inflammation, and the destruction of tissue, as well as the overwhelmed immune system.

The nutritional approach is often multifaceted and consists of nutrient support of the brain, thymus, adrenal, bone marrow, and upper respiratory system, enhancement of toxin elimination, and general support of the immune system.

Appropriate nutrients

Nutrition/gland therapy: Glandular adrenal, thymus, bone marrow, lung, intestines, and brain help to neutralize viral-induced inflammation, spare the involved organs, and nourish a compromised immune system (see Chapter 2, Gland Therapy, for additional information).

Note: Because canine distemper is a serious systemic disease, it is recommended that blood be analyzed both medically and physiologically to determine real and impending organ involvement and disease. This can help clinicians specifically formulate nutritional support based upon the animal's individual needs (Cima 2000, Goldstein 2000) (see Chapter 2, Nutritional Blood Testing, for additional information).

Sterols and sterolins: Animal studies have demonstrated that phytosterols have anti-inflammatory and antipyretic effects (Gupta 1980). Pegel (1997) feels that sterols are essential for a properly functioning immune system. In studies on cats with FIV, sterols are believed to have an immune-modulating effect and help to maintain proper lymphocyte levels (Bouic 1997). Treated cats showed a 20% mortality rate as compared to the nontreated cats (mortality rate of 75%). It was further reported that there were no deaths in these cats 3 years following treatment with the sterols. While the sterols have no direct antiviral properties, the balancing and stimulation of the immune system is enough to control the spread and effects of the virus.

N,N-Dimethylglycine (DMG): DMG has been shown to support immune function and improve toxin removal (Verdova 1965). DMG has immune-modulating ability and has been clinically proven to increase both tumor necrosis factor (TNF) and interferon production (Graber 1986, Kendall 2003, Reap 1990, Wang 1988).

Maitake mushrooms: Studies with maitake mushrooms have shown that they help enhance immune function and the ability to handle stressful conditions. They also help organ systems maintain balance and homeostasis (Nanba 1987).

Chinese herbal medicine
General considerations/rationale
Canine distemper is an external infectious pathogen. It is considered to be a febrile disease, mainly external Heat, Wind, and Toxins.

The external pathogenic factors that TCM alludes to are the canine distemper virus itself and any secondary bacterial invaders. The Heat is, of course, the inflammation, which is manifested as fever and purulent discharge. The Toxins are the inflammatory mediators. Wind can refer to the seizures in neurological disease or the manner by which the disease is "blown" into the body.

Canine distemper is treated according to the presenting signs. Initially there is an inflammatory febrile disease (Heat). This accompanies the gastrointestinal or respiratory disease. Gastrointestinal inflammation is due to toxic mediators and is evidenced by vomiting and diarrhea. Respiratory tract disease is manifested as coughing and dyspnea (pneumonia). These signs are caused by inflammation in the Lungs. Treatment is aimed at stopping the infection and secondary (bacterial) invaders. In addition, the specific signs such a coughing, seizures, vomiting, and diarrhea are addressed.

Appropriate Chinese herbs for pulmonary manifestations
Anemarrhena (Zhi mu): Has antibiotic effects (Yao Xue Qing Bao Tong Xun 1987).

Apricot seed (Xing ren): Promotes the phagocytic activity of Kupffer's cells and tracheal, bronchial, and lung alveoli macrophages in mice (Li 1991). It helps to clear phlegm and relieve cough (Zhang Wen Juan 1991).

Citrus (Chen pi): An effective expectorant (Huang Min 1999).

Fritillaria bulb (Bei mu): Helps decrease coughing (Zhu an Ni 1992) and has expectorant effects (Yao 1993, Li 1993).

Houttuynia (Yu xing cao): Has been used to treat humans with pneumonia with excellent results (Zhong Hua Nei Ke Za Zhi 1963).

Licorice (Gan cao): Decreases coughing and has expectorant effects (Zhong Yao Yao Li Yu Ying Yong 1983). It has been shown to inhibit the proliferation of several types of viruses and bacteria in vitro (Zhu 1996, Zhong Yao Zhi 1993).

Morus bark (Sang bai pi): Stops coughing (Zhong Yao Xue 1998).

Mulberry leaves (Sang ye): Has demonstrated antibacterial activity against several types of bacteria (Zhong Yao Yao Li Yu Ying Yong 1983).

Ophiopogon (Mai men dong): Enhances mucociliary transport velocity in quails and decreases respiratory tract mucus secretion (Tai 2002). It has antibacterial activity against several species of bacteria (Zhong Yao Xue 1998).

Pseudotellaria root (Tai zi shen): Has been used to treat pneumonia in children (Zhong Yao Lin Zheng Ying Yong 1980).

Poria (Fu ling): Enhances immunity. It increases the phagocytic abilities of macrophages (Lu 1990). It has antibiotic action against several types of bacteria (Zhong Yao Cai 1985).

Rhubarb (Da huang): Has been shown to be very effective against various bacteria and viruses (Zhao Man Jing 1999, Yang Shu Zhi 1997, Xie Yan Ying 1996). It has a protective effect on lung tissue. It has been shown to decrease lung damages caused by the excessive secretion of TNF-a, IL-1, and IL-6 (Miao 1998).

Trichosanthes (Tian hua feng): Has been shown to inhibit the growth of multiple bacteria and viruses (Zhong Yao Yao Li Yu Ying Yong 1983).

Appropriate Chinese herbs for gastrointestinal disease
Ash bark (Qin pi): An effective antibacterial herb (Zhong Yao Xue 1998).

Coptis (Huang lian): Has been used to stop vomiting induced by copper sulfate in a pigeon (Qin Cai Ling 1994). It also has antidiarrheal effects (Zhong Yao Xue 1998).

Pulsatilla root (Bai tou weng): Has activity against various bacteria (CA, 1948).

Appropriate Chinese herbs for neurological manifestations

Centipede (Wu gong): Has strong antiseizure effects. It has been shown to be effective in controlling seizures caused by various drugs (Zhong Yao Xue 1998).

Forsythia (Lian qiao): Has been demonstrated to have antiviral effects (Zhang 2002).

Grass-leaf sweet-flag root (Shi chang pu): Has demonstrated both sedative and antiseizure effects (Zhong Yao Xue 1998). One of the components of grass-leaf sweet-flag root, alpha-asarone, demonstrated an efficacy of approximately 85% in treating seizures in a group of 90 people (Yao Xue Tong Bao 1982).

Licorice (Gan cao): Helps to deal with the viral etiology of the neurological disease. Glycyrrhizin, an active component of licorice, has been shown to inhibit the proliferation of several viruses in vitro (Zhu 1996).

Red peony (Chi shao): One of the major active components of Chi shao, paeoniflorin, has demonstrated anticonvulsive and sedative effects in animals (Zhong Yao Xue 1998).

Scorpion (Quan xie): Has demonstrated usefulness in treating seizure disorders in several experiments and clinical studies. Seizures in mice induced by caffeine or megimide were controlled by scorpion (Shen Yang Yi Xue Yuan Xue Bao 1988). In rats with experimentally induced seizures, scorpion decreased the severity, duration, and recurrence rate of seizures (Shen Yang Yi Xue Yuan Xue Bao 1989). Seventy-five percent of humans with epilepsy had very good response when treated with scorpion, while another 16% had moderate response (Si Chuan Zhong Yi 1991).

Silkworm (Jiang can): Has been shown in multiple experiments to have antiseizure activity. It has been proven effective at decreasing seizure activity in mice with experimentally induced seizures (Zhong Cao Yao Xue 1980). In addition, it has synergistic effects with phenobarbital (Chang Yong Zhong Yao Cheng Fen Yu Yao Li Shou Ce 1994).

Uncaria (Gou teng): Has been proven to prevent seizures in animals (Hsieh 1999). In mice, one compound isolated from uncaria was shown to decrease spontaneous central nervous system activity, act synergistically with phentobarbital to enhance phenobarbital's sedative effect, and increase the content of 5-HT in the hypothalamus and the amygdaloid nucleus (Shi 1993).

Homotoxicology
General considerations/rationale

All viral infections constitute Impregnation Phase homotoxicoses in their initial stages. Canine distemper is a particularly vicious viral infection that quickly progresses to a Degeneration Phase disorder. Due to the author's practice location in an inner city area near a dog shelter, this disease is seen more frequently than in many U.S. veterinary practices, and many clients opt for treatment. Two of the employees in our practice have pets that have survived neurological canine distemper virus infection (Palmquist 2002).

Regressive vicariation is the goal in these cases. It is vital to understand that many symptoms and signs are actually the body's attempt to remove homotoxins—including impregnated viral particles—and these efforts need to be supported and not suppressed if a full recovery is to occur. Patients often suffer severe excretory or inflammatory dermatitis, gastroenteritis, and even urogenital inflammation (straining and discharge of mucus) during recovery. These signs can easily be missed and mistakenly treated with drugs that can cause progressive vicariation and worsening of the condition because they frequently occur several weeks to months after the primary clinical syndrome. Steroid medications should be avoided. Mild tics and seizures may be best handled homeopathically with reservation of anticonvulsants for only the most life-threatening manifestations.

A final word is in order regarding an antidistemper serum used by Alson Sears, DVM, of Lancaster, California. One of the authors worked with Dr Sears in the early 1980s and has personally witnessed many cases of canine distemper that were treated with Dr. Sears' antidistemper serum. There appears to be strong correlation between this serum and survival in naturally infected dogs. Parties interested in this serum and its method of production can visit the web site and learn more about the serum's method of production and utilization. It should be noted that this product must be applied early in the viral infection (first 4 days) to be effective (Sears 1999). Because this product requires handling and caring for live donor dogs, which may experience anaphylaxis during serum production, it is hoped that one day the serum will be commercially available from a blood laboratory or pharmaceutical company with an interest in helping these dogs.

Appropriate homotoxicology formulas

These cases may involve multiple systems, and as such, the practitioner must be able to monitor the entire case for current physical manifestations. Outpatient treatment is desirable in most cases. Therapeutic plans may need to be varied suddenly. See also protocols for epilepsy, dermatitis, pneumonia, bronchitis, and diarrhea for further recommendations. The authors treat all such cases with autosanguis therapy customized to the presenting state of the patient. Useful remedies include:

Aconitum homaccord: Treats early febrile phases. Aconitum is one of the most important homeopathic fever remedies, especially when the patient displays hot skin; great anxiety; rapid, tense pulse; strong and possibly irregular heartbeat; alternating fever and chills; possible hyperthermia with sudden onset of symptoms; and violence of the complaints. The restlessness and anguish are always seen, as are the redness of the mucosa and the sensation of distension, heaviness, pressure, and tension in the gastrointestinal tract. Stools contain mucus and bile. There is flatulent distension with small, frequent stools, and an urging to defecate, all of which are characteristic of the remedy. Low potencies are normally given in pyrexia and organic complaints, catarrhs, neuralgic symptoms with paresthesia, hyperthermia, and encephalitis with very high temperatures (e.g., post-vaccinial encephalitis or meningo-encephalitis) (Reckeweg 2002).

Atropinum compositum: Treats seizure and spasm and gastrointestinal cramping and upset.

Arsuraneel: Used intermittently in advanced cases that seem hopeless.

Belladonna homaccord: Indicated for seizures and screaming out at night. Violent delirium is characteristic of Belladonna, above all in fever. Belladonna's typical action on the eyes is also well-known, with cramps in the muscles of the eyes and eyelids, enlargement of the pupils, and, in particular, an inflammatory or irritative condition of the conjunctiva with great photophobia, lachrymation, and pain. Belladonna is indicated in incipient boils, tonsillitis, and surface inflammations such as erysipelas, conjunctivitis, scarlet fever, otitis, cholangitis, meningitis, and other inflammatory affectations. A delirious state occurs with a violent rise in temperature. There is considerably raised sensitivity of all the senses and a disproportionate sensitivity to touch, noises, light, and cold air, especially draughts and jarring as can be the case in meningitis. Along with nasal catarrhs, there may be catarrhs of the larynx and trachea with slight mucus, accompanied by a typical dry, rough, and barking cough with hoarseness. In the digestive organs, Belladonna affects acute gastric catarrhs (Reckeweg 2002).

Cerebrum compositum: Supports and detoxifies the brain. The component Hyoscyamus is indicated for symptoms of cerebral irritation with convulsions; muscle twitching; catalepsy; epileptiform spasms; eye conditions; conjunctivitis; spasmodic nocturnal attacks of cough with expectoration of green mucus on coughing; dryness in the throat, larynx, and lungs; stomach pains; and inflammation of the gastric mucosa and intestines with retching, vomiting, colic, and diarrhea (Reckeweg 2002).

Coenzyme compositum: The component Beta vulgaris reactivates cell respiration and can regenerate blocked respiratory enzymes, and is therefore indicated in all cellular phases (Impregnation, Degeneration, and Dedifferentiation). It is also indicated in viral diseases, viral influenza, and poliomyelitis (Reckeweg 2002).

Discus compositum: Used for the spinal, meningeal, and paralytic forms of canine distemper. It contains Ranunculus bulbosus to treat rheumatic and neuralgic symptoms. It also treats skin eruptions, particularly closely grouped crops of vesicles, coryza with a discharge of viscid mucus, and possibly ulceration of the nasal mucosa accompanied by the characteristic chest complaints with shortness of breath and a sense of constriction. These may be accompanied by gastric symptoms with purging, eructations, nausea, burning in the stomach, abdominal rumbling, and bleeding hemorrhoids. The skin eruptions are frequently present on the palms of the hands in the form of desquamating vesicular eruptions (Reckeweg 2002).

Distemper nosode: Given later to assist in recovery in all cases of known distemper. **Note:** Some advocate the use of distemper nosode to provide continuing immunity against the Distemper virus. At this time there is insufficient evidence to recommend this over routine puppy vaccination. While boostering intervals may be controversial, the authors cannot recommend Distemper nosode as an alternative option to vaccination. In the authors' opinion the use of vaccine titers is a far better way to evaluate the need for revaccination and is superior to automatic revaccination for this disease. Strong clinical evidence supports this opinion (Palmquist 2003).

Dulcamara homaccord: Symptoms are diarrhea, vomiting, colic, skin rash, convulsions, and paralysis. The complaints that indicate Dulcamara are aggravated by cold, damp weather as well as weather changes, especially in rainy weather. They are worse during hot days and cold nights. Increased mucosal secretions are also typical of Dulcamara. The nose is usually blocked as well (sinusitis), and the discharge being more copious in the warmth. The saliva is tough and soap-like. Additional indications: acute gastritis and enteritis, dysentery with violent stomach pains, colic, mucous, sour or dysenteric watery stools, pains persisting even after the stool, and associated with colic and rheumatic complaints (Reckeweg 2002).

Echinacea compositum: Stimulate host defenses, particularly against bacterial invaders. It contains many useful remedies, including Rhus toxicodendron, which is useful in a wide variety of inflammations. In the eyes there may be violent conjunctivitis with severe photophobia and a greenish-yellow, offensive nasal discharge. There may be gastroenteritis with watery, bloody, mucous stools and tenesmus; a tormenting, dry cough with bloody, purulent sputum; an eruption like measles all over the body or a vesicular eruption, and disturbances of consciousness such as occur in febrile conditions, e.g., dysentery, peritonitis, pneumonia, scarlatina, rheumatism, or diphtheria. Rhus toxicodendron is also indicated in myelitis with paresis (Reckeweg 2002).

Engystol N: Used in the early stages to improve defenses against viral infections.

Euphorbium compositum: Has antiviral properties and treats upper respiratory congestion.

Galium-Heel: Provides immune support and cellular detoxification in cellular phases. Assists in repair after survival of acute disease and damage from drugs that were administered to save the patient's life.

Gastricumeel: Treats vomiting early in the course of the disease (Heel 2003). Contains Antimonium crudum (Day 1990).

Gelsemium homaccord: Treats headache and neuralgia. Gelsemium is particularly indicated in states of paralysis, e.g., after apoplexy also in post-diphtheritic paralysis. The stools are copious and yellow, and influenzal catarrhs may be seen when there is thin, fluent nasal discharge and bloody mucus is blown out. A brief summary of symptoms includes nervous disorders, infectious diseases, paralysis, and spasmodic conditions (Reckeweg 2002). Gelsemium is common to *Echinacea compositum*.

Graphites homaccord: Treats nasal thickness and hard pad following acute phases.

Gripp-Heel: Used in early stages when upper respiratory and cold-like signs predominate. Also used for the characteristic persistent fevers. Contains Aconitum (see above).

Lymphomyosot: Provides immune support and lymph drainage. Myosotis arvensis particularly acts on the respiratory organs and the lungs. Characteristic symptoms include a cough with profuse mucopurulent expectoration, retching and vomiting while coughing, and aggravation during meals or immediately afterward.

Mucosa compositum: Supports mucous membranes throughout the body and the urogenital, respiratory, and gastrointestinal systems, especially during recovery after acute infection has waned.

Naso-Heel S: Treats nasal discharge.

Spascupreel: Treats tics, spasms, and headache.

Tonsilla compositum: Provides Impregnation Phase and Degeneration Phase support of the immune organs, particularly the spleen and bone marrow. Includes Mercurius Solubilis Hahnemanni for mucosal inflammations of the respiratory passages, the gastrointestinal tract, and the urinary and reproductive organs; skin diseases; inflammation of the tonsils, lymph glands, liver, and kidneys; inflammation of other glandular organs; ostealgia and rheumatism; enervating diseases; and cerebral angiosclerosis (Reckeweg 2002).

Ubichinon compositum: Used in Degeneration Phase disorders and after long courses of antibiotic therapy. Contains benzochinon. Another constituent, Parabenzoquinone, is a powerful remedy with certain protective functions against viral infections. One should always think of parabenzoquinone in almost incurable, unremitting dyspneas that may evolve into respiratory paralysis. It can also help with paresis occurring after poliomyelitis, meningeal irritation, encephalitis or vaccinations, where there is disturbance in neuromuscular coordination (Reckeweg 2002).

Authors' suggested protocols

Nutrition
Immune, brain/nerve, intestinal/IBD, and bronchus/lung support formulas: 1 tablet for each 25 pounds of body weight BID.

Betathyme: 1 capsule for each 35 pounds of body weight BID (maximum, 2 capsules BID).

Maitake DMG: 1 ml per 25 pounds of body weight BID.

Chinese herbal medicine
For pulmonary manifestations, the authors recommend H23 Pneumonia at a dose of 1 capsule per 10 to 20 pounds twice daily. In addition to the herbs mentioned above, H23Pneumonia also contains trichosanthes seeds (Gua luo ren), bamboo leaves (Zhu ye), gypsum (Shi gao), glehnia root (Sha shen), and perilla seeds (Su zi) to increase the efficacy of the formula.

For viral enteritis signs, the authors use the patent formula Bai tou weng tang at the dose recommended by the manufacturer. In addition to the herbs listed above, Bai tou weng tang contains Phellodendron (Huang bai).

For the manifestation of central nervous system disease, the authors recommend H90 Encephalitis at a dose of 1 capsule per 10 to 20 pounds twice daily. In addition to the herbs listed above, Encephalitis also contains bile treated arisaema (Dan nan xing), saussurea (Mu xiang), orange peel (Ju Hong), pinellia (Ban Xia), curcuma root (Yu Jin), salvia (Dan shen), lophatherum (Zhu ye), lonicera flower (Jin yin hua), isatis leaves (Da Qing ye), and gypsum (Shi gao). The additional herbs help support the functions of the herbs mentioned above.

Homotoxicology (Dose: 10 drops PO for 50-pound dog, 5 drops PO for small dog)
The authors treat all such cases with autosanguis therapy. Consider the following protocol for early cases:

Autosanguis (Give half of this orally or by injection as allowed by law, then place the other half into a cocktail of the symptom remedy): Gripp-Heel plus Euphorbium compositum, Engystol plus Lymphomyosot, Hepar compositum plus Tonsilla compositum OR Echinacea compositum, Coenzyme compositum.

Symptom remedy: Lymphomyosot, Galium-Heel, Aconitum homaccord plus relevant current symptom remedies (See pneumonia, bronchitis, seizures, etc.), QID initially to BID (chronic use) orally.

Product sources

Nutrition

Immune, brain/nerve, intestinal/IBD, and bronchus/lung support formulas: Animal Nutrition Technologies. **Alternatives:** Immune System and Enteric Support—Standard Process Veterinary Formulas; Immuno Support and NutriGest—Rx Vitamins for Pets; Immugen—Thorne Veterinary Products.

Betathyme: Best for Your Pet. **Alternative:** Moducare—Thorne Veterinary Products.

Maitake DMG: Vetri Science.

Chinese herbal medicine

H23 Pneumonia and H90 Encephalitis: White Crane Herbs by Natural Solutions, Inc.

Bai tou weng tang: Treasure of the East/Bluelight, Inc.

Homotoxicology
BHI/Heel Inc.

REFERENCES

Western medicine references

Appel MJG, Summers BA. Canine Distemper: Current Status. In: Recent Advances in Canine Infectious Diseases. International Veterinary Information Service (www.ivis.org), 1999.

Appel MJ. Canine distemper virus. In: Horzinek M, ed. Virus Infections of Carnivores. 1-Virus Infections of Vertebrates. Amsterdam: Elsevier Science Publishers, 1987; 133–159.

Durchfeld B, Baumgartner W, Herbst W, Brahm R. Vaccine-associated canine distemper infection in a litter of African hunting dogs (*Lycaon pictus*). *Zentralblatt für Veterinrmedizin* (1990) B 37: 203212.

Greene CE, Appel MJ. Canine Distemper. In: Greene CE, ed. Infectious Diseases of the Dog and Cat. 2nd ed. Philadelphia: WB Saunders Co, 1998; 9–22.

Montali RJ, Bartz CR, Teare JA, Allen JT, Appel MJG, Bush M. Clinical trials with canine distemper vaccines in exotic carnivores. *Journal of the American Veterinary Medical Association*, 1983.183: 1163–1167.

Spencer J, Burroughs R. Antibody response to canine distemper vaccine in African wild dogs. *Journal of Wildlife Diseases*, 1992. 28: 443–444.

van Heerden J, Swart WH, Meltzer DGA. Serum antibody levels before and after administration of live canine distemper vaccine to the wild dog *Lycaon pictus*. *Journal of the South African Veterinary Medical Association*, 1980. 51: 283–284.

IVM/nutrition references

Bouic PJD. Immunomodulation in HIV/AIDS: The Tygerberg Stellenbosch University experience. AIDS Bulletin published by the Medical Research Council of South Africa 6(3):18–20, Sept. 1997.

Cima J. Biochemical Blood Chemistry Evaluation, Palm Beach Gardens, FL., March 2000.

Goldstein R, et al. The BNA Handbook: A Working Manual for Veterinarians, Westport, CT: Animal Nutrition Technologies, 2000.

Graber G, Kendall R. N,N-Dimethylglycine and Use in Immune Response, US Patent 4,631,189, Dec 1986.

Gupta MB, Nath R, Srivastava N, et al. Anti-inflammatory and antipyretic activities of β-sitosterol. *Planta Medica* 1980;39:157–163.

Kendall RV. Building Wellness with DMG, Topanga, CA: Freedom Press, 2003.

Mani S, Whitesides J, Lawson J. Role of Dimethylglycine in Melanoma Inhibition—Abstract from Nutrition and Cancer Prevention: American Institute for Cancer Research, Sept 1999.

Nanba H, Hamaguchi AM, Kuroda H. The chemical structure of an antitumor polysaccharide in fruit bodies of *Grifola frondosa* (maitake). *Chem Pharm Bull* 1987;35:1162–8.

Pegel KH. The importance of sitosterol and sitosterolin in human and animal nutrition. *South African Journal of Science.* June 1997;93:263–268.

Reap E, Lawson J. Stimulation of the Immune Response by Dimethylglycine, a Non-toxic Metabolite. *Journal of Laboratory and Clinical Medicine.* 1990.115:481.

Verdova I, Chamaganova A. Use of vitamin B₁₅ for the treatment of certain skin conditions, Vitamin B₁₅ (Pangamic Acid) Properties, Functions and Use, Naooka, Moscow: Science Publishing, 1965.

Wang C, Lawson J. The Effects on the Enhancement of Monoclonal Antibody Production. Oct. 1988. Annual Meeting of the American Soc. of Microbiology.

Chinese herbal medicine/acupuncture references

CA, 1948; 42:4228a.

Chang Yong Zhong Yao Cheng Fen Yu Yao Li Shou Ce (A Handbook of the Composition and Pharmacology of Common Chinese Drugs), 1994; 1810: 1812.

China Journal of Chinese Medicine. 1994;19(7):427–429.

Hsieh CL, Tang NY, Chiang SV, Hsieh CT, Lin JG. Anticonvulsive and free radical scavenging actions of two herbs, Uncaria rhynchophylla (MIQ) Jack and Gastrodia elata Bl., in kainic acid-treated rats. *Life Sci* 1999; 65(20):2071–82.

Huang M, et al. *China Journal of Wild Botanic Resources.* 1999;18(1):36–37

Jiang Su Yi Yao (*Jiangsu Journal of Medicine and Herbology*), 1976;2:33.

Li CH, et al. Amygdalin's effect on mononuclear macrophages' phagocytotic function, *Journal of Shanxi College of Medicine.* 1991;22(1):1–3,79.

Li P, et al. *Journal of University of Pharmacology of China.* 1993;24(5):360–362.

Lu SC, et al. *Journal of No. 1 Military Academy.* 1990; 10(3):267.

Miao R, et al. *Journal of Chinese Materia Medica.* 1998;29(6): 395–397.

Pharmacology and Applications of Chinese Herbs, 1983.

Qin CL, et al. Research on Huang Lian Tang (Coptis decoction)'s preventive effects on experimental stomach mucosa injuries and suppression on vomiting. *China Journal of Chinese Medicine*. 1994;19(7):427–429.

Shen Yang Yi Xue Yuan Xue Bao (*Journal of Shenyang University of Medicine*), 1988; 5(2):110.

Shen Yang Yi Xue Yuan Xue Bao (*Journal of Shenyang University of Medicine*), 1989; 6(2):95.

Shi JS, et al. *China Journal of Pharmacology*. 1993;14(2): 114–117.

Si Chuan Zhong Yi (*Sichuan Chinese Medicine*) 1991; 9(11):12.

Tai S, Sun F, O'Brien D, Lee M, Zayaz J, King M. Evaluation of a Mucoactive Herbal Drug, Radix Ophiopogonis, in a Pathogenic Quail Model. *J of Herbal Pharmacotherapy* 2002;2(4):49–56.

Xie YY, et al. *Journal of Shandong Medical University*. 1996;34(2):166–169.

Yang SZ, et al. *Liaoning Journal of Traditional Chinese Medicine*. 1997;24(4):187.

Yao LN, et al. *Journal of Tongji Medical University*. 1993;22(1):47–49.

Yao Xue Qing Bao Tong Xun (*Journal of Herbal Information*), 1987; 5(4):62.

Yao Xue Tong Bao (Report of Herbology), 1982; 9: 50.

Zhang G, Song S, Ren J, Xu S. A New Compound from Forsythia suspense (Thunb.) Vahl with Antiviral Effect on RSV. *J of Herbal Pharmacotherapy*. 2002;2(3): 35–39.

Zhang WJ, et al. Processed Xing Ren: Its potency and acute toxicity. *Journal of Traditional Chinese Medicine Material*. 1991;14(8):38–40.

Zhao MJ, et al. *Zhejiang Journal of Traditional Chinese Medicine*. 1999;34(12):544.

Zhong Cao Yao Xue (Study of Chinese Herbal Medicine), 1980; 1423.

Zhong Hua Nei Ke Za Zhi (*Chinese Journal of Internal Medicine*), 1963;3:250.

Zhong Yao Cai (Study of Chinese Herbal Material), 1985; (2): 36.

Zhong Yao Lin Zheng Ying Yong (Clinical Applications of Chinese Herbs), 1980; 442.

Zhong Yao Xue (*Chinese Herbology*), 1998; 140:144.

Zhong Yao Xue (*Chinese Herbology*), 1998; 162:164.

Zhong Yao Xue (*Chinese Herbology*), 1998; 197:199.

Zhong Yao Xue (*Chinese Herbology*), 1998; 648:650.

Zhong Yao Xue (*Chinese Herbology*), 1998, 704:706.

Zhong Yao Xue (*Chinese Herbology*), 1998, 722:725.

Zhong Yao Xue (*Chinese Herbology*), 1998; 845:848.

Zhong Yao Yao Li Yu Ying Yong (Pharmacology and Applications of Chinese Herbs), 1983: 149.

Zhong Yao Yao Li Yu Ying Yong (Pharmacology and Applications of Chinese Herbs), 1983: 246.

Zhong Yao Zhi (*Chinese Herbology Journal*), 1993; 358.

Zhu AN, et al. *Journal of University of Pharmacology of China*. 1992;23(2):118–121.

Zhu LH. *China Journal of TCM Information*. 1996;3(3): 17–20.

Homotoxicology references

Day C. The Homeopathic Treatment of Small Animals: Principles and Practice. Saffron Walden, Essex: CW Daniel Company, LTD. 1990. p 117.

Heel. Veterinary Guide, 3rd English edition. Baden-Baden, Germany: Biologische Heilmettel Heel GmbH, 2003. pp 34–5, 50.

Palmquist R. Series of canine distemper cases treated and their outcomes. 2002.Unpublished case files.

Palmquist R. A survey of canine vaccine practices in contemporary veterinary clinics in the US. *JAHVMA*, July/Oct, 2003. 23:1, 2: pp 27–9.

Reckeweg H. Biotherapeutic Index: Ordinatio Antihomotoxica et Materia Medica, 5th ed. Baden-Baden, Germany: Biologische Heilmittel Heel GMBH, 2000. p 366.

Reckeweg H. Homeopathia Antihomotoxica Materia Medica, 4th ed. Baden-Baden, Germany: Aurelia-Verlag, 2002. p 120–1, 173–4, 177, 182, 282, 316, 352, 420, 431, 508–9, 514.

Sears A. Anti-Distemper Serum. 1999. http://www.edbond.com/antidistemper.html, Website, email address for author is AntiDistemper@aol.com.

CANINE PARVOVIRUS

Definition and cause

Caused by CPV-2 virus, canine parvovirus is characterized as a systemic disease in puppies that overwhelms the immune system and causes hemorrhagic enteritis (Carmichael 2003). Young puppies without proper maternal or vaccinal protection are the most likely to be infected with parvovirus. After the virus gains access to the alimentary canal, it rapidly infects gastrointestinal epithelial cells. Mucosa cells die after virus replication and the mucosal border becomes compromised, allowing virus particles to enter the submucosa and bloodstream. The virus gains access to the general circulation and replicates in the bone marrow and heart muscle as well. Immune suppression results as bacteria and bacterial toxins enter the systemic circulation.

Severe dehydration and electrolyte imbalance exacerbate this immune compromise in the infected puppy. In immuno-incompetent individuals this infection can progress to death, which occurs as a result of dehydration, electrolyte imbalance, secondary bacteria invasion, endotoxemia, sepsis, and systemic inflammatory response syndrome (Prittie 2004). In rare cases primary cardiac disease results from viral infection of the heart and these patients can suffer sudden death syndrome.

Properly vaccinating puppies can greatly reduce the risk of infection and is therefore recommended. Immune response is sufficient enough that most dogs establish sterile immunity as a result of vaccination. Certain breeds, however, such as Rottweilers and Doberman pinschers, may have an altered genetic ability to defend against this virus, and they may respond later or not at all to vaccination. Vaccination protection for most dogs is long term, and may last 3 to 10 years or longer in individual dogs; however, antibody levels may fall. In one author's practice fewer than 1% of dogs lose their protective vaccine titers in less than 2 years (Palmquist 2005).

In another study surveying vaccine practices, no clinical cases of parvovirus were reported in U.S. clinics that properly vaccinated puppies and then boostered immunity only as indicated by annual vaccine titers (Palmquist 2003, Twark 2000).

Twark and Dodds (2000) have reported similar data regarding immunity with 93.7% of dogs surveyed holding adequate vaccine titers for more than 2 years. Surviving natural infection generally gives long-term (potentially lifetime) immunity.

Medical therapy rationale, drug(s) of choice, and nutritional recommendations

Standard medical therapy consists of supportive aggressive fluid and electrolyte therapy, antibiotics, and antiemetics as needed for patient comfort. Antiemetics have been associated with prolonged hospitalizations in this condition and their use should be carefully considered before they are administered (Carmichael 2003, Mantione, 2005).

Parasites can increase mortality, so treatment with antiparasitacidal drugs may increase survival. One author routinely gives parvovirus puppies ivermectin (where breed tolerance is acceptable) and since instituting this has observed greatly reduced mortality (Palmquist 1986).

Anticipated prognosis

Proper vaccination protocols and prompt therapy are the best for increasing survival as well as preventing parvovirus disease. Prognosis can be good with intensive medical therapy, but is guarded in severely affected animals (Carmichael 2003).

Integrative veterinary therapies

Integrative modalities often improve patient survival rates for parvovirus infection. Integrative therapies can help reduce inflammation in the target organs such as the intestines and help to control diarrhea and bleeding. In many instances, adding therapeutic nutritional support and appropriate selected herbal and biological remedies helps with the viral infection.

Nutrition
General considerations/rationale
The addition of therapeutic nutrition takes into consideration support and protection of the gastrointestinal tract,

the immune system, and the viral-induced inflammation and destruction of tissue. The nutritional approach is multifaceted and consists of reduction of intestinal inflammation, nutrient support of the intestines, thymus, adrenal, lymph, and bone marrow, and enhancement of the elimination of toxins and metabolic wastes.

Appropriate nutrients
Nutrition/gland therapy: Glandular adrenal, thymus, bone marrow, lymph, and intestines help neutralize viral-induced inflammation, spare involved organs, and nourish the glands of a compromised immune system (see Chapter 2, Gland Therapy, for additional information).

Note: Because canine parvovirus is a serious, systemic disease, it is recommended that blood be analyzed both medically and physiologically to determine real and impending organ involvement and disease. This can help clinicians to specifically formulate nutritional support based upon the animal's individual needs (Cima 2000, Goldstein 2000) (see Chapter 2, Nutritional Blood Testing, for additional information).

Sterols and sterolins: Animal studies have demonstrated that phytosterols have anti-inflammatory and antipyretic effects (Gupta 1980). Pegel (1997) feels that sterols are essential for a properly functioning immune system. In studies on cats with FIV, sterols are believed to have an immune-modulating effect and help to maintain proper lymphocyte levels (Bouic 1997). Treated cats showed a 20% mortality rate as compared to nontreated cats' mortality rate of 75%. It was further reported that there were no deaths in these cats after a 3-year period with treatment with the sterols. While the sterols have no direct antiviral properties, the balancing and stimulation of the immune system is enough to control the spread and effects of the virus.

N,N-Dimethylglycine (DMG): DMG has been shown to support immune function and improve toxin removal (Verdova 1965). DMG has immune-modulating ability and has been clinically proven to increase both tumor necrosis factor (TNF) and interferon production (Graber 1986, Kendall 2003, Reap 1990, Wang 1988).

Maitake mushrooms: Studies with maitake mushrooms have shown that they help enhance immune function and the ability to handle stressful conditions while helping organ systems maintain balance and homeostasis (Nanba 1987).

Vitamin C: has been clinically proven as a potent antioxidant and immune-enhancing agent specifically against infectious agents (Pauling 1976). Vitamin C given parentally in large doses may help these puppies, but no controlled studies exist. Preservative-free vitamin C should be used if this is part of the treatment plan.

Glutamine: Glutamine is a nonessential and the most abundant amino acid present in dogs and cats. While glutamine is readily available in food and can be manufactured by the body, it has been discovered that during chronic periods of stress or disease, glutamine levels become depleted, negatively impacting health (O'Dwyer 1989). It is during these times of stress that glutamine becomes so important. It has also been shown that both low intracellular and plasma levels of glutamine can have adverse health consequences (Askanazi 1980, Souba 1992).

Besides improving immune function, glutamine is beneficial for the intestinal tract and can improve cellular integrity as well as permeability. This is especially important in immune-mediated disease conditions such as inflammatory bowel disease (Souba 1985, Windmueller 1982, Yoshimura 1993).

Chinese herbal medicine
General considerations/rationale
According to TCM, this type of diarrhea is caused by Heat, Dampness, and Toxins in the Blood. Heat refers to Blood in the diarrhea and Dampness to any pus. The toxins translate into the viral particles in modern terminology.

Appropriate Chinese herbs
Ash bark (Qin pi): Had an 80% success rate in treating people with bacterial dysentery (Zhong Yao Xue 1998).

Coptis root (Huang lian): Caused marked improvement in all participants in a study of 100 people with acute gastroenteritis (Si Chuan Yi Xue Yuan Xue Bao 1959).

Phellodendron bark (Huang bai): Has been used for chronic bacterial diarrhea (Zhong Yi Za Zhi 1959).

Homotoxicology
General considerations/rationale
Canine parvovirus, like all viral infections, initially constitutes an Impregnation Phase disorder that can rapidly lead to a Degeneration Phase condition. Parvovirus can cause vasculitis that negates the protective mechanisms of the blood-brain barrier, as well as concurrent infection with other viruses, particularly the canine distemper virus which can yield encephalitis. Such infections carry guarded prognoses and may cause increased medical problems later in life in dogs that survive. Once clinically recovered, puppies can shed parvovirus from the stool for several weeks. It is rare to see clinical cases in dogs older than 3 to 4 months. Another syndrome deserves mention here: accidental ingestion of modified live vaccine particles may cause gastrointestinal disease.

Biological therapeutic theory considers vomiting and diarrhea as effective methods for eliminating excess viral particles and other homotoxins. Many veterinarians are surprised to learn that antiemetics, which are considered a standard of care for parvovirus emesis, actually have

not been studied adequately to recommend their use in this situation. Intestinal stasis from ileus is quite common and allows for much greater absorption of homotoxins from dead cells as well as bacterial toxins.

Antibiotics can increase endotoxin levels: as intestinal bacterial masses perish and release endotoxins, they may contribute to the pathogenesis of systemic inflammatory response syndrome. Use of aggressive fluid and colloidal fluids and even enemas with electrolyte solution can assist some severely ill puppies by reducing homotoxin levels and promoting gastrointestinal motility. Many puppies become quite ill from ileus and a rapid improvement in their condition usually follows a large passing of toxic, malodorous stool as the bowel repairs and normal peristalsis returns.

Drugs that decrease intestinal motility should be strictly avoided because they aggravate this ileus condition. Prokinetic drugs may be associated with increased risk of intussusception. Parasites can increase mortality and treatment with antiphrastic drugs may increase survival.

Patients that survive parvovirus can undergo regressive vicariation immediately following infection, or they can rest physiologically and then have regressive vicariation at some future date. The clinician should be aware of the illness history for any patient undergoing biological therapy, so such regressive vicariations are recognized and treated biologically if possible. Use of antihomotoxic medications can help these patients to recover and can help handle signs which may occur from latent healing which manifests as regressive vicariation.

Appropriate homotoxicology formulas
BHI-Bleeding: Treats severe intestinal hemorrhage.

Cactus compositum: Used for coronary insufficiency, endocarditis, and myocarditis, and to improve circulation in febrile or septic conditions.

Coenzyme compositum: Provides metabolic assistance. Particularly useful in conjunction with *Engystol* to support mitochondrial function in viral diseases.

Cor compositum: Excellent for cardiac support in cases of collapse. Contains Carbo for shocky states, weakness, and collapse, as well as blood support.

Cor compositum: Provides cardiac support after injury.

Cralonin: Supports cardiac function.

Diarrheel: Used for profound diarrhea as a symptomatic agent. Not used in most cases.

Duodenoheel: Treats vomiting later in the course as the virus damages the duodenum and lower gastrointestinal tract. Used when the patient does not respond to *Gastricumeel*.

Echinacea compositum: Used against bacterial invasion.

Engystol N: Stimulates white blood cell activity through Vincetoxicum. This remedy is commonly used in viral infections to activate the host immune response. It is not specifically antiviral.

Gastricumheel: Used in cases of vomiting early in infection, especially when *Veratrum homaccord* has not been successful.

Mercurius-Heel: Treats ulcerative, erosive colitis. Has antibacterial activity, as compared to Vancomycin (Vestweber, et al. 1995).

Mucosa compositum: Helps the bowel to heal following trauma and Degeneration Phase disorders. Helps with leaky gut and may reduce sensitization to food items that can occur following parvovirus infection.

Nux vomica homaccord: Treats intestinal complaints.

Podophyllum compositum: Treats colitis. Contains mercurius.

Tanacet-Heel: Used for dysentery, nervous irritation during removal of nematodes, and gastrointestinal spasms associated with parasite removal.

Tonsilla compositum: Provides immune support in Impregnation and Degeneration phase conditions. Supports the spleen and bone marrow.

Ubichinon compositum: Provides mitochondrial resuscitation following antibiotics and is used as a phase remedy in Degeneration Phase homotoxicoses.

Veratrum homaccord: Indicated for bloody vomitus, rapid depression, collapse, and shock.

Authors' suggested protocols

Nutrition

Intestine and immune support formulas: 1 tablet for each 25 pounds of body weight BID.

Betathyme: 1 capsule for each 35 pounds of body weight BID (maximum, 2 capsules BID).

Maitake DMG: 1 ml per 25 pounds of body weight BID.

Glutimmune: One-fourth scoop per 25 pounds of body weight daily.

Vitamin C: 100 mgs per 10 pounds of body weight BID. Care should be taken because oral vitamin C may cause diarrhea in some animals and a lower dose adjustment may be required (see Chapter 2 for more information on the therapeutic use of vitamin C given intravenously).

Chinese herbal medicine

The authors recommend the patent formula Bai Tou Weng Tang, which contains pulsatilla (Bai tou weng), phellodenron bark (Huang bai), coptis root (Huang lian), and ash bark (Qin pi). This formula has strong antibacterial, antiviral, and antiparasitic effects. It also helps to control diarrhea and abdominal pain. It is available

through many herbal companies. It is dosed according to the label on the bottle.

Homotoxicology (Dose: 10 drops PO for 50-pound dog, 5 drops PO for small dog)

Symptom formula: Veratrum homaccord, Engystol N plus Coenzyme compositum, Echinacea homaccord, Cactus compositum, Cralonin, Podophyllum compositum, Mercurius-Heel, 6 to 8 times daily as needed, and then tapered to TID.

Detoxification following improvement: Galium-Heel, Mucosa compositum, Coenzyme compositum, Ubichinon compositum every 3 days for 2 to 3 weeks.

Product sources

Nutrition

Intestines and immune support formulas: Animal Nutrition Technologies. **Alternatives**: Immune System and Enteric Support—Standard Process Veterinary Formulas; Immuno Support and NutriGest—Rx Vitamins for Pets; Immugen—Thorne Veterinary Products.

Betathyme: Best for Your Pet. **Alternative**: Moducare—Thorne Veterinary Products.

Maitake DMG: Vetri Science.

Glutimmune: Well Wisdom. **Alternatives**: L-Glutamine powder—Thorne Veterinary Products.

Vitamin C: Over the counter. Intravenous vitamin C: McGuff Company.

Chinese herbal medicine

Bai Tou Weng Tang: Treasure of the East/Bluelight, Inc.

Homotoxicology

BHI/Heel Corporation.

REFERENCES

Western medicine references

Carmichael L. Parvoviral Infection—Dogs. In: Tilley L, Smith F. The 5-Minute Veterinary Consult: Canine and Feline, Blackwell Publishing, 2003.

Fenner FJ, Gibbs E, Paul J, Murphy FA, Rott R, Studdert MJ, White DO. Veterinary Virology, 2nd ed. 1993. Academic Press, Inc.

Mantione N, Otto C. Characterization of the use of antiemetic agents in dogs with parvovirus enteritis treated at the veterinary teaching hospital. *JAVMA*, 2005. Dec 1, 227(11): pp 1787–93.

Palmquist R. A survey of canine vaccine practices in contemporary veterinary clinics in the US. *JAHVMA*, 2003. 22(1, 2): pp 27–9.

Pollock RHV, Carmichael LE. Canine viral enteritis. In: Greene CE, ed. Infectious diseases of the dog and cat. Philadelphia: WB Saunders, 1990:268–279.

Pollock RHV, Parrish CR. Canine parvovirus. In: Olsen RG, Krakowa S, Blakeslee JR, eds. Boca Raton, FL: CRC Press, 1985:145–177.

Prittie J. Canine parvoviral enteritis: a review of the diagnosis, management, and prevention. *J Vet Emerg Crit Care*, 2004. 14: pp 167–176.

Twark L, Dodds W. Clinical use of serum parvovirus and distemper virus antibody titers in determining revaccination strategies in healthy dogs. *JAVMA*, 2000.217: pp 1021–4.

Zimmer JF. Clinical management of acute gastroenteritis including virus-induced enteritis. In: Kirk RW, ed. Current veterinary therapy—small animal practice, VIII., Philadelphia: Saunders, 1983:171–1177.

IVM/nutrition references

Askanazi J, Carpenter YA, Michelsen CB, et al. Muscle and plasma amino acids following injury: Influence of intercurrent infection. *Ann Surg* 1980;192:78–85.

Bouic PJD Immunomodulation in HIV/AIDS: The Tygerberg Stellenbosch University experience. AIDS Bulletin published by the Medical Research Council of South Africa 6(3):18–20, Sept. 1997.

Cima J. Biochemical Blood Chemistry Evaluation, Palm Beach Gardens, FL., March 2000.

Goldstein R, et al. The BNA Handbook: A Working Manual for Veterinarians, Westport, CT: Animal Nutrition Technologies, 2000.

Graber G, Kendall R. N,N-Dimethylglycine and Use in Immune Response, US Patent 4,631,189, Dec 1986.

Gupta MB, Nath R, Srivastava N, et al. Anti-inflammatory and antipyretic activities of β-sitosterol. *Planta Medica* 1980;39:157–163.

Kendall RV. Building Wellness with DMG, Topanga, CA: Freedom Press, 2003.

Mani S, Whitesides J, Lawson J. Role of Dimethylglycine in Melanoma Inhibition—Abstract from Nutrition and Cancer Prevention: American Institute for Cancer Research, Sept 1999.

Nanba H, Hamaguchi AM, Kuroda H. The chemical structure of an antitumor polysaccharide in fruit bodies of *Grifola frondosa* (maitake). *Chem Pharm Bull* 1987;35: 1162–8.

O'Dwyer S, et al. Maintenance of small bowel mucosa with glutamine-enriched parenteral nutrition, *Journal of Parenteral and Enteral Nutrition*, 1989;13:579.

Pegel KH. The importance of sitosterol and sitosterolin in human and animal nutrition. *South African Journal of Science* 1997; June 93:263–268.

Reap E, Lawson J. Stimulation of the Immune Response by Dimethylglycine, a non-toxic metabolite. *Journal of Laboratory and Clinical Medicine*. 1990.115:481,

Souba WW. Glutamine physiology, biochemistry, and nutrition in critical illness. Austin, TX: RG Landes Co; 1992.

Souba W et al. Glutamine metabolism in the intestinal tract: invited review, *JPEN* 1985;9:608–617.

Verdova I, Chamaganova A. Use of vitamin B$_{15}$ for the treatment of certain skin conditions, Vitamin B$_{15}$ (Pangamic Acid) Properties, Functions and Use, Naooka, Moscow: Science Publishing, 1965.

Wang C, Lawson J. The Effects on the Enhancement of Monoclonal Antibody Production. Annual Meeting of the American Soc. of Microbiology, Oct. 1988.

Windmueller HG, Glutamine utilization by the small intestine, *Adv. Enzymol* 1982;53:201–237.

Yoshimura K, et al. Effects of enteral glutamine administration on experimental inflammatory bowel disease, 1993; *JPEN* 17:235.

Chinese herbal medicine/acupuncture references

Si Chuan Yi Xue Yuan Xue Bao (*Journal of Sichuan School of Medicine*), 1959;1:102.

Zhong Yao Xue (*Chinese Herbology*), 1998;197:199.

Zhong Yi Za Zhi (*Journal of Chinese Medicine*), 1959;8:23.

Homotoxicology references

Mantione N, Otto C. Characterization of the use of antiemetic agents in dogs with parvovirus enteritis treated at the veterinary teaching hospital. *JAVMA*, 2005. Dec 1, 227(11): pp 1787–93.

Palmquist R. Doctor's Policy Manual: Parvovirus Protocol. Internal hospital training manual. Centinela Animal Hospital, Inc. 1986. Inglewood, CA.

Palmquist R. A survey of canine vaccine practices in contemporary veterinary clinics in the US. *JAHVMA*, 2003; 22(1, 2): pp 27–9.

Prittie J. Canine parvoviral enteritis: a review of the diagnosis, management, and prevention. *J Vet Emerg Crit Care*, 2004. 14: pp 167–176.

Twark L, Dodds W. Clinical use of serum parvovirus and distemper virus antibody titers in determining revaccination strategies in healthy dogs. *JAVMA*, 2000. 217: pp 1021–4.

Vestweber AM, Beuth J, Ko HL, Tunggal L, Buss G, Pulverer G. In vitro activity of Mercurius cyanatus complex against relevant pathogenic bacterial isolates [Article in German]. *Arzneimittelforschung*. 1995.;Sep;45(9):pp 1018–20.

INFECTIOUS HEPATITIS

Definition and cause

Canine infectious hepatitis is caused by an adenovirus (canine adenovirus type 1; CAV-1), which initially attacks specialized hepatic macrophages (Kupffer cells) that distribute the infection widely. Endothelial cells are also actively infected and this combination leads to massive viral release and damage to hepatocytes. The virus also targets other parenchymal organs and ocular tissues (resulting in classic anterior uveitis lesions known as "blue eye") (Center 2003, Greene 1998, Hoskins 2000, Swango 1989, Webster 2003).

Medical therapy rationale, drug(s) of choice, and nutritional recommendations

Medical therapy is supportive and includes fluid replacement plus dextrose, oral alimentation with a highly bioavailable diet, potassium supplementation, antimicrobial therapy, and antiemetics (Center 2003, Greene 1998, Hoskin 2000).

Anticipated prognosis

The prognosis is generally poor to guarded. Recovery is possible with a good antibody response against the virus; however, the animals can develop chronic liver conditions (Webster 2003).

Integrative veterinary therapies

Vaccination is recommended and is highly effective in preventing canine infectious hepatitis. The duration of immunity for canine adenovirus vaccination is not known; however, in the authors' practices no clinical cases have been seen in dogs that have received proper vaccination schedules as puppies, indicating that revaccination may not be required. At this time insufficient evidence exists to recommend nosodes for canine adenovirus type 1.

The integrative approach to infectious hepatitis focuses upon the inflammatory process and cellular destruction in the liver as well as the general immune function in relation to the viral infection. The addition of nutrients, nutriceuticals, medicinal herbs, and combination homeopathics that have anti-inflammatory, cellular, and organ-sparing properties may enhance liver cell regeneration. Immune system organs such as the thymus, adrenal, and spleen should also be supported and protected.

Nutrition
General considerations/rationale

Improving immune function against the virus, reducing inflammation, and eliminating toxins and metabolic wastes—along with appropriate medical therapy—can improve the prognosis. Glutathione binds and neutralizes various chemicals, toxins, herbicides, pesticides, heavy metals, etc. so they can pass through the liver and be excreted via the bile into the intestines or passed to the kidneys to be excreted in the urine (Sen 1997). Body glutathione levels can be raised by other nutrients such as vitamin C, whey protein, glutamine, methionine, S-adenosyl-L-methionine (SAMe), and alpha-lipoic acid (Amores-Sanchez 1999, Bounous 1989, Vendemiale 1989, Wang 1997). See chronic active hepatitis and cholangiohepatitis for more detailed information.

Antioxidants and phytonutrients can help reduce inflammation and neutralize compounds that the liver must deal with in its role as the body's filter and detoxifier.

Appropriate nutrients

Nutrition/gland therapy: Glandular liver helps to neutralize a cellular immune response and helps spare liver cells (see Gland Therapy in Chapter 2). Clinical trials using thymus extract have shown that it is beneficial in people with hepatitis B (Skotnicki 1989). Additional clinical studies with oral thymus extract showed that blood values related to liver function as well as the blood immune markers all improved (Galli 1985, Bortolotti 1988). Civereira (1989) showed similar results with hepatitis C.

Note: Infectious hepatitis can affect multiple organ systems, and therefore medical and physiological blood evaluations are recommended to assess general glandular health. This helps clinicians to formulate therapeutic nutritional protocols that address gland function and organ disease that may be present (Cima 2000, Goldstein 2000) (see Chapter 2, Nutritional Blood Testing, for additional information).

Lecithin/phosphatidylcholine: Lecithin/phosphatidylcholine has been shown to help prevent scar tissue from forming in inflammatory processes of the liver (Ma 1996).

Alpha-lipoic acid: Alpha-lipoic acid is an antioxidant that has been shown to reduce oxidation and inflammation. It increases the effectiveness of other antioxidants, such as vitamins C and E, Coenzyme Q10, and glutathione, making them more readily available for bodily function (Busse 1992, Lykkesfeldt 1998, Scholich 1989). In a study with people with liver disease who received an antioxidant-rich supplement containing 300 mg of alpha-lipoic acid, there was significant improvement of liver function (Berkson 1999).

S-adenosylmethionine (SAMe): SAMe is an antioxidant and has anti-inflammatory effects on the liver (Center 2000). SAMe has been shown to significantly improve survival and decrease the need for liver transplantation in people with liver disease. It has also been shown to improve liver function in less severe cases of cirrhosis (Gorbakov 1998, Mato 1999, Miglio 1975).

Vitamin B_{12} and folic acid: Vitamin B_{12} and folic acid have been shown to help people with hepatitis (Campbell 1952, 1955; Wallace 2001).

Chinese herbal medicine/acupuncture
General considerations/rationale

Infectious hepatitis is usually due to either Damp or Heat invading the Liver and Gallbladder, or infectious pathogens. This leads to Qi and Blood stagnation.

Infectious pathogens are of course any bacteria, virus, or fungus that attacks the liver or gallbladder. In the present case we are discussing canine adenovirus I. Damp and Heat can refer to inflammation and purulent debris. Qi and Blood stagnation refer to the abdominal pain that the patient experiences.

Appropriate Chinese herbs

Alisma (Ze xie): Enhances immunity and has anti-inflammatory effects (Dai 1991). It may decrease inflammation in the liver while avoiding immunosuppression.

Atractylodes (Bai zhu): Has been used for ascites from cirrhosis, infectious hepatitis, and cancer with good results (An Hui Zhong Yi Xue Yuan Xue Bao 1984). Although ascites is not commonly seen in CAV-I, it does indicate that this herb has a protective effect on the liver.

Cinnamon twigs (Gui zhi): Have shown antiviral effects against coxsackie virus B-1 and influenza (Zhong Yao Xue 1998; Chu 1998). It may have efficacy against other viruses, although more studies must be completed.

Crataegus (Shan zha): Enhances immunity. It seems to stimulate both the cellular and humoral immune system (Jin 1992). It also helps to control nausea (Zhong Xi Yi Jie He Za Zhi 1984).

Ginger (Gan jiang): Has been shown to decrease experimentally induced vomiting in dogs (Zhong Yao Xue 1998). It may help decrease vomiting in infectious hepatitis.

Licorice (Gan cao): Contains glycyrrhizin, which has demonstrated antiviral activity against multiple viruses, including human adenovirus II (Zhu 1996). It was 77% effective in treating 330 human patients with hepatitis B. It reduced inflammation, increased regeneration of hepatic cells, and decreased hepatic necrosis and cirrhosis (Zhong Yao Tong Bao 1987).

Malt (Mai ya): Has been used in patients with hepatitis. Symptoms improved in 85% of the cases of acute hepatitis and 57% of the cases of chronic hepatitis. Positive effects were defined as improved appetite, decreased pain, and decreased serum liver enzymes (Xin Yi Yao Tong Xun 1972).

Oriental wormwood (Yin chen hao): Reduces fevers. In rats with experimentally induced pyrexia, the duration of effect was 3 to 4 hours (Planta Med 1984). It has been shown to enhance phagocytosis in liver macrophages (Hu 1999). In one trial, 32 people with acute hepatitis were treated with yin chen hao for up to 2 weeks. In these patients, there was a significant decrease in hepatomegaly, icterus, and pyrexia (Fu Jian Zhong Yi Yao 1959).

Pinellia (Ban xia): Seems to have a centrally mediated antiemetic effect (Zhong Yao Yao Li Yu Ying Yong 1983). It may help control vomiting associated with infection.

Polyporus (Zhu ling): An immunostimulant (Zhong Guo Mian Yi Xue Za Zhi 1991). It also has hepatoprotective effects as demonstrated in rat experiments using CCL4 (Zhong Guo Yao Li Xue Tong Bao 1988).

Poria (Fu ling): Has hepatoprotective effects. In one experiment it protected hamster livers from carbon tetrachloride damage (Han 1977). It contains pachman, which has been shown to enhance the phagocytic function of macrophages in mice (Lu 1990). This indicates that it enhances the immune system.

Acupuncture

Acupuncture may help protect the liver. In one experiment 36 rats were treated with CCl4. The efficacy of acupuncture at St 36 and LI3 for hepatoprotection was investigated. The rats treated after exposure to CCl4 had lower AST and ALT levels, suggesting that acupuncture can protect the liver (Liu 2001). In one trial, 90 patients with hepatitis B were studied. Thirty received vitamin therapy, 30 received acupuncture at ST36, and 30 had electro-acupuncture at ST36. Hepatitis B surface antigen levels decreased in the acupuncture groups but not the vitamin group. IgG and C3 levels were increased in those patients receiving acupuncture (Chen 1999), which suggests that acupuncture may stimulate immunity and help clear viral hepatic infections.

Homotoxicology
General considerations/rationale
Viral diseases represent Impregnation Phase disorders and proper attention to phase remedy selections is helpful in such cases.

Due to the damage to tissue and endothelial barriers, both pathogenic and nonpathogenic bacteria may cause opportunistic infections and further tissue damage. This results in a Degeneration Phase in fairly rapid time. Compositae category antihomotoxic formulas may prove helpful in establishing cellular repair, organ drainage, and detoxification following recovery from infection.

The liver plays a critical role in the normal functioning of the body. Care should be taken to avoid strong detoxification remedies in early stages of hepatitis. Remedies that cause massive offload of toxins into the blood may overwhelm and further damage the compromised liver. Examples of strong detoxifiers/drainers are Thyroidea compositum, Testes compositum, and Ovarium compositum. Galium-Heel is useful but should be used intermittently to avoid excessive detoxification. For initial therapy concentrate on protecting the organ from further inflammation and free radical damage and providing adequate fluid and nutrient supplies for tissue repair to proceed.

Appropriate homotoxicology formulas
See also cholangiohepatitis and chronic active hepatitis protocols.

Coenzyme compositum: Supports the metabolism, and is helpful in cases of exhaustion from stress or disease.

Chelidonium homaccord: Supports the gallbladder.

Echinacea compositum: Supports immune function against bacteria and viral infections. Phase remedy for Inflammation and Impregnation phase homotoxicoses.

Engystol N: Supports nonspecific defenses against viral infection. The effect appears to be dose dependant.

Galium-Heel: Treats all cellular phases, hemorrhoids, and anal fissures, and is a detoxicant.

Gripp-Heel: An antiviral that also treats muscle aches and exhaustion.

Hepeel: Provides liver detoxification and drainage following infection. Can be combined with *Coenzyme compositum* and used every 3 days as needed until enzymes return to normal. Can be used concurrently with *Hepar compositum*, which is also given intermittently 1 to 3 times weekly.

Hepar compositum: Widely supports the liver (Hepar suis) and immune system (thymus suis) through detoxification, hepatocyte protection (Milk thistle), and metabolism (malic acid, fumaric acid, thioctic acid, lactic acid, alpha-ketoglutaric acid, and sodium oxalacetate). Sulfur and histamine in homeopathic dilution assist enzyme function and detoxification (Reckeweg 2000).

Lymphomyosot: Provides drainage and immune support.

Phosphor homaccord: Used in chronic cases or in those with petechial hemorrhages or frank bleeding.

Ubichinon compositum: Provides deeper support of metabolism than *Coenzyme compositum* and helps activate mitochondrial function after iatrogenic damage from antibiotics and other medicants.

Tonsilla compositum: Supports immunity broadly through the bone marrow, spleen, and tonsils.

Authors' suggested protocols

Nutrition

Liver and immune support formulas (thymus-enriched): 1 tablet for each 25 pounds of body weight BID.

Alpha-lipoic acid: 20 mg per 10 pounds of body weight daily.

SAMe: 10 to 20 mg/kg SID or follow manufacturer's dosing directions.

Lecithin/phosphatidylcholine: One-fourth teaspoon for each 25 pounds of body weight BID.

Folic acid: 50 micrograms for every 35 pounds of body weight (maximum, 200 micrograms).

Vitamin B$_{12}$: 50 micrograms for every 25 pounds.

Chinese herbal medicine

Formula H77 Cholangiohepatitis: 1 capsule per 10 to 20 pounds twice daily. For acute cases it may be necessary to use this supplement in conjunction with conventional supportive care, including antibiotics, fluid therapy, antiemetics, and so on. In addition to the herbs discussed above, H77 Cholangiohepatitis contains aconite (Fu zi) and leaven (Shen qu) to help increase the efficacy of the formula.

Acupuncture points that may help include BL18, BL19, BL20, GB34, LI3, PC6, ST36, and CV12.

Homotoxicology

See also cholangiohepatitis and chronic active hepatitis protocols.

Consider autosanguis therapy in these patients. In addition to excellent conventional Western medical support with nutritional support, fluids, antibiotics as needed, antiemetics only as needed, intestinal protectants (sucralfate), urodeoxycholic acid, and S-adenosylmethionine and vitamin E in most cases, consider the following: Phosphor homaccord, Chelidonium homaccord, Nux homaccord, Duodenoheel mixed together and given BID. Alternate Hepeel and BHI-Enzyme BID PO. Give Gastricumeel if vomiting and Engystol N for viral hepatitis. Galium-Heel, Lymphomyosot, Hepar compositum, and Solidago compositum should be given every 3 days. If there is diarrhea, consider adding Coenzyme compositum and Ubichinon compositum twice weekly.

Product sources

Nutrition

Liver and immune support formulas: Animal Nutrition Technologies. **Alternatives**: Immune System and Hepatic Support—Standard Process Veterinary Formulas; Immuno and Hepato Support—Rx Vitamins for Pets; Immugen and Hepagen—Thorne Veterinary Products.

Alpha-lipoic acid: Source Naturals.

SAMe: Nutramax Laboratories, Inc.

Lecithin/phosphatidylcholine: Designs for Health.

Vitamin B$_{12}$ and folic acid: Progressive Labs.

Chinese herbal medicine

Formula H77 Cholangiohepatitis: Natural Solutions, Inc.

Homotoxicology

BHI/Heel Corporation

REFERENCES

Western medicine references

Center SA. Hepatitis, Infectious Canine. In: Tilley L, Smith F. The 5-Minute Veterinary Consult: Canine and Feline, Blackwell Publishing, 2003.

Greene CE. Infectious canine hepatitis and canine acidophil cell hepatitis. In: Greene CE, ed. Infectious diseases of the dog and cat. 2nd ed. Philadelphia: Saunders, 1998:22–28.

Hoskins JD. Canine viral diseases. In: Ettinger SJ, Feldman EC, eds. Textbook of Veterinary Internal Medicine. Philadelphia: WB Saunders Co. 2000. pp. 418–419.

Swango LJ. Canine viral diseases. In: Ettinger SJ, ed. Textbook of Veterinary Internal Medicine. Philadelphia: WB Saunders Co. 1989. pp. 303–305.

Webster C. Hepatitis, Infectious Canine. In: Tilley L, Smith F. The 5-Minute Veterinary Consult: Canine and Feline, 3rd ed.

Philadelphia: Lippincott Williams and Wilkins, 2003. pp 570–71.

IVM/nutrition references

Amores-Sanchez MI, Medina MA. Glutamine, as a precursor of glutathione, and oxidative stress. *Mol Genet Metab* 1999;67: 100–5.

Berkson BM. A conservative triple antioxidant approach to the treatment of hepatitis C. Combination of Alpha lipoic acid (thioctic acid), silymarin, and selenium: three case histories. *Med Klin* 1999;94 Suppl 3:84–9.

Bortolotti F, Cadrobbi P, Crivellaro C, et al. Effect of an orally administered thymic derivative, thymomodulin, in chronic type B hepatitis in children. *Curr Ther Res* 1988;43:67–72.

Bounous G, Gervais F, Amer V, et al. The influence of dietary whey protein on tissue glutathione and the diseases of aging. *Clin Invest Med* 1989;12:343–9.

Busse E, Zimmer G, Schorpohl B, et al. Influence of alpha-lipoic acid on intracellular glutathione in vitro and in vivo. *Arzneimittelforschung* 1992;42:829–31.

Campbell RE, Pruitt FW. Vitamin B$_{12}$ in the treatment of viral hepatitis. *Am J Med Sci* 1952;224:252–62.

Campbell RE, Pruitt FW. The effect of vitamin B$_{12}$ and folic acid in the treatment of viral hepatitis. *Am J Med Sci* 1955;229: 8–15.

Center SA. S-adenosyl-methionine an antioxidant and anti-inflammatory nutraceutical. Proceedings of the 18th ACVIM, Seattle, WA. 2000. 550–552.

Cima J. Biochemical Blood Chemistry Evaluation, Palm Beach Gardens, FL., March 2000.

Civeira MP, Castilla A, Morte S, et al. A pilot study of thymus extract in chronic non-A, non-B hepatitis. *Aliment Pharmacol Ther* 1989;3:395–401.

Galli M, Crocchiolo P, Negri C, et al. Attempt to treat acute type B hepatitis with an orally administered thymic extract (thymomodulin): Preliminary results. *Drugs Exp Clin Res* 1985;11:665–9.

Goldstein R, et al. The BNA Handbook: A Working Manual for Veterinarians, Westport, CT: Animal Nutrition Technologies, 2000.

Gorbakov VV, Galik VP, Kirillov SM. Experience in heptral treatment of diffuse liver diseases. *Ter Arkh* 1998;70:82–6.

Lykkesfeldt J, Hagen TM, Vinarsky V, Ames BN. Age-associated decline in ascorbic acid concentration, recycling, and biosynthesis in rat hepatocytes—reversal with (R)-alpha-lipoic acid supplementation. *FASEB J* 1998;12:1183–9.

Ma X, Zhao J, Lieber CS. Polyenylphosphatidylcholine attenuates non-alcoholic hepatic fibrosis and accelerates its regression. *J Hepatol* 1996;24:604–13.

Mato JM, Camara J, Fernandez de Paz J, et al. S-adenosylmethionine in alcoholic liver cirrhosis: a randomized, placebo-controlled, double-blind, multicenter clinical trial. *J Hepatol* 1999;30:1081–9.

Miglio F, Stefanini GF, Corazza GR, et al. Double-blind studies of the therapeutic action of S-Adenosylmethionine (SAMe) in oral administration, in liver cirrhosis and other chronic hepatitides. *Minerva Med* 1975;66:1595–9 [In Italian].

Scholich H, Murphy ME, Sies H. Antioxidant activity of dihydrolipoate against microsomal lipid peroxidation and its

dependence on alpha-tocopherol. *Biochem Biophys Acta* 1989;1001:256–61.

Sen CK. Nutritional biochemistry of cellular glutathione. *Nutr Biochem* 1997;8:660–72.

Skotnicki AB. Therapeutic application of calf thymus extract (TFX). *Med Oncol Tumor Pharmacother* 1989;6:31–43.

Vendemiale G, Altomare E, Trizio T, et al. Effects of oral S-adenosyl-L-methionine on hepatic glutathione in patients with liver disease. *Scand J Gastroenterol* 1989;24:407–15.

Wallace AE, Weeks WB. Thiamine treatment of chronic hepatitis B infection. *Am J Gastroenterol* 2001;96:864–8.

Wang ST, Chen HW, Sheen LY, Lii CK. Methionine and cysteine affect glutathione level, glutathione-related enzyme activities and the expression of glutathione S-transferase isozymes in rat hepatocytes. *J Nutr* 1997;127:2135–41.

Chinese herbal medicine/acupuncture references

An Hui Zhong Yi Xue Yuan Xue Bao (*Journal of Anhui University School of Medicine*), 1984;2:25.

Chen J, Chen M, Zhao B, Wang Y. Effects of acupuncture on the immunological functions in hepatitis B virus carriers. *J Tradit Chin Med.* 1999;19: 268–272.

Chu XH, et al. *China Journal of New Herbal Medicine and Clinical Practice.* 1998;17(60):327–328.

Dai Y, et al. *China Journal of Chinese Medicine.* 1991;16(10): 622.

Fu Jian Zhong Yi Yao (*Fujian Chinese Medicine and Herbology*), 1959;7:42.

Han DW, et al. *China Journal of Internal Medicine.* 1977;2(1):13.

Hu YQ, et al. The extraction and separation of Yin Chen polypeptides and their liver-protecting effects in mice. *Journal of Chinese Materia Medica.* 1999;30(12):894–896.

Jin ZC, et al. Effects of Shan Zha injection solution on immune functions. *Journal of Chinese Materia Medica.* 1992;23(11), 592–593.

Lu SC, et al. *Journal of No. 1 Military Academy.* 1990;10(3):267.

Liu HJ, Hsu SF, Hsieh CC, Ho TY, Hsieh CL, Tsai CC, Lin JG. The Effectiveness of Tsu-San-Li and Tai-Chung Acupoints for Treatment of Acute Liver Damage in Rats. *American Journal of Chinese Medicine*, Spring, 2001.

Planta Med, 1984; 46(1):84.

Xin Yi Yao Tong Xun (*Journal of New Medicine and Herbology*), 1972; 1:21.

Zhong Guo Mian Yi Xue Za Zhi (*Chinese Journal of Immunology*), 1991; 7(3):185.

Zhong Guo Yao Li Xue Tong Bao (*Journal of Chinese Herbal Pharmacology*), 1988; 9(4):345.

Zhong Xi Yi Jie He Za Zhi (*Journal of Integrated Chinese and Western Medicine*), 1984; 5: 315.

Zhong Yao Tong Bao (*Journal of Chinese Herbology*), 1987;9:60.

Zhong Yao Xue (*Chinese Herbology*), 1998;65:67.

Zhong Yao Xue (*Chinese Herbology*), 1998; 378–380.

Zhong Yao Yao Li Yu Ying Yong (Pharmacology and Applications of Chinese Herbs), 1983:383.

Zhu LH. *China Journal of TCM Information.* 1996;3(3): 17–20.

Homotoxicology reference
Reckeweg H. Biotherapeutic Index: Ordinatio Antihomotoxica et Materia Medica, 5th ed. Baden-Baden, Germany: Biologische Heilmittel Heel GMBH, 2000. pp 347–50.

INFECTIOUS TRACHEOBRONCHITIS (PARAINFLUENZA)

Definition and cause

Infectious tracheobronchitis is a contagious, upper respiratory infection of dogs caused by a number of different viruses and bacteria such as *Bordetella bronchiseptica*. The underlying process is inflammatory. Depending upon the viral infectious agents, parainfluenza is usually self-limiting (Ford 1990, Hoskins 2003).

Medical therapy rationale, drug(s) of choice, and nutritional recommendations

Rest and isolation is recommended. If therapy is chosen it is usually antibiotics, cough suppressants, and bronchodilators (Hoskins 1994).

Anticipated prognosis

Infectious bronchitis is generally self-limiting, with healing occurring in 10 to 14 days. With more severe disease, the course may be 4 to 6 weeks and severely immune suppressed animals can die of complications such as pneumonia (Hoskins 2003).

Integrative veterinary therapies

While the target tissue is the upper respiratory system, the integrative approach also takes into consideration the immune system and its response to the invading organism. In addition, if medications are chosen, nutritional and biological therapies help minimize side effects.

Nutrition
General considerations/rationale
The nutritional approach to infectious tracheobronchitis consists of nutrient support of the upper respiratory and immune systems, as well as helping to decrease the inflammatory process that incites the coughing.

Appropriate nutrients
Nutritional/gland therapy: Glandular adrenal, thymus, lung, and bronchus help to neutralize viral-induced inflammation (see Chapter 2, Gland Therapy, for additional information).

Quercetin: Quercetin is a potent antioxidant that helps to reduce cellular inflammation (Knekt 2002). Quercetin also functions like an antihistamine, by inhibiting cells from releasing histamines (Middleton 1986, Ogasawara 1985). Therefore, quercetin is beneficial in the treatment of inflammation of the upper respiratory system.

Sterols and sterolins: Animal studies have demonstrated that phytosterols have anti-inflammatory and antipyretic effects (Gupta 1980). Pegel (1997) feels that sterols are essential for a properly functioning immune system.

Vitamin C: Vitamin C has been clinically proven as a potent antioxidant and immune enhancing agent, specifically against infectious agents (Pauling 1976).

Chinese herbal medicine/acupuncture
General considerations/rationale
Parainfluenza is an infectious pathogen that invades the body and attacks the Lung. It is most likely to occur during the change of seasons or under stressful conditions.

As in Western understanding, parainfluenza is an infectious pathogen. The presenting signs are respiratory as it attacks the Lungs. Both schools of thought recognize the importance of stress on repelling the virus. Therapy is aimed at repelling the virus, strengthening the immune system, preventing secondary infections, and controlling signs of disease.

Appropriate Chinese herbs
Apricot (Xing ren): An effective expectorant and cough suppressant (Zhang 1991).

Codonopsis (Dang shen): An immunostimulant. It can increase the leukocyte count (Huang 1994), which may help the patient clear infection faster.

Forsythia fruit (Lian qiao): Contains rengynic acid, which inhibits viruses (Zhang 2002). In addition, it has antibacterial properties that may help prevent secondary bacterial infections (Ma 1982).

Gypsum (Shi gao): Increases the phagocytic activity of macrophages (Zhong Yao Xue 1998), which may help stimulate immunity to help the patient recover more quickly.

Honeysuckle (Jin yin hua): Has antibacterial activity (Xin Yi Xue 1975, Jiang Xi Xin Yi Yao 1960). This may help prevent secondary bacterial infections.

Isatis root (Ban lan gen): Has antiviral effects. Its effects are similar to that of ribavirin (Jiang 1992, Zhu 1999, Li 2000).

Licorice (Gan cao): Contains glycyrrhizin, which has antiviral properties (Zhu 1996).

Mint (Bo he): Inhibits viruses and bacteria (Wang 1983).

Pinellia (Ban xia): Has antitussive activity (Gui 1998).

Platycodon root (Jie geng): Decreases coughing (Zhong Yao Yao Li Yu Ying Yong 1983).

Poria (Fu ling): Inhibits bacterial growth (Nanjing College of Pharmacy 1976).

Scutellaria (Huang qin): Contains baicalin, which has antibiotic activity against multiple bacteria (Zhong Yao Xue 1988).

White atractyloides (Bai zhu): Increases the T helper cell count (Xu 1994). It may help stimulate the immune system to help clear the virus.

Acupuncture

Sinusitis, rhinitis, and the common cold are all on the World Health Organization's list of disorders responsive to acupuncture (World Health Organization 10/15/2006). Although parainfluenza virus was not specifically studied by the WHO, the inclusion of viral upper respiratory diseases on the list indicates that acupuncture may be effective in treating viral conditions such as parainfluenza.

Homotoxicology
General considerations/rationale

This is an Impregnation homotoxicosis. Caused by many different viral agents, these infections are often self-limiting and no therapy may be needed in many cases. Secondary bacterial infections can occur and may assist the patient in the removal of homotoxins by bacterial action. Treating with antibiotics is common, but some biological therapists feel that such treatment may predispose the patient to a worsening of the homotoxicosis. Use of antibiotics should be carefully considered. With homotoxicology, herbal medicines, nutritional therapy, and classical homeopathy, many cases can be successfully treated without antibiotic or other drug therapy.

Patients frequently have a deep and productive cough following recovery from the acute viral state. This is actually a cleansing effect as the mucosal border repairs itself and leads to discharge of dead cellular debris and homotoxins trapped within the lungs and bronchial areas. Drinking adequate water, taking antioxidants, and getting gentle exercise are beneficial in assisting this natural detoxification and repair cycle. Suppressing such symptoms with cough medication, decongestants, and other pharmaceutical agents traps the material in the lung and leads to progressive vicariation. If at all possible the veterinarian should attempt to assist this natural and desirable cleansing process.

Appropriate homotoxicology formulas

For more in-depth descriptions of these formulas, see the protocols for other respiratory diseases such as bronchitis, pneumonia, and feline upper respiratory disease.

Aconitum homaccord: Used in the early stages of catarrhal infections and for influenza-like conditions.

Belladonna homaccord: Treats bronchitis and sinusitis.

BHI-Bronchitis: Treats both extremely wet and dry coughs; rattling mucus; and cough after wet, cold weather that worsens in warm rooms.

BHI-Chest: Treats deep cough.

BHI-CoughFree: A natural, lemon flavored cough syrup and expectorant.

BHI-Sinus: Treats sinusitis and otitis media.

Bronchalis-Heel: Treats coughing upon entering a warm room, bronchitis, smoker's lung, barking cough, laryngopharyngitis, and cough with nausea.

Bryaconeel: Treats influenzal infections, bronchopneumonia, bronchitis caused by chill, and rheumatism. The symptoms are worse after exercise or motion, and better when the patient lies still or holds its head up.

Droperteel: Used for congestive bronchitis, globus hystericus, spasmodic cough, asthma, and bluish red tonsilar swelling, and as a cardiac tonic (especially in older pets).

Drosera: Treats bronchogenic asthma, whooping cough, bronchitis, dypsnea and difficult respiration, and hay-fever-like signs.

Dulcamara homaccord: Used for productive coughs aggravated by damp, cold weather and vomiting white tenacious mucus after activity.

Echinacea compositum: Supports immunity in bacterial infections. Can be used instead of antibiotics in some cases, such as influenza-like conditions.

Engystol N: An antiviral that increases white blood cell numbers.

Euphorbium compositum: Treats rhinitis, sinusitis, catarrh of ear passages, otitis media, and mostly upper respiratory membranes. An antiviral agent that helps with respiratory signs and limits viral numbers in initial exposures (Glatthaar-Saalmüller 2001).

Galium-Heel: Activates the immune system in several phases, and provides cellular detoxification and drainage.

Gripp-Heel: An antiviral used for cold and flu-like symptoms (Rabe, Weiser, Klein 2004).

Husteel: Treats dry coughs, bronchopneumonia, deep coughs that worsen at night, coughs when lying down, and catarrh of the respiratory tract.

Lymphmyosot: Provides immune support and lymph drainage.

Mucosa compositum: Rehabilitates the mucosa following disease.

Phosphor homaccord: Used with friendly dispositioned dogs for vomiting and coughing, laryngitis with or without possible hemorrhages, ecchymoses, or when petechiae is noted.

Tartephadreel: Treats catarrh of the respiratory tract, asthmatic complaints, deep "whooping cough-like" affectations, and cough with nausea and vomiting.

Tonsilla compositum: Supports endocrine and reticu-loendothelial defenses.

Authors' suggested protocols

Nutrition

Immune and bronchus/lung support formulas: 1 tablet for each 25 pounds of body weight BID.

Betathyme: 1 capsule for each 35 pounds of body weight BID (maximum, 2 capsules BID).

Quercetin tablets: 35 mg for each 10 pounds of body weight SID.

Chinese herbal medicine/acupuncture

Ban Lan Gen Tang Jia Wei, a patent formula, at the manufacturer's recommended dose.

The traditional formula contains the herbs in the following ratio: isatis root 20 g, honeysuckle 10 g, chrysanthemum flower 7 g , forsythia fruit 10 g, codonopsis 10 g, poria 10 g, mint 7 g, platycodon root 7 g, bitter apricot 7 g, pinellia 7 g, scutellaria 7 g, white atractyloides 7 g, licorice root 7 g, gypsum 40 g (Modern Complete Works of Traditional Chinese Veterinary Medicine 2000).

Commonly used acupuncture points include LI4, GV14, LI11, and LU7 (Handbook of TCM Practitioners 1987).

Product sources

Nutrition

Immune and bronchus/lung support formulas: Animal Nutrition Technologies. **Alternatives:** Immune System Support—Standard Process Veterinary Formulas; Immuno Support—Rx Vitamins for Pets; Immugen—Thorne Veterinary Products.

Betathyme: Best for Your Pet. **Alternative:** Moducare—Thorne Veterinary Products.

Quercetin: Source Naturals; Quercitone—Thorne Veterinary Products.

Chinese herbal medicine

Ban Lan Gen Tang Jia Wei: Mayway Corporation.

Homotoxicology

BHI/Heel Corporation

REFERENCES

Western medicine references

Ford RB, Vaden SL. Canine infectious tracheobronchitis. In: Greene CE, ed. Infectious diseases of the dog and cat. Philadelphia: Saunders, 1990:259–265.

Hoskins JD, Taboada J. Specific treatment of infectious causes of respiratory disease in dogs and cats. *Vet Med* 1994;89: 443–452.

Hoskins JD. Tracheobronchitis, Infectious—Dogs. In: Tilley L, Smith F. The 5-Minute Veterinary Consult: Canine and Feline, Blackwell Publishing, 2003.

IVM/nutrition references

Gupta MB, Nath R, Srivastava N, et al. Anti-inflammatory and antipyretic activities of β-sitosterol. *Planta Medica* 1980;39: 157–163.

Knekt P, Jarvinen R, Seppanen R, et al. Dietary flavonoids and the risk of lung cancer and other malignant neoplasms. *Am J Epidemiol* 1997;146:223–30.

Middleton E Jr. Effect of flavonoids on basophil histamine release and other secretory systems. *Prog Clin Biol Res.* 1986;213:493–506.

Ogasawara H, Middleton E Jr. Effect of selected flavonoids on histamine release (HR) and hydrogen peroxide (H2O2) generation by human leukocytes [abstract]. *J Allergy Clin Immunol.* 1985;75(suppl):184.

Pegel KH. The importance of sitosterol and sitosterolin in human and animal nutrition. *South African Journal of Science* June 1997;93:263–268.

Chinese herbal medicine/acupuncture references

Gui CQ, et al. *Journal of Pharmacology and Clinical Application of TCM.* 1998;14(4):27–28.

Handbook of TCM Practitioners, Hunan College of TCM, Shanghai Science and Technology Press, Oct 1987, p 154–156.

Huang T, et al. Pharmacology research on Ming Dang Shen decoction solution and polysaccharides. *Journal of Chinese Patented Medicine.* 1994;16(7):31–33.

Jiang Xi Xin Yi Yao (*Jiangxi New Medicine and Herbology*), 1960 (1):34.

Jiang XY, et al. Comparison between 50 kinds of Chinese herbs that treat hepatitis and suppress in vitro HBAg activity. *Journal of Modern Applied Pharmacy.* 1992;9(5):208–211.

Li S, et al. Various Ban Lan Gen and Da Qing Ye's effect in antagonizing influenza A virus. *Journal of Second Military Medical College.* 2000;21(3):204–206.

Ma Zhen Ya. *Shannxi Journal of Traditional Chinese Medicine and Herbs.* 1982;(4):58.

Yu C, Chen ZB. Modern Complete Works of Traditional Chinese Veterinary Medicine. Guangxi Science and Technology Press, March 2000, 601–602.

Nanjing College of Pharmacy. Materia Medica, vol. 2. Jiangsu: People's Press; 1976.

Xin Yi Xue (*New Medicine*), 1975; 6(3): 155.

Xu SC, et al. *Shanghai Journal of Immunology.* 1994;14(1): 12–13.

Wang YS. Application and Pharmacology of TCM. Beijing: People's Health Press; 1983.

World Health Organization list of common conditions treatable by Chinese Medicine and Acupuncture. Available at: http//tcm/health-info.org/WHO-treatment-list.htm accessed 10/15/2006.

Zhang G, Song S, Ren J, Xu S. A New Compound from Forsythia suspense (Thunb.) Vahl with Antiviral Effect on RSV. *J of Herbal Pharmacotherapy.* 2002;2(3): 35–39.

Zhang WJ, et al. Processed Xing Ren: Its potency and acute toxicity. *Journal of Traditional Chinese Medicine Material.* 1991;14(8):38–40.

Zhong Yao Xue (*Chinese Herbology*), 1988; 137:140.

Zhong Yao Xue (*Chinese Herbology*), 1998, 115: 119.

Zhong Yao Yao Li Yu Ying Yong (Pharmacology and Applications of Chinese Herbs); 1983; 866.

Zhu LA, et al. Research on Ban Lan Gen's preventive effects on cardiac cells in experimental cyocarditis models. *China Journal of Cardiovascular Disease.* 1999;27(6):467–468.

Zhu LH. *China Journal of TCM Information.* 1996;3(3): 17–20.

Homotoxicology references

Glatthaar-Saalmüller B, Fallier-Becker P. Antiviral Action of Euphorbium compositum® and its Components. *Forsch Komplementärmed Klass Naturheilkd,* 2001.8:pp 207–212.

Rabe A, Weiser M, Klein P. Effectiveness and tolerability of a homeopathic remedy compared with conventional therapy for mild viral infections. *International Journal of Clinical Practice,* 2004.58(9): pp 827–832.

FELINE UPPER RESPIRATORY DISEASES

Definition and cause

Feline upper respiratory diseases are common upper respiratory viral infections in cats that result in sneezing, sinusitis, rhinitis, conjunctivitis, fever, and potentially pneumonia. The cause is feline herpes virus (FHV-1) (Ford 1994, Gaskell 1998, Norsworthy 2003, Pederson 1988, Scott 2003).

Medical therapy rationale, drug(s) of choice, and nutritional recommendations

Antiviral drugs are generally ineffective. Broad-spectrum antibiotics are recommended for secondary bacterial infection along with topical eye ointments (Norsworthy 2003, Scott 2003).

Anticipated prognosis

Generally the prognosis for recovery is good; however, chronic tearing or rhinitis is possible. The prognosis is more guarded if the disease progresses to pneumonia. Some animals become carriers for the virus (Norsworthy 2003, Scott 2003).

Integrative veterinary therapies

An integrative approach to feline upper respiratory viral infections takes into consideration the target respiratory system as well as supporting general immune function against the virus. The use of therapeutic nutrients, medicinal herbs, and combination homeopathics that are anti-inflammatory, tissue-protective and immune enhancing can help speed recovery and prevent recurrences.

Nutrition
General considerations/rationale

While medical therapy is focused upon secondary bacterial infection, therapeutic nutrition adds glandular support for the tissue and organs of the respiratory and immune systems.

Appropriate nutrients

Nutritional/gland therapy: Glandular lung, adrenal, thymus, and bone marrow supply intrinsic nutrients that help to reduce cellular inflammation and improve immune organ function (see Gland Therapy in Chapter 2 for a more detailed explanation).

N,N-Dimethylglycine (DMG): N,N-Dimethylglycine has been widely researched in both humans and animals. It has been found to increase energy and enhance immune function (Barnes 1979, Graber 1981, Kendall 2000, Reap 1990, Walker 1988). In a double-blind study, Graber (1981) showed that DMG has a protective and therapeutic effect in people with pneumonia. Also, DMG can help the body to eliminate toxins that may predispose and cause the upper respiratory infections (Kendall 2003).

Betasitolsterol: Plant-derived sterols have been shown to have anti-inflammatory and antipyretic properties which appear to be similar to corticosteroids and aspirin (Gupta 1980). In addition, sterols have been proven to enhance immune function (Bouic 1996). Sterols have been found to be able to enhance T- lymphocyte production and moderate B cell activity, thereby helping to balance the immune response and indirectly reducing the risk of an autoimmune reaction (Bouic 1996).

Studies on cats with FIV indicate that sterols are believed to have an immune-modulating effect and help to maintain proper lymphocyte levels (Bouic 1997). Treated cats showed 20% mortality as compared to the nontreated cats' mortality of 75%. While the sterols have no direct antiviral properties, the balancing and stimulation of the immune system is enough to control the spread and effects of the virus.

Maitake mushrooms: Studies have shown that maitake mushrooms help enhance immune function and help organ systems maintain balance and homeostasis, and they improve the ability to handle stressful conditions (Nanba 1987).

L-Lysine: The herpes virus requires arginine to replicate. Lysine, which is an arginine antagonist, can reduce viral access and replication. It has been shown that l-lysine, taken orally, may be helpful in early treatment for FHV-1 infection and can reduce the severity of the disease. It is also thought that lysine can reduce viral shedding, especially in cats in stressful conditions such as a change in housing (Maggs 2003, Stiles 2002).

Chinese herbal medicine/acupuncture
General considerations/rationale
Feline upper respiratory disease is caused by infectious pathogens invading the body, especially during seasonal changes or under stressful conditions. The primary organ involved is the Lung. Because the Lung controls the Throat and Respiratory Tract, major signs seen in this condition include wheezing, pneumonia, and nasal discharge. The pathogen and immune system battle on the surface of the body, producing ocular and nasal discharges and fever. Treatment is aimed at decreasing nasal and ocular discharge, reducing fever, and combating the pathogen.

Appropriate Chinese herbs
Anemarrhena (Zhi mu): Possesses antibacterial properties (Yao Xue Qing Bao Tong Xun 1987). It also decreases fevers (Zhong Yao Xue, 1998).

Basket fern (Guan Zhong): A very effective antiviral herb (Zhong Yao Xue 1998).

Bupleurum (Chai hu): Has both antiviral and antibiotic properties (Wang Sheng Chun 1998, Zhong Yao Xue 1988). It stimulates both humoral and cellular immunity in mice (Shang Hai Yi Ke Da Xue Xue Bao 1986), which suggests it may help affected cats control the pathogen. Finally it was shown to be effective at decreasing fevers caused by 2, 4-dinitrophenol, yeast, or illness (Zhang Qing Ye 1997).

Chrysanthemum (Ju hua): Has demonstrated antibacterial effects (Yi Xue Ji Shu Zi Liao 1974).

Forsythia (Lian qiao): Contains rengynic acid, which has shown antiviral effects (Zhang 2002). Forsythia also inhibits the growth of bacteria (Ma 1982).

Gypsum (Shi gao): Has antipyretic effects. In one study of 200 patients with fevers, 90% experienced significant reduction of temperature (Xin Zhong Yi 1980). It increases the phagocytic activity of macrophages (Zhong Yao Xue 1998), which may help the patients fight off infection.

Honeysuckle (Jin yin hua): Has chlorogenic acid and isochlorogenic acid. These compounds have demonstrated the ability to inhibit the growth of various bacteria (Xin Yi Xue 1975, Jiang Xi Xin Yi Yao 1960). It has shown anti-inflammatory and antipyretic effects (Shan Xi Yi Kan 1960).

Isatis leaves (Da qing ye): Have antiviral and antibiotic properties (Zhong Yao Xue 1998, Fu Jian Zhong Yi Yao 1998). Furthermore, they stimulate immunity by increasing the phagocytic activity of macrophages (Li 1996).

Pueraria (Ge gen): Reduces fevers. Pueraria decreased body temperature in rabbits with typhoparatyphoid vaccine-induced fever (Modern TCM Pharmacology 1997).

Acupuncture
Sinusitis, rhinitis and the common cold are all on the World Health Organization's list of disorders that respond to acupuncture (World Health Organization 2006).

Homotoxicology
General considerations/rationale
Viral infections all fall into the Impregnation Phase. Full recovery can occur if the immune system can defeat the virus and eliminate the associated homotoxins. Many feline viruses cause persistent carrier state infections, and an active infection can occur following immunosuppressive events (stress, pregnancy, medications, etc.). Chronic viral infections can activate chronic, recurrent inflammatory conditions, which are a hallmark of Impregnation Phase diseases. Conditions such as chronic stomatitis, pharyngitis, asthma, and dental cervical neck lesions may have roots in Impregnation Phase homotoxicoses. As the circumstances progress, they can lead to Degeneration Phase and Dedifferentiation Phase conditions. Antibiotics may disturb the immune system and lead to progressive vicariation. Therefore, clinicians should attempt to handle such conditions naturally wherever possible, and should be aware of signs of regressive vicariation following recovery from these infections. L-lysine is particularly helpful in the treatment of feline herpes virus infections and recurrences (Norsworthy 2004). Properly handling regressive vicariation may prevent or delay the development of other chronic diseases in these patients.

Vaccination is a helpful tool in avoiding respiratory infections in cats, but it is advisable to avoid overvaccination because vaccinations lead directly to Impregnation Phase homotoxicoses. Many practitioners routinely administer booster vaccinations for feline upper respiratory diseases every three years instead of annually, as recommended by most pharmaceutical vaccine manufacturers.

Appropriate homotoxicology formulas
There is no specific research with feline viral infections, but extrapolation of human data makes this theoretically useful data. The authors have used these remedies frequently, especially in hard-to-control sinus and upper respiratory cases. The clinical results indicate that further research is desirable. For treatment plans in which biological therapy is desired, consider the following formulas:

Aconitum homaccord: Use in early febrile phases. This remedy is common to *Barijodeel, Bryaconeel, Echinacea compositum, Gripp-Heel, Rhododendroneel, Spascupreel, Strophanthus compositum, Traumeel, BHI-Chamomilla Complex,* and *BHI-FluPlus,* among others. Aconitum is one of the most important homeopathic fever remedies, especially when the patient displays hot skin; great anxiety;

rapid, tense pulse; strong and possibly irregular heartbeat; alternating fever and chills; possible hyperthermia with sudden onset of symptoms; and violence of the complaints. The restlessness and anguish are always seen, as are redness of the mucosa, and the sensation of distension, heaviness, pressure, and tension in the gastrointestinal tract. Stools contain mucus and bile. There is flatulent distension with small, frequent stools, and an urging to defecate, all of which are characteristic of the remedy. Low potencies are normally given in pyrexia and organic complaints, catarrhs, neuralgic symptoms with paraesthesia, hyperthermia, and encephalitis with very high temperatures (e.g., post-vaccinial encephalitis or meningo-encephalitis (Reckeweg 2002).

Apis homaccord: Helps to remove excess fluid accumulations such as edema and ascites when combined with *Lymphomyosot*.

Belladonna homaccord: Treats seizures and screaming out at night. Violent delirium is characteristic of Belladonna, above all in fever. Belladonna's typical action on the eyes is also well-known, with cramps in the muscles of the eyes and eyelids, enlargement of the pupils, and, in particular, an inflammatory or irritative condition of the conjunctiva with great photophobia, lachrymation, and pain. Belladonna is indicated in incipient boils; tonsilitis; and surface inflammations such as erysipelas, conjunctivitis, and scarlet fever. It is also indicated in otitis, cholangitis, meningitis, and other inflammatory affections. A delirious state occurs with a violent rise in temperature with considerably raised sensitivity of all the senses and a disproportionate sensitivity to touch, noises, light, and cold air—especially draughts and jarring—as can be the case in meningitis. Along with nasal catarrhs, there may be catarrhs of the larynx and trachea with slight mucus, accompanied a typical dry, rough, and barking cough with hoarseness.

In the digestive organs, Belladonna affects acute gastric catarrhs (Reckeweg 2002). The classical remedy, Dulcamara, is used for cases manifesting symptoms of diarrhea, vomiting, colic, skin rash, convulsions, and paralysis; death is a possible outcome. The complaints of Dulcamara-type cases are aggravated by cold, damp weather and weather changes, especially rainy weather. Increased mucosal secretions are also typical of Dulcamara-type symptoms. The nose is usually blocked (sinusitis), and the discharge is more copious in the warmth. The saliva is tough and soap-like. Acute gastritis and enteritis; dysentery with violent stomach pains; colic; mucous, sour, or dysenteric watery stools; pains persisting even after the stool that are associated with colic; and rheumatic complaints signal the possible need for this remedy (Reckeweg 2002).

BHI-Sinus: Used for sinusitis, this remedy contains Echinacea angustifolia, Aconitum, Sanguinaria, Baptisia, Eupatorium perfoliatum, Pulsatilla, Thuja, Phytolacca, Rhus toxicodendron, Arnica, Bryonia, Gelsemium, and Euphorbium.

Bronchalis: Treats bronchial complaints.

Causticum compositum: Causticum (also in *Barijodeel, Husteel, BHI-Throat*, etc.) symptoms are often brought on by dry cold, e.g., cases with hoarseness and laryngitis, dryness and rawness in the throat, and pain on coughing. Typical symptoms include tiredness, painful/battered sensations, and pain in the chest; thus Causticum is an excellent remedy in influenza along with Eupatorium perfoliatum, Rhus toxicodendron, Aconitum, and others (Reckeweg 2002). This remedy also contains Aconitum (see *Aconitum homaccord*) and Fumaricum acidum (common to *Coenzyme compositum, Cor compositum, Hepar compositum, Thyroidea compositum, BHI-Enzyme*, etc.). Symptoms from this proving are noted for their effect on the upper respiratory system. Hoarseness, dry cough, sore and raw throat, sneezing, catarrh, head heaviness, difficultly breathing, sneezing, and catarrh extending to the frontal sinuses and associated with a post-nasal drip from allergies are noted. Histamine is used for its obvious signs in various allergic and inflammatory conditions (it is contained in *Hepar compositum, Histamin-Heel, Luffa compositum-Heel nasal spray, and Ubichinon compositum*).

Cerebrum compositum: Supports and detoxifies the brain. Hyoscyamus is included for symptoms of cerebral irritation with convulsions, muscle twitching; catalepsy; epileptiform spasms; eye conditions; conjunctivitis; spasmodic nocturnal attacks of cough; with expectoration of green mucus on coughing; dryness in the throat, larynx, and lungs; stomach pains; and inflammation of the gastric mucosa and intestines with retching, vomiting, colic, and diarrhea (Reckeweg 2002).

Coenzyme compositum: Provides energy metabolism support for exhausted tissues and helps to reverse some effects of antibiotic therapy. The component Beta vulgaris reactivates cell respiration and can regenerate blocked respiratory enzymes, and is therefore indicated in all cellular phases (Impregnation, Degeneration, and Neoplasm), and in viral diseases, viral influenza, and poliomyelitis in humans (Reckeweg 2002). Beta vulgaris has been the subject of research concerning mitochondrial elements, and while the mechanism of action is not known, plant extracts contain many mitochondrial enzymes and energy production catalysts, which may be involved in its observed action.

Alpha-ketoglutaricum acidum, which is also contained in *Cor compositum, Cutis compositum, Hepar compositum, Syzygium compositum, Thyroidea compositum*, and *BHI-Enzyme*, is an active factor in the citric acid cycle and in redox systems. It is used in all kinds of impregnation phases, and to improve cell respiration.

Alpha-ketoglutaric acid, among all the catalysts of the citric acid cycle, has a particularly prominent symptom: the patient always gets too little air, both in asthma and in emphysema, as well as in such conditions as allergic rhinitis and influenza.

Natrium oxalaceticum (contained in *BHI-Enzyme, Cor compositum, Ginseng compositum, Hepar compositum, Mucosa compositum, Thyroidea compositum, Ubichinon compositum,* etc.) is another active factor of the citric acid cycle and redox systems. It is used in Impregnation Phases of all kinds and to improve cell respiration. Special indications for this component include asthmatic bronchitis; sinusitis; otitis media; and all acute and chronic inflammations of the nasopharynx, lungs, and bronchi. In many cases Natrum oxalaceticum can cut short the acute common cold.

This remedy contains the following minerals: Mercurius sublimatus corrosivus, Phosphorus, Zincum metallicum, Hepar sulfuris, Arsenicum album, Argentum nitricum, and Sulphur. It contains the following nosodes: Grippe-nosode, Streptococcinum, Staphylococcinum, and Pyrogenium. It contains the zoological component Lachesis (snake venom) and the homeopathically prepared allopathic drug Cortison acetate.

Discus compositum: Used for the spinal, meningeal, and paralytic forms of this disease. It contains Ranunculus rulbosus to treat rheumatic and neuralgic symptoms, skin eruptions—particularly closely grouped crops of vesicles—coryza with a discharge of viscid mucus, and possibly ulceration of the nasal mucosa that is accompanied by the characteristic chest complaints with shortness of breath and a sense of constriction. These may be accompanied by gastric symptoms with purging, eructations and nausea, burning in the stomach, abdominal rumbling, and bleeding hemorrhoids. The skin eruptions are frequently present on the palms of the hands in the form of desquamating vesicular eruptions (Reckeweg 2002).

Droperteel: Treats bronchitis, deep cough, and asthma.

Drosera homaccord: Treats bronchiolitis, "whooping" cough-like disorders, and asthma.

Echinacea compositum: This terribly important formula deserves more extensive consideration because it can stimulate host defenses, particularly against bacterial invaders. It is the homotoxicologist's "antibiotic," and while it provides no antibacterial activity, its action stimulates host defenses against bacterial infections. It contains, among many other useful remedies, Echinacea angustifolia (also in *Belladonna homaccord, Euphorbium compositum, Mercurius-Heel, Tonsilla compositum,* and *Traumeel*) and Rhus toxicodendron (also in *Aesculus compositum, Arnica-Heel, Echinacea compositum, Gelsemium homaccord, NeuralgoRheum, BHI-Headache, BHI-Inflammation,* and many others). It is characteristically used in a

wide variety of inflammations, e.g., violent conjunctivitis with severe photophobia; greenish-yellow, offensive nasal discharge; gastroenteritis with watery, bloody, mucous stools and tenesmus; a tormenting, dry cough with bloody, purulent sputum; skin eruptions like measles or vesicular eruptions all over the body; and disturbances of consciousness in febrile conditions (Reckeweg 2002).

It contains Hepar sulphuris calcareum (also in *Belladonna homaccord, Cantharis compositum, Coenzyme compositum, Euphorbium compositum, Mercurius-Heel, Solidago compositum, Traumeel, BHI-Chamomilla Complex, BHI-Enzyme, BHI-Infection, BHI-Inflammation,* and others). Hepar sulph is the remedy for chronic catarrhs of the respiratory organs with expectoration of purulent sputum, croupy cough with rattling mucus but difficulty in expectorating. Here, Hepar sulph is more frequently indicated after Aconitum or Spongia. Because of its action in suppurations, Hepar sulph (along with *Graphites homaccord* and other remedies) is the main remedy in protracted pneumonia with the risk of abscess formation, abscesses of the tonsils, and purulent, offensive discharge from the ears. Hepar sulph also may help where there is a chronic tendency to catch cold (cf. Thuja). The component Argentum nitricum (also common to *Atropinum compositum, Euphorbium compositum, Mucosa compositum, Pectus-Heel, Phosphor homaccord, BHI-Inflammation,* and *BHI-Throat*) is indicated in hoarseness with roughness and scratching in the throat; polyps of the vocal cords; and catarrh of the pharynx, ears, and conjunctiva.

Echinacea compositum includes Arnica (common to *Aesculus compositum, Arnica-Heel, Aurumheel, Barijodeel, Belladonna compositum, Causticum compositum, Pectus-Heel, Traumeel, BHI-Allergy, BHI-Inflammation, BHI-Throat,* and many others), which has indications for septic states and coughing with chest pain. It also contains Arsenicum album (also in *BHI-Chest, BHI-Cough, Arsuraneel, Atropinum compositum, Causticum compositum, Pectus-Heel, Traumeel,* etc.) for asthma—particularly at night—excoriating discharges, burning coryza, and conjunctivitis with burning secretion. Cortisone (common to *Pulsatilla compositum, Thyroidea compositum, Tonsilla compositum,* etc.) treats inflammation of the mucosae of the eye and of the respiratory organs, as well as asthma. Influenzinum (also in *Ginseng compositum*) treats hoarseness, bronchial asthma, chronic polysinusitis and other sequelae of influenza, iatrogenic damage, and parainfluenzal diseases. Lachesis (also in *Gripp-Heel, Klimakteel, Mercurius-Heel, Mucosa compositum,* and *BHI-Inflammation*) is suited to septic illnesses and decomposition of the blood, as well as thrombocytopaenic purpura, asthma, influenza, laryngitis, sore throat, uveitis, nasal catarrh with discharge, otitis media, etc.

Phosphorus (also in *Apis homaccord, Galium-Heel, Gripp-Heel, Mucosa compositum, Nasoheel, Pectus-Heel, Phosphor homaccord, Secale compositum, BHI-FluPlus, BHI-Sinus, BHI-Throat*, etc.) is an effective hemorrhage remedy; it is indicated in purpura, bruises, petechiae, and hematoma. It is also indicated in inflammation of the respiratory organs, severe infectious diseases, disorders in convalescence, conditions of exhaustion, in bronchial pneumonia, colds which proceed from the nose downward into the trachea and bronchi, and pneumonia. Phosphorus is given orally or injected, in the potencies 10 X, 30 X, 200 X, and 1,000 X. The component Sanguinaria is a routine remedy for coryza and colds, because of its relationship to chest complaints and colds. There is pain and burning in the mouth, chest, larynx, and trachea when coughing and breathing, that is worse at night. It is used against pharyngitis, tracheitis, and nasal polypi, along with a constitutional remedy such as Calcium carbonicum. It is excellent in influenzal, feverish, and catarrhal conditions when combined with Aconitum, Bryonia, Eupatorium perfoliatum and others. The typical descending, burning sensation in all the mucosa of the respiratory tract should bring Causticum to mind (see *Causticum compositum*, above.) Sanguinaria can be used in pneumonia, particularly in the lower lobes, where it rivals Chelidonium sanguinaria (in the 30 X potency). It has been used in many cases of bronchiectasis with tough, thick, offensive expectoration.

Thuja (common to *Atropinum compositum, Galium-Heel, Psorinoheel, BHI-Allergy, BHI-Inflammation,* and *BHI-Sinus*) treats asthmatic bronchitis with copious expectoration at night, and vaccination reactions (Reckeweg 2002). This also contains Gelsemium (see *Gelsemium homaccord*), Aconitum (see *Aconitum homaccord*), Euphorbium (see *Euphorbium compositum*), Pulsatilla, Sulphur (see *Causticum compositum*), Mercurius corrosives, and Eupatorium (see *BHI-FluPlus*).

Echinacea compositum also contains Euphorbium(also in *BHI-Sinus*), with indications for inflammation of the respiratory passages and irritation of mucous membranes leading to catarrhs of the eyes, nose, larynx. It is also indicated for eustachian catarrh with swelling of the middle ear and a sensation of complete deafness in the affected ear. It is a supporting remedy in nasal ulceration, and it is indicated for pharyngitis, sinusitis, and catarrhs of various sinuses.

Mucosa nasalis suis (also in *Mucosa compositum*) treats the nasal mucous membrane. The main indications are chronic sinusitis, polysinusitis—often with offensive nasal discharges along with nasal polypi—and mucus in the throat. Sinusitis nosode is used in acute and chronic suppuration of the sinuses or bloody discharge. Other symptoms include itching and tickling of the internal sinuses with obstruction and sneezing; lymphadenopathy;

nasal ulcers; asthma; rough, scratchy throat associated with mucus and expectoration of phlegm; and illnesses which may be influenced from the nasal mucosa, e.g. (experimentally) in duodenal and gastric ulcer, etc. It is also used for conjunctivitis with sticky mucus and pus and burning irritation with tear formation (Reckeweg 2002). This remedy also contains Hepar sulph, Argentum, (see Echinacea comp), and Pulsatilla (see *Causticum compositum*).

Engystol N: Stimulates the immune system (Ben-Yakir 2004). This remedy has been used for viral infections for many years (Fimiani 2000, Oberbaun 2005); It is a combination preparation containing Vincetoxicum hyrundinaria in 6X, 10X, and 30X potencies. Vincetoxicum (Asclepias vincetoxicum) has the main indications of acute febrile reaction phases, glandular fever, lymphadenitis, and viral diseases (Reckeweg 2002). *Engystol N* also has Sulphur (see *Causticum compositum*) in 4 X and 10 X potencies, which has been studied extensively. It has been used to treat bronchitis, sinusitis, pharyngitis, herpes, sore throat, laryngitis, and other infections. It was studied in 1,479 patients in Europe with very good results and excellent tolerance in flu and febrile conditions (Herzberger, Weiser 1997). Another study assessing *Engystol* as a prophylactic remedy indicated that it appeared to affect only the humoral phase of immunodefense, and the authors theorized that 1 injection per week would be best suited for prophylactic immunostimulation (Heilman 1994).

Euphorbium compositum: An antiviral agent that helps with respiratory signs and limiting viral numbers in initial exposures. It has demonstrated in vitro viral inhibition for the following viruses: influenza A, respiratory syncytial virus, and type I herpes simplex virus (HSV1) (Glatthaar-Saalmüller 2001).

FluPlus: Contains the ingredient Anas barabriae, hepatis et cordis extractum, a nosode made from duck liver, which is a source of flu virus (also known as Oscillococcinum). Use at the onset of a flu-like illness. The component Eupatorium perfoliatum (common to *Echinacea compositum* and *Gripp-Heel*) is said to complement Anas barabariae and hepatis et cordis extractum (Chavanon 1935, Schmid et al.) It is indicated for headache with a chill; aversion to light; coryza with aching in every bone; dry throat so the patient can hardly talk; difficult breathing; perspiration; hard, dry cough; soreness in the chest; intense ache in the back and limbs; stiffness of the arms and fingers; sleeplessness with fever; chill with thirst; fever preceded by thirst; remittent fever; dengue fever (Hering 1983); catarrhal fevers; influenza with pains in the limbs; influenza; parainfluenzal feverish diseases; and rheumatism (Reckeweg 2002).

Mercurius sublimatus corrosivus (common to Echinacea compositum, et al.) has characteristic mercurial action in tonsilitis, affections of the mucosa, salivation, fluent coryza, keratitis, iritis, gingivitis, and influenza, i.e. highly acute inflammations of the mucosae of the eyes, oral cavity, and tonsils (Reckeweg 2002). Zincum metallicum is indicated in classical homeopathy for the treatment of fever and chills (Clarke). Zinc deficiency has been found in immunodeficiencies (Yoffe 1986), including those in which zinc decreases in a parallel fashion to the evolution of the disease (Dousset et al. 1994). Zinc gluconate in homeopathic dilution appeared beneficial in a randomized, double-blind, placebo-controlled study to control viral flu (Nossas et al. 1996). Zinc chloride associated with Sanguinaria has demonstrated antimicrobial properties in vitro (Gomez 1987). Also contains Lachesis, Phosphorus (see *Echinacea compositum*), Pulsatilla, Sulphur (see *Causticum compositum*), and Aconitum (see *Aconitum Homaccord*).

Galium-Heel: Provides cellular detoxification and repair, activation of the nonspecific host defenses, support in vaccine reactions, and renal tubular support. Phase remedy in Deposition, Degeneration, and Dedifferentiation phase conditions.

Gelsemium homaccord: Treats headache and neuralgia. Gelsemium is quite particularly indicated in states of paralysis, e.g., after apoplexy and also in post-diphtheritic paralysis. The stools are copious and yellow, and influenzal catarrhs may be seen when thin, fluent nasal discharge and bloody mucus is blown out. A brief summary includes nervous disorders, infectious diseases, paralysis, and spasmodic conditions (Reckeweg 2002). Gelsemium is common to *Echinacea compositum*.

Ginseng compositum: See *Causticum compositum* for common remedies.

Ginseng compositum: Provides constitutional improvement during chronic disease (Reckeweg 2000).

Gripp-Heel: An antiviral for cold and flu-like symptoms (Rabe 2004). Aconitum acts in *Gripp-Heel* (in D4) specifically against colds (also see *Aconitum homaccord*); also contains Eupatorium perfoliatum (see *FluPlus*), Lachesis (see *Echinacea compositum*) for hot flushes, sore throat, septic course); Bryonia for pleuritis, dry cough, and thirst; and Phosphorus (see *Echinacea compositum*) when there is a risk of pneumonia or bronchopneumonia. One of 170 German soldiers compared acetylsalicylic acid to *Gripp-Heel* and found that the homeopathic preparation was comparable to acetylsalicylic acid in the beneficial changes in the clinical findings and in the length of time the patients were unable to work (Maiwald et al. 1993).

Gripp-Heel is most effective if given early in the disease process. Endogenous immunity can no longer be adequately activated once the illness has advanced. In uncomplicated cases the viral infection lasts only a few days, unless secondary infections arise, which may result in

persistence, particularly with immunsuppressed patients. Antiphlogistic and antipyretic medicines repress the symptoms but delay healing, because they interfere with normal biological functions. *Gripp-Heel* is mentioned in medical literature as early as 1954; it has been said that the total effect corresponds to an acceleration of mesenchymal immune reaction (Till 1986).

Hepar compositum: Provides liver drainage and detoxification.

Husteel: Treats dry, hacking coughs.

Lymphomyosot: Provides lymph drainage and detoxification, hormonal support, and immune support. Myosotis arvensis acts particularly on the respiratory organs and the lungs. Characteristic symptoms include a cough with profuse mucopurulent expectoration, retching and vomiting while coughing, and aggravation during meals or immediately afterward.

Mercurius-Heel: Has antiviral elements and treats stomatitis and peritonsillar inflammation.

Mezereum homaccord: Treats vesicular lesions associated with herpes infections in humans and itching associated with herpes virus impregnation. Feline herpes virus type 1 infections can cause ulcerations near the nasal openings; and *Mezereum homaccord* and *Lamioflur* may help these cats.

Molybdan compositum: Can supply trace minerals that may prove helpful in supporting recovery due to the poor nutritional state that is often characteristic of this disease (Reckeweg 2000).

Mucosa compositum: Provides repair, detoxification, and drainage of mucosal tissues throughout the body in the Degeneration Phase and in recovery periods following other illnesses or iatrogenic damage such as that which follows antibiotic of NSAID therapy. Supports mucous membranes throughout the body, including the urogenital, respiratory, and gastrointestinal systems, and especially during recovery after the acute infection has waned.

Nasoheel: Treats acute and chronic rhinitis and sinusitis (Reckeweg 2000). Contains Ammonium carbonicum for chronic and acute colds, mucus in chest with coughs but no expectoration and infectious diseases with circulatory insufficiency and inflammations of the oral cavity and of the respiratory passages. Cistus canadensis is indicated in dryness of the oral and pharyngeal mucosa, colds that settle in the throat, lymphadenitis, and pulmonary diseases. Kali bichromicum (also in *Mucosa compositum*, *BHI-Sinus*, etc.) can be helpful in a few characteristic symptoms, e.g., catarrhal conditions of the mucosa of the respiratory passages and migratory pains with possible alternation of catarrhal and rheumatic complaints. Especially characteristic of Kali bichromicum are the tough, stringy mucous secretions that occur with catarrhs of the sinuses, nose, bronchi, etc. Inflammations of the eyelids and conjunctivitis also occur, sometimes with corneal ulcers with a punched-out appearance. These ulcerations may be found on the gums, tongue, and lips, and in gastric and duodenal tissues.

Lemna minor is included for anosmia (a symptom that is hard to identify in cats but may manifest as anorexia); scabby, purulent, offensive, and bloody nasal catarrhs; that sometimes appear with polyps and pharyngeal catarrh; and chronic sniffles. Melilotus officinalis is included for blood congestion, not only of the brain, but also of the lungs and rectum; that symptom is associated with epistaxis and hemoptysis. The component Natrum nitricum is mainly indicated for asthma, dyspnea with hemorrhagic tendencies, infections, rheumatism, and conditions of weakness (Reckeweg 2002). This remedy also contains Phosphorus (see *Echinacea compositum*).

Natrium homaccord: Treats catarrh of the mucous membranes, sudden chills, and croupy inflammation with a tendency toward hemorrhage.

Phosphor homaccord: Treats laryngitis, pharyngitis, hemorrhages or petechial bleeding, and bruising.

Pulsatilla compositum: Used for chronic, nonresponsive cases with regulation rigidity. Pulsatilla (common to *Abropernol, Coenzyme compositum, Cruroheel, Echinacea compositum, Euphorbium compositum, Ginseng compositum, Mucosa compositum, Pulsatilla compositum, Rhododendroneel, Thyroidia compositum, Tonsilla compositum, Viburcol, BHI-Chamomilla Complex, BHI-Cold, BHI-Enzyme, BHI-FluPlus, BHI-Inflammation,* and *BHI-Sinus*) is indicated for yellowish-green secretions, particularly in the mornings and in the evenings. Often the discharges are thin and runny. There is catarrh in the larynx and air passages, coughing with tenacious mucus, and bronchitis and broncho-pneumonia.

Solidago compositum: Provides drainage and support of the urogenital tract.

Spascupreel: Treats spasmodic cough.

Tartephedreel: Used for bronchial catarrh and severe, unrelenting coughs, as well as catarrhal respiratory tract involvement.

Thyroidea compositum: Used in recovery phases to normalize the hormonal axis and cleanse the deep matrix. Provides hormonal support and detoxification of matrix elements.

Tonsilla compositum: Provides Impregnation Phase and Degeneration Phase support of immune organs, particularly the spleen and bone marrow. Activates reticuloendothelial elements in deeper homotoxicoses. Contains Mercurius solubilis Hahnemanni for mucosal inflammations of the respiratory passages, gastrointestinal tract, and urinary and reproductive organs; skin diseases; inflammation of the tonsils, lymph glands, liver, and kidneys; inflammation of other glandular organs; osteal-

gia and rheumatism; enervating diseases; and cerebral angiosclerosis (Reckeweg 2002).

Traumeel S: Used for gingivitis, stomatitis, modulation of inflammation, and in regulation rigidity cases to activate sulfur-containing enzyme systems. Traumeel S treats Impregnation Phases and retoxications of all kinds, as well as allergic illnesses, bronchial asthma, and vasomotor rhinitis. Histamine, which is common to *Hepar compositum* and *BHI-Allergy*, is used in Inflammation phases. Histamine is decisively important for the initial phase of Inflammation. It widens the capillaries to allow an infusion of plasma into the tissues, resulting in the consecutive symptoms of pain, swelling, heat, and redness. Histamine becomes especially biologically dangerous if such inflammations are suppressed.

Ubichinon compositum: Used for mitochondrial energy metabolism, in Degeneration Phase disorders, and after long courses of antibiotic therapy. *Ubichinon compositum* provides deeper support of metabolism than *Coenzyme compositum* and helps activate mitochondrial function after iatrogenic damage from antibiotics and other medicants. Benzochinon parabenzoquinone is a powerful remedy in this combination, with certain protective functions against viral infections and other chronic disease. One should always think of parabenzoquinone in almost an incurable, unremitting dyspnea that has the possibility of transition into respiratory paralysis. It can also help with a state of paresis occurring after poliomyelitis, meningeal irritation, encephalitis or vaccinations, and where there is disturbance in neuromuscular coordination (Reckeweg 2002).

The important component, Sulphur, is successful in acute and chronic cases. It reactivates enzyme-based detoxifying procedures, particularly when well-indicated remedies are not working. Suppression of eliminations—whether they are an Excretion Phase or some inflammation, which cleanse the body of homotoxins—occurs when enzyme systems are entrusted with this detoxifying function and are inhibited or destroyed. Enzyme damage creates an Impregnation Phase or deeper phase. Because Sulphur is one of the most important components of tissue in the body, the basic substance of the mesenchyme in all cases which do not respond to well-indicated biotherapeutic or antihomotoxic remedies, Sulphur-containing formulas (also in *Cerebrum compositum, Coenzyme compositum, Echinacea compositum, Engystol, Ginseng compositum, Hepar compositum, Molybdan compositum, Mucosa compositum, Psorinoheel, Pulsatilla compositum, Spigelon, Sulfur-Heel, Thyroidea compositum, Tonsilla compositum, Ubichinon compositum, BHI-Allergy, BHI-Asthma, BHI-Chest, BHI-Cold, BHI-Enzyme, BHI-FluPlus, BHI-Hayfever,* and many others) should be given intercurrently, e.g. as an intravenous injection, e.g. in acute pneumonia, tuberculosis in its various forms, or any one of numerous cellular phases, and in acute and chronic inflammations of the respiratory organs (Reckeweg 2002). Also contains Arnica and Arsenicum album (see *Echinacea compositum*).

Authors' suggested protocols

Nutrition

Bronchus/lung and immune support formulas: 1 to 2 tablets BID.

Betathyme: One-half capsule BID.

Maitake DMG: One-half to 1 ml BID.

L-lysine: 250 mgs SID.

Chinese herbal medicine/acupuncture

Formula H40 Antiviral/Papillomas: 1 capsule per 10 pounds twice daily. In addition to the herbs discussed above, H40 Antiviral/Papillomas contains phragmites (Lu gen) and sweet wormwood (Qing hao) to help increase the efficacy of the formula.

Commonly recommended acupuncture points are LI4, GV14, LI11, and LU7 (Handbook of TCM Practitioners 1987).

Homotoxicology (Dose: 5 to 7 drops PO for cats)

Echinacea compositum IV, if possible, to start, combined with Coenzyme compositum. Lymphomysot, Engystol N, Gripp-Heel, and Echinacea compositum, combined and given orally 4 to 5 times daily the first 24 hours and then BID. Some cases may respond to Natrium homaccord as a single agent.

Broadfoot uses Nasoheel plus Euphorbium compositum BID-TID, with Engystol plus Gripp Heel or Echinacea compositum, as needed. Causticum and Ginseng also may be powerful adjuncts if indicated by symptoms.

Product sources

Nutrition

Bronchus/lung and immune support formulas: Animal Nutrition Technologies. **Alternatives:** Immune System Support—Standard Process Veterinary Formulas; Immuno Support—Rx Vitamins for Pets; Immugen—Thorne Veterinary Products.

Betathyme: Best for Your Pet. **Alternative:** Moducare—Thorne Veterinary Products.

Maitake DMG: Vetri Science.

L-lysine: Over the counter.

Chinese herbal medicine

Formula H40 Antiviral/Papillomas: Natural Solutions, Inc.

Homotoxicology

BHI/Heel Corporation

REFERENCES

Western medicine references

Ford RB, Levy JK. Infectious diseases of the respiratory tract. In: Sherding RG, ed. The cat: diseases and clinical management. New York: Churchill Livingstone, 1994:489–500.

Gaskell R, Dawson S. Feline respiratory disease. In: Greene CE, ed. Infectious diseases of the dog and cat. Philadelphia: Saunders, 1998:97–106.

Norsworthy, GD. Feline Rhinotracheitis Virus. In: Tilley L, Smith F. The 5-Minute Veterinary Consult: Canine and Feline, Blackwell Publishing, 2003.

Pedersen NC. Feline calicivirus infection. In: Pratt PW, ed. Feline infectious diseases. Goleta, CA: American Veterinary, 1988:61–67.

Scott FW. Calici Virus—Cats. In: Tilley L, Smith F. The 5-Minute Veterinary Consult: Canine and Feline, Blackwell Publishing, 2003.

IVM/nutrition references

Barnes L. B15: The politics of ergogenicity. *Physicians and Sports Medicine.* 1979;7(#11):17.

Bouic PJD, et al. Beta-sitosterol and beta-sitosterol glucoside stimulate human peripheral blood lymphocyte proliferation: Implications for their use as an immunomodulatory vitamin combination. *International Journal of Immunopharmacology* 1996;18:693–700.

Bouic PJD. Immunomodulation in HIV/AIDS: The Tygerberg Stellenbosch University experience. AIDS Bulletin published by the Medical Research Council of South Africa 6(3):18–20, Sept. 1997.

Graber G, Goust J, Glassman A, Kendall R, Loadholt C. Immunomodulating Properties of Dimethylglycine in Humans. *Journal of Infectious Disease.* 1981;143:101.

Gupta MB, Nath R, Srivastava N, et al. Anti-inflammatory and antipyretic activities of β-sitosterol. *Planta Medica* 1980;39: 157–163.

Kendall R, Lawson JW. Recent Findings on N,N-Dimethylglycine (DMG): A Nutrient for the New Millennium, *Townsend Letter for Doctors and Patients*, May 2000.

Kendall RV. Building Wellness with DMG. Topanga, CA: Freedom Press, 2003.

Maggs DJ, Nasisse MP, Kass PH. Efficacy of oral supplementation with L-lysine in cats latently infected with feline herpes virus, *American Journal of Veterinary Research*, 2003, 64(1): pp 37–42.

Reap E, Lawson J. Stimulation of the Immune Response by Dimethylglycine, a non-toxic metabolite. *Journal of Laboratory and Clinical Medicine.* 1990;115:481.

Stiles J, Townsend WM, Rogers QR, Krohne SG. Effect of oral administration of L-lysine on conjunctivitis caused by feline herpes virus in cats, *American Journal of Veterinary Research*, 2002, 63(1) pp99–103.

Walker M. Some Nutri-Clinical Applications of N,N-Dimethylglycine. *Townsend Letter for Doctors.* June 1988.

Nanba H, Hamaguchi AM, Kuroda H. The chemical structure of an antitumor polysaccharide in fruit bodies of Grifola frondosa (maitake). *Chem Pharm Bull* 1987;35:1162–1168.

Chinese herbal medicine/acupuncture references

Fu Jian Zhong Yi Yao (*Fujian Chinese Medicine and Herbology*), 1998;174:175.

Handbook of TCM Practitioners, Hunan College of TCM, Shanghai Science and Technology Press, Oct 1987, p154–156.

Jiang Xi Xin Yi Yao (*Jiangxi New Medicine and Herbology*), 1960 (1):34.

Li MZ, et al. The pharmadynamics of Re Du Qing Injection. *China Journal of Experimental Recipes.* 1996;2(6):24–30.

Ma ZY. *Shannxi Journal of Traditional Chinese Medicine and Herbs.* 1982;(4):58.

Modern TCM Pharmacology. Tianjin: Science and Technology Press; 1997.

Shan Xi Yi Kan (*Shanxi Journal of Medicine*), 1960; (10):32.

Shang Hai Yi Ke Da Xue Xue Bao (*Journal of Shanghai University of Medicine*), 1986; 13(1): 20.

Wang SC, et al. *Journal of Shizhen Medicine.* 1998;9(5): 418–419.

World Health Organization list of common conditions treatable by Chinese Medicine and Acupuncture. Available at: http//tcm/health-info.org/WHO-treatment-list.htm accessed 10/15/2006.

Xin Yi Xue (*New Medicine*), 1975; 6(3): 155.

Xin Zhong Yi (*New Chinese Medicine*), 1980;6:28.

Yao Xue Qing Bao Tong Xun (*Journal of Herbal Information*), 1987; 5(4):62.

Yi Xue Ji Shu Zi Liao (*Resource of Medical Techniques*), 1974;(1:2):113.

Zhang G, Song S, Ren J, Xu S. A New Compound from Forsythia suspense (Thunb.) Vahl with Antiviral Effect on RSV. *J of Herbal Pharmacotherapy.* 2002;2(3): 35–39.

Zhang QY, et al. *Journal of Traditional Chinese Medicine Material.* 1997;20(3):147–149.

Zhong Yao Xue (*Chinese Herbology*), 1988;103: 106.

Zhong Yao Xue (*Chinese Herbology*), 1998; 115: 119.

Zhong Yao Xue (*Chinese Herbology*), 1998; 174: 175.

Zhong Yao Xue (*Chinese Herbology*), 1998; 459: 462.

Homotoxicology references

Ben-Yakir S. Primary evaluation of homeopathic remedies injected via acupuncture points to reduce chronic high somatic cell counts in modern dairy farms. *Veterinary Acupuncture Newsletter*, 2004;Feb;27(1): pp 19–21.

Chavanon P. Therapeutique O.R.L. (E.N.T.) homeopathique. Imprimerie Saint-Denis. 1935.

Clarke JH. Dictionary and Materia Medica. Vol. 3:1595.

Dousset B, May T, Duboit F, Allavena C, Rabaud C, Nabet-Belleville F, Canton P. Relations of trace element status to immunological activity markers and progression of human immunodeficiency virus infection. Int Conf AIDS. Aug 1994; 7–12;10(1):p 159.

Fimiani V, Cavallaro A, Ainis O, Bottari C. Immunomodulatory effect of the homeopathic drug Engystol-N on some activities of isolated human leukocytes and in whole blood. *Immunopharmacol Immunotoxicol.* 2000.Feb;22(1): pp 103–15.

Glatthaar-Saalmüller B, Fallier-Becker P. Antiviral action of euphorbium compositum®and its components. *Forsch Komplementärmed Klass Naturheilkd.* 2001. 8:pp 207–212.

Gomez S, Baum RH. Antimicrobial properties of sanguinaria, stannous fluoride and zinc chloride on the growth and acid production of streptococcus mutans (*in vitro*). *Odontol Chil* 1987. Dec;35(2):pp 89–94.

Heilmann A. Combination injection preparation as a prophylactic for flu and common colds. *Bio Ther.* 1994;Oct; 12 (40):pp 249–253.

Hering C. Condensed Materia Medica. Jain Publishing Reprint, 1983.pp 405–408.

Herzberger G, Weiser M. Homeopathic treatment of infections of various origins: a prospective study. *Biol Med.* 1997. April: pp 73–77.

Maiwald L, et al. The therapy of the common cold. *Bio Ther.* 1993; Jan;11(1):pp 2–8.

Norsworthy G. Feline Rhinotracheitis Infection. In: Tilley L, Smith F. The 5-Minute Veterinary Consult: Canine and Feline, 3rd edition, Philadelphia: Lippincott Williams and Wilkins, 2004. pp 470–1.

Nossas SB, Macknin ML, Meddendorp SV, Mason P. Zinc gluconate lozenges for treating the common cold: double-blind, placebo-controlled study. *Ann Inter Med.* 1996;125:pp 81–88.

Oberbaum M, Glatthaar-Saalmuller B, Stolt P, Weiser M. Antiviral activity of Engystol: an in vitro analysis. *J Altern Complement Med.* 2005;Oct;11(5): pp 855–62.

Rabe A, Weiser M, Klein P. Effectiveness and tolerability of a homeopathic remedy compared with conventional therapy for mild viral infections. *International Journal of Clinical Practice*, 2004;58(9): pp 827–832.

Reckeweg H. Aconitum Napelus (Monkshood) homeopathic single remedy: Aconitum as an active factor in antihomotoxic biotherapeutics. *Biol Ther.* 1987;5(1).

Reckeweg H. Biotherapeutic Index: Ordinatio Antihomotoxica et Materia Medica, 5th ed. Baden-Baden, Germany: Biologische Heilmittel Heel GMBH, 2000. pp 366, 371–2.

Reckeweg H. Homeopathia Antihomotoxica Materia Medica, 4th ed. Baden-Baden, Germany: Aurelia-Verlag, 2002. p 120–1, 132, 147, 148–9, 152, 172–5, 176–9, 182, 217–20, 240, 293–4, 282–4, 307–8, 315–6, 340–2, 343–4, 350–2, 358, 366, 373, 382, 386, 412, 420, 426–7, 431, 445, 446, 489–90, 505, 508–9, 512–4, 521–2, 536–8, 555–60, 572, 597.

Schmid F, Rimpler M, Wemmer U. *Medicina Antihomotoxica*: 329.

Till MW. The effective principle of gripp-heel. *Biol Ther.* 1986. 4(3/4):pp 47, 52.

Yoffe B, Pollack S, Ben-Porath E, Zinder O, Barzilai D, Gershon H. Natural killer cell activity in post-necrotic cirrhotic patients as related to hepatitis-B virus infection and plasma zinc levels. *Immunol Lett.* 1986; Nov 17; 14(1):pp 15–19.

FELV, FIV, AND FIP

Definition and cause

Feline Immunodeficiency virus (FIV) is caused by a retrovirus from the same subfamily of viruses that causes HIV in people (lentiviruses). The virus is most commonly passed via a bite wound. The virus directly compromises the immune system, eventually leading to secondary infections and disease. The animal's immune function (both humoral and cellular) directly controls the activation of the virus and the inherent secondary infections such as persistent elevated fever, loss of appetite, anemia, respiratory infections, chronic gingivitis, chronic diarrhea, periodontal disease, loss of weight, neurological disorders, upper respiratory and lower urinary infections, and cancer (Barr 1993, 1995, 1997; English 1992; Hopper 1994; Macy 1994; Sherding 1994; Sparger 1991).

Feline leukemia (FeLV) is caused by a retrovirus. FeLV is spread by contact with infected cats and is similar to FIV in that it causes an immune suppression disease (See Section 5 Cancer, for more detailed information about cancer protocols) (Barr 2003, Rojko 1994).

Feline infectious peritonitis (FIP) is caused by a coronavirus that can incubate within the cat for years. Activation of the virus causes immune suppression resulting in a systemic disease with multiple secondary infections. Symptoms can include persistent fevers, infections in various organ systems such as lymphadenopathy, vomiting, diarrhea, fluid accumulation in the chest and/or abdomen, and pyogranulomas. The cause is feline coronavirus 1 and 2 (FCoV 1 and 2). Vaccinations for FIP are unreliable (McReynolds 1997, Norsworthy 1998, Scott 1997, Stoddart 1994, Weiss 1994).

Medical therapy rationale, drug(s) of choice, and nutritional recommendations

Medical therapy for FIV is directed toward the secondary infections and diseases. Antibiotics, corticosteroids, fluid therapy and immunomodulatory drugs such as immunoregulan, acemannan, and alpha interferon are normally recommended for therapy (Barr 1997, Hooper 1994, Macy 1994, Sherding 1994).

Medical therapy for FeLV includes immunomodulatory drugs such as alpha interferon. If neoplasia (lymphoma) is present, chemotherapy and immune-suppressing drugs such as corticosteriods are recommended (Barr 2003).

Medical therapy for FIP includes supportive care, fluid therapy, antibiotics, cortisone, immune-modulating drugs such as alpha interferon, and high-quality nutrition and vitamins (Norsworthy 1997, Scott 1997).

Anticipated prognosis

It is estimated that 20% of cats with FIV will die within 1 to 2 years of exposure and infection. Cats with a stronger immune system can live a normal life and remain free of symptoms of other secondary diseases (Barr 1997, Hooper 1994, Sparger 1991). Patients may convert to negative status, but this is rare. It is estimated that 50% of FeLV-positive cats die within 1 to 2 years (Barr 2003).

Both the wet and dry forms of FIP are most often fatal (McReynolds 1997, Scott 1997).

Integrative veterinary therapies

Conventional treatment offers supportive care along with immunomodulating drugs. The addition of integrative modalities can often improve immune competence and day-to-day quality of life. The addition of nutrients, nutriceuticals, medicinal herbs, and combination homeopathics that have anti-inflammatory and immune enhancing effects on the cells and organ systems can often improve clinical signs and further modulate immune function and the ability to control the spread of the virus.

Nutrition
General considerations/rationale
The nutritional approach adds glandular support for the organs of the immune system as well as nutrients to help decrease cellular inflammation.

Appropriate nutrients
Nutritional/gland therapy: Glandular adrenal, thymus, bone marrow, and spleen supply intrinsic nutrients that help to improve immune organ function (see Gland Therapy in Chapter 2 for a more detailed explanation).

Because feline viral diseases are systemic, it is recommended that blood be analyzed both medically and physiologically to determine real and impending organ involvement and disease. This helps clinicians to formulate therapeutic nutritional protocols that are specific for the cat (Cima 2000, Goldstein 2000) (see Chapter 2, Nutritional Blood Testing, for additional information).

Betasitolsterol: Plant-derived sterols have been shown to have anti-inflammatory and antipyretic properties (Gupta 1980). Sterols have been proven to enhance immune function and T- lymphocyte production, and moderate B cell activity, thereby helping to balance the immune response (Bouic 1996). In studies on cats with FIV, sterols are believed to have an immune-modulating effect and help to maintain proper lymphocyte levels (Bouic 1997). Treated cats showed a 20% mortality rate as compared to the nontreated cats' mortality rate of 75%. While the sterols have no direct antiviral properties, the balancing and stimulation of the immune system is enough to control the spread and effects of the virus.

Maitake mushrooms: Studies with maitake mushrooms have shown that they enhance immune function and the ability to handle stressful conditions, while helping organ systems maintain balance and homeostasis (Nanba 1987).

N,N-Dimethylglycine (DMG): DMG has been widely researched in both humans and animals. It has been found to increase energy and enhance immune function (Barnes

1979, Graber 1981, Kendall 2000, Reap 1990, Walker 1988). In a double-blind study, Graber (1981) showed that DMG has a protective and therapeutic effect in people. Also, DMG can help the body to eliminate toxins that may predispose and cause infections (Kendall 2003).

Vitamin C: Numerous papers, clinical trials, and books have been written about vitamin C's effects as an antioxidant, general stimulant for the immune system as well as its properties such as stimulating interferon production, activating natural killer cells (NK), and improving day-to-day quality of life. de la Fuente (1998) and Penn (1991) showed that vitamin C in combination with other vitamins significantly improved immune function as compared with placebos.

Chinese herbal medicine
General considerations/rationale
Both TCM and Western etiologies are similar. According to Traditional Chinese Medicine, these 3 diseases are external infectious pathogens. In addition to treating the cause (the external pathogen, or the virus), doctors recommend treating symptoms caused by the virus such as fever. In the cases of FeLV and FIV, immunodeficiency (Wei Qi deficiency) is a component of the diseases; therefore, stimulation of the immune system is beneficial.

Appropriate Chinese herbs
Anemarrhena (Zhi mu): Reduces fever (Zhong Yao Xue 1998).

Bupleurum (Chai hu): Well suited for use with viral illnesses. It is an immune stimulant. In experiments it has been shown to enhance the both humoral and cellular immunity in mice (Shang Hai Yi Ke Da Xue Xue Bao 1986). It has also demonstrated antiviral effects against several viruses. One investigation found activity against chick embryo flu virus and pneumonia virus in mice (Wang 1998). In humans it has an inhibitory effect on respiratory syncytial virus (RSV) (Liao 1999). Another study found antiviral effects against some influenza viruses, poliomyelitis virus, and hepatitis virus (Zhong Yao Xue 1998).

Dryopteris root (Guan zhong): Has demonstrated antiviral effects against influenza, adenovirus, encephalitis, and herpes B (Zhong Yao Xue 1998, Zhong Cao Yao Tong Xun, 1973).

Forsythia (Lian qiao): Contains rengynic acid, which has antiviral effects. It has been shown to inhibit RSV in vitro (Zhang 2002).

Gypsum (Shi gao): Rapidly decreases fevers. In one study of 200 patients with fevers, 90% experienced significant reduction of temperature (Xin Zhong Yi 1980). In addition it has immunostimulatory effects. It increases

the phagocytic activity of macrophages (Zhong Yao Xue 1998).

Honeysuckle (Jin yin hua): Has been shown to decrease the body temperature in rabbits with endotoxin-induced fever (Yang Lin 1998).

Isatis leaves (Da Qing ye): Enhance immunity. In mice they have been shown to enhance the phagocytic ability of macrophages and increase the content of serum lysozyme (Li 1996). In addition they have antiviral activity. They have been shown to have efficacy against influenza, measles, and encephalitis B (Fu Jian Zhong Yi Yao, 1998, Shang Hai Zhong Yi Yao Za Zhi 1963, Fu Jian Zhong Yi Yao, 1965).

Pueraria (Ge gen): Has antipyretic effects (Modern TCM Pharmacology, 1997).

Homotoxicology
General considerations/rationale
All viral infections constitute Impregnation Phase disorders. Because of the actual damage done to tissues, these 3 conditions frequently develop into Degeneration Phase homotoxicoses. In FeLV and FIV, progressive vicariation can lead to Dedifferentiation Phase disease.

FIV retrovirus infects local tissues and then spreads via lymphocytes and macrophages. Both CD4 and CD8 T-lymphocytes are infected. A gradual decrease in CD 4 T-cells occurs as the disease advances. FIV can further infect astrocytes and microglial cells in the brain. Drug therapy exists to slow advancement of the virus.

The FIP coronavirus attacks epithelial cells directly, is picked up by macrophages, and is carried to all parts of the body. Diseased cats develop a pyogranulamatous lesion, which destabilizes normal tissue leading to the 2 forms of the disease (dry and wet). There is no effective therapy for this condition once the chronic form develops.

FeLV retrovirus initially infects the tonsils and regional lymph nodes. Infection of B-lymphocytes spreads the disease systemically. FeLV is an RNA-containing virus with reverse transcriptase. This allows the RNA to encode DNA, which can be inserted into the host cat's genome. Altered DNA results in the development of lymphoid neoplasia and allows the virus to be transmitted genetically to offspring. The chronic forms of these diseases are treated symptomatically; homotoxicology attempts to normalize immune function, reduce homotoxin levels, promote repair of damaged tissues, and assist in managing symptoms of disease.

Appropriate homotoxicology formulas
Little feline-specific antihomotoxic research has been conducted; therefore, practitioners considering use biological therapy on these patients should inform clients of its unproven nature and then proceed as indicated. Remedy formulas to consider include:

Aconitum compositum: Used for fever and aches and flu-like symptoms.

Apis homaccord: When combined with Lymphomyosot is helpful in removing excess fluid accumulations such as edema and ascites.

Coenzyme compositum: Assists energy metabolism.

Echinacea compositum: Treats fever and bacterial infections.

Engystol N: Stimulates the immune system, although it is not directly antiviral (Ben-Yakir 2004). This remedy has been used for viral infections for many years (Fimiani 2000, Oberbaun 2005). There is a simple published protocol for regularly administering *Engystol N* and *Echinacea compositum* for FeLV-infected cats, but no there is no data regarding its efficacy (Serrentino 2002).

Euphorbium compositum: An antiviral agent that helps with respiratory signs and limits viral numbers in initial exposures (Glatthaar-Saalmüller 2001). There is no specific research with FeLV, FIV, or FIP, but extrapolation of human data makes this theoretically useful data. The authors have used this remedy frequently, especially in hard-to-control sinus and upper respiratory cases with the appearance of clinical result, making further research desirable.

Galium-Heel: Provides cellular detoxification and repair, activation of the nonspecific host defenses, support in vaccine reactions, and renal tubular support. Phase remedy in Deposition, Degeneration, and Dedifferentiation phase conditions.

Gripp-Heel: Antiviral for cold and flu-like symptoms (Rabe 2004).

Hepar compositum: Provides liver drainage and detoxification.

Lymphomyosot: Provides lymph drainage and detoxification.

Solidago compositum: Drains and supports the urogenital tract.

Thyroidea compositum: Provides hormonal support and detoxification of matrix elements.

Tonsilla compositum: Activates reticuloendothelial elements in deeper homotoxicoses.

Ubichinon compositum: Used for mitochondrial energy metabolism.

Viburcol: Useful in febrile stages, to moderate the patient, and improve the comfort level.

Authors' suggested protocols

Nutrition

Immune and blood/bone marrow support formulas: One-half to 1 tablet BID.

Betathyme: One-half capsule BID.
Maitake DMG: One-half ml BID.
Vitamin C: 250 mgs BID.

Chinese herbal medicine

H40 Antiviral/Papilloma: 1 capsule per 10 to 20 pounds twice daily to effect. In addition to the herbs listed above, H40 Antiviral/Papilloma contains chrysanthemum (Ju hua), phragmites (Lu gen), and sweet wormwood (Qing hao). In general, cats with FeLV and FIV respond better than those with FIP. Cats with FIP usually do not show marked or prolonged response.

Homotoxicology (Dose: 5 drops PO for cat)

Autosanguis therapy can prove helpful in these cases.

FeLV and FIV protocol: Engystol N, Gripp-Heel, AND/OR Euphorbium compositum, Lymphomyosot, Galium-Heel, mixed together and given orally BID. Tonsilla compositum, Coenzyme compositum, Ubichinon compositum mixed together and given orally every 3 days.

FIP protocol: Engystol N, Euphorbium compositum, Lymphomyosot, Galium-Heel, Mucosa compositum, Ranunculus homaccord, Merezeum Homaccord, and Ginseng compositum mixed together and given orally BID. In wet FIP add Apis homaccord to the BID mixture. For tissue support, give the following formula orally every 3 days: Tonsilla compositum, Coenzyme compositum, and Ubichinon compositum mixed together.

Product sources

Nutrition

Immune and blood/bone marrow support formulas: Animal Nutrition Technologies. **Alternatives:** Immune System Support—Standard Process Veterinary Formulas; Immuno Support—Rx Vitamins for Pets; Immugen—Thorne Veterinary Products.

Betathyme: Best for Your Pet. **Alternative:** Moducare—Thorne Veterinary Products.

Maitake DMG: Vetri Science.

Vitamin C: Over the counter.

Chinese herbal medicine

Formula H40 Antiviral/Papilloma: Natural Solutions, Inc.

Homotoxicology

BHI/Heel Corporation

REFERENCES

Western medicine references for FIV

Barr MC, Olsen CW, Scott FW. Feline viral diseases. In: Ettinger SJ, Feldman EC, eds. Textbook of Veterinary Medicine. Philadelphia: WB Saunders Co. 1995: 409–435.

Barr MC. Feline immunodeficiency virus. In: Tilley L, Smith F. The 5 Minute Veterinary Consult: Canine and Feline. Baltimore: Williams and Wilkins 1997: 584–5.

Barr MC. Feline Immunodeficiency Virus Tests and their Interpretation, Feline Colloquium on FeLV/FIV: Tests and Vaccination, *J Amer Vet Med Assoc* 1991;199(10).

English RV. Feline immunodeficiency virus. In: Bonagura JD, ed. Current Veterinary Therapy XII. Philadelphia: WB Saunders Co. 1992: 280–286.

Health Topics for Veterinarians, Cornell Feline Health Center 8(3), 1993.

Hopper CD, Sparkes AH, Harbour DA. Feline Immunodeficiency Virus. In: Chandler EA, Gaskell CJ, Gaskell RM, eds. Feline Medicine and Therapeutics. Cambridge, MA: Blackwell Scientific Publications. 1994: 506–514.

Macy D. Feline Immunodeficiency Virus. In: The Cat: Diseases and Clinical Management, 2nd ed. Sherding R, ed. NY: Churchill Livingstone 1994.

Sherding RG. Feline immunodeficiency virus. In: Birchard SJ, Sherding RG, eds. Saunders Manual of Small Animal Practice. Philadelphia: WB Saunders Co. 1994: 91–3.

Sparger E. Feline Immunodeficiency Virus. In: Consultations in Feline Internal Medicine, August J, ed. Philadelphia: WB Saunders Co, 1991.

Western medicine references for FeLV

Barr MC. Feline Leukemia Virus (FeLV). In: Tilley L, Smith F. The 5-Minute Veterinary Consult: Canine and Feline, Blackwell Publishing, 2003.

Rojko JL, Hardy WD Jr. Feline leukemia virus and other retroviruses. In: Sherding RG, ed. The cat: diseases and clinical management. 2nd ed. New York: Churchill Livingstone, 1994:63–432.

Western medicine references for FIP

Fehr D, Holznagel E, Bolla S, et al. Placebo-controlled evaluation of a modified live virus vaccine against feline infectious peritonitis: Safety and efficacy under field conditions. *Vaccine.* 1997;15(10):1101–1109.

Foley JE, Pedersen NC. The inheritance of susceptibility to feline infectious peritonitis in purebred catteries. *Fel Pract* 1996;24(1): 14–22.

Foley JE, et al. Patterns of feline coronavirus infection and fecal shedding from cats in multiple-cat environments. *J Amer Vet Med Assoc* 1997; 210(9): 1307–1312.

Hoskins JD. FIP vaccination. *J Amer Vet Med Assoc* 1997. 210(9): 1307–1312.

McReynolds C, Macy D. Feline infectious peritonitis. Part I. Etiology and Diagnosis. *Compendium of Continuing Education for the Practicing Veterinarian.* 1997;19(9):1007–1016.

Norsworthy GD. Feline infectious peritonitis. In: Norsworthy GD, et al, ed. The Feline Patient: Essentials of Diagnosis and Treatment, Baltimore: Williams and Wilkins, 1998, pp. 200–203.

Scott FW. Evaluation of risks and benefits associated with vaccination against coronavirus infections in cats. *Advances Vet Med* 1999;41:347–358.

Scott FW. Feline infectious peritonitis. In: Tilley L, Smith F. The 5 Minute Veterinary Consult: Feline and Canine. Baltimore: Williams and Wilkins. 1997;586–7.

Stoddart ME, Bennett M. Feline coronavirus infection. In: Chandler EA, Gaskell CJ, Gaskell RM, eds. Feline Medicine and Therapeutics. Blackwell Scientific Publications. 1994;506–514.

Weiss RC. Feline infectious peritonitis and other coronaviruses. In: Sherding RG, ed. The Cat: Diseases and Clinical Management, 2nd ed. Philadelphia: WB Saunders Co. 1994, pp. 449–477.

IVM/nutrition references

Barnes L. B15: The politics of ergogenicity. *Physicians and Sports Medicine.* 1979;7(#11):17.

Bouic PJD, et al. Beta-sitosterol and beta-sitosterol glucoside stimulate human peripheral blood lymphocyte proliferation: Implications for their use as an immunomodulatory vitamin combination. *International Journal of Immunopharmacology* 1996;18:693–700.

Bouic PJD. Immunomodulation in HIV/AIDS: The Tygerberg Stellenbosch University experience. AIDS Bulletin published by the Medical Research Council of South Africa 6(3):18–20, Sept. 1997.

Cima J. Biochemical Blood Chemistry Evaluation, Palm Beach Gardens, FL., March 2000.

de la Fuente M, Ferrandez MD, Burgos MS, et al. Immune function in aged women is improved by ingestion of vitamins C and E. Can J Physiol Pharmacol 1998;76:373–80.

Goldstein R, et al. The BNA Handbook: A Working Manual for Veterinarians, Westport, CT: Animal Nutrition Technologies, 2000.

Graber G, Goust J, Glassman A, Kendall R, Loadholt C. Immunomodulating Properties of Dimethylglycine in Humans. *Journal of Infectious Disease.* 1981;143:101.

Gupta MB, Nath R, Srivastava N, et al. Anti-inflammatory and antipyretic activities of β-sitosterol. *Planta Medica* 1980; 39:157–163.

Kendall R, Lawson JW. Recent Findings on N,N-Dimethylglycine (DMG): A Nutrient for the New Millennium, Townsend Letter for Doctors and Patients, May 2000.

Kendall RV. Building Wellness with DMG, Topanga, CA: Freedom Press, 2003.

Nanba H, Hamaguchi AM, Kuroda H. The chemical structure of an antitumor polysaccharide in fruit bodies of Grifola frondosa (maitake). *Chem Pharm Bull* 1987;35:1162–8.

Penn ND, Purkins L, Kelleher J, et al. The effect of dietary supplementation with vitamins A, C and E on cell-mediated immune function in elderly long-stay patients: a randomized controlled trial. *Age Ageing* 1991;20:169–74.

Reap E, Lawson J. Stimulation of the Immune Response by Dimethylglycine, a Non-toxic Metabolite. *Journal of Laboratory and Clinical Medicine.* 1990.115:481.

Walker M. Some Nutri-Clinical Applications of N,N-Dimethylglycine. Townsend Letter for Doctors. June 1988.

Chinese herbal medicine/acupuncture references

Fu Jian Zhong Yi Yao (*Fujian Chinese Medicine and Herbology*), 1965;4:11.

Fu Jian Zhong Yi Yao (*Fujian Chinese Medicine and Herbology*), 1998;174:175.

Li MZ, et al. The pharmadynamics of Re Du Qing Injection. *China Journal of Experimental Recipes.* 1996;2(6):24–30.

Liao CS, et al. *Shenzhen Journal of Integrated Medicine.* 1999;9(2):20–21.

Modern TCM Pharmacology. Tianjin: Science and Technology Press; 1997.

Shang Hai Yi Ke Da Xue Xue Bao (*Journal of Shanghai University of Medicine*), 1986; 13(1):20.

Shang Hai Zhong Yi Yao Za Zhi (*Shanghai Journal of Chinese Medicine and Herbology*), 1963;2:23.

Wang SC, et al. *Journal of Shizhen Medicine.* 1998;9(5): 418–419.

Xin Zhong Yi (*New Chinese Medicine*), 1980;6:28.

Yang L. *Zhejiang Journal of Traditional Chinese Medicine.* 1998;33(6):282.

Zhang G, Song S, Ren J, Xu S. A New Compound from Forsythia suspense (Thunb.) Vahl with Antiviral Effect on RSV. *J of Herbal Pharmacotherapy.* 2002;2(3):35–39.

Zhong Cao Yao Tong Xun (*Journal of Chinese Herbal Medicine*), 1973; 6:40.

Zhong Yao Xue (*Chinese Herbology*), 1988; 103:106.

Zhong Yao Xue (*Chinese Herbology*), 1998; 115:119.

Zhong Yao Xue (*Chinese Herbology*), 1998; 459:462.

Homotoxicology references

Ben-Yakir S. Primary evaluation of homeopathic remedies injected via acupuncture points to reduce chronic high somatic cell counts in modern dairy farms. *Veterinary Acupuncture Newsletter,* 2004. Feb;27(1): pp 19–21.

Fimiani V, Cavallaro A, Ainis O, Bottari C. Immunomodulatory effect of the homeopathic drug Engystol-N on some activities of isolated human leukocytes and in whole blood. *Immunopharmacol Immunotoxicol.* 2000. Feb;22(1): pp 103–115.

Glatthaar-Saalmüller B, Fallier-Becker P. Antiviral Action of Euphorbium compositum®and Its Components. *Forsch Komplementärmed Klass Naturheilkd* 2001. (8): pp 207–212.

Oberbaum M, Glatthaar-Saalmüller B, Stolt P, Weiser M. Antiviral activity of Engystol: an in vitro analysis. *J Altern Complement Med.* 2005.Oct;11(5): pp 855–862.

Rabe A, Weiser M, Klein P. Effectiveness and tolerability of a homeopathic remedy compared with conventional therapy for mild viral infections. *International Journal of Clinical Practice,* 2004. 58(9): pp 827–832.

Serrentino J. Veterinary Homotoxicology: The Antiviral Capacity of Engystol. *J Biomed Therapy.* 2002. Spring: p 8.

HERPES STOMATITIS

Definition and cause

Feline herpes virus causes upper respiratory infections in cats that include the eyes, oral cavity, sinuses, bronchus, and lungs. This section covers stomatitis. For recommendations for upper respiratory infections, corneal ulcers, or sinusitis/rhinitis, see the appropriate disease protocols.

It is possible that this virus is a cofactor or predisposing causal agent in other chronic diseases. No cure is known. Vaccination prevents clinical infections in many patients, but immunity is short lived (3 years or less). Support of the patient's native immunity through immunosupportive therapy may be helpful in shortening the disease.

Medical therapy rationale, drug(s) of choice, and nutritional recommendations

Treatment of viral stomatitis focuses upon inflammation and secondary infection. Broad spectrum antibiotics are commonly prescribed in combination with prednisone (Baker 2003).

L-lysine interferes with arginine absorption, which is essential for herpes viral replication. Use of l-lysine has been shown to assist cats in recovery from clinical disease, lessen the severity, and reduce shedding of the virus after a stressful episode such as rehousing (Maggs 2003, Stiles 2002).

Anticipated prognosis

Prognosis is generally good when there are no secondary infections of complicating diseases. Stomatitis can become recurrent and chronic and require ongoing medication (Norsworthy 2003).

Integrative veterinary therapies

Other concurrent issues may be present in these cats such as genetic defects, nutritional issues, emotional stressors, toxin exposure, iatrogenic factors, concurrent dental disease, allergies, and infectious diseases (FeLV, FIV, Bartonella). Attempts should be made to identify these and eliminate or improve them where possible. These cases can be extremely frustrating to manage.

The integrative approach to viral stomatitis is to focus both locally and systemically on the virus. The use of therapeutic nutrition, medicinal herbs, and homotoxicology remedies either alone or in combination with medications such as antibiotics and cortisone may be required. These combination therapies give the clinician the opportunity to not only control local disease but also to prevent and control secondary disease and autoimmune processes that result from the inflammatory process in the mouth.

Nutrition
General considerations/rationale
Therapeutic nutrition should address the inflammatory process in the mouth along with immune system support to help control viral replication.

Appropriate nutrients
Nutrition/gland therapy: Glandular adrenal, thymus, and bone marrow help to balance immune system organs, provide antioxidants and nutrients to help reduce inflammation, and prevent or control infection (see Gland

Therapy in Chapter 2 for more details). The addition of L-Lysine can also be beneficial for the treatment and control of herpes infection (Maggs 2003, Stiles 2002).

Note: Because viral infections are systemic in that they are allowed to progress based upon the competence of the immune system, it is recommended that the clinician evaluate the blood both medically and physiologically to determine other organ weaknesses and disease (Cima 2000, Goldstein 2000)(see Chapter 2, Nutritional Blood Testing, for additional information).

Coenzyme Q10: CoQ10 is a strong antioxidant that helps to reduce the associated inflammation that is the precursor to many chronic diseases. It has indications in the prevention and treatment of common diseases such as gingivitis and periodontal disease, heart disease, arthritis, diabetes, and many types of cancer (Gaby 1998, Shigeta 1966).

With regards to periodontal disease, double-blind clinical trials shows that people who supplemented with CoEnzyme Q10 had improved results as compared to those taking only a placebo (Gaby 1998). Research suggests that periodontal disease is directly linked to a Coenzyme Q10 deficiency (Nakamura 1973). In addition, double-blind studies show that administering 50 mgs daily for 3 weeks led to a significant reduction in the symptoms of periodontal disease (Wilkinson 1976).

Vitamin C: Vaananen (1993) showed that people who are deficient in vitamin C are more prone to periodontal disease. Aurer-Kozelj (1982) showed that increasing the daily dose of vitamin C from 20 to 35 mg to 70 mgs showed a significant improvement in periodontal disease.

Folic acid: Folic acid, both as a topical rinse and taken systemically, has been clinically proven to be beneficial in reducing inflammation and helping to stop bleeding in people with gingivitis and periodontal disease (Pack 1984; Vogel 1976, 1978).

Sterols: Plant-derived sterols such as betasitosterol show anti-inflammatory properties that appear to be similar to corticosteriods (Gupta 1980). A cortisone-like effect without the associated immune-suppressing effects is beneficial in immune-mediated conditions (Bouic 1996).

Colostrum: Colostrum has been shown to improve intestinal health and digestion and help balance intestinal flora. In addition, colostrum can improve the immune status of the intestinal tract, which can, via intestinal production of globulins, help the overall immune competency of the body (Blake 1999).

Chinese herbal medicine/acupuncture
General considerations/rationale
Herpes stomatitis is due to Wind, Heat, and Toxin accumulation, with Stomach Fire rising up.

Wind blows the pathogen into the body. This causes Heat and Toxin accumulation, which translates into severe inflammation. Because the Stomach opens to the Mouth, Fire in the Stomach can sear the oral mucous membranes. This leads to ulceration. Treatment is aimed at controlling the inflammation, minimizing the ability of the virus to cause pathology, and treating bacterial overgrowth.

Appropriate Chinese herbs
Alisma (Ze xie): Has dual functions of enhancing immunity and decreasing inflammation (Dai 1991). The increased immune defense may help to control the virus as well as decrease secondary infections by oral bacteria.

Anemarrhena (Zhi mu): Increases the corticosterone level in serum and decreases inflammation (Chen 1999). Cortisols are often used to control the inflammation of the gingiva.

Angelica (Dang gui): Has anti-inflammatory action (Yao Xue Za Zhi 1971) yet does not cause immunosuppression. In fact, it increases phagocytic activity of macrophages (Zhong Hua Yi Xue Za Zhi 1978). This is ideal for a condition wherein inflammation must be addressed but the primary pathogen is a virus and immunosuppression may increase viral replication.

Cinnamon (Rou gui): Normalizes the immune system. It decreases production of nonspecific antibiodies (Zeng 1984). At the same time it increases the reticuloendothelial system's ability to phagocytize foreign material (You 1990). It has been proven to have anti-inflammatory effects on both acute and chronic inflammatory conditions (Li 1989).

Crataegus (Shan zha): Enhances immunity. It increases serum lysozyme levels, serum antibody levels, and T cell activity (Jin 1992). In addition to its effects on immunity it has direct antibiotic activity on some bacteria (Guang Xi Zhong Yi Yao 1990, Hao 1991).

Forsythia (Lian qiao): Reduces edema and inflammation by decreasing capillary permeability (Ke 1982). It has demonstrated antiviral and antibacterial effects (Zhang 2002, Ma 1982). This is especially useful in the case of a viral etiology.

Honeysuckle (Jin yin hua): Has antibacterial activity, mainly due to chlorogenic acid and isochlorogenic acid (Xin Yi Xue 1975, Jiang Xi Xin Yi Yao 1960). Anti-inflammatory effects have been demonstrated experimentally in rabbits and mice (Shan Xi Yi Kan 1960).

Isatis root (Ban lan gen): Has antiviral activity (Wang 1997, Jiang Xi Yi Yao 1989, Li 2000). In some cases it is as effective as ribavirin (Jiang 1992). It also has antibacterial efficacy (Zhong Cheng Yao Yan Jiu 1987). In addition to direct effects on pathogens, isatis root also stimulates the immune system. It seems to affect both humoral and cellular immunity (Xu 1991).

Licorice (Gan cao): Contains glycyrrhizin and glycyrrhetinic acid. These chemicals have approximately 10% of the steroid effects of cortisone (Zhong Cao Yao 1991). In addition, glycyrrhizin has shown activity against several viruses and therefore may be useful in viral-mediated stomatitis (Zhu 1996).

Ophiopogon (Mai dong): Has demonstrated the ability to inhibit several types of bacteria (Zhong Yao Xue 1998). This may decrease the role of bacteria in the pathology of the disease.

Oriental wormwood (Yin chen): Contains capillarin, which has anti-inflammatory properties (Wan 1987, Shan 1982).

Phellodendron (Huang bai): Has antibacterial actions against a variety of bacteria (Zhong Yao Xue 1998, Zhong Yao Da Ci Dien 1977, Zhong Cao Yao 1985). This may control the secondary bacterial infections.

Plantain seeds (Che qian zi): Decrease inflammation by decreasing capillary permeability (Zhang 1996).

Red peony (Chi shao): Stimulates cellular immunity by enhancing proliferation of T cells (Fan 1992). This may help the body control the herpes virus.

Rehmannia (Sheng di huang): Increases the plasma levels of adrenocortical hormone (Zhong Yao Xue 1998). This may increase the amount of cortisol in circulation, and corticosteroids are commonly used to treat stomatitis by Western practitioners. Rehmannia has been shown to reduce swelling and inflammation (Zhong Yao Yao Li Yu Ying Yong 1983).

Scrophularia (Xuan shen): Inhibits many strains of bacteria (Chen 1986, Zheng 1952). This may control secondary infections.

Sophora root (Shan dou gen): Stimulates the humoral immune system, resulting in increased levels of IgM and IgG (Guo Wai Yi Xue Zhong Yi Zhong Yao Fen Ce 1989). It also has activity against several types of bacteria (Xian Dai Shi Yong Yao Xue 1988). This may help cover secondary bacterial infections as well as control the viral etiology.

Acupuncture

Gingivitis is on the World Health Organization's list of conditions responsive to acupuncture (World Health Organization 10/15/2006). Many studies demonstrate acupuncture's efficacy in treating dental pain (Rosted 1998, Sung 1977). Other studies have demonstrated the ability of acupuncture to stimulate the immune system and help treat infections (Xu 1986).

Homotoxicology
General considerations/rationale

As a viral infection, herpes virus is an Impregnation Phase disorder. Acute exacerbations can represent regressive vicariation to the Inflammation Phase or progressive vicariation and deterioration of the case (often associated with stress or other homotoxin damage).

Appropriate homotoxicology formulas

See also feline upper respiratory disease, bronchitis, pneumonia, parainfluenza, stomatitis, and corneal ulcer protocols for more in-depth discussions of these pathologies and therapeutic agents.

Belladonna homaccord: Treats focal, intense inflammatory reactions and intensely red and swollen eyes or gums.

BHI-Sinus: Treats sinusitis.

Echinacea compositum: Provides immune support during infections.

Engystol N: Supports natural defenses in viral infections.

Euphorbium compositum: Antiviral agent. Helps with respiratory signs and limiting viral numbers in initial exposures (Glatthaar-Saalmüller 2001).

Lamioflur: Treats chronic rhinitis and sinusitis and diseases involving mucous membranes and skin.

Mercurius Heel: An antiviral that is useful in some cases of stomatitis.

Mezereum homaccord: Treats vesicular eczema, herpetic skin lesions, and itching and irritated skin (Reckeweg 2000).

Mucosa compositum: Supports mucosal elements in Degeneration Phase disorders and in periods of repair following infection and allopathic therapy.

Nux vomica homaccord: Used for gastrointestinal support, stomatitis, and following antibiotic damage to the mucosal elements and flora of the bowel.

Oculoheel: Supports ocular tissues.

Ranunculus homaccord: Used in human medicine for *Herpes zoster* and shingles signs, intercostals pain, and neuralgia.

Tonsilla compositum: Provides immune and endocrine support in Impregnation and Dedifferentiation phase disorders.

Traumeel S: Has anti-inflammatory and antiviral effects, activates sulfur-containing enzyme systems, and assists in regulation rigidity in chronic diseases.

Authors' suggested protocols

Nutrition

Immune and gingival/mouth support formulas: One-half to 1 tablet BID.

Betathyme: One-half capsule BID.

Coenzyme Q10: 25 mgs for every 10 pounds of body weight BID.

Additional vitamin C: 50 mgs for each 10 pounds of body weight BID.

Folic acid: 25 to 50 micrograms SID.

Colostrum: One-third teaspoon of powdered formula BID.

L-Lysine: 250 mgs SID.

Chinese herbal medicine/acupuncture

Formula H80, Gingival Stomatitis/Chronic: 1 capsule per 10 to 20 pounds twice daily. This formula is useful for acute or chronic gingival stomatitis of bacterial, viral, or immune-mediated etiology. In addition to the herbs cited above, H80 Gingival Stomatitis/Chronic contains aurantium fruit (Zhi qiao), dendrobium (Shi hu), imperata (Bai mou gen), malt (Mai ya), melia (Chuan lian zi), polyphorus (Zhu ling), and sweet wormwood (Qing hao). These additional herbs increase the efficacy of the formulation.

The acupuncture points used include LI4, ST6, and ST7 (Handbook of TCM Practitioners 1987).

Homotoxicology (Dose: 5 to 7 drops PO for cats)

The following combinations are used commonly but have not been evaluated for efficacy. They are offered as a starting point for therapy in these cats:

General herpes infections in cats: Traumeel S, Engystol N, Ranunculus homaccord, Lamioflur, and Mezereum homaccord mixed together and given TID to BID. Euphorbium nasal spray used topically BID. Consider Tonsilla compositum every 3 days.

Stomatitis: Echinacea compositum and Mucosa compositum mixed together and given every 3 days. Traumeel S and Engystol N given BID to TID PO. Consider Belladonna homaccord given BID in acute cases. Nux vomica may help due to its draining effects and is worthy of consideration in the Detox Kit (Lymphomyosot, Nux vomica homaccord, and Berberis homaccord) given for 30 to 60 days 2 to 3 times yearly (Heel 2003).

Corneal ulcers: Traumeel S, Engystol N, Ranunculus homaccord, Lamioflur, Mezereum Homaccord, and Oculoheel mixed together and given TID to BID. Ubichinon BID. Also consider Mercurius-Heel for corneal ulceration. Tonsilla compositum and Mucosa compositum given every 3 to 7 days. Euphorbium nasal spray used topically (nasally) BID. Consider Tonsilla compositum every 3 days.

Product sources

Nutrition

Immune and gingival/mouth support formulas: Animal Nutrition Technologies. **Alternatives:** Immuno Support—Rx Vitamins for Pets; Immungen—Thorne Veterinary Products; Immune System Support—Standard Process Veterinary Formulas.

Betathyme: Best for Your Pet. **Alternative:** Moducare Thorne Veterinary Products.

Coenzyme Q10: Vetri Science; Rx Vitamins for Pets; Integrative Therapeutics; Thorne Veterinary Products.

Vitamin C, folic acid, and L-lysine: Over the counter.

Colostrum: New Life Foods, Inc.; Saskatoon Colostrum Company.

Chinese herbal medicine

Formula H80-Gingival Stomatitis/Chronic: Natural Solutions, Inc.

Homotoxicology

BHI/Heel Corporation

REFERENCES

Western medicine references

Baker L. Stomatitis. In: Tilley L, Smith F. The 5-Minute Veterinary Consult: Canine and Feline, Blackwell Publishing, 2003.

Maggs DJ, Nasisse MP, Kass PH. Efficacy of oral supplementation with L-lysine in cats latently infected with feline herpes virus. *American Journal of Veterinary Research*, January 2003, 64:37–42.

Norsworthy GD. Feline Rhinotraxcheitis Virus. In: Tilley L, Smith F. The 5-Minute Veterinary Consult: Canine and Feline, Blackwell Publishing, 2003.

Stiles J, Townsend WM, Rogers QR, Krohne SG. Effect of oral administration of L-lysine on conjunctivitis caused by feline herpes virus in cats. *American Journal of Veterinary Research*, January 2002, vol. 63, no. 1.

IVM/nutrition references

Blake SR. Bovine Colostrum, The Forgotten Miracle. *Journal of the American Holistic Veterinary Medical Association*; July 1999, Volume 18, Number 2, pp 38–39.

Bouic PJD. et al. Beta-sitosterol and beta-sitosterol glucoside stimulate human peripheral blood lymphocyte proliferation: Implications for their use as an immunomodulatory vitamin combination. *International Journal of Immunopharmacology* 1996;18:693–700.

Cima J. Biochemical Blood Chemistry Evaluation, Palm Beach Gardens, FL., March 2000.

Gaby AR. Coenzyme Q10. In: Pizzorno JE, Murray MT. *A Textbook of Natural Medicine*. Seattle: Bastyr University Press, 1998, V:CoQ10-1-8.

Goldstein R, et al. The BNA Handbook: A Working Manual for Veterinarians, Westport, CT: Animal Nutrition Technologies, 2000.

Gupta MB, Nath R, Srivastava N, et al. Anti-inflammatory and antipyretic activities of β-sitosterol. *Planta Medica* 1980;39:157–163.

Nakamura R, Littarru GP, Folkers K. Deficiency of coenzyme Q in gingiva of patients with periodontal disease. *Int J Vitam Nutr Res* 1973;43:84–92.

Pack ARC. Folate mouthwash: effects on established gingivitis in periodontal patients. *J Clin Periodontol* 1984;11:619–28.

Shigeta Y, Izumi K, Abe H. Effect of coenzyme Q7 treatment on blood sugar and ketone bodies of diabetics. *J Vitaminol* 1966;12:293–8.

Vogel RI, Fink RA, Frank O, Baker H. The effect of topical application of folic acid on gingival health. *J Oral Med* 1978;33(1):20–2.

Vogel RI, Fink RA, Schneider LC, et al. The effect of folic acid on gingival health. *J Periodontol* 1976;47:667–8.

Vaananen MK, Markkanen HA, Tuovinen VJ, et al. Periodontal health related to plasma ascorbic acid. *Proc Finn Dent Soc* 1993;89:51–9.

Wilkinson EG, Arnold RM, Folkers K. Bioenergetics in clinical medicine. VI. Adjunctive treatment of periodontal disease with coenzyme Q10. *Res Commun Chem Pathol Pharmacol* 1976;14:715–9.

Chinese herbal medicine/acupuncture references

Chen SY, et al. *Fujian Journal of Chinese Medicine.* 1986;17(4):57.

Chen WS, et al. *Journal of Second Military Medical College.* 1999;20(10):758–760.

Dai Y, et al. *China Journal of Chinese Medicine.* 1991;16(10): 622.

Fan LQ, et al. *Zhejiang Journal of Traditional Chinese Medicine.* 1992;27(3):123–125.

Guang Xi Zhong Yi Yao (*Guangxi Chinese Medicine and Herbology*), 1990; 13(3):45.

Guo Wai Yi Xue Zhong Yi Zhong Yao Fen Ce (*Monograph of Chinese Herbology from Foreign Medicine*), 1989; 11(2):59.

Hao QG, et al. Study on antibiotic function of ten commonly used herbs. *Shandong Journal of TCM.* 1991;10(3):39–40.

Handbook of TCM Practitioners, Hunan College of TCM, Shanghai Science and Technology Press, Oct 1987, p 796.

Jiang Xi Xin Yi Yao (*Jiangxi New Medicine and Herbology*), 1960(1):34.

Jiang Xi Yi Yao (*Jiangxi Medicine and Herbology*), 1989; 24(5):315.

Jiang XY, et al. Comparison between 50 kinds of Chinese herb that treat hepatitis and suppress in vitro HBAg activity. *Journal of Modern Applied Pharmacy.* 1992;9(5):208–211.

Jin ZC, et al. Effects of Shan Zha injection solution on immune functions. *Journal of Chinese Materia Medica.* 1992;23(11), 592–593.

Ke Yan Tong Xun (*Journal of Science and Research*), 1982;(3):35.

Li JD. *Journal of Foreign Medicine*, vol. of Traditional Chinese Medicine. 1989;11(1):1.

Li S, et al. Various Ban Lan Gen and Da Qing Ye's effect in antagonizing influenza A virus. *Journal of Second Military Medical College.* 2000;21(3):204–206.

Ma ZY. *Shannxi Journal of Traditional Chinese Medicine and Herbs.* 1982;(4):58.

Rosted P. The use of acupuncture in dentistry: a systematic review. *Acupuncture Medicine*, 1998 16(1):43–48.

Shan Xi Yi Kan (*Shanxi Journal of Medicine*), 1960; (10):32.

Shan YTE, et al. *Journal of Pharmacy.* Japan. 1982;102(3): 285.

Sung YF, et al. Comparison of the effects of acupuncture and codeine on postoperative dental pain. *Anesthesia and Analgesia*, 1977, 56:473–378.

Wan YD. The antipyretic effects of capillarin. *Pharmacy Bulletin.* 1987;(10):590–593.

Wang SD. Therapeutic observations on treating herpes simplex with Ban Lan Gen Injection. *China Journal of Village Medicine.* 1997;25(10):24–25.

World Health Organization list of common conditions treatable by Chinese Medicine and Acupuncture. Available at: http//tcm/health-info.org/WHO-treatment-list.htm accessed 10/15/2006.

Xian Dai Shi Yong Yao Xue (*Practical Applications of Modern Herbal Medicine*), 1988; 5(1):7.

Xin Yi Xue (*New Medicine*), 1975; 6(3):155.

Xu BQ, et al. (Experimental studies on acupuncture treatment of acute bacillary dysentery-the role of humoral immune mechanism.) Zhang XT, ed. (Researches on acupuncture-moxibustion and acupuncture-anesthesia.) Beijing Science Press, 1986:573–578 [in Chinese].

Xu YM, et al. Experimental research on Ban Lan Gen polysaccharide's effect in promoting immune functions. *Journal of Integrated Medicine.* 1991;11(6):357–359, 325.

Yao Xue Za Zhi (*Journal of Medicinals*), 1971;(91):1098.

You TZS, et al. *Journal of Foreign Medicine*, vol. of Traditional Chinese Medicine. 1990;12(6):373.

Zeng XY, et al. *Guangxi Journal of Medicine* 1984;6(2):62.

Zhang G, Song S, Ren J, Xu S. A New Compound from Forsythia suspense (Thunb.) Vahl with Antiviral Effect on RSV. *J of Herbal Pharmacotherapy.* 2002;2(3): 35–39.

Zhang ZQ, et al. Che Qian Zi pharmaceutical effects. *Journal of Traditional Chinese Medicine Material.* 1996;19(2): 87–89.

Zheng WF, et al. *China Journal of Medicine.* 1952;38(4): 315.

Zhong Cao Yao (*Chinese Herbal Medicine*), 1985;16(1):34.

Zhong Cao Yao (*Chinese Herbal Medicine*) 1991;22(10): 452.

Zhong Cheng Yao Yan Jiu (*Research of Chinese Patent Medicine*), 1987; 12:9.

Zhong Hua Yi Xue Za Zhi (*Chinese Journal of Medicine*), 1978;17(8):87.

Zhong Yao Da Ci Dien (Dictionary of Chinese Herbs), 1977:2032.

Zhong Yao Xue (*Chinese Herbology*), 1998;144:146.

Zhong Yao Xue (*Chinese Herbology*), 1998;845:848.

Zhong Yao Yao Li Yu Ying Yong (Pharmacology and Applications of Chinese Herbs), 1983:400.

Zhu Li Hong. *China Journal of TCM Information.* 1996;3(3):17–20.

Homotoxicology references

Glatthaar-Saalmüller B, Fallier-Becker P. Antiviral Action of Euphorbium compositum® and its Components. *Forsch Komplementärmed Klass Naturheilkd*, 8: 2001. pp 207–212.

Heel. Veterinary Guide, 3rd English edition. Baden-Baden, Germany: Biologische Heilmettel Heel GmbH. 2003. p 63.

TICK-BORNE DISEASES: LYME, EHRLICHIA, ROCKY MOUNTAIN SPOTTED FEVER

Definition and cause

Rickettsial organisms enter the body following a tick bite. They adhere to cell surfaces and then gain access into various target cells. Once inside, the pathogen multiplies and escapes through one of several mechanisms, which ultimately damage cell integrity.

Autoimmune pathology can develop as antigen-antibody complexes are deposited in tissues such as kidney, joints, and eyes, where they can contribute to more chronic forms of disease pathology (Impregnation and Degeneration phases) (Harrus 1997). *Borrelia* organisms in Lyme disease replicate in endothelial cells, whereas *Ehrlichia* organisms also target macrophages. The organisms replicate in mononuclear cells within the lymph nodes, spleen, bone marrow, and liver, which leads to hyperplasia of the cell lines and organomegaly of the affected organs (Paddock, et al. 2003).

Typical bloodwork shows nonregenerative anemia and thrombocytopenia due to peripheral destruction of red blood cells and platelets. Also seen is leukopenia or pancytopenia due to hypoplastic bone marrow, particularly in German Shepherds. This finding carries a grave prognosis in affected dogs. Also seen are monoclonal gammopathies or lymphocytosis, hyperproteinemia, hyperglobulinemia, hypoalbuminemia, increases in serum alanine transaminase (ALT) and serum alkaline phophatase (SAP), proteinuria, hematuria, increased bleeding times (even with normal platelet counts), and cerebrospinal fluid in dogs and humans with CNS signs manifesting in similar fashion to a viral infection, e.g., lymphocytic pleocytosis, and increased proteins. Though not commonly reported, Broadfoot has seen some consistent elevations in the eosinophilic fraction of the white cell lines.

The acute phase may last 1 to 4 weeks and either results in complete recovery, or the dog enters an asymptomatic phase that can persist for months to years. In some cases, the only clue that may be present is a permanent mild thrombocytopenia. The factors responsible for the induction of the chronic phase of the disease remain unknown, since dogs can remain healthy for several years following exposure, and there may be some specific breed predilections. The common manifestations of the chronic phase are due to mononuclear phagocytic system hyperplasia and encompass mild to severe clinical signs: weight loss, fever, bleeding, pale mucous membranes, generalized lymphadenopathy, hepatosplenomegaly, uveitis (anterior or posterior, particularly associated with *E. platys*), changes in eye color, blindness, retinal disease (papill-

edema, chorioretinitis, retinal hemorrhage, retinal detachment), neurological signs due to meningoencephalomyelitis, and peripheral limb edema (Paddock 2003).

Other disease processes may be involved and signs of thrombocytopenia, coagulation defects, electrolyte disturbances, encephalitis, hypotension, hypoalbuminemia, anterior uveitis, and other osmotic injuries may require other supportive therapies (Oria 2004). Further complications may manifest in other organ systems, e.g., in splenomegaly, and conditions of rapidly developing icterus. For these cases, refer to the chapters on liver therapies. A central set of symptoms includes lymphadenopathy, conjunctivitis, anemia, critical thrombocytopenia, autoaggression, appetite dyscrasias, rheumatic and joint pains, and neurological deficits to the point of paresis/paralysis. These complications must be addressed. This is a "mimic" disease, and can easily be missed, because it has a myriad of presentations (Appel 2003, Barr 2003).

Medical therapy rationale, drug(s) of choice, and nutritional recommendations

Conventional therapy consists of suppressing the organism with antibiotics such as doxycycline or chloramphenicol. These are rickettsiostatic and not rickettsiacidal; therefore, full recovery depends upon a properly functioning host defense system. *Ehrlichia* species are susceptible to tetracyclines and their derivatives; many other pathogens, including rickettsiae, chlamydiae, borreliae, mycoplasmas, *Actinomyces* spp., *Vibrio* spp., *Bartonella* spp., and some *Mycobacterium* spp. and protozoa, are also susceptible to tetracyclines. These drugs, particularly doxycycline, represent the treatment of choice for many clinicians. As an alternative or supplement to doxycycline, imidocarb dipropionate (5 mg/kg IM, 2 injections at 14-day intervals) may be used. As with all pharmaceuticals, astute clinicians should be well versed in potential adverse reactions associated with doxycycline and other tetracycline drugs. This is particularly important because some of these adverse reactions are similar to those encountered from the primary rickettsial diseases discussed here (Appel 2003, Barr 2003, Green 1998, Breitschwerdt 1991).

The following serious adverse reactions to doxycycline are reported in humans: "tooth discoloration (pediatric), photosensitivity, superinfection, anaphylaxis, angioedema, lupus-like syndrome, serum sickness-like reaction, vasculitis, pericarditis, hepatitis, autoimmune hepatotoxicity (rare) nephrotoxicity, pseudomembranous colitis (rare) esophagitis (rare, with capsule forms), esophageal ulcer (rare, with capsule forms), pancreatitis, erythema multiforme, exfoliative dermatitis (rare), Stevens-Johnson syndrome (rare), thrombocytopenia, neutropenia, hemolytic anemia, pseudotumor cerebri, bulging fontanels (infants), Jarisch-Herxheimer reaction (brucellosis/spirochetal infections), and fetal harm (in utero exposure)" (Epocrates.com 2006).

Anticipated prognosis

Tick-borne diseases that are diagnosed early and receive appropriate antibiotic therapy respond well and the patients return to health. Recurrences are common, however. The prognosis is poor when there is secondary disease such as autoimmune reactions, arthritis, CNS disease, and bone marrow suppression (Appel 2003, Barr 2003, Green 1998).

Integrative veterinary therapies

The literature specifically links tick-borne diseases to specific rickettsial causes and describes specific antimicrobial agents as the therapy. Symptoms in Lyme disease, for example, can range from mild lameness to immune-mediated glomerular nephritis. What is most often left out of the literature is the immune system's role in the development of tick-borne diseases. Littman (1997), in her "Why I Don't Use Lyme Disease Vaccine" discussion, states that in endemic areas, that less than 5% of those animals who are positive for Lyme show any joint disease, fever, lethargy, etc. Similarly, the same percentage of seronegative dogs also demonstrated the same symptoms. That means that approximately 95% of those exposed have immune systems that stop the development of the disease or the associated symptoms.

Integrative therapies therefore should work along with medical therapies to enhance immune function and not only improve healing of current diseases but also prevent future recurrences.

Nutrition

General considerations/rationale
The nutritional approach to tick-borne diseases should be threefold: nutritionally support the target organ (for example, joints, eyes, kidneys); help reduce cellular inflammation; and reduce free radical production and support general immune function and organ integrity.

Appropriate nutrients
Nutrition/gland therapy: Glandular kidney, adrenal, thymus, eye, and bone marrow are often recommended when treating tick-borne disease.

Note: Because tick-borne disease can range in severity from simple limping to serious organ failure it is recommended that blood be analyzed both medically and physiologically to determine real and impending organ involvement and disease, such as glomerular nephritis, and to more specifically formulate the nutritional support

protocol (Cima 2000, Goldstein 2000) (see Chapter 2, Nutritional Blood Testing, for additional information).

Quercetin: Quercetin is a potent antioxidant that helps to reduce cellular inflammation (Knekt 2002).

Vitamin C: Vitamin C has been clinically proven as a potent antioxidant and immune-enhancing agent; it works specifically against infectious agents (Pauling 1976).

Plant sterols: Betasitosterol is a plant sterol and immune modulating agent that has immune-enhancing and anti-inflammatory effects (Bouic 1996, 1999; Gupta 1980; Vanderhaeghe 1999).

N,N-Dimethylglycine: DMG has been shown to support immune function and improve toxin removal (Verdova 1965). DMG has immune modulating ability and has been clinically proven to increase both tumor necrosis factor (TNF) and interferon production (Graber 1986, Kendall 2003, Reap 1990, Wang 1988).

Chinese herbal medicine/acupuncture
General considerations/rationale
In TCM theory, tick-borne illnesses are due to infectious pathogens that allow Wind, Heat and Damp to invade the body. Wind blows the pathogen into the body. If the Wind blows the pathogen into the joint, it causes Heat (inflammation) and Damp (stiffness). The Wind may also blow the pathogen into the Kidney, resulting in renal disease.

Treatment varies depending upon which organ is affected by the pathogen. If it is a musculoskeletal presentation, controlling the pathogen, decreasing pain, and increasing mobility are the goals. If the Kidney is affected, the objectives include repelling the pathogen and supporting renal function as well as treating anemia and/or hypertension secondary to renal pathology. The treatment varies depending upon whether it is an acute infection with much heat and swelling and possibly fever or a more chronic manifestation with more stiffness and dull pain.

Appropriate Chinese herbs for musculoskeletal manifestations
Aconite (Fu zi): Decreases pain (Zhong Guo Zhong Yao Za Zhi 1992). It has been shown to reduce swelling and inflammation in joints (Zhong Yao Tong Bao 1988).

Allium (Cong bai): Has antipyretic effects (Zhong Yao Xue 1998). This may be useful during pyretic phases of the disease process.

Anemarrhena (Zhi mu): Decreases inflammation. The polysaccharides in anemarrhena can raise the plasma corticosterone level in rats (Chen 1999).

Angelica (Bai zhi): Has shown anti-inflammatory, analgesic, and antipyretic effects (Zhong Guo Zhong Yao Za Zhi 1991).

Atractylodes (Bai zhu): Regulates the immune system. It can increase the T helper cell count and the TH/TS ratio

(Xu 1994). This action may help the body to control the pathogen.

Bupleurum (Chai hu): Has dual actions. It contains saikosaponin, which has analgesic and antipyretic properties (Shen Yang Yi Xue Yuan Bao 1984). In addition, it stimulates both humoral and cellular immunity (Shang Hai Yi Ke Da Xue Xue Bao 1986). Finally, it has demonstrated antibiotic effects (Zhong Yao Xue 1988).

Cinnamon twigs (Gui zhi): Have analgesic effects (Zhong Yao Xue 1998). Thirty people with arthritis were treated with a formula containing gui zhi and other herbs. There was complete recovery in 50%, marked improvement in 20%, and some improvement in 17%. Thirteen percent did not respond (Shi Zhen Gua Yao Yan Jiu 1991).

Cnidium (Chuan xiong): Can increase the phagocytic function of macrophages (Lang 1991, Zhao 1993).

Ginger (Sheng jiang): Has anti-inflammatory effects. It can inhibit dimethylbenzene-induced ear swelling in mice and egg-white-induced swelling in rats (Zhang 1989). It has been used effectively to treat arthritis (He Bai Xin Yi Yao 1972, Chi Jiao Yi Shi Za Zhi 1077).

Licorice (Gan cao): Can help to control pain (Zhong Yao Xue 1998). It also has antibacterial efficacy (Zhong Yao Zhi 1993).

Jujube fruit (Da zao): An anti-inflammatory. It decreases dimethylbenzene-induced ear swelling in mice and egg-white-induced toe swelling in rats (Li 1997).

Notopterygium (Qiang huo): Has anti-inflammatory and analgesic effects. It decreases xylol-induced ear swelling and carrageenin- and dextravan-induced foot swelling in mice. It also increases the thermal pain threshold. Experimentally, it was shown to decrease pyrexia in rats with induced hyperthermia (Xu 1991). Notopterygium also inhibits the growth of various bacteria (Jin 1981).

Peucedanum (Qian hu): Has demonstrated antibiotic efficacy (Zhong Yao Xue 1998).

Platycodon (Jie geng): Contains platycodin, which counteracts temperature rise in rats (Li 1984, Zhang 1984).

Poria (Fu ling): Inhibits the growth of various bacteria (Nanjing College of Pharmacy 1976). It also increases the phagocytic function of macrophages (Lu 1990).

Pubescent angelica root (Du huo): Has analgesic and anti-inflammatory effects (Zhong Yao Yao Li Yu Ying Yong 1983).

Siler (Fang feng): Decreases fever (Zhong Yi Yao Xin Xi 1990). It also possesses antibiotic properties (Zhong Yao Tong Bao 1988).

White peony: Contains paeoniflorin, which is a strong antipyretic and anti-inflammatory (Zhong Yao Zhi 1993).

Appropriate Chinese herbs for renal manifestations

Achyranthes (Niu xi): Has anti-inflammatory effects. It decreases egg-white-induced foot swelling in rats (Xong 1963).

Angelica root (Dang gui): As strong as aspirin at decreasing inflammation (Yao Xue Za Zhi 1971). In addition it has antibacterial properties (Hou Xue Hua Yu Yan Jia 1981). This may be useful in infection.

Astragalus (Huang qi): Can increase serum albumin and decrease proteinuria, which in turn helps to preserve amino acids, and improves the dysfunctional protein metabolism in glomerulopathies (Zhou 1999). It has demonstrated the ability to lower the blood pressure of animals under anesthesia (Xu 1999, Luo 1999). It may help control renal hypertension.

Cnidium (Chuan xiong): Dilates blood vessels and reduces blood pressure (Zhong Yao Yao Li Yu Ying Yong 1989).

Codonopsis (Dang shen): Can increase the hematocrit and lowers blood pressure (Zhong Yao Xue 1998). This herb may counteract the anemia and hypertension that often accompany renal pathology.

Corn silk (Yu mi xu): Has been shown to lower blood pressure in dogs (Zhong Yao Da Chi Dien 1037). In a trial involving 9 people with chronic nephritis, 3 recovered completely and 2 improved after 2 weeks to 6 months. Kidney function improved, edema was reduced, and proteinuris decreased (Zhong Hua Yi Xue Za Zhi 1956).

Eucommia bark (Du Zhong): Lowers blood pressure. In humans, the zinc:copper ratio in RBC is elevated in hypertensive people as compared to individuals with normal blood pressure. Eucommia can lower the zinc:copper ratio and the blood pressure (Wang 1997). One component, chlorogenic acid, has antibacterial effects (Wang 1993).

Fleece flower root (He shou wu): Has antibacterial properties (Zhen 1986).

Giant knotweed root (Hu zhang): Lowers blood pressure (Xi An Yi Ke Da Xue Xue Bao 1982) and has anti-inflammatory properties (Zhong Guo Yi Yuan Yao Xue Za Zhi 1988).

Honeysuckle (Jin yin hua): Contains chlorogenic acid and isochlorogenic acid. These compounds have antibacterial functions (Xin Yi Xue 1975, Jiang Xi Xin Yi Yao 1960). It has demonstrated anti-inflammatory effects in mice and rabbits (Shan Xi Yi Kan 1960).

Imperata (Bai mao gen): Has been used to treat renal inflammation. In one trial 11 children with acute nephritis were treated with imperata. Nine recovered completely and 2 showed moderate improvement. Edema and hypertension resolved and hematuria and proteinuria cleared (Guang Dong Yi Xue 1965).

Isatis root (Ban lan gen): Has demonstrated antibacterial properties in numerous studies (Xu 1987, Li 1994).

Leonurus (Yi mu cao): Protects the kidneys. In one experiment it was shown to decrease renal damage in gentamicin-induced acute renal failure in rats (Xia 1997).

Moutan (Mu dan pi): Inhibits bacterial proliferation (Zhong Yao Cai 1991). It also possesses anti-inflammatory properties. In mice, it can prevent dimethylbenzene-induced ear inflammation and carrageenin-, formaldehyde-, or egg-white-induced foot swelling (Wu 1990). Moutan can decrease blood pressure (Yao Xue Xue 8).

Ophiopogon (Mai dong): Has antibiotic properties (Zhong Yao Xue 1998).

Phellodendron (Huang bai): Has antibacterial effects (Zhong Yao Da Ci Dien 1977, Zhong Cao Yao 1985). It also decreases blood pressure (Zhong Guo Yao Li Xue Tong Bao 1989).

Poria (Fu ling): Has antibacterial effects (Nanjing College of Pharmacy 1976).

Rehmannia (Sheng di huang): Lowers blood pressure (Zhong Yao Xue 1998).

Salvia (Dan shen): Controlled the signs of 70% of 48 patients with chronic nephritis in one study (Shang Hai Yi Yao Za Zhi 1981). It also reduces blood pressure (Guo Wai Yi Xue Zhong Yi Zhong Yao Fen Ce 1991).

Scrophularia (Xuan shen): Can lower blood pressure (Zhang 1959, Gong 1981). It also inhibits bacteria (Chen 1986, Zheng 1960).

White atractylodes (Bai zhu): Can increase the proliferation rate of CFU-E and BFU-E colonies (Hou 1999). This may make it useful for treating the anemia associated with renal disease. It also decreases the degeneration rate of the kidney (Jing 1997). This effect may help protect the kidney from damage from the immune complex deposition.

Wolfberry (Gou qi zi): Has several functions in an herbal supplement designed for renal disease. It increases the production of red blood (Zhong Yao Xue 1998), decreases blood pressure (Zhong Yao Zhi 1984), and has antibacterial effects (Jin 1995).

Appropriate Chinese herbs for chronic Lyme disease

Angelica root (Dang gui): Increases the phagocytic activity of macrophages (Zhong Hua Yi Xue Za Zhi 1978).

Astragalus (Huang qi): Stimulates the cellular and humoral immune systems. It contains astragalan, which enhances phagocytic activity of macrophages and antibody synthesis (Jiao 1999).

Codonopsis (Dang shen): Enhances the immune system by increasing the weight of the spleen and thymus and the total number of white blood cells and lymphocytes (Huang 1994).

Dioscorea (Shan yao): Enhances both the cellular and humoral immune systems (Miao 1996).

Fleece flower root (He shou wu): Increases the total white cell count, especially the T cells, and increases the phagocytic activity of macrophages (Zhong Yao Yao Li Yu Lin Chuang 1989).

Licorice (Gan cao): Can enhance the phagocytic activity of macrophages (Zhong Yao Xue 1998).

Lotus seed (Lian zi): Was shown to increase the number of T cells in the thymuses in mice (Ma 1995). This implies that it may be useful in treating immunosuppression.

Poria (Fu ling): Contains pachman, which increases the phagocytic function of macrophages (Lu 1990).

Psoralea (Bu gu zhi): Stimulates the phagocytic actions of macrophages (Wang 1990).

Rehmannia (Shu di huang): Increases the phagocytic activity of macrophages (Cao 1989).

Schizandra (Wu wei zi): Can prevent cyclophosphamide-induced decrease in the white blood count (Li 1995, Qu 1996). It seems to support the production of leukocytes, which may help to strengthen the immune system.

White atractylodes (Bai zhu): Increases the TH cell count and the TH:TS ratio (Xu 1994). It increases the phagocytic function of macrophages (Tang 1998).

Wolfberry (Gou qi zi): Increases the phagocytic activity of macrophage and raises the total T cell count (Zhong Cao Yao 19(7).

Zizyphus (Suan zao ren): Enhances cellular and humoral immunity (Lang 1991).

Acupuncture

The World Health Organization has listed pain as a condition that is responsive to acupuncture (World Health Organization 2006). Acupuncture has also been reported to help treat joint inflammation and immune system dysregulation (Ruchkin 1987, Xiao 1992).

Homotoxicology
General considerations/rationale

Localized infection leads to small eschars. Infection of endothelial cells leads to vasculitis, sepsis (Inflammation Phase), and thrombosis (Deposition and Impregnation phases).

Subsequent development of endovasculitis and blockage of vessels can cause gangrenous changes in various tissues (Degeneration Phase) and secondary disease processes. Inflammation Phase symptoms occur as the body attempts to eliminate homotoxins associated with these diseases. The goal of biological therapy in these conditions is to improve immune function, support cellular healing, and excrete homotoxins.

Symptoms often disappear within 3 days of beginning antibiotic therapy in acute cases, but autoaggressive and other damage in more chronic forms may result in slower recovery rates.

Prevention is through avoidance of tick bites and vaccination. Several vaccinations exist for protection against *Borrelia* in Lyme disease, and as with all such products, adverse reactions to vaccination can occur and no vaccine is protective of 100% of vaccinates. The clinician should carefully weigh the patient's risk of disease and risk of adverse effect prior to selecting a vaccination. Biological therapy can also be used to assist with management of adverse reactions to vaccination such as pain at the site of injection, arthritis, dermatitis, fever of unknown origin, headache, numbness, inappetence, and dizziness.

There are no controlled studies regarding antihomotoxic agents for dogs suffering from tick-borne diseases. The following protocols are theoretical and have been used in the management of patients suffering from these diseases (Broadfoot 2005).

Appropriate homotoxicology formulas

See also anemia, arthritis, autoimmune arthritis, autoimmune anemia/ITP, and other related disorders.

Aconitum homaccord: Treats polyarthritis, particularly when combined with *Rhododendroneel S* and *Bryaconeel*.

Apis compositum: Formerly known as *Albumoheel*, this is a major remedy for renal disease (especially albuminuria and edema). It is also used for glomerulonephritis (acute and chronic), nephrosis, and bleeding from the kidney and bladder (Nux moschata). This agent may modify mast cell activity; if so, that might be a theoretical explanation of its mechanism of action.

BHI-Arthritis: Treats swollen, painful joints and muscle stiffness. Particularly useful for those patients that are more affected in cold, wet weather (Heel 2002). This is often the remedy of first choice, because it contains Bryonia (common to many other arthritis remedies such as *Arnica-heel, Atropinum compositum, Bryaconeel, Echinacea compositum, Rheuma-Heel, BHI-Inflammation,* and *BHI-Spasm-Pain*). Bryonia is good for acute inflammation of the temporo-mandibular joint, acute rheumatic inflammatory illness—e.g., rheumatic pains in the elbow, wrists, and intercostals muscles—pain in the sacrum and loins, arthritis of the knee joint, and inflammatory pains in the ankle and toe joints, as well as when the synovial membrane and fibrous tissue are also involved. It is an important remedy in acute polyarthritis and acute muscular rheumatism, particularly when ameliorated by pressure.

Ferrum phosphoricum is included for exhaustion, rheumatic conditions, acute rheumatism (which makes its presence felt particularly at night) and especially rheumatic diseases of the spine and shoulder joints (Reckeweg

2002). Also contains Berberis (see *Aesculus compositum*), Arnica (see *BHI-Injury*), Causticum (see *Causticum compositum*), Colchicum (see *Aesculus compositum*), Colocynthis (see *Colocynthis homaccord*), Dulcamara (see *Dulcamara homaccord*), Ledum (see *Discus compositum*), Ranunculus bulbosus (see *Discus compositum*), Rhododendron (see *Rhododendroneel*), Rhus toxicodendron (also in *BHI-Back, BHI-Inflammation* and *BHI-Injury*), and Sulphur (see *BHI-Injury*).

BHI-Bleeding: Contains Bursa pastoris, which has specific indications for hemorrhages, hematuria, and epistaxis. The component Crotalus horridus is indicated for hemorrhages of dark, fluid blood from the eyes, ears, nose, and any other organ; yellow fever; typhus; viral hepatitis; inflammations with gangrene and sepsis; weak heart; toxic icterus; acute yellow atrophy of the liver; rectal hemorrhage; possibly hemophilia; a tendency to general blood poisoning; and paralysis.

Erigeron canadensis (also in *Hormeel*) is used for bright red spurting hemorrhages, hemoptysis, burning and pain in the eyes, increased mucous secretion from the nose, epistaxis (of bright red blood), hemorrhages in the gums, and rheumatic type pains. Another valuable component of this combination is Hamamelis (also in *Aesculus compositum, Cinnamomum compositum, Cruroheel, Hamamelis homaccord, Traumeel,* and *BHI-Injury*, etc). Hamamelis is particularly suited for the veins, and is used in venous stasis, varicose veins, and passive hemorrhages of dark blood. There is often pain, as if bruised, in both venous stasis and rheumatism. It can be used for hematemesis with vomiting of dark blood. If there is hematuria, it is usually accompanied by a dull pain in the renal area. Epistaxis, hemoptysis, and bleeding of the skin and mucosae are additional indications.

Ipecacuanha (also in *Aconitum homaccord, Mucosa compositum, BHI-FluPlus, BHI-Nausea,* and others.) is suggested in bright red, gushing hemorrhages that occur both acutely and profusely from the rectum, lungs, nose, bladder, or any other orifice. It is also used for mucosal bleeding and circulatory disorders. Phosphorus (also contained in *Echinacea compositum, Galium-Heel, Gripp-Heel, Hepeel, Leptandra compositum, Molybdan compositum, Mucosa compositum, Phosphor homaccord, Secale compositum, BHI-Exhaustion, BHI-FluPus,* etc.) is indicated for visual and hearing difficulties; exhaustion after acute illness; loss of vital fluids; Lobar pneumonia; coughing with mucus; blood-streaked, rusty-colored, and possibly salty sputum; purpura; bruises; petechiae; thrombocytopenia; and hematomas. Higher potencies must be used where there is a hemorrhagic tendency. Phosphorus is indicated in hepatitis with jaundice and in other kinds of Impregnation and Degeneration phases (e.g., myocardial damage, endocarditis, fatty degeneration of the heart, typhoid anemia, and suppurations of connective tissues and glands. Clear states of exhaustion require Phosphorus in low potency. Phosphorus is useful in pneumonia, (orally or injected, in the potencies 10 X, 30 X, 200 X and 1,000X). Damage to the parenchyma of the kidneys can occur with albuminuria and nephrosis, and thus, should be considered in these tick diseases with their constellation of damage.

BHI-Infection: Contains Echinacea angustifolia (see *Echinacea compositum* and *Echinacea purpurea*). The indications are as for Echinacea angustifolia. Used as adjuvant therapy for serious and feverish infections.

Bryaconeel: Treats polyarthritis, particularly when combined with *Rhododendroneel S* and *Aconitum homaccord*.

Coenzyme compositum: Provides metabolic support and energy. It is used in cases of exhaustion, and it may assist in reversing antibiotic-induced damage to mitochondrial elements by activating blocked enzymes.

Colnadul: Used for arthritis worsened by cold, wet weather (Solanum dulcamara). Treats stabbing pains and neuralgia (Citrullus colocynthis).

Colocynthis homaccord: Useful for pain in the lumbosacral and hip area. Also treats stabbing pains and neuralgia (Citrullus colocynthis).

Echinacea compositum: Supports immune function against bacteria and viral infections. Phase remedy for Inflammation and Impregnation phase homotoxicoses. It is named primarily for Echinacea angustifolia (common to *Aesculus compositum, Arnica homaccord, Belladonna compositum, Galium-Heel, Mercurius-Heel, Tonsilla compositum, Traumeel, BHI-Infection,* and *BHI-Injury*). This useful component is indicated in fever, sepsis, and inflammations of every kind. It is considered an "internal antiseptic" that acts on the lymphatic system, and thus may be useful in diseases whose symptom pictures include lymphadenopathy. There may be fever-type symptoms with a sensation of fullness in the head, a red face, and rapid pulse. Many patients also complained of weakness and sharp, neuralgic pains moving here and there, which fits the migrating pain that is sometimes seen. In addition, a decrease in the red blood corpuscles may occur. This remedy is broadly used for many other symptoms, including adynamic feverish states and blood poisoning. The duration of Lyme disease was reduced when this agent was used (Baselga, 1998). Echinacea is also used for the negative consequences of vaccination or when a malignant degeneration begins in the course of acute or subacute illnesses.

Eupatorium perfoliatum (also found in *Echinacea compositum, Gripp-Heel, BHI-FluPlus*) is included for catarrhal fevers, influenza with pain in the limbs (especially the shin-bones), vomiting of bile, remittent fevers, feverish diseases of the hepatobiliary system; and rheumatism (Reckeweg 2002). Finally, this remedy also includes

Lachesis (see *Klimakteel*) and Phosphorous (see *BHI-Bleeding*).

Engystol N: Stimulates cellular immunity. When used in combination with Gripp-Heel, there is a demonstrable synergistic increase in phagocytic activity of the immune system, in addition to subjective improvements in the course of the disease (Wagner, et al. 1993).

Ferrum homaccord: Contains Phosphorus (see *Klimakteel*) for fever, inflammatory conditions with shoulder pain, patients that seek heat and worsen when cold, and anemia.

Galium-Heel: Provides support of chronic disease states and is a cellular phase remedy.

Ginseng compositum: Increases energy and awareness in geriatric pets, or any others suffering great fatigue. Contains China (also in *China homaccord*, another good remedy for exhaustion). Cinchona succirubra is well-known as one of the most important remedies from which quinine is obtained. It was formerly used as a specific against malaria. It was also used for fever, particularly undulating fever, and states of exhaustion. In homeopathy, China is used less as a fever remedy and more in states of weakness and anemia after losses of vital fluids of all kinds. Substantial loss of blood is a common indication. China symptoms are characterized by a pale, yellowish face with sunken eyes. There is also a tendency to profuse hemorrhage of dark blood from various organs; however, it is often expedient to initially treat the hemorrhage symptomatically (e.g. with preparations of *Cinnamomum*) and only to use China later on to remove the secondary anemia. Additional indications are disturbances of liver function with loss of appetite, emaciation, sensation of a lump beneath the sternum, abdominal distension, loss of appetite after a few mouthfuls, and icterus. Whereas the episodes of fever, such as those that periodically occur in malaria, may be cured in rare cases by China tincture, a suppression of the fever can possibly be achieved with Chininum sulphuricum in allopathic dosage. Symptoms that progressively worsen from day to day are characteristic not only of the fever, but also of other conditions that occur in a daily-changing rhythm. There may also be sensitivity in the left hypogastrium, corresponding roughly to the position of the spleen with hepatomegaly and splenomegaly, possibly with icterus (Reckeweg 2002). This also contains Hydrastis (see *Mucosa compositum*) and a number of other components to improve body energetics. Clinically, this is a valuable adjunctive remedy (Broadfoot 2005).

Glyoxal compositum: Supports the metabolism and unblocks receptors and enzymes.

Hormeel: Contains several bleeding remedies that are profiled in *BHI-Bleeding*, including Bursa pastoris, Erigeron canadensis, and Ignatia.

Kalmia compositum: Treats right-sided neuralgia and joint pain; red, hot joints; pain in the index finger, and long bone pain.

Klimakteel: Contains Cedron for neuralgias and intermittent fevers, malaria with tumor of the spleen, anemia and dropsical symptoms, neuralgic complaints that accompany iritis and glaucoma, and particularly fevers which recur daily between 13:00 and 18:00. It has Ignatia for intermittent fever, articular pains, possibly weakness in the lower limbs as in incipient primary chronic polyarthritis, jaundice, and febrile attacks similar to malaria.

The constituent Lachesis (also in *Ceanothus homaccord*, *Echinacea compositum*, *Gripp-Heel*, *Mucosa compositum*, *BHI-Inflammation*, *BHI-Pancreas*, and *BHI-Recovery*) is suitable in widely varying illnesses, both functional and organic. Above all, it is suited to septic illnesses and decomposition of the blood, but it is also indicated for thrombocytopenic purpura or hemorrhagic diathesis, stroke, uveitis, nasal catarrh with discharge, malaria, and kidney diseases with edematous swellings. Lachesis is often indicated not only in serious blood dyscrasias but also in disorders of hormonal function. It usually works particularly well in the form of injections, since this is most similar to the natural toxic action of snake venoms. It also treats malignant infectious diseases, acute infections, kidney disorders with albuminuria and dysuria, and skin diseases with exfoliation and hemorrhagic tendency (Reckeweg 2002).

Lymphomyosot: Provides lymph drainage. Aranea diadema, also known as Diadem spider(also present in *Dulcamara homaccord*, *Osteoheel*, *BHI-Bone*, *BHI-Lymphatic*, and *BHI-Migraine*) is indicated in lack of vital heat, chilliness, complaints aggravated by wet and cold, neuralgia of the upper jaw, feeling of ice in bones, hemorrhagic tendency, and colitis with bleeding. It is useful for periodic neuralgia, intermittent fever, paralgesia, and painful articular disease. Aranea is also said to be indicated in malarial cachexia with considerable enlargement of the spleen, periodically occurring neuralgia, intermittent episodes of fever, paralgesia, and painful articular disease (Reckeweg 2002).

Mucosa compositum: Normalizes mucosal elements. Ceanothus americanus (also in *BHI-Pancreas*) is indicated for complaints of the spleen and a tangled sensation in the left hypochondrium with airhunger. Also has Hydrastis for epistaxis, great weakness, gastrointestinal ulceration, liver conditions with jaundice, cystitis, general physical weakness and exhaustion, and rheumatic muscular and nervous pains. Also contains Ipecacuanha (see *BHI-Bleeding*), Lachesis, and phosphorus (see *Klimakteel*).

Osteoheel: Treats ankle pain. Contains Hekla lava (also in *BHI-Bone*) for a wide variety of bone diseases includ-ing osteosarcoma, tubercular and syphilitic osteitis, and exostosis. Thus, it is useful in inflammation of bones and periosteum and exostosis. Also contains Calcium phosphoricum (see *Discus compositum*), Kali iodatum for nightly pains in the bones and soft-tissue rheumatism, and Mercurius praecipitatus ruber (see *Discus compositum*) (Reckeweg 2002).

Phosphor homaccord: Treats petechial bleeding and diseases of the liver, kidney, and spleen. Its primary remedy is Phosphorus (see *BHI-Bleeding*).

Psorinoheel: Used for syphilitic miasm and constitutional and miasmic considerations. A miasm is a particular term signifying a cluster of signs and symptoms that fit a particular disease presentation, which in this case is that of syphilis (Vermulen 1992). Syphilinum has a symptom picture that is often associated with patients suffering from Lyme disease. Hahnneman (1997) called this symptom group the "syphilitic miasm." Natrum muriaticum is used for edema, hypertension, and possibly a state of anemia. Natrum muriaticum has been found to be a great remedy for intermittent fever, malaria, complaints of the alimentary tract and the skin, and sensations of intense weakness. According to Reckeweg (2002), Nash describes Natrum muriaticum as one of the best remedies for anemia, no matter whether it is a result of loss of vital fluids or other physical influences. Pallor and emaciation are usually present, although the patient eats well. *Natrum muriaticum* can be a very good remedy in intermittent fever, and it works better in high potencies. It also is indicated in rheumatic complaints with coldness of the legs, giving-way of the joints, and nervous twitching during sleep. Natrum muriaticum should also be tried in neuralgias, if other symptoms agree (e.g., emaciation, anemia, long-standing rheumatism, gouty or rheumatic arthritis). *Natrum muriaticum* is also indicated in infiltration of cellular tissue and the glands, where there are exudates and transudates that are not easily reabsorbed, and palpitations with arrhythmias, especially at rest (Reckeweg 2002).

Rheuma-Heel: Treats left sided arthritis of the shoulder or knee.

Rhododendroneel S: Treats polyarthritis, particularly when combined with *Bryaconeel* and *Aconitum homaccord*. Contains Rhododendron, which is said to be used for pains in bones, muscles, and joints, as well as heart complaints (the heart beat often becoming stronger). In many cases these symptoms are typified by an aggravation of complaints before a change occurs in the weather. Because the nervous system is also affected, Rhododendron may also be used in sleeplessness when it has a rheumatic cause. In general, Rhododendron is an antirheumatic, but it can be used where there are gouty deposits, particularly in primary chronic arthritis. It is a chief remedy for arthritis, especially when there is deformity of the small interphalangeal joints. It also has amelioration from movement (cf. Rhus toxicodendron), but the pains associated with Rhododendron are deeper and localized in the periosteum. Other components of this wonderful combination are Benzoicum acidum resina (see *Aesculus compositum*), Dulcamara (see *Dulcamara homaccord*), Ledum and Pulsatilla (see *Discus compositum*), Spiraea ulmaria (also in *Ferrum homaccord* and *Neuralgo-Rheum*) for shifting rheumatism, epicondylitis for local infiltration, and stellaria media that is called for in gout and rheumatism of the joints of the feet (possibly in psoriasis) and hepatic disorders (Reckeweg 2002).

Thyroidea compositum: Provides matrix drainage and support of endocrine a2nd immune function. Phase remedy for Impregnation Phase diseases.

Tonsilla compositum: Stimulates function of the spleen and immune elements, and is a Degeneration Phase remedy. This remarkable remedy contains Echinacea angustifolia (see *Echinacea compositum*) and Splen suis (also in *Thyroidea and Cutis compositum*) for leukemia, anemia, or agranulocytosis (Reckeweg 2002). It has a wide ranging set of components for revitalization and system support, and is often used in an autosanguis (Broadfoot 2005).

Traumeel: An inflammatory mediator and nonsteroidal anti-inflammatory agent. It activates blocked enzymes. *Traumeel* contains Aconitum napellus for inflammatory rheumatic complaints, chills, and fever; Arnica Montana for soft tissue and joint pain, analgesia, and hemostasis; Belladonna for hot, red lesions; Echinacea angustifolia to activate mesenchymal defenses, inhibit hyaluronidase, and serve as an anti-inflammatory; and Echinacea purpurea to activate the immune response.

Ubichinon compositum: Provides support of deep metabolism and cytochrome oxidase system. Also provides mitochondrial support. Contains para benzochinonum (p-benzoquinone), which is indicated in all cellular phases, leukemia, asthma, organic diseases of the nerves, pre-cancerous states, neoplastic phases, hepatitis and other conditions such as in damage to the spleen with changes in the blood composition or states arising from splenectomy, and in pancreatic insufficiency with enzyme disturbance and consequent respiratory problems.

Used in combination with Malicum acidum, Fumaricum acidum, and Natrum oxalaceticum, it is helpful in serious toxic states and in reaction phases. Parabenzoquinone may well have an effect in albumin poisoning in which auto-antigens (wild peptides) are involved; auto-immune diseases (e.g. primary chronic polyarthritis, endocarditis, and other auto-immune diseases); and after blood transfusions. Hydroquinone is also indicated in right-sided epistaxis, toxicity of the liver (e.g. in jaundice

from various causes) and visual disturbances such as photophobia that causes squinting, foggy vision, and incoordination. A leading symptom in these tick diseases is decreased appetite, sensation of fullness, or loss of appetite after only a few bites. Also contains Hydrastis (see *Mucosa compositum*).

Authors' suggested protocols

Nutrition

Immune support formula: 1 tablet for each 25 pounds of body weight BID.

Eye and kidney support formulas: One-half tablet for each 25 pounds of body weight BID.

DMG: 5 mg/pound of body weight daily.

Quercetin: 35 mgs for each 10 pounds of body weight SID.

Betathyme: 1 capsule for each 35 pounds of body weight BID (maximum, 2 capsules BID).

Chinese herbal medicine/acupuncture

Depending upon the presentation, tick-borne illnesses are treated differently. The following formulas can be combined if the patient's condition warrants such therapy.

For musculoskeletal manifestations, the authors use H78 JointGuard at a dose of 1 capsule per 10 to 20 pounds twice daily in conjunction with antibiotics. In addition to the herbs cited above, H78 JointGuard contains aurantium fruit (Zhi qiao) to help increase efficacy of the formula.

The authors use the following points for joint pain: GB20, LI11, GV14, ST36, GB34, LI4, Baihui, SP6, and SP9.

For renal disease, the authors recommend H87 Shar pei Fever at a dose of 1 capsule per 10 to 20 pounds twice daily. This supplement is designed for renal disease with an immune component. In addition to the herbs above, H87 also contains areca peel (Da fu pi), ciborium (Gou ji), fossil bones (Long gu), oldenlandia (Bai hua she cao), oyster shell (Mu li), pyrola (Lu xian cao), and tortoise plastron (Gui ban) and carapace (Bie jia). The additional herbs improve the function of the formula.

For chronic disease, the authors recommend H7 ImmuneStimulator at a dose of 1 capsule per 10 to 20 pounds twice daily. In addition to the herbs mentioned above, ImmuneStimulator also contains euryale (Qian shi), longan fruit (Long yan rou), saussurea (Mu xiang), and white peony (Bai shao). These herbs increase the efficacy of the formula.

Homotoxicology

Due to the wide variety of clinical symptoms associated with rickettsial infections, the following represent starting points only, and must be adjusted to the clinical syndromes present in the particular patient being evaluated.

Autosanguis according to Broadfoot: Traumeel plus Lymphomyosot; Engystol-N plus Galium-Heel; Mucosa compositum; Tonsilla compositum; and Coenzyme compositum plus Ubichinon compositum. Inject half the material into the patient subcutaneously or into relative acupuncture points, and place the remaining solution into the symptom remedy below.

Symptom remedy: Gingseng compositum, Rhododendroneel, Kalmia compositum, Apis homaccord, and Psorinoheel mixed together and given BID to TID. Consider Phosphor homaccord and Ferrum homaccord for anemia, and BHI-Arthritis for arthritic signs.

Symptom remedy for Lyme arthritis: Rhodondendroneel and Bryaconeel given TID. Add the following depending upon location of affected joints: Ferrum homaccord (shoulder), Rheuma-Heel (left stifle), Colnadul (right stifle), Colocynthis homaccord (hip), and Osteoheel (ankle). Echinacea compositum and Traumeel should be given at rate of 1 vial 3 times weekly. Traumeel ointment or gel can be used topically for overnight wraps. Although at first glance an unlikely candidate for this cluster of diseases, the remedy Klimakteel may prove to be a valuable adjunct in patient care.

Detoxification therapy: Galium-Heel, Lymphomyosot, Hepar compositum, Solidago compositum, Thyroidea compositum, Coenzyme compositum, and Ubichinon compositum mixed together and given twice weekly for 3 to 4 months. Also give Glyoxal compositum (1 tablet per week) to jump start regulatory functions.

Product sources

Nutrition

Immune, eye, and kidney support formulas: Animal Nutrition Technologies. **Alternatives:** Immune System Support—Standard Process Veterinary Formulas; Immuno Support—Rx Vitamins for Pets; Immugen—Thorne Veterinary Products; Renal support—Standard Process Veterinary Formulas; Renal Essentials—Vetri Science Laboratories.

DMG: Vetri Science Labs.

Quercetin: Source Naturals; Quercitone—Thorne Veterinary Products.

Betathyme: Best for Your Pet; Moducare—Thorne Vetermary Products

Chinese herbal medicine
Formulas H78 JointGuard, H87 Shar pei Fever, and H7 Immune Stimulator: Natural Solutions, Inc.

Homotoxicology
BHI/Heel Corporation

REFERENCES

Western medicine references

Appel M. Lyme disease, In: Tilley L, Smith F. The 5-Minute Veterinary Consult: Canine and Feline, Blackwell Publishing, 2003.

Barr SC. Ehrlichiosis. In: Tilley L, Smith F. The 5-Minute Veterinary Consult: Canine and Feline, Blackwell Publishing, 2003.

Barr SC. Rocky Mountain Spotted Fever. In: Tilley L, Smith F. The 5-Minute Veterinary Consult: Canine and Feline, Blackwell Publishing, 2003.

Breitschwerdt EB, Davidson MG, Aucoin DP, et al. Efficacy of chloramphenicol, enrofloxacin, and tetracycline for treatment of experimental Rocky Mountain spotted fever in dogs. *Antimicrob Agents Chemother* 1991;35:2375–2381.

Epocrates.com. 2006. Doxycycline Adverse Effects. www.online.epocrates.com/front porch/.

Greene CE, Appel MJG, Straubinger RK. Lyme borreliosis. In: Greene CE, ed. Infectious diseases of the dog and cat. Philadelphia: Saunders, 1998:282–293.

Greene CE, Breitschwerdt EB. Rocky Mountain spotted fever, Q fever, and typhus. In: Greene CE, ed. Infectious diseases of the dog and cat. 2nd ed. Philadelphia: Saunders, 1998;155–165.

Harrus S, Bark H, Waner T. Canine monocytic ehlichiosis: an update. *Compendium Contin Ed Prac Vet.* 1997. 5(1):pp 9–16.

Levy SA, Barthold SW, Daubach DM, et al. Canine Lyme borreliosis. *Compend Contin Educ Pract Vet* 1993;15:833–848.

Oria A, Pereira P, Laus J. Uveitis in dogs infected with Ehrlichia canis. Cienc Rural. [online]. 2004.34(4):pp 1289–1295. http://www.scielo.br/scielo.php?script=sci_arttextandpid=S0103-84782004000400055andlng=enandnrm=iso. ISSN 0103–8478. doi: 10.1590/S0103–84782004000400055.

Paddock C, Childs J. Ehrlichia chaffeensis: a prototypical emerging pathogen. *Clin Micro Rev*, 2003.January, 16(1):pp 37–64. CDC Viral and Rickettsial Zoonoses Branch, Division of Viral and Rickettsial Diseases, National Center for Infectious Diseases, Centers for Disease Control and Prevention, Atlanta, Georgia.

Integrative veterinary medicine reference

Littman MP. Perspectives in Veterinary Medicine, *Compend Contin Educ Pract Vet* Nov 1997;19[11]:1269;1272–1275.

Nutrition references

Bouic PJD. Plant sterols and sterolins: a review of their immune-modulating properties. *Altern Med Rev* 1999;4:170–177.

Bouic PJD, Etsebeth S, Liebenberg RW, et al. Beta-sitosterol and beta-sitosterol glycoside stimulate human peripheral blood lymphocyte proliferation: implications for their use as an immunomodulatory vitamin combination. *Int J Immunopharmacol* 1996:18:693–700.

Cima J. Biochemical Blood Chemistry Evaluation, Palm Beach Gardens, FL., March 2000.

Goldstein R, et al. The BNA Handbook: A Working Manual for Veterinarians, Westport, CT: Animal Nutrition Technologies, 2000.

Graber G, Goust J, Glassman A, Kendall R, Loadholt C. Immunomodulating Properties of Dimethylglycine in Humans. *Journal of Infectious Disease.* 1981;143:101.

Graber G, Kendall R. N,N-Dimethylglycine and Use in Immune Response, US Patent 4,631,189, Dec 1986.

Gupta MB, Nath R, Srivastava N, et al. Anti-inflammatory and antipyretic activities of Beta sitosterol *Planta Medica* 1980; 39: 157–163.

Kendall RV. Building Wellness with DMG, Topanga, CA: Freedom Press, 2003.

Knekt P, Kumpulainen J, Jarvinen R, et al. Flavonoid intake and risk of chronic diseases. *Am J Clin Nutr.* 2002;76(3): 560–568.

Pauling L. Vitamin C: The common cold and the flu, San Francisco: WH Freeman, 1976.

Reap E, Lawson J. Stimulation of the Immune response by Dimethylglycine, a non-toxic metabolite. *Journal of Laboratory and Clinical Medicine.* 1990;115:481.

Vanderhaeghe LR, Bouic PJD. The Immune System Cure: Optimize Your Immune System in 30 Days—The Natural Way! New York City: Kensington Books, 1999, p. 205.

Chinese herbal medicine/acupuncture references for musculoskeletal manifestations

Chen WS, et al. *Journal of Second Military Medical College.* 1999;20(10):758–760.

Chi Jiao Yi Shi Za Zhi (*Journal of the Barefoot Doctors*), 1077; 11:13.

He Bai Xin Yi Yao (*Hebei New Medicine and Herbology*), 1972; 3:31.

Jin SF, et al. Pharmacology of Qiang Huo Injection. *Journal of Chinese Patented Medicine Research.* 1981;(12):41.

Lang XC, et al. *Journal of Hebei Medical College.* 1991;12(3):140.

Li XM, et al. *Journal of Shizhen Medicinal Material Research.* 1997;8(4):373–374.

Li YF (translator). *Foreign Medicine,* vol. of TCM. 1984;6(1):15–18.

Lu SC, et al. *Journal of No. 1 Military Academy.* 1990;10(3): 267.

Nanjing College of Pharmacy. Materia Medica, vol. 2. Jiangsu: People's Press; 1976.

Shang Hai Yi Ke Da Xue Xue Bao (*Journal of Shanghai University of Medicine*), 1986; 13(1): 20.

Shen Yang Yi Xue Yuan Bao (*Journal of Shenyang University of Medicine*), 1984; 1(3):214.

Shi Zhen Gua Yao Yan Jiu (*Research of Shizen Herbs*), 1991; 5(4):36.

Xu HB, et al. Pharmacology of Qiang Huo volatile oil. *Journal of Chinese Materia Medica.* 1991;22(1):28–30.

Xu SC, et al. *Shanghai Journal of Immunology.* 1994;14(1):12–13.

Zhang SC, et al. *Journal of Chinese Patent Medicine Research.* 1984;(2):37.

Zhang ZX, et al. *Journal of Chinese Materia Medica.* 1989;20(12):544, 545–546.

Zhao ZB, et al. *Sichuan Journal of Traditional Chinese Medicine.* 1993;11(11):13.

Zhong Guo Zhong Yao Za Zhi (*People's Republic of China Journal of Chinese Herbology*), 1991; 16(9):560.

Zhong Guo Zhong Yao Za Zhi (*People's Republic of China Journal of Chinese Herbology*), 1992; 17(2):104.

Zhong Yao Tong Bao (*Journal of Chinese Herbology*), 1988; 13(6):40.

Zhong Yao Tong Bao (*Journal of Chinese Herbology*), 1988:13(6):364.

Zhong Yao Xue (*Chinese Herbology*), 1998; 65:67.

Zhong Yao Xue (*Chinese Herbology*), 1998; 85:88.

Zhong Yao Xue (*Chinese Herbology*), 1988; 103:106.

Zhong Yao Xue (*Chinese Herbology*), 1998; 617:618.

Zhong Yao Xue (*Chinese Herbology*), 1998; 759:765.

Zhong Yao Zhi (*Chinese Herbology Journal*), 1993:183.

Zhong Yao Zhi (*Chinese Herbology Journal*), 1993;358.

Zhong Yi Yao Xin Xi (*Information on Chinese Medicine and Herbology*), 1990; (4):39.

Chinese herbal medicine/acupuncture references for renal manifestations

Chen SY, et al. *Fujian Journal of Chinese Medicine.* 1986;17(4):57.

Gong WG, et al. *Zhejiang Journal of Medicine.* 1981;3(1):11.

Guang Dong Yi Xue (*Guangdong Medicine*), 1965; 3:28.

Guo Wai Yi Xue Zhong Yi Zhong Yao Fen Ce (*Monograph of Chinese Herbology from Foreign Medicine*), 1991; 13(3):41.

Hou D, et al. *Journal of Jiangxi College of TCM.* 1999;11(1):28.

Hou Xue Hua Yu Yan Jia (Research on Blood-Activating and Stasis-Eliminating Herbs), 1981:335.

Jiang Xi Xin Yi Yao (*Jiangxi New Medicine and Herbology*), 1960 (1):34.

Jin ZC, et al. Antibacterial effects of Gou Qi Zi extract. *Inner Mongolia Journal of Medicine.* 1995;15(4):203.

Jing WZ, et al. *China Journal of Geriatrics.* 1997;17(6): 365–367.

Li WW. Ban Lan Gen's effect on nephritic syndrome. *Hunan Journal of Medicine.* 1994;11(3):168.

Luo XP, et al. *China Journal of Pathology and Physiology.* 1999;15(7):639–643.

Nanjing College of Pharmacy. Materia Medica, vol.2. Jiangsu: People's Press; 1976.

Shan Xi Yi Kan (*Shanxi Journal of Medicine*), 1960; (10):32.

Shang Hai Yi Yao Za Zhi (*Shanghai Journal of Medicine and Herbology*), 1981; 1:17.

Wang CL, et al. *Journal of Trace Elements and Health Research.* 1997;14(4):33–34.

Wang JL, et al. *Journal of Chinese Materia Medica.* 1993;24(12):655–656.

Wu GZ, et al. *Journal of University of Pharmacology of China.* 1990;21(4).

Xi An Yi Ke Da Xue Xue Bao (*Journal of Xian University School of Medicine*), 1982; 3(4):941.

Xia XH, et al. *China Journal of Pathology and Physiology.* 1997;13(2):183–187.

Xin Yi Xue (*New Medicine*), 1975; 6(3): 155.

Xong ZY, et al. *Journal of Pharmacology.* 1963;10(12):708.

Xu SA, et al. *China Journal of Pharmacy.* 1999;34(10)663–665.

Xu ZC, et al. Assessment of antibacterial effects of the Chinese herb Ban Lan Gen. *Journal of Chinese Patented Medicine Research.* 1987;11(12):9–11.

Yao Xue Xue Bao (*Journal of Herbology*), 8 (6):250.

Yao Xue Za Zhi (*Journal of Medicinals*), 1971;(91):1098.

Zhang Bao Heng. *Journal of Beijing Medical College.* 1959;(1):59.

Zhen HC, et al. *Chinese Medicine Bulletin.* 1986;(3):53.

Zheng QY, et al. *Pharmacy Bulletin.* 1960;8(2):57.

Zhong Cao Yao (*Chinese Herbal Medicine*), 1985;16(1):34.

Zhong Guo Yao Li Xue Tong Bao (*Journal of Chinese Herbal Pharmacology*), 1989; 10(5):385.

Zhong Guo Yi Yuan Yao Xue Za Zhi (*Chinese Hospital Journal of Herbology*), 1988; 8(5):214.

Zhong Hua Yi Xue Za Zhi (*Chinese Journal of Medicine*), 1956; 10:922.

Zhong Yao Cai (*Study of Chinese Herbal Material*), 1991; 14(2):41.

Zhong Yao Da Chi Dien (Dictionary of Chinese Herbs), 1037.

Zhong Yao Da Ci Dien (Dictionary of Chinese Herbs), 1977:2032.

Zhong Yao Xue (Chinese Herbology), 1998; 156:158.

Zhong Yao Xue (Chinese Herbology), 1998; 739:741.

Zhong Yao Xue (Chinese Herbology), 1998; 845:848.

Zhong Yao Xue (Chinese Herbology), 1998; 860:862.

Zhong Yao Yao Li Yu Ying Yong (Pharmacology and Applications of Chinese Herbs), 1989; (2):40.

Zhou Q. Journal of Chinese Materia Medica. 1999;30(5):386–388.

Chinese herbal medicine/acupuncture references for chronic Lyme disease

Cao ZL, et al. *Henan Journal of TCM.* 1989;9(3):86.

Huang TK, et al. Pharmacology research on Ming Dang Shen decoction solution and polysaccharides. *Journal of Chinese Patented Medicine.* 1994;16(7):31–33.

Jiao Y, et al. *China Journal of Integrated Medicine.* 1999;19(6): 356–358.

Lang XC, et al. The effects of Suan Zao Ren on immunity and radiation damages of mice. *China Journal of Chinese Medicine.* 1991;16(6):366–368.

Li Y, et al. Journal *of Norman Bethune Medical University.* 1995;21(6):583–385.

Lu SC, et al. *Journal of No. 1 Military Academy.* 1990;10(3):267.

Ma ZJ, et al. Experimental research on anti-aging effects of Lian Zi. *Journal of Chinese Materia Medica.* 1995;26(2):81–82.

Miao MS. *Henan Journal of TCM.* 1996;16(6):349–50.

Qu SC, et al. *Jilin Journal of Chinese Medicine.* 1996;(2): 41–42.

Tang XH. *Journal of Research in Traditional Chinese Medicine.* 1998;11(2):7–9.

Wang BL, et al. *Journal of Bethune Medical University.* 1990;16(4):325–328.

Xu SC, et al. *Shanghai Journal of Immunology.* 1994;14(1): 12–13.

Zhong Cao Yao (*Chinese Herbal Medicine*), 19(7):25.

Zhong Hua Yi Xue Za Zhi (*Chinese Journal of Medicine*), 1978;17(8):87.

Zhong Yao Xue (*Chinese Herbology*), 1998; 759:766.

Zhong Yao Yao Li Yu Lin Chuang (*Pharmacology and Clinical Applications of Chinese Herbs*), 1989; 5(1):24.

Acupuncture references

Ruchkin IN, et al. auriculo-electropuncture in rheumatoid arthritis (a double blind study). *Terapevticheskii Arkhiv,* 1987, 59(12):26–30 [in Russian].

World Health Organization list of common conditions treatable by Chinese Medicine and Acupuncture. Available at http://tcm.health-info.org/WHO-treatment-list.htm. Accessed 10/20/2006.

Xiao J, et al. (Analysis of the therapeutic effect on 41 cases of rheumatoid arthritis treated by acupuncture and the influence on interleukin-2). *Chinese Acupuncture and Moxibustion,* 1992, 12(6):306–308 [in Chinese].

Homotoxicology references

Baselga J. Lyme disease in dogs. *Biomed Ther.* 1998.16(3):p 241.

Broadfoot, P. Unpublished personal communication regarding clinical applications of antihomotoxic agents in canine rickettsial diseases. 2005.

Hahnemann S. Hahnemann's Organon of Medicine, 6th ed. Homeopathy Home, 1997, 78–79. http://www.homeopathyhome.com/reference/organon/organon.html

Heel. BHI Homeopathic Therapy: Professional Reference. Albuquerque, NM: Heel Inc. 2002. pp 31, 34.

Reckeweg H. Biotherapeutic Index: Ordinatio Antihomotoxica et Materia Medica, 5th ed. Baden-Baden, Germany: Biologische Heilmittel Heel GMBH, 2000. pp 422–3.

Reckeweg H. Homeopathia Antihomotoxica Materia Medica, 4th ed. Baden-Baden, Germany: Aurelia-Verlag GMBH, 2002. pp 124, 141–2, 145, 148–9, 150–3, 177–8, 180–1, 186–9, 190, 191, 195–6, 213–5, 217–20, 221, 222–5, 228–30, 236–7, 246–9, 249–50, 252–3, 263–4, 265, 267, 279, 283–4, 285, 286, 291, 296–99, 310–11, 322, 329, 334, 335–6,347–8, 352, 355–7, 369, 377, 380–2, 386, 388, 407–9, 410–11, 417, 418–21, 442–444, 446, 456–8, 488–50, 494, 504–6, 508–9, 511–12, 512–13, 531–3, 525–6, 534–6, 542, 546, 555–9, 563, 591–2.

Wagner H. The effect of homeopathic pharmaceuticals on the phagocytic activity of granulocytes. *Biomed Ther J.* 1993. 11(2):pp 43–49.

SECTION 4

Western Herbal Disease Protocols

INTRODUCTION

This section addresses some of the veterinary conditions that are sometimes problematic for conventional medicine. Either they are poorly responsive, treatment options are limited, or the medications have undesirable side effects. The list of conditions is not exhaustive, and it is designed to show the breadth and depth of Western herbal medicine. Veterinarians who are seriously interested in treating with herbal medicine are urged to study the subject because it takes dedicated study and several years to master the complexity of the medicines. Herbal medicine can be reduced to biomedical action, which is largely what this section is about, but it has infinitely more power to restore health when combined with a knowledge of individual herbs, their energetics, and breadth of activity, as well as combinations of herbs.

The following section outlines herbs that are supported by science or traditions for particular conditions. The formulas and products suggested are based on diagnoses and are only starting points. However, the patient prescription should ideally NOT be formulated on the basis of the diagnosis, but on the underlying pathophysiology, constitution, and predisposing and perpetuating factors of the individual patient. In this way chronic disease can be treated effectively.

Note that the most effective herbal formula is not based on a shotgun approach but by formulating a synergistic combination of herbs according to presenting signs, pathophysiology of the condition, and energetics of the patient.

See Table 31.1 at the end of this section for a list of herbal products (including ingredients) as well as their suppliers and the conditions that they treat.

Chapter Nineteen

Diseases of the Blood and Lymph

When herbalists think of chronic disease they often think of blood cleansers and blood purifiers; however, veterinarians and doctors immediately argue there is no such thing (apart from dialysis and chelation). Nevertheless, alteratives and depuratives are terms that were common in the early veterinary literature until the mid 1900s, and were defined as drugs that effected "gradual change and corrected the morbid condition of organs" (Banham 1935). Herbalists still know them as blood cleansers and blood purifiers. These herbs improve metabolic processes and waste elimination, so they are often mild in action and may have laxative, cholagogue, or diuretic action. This is how they improve general health and it illustrates how these herbs may be thought of as cleansing or purifying.

Herbs that have traditionally been used as alteratives include Burdock, Neem, Oregon grape, Barberry, Gotu kola, Fumitory, Cleavers, Blue flag, Yellow dock, Sarsaparilla, Red clover, and Heartsease. Alteratives should be considered in a formula for any chronic condition as a means of improving overall health from a traditional perspective.

Blood tonics are another traditional category of herbs; they treat anemia or constitutional weakness. Traditional blood tonics include Codonopsis, Polygonum, Dandelion, Alfalfa, Parsley, Nettle, Yellow dock, and others. A number of herbs have demonstrated hematinic effects on erythrocytes and hemoglobin counts. *Angelica sinensis* is a Chinese herb that improves integrity and deformability of erythrocytes (Wang 2001). Human volunteers given Withania (*Withania somnifera*) (3 g/day) showed increases in hemoglobin and red blood cell counts (Kuppurajan 1980). In a double-blind study of 60 healthy children, after 30 days the Withania-treated group had a significant increase in hemoglobin (Venkataraghaven 1980). A double-blind, placebo-controlled, crossover trial in horses showed that Echinacea supplementation for 42 days increased the size and concentration of peripheral red blood cells, hemoglobin, and packed cell volume (O'Neill 2002). *Rehmannia glutinosa* was shown in one study to improve symptoms and recovery of people with aplastic anemia (Yuan 1998).

"Lymphatic" herbs are also frequently used in chronic disease as well as for conditions affecting the lymphatic system. These include Wild Indigo, Poke root, Cleavers and Calendula. In lymphatic disorders, plants high in rutin may help improve capillary fragility and help prevent edema. These include St. John's wort, Meadowsweet, Hawthorn, Buchu, Calendula, Cornsilk, Golden Rod, and Sheep sorrel. Edema can be treated with Bilberry, Cleavers, Cornsilk, Dandelion, Echinacea, Feverfew, Gotu kola, Grape seed, and Horsetail. A Bilberry (*V. myrtillus*) preparation (25% anthocyanidins) in rabbits demonstrated significant vasoprotective and anti-edema properties, and it was more active and longer lasting than preparations of rutin or mepiramine (Lietti 1976). Animal models suggest Echinacea may reduce inflammation and edema, possibly by inhibiting cyclo-oxygenase and lipoxygenase (Muller-Jakic 1994). Gotu kola (*Centella asiatica*) appears to improve microcirculation and reduce capillary fragility, and it helps prevent microangiopathy in people with hypertension or diabetes (De Sanctis 2001). Grape seed proanthocyanidins (PAs) have demonstrated anti-inflammatory effects on experimental studies in rats and mice (Li 2001) and stabilized capillary walls and prevented the increase in capillary permeability caused by induced toxicity (Zafirov 1990). They significantly increased the rate of disappearance of postoperative edema (Baruch 1984).

Prescription for anemia

The underlying pathophysiology of the anemia must be addressed. Anemia is caused by blood loss (external such as trauma; internal such as tumor, ruptured spleen, anticoagulant toxicity), reduced production of red blood cells (primary bone marrow disease, chronic renal failure, infectious disease, chronic disease), or hemolysis (blood-borne parasites, immune disease, drug-induced).

Therefore, herbal therapy is secondary to diagnosis and treatment of the underlying cause.

Strategy

Blood tonics may be useful to stimulate hematopoesis and support the patient, particularly in patients with mild anemia secondary to chronic disease. The use of adaptogens (such as Withania) assists the patient in coping with physical stress. Mineral-rich herbs can enhance nutrition. Herbs that address the cause are important (for example, anticancer herbs or herbal support for renal disease).

Herbal anemia support formula

The following herbs provide the best results when used in alcohol or glycetract tinctures. Alternatively, teas can be used.

Withania: Tonic, adaptogen, nervine, sedative, anti-inflammatory; 2 parts.

Codonopsis: Adaptogen, immune enhancer, blood tonic, mild vasodilator; 1 part.

Nettle: Nutritive, hemostatic, circulatory stimulant; 1 part.

Dong guai, rehmannia, or parsley: Blood tonics; 1 part.

For tinctures, give 1 ml per 10 pounds twice daily in food. For teas, give one-fourth cup per 10 pounds twice daily in food.

Prescription for chylothorax

Chylothorax is a frustrating and potentially devastating condition. The clinician should attempt to determine the etiology. Often a cause cannot be found and the clinician is left with a diagnosis of idiopathic chylothorax. An herbal formula does not treat chylothorax per se; however, it can be very useful to treat the debility associated with loss of chyle following pleural drainage. Drainage often results in losses of protein, fat, fat-soluble vitamins, antibodies, and lymphocytes into the pleural cavity as well as dehydration and electrolyte imbalances. Along with aggressive nutritional support (low-fat diet and supplementation with fat-soluble vitamins) an herbal prescription might support the patient during treatment and recovery. Surgical management may also be necessary. Other appropriate herbs can be chosen if the underlying cause is known. Potential complications include plueritis.

Strategy

Give Rutin (50 to 100 mg/kg, PO, TID) and consider herbs that contain Rutin. Add immune-supporting herbs and supply adaptogens to assist with physical stress. Consider nervines if the patient is hospitalized and stressed.

If the underlying etiology is known, give herbs that treat that condition. Herbs that are high in proanthocyanidins such as Hawthorn or Grapeseed should be given. Finally, anti-inflammatory herbs and those that support the respiratory system may help.

Herbal chylothorax support formula

The following herbs provide the best results when used in alcohol or glycetract tinctures. Alternatively, teas can be used.

Withania: Tonic, adaptogen, nervine, sedative, anti-inflammatory; 2 parts.

Hawthorn: Cardiotonic, antioxidant, vasodilator, hypotensive; 1 part.

Echinacea: Immunostimulant, anti-inflammatory, antiviral, vulnery, antibacterial; 1 part.

Bilberry: Vasoprotective, anti-edema, anti-inflammatory, antioxidant, astringent; 1 part.

For tinctures, give 1 ml per 10 pounds twice daily in food. For teas, give one-fourth cup per 10 pounds twice daily in food.

REFERENCES

Banham G. Table of veterinary posology and therapeutics . . . for the use of students and practitioners. 1935. New York: WR Jenkins.

Baruch J. Effect of Endotelon in postoperative edema. Results of a double-blind study versus placebo in 32 female patients. *Ann Chir Plast Esthet* 1984;29:393–395.

De Sanctis MT, Belcaro G, Incandela L, Cesarone MR, Griffin M, Ippolito E, Cacchio M. Treatment of edema and increased capillary filtration in venous hypertension with total triterpenic fraction of *Centella asiatica*: a clinical, prospective, placebo-controlled, randomized, dose-ranging trial. *Angiology*. 2001 Oct;52 Suppl 2:S55–9.

Kuppurajan K, Rajagopalan SS, Sitaraan RV. Effect of Aswagandha (*Withania somnifera dunal*) on the process of aging in human volunteers. *J. Res. Ayurveda Siddha* 1980 247–258.

Li WG, Zhang XY, Wu YJ, Tian X. Anti-inflammatory effect and mechanism of proanthocyanidins from grape seeds. *Acta Pharmacol Sin*. 2001 Dec;22(12):1117–20.

Lietti A, Cristoni A, Picci M. Studies on *Vaccinium myrtillus* anthocyanosides. I. Vasoprotective and anti-inflammatory activity. *Arzneimittelforschung* 1976;26:829–832.

Muller-Jakic B, Breu W, Probstle A, Redl K, Greger H, Bauer R. In vitro inhabitation of cyclooxygenase and 5-lipoxygenase by alkamides from Echinacea and Achillea species. *Planta Med.* 1994;60:37–40.

O'Neill W, McKee S, Clarke AF. Immunological and haematinic consequences of feeding a standardised Echinacea (Echinacea angustifolia) extract to healthy horses. *Equine Vet J.* 2002 May;34(3):222–7.

Venkataraghaven S, Seshadri C, Sundaresan TP, et al. The comparative effect of milk fortified with ashwaghanda and punarnava in children—a double blind study. *J Res Ayur Sid* 1980;1:370–385.

Wang X, Wei L, Ouyang JP, et al. Effects of an angelica extract on human erythrocyte aggregation, deformation and osmotic fragility. *Clin Hemorrheol Microcirc* 2001;24:201–205.

Yuan CS, Attele AS, Wu JA, Liu D. Modulation of American

ginseng on brainstem GABAergic effects in rats. *J Ethnopharmacol.* 1998 Oct;62(3):215–22.

Zafirov D, Bredy-Dobreva G, Litchev V, Papasova M. Antiexudative and capillaritonic effects of procyanidines isolated from grape seeds *(V. vinifera). Acta Physiol Pharmacol Bulg* 1990;16:50–54.

Chapter Twenty

Emotional and Behavioral Conditions

HERBS FOR BEHAVIORAL CONDITIONS

Most behavioral conditions in small animals arise from stress and anxiety. These include aggression, inappropriate urination, lick granuloma, separation anxiety, and storm and other phobias. Herbal medicines provide a number of interesting alternatives to conventional veterinary mood-modifying drugs. The approach depends upon the nature of the behavioral disturbance and the severity and duration of the condition. Other perpetuating factors and health issues such as pain or endocrine disturbances, which can contribute to aggression and anxiety, must be considered.

Nervines are the traditional class of herbs employed for emotional conditions in humans, and they have applications in veterinary medicine, too. Nervines can be further classified. Nervine relaxants have anxiolytic, sedating, or hypnotic activity. They include herbs such as Valerian, Hops, Lavender, Lemon balm, and Passion flower, and may be prescribed for anxiety, hyperactivity, restlessness, and irritability. Nervine stimulants are perhaps the least used group in veterinary medicine, but they may be beneficial for a depressed or hypoactive nervous system. They may be used extensively by veterinary staff in the form of tea and coffee. Others, such as Kola nut and Guarana, can induce anxiety and tension. Perhaps the most useful one in practice is St. John's wort (*Hypericum performatum*), which can be helpful in mild depression. Adaptogens should also be considered for animals where stress is a cause or outcome of the condition.

What is most surprising about herbal medicine is the fact that herbs have actives that just happen to bind to and interact with neurotransmitter receptors in animals (and humans). For example, American ginseng extracts may regulate GABA-ergic neurotransmission (Yuan 1998). Withania extract contains a constituent with GABA-mimetic activity (Mehta 1991). Chamomile oil also affects GABA-ergic activity (Yamada 2000). In Chinese medicine, Dan Shen is used to "Nourish the Heart and Calm the Spirit" and has been shown to bind to the same sites as benzodiazepines on the γ-aminobutyric acid (GABA) receptor complex (Lee 1991). Baicalin and Baicalein in Baical skullcap (*Scutellaria baicalensis*) and Skullcap (*Scutellaria lateriflora*) are also known to bind to the benzodiazepine site of GABA-A (Awad 2003).

The lignan hydroxypinoresinol, a constituent of Valerian, binds benzodiazepine receptors and Valerenic acid inhibits the breakdown of GABA (Houghton 1999). Aqueous extracts of valerian root contain significant amounts of GABA, though oral bioavaibility of this neurotransmitter is unknown. St. John's wort has a number of constituents thought to be active neurochemicals. Hypericum extract is theorized to indirectly activate sigma receptors (Mennini 2004). Hyperforin leads to nonselective inhibition of uptake of many neurotransmitters, as well as interaction with dopamine and opioid receptors (Butterweck 2003, Simmen 2001).

In addition to appropriate behavioral modification, the following herbs can help address behavioral conditions in veterinary practice.

Ashwaganda (*Withania somnifera*)

Withania is a very useful adaptogen for animals suffering from stress of any kind. The species name somnifera refers to the Latin word for sleep; it is a relaxing nervine. Several studies support the use of Withania in nervous exhaustion due to stress and in cachexia to increased body weight (Mishra 2000). The use of withania as a mood stabilizer in clinical conditions of anxiety and depression has been supported by studies (Bhattacharya 2000). Withania alkaloids have exhibited a taming effect and a mild depressant (tranquilizer) effect on the central nervous system in cats, dogs, monkeys, rats, and mice (Malhotra 1965b, Bhattacharya 1997).

Bacopa (*Bacopa monniera*)

Bacopa reduces anxiety, pain, and depression in laboratory animals. In rats, a standardized extract of bacopa (5, 10, and 20 mg/kg) was found to be comparable to the anxiolytic activity of lorazepam at 0.5 mg/kg IP (Bhattacharya 1998). It was also comparable to the antidepressant activity of imipramine in a rat model of depression using a standardized methanolic extract of bacopa (bacoside A) at 20 and 40 mg/kg PO once daily for 5 days (Sairam 2002). Significant improvements in visual information processing, learning rate, anxiety, and memory consolidation were found following bacopa administration in a double-blind, placebo-controlled clinical trial of people. They were tested after 5 and 12 weeks of administration of 300 mg of bacopa or placebo daily (Stough 2001).

Skullcap (*Scutellaria lateriflora*) and Baical skullcap (*Scutellaria baicalensis*)

Traditionally, Skullcap has been used to treat epilepsy and nervousness. Both species of Skullcap have the constituents baicalin and baicalein. *S. lateriflora* demonstrated anxiolytic effects in rats in an observation study in which they spent more time in the center of an "open-field arena" in a maze test, indicating reduced anxiety (Awad 2003). A double-blind, placebo-controlled study of healthy human subjects showed that the effect of Skullcap on anxiety was pronounced, and results were superior to the placebo (Wolfson 2003). The flavonoids Baicalein, Baicalin, and Wogonin (in Baical skullcap) have anxiolytic effects similar to diazepam but without the typical adverse effects (sedative and myorelaxant) of benzodiazepines (Hui 2002).

Chamomile (*Matricaria recutita*)

In mice, the constituent Apigenin showed anxiolytic activity without sedation, muscle relaxant effects, or anticonvulsant action. A mild sedative effect was gained with a 10-fold increase in dosage (Viola 1995). The oil had significant sedative effects in mice (Wakame 2003), and inhaling Chamomile oil vapor decreased stress-induced increases in the plasma adrenocorticotropic hormone (ACTH) level in rats (Yamada 1996).

Lemon balm (*Melissa officinalis*)

A randomized, placebo-controlled, double-blind, balanced crossover study in healthy, young human subjects using a high dose (1,600 mg) suggests that Lemon balm can improve cognitive performance and mood; the most notable effects were improved memory and increased calmness (Kennedy 2003). 42 patients with mild to moderate Alzheimer's disease in a 4-month, parallel-group, placebo-controlled trial were given 60 drops daily (equivalent to 1,500 mg per mL) of an extract in 45% alcohol. Compared to the placebo, the Lemon balm extract pro-

duced a significantly better outcome in terms of cognitive function, and agitation was more common in the placebo group (Akhondzadeh 2003). The essential oil of Lemon balm was investigated for agitation in people with severe dementia in a placebo-controlled trial. Seventy-two people with clinically significant agitation with severe dementia were randomly assigned to aromatherapy with Melissa essential oil or placebo (sunflower oil). Sixty percent of the active treatment group and 14% of the placebo-treated group experienced a 30% reduction in agitation, and quality of life indices were significantly greater in the treatment group (Ballard 2003).

Passion flower (*Passiflora incarnata*)

Passion flower is a traditional herb used to treat patients with nervous disorders. The methanol leaf extract of *P. incarnata* exhibited significant sedative, anticonvulsant, and CNS-depressant activities at 200 mg/kg, as well as analgesic and anti-inflammatory activities in mice (Kamaldeep 2003). Anxiolytic effects were demonstrated with methanol extracts of leaves, stems, flowers, and whole plants at 100, 125, 200, and 300 mg/kg, respectively. Roots were practically devoid of anxiolytic effects (Dhawan 2001). Passion flower (45 drops per day) had comparable anxiolytic effects to oxazepam (30 mg/day) in a double-blind, randomized trial of 36 humans with generalized anxiety disorder. Oxazepam provided a more rapid onset of action but a significantly greater number of adverse effects related to impaired job performance. This study suggests that Passion flower is an effective treatment for the management of generalized anxiety disorder (Akhondzadeh 2001).

Kava kava (*Piper methysticum*)

In the Pacific Islands there is a long tradition of Kava consumption for its mind-altering effects. A meta-analysis reviewing the effectiveness and safety of Kava extract for treating anxiety suggested a significant reduction in anxiety in patients receiving Kava extract compared with placebo. Adverse events were mild, transient, and infrequent. It was concluded that Kava extract is an effective symptomatic treatment option for anxiety and is relatively safe for short-term treatment (Pittler 2003). In 50 patients with nonpsychotic anxiety, a placebo-controlled double-blind outpatient trial showed Kava at 50 mg 3 times daily was a safe and effective treatment and was well tolerated (Geier 2004). A randomized, reference-controlled, double-blind, multicenter clinical trial concluded that Kava kava is as effective as buspirone and opipramol in the acute treatment of generalized anxiety disorder and is well tolerated (Boerner 2003). In mice,

Kava extract demonstrated anxiolytic-like activity and a reduced locomotor activity (Garrett 2003).

St. John's wort (*Hypericum perforatum*)

St. John's wort was found to produce significant positive responses for mild to moderate depression in a meta-analysis that reviewed 37 randomized, double-blind, controlled trials. St. John's wort was more effective than a placebo but not for severe depression. However, it was as effective as conventional antidepressants for mild to moderate depression (Linde 2005). In another review of 38 trials, representing 34,804 patients, adverse events were mild and transient in almost all cases (Schulz 2006). In a study of 12 people with obsessive compulsive disorder, treatment with 450 mg of 0.3% hypericin twice daily for 12 weeks, 5 of 12 patients were much or very much improved, 6 were minimally improved, and 1 exhibited no change. Significant change was noted at 1 week and continued to increase in the responsive patients (Taylor 2000).

Valerian (*Valeriana officinalis*)

Valerian has traditionally been used for insomnia, anxiety, maniacal and aggressive behavior, and seizures. A constituent of Valerian binds the 5-hydroxy tryptamine receptor area of the brain implicated in the sleep-wake cycle (Dietz 2005). A review of Valerian for insomnia concluded that studies were inconsistent and that Valerian needs further study (Stevinson 2000). One trial showed equal efficacy for Valerian (600 mg/day) when compared to oxazepam for the treatment of insomnia (Dorn 2000). When Valerian is used for insomnia, it does not work immediately. The onset of action is generally 2 to 3 weeks after beginning supplementation (Wheatley 2005). In a double-blind trial, adults who were given Valerian in laboratory social stress tests reported reduced symptoms of anxiety (Kohnen 1988). In another randomized, double-blind study, 270 mg daily of a standardized Valerian extract was as effective and well tolerated as clobazapam in people with various anxiety syndromes (Sousa 1992). Cats administered Valerian extract (10 mg/kg) by gastric lavage showed significant decreases in restless, fearful, and aggressive behaviors (von Eickstedt 1969).

California poppy (*Eschscholzia californica*)

California poppy has anxiolytic effects in mice at doses of 25 mg/kg (Rolland 1991) and has an affinity for benzodiazepine receptors and peripheral analgesic effects (Rolland 2001).

PRESCRIPTIONS FOR BEHAVIORAL CONDITIONS

Prescriptions for conditions with anxiety as an underlying feature such as aggression, inappropriate urination, separation anxiety, storm and other phobias, and psychogenic self trauma (lick granulomas and overgrooming) may benefit from the following prescriptions.

Strategy

Consider early, appropriate conventional medication if necessary. Implement appropriate behavioral modification, stress reduction, consistent routine, quality play time, and client education (avoid punishment). Consider pheromones and dietary manipulation. Use adaptogens to reduce the impact of stress and use nervines to reduce nervous tension. Also use herbs with anxiolytic activity. Finally, consider the influence of other health issues such as pain on anxiety.

Chamomile tea (carminative, bitter, spasmolytic, anti-anxiety, anti-inflammatory, spasmolytic) should be given for mild anxiety. One-fourth cup per 10 pounds twice daily in food is an easy first choice as adjunctive therapy for mild conditions.

For separation anxiety, give Kava kava (anxiolytic, sedative, antispasmodic). The dried herb should be given at 25 to 75 mg/kg, divided daily (optimally TID). The tincture (60% ethanol) should be given at a ratio of 1:2 to 1:3:0.5 to 1.5 mL per 10 kg (20 pounds) divided daily (optimally TID) and diluted or combined with other herbs.

Cats may be given Valerian (sedative, hypnotic, carminative, hypotensive, antispasmodic). The dried herb should be given at a dose of 25 to 75 mg/kg divided daily (optimally TID) if extracted and dried; the dose should be tripled or quadrupled if an unprocessed herb is used. The tincture is difficult to give on its own. The tincture usually is made up of 45% to 55% ethanol. It should be given at a ratio of 1:2 to 1:3:0.25 to 0.75 mL per 5 kg (10 pounds) divided daily (optimally TID) and diluted or combined with other herbs.

Herbal anxiety support

Use alcohol or glycetract tinctures for best results. Alternatively, teas may be given.

Withania: Tonic, adaptogen, nervine, sedative, anti-inflammatory; 2 parts.

Chamomile: Carminative, bitter, spasmolytic, anti-anxiety, anti-inflammatory; 1 part.

Lemon balm: Anxiolytic, sedative, carminative, antispasmodic; 1 part.

Passion flower: Anxiolytic, sedative, hypnotic, antispasmodic, anodyne; 1 part.

For tinctures, give 1 ml per 10 pounds twice daily in food. For teas, give one-fourth cup per 10 pounds twice daily in food.

OR use the following herbs in alcohol or glycetract tinctures for best results; alternatively, teas may be given.

Elutherococcus: Adaptogenic, immunomodulatory; 1 part.

Chamomile: Carminative, bitter, spasmolytic, antianxiety, anti-inflammatory; 1 part.

Lemon balm: Anxiolytic, sedative, carminative, antispasmodic; 1 part.

St. John's wort: Antidepressant, nervine tonic, antiinflammatory; 1 part.

Passion flower: Anxiolytic, sedative, hypnotic, antispasmodic, anodyne; 1 part.

For tinctures, give 1 ml per 10 pounds twice daily in food. For teas, give one-fourth cup per 10 pounds twice daily in food.

Prescription for compulsive disorder

Use alcohol or glycetract tinctures for best results; alternatively, teas may be given.

Elutherococcus: Adaptogenic, immunomodulatory; 1 part.

St. John's wort: Antidepressant, nervine tonic, antiinflammatory; 2 parts.

Lemon balm: Anxiolytic, sedative, carminative, antispasmodic; 1 part.

Chamomile: Carminative, bitter, spasmolytic, antianxiety, anti-inflammatory; 1 part.

For tinctures, give 1 ml per 10 pounds twice daily in food. For teas, give one-fourth cup per 10 pounds twice daily in food.

REFERENCES

Akhondzadeh S, Naghavi HR, Vazirian M, Shayeganpour A, Rashidi H, Khani M. Passionflower in the treatment of generalized anxiety: a pilot double-blind randomized controlled trial with oxazepam. *J Clin Pharm Ther* 2001;26:363–367.

Akhondzadeh S, Noroozian M, Mohammadi M, Ohadinia S, Jamshidi AH, Khani M. *Melissa officinalis* extract in the treatment of patients with mild to moderate Alzheimer's disease: a double blind, randomised, placebo controlled trial. *J Neurol Neurosurg Psychiatry* 2003;74:863–866.

Awad R, Arnason JT, Trudeau V, et al. Phytochemical and biological analysis of skullcap (*Scutellaria lateriflora* L.): a medicinal plant with anxiolytic properties. *Phytomedicine* 2003;10:640–649.

Ballard CG, O'Brien J, Reichelt K, et al. Aromatherapy as a safe and effective treatment for the management of agitation in severe dementia: the results of a double-blind, placebo-controlled trial with Melissa. *J Clin Psychiatry* 2003;64:732.

Bhattacharya SK, Satyan KS, Ghosal S. Antioxidant activity of glycowithanolides from *Withania somnifera*. *Indian J Exp Biol* 1997;35:236–239.

Bhattacharya SK, Ghosal S. Anxiolytic activity of a standardized extract of *Bacopa monniera*: an experimental study. *Phytomedicine* 1998;5:77–82.

Bhattacharya SK, Bhattacharya A, Sairam K, Ghosal S. Anxiolytic-antidepressant activity of *Withania somnifera* glycowithanolides: an experimental study. *Phytomedicine* 2000;7:463–469.

Boerner RJ, Sommer H, Berger W, Kuhn U, Schmidt U, Mannel M. Kava-kava extract LI 150 is as effective as opipramol and buspirone in generalised anxiety disorder—an 8-week randomized, double-blind multi-centre clinical trial in 129 out-patients. *Phytomedicine* 2003;10(suppl):38–49.

Butterweck V. Mechanism of action of St John's wort in depression : what is known? *CNS Drugs.* 2003;17(8):539–62.

Dhawan K, Kumar S, Sharma A. Anxiolytic activity of aerial and underground parts of *Passiflora incarnata*. *Fitoterapia* 2001;72:922–926.

Dietz BM, Mahady GB, Pauli GF, Farnsworth NR. Valerian extract and valerenic acid are partial agonists of the 5-HT5a receptor in vitro. *Brain Res Mol Brain Res.* 2005 Aug 18;138(2):191–7.

Dorn M. Efficacy and tolerability of Baldrian versus oxazepam in non-organic and non-psychiatric insomniacs: a randomised, double-blind, clinical, comparative study. [Article in German] *Forsch Komplementarmed Klass Naturheilkd* 2000;7:79–84.

Garrett KM, Basmadjian G, Khan IA, Schaneberg BT, Seale TW. Extracts of kava (*Piper methysticum*) induce acute anxiolytic-like behavioral changes in mice. *Psychopharmacology* (Berl) 2003;170:33–41.

Geier FP, Konstantinowicz T. Kava treatment in patients with anxiety. *Phytother Res* 2004;18:297–300.

Hui KM, Huen MS, Wang HY, et al. Anxiolytic effect of wogonin, a benzodiazepine receptor ligand isolated from Scutellaria baicalensis Georgi. *Biochem Pharmacol* 2002; 64:1415–1424.

Houghton PJ. The scientific basis for the reputed activity of Valerian. *J Pharm Pharmacol.* 1999 May;51(5):505–12.

Kamaldeep D, Suresh K, Anupam S. Evaluation of central nervous system effects of *Passiflora incarnata* in experimental animals. *Pharmaceut Biol* 2003;41:2,87–91.

Kennedy DO, Wake G, Savelev S, et al. Modulation of mood and cognitive performance following acute administration of single doses of Melissa officinalis (Lemon balm) with human CNS nicotinic and muscarinic receptor-binding properties. *Neuropsychopharmacology* 2003;28:1871–1881.

Kohnen R, Oswald WD. The effects of valerian, propranolol, and their combination on activation, performance, and mood of healthy volunteers under social stress conditions. *Pharmacopsychiatry.* 1988 Nov;21(6):447–8.

Lee CM, Wong HN, Chui KY, Choang TF, Hon PM, Chang HM. Miltirone, a central benzodiazepine receptor partial agonist from a Chinese medicinal herb *Salvia miltiorrhiza*. *Neurosci Lett* 1991;127:237–241.

Linde K, Mulrow CD, Berner M, Egger M. St John's wort for depression. *Cochrane Database Syst Rev.* 2005 Apr 18;(2): CD000448.

Malhotra CL, Mehta VL, Das PK, Dhalla NS. Studies on Withania-ashwagandha, Kaul. The effect of total alkaloids (ashwagandholine) on the central nervous system. *Indian J Physiol Pharmacol* 1965;9:127–136.

Mehta AK, Binkley P, Gandhi SS, Ticku MK. Pharmacological effects of *Withania somnifera* root extract on GABAA receptor complex. *Indian J Med Res* 1991;94:312–315.

Mennini T, Gobbi M. The antidepressant mechanism of Hypericum perforatum. *Life Sci.* 2004 Jul 16;75(9):1021–7.

Mishra LC, Singh BB, Dagenais S. Scientific basis for the therapeutic use of Withania somnifera (ashwagandha): a review. *Altern Med Rev* 2000;5:334–346.

Pittler MH, Ernst E. Kava extract for treating anxiety. The *Cochrane Database of Systematic Reviews* 2003.

Rolland A, Fleurentin J, Lanhers MC, et al. Behavioural effects of the American traditional plant *Eschscholzia californica*: sedative and anxiolytic properties. *Planta Med.* 1991;5:212–216.

Rolland A, Fleurentin J, Lanhers MC, Misslin R, Mortier F. Neurophysiological effects of an extract of *Eschscholzia californica* Cham (Papaveraceae). *Phytother Res* 2001;15: 377–381.

Sairam K, Dorababu M, Goel RK, Bhattacharya SK. Antidepressant activity of standardized extract of *Bacopa monniera* in experimental models of depression in rats. *Phytomedicine* 2002;9:3,207–211.

Schulz V. Safety of St. John's Wort extract compared to synthetic antidepressants. *Phytomedicine.* 2006 Feb;13(3):199–204.

Simmen U, Higelin J, Berger-Buter K, et al. Neurochemical studies with St. John's wort in vitro. *Pharmacopsychiatry* 2001;34(suppl 1):S137–S142.

Sousa MP, Pacheco P, Roldao V. Double Blind Comparative Study of Efficacy and Safety of Valerian versus Clobazapam. *Kal Chemie Medical Research and Information*; 1992.

Stevinson C, Ernst E. Valerian for insomnia: a systematic review of randomized clinical trials. *Sleep Med.* 2000 Apr 1;1(2): 91–99.

Stough C, Lloyd J, Clarke J, et al. The chronic effects of an extract of *Bacopa monniera* (Brahmi) on cognitive function in healthy human subjects. *Psychopharmacology* (Berl) 2001;156: 481–484.

Taylor LH, Kobak KA. An open-label trial of St. John's Wort *(Hypericum perforatum)* in obsessive-compulsive disorder. *J Clin Psychiatry* 2000;61:575–578.

Viola H, Wasowski C, Levi de Stein M, et al. Apigenin, a component of Matricaria recutita flowers, is a central benzodiazepine receptor-ligand with anxiolytic effects. *Planta Med* 1995;61:213–216.

von Eickstedt KW, Rahman S. Psychopharmacologic effect of valepotriates; *Arzneimittelforschung.* 1969 Mar;19(3): 316–9.

Wakame K, Wagatsuma C, Miura T. Sedative, analgesic, and sleep-prolonging effects to the mouse of commercial essential oils [in Japanese]. *Aroma Res* 2003;4:3,249–252.

Wheatley D. Medicinal plants for insomnia: a review of their pharmacology, efficacy and tolerability. *J Psychopharmacol.* 2005 Jul;19(4):414–21.

Wolfson P, Hoffmann DL. An investigation into the efficacy of *Scutellaria lateriflora* in healthy volunteers. *Altern Ther Health Med* 2003;9:74–78.

Yamada K, et al. Effect of inhalation of chamomile oil vapour on plasma ACTH level in ovariectomized-rat under restriction stress. *Biol Pharm Bull.* 1996 Sep;19(9):1244–6.

Yamada K, et al. Effect of psychotopic drugs and essential oil on plasma ACTH level of menopausal model rats under restriction stress. [in Japanese] *Aroma Research.* 2000. 1: 1, 24–28.

Yuan CS, Attele AS, Wu JA, Liu D. Modulation of American ginseng on brainstem GABAergic effects in rats. *J Ethnopharmacol.* 1998 Oct;62(3):215–22.

Chapter Twenty-One

Diseases of the Cardiovascular System

HERBS FOR DISEASES OF THE CARDIOVASCULAR SYSTEM

Herbs considered important for the cardiovascular system are classified according to traditional actions of cardioactive, cardioprotective, cardiotonic, and circulatory stimulants. Anticoagulants are a more modern application of herbs to cardiovascular disease and nervines and diuretic herbs are traditionally included in formulas. The diseases that are indicated for these herbs include cardiomyopathy (dilatative and hypertrophic), congestive heart failure/valvular disease, heartworm disease, and hypertension.

Cardioactive herbs

Cardioactive herbs are some of the most potentially toxic herbs. Many of these contain cardioactive glycosides such as Foxglove (*Digitalis purpurea*) and Lily of the Valley (*Convallaria majalis*), which are ionotropic and lead to a more efficient and coordinated cardiac contraction. Perhaps the most useful from a veterinary perspective is Bugleweed (*Lycopus europaeus, L. virginicus*). It does not contain cardiac glycosides but is still cardioactive. *L. virginicus* was recognized by the early Eclectics as an excellent sedative with properties similar to digitalis but without adverse side effects. *L. europaeus* may have applications in feline hyperthyroidism as well as cardiovascular disease. *L. europaeus* was compared to atenolol in hyperthyroid rats (induced with thyroxine). Lycopus extract and atenolol reduced the increased heart rate and blood pressure. The cardiac hypertrophy was alleviated significantly by both treatment regimes. The Lycopus extract or the beta-blocking agent showed an almost equal efficacy in terms of significantly reduced beta-adrenoceptor density in heart tissue. Although the mode of action remains unclear, these organo-specific antithyroid effects may help patients with latent hyperthyroidism (Vonhoff 2006).

Cardioprotective herbs

Cardioprotective herbs are used by herbalists to reduce the risk of damage due to ischemia or toxins. Potential actions include increasing cardiac blood flow, raising intracellular levels of cAMP, reducing capillary fragility, reducing peripheral vascular resistance through vasorelaxant activity, reducing cholesterol, and reducing hypertension. These herbs are generally rich in flavonoids, providing antioxidant benefits for systems undergoing oxidative stress. Perhaps the best known and used cardioprotective herb is Hawthorn (*Crataegus* spp), although it is also mildly cardiotonic and possibly even mildly cardioactive. Its activity has been attributed to the flavonoid components, particularly the procyanidins. The beta–adrenoceptor blocking activity of flower, leaf, and fruit extracts (standardized for their procyanidin content) have been demonstrated in vivo in the dog and in vitro in the frog heart (Rácz 1980). Hawthorn has demonstrated hypotensive activity due to a vasodilation action rather than via adrenergic, muscarinic, or histaminergic receptors (Abdul-Ghani 1987). Extracts increased coronary blood flow in vivo (in the dog, cat, and rabbit), reduced blood pressure in vivo (in the dog, cat, rabbit, and rat), increased (skeletal muscle, kidney, head) and reduced (gastrointestinal tract, skin) peripheral blood flow in vivo (in the dog), and reduced peripheral resistance in vivo (in the dog) (Rácz 1980; Abdul-Ghani 1987; Ammon 1981a,b,c; Lièvre 1985; Petkov 1979).

A crude extract of *Crataegus* has been reported to exert a protective action on experimental ischemic myocardium in anesthetized dogs (Lianda 1984a). It was shown to decrease left ventricular work, decrease the consumption of oxygen index, and increase coronary sinus blood oxygen concentrations, resulting in a decrease in oxygen consumption and balance of oxygen metabolism. An increase in coronary blood flow was not observed, in contrast to other studies. The opposing results were attributed by the authors to variation in concentrations of active constituents in different plant parts.

Several clinical studies in humans support the use of Hawthorn. In mildly hypertensive humans, 500 mg daily of Hawthorn extract led to a reduction in diastolic blood pressure (Walker 2002). In a randomized, double–blind, placebo–controlled trial involving 40 patients with chronic heart failure, a commercial Hawthorn/Passion flower extract (standardized on flavone and proanthocyanidin content) given at a dose of 6 mL daily for 42 days demonstrated significant improvements for the treatment group, compared with the placebo with regards to exercise capacity, heart rate at rest, diastolic blood pressure at rest, and concentrations of total plasma cholesterol and low–density lipids (von Eiff 1994). In a randomized, double–blind, controlled trial in 60 patients with stable angina, 60 mg of Hawthorn 3 times daily was reported to increase coronary perfusion and reduce myocardial oxygen consumption (Hanak 1983). Thirty mg of Hawthorn extract (standardized to 1 mg procyanidin) was assessed in a double–blind, placebo–controlled study involving 80 patients. Compared to the placebo, treated patients showed greater overall improvement of cardiac function and symptoms such as dyspnea and palpitations, although there was no significant difference in ECG between the 2 groups (Iwamoto 1981). Most trials demonstrate the greatest effect after 6 to 8 weeks of use, and it may enhance the effects of cardiac glycosides (Jellin 1999).

Arjun tree (*Terminalia arjuna*) also reduced blood pressure and demonstrated positive inotropic activity and β-2-adrenergic activity in an uncontrolled study in dogs (Nammi 2003). Astragalus *(Astragalus membranaceus)* can control a rise in blood pressure and lower the blood pressure of cats, dogs, and rats under anesthesia, and can increase coronary blood flow and decrease coronary circulation resistance (Modern TCM Pharmacology 1997). Garlic *(Allium sativum)* has mild antihypertensive properties in humans, rats, and dogs (Wilburn 2004, Sharifi 2003a,b, Pantoja 1991, Malik 1981). Garlic reduced diastolic blood pressure and heart rate in a study in dogs (Martin 1992, Nagourney 1998).

Valerian *(Valeriana officinalis)*, which is better known for its mild sedating properties, dilated pulmonary vascular smooth muscle in cats, probably via nonselective γ-aminobutyric acid (GABA)-mediated mechanism (Fields 2003). Dan Shen *(Salvia miltiorrhiza)* has traditionally been used in China for cardiovascular and cerebrovascular disease; and is contemporarily used in Chinese hospitals to treat angina, acute heart attacks, and hypertension and to assist in recovery from stroke (Chang 1986). It improves coronary blood flow in dogs with experimental acute myocardial infarction. This may be a result of it improving the opening and formation of coronary collateral circulation, thereby protecting myocardia from ischemia (Liu 1999). Korean ginseng (*Panax ginseng*) saponins

have different actions on cardiac hemodynamics, including increasing and decreasing cardiac performance. They also have calcium antagonist activity and a protective effect on experimental myocardial infarction in rabbits (Manren 1987). Tienchi ginseng (*Panax notoginseng*) increased coronary blood flow and had a positive inotropic effect in vitro (Lei 1986).

Cardiotonic herbs

Cardiotonic herbs, like cardioprotective herbs, have a gentle action on the heart compared to the cardioactive herbs which have a much more profound action. Withania (*Withania somnifera*) is a very useful cardiotonic and general tonic for geriatric animals. The effect of Withania was studied on the cardiovascular and respiratory systems in dogs. The alkaloids had a prolonged hypotensive, bradycardiac activity and stimulated the vasomotor and respiratory centers in the brainstem of dogs. The cardioinhibitory action in dogs appeared to be due to ganglion blocking and direct cardiodepressant actions (Malhotra 1981). Withania extract induced a significant decrease in arterial and diastolic blood pressure in normotensive pentobarbital-anesthetized dogs (Ahumada 1991); 5 mg/kg of Withania extract caused a blood pressure drop in dogs (blocked by atropine, not by mepyramine or propranolol) (Budhiraja 1983). Motherwort *(Leonurus cardiaca)* is traditionally used for palpitations, arrhythmias, and anxiety. One of its constituents, lavandulifolioside, causes decreased blood pressure, significant negative chronotropism, and prolongation of the P-Q and Q-T intervals and the QRS complex (Milkowska-Leyck 2002).

Circulatory stimulants

Circulatory stimulants are traditionally used to "warm" the circulation when there is stagnation of circulation or where blood flow is compromised. Ginkgo leaf extract *(Ginkgo biloba)* has been studied in normal rats and those with ischemic brain damage, and Ginkgo extract given at a dose of 100 mg/kg orally was reported to increase cerebral blood flow in normal rats. The increase was less marked in rats with cerebral artery occlusion, however (Zhang 2000). Dong guai (Angelica sinensis) (2 g/kg body weight) given intravenously to anesthetized dogs increased coronary blood flow from 88 ml before administration to 128 ml (per 100 g cardiac muscle/minute post-injection). Both coronary vascular resistance and myocardial oxygen consumption were reduced, while the heart rate decreased or remained unchanged (Chou 1979). Dong guai injection also has a therapeutic effect in treating acute cerebral infarction in people (Liu 2004b). In rabbits with peripheral circulatory disturbances, Dan Shen (*Salvia miltiorrhiza*) tanshinone derivatives improved blood flow, de-aggregated red blood cells, and inhibited platelet activity (Chang 1986). Dan Shen also provided good results in disseminated intravascular coagulation (Chang 1986).

Nervines may be useful in animals with restlessness, insomnia, and anxiety associated with cardiovascular disease. Valerian (*Valeriana officinalis*), when compared to a placebo, significantly attenuated heart rate and blood pressure changes in people (Cropley 2002). Others include Lemon balm (*Melissa officinalis*), Motherwort (Leonurus cardiaca), and Linden *(Tilia platyphyllos).*

Many herbs, including the cardioactive herbs, have traditionally been used to treat "dropsy;" there are too many to list here. Herbs such as Parsley *(Petroselinum crispum)* and Dandelion are frequently included in formulas for heart disease. Dandelion leaf (*Taraxacum officinale*) extracts given orally had a diuretic effect in rats and mice, and the effect was assessed as equal to that of furosemide and stronger than Juniper berry and Horsetail (Bisset 1994). However, diuretic activity was not observed in another study after oral or intraperitoneal administration (Tita 1993).

Anticoagulant herbs are a more modern application and probably have more use in human medicine; however, their use may be important in conditions associated with thrombosis. Garlic (*Allium sativum*) inhibits platelet aggregation (Rahman 2000); however, its potential for red blood cell toxicity in cats and dogs may limit its use. In this author's experience, the tincture does not appear to cause this problem. Ginkgo extract *(Ginkgo biloba)* containing ginkgolides inhibits platelet aggregating factors (PAF); this may have additive effects for human patients or cats taking anticoagulants to prevent thrombosis (Wynn 2006). Dan Shen (*Salvia miltiorrhiza*) inhibits platelet activity, has antithrombin III–like activity, and promotes fibrinolysis (Chan 2001). In rats fed a high-cholesterol diet, Korean ginseng (*Panax ginseng*) reduced serum cholesterol and triglycerides, decreased platelet adhesiveness, and decreased fatty changes to the liver (Yamamoto 1982). Ginseng has also been shown to reduce blood coagulation and enhance fibrinolysis (Kuo 1990).

FORMULAS FOR CARDIOVASCULAR CONDITIONS

Strategy

Implement appropriate lifestyle changes and appropriate diet. Monitor patients regularly, particularly if herbs are used as the sole treatment for early cases or if the patients are on conventional medication. Doses can be adjusted upwards if changes of less than 20% have been observed per week. The doses of conventional medicines may need to be reviewed 1 to 2 weeks after beginning treatment with herbs. It is assumed that conventional medicines will be used for diagnosed cardiac disease, whenever good evidence exists for efficacy. In most cases these formulas provide adjunctive care. The formulas below can be made as per the recipe or adapted from other recipes according to patient needs. They are formulated to allow substitution.

Hypertrophic cardiomyopathy

Astragalus: Immune-enhancing, tonic, cardiotonic, nephroprotective, diuretic, hypotensive; 1 part.

Bugleweed: Cardioactive, diuretic, reduced heart rate, sedative, thyroxine antagonist; 1 part.

Motherwort: Sedative, antispasmodic, cardiac tonic; 1 part.

Ginkgo: PAF inhibitor, antioxidant, circulatory stimulant, cognitive enhancer; 1 part.

Dandelion leaf: Diuretic, laxative, cholagogue, antirheumatic; 1 part.

For tinctures, give 1 ml per 10 pounds twice daily in food. For teas, give one-fourth cup per 10 pounds twice daily in food.

Dilated cardiomyopathy

Hawthorn: Cardiotonic, coronary vasodilator, hypotensive, antioxidant; 1 part.

Panax ginseng: Adaptogen, anti-arrhythmic, cardioprotective, circulatory stimulant; 1 part.

Dan Shen: Cardioprotective, hypotensive, anticoagulant, antiplatelet, hepatoprotective; 1 part.

Ginkgo: PAF inhibitor, antioxidant, circulatory stimulant, cognitive enhancer; 1 part.

Lemon balm: Carminative, antispasmodic, sedative; 1 part.

For tinctures, give 1 ml per 10 pounds twice daily in food. For teas, give one-fourth cup per 10 pounds twice daily in food.

Mild congestive heart failure

Hawthorn: Cardiotonic, coronary vasodilator, hypotensive, antioxidant; 2 parts.

Korean ginseng: Adaptogen, anti-arrhythmic, cardioprotective, circulatory stimulant; 1 part.

Dandelion leaf: Diuretic, laxative, cholagogue, antirheumatic; 1 part.

Lemon balm: Carminative, antispasmodic, sedative; 1 part.

For tinctures, give 1 ml per 10 pounds twice daily in food. For teas, give one-fourth cup per 10 pounds twice daily in food.

Heartworm disease

Black walnut hull is commonly advocated for the prevention and treatment of heartworm in dogs; however, there is no traditional or scientific basis for this use to date. In 1 study dogs naturally infected with *Dirofilaria immitis* were treated with alcoholic extracts of Ginger. Ginger at 100 mg/kg administered by 12 subcutaneous injections reduced microfilarial concentration in blood by a maximum of 98%. After the last injection (day 55), an 83% reduction in microfilarial concentration was recorded, suggesting that partial destruction of adult worms had occurred (Datta 1987). A decoction of *Andrographis paniculata* leaves killed the microfilaria of *Dipetalonema reconditum* in 40 minutes in an in vitro study. Infected dogs were given 3 subcutaneous injections of the extract (0.06 mL per kg), which reduced microfilariae by more than 85%. While further injections did not eliminate the infection, the reduced level of microfilaria persisted. Lethargy was observed for 1 week following treatment (Dutta 1982).

Heartworm disease support is indicated during treatment and post treatment. Conventional monthly preventatives are recommended during transmission risk periods. Support protocols include:

Hawthorn: Cardiotonic, coronary vasodilator, hypotensive, antioxidant; 2 parts.

Korean ginseng: Adaptogen, anti-arrhythmic, cardioprotective, circulatory stimulant; 1 part.

Andrographis: Immunostimulant, bitter, anti-inflammatory, hepatoprotective; 1 part.

Ginger: Carminative, antispasmodic, antiplatelet, anti-inflammatory; 1 part.

For tinctures, give 1 ml per 10 pounds twice daily in food. For teas, give one-fourth cup per 10 pounds twice daily in food.

Hypertension

Hawthorn: Cardiotonic, coronary vasodilator, hypotensive, antioxidant; 1 part.

Yarrow: Antispasmodic, mild vasodilator, hypotensive, bitter; 1 part.

Astragalus: Immune-enhancing, tonic, cardiotonic, nephroprotective, diuretic, hypotensive; 1 part.

Withania: Tonic, adaptogen, nervine, sedative, anti-inflammatory; 2 parts.

For tinctures, give 1 ml per 10 pounds twice daily in food. For teas, give one-fourth cup per 10 pounds twice daily in food.

Feline hypertension

Lemon balm: Carminative, antispasmodic, sedative; 1 part.

Bugleweed: Cardioactive, diuretic, reduces heart rate, sedative, thyroxine antagonist; 1 part.

Motherwort: Sedative, antispasmodic, cardiac tonic; 1 part.

Hawthorn: Cardiotonic, coronary vasodilator, hypotensive, antioxidant; 2 parts.

For tinctures, give 1 ml per 10 pounds twice daily in food. For teas, give one-fourth cup per 10 pounds twice daily in food.

REFERENCES

Abdul-Ghani A-S, et al. Hypotensive effect of *Crateagus oxyacantha*. *Int J Crude Drug Res* 1987; 25: 216–220.

Ahumada F, Aspee F, Wikman G, Hancke J. Withania somnifera extract. Its effect on arterial blood pressure in anaethetised dogs. *Phytotherpay Research* 1991 5(3):111.

Ammon HPT, Händel M. Crataegus, toxicology and pharmacology. Part I: Toxicity. *Planta Med* 1981a43: 105–120.

Ammon HPT, Händel M. Crataegus, toxicology and pharmacology. Part II: Pharmacodynamics. *Planta Med* 1981b 43: 209–239.

Ammon HPT, Händel M. Crataegus, toxicology and pharmacology. Part III: Pharmacodynamics and pharmacokinetics. *Planta Med* 1981c43: 313–322.

Bisset NG. Herbal Drugs and Phytopharmaceuticals (Wichtl M, ed. [German edition]). Stuttgart: Medpharm; 1994.

Budhiraja RD, Sudhir S, Garg KN. Cardiovascular effects of a withanolide from Withania coagulans, dunal fruits. *Indian J Physiol Pharmacol.* 1983 Apr–Jun;27(2):129–34.

Chan TY. Interaction between warfarin and danshen (*Salvia miltiorrhiza*). *Ann Pharmacother* 2001;35:501–504.

Chang HM, But PPH. Pharmacology and Applications of Chinese Materia Medica, vol 1. Singapore: World Scientific Publishing; 1986.

Chou YP. The effect of Angelica sinensis on hemodynamics and myocardiac oxygen consumption in dogs. *Acta Pharmaceutica Sinica*, 1979, 14:156–160.

Cropley M, Cave Z, Ellis J, Middleton RW. Effect of kava and valerian on human physiological and psychological responses to mental stress assessed under laboratory conditions. *Phytother Res* 2002;16:23–27.

Datta A, Sukul NC. Antifilarial effect of *Zingiber officinale* on *Dirofilaria immitis*. *J Helminthol* 1987;61:268–270.

Dutta A, Sukul NC. Filaricidal properties of a wild herb, Andrographis paniculata. *J Helminthol* 1982;56:81–84.

Fields AM, Richards TA, Felton JA, et al. Analysis of responses to valerian root extract in the feline pulmonary vascular bed. *J Altern Complement Med* 2003;9:909–918.

Hanak TH, Brückel M-H. Behhandlung von leichten stabilen Formen der Angina pectoris mit Crataegutt novo. *Therapiewoche* 1983; 33; 4331–4333.

Iwamoto M, et al. Klinische Wirkung von Crataegutt bei Herzerkrankungen ischämischer und/oder hypertensiver Genese. *Planta Med* 1981; 42: 1–16.

Jellin JM, Batz F, Hitchens K. Pharmacists Letter/Prescribers Letter Natural Medicines Comprehensive Database. Stockton, Calif: Therapeutic Research Faculty; 1999.

Kuo S-C, et al. Antiplatelet components in *Panax ginseng*. *Planta Med* 1990; 56: 164–167.

Lei X-L, et al. Cardiovascular pharmacology of *Panax notoginseng* (Burk) F.H. Chen and *Salvia militiorrhiza*. *Am J Chin Med* 1986; 14: 145–152.

Lianda L, et al. Studies on hawthorn and its active principle. I. Effect on myocardial ischemia and hemodynamics in dogs. *J Trad Chin Med* 1984; 4: 283–288.

Lièvre M, Andrieu JL, Baconin A. Cardiovascular effects of hyperoside extracted from hawthorn in anesthetized dogs. *Ann Pharm Fr.* 1985;43(5):471–7. [Article in French]

Liu Q, Lu Z. Effect of Salvia Miltiorrhiza on coronary collateral circulation in dogs with experimental acute myocardial infarction. *J Tongji Med Univ.* 1999; 19(1): 40–1, 69.

Liu YM, Zhang JJ, Jiang J. Observation on clinical effect of Angelica injection in treating acute cerebral infarction. [Chinese] *Chinese Journal of Integrated Traditional and Western Medicine/Zhongguo Zhong Xi Yi Jie He Xue Hui, Zhongguo Zhong Yi Yan Jiu Yuan Zhu Ban.* 2004 Mar. 24(3):205–8.

Malhotra CL, Das PK, Dhalla NS, Prasad K. Studies on Withania ashwagandha, Kaul. III. The effect of total alkaloids on the cardiovascular system and respiration. *Indian J Med Res* 1981;49:448–460.

Malik ZA, Siddiqui S. Hypotensive effect of freeze dried garlic *(Allium sativum)* sap in dog. *J Pak Med Assoc* 1981;31: 12–13.

Manren R, et al. Calcium antagonistic action of saponins from *Panax notoginseng* (sanqi–ginseng). *J Trad Chin Med* 1987; 7: 127–130.

Martin N, Bardisa L, Pantoja C, Roman R, Vargas M. Experimental cardiovascular depressant effects of garlic *(Allium sativum)* dialysate. *J Ethnopharmacol* 1992;37:145–149.

Milkowska-Leyck K, Filipek B, Strzelecka H. Pharmacological effects of lavandulifolioside from *Leonurus cardiaca*. *J Ethnopharmacol* 2002;80:85–90.

Modern TCM Pharmacology. Tianjin: Science and Technology Press; 1997.

Nagourney RA. Garlic: medicinal food or nutritional medicine? *J Medicinal Foods* 1998;1:13–28.

Nammi S, Gudavalli R, Babu BS, Lodagala DS, Boini KM. Possible mechanisms of hypotension produced 70% alcoholic extract of Terminalia arjuna (L.) in anaesthetized dogs. *BMC Complement Altern Med.* 2003 Oct 16;3:5.

Pantoja CV, Chiang LC, Norris BC, Concha JB. Diuretic, natriuretic and hypotensive effects produced by *Allium sativum* (garlic) in anaesthetized dogs. *J Ethnopharmacol* 1991;31: 325–331.

Petkov V. Plants with hypotensive, antiatheromatous and coronarodilatating action. *Am J Chin Med* 1979;7:197–236.

Rácz-Kotilla E, et al. Hypotensive and beta–blocking effect of procyanidins of *Crataegus monogyna*. *Planta Med* 1980; 39: 239.

Rahman K, Billington D. Dietary supplementation with aged garlic extract inhibits ADP-induced platelet aggregation in humans. *J Nutr* 2000;130:2662–2665.

Sharifi AM, Darabi R, Akbarloo N. Investigation of antihypertensive mechanism of garlic in 2K1C hypertensive rat. *J Ethnopharmacol* 2003a;86:219–224.

Sharifi AM, Darabi R, Akbarloo N. Study of antihypertensive mechanism of *Tribulus terrestris* in 2K1C hypertensive rats: role of tissue ACE activity. *Life Sci* 2003b;73:2963–2971.

Tita B, et al. BMC complementary and alternative medicine: pharmacological effect of ethanol extract. *Pharmacol Res* 1993;27:23–24.

von Eiff M, et al. Hawthorn/Passionflower extract and improvement in physical exercise capacity of patients with dyspnoea Class II of the NYHM functional classification. *Acta Ther* 1994; 20: 47–66.

Vonhoff C, Baumgartner A, Hegger M, et al. Extract of Lycopus europaeus L. reduces cardiac signs of hyperthyroidism in rats. *Life Sci.* 2006 Feb 2;78(10):1063–70.

Walker AF, Marakis G, Morris AP, Robinson PA. Promising hypotensive effect of hawthorn extract: a randomized double-blind pilot study of mild, essential hypertension. *Phytother Res* 2002;16:48–54.

Wilburn AJ, King DS, Glisson J, Rockhold RW, Wofford MR. The natural treatment of hypertension. *J Clin Hypertens* (Greenwich) 2004;6:242–248.

Wynn S, Fougere B. Veterinary Herbal Medicine. Oxford, UK: Elsevier, 2006.

Yamamoto M, Kumagai M. Anti-atherogenic action of *Panax ginseng* in rats and in patients with hyperlipidemia. *Planta Med* 1982; 45: 149–166.

Zhang WR, et al. Protective effect of Ginkgo extract on rat brain with transient middle cerebral artery occlusion. *Neurol Res* 2000;22:517–521.

Chapter Twenty-Two

Diseases of the Skin

HERBS FOR DISEASES OF THE SKIN

Herbal treatment of skin disorders—allergic dermatitis/atopy/flea bite dermatitis, alopecia, chronic pyoderma, and mange (demodectic/sarcoptic)—draws on some traditional concepts that need explanation. The skin is considered to be an outer manifestation of internal health; therefore, skin disease is considered to be a sign of a deeper disease process. Topical herbs are a superficial approach (but can be very useful) and as in conventional medicine, a diagnosis is imperative. There is no point treating a flea allergy dermatitis just with herbs! In most chronic skin conditions the skin lesion is thought to be an effort by the body to release, discharge, or remove toxic substances; therefore, medications that suppress signs (such as corticosteroids) are thought to drive the process deeper over time.

Consideration must be given to the organs of detoxification, and hence in human herbal medicine it is common to hear at least the principle of "detoxification" in order to "cleanse" skin. Even in veterinary medicine, in the early part of the 20th century there were references to Aloes for horses and Jalap for dogs for eczema, as well as alteratives for urticaria. Barbadoes aloe, Aniseed, Ginger, Gentian, Fenugreek, Fennel, and Linseed meal were common ingredients in alterative "physick" balls to improve general condition, including coat condition in horses (Leeney 1921).

When eliminative organs are impaired, toxemia, or the accumulation of toxic metabolites, occurs. In chronic skin disease, the digestive system is the eliminative process most likely to be impaired. The goals of herbal therapy are to remove toxins by enhancing and supporting the eliminatory functions of the body, and alteratives are considered to be fundamental. This group of herbs is thought to effect a change in metabolic processes through mild laxative, diuretic, or cholagogue activity, thus aiding elimination. While the theory of toxemia is a traditional one, there is some scientific support for it. We know that incomplete digestion, inflammation, and a failure of the

local immune response (for systemic tolerance) facilitate the absorption of macromolecules with high antigenicity in animals (Halliwell 1995), leading to the development of food sensitivities and allergies.

There is also increasing evidence to suggest that a leaky gut or a more permeable bowel wall may lead to translocation of bacteria and/or endotoxins, which may be an important stimulus for inflammatory cytokine activation (Krack 2005), as well as increased toxic insult to the liver. Permeability is increased in a number of gastrointestinal diseases (parasitical, infection, inflammation) and by trauma, burns, and nonsteroidal anti-inflammatory drugs (Hollander 1999). Gastrointestinal herbs may correct the leaky gut and can improve overall health and reduce allergies and chronic disease.

Dysbiosis is also thought to be a major contributing factor to chronic disease, including skin disorders and food allergies (Fratkin 1996). It follows the use of antibiotics, other medications, or diets that adversely alter the normal flora; or conditions that allow pathogenic microbes to multiply, producing endotoxins that challenge and deplete the immune system and increase gut permeability (thus predisposing to food allergies and sensitivities). Attention to correcting a suspected dysbiosis is worthwhile and relatively straightforward.

The key principle in addressing chronic skin disease, whether autoimmune, atopic, pyodermic, or simply chronic, is to consider the perpetuating factors such as leaky gut syndrome, dysbiosis, and toxemia, as well as the diet, stress levels, drug use, etc. Emphasis is placed on improving systemic health, not just skin health.

ALTERATIVES OR DEPURATIVES

Alteratives or depuratives, otherwise known as blood cleansers, are used to effect a gradual change in chronic disease states, including skin diseases, and are the foundation of any skin formula. There is a dearth of scientific research to support the use of alteratives; however, traditional use and indications are based on empirical observations in people and may have application in animals.

Cleavers (*Galium aparine*) are used for dry skin conditions, eczema, seborrhoea, and psoriasis. The iridoid glycoside constituents are mildly laxative. Burdock root (*Articum lappa*) is one of the best known alteratives for eczema and chronic inflammatory states. One of its constituents, inulin, works as a gentle laxative. It is traditionally recommended for dry, red, scaly skin with hair loss (Wood 2004). Oregon grape (*Mahonia aquifolium*) is used for rough, dry, scaly skin and dandruff. Red clover flowers (*Trifolium pratense*) and Yellow dock root (*Rumex crispus*) are used for chronic skin disease. Cholaretic herbs are also considered to have depurative activity. These include Dandelion (*Taraxacum officinale*), Fumitory (*Fumaria officinalis*), Barberry (*Berberis vulgaris*), and Globe artichoke (*Cynara scolymus*). Similarly diuretic herbs that increase detoxification through the urinary tract might be useful; these include Dandelion leaf (*Taraxacum officinale*), Cleavers (*Gallium aparine*), Burdock (*Arctium lappa*), and Red clover (*Trifolium pratense*). Herbs with activity on the immune system are also regarded as possessing depurative activity and include Echinacea (*Echinacea purpurea*), which is indicated in bacterial and viral infections, mild septicemia, furunculosis, boils, carbuncles, abscesses (Bradley 1992, BHP 1983), and poke root (*Phytolacca decandra*), a toxic herb.

It is sensible to use anti-inflammatory herbs while longer-term alterative strategies take effect. Chamomile (*Matricaria recutita*) and its antipuritic effects were tested in mice fed a diet containing 1.2 w/w% of ethyl acetate extract of dried flower of German chamomile for 11 days. Induced scratching behavior was significantly suppressed without affecting body weight. The inhibitory effects of the dietary intake of the German chamomile extracts were comparable to those of an anti-allergic agent (Kobayashi 2003). Green tea (*Camellia sinensis*) catechin may be useful in the treatment of atopic dermatitis (Hisano 2003). Others include Rehmannia (*Rehmannia glutinosa*); evening primrose oil (*Oenothera biennis*); turmeric (*Curcuma longa*)—which, at low levels the constituent cucurmin is a prostaglandin inhibitor and at higher levels it stimulates the adrenal glands to secrete cortisone—(Srivastava 1985); and Bupleurum (*Bupleurum falcatum*)—which inhibits arachidonic acid metabolism (Bermejo 1998) and the potency of the anti-inflammatory saikosaponins and is similar to that of prednisolone (Chang 1987).

Gotu kola (*Centella asiatica*) triterpenoids are reported to possess wound–healing ability and its constituents Asiaticoside and Madecassoside are documented to be anti–inflammatory (Jacker 1982). Oregon grape (*Berberis aquifolium*) alkaloids were tested in vitro and found to inhibit lipid peroxide substrate accumulation, either by direct reaction with peroxide or by scavenging lipid-derived radicals (Bezakova 1996). Licorice (*Glycyrrhiza glabra*) contains saponins with anti-inflammatory activity; it is shown to inhibit the activity of proinflammatory prostaglandins and leukotrienes and appears to have a cortisone-like effect, making it useful as an anti-inflammatory (Okimasu 1983).

Other anti-allergy herbs also have a role to play. An ethanol extract of Astragalus (*Astragalus membranaceus*) was tested on both in vitro and in vivo murine CD4 T cells and their differentiation into Th1 and Th2 subsets. The data indicated that Astragalus selectively alters Th1/Th2 cytokine secretion patterns and provides the pharmacological basis for its clinical applications (Kang 2004).

Astragalus was given to 106 people with herpes virus keratitis; it modulated the imbalance state of Th1/Th2 in these patients and improved their immune function disturbance (Mao 2004). Other anti-allergy herbs include nettles (*Urtica dioica*), Albizzia (*Albizzia lebbeck*), and *Albizzia kalkora*, also known as mimosa. Studies on a bark extract of Albizzia showed anti-allergy activity against anaphylaxis and atopic allergy (Tripathi 1979). Albizzia has been shown to stabilize mast cell degranulation, depress levels of anti-allergy antibodies, and decrease the overaggressive action of T and B lymphocytes (Bone 1996).

Baical skullcap root (*Scutellaria baicalensis*) contains the flavonoids baicalin and wogonin (similar to quercetin in mechanism of action), both of which have anti-allergy and free radical scavenging activity (Bochorakova 2003, Lin 1996). Another constituent, baicalein, is also anti-inflammatory and anti-allergy; it reduces leukotriene B4 and C4 production by inhibiting lipooxygenase (Chang 1987). Quercetin is an active flavonoid found abundantly in many plants. Degranulation of mast cells is an active process that requires the influx of calcium. Quercetin prevents this influx into the cell (Nishino 1984). Quercetin also inhibits many steps along the eicosanoid membrane pathway, including phospholipase A2 and lipooxygenase (Yoshimoto 1983). It is a strong inhibitor of basophil and mast cell degranulation (Amellal 1985).

Quercetin is found in *Ginkgo biloba*, Evening primrose leaf (*Oenothera biennis*), Green tea (*Camellia sinensis*), Neem (*Azadirachta indica*), Oats (*Avena sativa*), Apple (*Malus domestic*), Cranberry (*Vaccinium macrocarpon*), Nettle (*Urtica dioca*), and Brassica vegetables. Licorice (*Glycyrrhiza glabra*) is anti-allergic (Baltina 2003) and Rehmannia (*Rehmannia glutinosa*) demonstrated anti-allergic effects on induced allergic reactions in vivo and in vitro by reducing plasma histamine levels in a dose-dependent manner. It also dose-dependently inhibited the histamine release from the rat peritoneal mast cells (Kim 1998).

Licorice helps to reduce oxidative damage associated with inflammation. Other herbs to consider include Ginger (*Zingiber officinale*), Ginkgo biloba, Grape seed (*Vitis vinifera*), Green tea (*Camellia sinensis*), Reishi (*Gandoderma lucidium*), Rosemary (*Rosmarinus officinale*), Skullcap (*Scutellaria lateriflora*), Milk thistle (*Silybum marianum*), and Turmeric (*Curcuma longa*).

Adaptogens should be considered if the patient is stressed, anxious, or depressed, and for convalescence. This type of adaptogens includes Ashwaganda *(Withania somnifera)*, Bupleurum *(Bupleurum falcatum)*, Licorice *(Glycyrrhiza glabra)*, Rehmannia *(Rehmannia glutinosa)*, Siberian ginseng *(Elutherococcus senticosus)*, and Gotu kola *(Centella asiatica)*. Likewise, nervine herbs can be beneficial. Consider Skullcap (*Scutellaria lateriflora*), Oats (*Avena sativa*), and St. John's wort (*Hypericum perforatum*).

PRESCRIPTIONS FOR SKIN DISEASES

The following prescriptions are suggested as a starting point. Herb selection depends on pathophysiology, the patient, the herbs most suited to the individual, and the actions of the herbs.

General strategies

Consider regulating or enhancing specific body systems, organs, or tissues, and using alteratives to correct imbalances. The gut-skin connection is a central consideration. While the action of alteratives is unclear, they are invaluable in the treatment of chronic allergic skin disease. Optimize nutrition, and improve vitality by using tonics and adaptogens. Concurrent conventional therapy may be required initially, and doses may need to be reduced after 4 to 6 weeks. Continue herbal therapy for a minimum of 3 months.

Atopy and skin allergies

Reduce exposure to known allergens. Consider an elimination diet, as well as herbs that modulate immunity (those that down regulate TH2 cells). Use herbs to reduce allergic pruritis and those with anti-inflammatory action. Also consider herbs that inhibit mast cell release of histamine.

For allergic dermatitis with either dry or moist skin lesions, give:

Burdock: Depurative, mildly laxative, nutritive; 1 part.

Red clover: Alterative; 1 part.

Cleavers: Diuretic, astringent; 1 part.

Nettle leaf: Nutritive, circulatory stimulant, anti-inflammatory, diuretic; 1 part.

Astragalus: Immune modulating, tonic, diuretic; 1 part.

For tinctures, give 1 ml per 10 pounds twice daily in food. For teas, give one-fourth cup per 10 pounds twice daily in food.

For atopic dermatitis, give:

Baical skullcap: Anti-allergy, anti-inflammatory, anti-bacterial, mild sedative, diuretic, bitter; 1 part.

Nettle leaf: Nutritive, circulatory stimulant, anti-inflammatory, diuretic; 1 part.

Burdock: Depurative, mildly laxative, nutritive; 1 part.

Licorice: Anti-inflammatory, adaptogen, laxative, taste improver; 1 part.

Astragalus: Immune modulating, tonic, diuretic; 1 part.

For tinctures, give 1 ml per 10 pounds twice daily in food. For teas, give one-fourth cup per 10 pounds twice daily in food.

For alopecia, dry skin, dry or coarse coat, and brittle nails, give:

Horsetail: Contains minerals, including silica; 1 part.

Bladderwrack: Contains iodine, may be useful in subclinical hypothyroid; 1 part.

Red clover: Alterative; 1 part.

Burdock: Alterative, mildly laxative, contains linoleic acid; 1 part.

Rehmannia: Adaptogen, blood tonic; 1 part.

For tinctures, give 1 ml per 10 pounds twice daily in food. For teas, give one-fourth cup per 10 pounds twice daily in food,

For alopecia, substitute Panax ginseng for Red clover. A methanol extract of Panax red ginseng promoted hair growth on mouse vibrissal follicles in organ culture. This indicated that Ginseng radix possesses hair-growth-promoting activity and its bioactive components are partially attributable to the Ginseng saponin components (Matsuda 2003).

Chronic pyoderma

Improve systemic health. Use herbs that improve immunity, reduce bacterial load, and support the lymphatic system. Use alteratives to improve metabolism. The following are suggested:

Echinacea: Immune modulating, anti-inflammatory, antibacterial, antiviral, vulnery; 1 part.

Cleavers: Diuretic, astringent, lymphatic; 1 part.

Astragalus: Immune modulating, tonic, diuretic; 1 part.

Calendula: Lymphatic, anti-inflammatory, astringent, vulnery, cholagogue; 1 part.

Withania: Tonic, adaptogen, nervine, sedative, anti-inflammatory; 1 part.

Poke root: Immune enhancing, lymphatic; add 1/20th of volume of formula.

For tinctures, give 1 ml per 10 pounds twice daily in food. For teas, give one-fourth cup per 10 pounds twice daily in food.

Chronic demodex

Consider using conventional treatment, which may relieve suffering much faster than herbal treatment. If these treatments are ineffective or inappropriate for the patient, however, consider herbs to improve immunity, reduce secondary bacterial load, improve systemic health (especially GIT health), and nourish skin.

Echinacea: Immune modulating, anti-inflammatory, antibacterial, antiviral, vulnery; 1 part.

Burdock: Depurative, mildly laxative, nutritive; 1 part.

Panax ginseng: Adaptogen, thymoleptic, tonic, immunostimulant, hepatoprotective; 1 part.

Baptisia: Antimicrobial, antipyretic, antiseptic; 1 part.

Calendula: Lymphatic, anti-inflammatory, astringent, vulnery, cholagogue 1 part.

For tinctures, give 1 ml per 10 pounds twice daily in food. For teas, give one-fourth cup per 10 pounds twice daily in food.

Consider adding poke root at 5% of the formula for sarcoptic mange. It has been suggested that sarcoptic mange in dogs is susceptible to local application of crude extracts of Garlic, Neem, and Sitaphalas, 1:10 (v/w), resulting in recovery rates of 54%, 67%, and 44%, respectively. The average numbers of days required for complete cure were 22 ± 0.6, 27 ± 1.7, and 28 ± 1.9 days. All treatments were ineffective in treating *Demodex* species infection (Dakshinkar 1997).

REFERENCES

Amellal M, Bronner C, Briancon F et al. Inhibition of Mast Cell Histamine Release by Flavonoids and BioFlavonoids. *Planta Medica*, 1985;51:16–20.

Baltina LA. Chemical modification of glycyrrhizic acid as a route to new bioactive compounds for medicine [Review]. *Curr Med Chem* 2003;10:155–171.

Bermejo Benito, P. et al. In vivo and in vitro anti-inflammatory activity of saikosaponins. *Life Sciences*. 1998. 63: 13, 1147–1156.

Bezakova L, Misik V, Malekova L, Svajdlenka E, Kostalova D. Lipoxygenase inhibition and antioxidant properties of bisbenzylisoqunoline alkaloids isolated from *Mahonia aquifolium*. *Pharmazie* 1996;51:758–761.

British Herbal Pharmacopoeia. Keighley, U.K.: British Herbal Medicine Association. 1983.

Bochorakova H, Paulova H, Slanina J, et al. Main flavonoids in the root of *Scutellaria baicalensis* cultivated in Europe and their comparative antiradical properties. *Phytother Res.* 2003 Jun;17(6):640–4

Bone K. Clinical Applications of Ayurvedic and Chinese Herbs—Monographs for the Western Herbal Practitioner. Warwick, Queensland, Australia: Phytotherapy Press; 1996:94.

Bradley PR. British Herbal Compendium, vol 1. Bournemouth: British Herbal Medicine Association, 1992.

Chang HM, But PPH. Pharmacology and Applications of Chinese Materia Medica, vol 2. Singapore: World Scientific Publishing; 1987.

Dakshinkar N, Sarode D. Therapeutic evaluation of crude extracts of indigenous plants against mange of dogs: ethnoveterinary medicine: alternatives for livestock development. In: Ethnoveterinary Medicine: Alternatives for Livestock Development Proceedings of an International Conference; November 4–6, 1997; Pune, India (available at: http://www.vetwork.org.uk/pune20.htm).

Fratkin J. Leaky gut syndrome: treating intestinal candidiasis and dysbiosis. Proceedings of the American Holistic Medical Association Conference; New York, NY. May 1996.

Halliwell RE. Dietary allergy and intolerance in the dog: new concepts. ASAVA Dermatology 1995 AVA Annual Conference Proceedings.

Hisano M, et al. Inhibitory effect of catechin against the superantigen staphylococcal enterotoxin B (SEB). Archives of Dermatological Research. Berlin, Germany: Springer-Verlag, 2003. 295: 5, 183–189.

Hollander D. Intestinal permeability, leaky gut, and intestinal disorders. *Curr Gastroenterol Rep.* 1999 Oct;1(5):410–6.

Jacker H-J, et al. Zum antiexsudativen Verhalten einiger Triterpensaponine. *Pharmazie* 1982;37:380–382.

Kang H, Ahn KS, Cho C, Bae HS. Immunomodulatory effect of *Astragali radix* extract on murine TH1/TH2 cell lineage development. *Biol Pharm Bull* 2004;27:1946–1950.

Kim H, Lee E, Lee S, Shin T, Kim Y, Kim J. Effect of *Rehmannia glutinosa* on immediate type allergic reaction. *Int J Immunopharmacol* 1998;20:231–240.

Kobayashi Y, Nakano Y, Inayama K, Sakai A, Kamiya T. Dietary intake of the flower extracts of German chamomile *(Matricaria recutita* L.) inhibited compound 48/80-induced itch-scratch responses in mice. *Phytomedicine* 2003;10:657–664.

Krack A, Sharma R, Figulla HR, Anker SD. The importance of the gastrointestinal system in the pathogenesis of heart failure. *Eur Heart J* 2005;26:2368–2374.

Leeney H. Home Doctoring for Animals. London: MacDonald and Martin; 1921.

Lin CC, Shieh DE. The anti-inflammatory activity of *Scutellaria rivularis* extracts and its active components, baicalin, baicalein and wogonin. *Am J Chin Med* 1996;24:31–36.

Mao SP, Cheng KL, Zhou YF Modulatory effect of *Astragalus membranaceus* on Th1/Th2 cytokine in patients with herpes simplex keratitis. Zhongguo Zhong Xi Yi Jie He Za Zhi 2004;24:121–123.

Matsuda H, Yamazaki M, Asanuma Y, Kubo M. Promotion of hair growth by *Ginseng radix* on cultured mouse vibrissal hair follicles. *Phytother Res* 2003;17:797–800.

Nishino H, Naitoh E, Iwashima A, et al. Quercetin interacts with calmodulin (a calcium regulatory protein). *Experentia* 1984;40:184–5.

Okimasu E, Moromizato Y, Watanabe S, et al. Inhibition of phospholipase A2 and platelet aggregation by glycyrrhizin, an anti-inflammation drug. *Actu Med Okayama* 1981;37:457–463.

Srivastava R, Srimal RC. Modification of certain inflammation induced biochemical changes by curcumin. *Indian J Med Res* 1985;81:215–223.

Tripathi RM, Sen PC, Das PK. Further studies on the mechanism of the anti-anaphylactic action of Albizzia lebbeck, an Indian indigenous drug. *J Ethnopharmacol* 1979;1:397–400.

Wood M. Herbalism: Basic Doctrines, Energetics, and Classification. Berkeley, CA: North Atlantic Books; 2004.

Wynn S, Marsden S. Manual of Natural Veterinary Medicine. Sydney: Mosby; 2003.158.

Yoshimoto T, Furukawa M, Yamamoto S, et al. Flavonoids: potent inhibitors of arachidonate 5-lipoxygenase. *Biochem Biophys Res Commun* 1983;116:612–618.

Chapter Twenty-Three

Diseases of the Digestive System

In herbal medicine, there is a recognized fundamental linkage between the gut and systemic health in conditions as widely ranging as asthma, atopy, autoimmune disease, and even arthritis. This is important, considering that the gut plays a significant role in immune function. Herbalists emphasize the health of the digestive system, bowel movements, and any symptoms related to gut function—even mild digestive disturbances such as burping, mild constipation, inconsistent stools, or excessive flatulence are always considered significant, even if not the reason for presentation for consultation.

The herbs outlined below are useful in gastrointestinal health and disease management and are supported by traditional use or research. The lists are by no means complete, and there are differences in the potency of the actions of the individual herbs. However, by knowing the particulars of the patient, an herb might be chosen for its breadth of action when more than 1 system is involved or for a particularly strong action that is needed. Sometimes only a gentle stimulation, triggering an appropriate reflex response or dampening a response, may be all that's needed to reach equilibrium again. The beauty and art of herbal medicine is in the selection of herbs that have appropriate action and yet are tailored for the whole health of the individual patient.

Bitters

Bitters, sialogogues, and stomachics refer to herbs that improve digestive function either by increasing saliva production (sialogogue) or increasing gastric secretion (stomachic). They are frequently bitter tasting, hence "bitters." Some early work carried out in cachectic dogs showed that a tincture of Gentian (*Gentiana lutea*) given by mouth increased appetite, gastric secretion and acid, and pepsin content. It is suggested that the bitter taste has a priming effect on upper digestive function, particularly when digestion is suboptimal (Moorhead 1915). This is possibly mediated via a reflex vagal stimulation from bitter taste buds, causing increases in gastric acid secretion, gastrin, and gallbladder motility, and priming the pancreas (ACP 1999).

Traditionally, bitters have been an essential component of any digestive tract formula in which upper digestive tract function is impaired. Many herbs have bitter principals, including many of the alteratives, depuratives, and cholaretics. They include Oregon grape (*Berberis aquifolium*), Barberry (*Berberis vulgaris*), Bupluerum (*Bupleurum falcatum*), Golden seal (*Hydrastis canadensis*), Chamomile (*Matricaria recutita*), Picrorrhiza (*Picrorrhiza kurroa*), Baical skullcap (*Scutellaria baicalensis*), Dandelion (*Taraxacum officinale*), Thyme (*Thymus vulgaris*), and Ginger (*Zingiber officinale*).

Carminatives

Carminatives help reduce and dispel gas, and they are a feature of herbs that contain mainly volatile compounds or essential oils. Fennel (*Foeniculum vulgare*) has long been used to relieve the pain of intestinal spasm and gas and is an ingredient of "gripe water" that is used in infant colic. Fennel and other carminatives are thought to relax smooth muscle spasms that occur in response to gaseous distension, leading to relief of intestinal cramping. A fennel infusion in animals reduced peristalsis tone and amplitude 2 to 30 minutes after administration. In vitro studies and animal models indicate that fennel extracts modulate calcium availability and metabolism. In a multicenter, randomized, placebo-controlled trial, Fennel significantly relieved symptoms of infant colic (defined as a decrease in the number of hours spent crying weekly) compared with a placebo (Alexandrovich 2003). Other carminatives include Ginger (*Zingiber officinale*), Peppermint oil (*Mentha x piperita*), Chamomile (*Matricaria recutita*), Thyme (*Thymus vulgaris*), Cinnamon (*Cinnamomum zeylanicum*), Lavender (*Lavendula officinalis*), Lemon balm (*Melissa officinalis*), Catnip (*Nepeta cataria*),

Rosemary (*Rosmarinus officinalis*), Valerian (*Valeriana* spp.), Parsley (*Petroselinum crispum*), and Aniseed (*Pimpinella anisum*).

Spasmolytics

Most of the carminative herbs have spasmolytic activity. They act in various ways; for example, Chamomile's (*Matricaria recutita*) activity has been attributed to apigenin, apigenin-7-O-glucoside, and a-bisabolol, which act similarly to papaverine (Bruneton 1995, Della Loggia 1990). Peppermint oil has been shown to decrease the gut contractile response to histamine, serotonin, acetylcholine, and substance P (Hills 1991) and was shown to suppress gastric spasms in people during upper gastrointestinal endoscopy (Hiki 2003). *Corydalis ambigua* is a traditional anodyne for visceral pain. Others include Cramp bark (Viburnum opulus), Wild yam (Disocorea villosa), and Calendula (Calendula officinalis).

Antacid, anti-ulcerogenic, and anti-inflammatory herbs

Several plants help protect gastric mucosa and heal ulcers. Meadowsweet (*Filipendula ulmaria*), which contains salicylates administered at rates of 0.7 and 1.25 ml/kg, was shown to reduce ulceration (induced by aspirin) in an in vivo study by 25.4% and 26.2%, respectively (Gorbacheva 2002). Licorice given orally for 3 days protected rats against induced duodenal ulcers but was ineffective against acute aspirin-induced gastric ulcers. The effect of Licorice may be due to inhibition of acid-pepsin secretion and augmentation of mucosal defensive factors. These mucosal defense factors may include enhanced mucin secretion and decreased cell shedding or acceleration of mucin excretion via Licorice increasing the synthesis of glycoprotein at the gastric mucosa, prolonging the life of the epithelial cells and antipepsin activity (Dehpour 1995). Oral administration of deglycyrrhizinated Licorice (380 mg, 3 times daily) to 169 patients with chronic duodenal ulcers was as effective as antacid or cimetidine treatments, indicating that constituents other than glycyrrhetic acid contribute to its anti-ulcer activity (Kassir 1985).

Turmeric extracts (water or ethanol) reduced gastric secretion in rabbits (Sakai 1989) and increased the mucin content of gastric juice (Rafatullah 1990). Extracts from Lemon balm (*Melissa officinalis*), Chamomile (*Matricaria recutita*), Peppermint (*Mentha x piperita*), Licorice (*Glycyrrhiza glabra*), Angelica root (*Angelica archangelica*), Milk thistle (*Silybum marianum*), and greater Celadine (*Chelidonium majus*), singly and combined, produced a dose-dependent anti-ulcerogenic activity associated with reduced acid output and increased mucin secretion,

increased prostaglandin E2 release, and decreased leukotrienes (Khayyal 2001). An ethanolic extract of Parsley (*Petroselinum crispum*) protected gastric mucosa against induced ulcers in rats (Al-Howiriny 2003). Other anti-ulcerogenic herbs include Gotu kola (*Centella asiatica*) and Chamomile (*Matricaria recutita*), and anti-inflammatory herbs include Dong guai (*Angelica sinensis*), Baical skullcap (*Scutellaria baicalensis*), Calendula (*Calendula officinalis*), Wild yam (*Dioscorea villosa*), Slippery elm (*Ulmus rubra*), and Marshmallow (*Althaea officinalis*).

Demulcents and mucilages

Demulcents are used to soothe and protect an alimentary mucous membrane (buccal, pharyngeal, oesophageal, and gastric mucosa), whereas mucilages refer to plants that contain mucilaginous substances, which cause demulcency. Marshmallow (*Althaea officinalis*) is a mucilage and has a demulcent action due to its high content of polysaccharide hydrocolloids, which form a protective coating on the oral and pharyngeal mucosa, soothing local irritation and inflammation (Franz 1989).

Adhesion of constituents varies between plants. Polysaccharides from *Althaea officinalis*, *Plantago lanceolata*, *Malva moschata*, or *Tilia cordata* showed moderate bioadhesion to epithelial tissue compared to polysaccharides from *Fucus vesiculosus* and *Calendula officinalis*, which were concentration-dependent. Histological studies of membranes indicated the presence of distinct polysaccharide layers on the apical membrane surface, which account (in part) for the therapeutic effects of mucilage-containing plants in the treatment of irritated membranes (Schmidgall 2000). Demulcent action is found in Marshmallow (*Althaea officinalis*), Slippery elm (*Ulmus fulva*), Sarsaparilla (*Smilax ornate*), Licorice (*Glycyrrhiza glabra*), Bladderwrack (*Fucus vesiculosus*), Fenugreek (*Trigonella foenum-graecum*), Mullein (*Verbascum thapsus*), Calendula (*Calendula officinalis*), and Corn silk (*Zea May*).

Intestinal astringents

Intestinal astringents are most useful in acute diarrhea. Most of these herbs contain tannic acid, which precipitates protein on the mucosal surface. This acts as a barrier between tissue and irritant, and the protecting and soothing effect is enhanced by an astringent action on any exposed nerve endings so that pain is lessened. Herbs that are high in tannins are ideally used for short periods only, and they can interact with or limit absorption of some alkaline drugs. Intestinal astringents including Agrimony (*Agrimonia eupatoria*), Tormentil (*Potentilla tormentilla*), Blackberry (*Rubus fructosis*), and stewed Tea (*Camellia sinensis*).

Laxatives

Herbs with laxative action contain aperients, which promote a natural movement of the bowels rather than provoking them forcibly. These safe-to-use laxatives include Psyllium, Linseed, and dietary fibers, as well as Burdock (*Articum lappa*), Oregon grape (*Berberis aquifolium*), Barberry (*Berberis vulgaris*), Licorice (*Glycchyriza glabra*), Rehmannia (*Rehmannia glutinosa*), and Dandelion (*Taraxacum officinalis*).

Aloe (*Aloe barbadensis*) was a popular anthracene purgative until synthetic anthraquinones were introduced in veterinary medicine. Cascara (*Rhamnus purshiana*) was also used in cats and dogs. It has been suggested that Cascara and Buckthorn (*Rhamnus frangulara*) may be the preferred herbs of choice for constipation in cats (Wynn 2003). Senna pod (*Cassia angustifolia*) produces sublaxative effects at low doses, whereby the bowel motions are made comfortable, normal, and soft. Other laxatives include Fringe tree (*Chionanthus virginicus*), Fumitory (*Fumaria officinalis*), Licorice (*Glycyrrhiza glabra*), Butternut (*Juglans cinerea*), Yellow dock (*Rumex crispus*), and Fenugreek (*Trigonella foenum-graecum*).

Anti-emetics

When emesis is centrally initiated, the cause must be diagnosed. Conventional medications should be considered, although herbs can be given via enema. Administering herbs to a vomiting animal is not recommended; However, for chronic gastritis, demulcents (which coat, protect, lubricate, and soothe the gastric mucosa) and local gastric sedatives (antacids and stomachics) might be helpful to suppress the vomiting reflex.

Ginger (*Zingiber officinale*) significantly reduced the number of vomiting episodes in healthy dogs with cisplatin-induced emesis (3 mg/kg IV), at doses as low as 25 mg/kg per os. The highest dose tested for both ethanol and acetate extracts was 200 mg/kg, which led to the fewest vomiting episodes but a shorter latency in minutes to the first episode. These doses were comparable with the anti-emetic efficacy of granisetron. Because Ginger was ineffective in inhibiting apomorphine-induced emesis (which was mediated through a dopaminergic mechanism), the authors hypothesized that 5-HT$_3$ receptors may be involved in the activity of ginger (Sharma 1997). The emetic action of the peripherally acting agent copper sulfate was also inhibited in dogs given an intragastric dose of Ginger extract (Zhou 1960). Ginger's anti-emetic activity is peripheral (it does not involve the central nervous system) and has been attributed to the combined action of zingerones and shogaols (Ghazanfar 1994).

Antimicrobials

Many herbs have direct antimicrobial activity in the gastrointestinal tract. Berberine (in several herbs) and hydrastine (in golden seal) are some of the best studied for GIT infections. The isolated alkaloid berberine has been shown to inhibit intestinal fluid accumulation and smooth muscle contraction, reduce inflammation, and suppress bacterial enterotoxin formation. Tormentil root (*Potentilla erecta*) extract in controlled doses shortened the duration of rotavirus diarrhea and decreased the requirement for rehydration solutions in children suffering from rotavirus diarrhea (Subbotina 2003). It also may be useful in rotaviral infections in animals.

Consider immune-modulating herbs such as Echinacea, Astragalus, Andrographis, and Picrorrhiza in microbial infections. Most herbs with antimicrobial activity have other properties, which should be considered, depending on the nature of the condition. Just some of the herbs to consider include Chamomile (*Matricaria recutita*), Thyme (*Thymus vulgaris*)—especially against helicobacter—Picrorrhiza (*Picrorrhiza kurroa*), Oregon Grape (*Berberis aquifolium*), Barberry (*Berberis vulgaris*), Golden seal (*Hydrastis sinensis*), Fennel (*Foeniculum vulgare*), and Citrus seed extract (*citrus spp.*).

Parasiticides

Many herbs have well researched activity against parasites. The traditional approach in veterinary medicine prior to modern anthelmintics was to use fairly toxic herbs and to purge parasites, often leading to cramping and diarrhea. Current anthelmintics pose little risk and work well; however, some people prefer not to use drugs and desire herbal options. Garlic is frequently mentioned as an effective worming agent. It has some activity against roundworm (*Ascaris strongyloides*) and hookworm (*Ancylostoma caninum* and *Necator americanus*). Allicin appears to be an anthelmintic constituent, but diallyl disulphide was not effective (Kempski 1967, Soh 1960). However, garlic (whole clove) efficacy has not been well documented and may in fact be ineffective for parasite control (Abells 1999).

The alkaloid berberine (in Barberry and Orgeon grape, among others) showed strong nematocidal activity against *Toxocara canis* in vitro (Satou 2002). Hydrastine (in Golden seal) has been studied on the protoscolices of the tapeworm (*Echinococcus granulosus*) in vitro and in vivo. Hydrastine at 0.3% concentration produced 70% mortality of the larvae in both experiments (Chen 1991). Cucurbitine contained in crushed pumpkin seeds is 55% efficacious against *Taenia saginata* (Pawlowski 1970).

Herbs that have been traditionally used for their anthelmintic activity in humans and animals include

Wormwood (*Artemesia absinthium*), Butternut (*Juglans cinerea*), Thyme (*Thymus vulgaris*), and Ginger (*Zingiber officinale*). A number of herbs have shown antiprotozoal activity; they include Oregano (*Oreganum vulgare*), Propolis, Sweet Annie (*Artemesia annua*), and berberine-containing herbs. Essential oils may also be effective, preventive, or curative treatments against several flagellated parasites; however, efficacy is not well documented and conventional treatment is more likely to be curative.

Liver and gallbladder herbs

Cholagogues, which stimulate the release and flow of bile already formed in the liver, and choleretics, which stimulate bile production by hepatocytes, are often found in bitter herbs. Cholagogues are used to improve the "cleansing of the liver" by improving bile excretion. Cholagogues include Agrimony (*Agrimonia eupatoria*), Oregon grape (*Berberis aquifolium*), Calendula (*Calendula officinalis*), Greater celandine (*Chelidonium majus*), Fringe tree (*Chionanthus virginicus*), Turmeric (*Curcuma longa*), Globe artichoke (*Cynara scolymus*), Wormwood (*Artemesia absinthium*), Picrorrhiza (*Picrorrhiza kurroa*), Yam (*Dioscorea spp*), Gentian (*Gentiana lutea*), Chamomile (*Matricaria recutita*), Yellow dock (*Rumex crispus*), Milk thistle (*Silybum marianum*), and Dandelion (*Taraxacum officinale*). They are often combined with laxatives in the treatment of liver disease and wider liver dysfunction (Mills 1989).

Choleretic herbs improve liver function and are particularly indicated if digestive symptoms are predominant. Most of the hepatoprotective herbs have choleretic activity. Contraindications for choleretic and cholagogues include obstructed bile ducts (e.g., bile duct or pancreas cancer), jaundice following hemolytic diseases, acute or severe hepatocellular disease (e.g., viral hepatitis, septic cholecystitis, intestinal spasm or ileus), or liver cancer. Strongly choleretic herbs include Hydrastis (*golden seal*), Berberis vulgaris (*Barberry*), and Bhelidonium (*greater celandine*). Bitter herbs can cause nausea in patients with liver damage so they should be avoided after hepatic restoratives have been used. Choleretics include *Artemesia absinthium*, *Berberis vulgaris*, *Calendula officinalis*, *Chelidonium majus*, *Glycyrrhiza glabra*, *Hydrastis canadensis*, *Mentha x piperita*, *Silybum marianum*, and *Zingiber officinale*.

Hepatotonic herbs include those with choleretic, cholagogue, hepatoprotective, or hepatorestorative properties. They include Andrographis (*Andrographis panniculata*), Oregon grape (*Berberis aquifolium*), Barberry (*Berberis vulgaris*), Bupleurum (*Bupleurum falcatum*), Fringe tree (*Chionanthus virginicus*), Globe artichoke (*Cynara scolymus*), *Panax ginseng*, Phyllanthus (*Phyllanthus amarus*), Picrorrhiza (*Picrorrhiza kurroa*), Dan Shen (*Salvia multirrhiza*), Schisandra (*Schisandra chinensis*), Milk thistle (*Silybum marianum*), and Dandelion (*Taraxacum officinale*). Hepatorestorative herbs restore liver paranechyma. *Panax ginseng* (250 500 mg/kg) accelerates liver regeneration and ameliorates liver injury after hepatectomy in dogs (Kwon 2003). In studies relating to regeneration of livers of rats subjected to partial hepatectomy, silybin from Milk thistle (*Silybum marianum*) increased mitotic activity of Kupffer's cells (Magliulo 1979). Globe artichoke (Cynara scolymus) is also considered to be regenerative.

The hepatoprotective herb Milk thistle (*Silybum marianum*) is one of the best known liver herbs. It protected against Amanita phalloides poisoning in Beagles and prevented deaths in all of the silibinin-treated dogs compared to controls (Vogel 1984). Silymarin was tested in dogs suffering from CCl4 intoxication of the liver and treated dogs had significantly lower AST and ALT compared with the control CCl4-intoxicated group (Paulova 1990). Other herbs with hepatoprotective properties include Burdock (*Articum lappa*), Andrographis (*Andrographis panniculata*), Bupleurum (*Bupleurum falcatum*), Tumeric (*Curcuma longa*), Globe artichoke (*Cynara scolymus*), Asian Ginseng (*Panax ginseng*), Phyllanthus (*Phyllanthus amarus*), Picrorrhiza (*Picrorrhiza kurroa*), Dan Shen (*Salvia multirrhiza*), Schisandra (*Schisandra chinensis*), and Dandelion (*Taraxacum radix*).

Pancreatic herbs

A number of herbs have traditional indications for pancreatic disorders; some have been supported by research. Fringe tree (*Chionanthus virginicus*) is one of the best known traditional herbs advocated for pancreatic disease, inflammatory or otherwise, and for diabetes (Felter 1898). Gymnema (*Gymnema silvestre*) doubled the number of islet cells and beta cells in diabetic rats after 60 days of administration. It was suggested that it could bring about blood glucose homeostasis through increased serum insulin levels provided by repair/regeneration of the endocrine pancreas (Shanmugasundaram 1990).

Emodin (in *Aloe vera* and other herbs) is a potent agent in the management of clinical and experimental acute pancreatitis. In experiments of induced pancreatitis in rats, the emodin-treated group had significantly lower serum amylase levels compared to controls. Emodin might upregulate gene expression, which subsequently increases DNA synthesis and protein content and then accelerates pancreatic repair and regeneration (Gong 2002). Emodin in combination with baicalein has significant therapeutic benefits in severe acute pancreatitis in rats (Zhang 2005). Dandelion (*Taraxacum officinale*) showed insulin secretagogue activity (Hussain 2004), and in a study of induced pancreatitis in rats, it (10 mg/kg PO) reduced IL-6, a principal mediator of acute phase response, and TNF-α production during cholecystokinin-induced acute pancreatitis (Seo 2005).

FORMULAS FOR GASTROINTESTINAL CONDITIONS

The formulas below are indicated for gingivitis, stomatitis, and periodontal disease; food allergy gastritis and enteritis; gastritis and vomiting; immune-mediated inflammatory bowel disease; internal parasites (coccidia, giardia, roundworms, hookworms, whipworms, and tapeworms); chronic active hepatitis and cholangiohepatitis; and acute and chronic pancreatitis.

Strategy

Implement appropriate lifestyle changes and appropriate diet. Monitor patients regularly, particularly if herbs are used as the sole treatment for early cases or if the animals are on conventional medication. Doses can be adjusted upwards if no changes of 20% per week have been observed. Doses of conventional medicines may need to be reviewed 1 to 2 weeks after commencing treatment with herbs.

These formulas can be made as per the recipe or adapted from other recipes according to patient needs. They are formulated to allow substitution.

Gingivitis and periodontal disease and stomatitis

Implement dental prophylaxis and teeth cleaning. Use vulnery (wound healing), anti-inflammatory, and antimicrobial herbs, and consider immune-supporting herbs. Improve peripheral circulation and control pain. Use Coenzyme Q10 (30 to 100 mg).

There is some research to support the use of the following herbs for gingivitis and periodontal disease: Calendula (*Calendula officinalis*) (Krazhan 2001), Green tea (*Camellia sinensis*) (Yun 2004), Gotu kola (*Centella asiatica*), and Pomegranate (*Punica granatum*) (Sastravaha 2003). Others include Chinese basil (*Perilla frutescens*), Witch hazel (*Hamamelis virginiana*), Marshmallow (*Althaea officinalis*), Propolis, and berberine-containing herbs and *Aloe vera* gel. Other classics include Myrrh (*Commiphora myrrha*), Golden seal (*Hydrastis canadensis*), Coptis (*Coptis chinensis*), and Sage (*Salvia officinalis*). If gums are bleeding consider Bilberry (*Vaccinium myrtillus*) or Yunnan pai yao.

Calendula: Antiseptic, anti-inflammatory, astringent, vulnery; 1 part.

Echinacea: Immunostimulant, anti-inflammatory, antimicrobial, vulnery: 1 part.

Baptisia: Antimicrobial, antiseptic, antipyretic; 1 part.

Gotu kola: Adaptogen, connective tissue regenerator, nerve tonic, alterative; 1 part.

Bilberry: Anti-edema, antioxidant, anti-inflammatory, astringent; 1 part.

For tinctures, give 1 ml per 10 pounds twice daily in food. For teas, give one-fourth cup per 10 pounds twice daily in food.

Food allergy, gastritis, vomiting, and enteritis

Identify the cause by using a food elimination trial or single protein source diet or by giving frequent small meals. Use conventional medications as necessary for symptomatic relief of pain and discomfort. Use demulcent herbs and anti-inflammatory herbs, and consider carminative and spasmolytic herbs.

Chamomile: Carminative, anti-inflammatory, bitter tonic, cholagogue, anti-allergic, mild sedative, spasmolytic; 2 parts.

Milk thistle: Antioxidant, hepatoprotective, hepatatonic; 1 part.

Globe artichoke: Bitter tonic, cholagogue, choleretic, hepatoprotective; 1 part.

Marshmallow: Demulcent, vulnery, diuretic; 1 part.

For tinctures, give 1 ml per 10 pounds twice daily in food. For teas, give one-fourth cup per 10 pounds twice daily in food.

Inflammatory bowel disease

Identify the cause. Address possible food sensitivity and allergy, as well as stress. Use conventional medications as necessary for symptomatic relief of pain and discomfort. Use demulcent herbs and anti-inflammatory herbs, and consider carminative and spasmolytic herbs.

Oral aloe vera gel was assessed in vitro on the production of reactive oxygen metabolites, eicosanoids, and interleukin-8, all of which may be pathogenic in inflammatory bowel disease. The results indicated that it may have a therapeutic effect in inflammatory bowel disease (Langmead 2004a,b).

Chamomile: Carminative, anti-inflammatory, bitter tonic, cholagogue, anti-allergic, mild sedative, spasmolytic; 1 part.

Calendula: Antiseptic, anti-inflammatory, astringent, spasmolytic, vulnery, cholagogue; 1 part.

Meadowsweet: Anti-ulcerogenic, antacid, anti-inflammatory, astringent; 1 part.

Marshmallow: Demulcent, vulnery, diuretic: 1 part.

Astragalus: Immune modulating; 1 part.

For tinctures, give 1 ml per 10 pounds twice daily in food. For teas, give one-fourth cup per 10 pounds twice daily in food.

Parasites

Conventional treatment is safe and effective. When considering herbal treatment, fecal floats prior to and post herbal treatment are useful to monitor efficacy. Long-term use of herbal formulas is generally required for treatment. If animals are predisposed to parasites, consider improving the diet and use herbs to improve digestive function and immunity.

Calendula: Antiseptic, anti-inflammatory, astringent, spasmolytic, vulnery, cholagogue; 1 part.

Astragalus: Immune modulating; 1 part.

Oregon grape: Cholagogue, mild laxative, bitter tonic, alterative, 1 part.

Thyme: Carminative, antispasmodic, anthelmintic, astringent; 1 part.

Wormwood: Bitter tonic, anthelmintic, choleretic; 1 part.

For tinctures, give 1 ml per 10 pounds twice daily in food.

Chronic active hepatitis and cholangiohepatitis

It is important to determine the underlying pathophysiology of particular hepatic disorders to tailor treatment for the individual case. Antimicrobial, antiviral, and immune-enhancing herbs may be necessary. Where fibrosis is a concern, hepatotrophorestorative herbs are an important part the of strategic treatment. Consider hepatoprotective herbs to minimize liver damage and consider using silybum and schisandra in more concentrated forms, perhaps by adding tablet forms alongside a formula. Consider immune-enhancing herbs such as Astragalus (*Astragalus membranaceus*) for chronic infection, as well as Picrorrhiza. For more acute infections consider Echinacea or Andrographis. In acute infections and viral infections consider St. John's wort (*Hypericum performatum*) and Phyllanthus (*Phyllanthus amarus*). Consider hepatic trophorestoratives such as *Panax ginseng*. For toxic insults to the liver consider Milk thistle (*Schisandra chinensis*) and Silybum (*Silybum marianum*).

Bupluerum: Hepatoprotective, anti-inflammatory, tonic; 1 part.

Schisandra: Hepatoprotective, nervine tonic, adaptogen; 1 part.

Milk thistle: Hepatotonic, hepatoprotective, antioxidant; 1 part.

Panax ginseng: Adaptogen, anti-inflammatory, anti-allergic, immune enhancing, hepatorestorative; 1 part.

Astragalus: Immune modulating; 1 part.

For tinctures, give 1 ml per 10 pounds twice daily in food. For teas, give one-fourth cup per 10 pounds twice daily in food.

Pancreatitic disease

Conventional treatment of acute pancreatitis is needed while vomiting is occurring (alternatively, administer herbs via enema). Use herbs that improve pancreatic function and protect against possible sequelae. Improve overall digestive function using bitters and anti-inflammatory herbs. Use immune modulation when autoimmune disease is present. Consider lipid-lowering herbs.

Fringe tree: Laxative, anti-emetic, liver tonic, cholagogue; 1 part.

Gymnema: Pancreatic trophorestorative, mildly diuretic, hypoglycemic; 1 part.

Dandelion: Diuretic, laxative, pancreatic secretagogue, cholagogue; 1 part.

Chamomile: Carminative, anti-inflammatory, bitter tonic, cholagogue, anti-allergic, mild sedative, spasmolytic; 1 part.

Astragalus: Immune modulating; 1 part.

For tinctures, give 1 ml per 10 pounds twice daily in food. For teas, give one-fourth cup per 10 pounds twice daily in food.

REFERENCES

Al-Howiriny T, Al-Sohaibani M, El-Tahir K, Rafatullah S. Prevention of experimentally-induced gastric ulcers in rats by an ethanolic extract of "Parsley" Petroselinum crispum. *Am J Chin Med.* 2003;31(5):699–711.

Abells SG, Haik R. Efficacy of garlic as an anthelmintic in donkeys. *Israel J Vet Med* 1999;54:1 (available online at: http://www.isrvma.org/article/54_1_5.htm) accessed July 2005.

ACP Australian College Phytotherapy. Course Notes, Module 4, Gastrointestinal System, 1999.

Alexandrovich I, Rakovitskaya O, Kolmo E, Sidorova T, Shushunov S. The effect of fennel (*Foeniculum vulgare*) seed oil emulsion in infantile colic: a randomized, placebo-controlled study. *Altern Ther Health Med* 2003;9:58–61.

Bruneton J. Pharmacognosy, Phytochemistry, Medicinal Plants. Paris: Lavoisier Publishing; 1995:604.

Chen QM, Ye YC, Chai FL, Jin KP. Protoscolicidal effect of some chemical agents and drugs against *Echinococcus granulosus*. Zhongguo Ji Sheng Chong Xue Yu Ji Sheng Chong Bing Za Zhi 1991;9:137–139.

Dehpour AR, et al. Anti-ulcer activities of licorice and its derivatives in experimental gastric lesion induced by ibuprofen in rats. *Int J Pharmaceut* 1995;119:133–138.

Della Loggia R. Evaluation of the anti-inflammatory activity of chamomile preparations. *Planta Med* 1990;56:657–658.

Felter HW, Lloyd JU. King's American Dispensatory, 1898.

Franz G. Polysaccharides in pharmacy: current applications and future concepts. *Planta Medica*, 1989, 55:493–497.

Ghazanfar SA. Handbook of Arabian medicinal plants. Boca Raton, FL: CRC Press, 1994.

Gong Z, Yuan Y, Lou K, Tu S, Zhai Z, Xu J. Mechanisms of Chinese herb emodin and somatostatin analogs on pancreatic regeneration in acute pancreatitis in rats. *Pancreas* 2002;25: 154–160.

Gorbacheva AV, et al. Anti-ulcerogenic characteristics of Filipendula ulmaria (L.) Maxim. [In Russian] Rastitel'nye Resursy. Nauka, Sankt-Peterburg, St. Petersburg, Russia: 2002. 38:2, 114–119.

Hiki N, Kurosaka H, Tatsutomi Y, Shimoyama S, Tsuji E, Kojima J, Shimizu N, Ono H, Hirooka T, Noguchi C, Mafune K, Kaminishi M. Peppermint oil reduces gastric spasm during upper endoscopy: a randomized, double-blind, double-dummy controlled trial. *Gastrointest Endosc* 2003;57:475–482.

Hills JM, Aaronson PI. The mechanism of action of peppermint oil on gastrointestinal smooth muscle. *Gastroenterology* 1991;101:55–65.

Hussain Z, Waheed A, Qureshi RA, et al. The effect of medicinal plants of Islamabad and Murree region of Pakistan on insulin secretion from INS-1 cells. *Phytother Res* 2004;18:73–77.

Kassir ZA. Endoscopic controlled trial of four drug regimens in the treatment of chronic duodenal ulceration. *Irish Med J* 1985;78:153–156.

Kempski H. Zur kausalen Therapie chronischer Helminthien-Bronchitis Medizinische Klinik 1967;62:259–260.

Khayyal MT, el-Ghazaly MA, Kenawy SA, Seif-el-Nasr M, Mahran LG, Kafafi YA, Okpanyi SN. Anti-ulcerogenic effect of some gastrointestinally acting plant extracts and their combination. *Arzneimittelforschung.* 2001;51(7):545–53.

Krazhan IA, Garazha NN. Treatment of chronic catarrhal gingivitis with polysorb-immobilized calendula. *Stomatologia* (Mosk). 2001;80(5):11–3.

Kwon YS, Jang KH, Jang IH. The effects of Korean red ginseng (ginseng radix rubra) on liver regeneration after partial hepatectomy in dogs. *J Vet Sci.* 2003 Apr;4(1):83–92.

Langmead L, Feakins RM, Goldthorpe S, et al. Randomized, double-blind, placebo-controlled trial of oral aloe vera gel for active ulcerative colitis. *Aliment Pharmacol Ther* 2004a;19: 739–747.

Langmead L, Makins RJ, Rampton DS. Anti-inflammatory effects of aloe vera gel in human colorectal mucosa in vitro. *Aliment Pharmacol Ther* 2004b;19:521–527.

Magliulo E, Scevola D, Carosi GP. Investigations on the actions of silybin on regenerating rat liver. Effects on Kupffer's cells. *Arzneimittelforschung* 1979;29:1024–1028.

Mills S. The Complete Guide to Modern Herbalism. London: Thorsons; 1989:22.

Moorhead LD. Contributions to the physiology of the stomach. XXVIII. Further studies on the action of the bitter tonic on the secretion of gastric juice. *J Pharmacol Exp Ther* 1915; 7:577–589.

Paulova J, Dvorak M, Kolouch F, Vanova L, Janeckova L. [Verification of the hepatoprotective and therapeutic effect of silymarin in experimental liver injury with tetrachloromethane in dogs]: overeni hepatoprotektivniho a terapeutickeho ucinku silymarinu pri experimentalnim poskozeni jater tetrachlormetanem u psu. *Vet Med* (Praha) 1990;35:629–635.

Pawlowski Z, Chwirot E. 5th Int Knogr Infektionskr. 1970. 277.

Rafatullah S, Tariq M, Al-Yahya MA, Mossa JS, Ageel AM. Evaluation of turmeric (Curcuma longa) for gastric and duodenal antiulcer activity in rats. *J Ethnopharmacol.* 1990 Apr;29(1):25–34.

Sakai K, Miyazaki Y, Yamane T, et al. Effect of extracts of Zingiberaceae herbs on gastric secretion in rabbits. *Chem Pharm Bull* (Tokyo). 1989 Jan;37(1):215–7.

Sastravaha G, Yotnuengnit P, Booncong P, Sangtherapitikul P. Adjunctive periodontal treatment with *Centella asiatica* and *Punica granatum* extracts. A preliminary study. *J Int Acad Periodontol* 2003;5:106–115.

Satou T, Akao N, Matsuhashi R, Koike K, Fujita K, Nikaido T. Inhibitory effect of isoquinoline alkaloids on movement of second-stage larvae of *Toxocara canis. Biol Pharm Bull* 2002;25:1651–1654.

Schmidgall J, Schnetz E, Hensel A. Evidence for bioadhesive effects of polysaccharides and polysaccharide-containing herbs in an ex vivo bioadhesion assay on buccal membranes. *Planta Med.* 2000 Feb;66(1):48–53.

Seo SW, Koo HN, An HJ, et al. Taraxacum officinale protects against cholecystokinin-induced acute pancreatitis in rats. *World J Gastroenterol.* 2005 Jan 28;11(4):597–9.

Shanmugasundaram ER, et al. Possible regeneration of the islets of Langerhans in streptozotocin-diabetic rats given Gymnema sylvestre leaf extracts. *J Ethnopharmacol* 1990;30:265–279.

Sharma SS, Kochupillai V, Gupta SK, Seth SD, Gupta YK. Antiemetic efficacy of ginger (*Zingiber officinale*) against cisplatin-induced emesis in dogs. J ethnopharmacol 1997;57:93–96.

Soh C. The effects of natural food preservative substances on the development and survival of intestinal Helminth eggs and larvae II action on Ancylostoma caninum larvae. *American Journal of Tropical Medicine and Hygiene* 1960 9:8–10.

Subbotina MD, Timchenko VN, Vorobyov MM, Konunova YS, Aleksandrovih YS, Shushunov S. Effect of oral administration of tormentil root extract (Potentilla tormentilla) on rotavirus diarrhea in children: a randomized, double blind, controlled trial. *Pediatr Infect Dis J.* 2003 Aug;22(8):706–11.

Vogel G, Tuchweber B, Trost W, Mengs U. Protection by silibinin against *Amanita phalloides* intoxication in beagles. *Toxicol Appl Pharmacol* 1984;73:355–362.

Wynn S, Fougere B. Veterinary Herbal Medicine. Oxford, UK: Elsevier, 2006.

Wynn S, Marsden S. Manual of Natural Veterinary Medicine. Sydney: Mosby; 2003:158.

Yun JH, Pang EK, Kim CS, et al. Inhibitory effects of green tea polyphenol (-)-epigallocatechin gallate on the expression of matrix metalloproteinase-9 and on the formation of osteoclasts. *J Periodontal Res* 2004;39:300–307.

Zhang XP, Li ZF, Liu XG, et al. Effects of emodin and baicalein on rats with severe acute pancreatitis. *World J Gastroenterol* 2005;11:2095–2100.

Zhou JG. *Tianjin Medical Journal*, 1960, 2:131.

Chapter Twenty-Four

Diseases of the Eye and Ear

HERBS FOR DISEASES OF THE EYE AND EAR

A number of eye and ear diseases may be treated with herbal therapy. They include cataracts, conjunctivitis, corneal ulcers, glaucoma, keratoconjuntivitis sicca, and otitis (chronic and acute).

Many of today's ophthalmic preparations have origins in ethnobotanical history. Atropine has been derived from solanaceous plants, physostigmine was used as a poison, and pilocarpine was used by Amazonians as a panacea (Packer 1992). For chronic or serious eye problems, referral to an ophthalmologist is always recommended. For mild conditions or as adjunctive therapy herbs can be used as eye washes or eye drops. Fresh herbal tea should be made fresh daily and kept refrigerated when not in use. Sterile saline can be used to infuse the herb.

Consider the systemic implications or associations of eye conditions and consider herbal treatment for pain relief, immune modulation, vulnery (healing) action, anti-inflammatory effects, and health support.

CATARACTS

Strategy

Cataracts can be caused by toxic insult (chemotherapy), nutritional deficiencies, heredity, genetic predisposition, or diabetes, as well as endogenous causes such as uveitis, retinal degeneration (PRA), and glaucoma. Referral to a veterinary ophthalmologist and possible surgical treatment is warranted, but if that is not possible then herbal support may be beneficial.

Use herbs that are high in antioxidants and that improve circulation. Botanicals such as Bilberry (*Vaccinium myrtillus*) may be helpful. In diabetic cataracts, flavonoids, particularly Quercetin, are potent inhibitors of aldose reductase (Head 2001). In a study of people with senile cataracts, a combination of Bilberry (standardized to 25% anthocyanosides; given at a dose of 180 mg twice daily) and vitamin E (100 mg twice daily) that was given for 4 months halted progression in 96% of patients com-

pared to 76% of the control group (Bravetti 1989). In a study in rats with early senile cataract and macular degeneration, the effect of Bilberry was investigated over 1.5 to 3 months. The treatment group was given a diet supplemented with 25% Bilberry extract (20 mg/kg, including 4.5 mg of antocianidin) or vitamin E (40 mg/kg). At the end of the study, more than 70% of the control rats (unsupplemented) had cataracts and macular degeneration compared to the treated group, which completely prevented impairments in the lenses and retina. The vitamin E had no significant effects but both antioxidants decreased lipid peroxides in the retina and serum of the rats. This suggests that long-term supplementation with Bilberry is effective in prevention of macular degeneration and cataracts (Fursova 2005).

Oral dose: Aqueous extract standardized to 25% anthocyanosides, 2 to 4 mg/kg TID; tincture, 1:2 to 1:3 : 0.5 to 1.5 mL per 10 kg (20 pounds) divided daily (Wynn 2006).

Turmeric and Curcumin were investigated on streptozotocin-induced diabetic cataracts in rats in a placebo-controlled study. The treatment groups received 0.002% and 0.01% curcumin and 0.5% turmeric in their diets, respectively, for 8 weeks. Although neither Curcumin nor Turmeric prevented streptozotocin-induced hyperglycemia, slit lamp microscope observations indicated that these supplements delayed the progression and maturation of cataracts and the results indicate that Turmeric and Curcumin might prevent or delay the development of cataracts (Suryanarayana 2005).

Curcumin dose: Canine, 0 to 250 mg TID; feline, 50 to 100 mg SID (Silver 1997); dried herb, 50 to 150 mg/kg divided daily if extracted and dried; triple or quadruple dose for unprocessed herb (to maximum palatability tolerance); tincture, 1:2 to 1:3 : 1 to 3 mL per 10 kg (20 pounds) divided daily (Wynn 2006).

Ginkgo biloba was investigated in a placebo-controlled study in preventing radiation-induced cataracts in the lens after total-cranium irradiation of rats with a single radiation dose of 5 Gy. The results suggested that Ginkgo biloba is an antioxidant that protects the rat lens from radiation-induced cataracts (Ertekin 2004).

Dose: Standardized extract, (50:1) 10 to 50 mg per 10 kg divided BID or TID; tincture, 1:2 to 1:3 : 0.5 to 1 mL per 10 kg (20 pounds) divided daily (Wynn 2006).

The anticataract activity of a Grapeseed extract (containing 38.5% procyanidins) was investigated in hereditary cataractous rats. The rats were fed a standard diet that contained 0% or 0.213% GSE (0.082% procyanidins in the diet (w/w)) for 27 days. Results suggested that procyanidins and their antioxidative metabolites prevented the progression of cataract formation by their antioxidative action (Yamakoshi 2002).

Canine dose: 1 to 2 mg per kg of extract daily (Wynn 2006).

In rats with cataracts induced by subcutaneous injection of selenite, administration of aqueous extracts of green and black tea led to a retardation of the progression of lens opacity, suggesting the potential cataractostatic ability of tea (Thiagarajan 2001).

Dose: Standardized extract containing 80% polyphenols, 25 to 75 mg/kg divided daily. Green tea can be added easily to moist food and in water (one-half to 1 cup per 10 kg per day) (Wynn 2006).

Other herbs have been investigated for their protective action. In streptozotocin-induced diabetic rats, dried leaf powder of Mulberry (*Morus indica* L.) given at a dose of 25% of the diet for 8 weeks resulted in controlled hyperglycemia, glycosuria, and albuminuria, and it retarded the onset of retinopathy. The control rats showed the hallmarks of diabetes and developed lenticular opacity after 8 weeks of study (Andallu 2002). Evidence suggests that lutein consumption is inversely related to eye diseases such as age-related macular degeneration and cataracts in people (Alves-Rodrigues 2004). Lutein can be obtained from the diet in several different ways, including supplements, and some pet foods.

A crude extract of Corydalis inhibited aldose reductase, which may help prevent cataracts associated with diabetes (Kubo 1994a). Oral Wheat sprout extract (dose not provided) was investigated for its effect on cataracts in dogs. Older dogs were treated for a month and the lens opacity was analyzed before and after the treatment. Results showed a reduction of 25% to 40% of lens opacity. The efficacy of Wheat sprouts in the recovery of age-related alterations and in treating age-associated pathologies is possibly due to the presence of small regulatory acid peptides, phosphoric radicals, and antioxidants (Basso 2005).

CORNEAL ULCERS

Strategy

Trauma to the cornea must occur for microbial colonization to occur. Consider herpes virus infection in cats with corneal ulcers. Topical Aloe gel (*Aloe vera*) has been advocated for the treatment of corneal ulcers and keratitis (de Bairacli Levy 1963).

A study using pig cornea showed that biologically active Aloe substances could not penetrate this biological barrier. Therefore, eye drops that contain Aloe and neomycin sulfate may be useful for the treatment of inflammation and infection of external parts of the eye, such as the conjuctiva, eyelid edges, lacrimal sac, and cornea (Kodym 2002).

Consider herbs that reduce anxiety and relieve pain (conventional pain relief may be necessary).

GLAUCOMA

Strategy

Glaucoma is characterized by increased intraocular pressure (IOP) in most cases. Some patients have normal IOP but poor circulation with damage to the optic nerve. Therapy is either medical or surgical. An immediate referral to a veterinary ophthalmologist is recommended if the clinician is not completely comfortable managing a case, because marked increases in IOP may result in irreversible damage to the retina and optic nerve in 24 to 48 hours. For controlled glaucoma, herbal medicine may be supportive and therapeutic, but should not be used as the sole treatment. Consider herbal treatment post surgery or as supportive care for conventional treatment.

Ginkgo biloba increases circulation to the optic nerve and has been linked with improvements in pre-existing field damage in some patients with normal tension glaucoma (Head 2001, Bartlett 2004). It is claimed that *Ginkgo biloba* extract has numerous properties that theoretically should be beneficial in treating non-IOP-dependent mechanisms in glaucoma. The actions of relevance include increased ocular blood flow, antioxidant activity, platelet activating factor inhibitory activity, nitric oxide inhibition, and neuroprotective activity. Together, these suggest that *Ginkgo biloba* could be valuable in the treatment of glaucoma (Ritch 2005).

Dose: Standardized extract (50:1), 10 to 50 mg per 10 kg (20 pounds) divided BID or TID; tincture, 1:2 to 1:3 : 0.5 to 1 mL per 10 kg (20 pounds) divided daily (Wynn 2006).

Other herbs and constituents have been studied. Forskolin (an extract from *Coleus forskohlii*) has been used successfully as a topical agent to lower intraocular pressure.

Dose: 4 to 8 drops 1:1 extract in an eye bath (Bone 1996). Eye baths should be sterile and well filtered.

Salvia miltiorrhiza (by IM injection) has shown benefits in improving visual acuity and peripheral vision in people with glaucoma (Head 2001). Cannabinoids effectively lower IOP and have neuroprotective actions, so they could potentially be useful in the treatment of glaucoma (Tomida 2004).

CONJUNCTIVITIS

Strategy

Diagnosis and appropriate treatment is important. For example, if the cause is allergic, use herbs that treat the allergy. Conjunctivitis in cats is nearly always caused by a primary pathogen—Chlamydia and feline herpes virus are common causes. Consider antiviral herbs for herpes virus infections and L-lysine administration.

Herbal teas are useful for noncomplicated conjunctivitis. The potential for contamination by bacteria that can colonize the eye should be considered. Herbal teas traditionally used for conjunctivitis include Chamomile, Comfrey, Coptis, Fennel, and Golden seal. *Aloe vera* gel has also been used.

An uncontrolled trial investigated the efficacy and tolerability of *Euphrasia* eye drops in humans with conjunctivitis. It yielded positive results in all but 1 of 65 patients. The authors recommend 1 drop TID in the affected eyes (Stoss 2000).

KERATOCONJUCNTIVITIS SICCA

Strategy

Treatment is directed toward stimulating tear production, replacing tears, and correcting any underlying cause. Consider herbs if immune-mediated disease is the cause. Also consider anti-inflammatory herbs.

In a randomized study of 80 dry eye patients, a Chinese herb formula, Chi-Ju-Di-Huang-Wan, was shown to be an effective stabilizer of tear film and it decreased the abnormality of corneal epithelium, providing an alternative choice for dry eye treatment (Chang 2005).

HERBAL EYE TONIC FORMULA

Use alcohol or glycetract tinctures for best results; alternatively, use teas. This formula is taken orally.

Bilberry: Asoprotective, anti-edema, antioxidant, anti-inflammatory; 2 parts.

Gingko: Antioxidant, circulatory stimulant; 1 part.

Eyebright: Anticatarrhal, anti-inflammatory, astringent; 1 part.

Adaptogen: Withania, eluethero, or *Panax ginseng*; 1 part.

For tinctures, give 1 ml per 10 pounds twice daily in food for 3 weeks. For teas, give 1 dessert spoon full twice daily in food for 3 weeks. Repeat if necessary.

Otitis

Strategy

Consider ear cytology to identify disease processes and type of disease organisms present. Diagnosis of underlying etiology is important; the herbal strategy usually requires attention to the immune system (allergies, infections) and overall health. Consider products that flush exudates and disinfect the ear canal prior to instilling herbal products. Consider the primary causes of ear disease, such as foreign bodies, hypothyroidism, seborrheic diseases, and underlying pruritic disease (atopy, food hypersensitivity, parasites), as well as other dermatological conditions that affect the ear canal, such as autoimmune diseases, keratinization disorders, and drug reactions. Consider predisposing causes of ear disease such as breed predilection for more cerumen glands that result in yeast, as well as excess moisture from bathing or swimming and trauma from overzealous cleaning or plucking. Consider perpetuating factors that keep the process going, such as contact allergies to otic preparations and overtreatment with cleaners or inappropriate therapy.

In a randomized study, an herbal formula (*Allium sativum, Verbascum thapsus, Calendula flores*, and *Hypericum perforatum* in olive oil) was compared with a commercial ear preparation (ametocaine and phenazone in glycerin) for the management of ear pain associated with acute otitis media in 103 children. The formula was shown to be as effective as the commercial preparation and was proven appropriate for the management of ear pain associated with acute otitis media (Sarrell 2001).

In humans, fungal ear infections represent a small percentage of clinical external otitis. One in vitro study examined the efficacy of garlic extracts against aspergillus, which is the most common cause of this infection. Aqueous Garlic extract (AGE) and concentrated Garlic oil (CGO) were found to have antifungal activity with similar or better inhibitory effects than the pharmaceutical preparations and with similar minimum inhibitory concentrations (Pai 1995).

Borneol walnut oil was investigated against neomycin in a controlled study for the treatment of purulent otitis media. One hundred seventy patients were treated with Borneol walnut oil of various concentrations, and controls (108 patients) were treated with neomycin compound. The total effective rates were 98.06% and 84.26%, respectively (Liu 1990).

Andrographis paniculata extract is traditionally used as a medicine to treat otitis media (WHO 1999). Other herbs used topically include Bloodroot, Goldenseal, Mullein, Neem, and Thuja.

HERBAL EAR ORAL FORMULA

Use alcohol or glycetract tinctures for best results; alternatively, use teas. This formula is taken orally.

Burdock: Alterative, mild laxative, mildly antiseptic, diuretic; 1 part.

Echinacea: Immune stimulating, anti-inflammatory, antibacterial, vulnery; 1 part.

Calendula: Antiseptic, lymphatic, anti-inflammatory, astringent, vulnery, cholagogue, spasmolytic; 1 part.

Pau d'aco: Antibacterial, antifungal, antiviral; 1 part.

St. John's wort: Vulnery, anti-inflammatory, antidepressant, nervine; 1 part.

For tinctures, give 1 ml per 10 pounds twice daily in food for 3 weeks. For teas, give 1 dessert spoon full twice daily in food for 3 weeks. Repeat if necessary.

REFERENCES

Alves-Rodrigues A, Shao A. The science behind lutein. *Toxicol Lett.* 2004 Apr 15;150(1):57–83.

Andallu B, Varadacharyulu NCH. Control of hyperglycemia and retardation of cataract by mulberry (*Morus indica L.*) leaves in streptozotocin diabetic rats. *Indian J Exp Biol.* 2002 Jul;40(7):791–5.

Bartlett H, Eperjesi F. An ideal ocular nutritional supplement? *Ophthalmic Physiol Opt.* 2004 Jul;24(4):339–49.

Basso A, Rossolini G, Piantanelli A, Amici D, Calzuola I, Mancinelli L, Marsili V, Gianfranceschi GL. Aging reversibility: from thymus graft to vegetable extract treatment—application to cure an age-associated pathology. *Biogerontology.* 2005;6(4):245–53.

Bone K. Clinical Applications of Ayurvedic and Chinese Herbs—Monographs for the Western Herbal Practitioner. Warwick, Queensland, Australia: Phytotherapy Press; 1996:94.

Bravetti G. preventative medical treatment of senile cataract with vitamin E and anthocyanosides: clinical evaluation. *Ann Ottalmol Clin Ocul* 1989;115:109.

Chang YH, Lin HJ, Li WC. Clinical evaluation of the traditional Chinese prescription Chi-Ju-Di-Huang-Wan for dry eye. *Phytother Res.* 2005 Apr;19(4):349–54.

de Bairacli Levy J. Herbal Handbook for Farm and Stable. London: Faber and Faber Limited; 1963.

Elhajili M, Baddouri K, Elkabbaj S, Meiouat F, Settaf A. Diuretic activity of the infusion of flowers from *Lavendula officinalis*. (In French) *Reprod Nutr Dev* 2001;41:393–399.

Ertekin MV, Kocer I, Karslioglu I, Taysi S, Gepdiremen A, Sezen O, Balci E, Bakan N. Effects of oral Ginkgo biloba supplementation on cataract formation and oxidative stress occurring in lenses of rats exposed to total cranium radiotherapy. *Jpn J Ophthalmol.* 2004 Sep–Oct;48(5):499–502.

Fursova AZH, Gesarevich OG, Gonchar AM, et al. Dietary supplementation with bilberry extract prevents macular degeneration and cataracts in senesce-accelerated OXYS rats. *Adv Gerontol.* 2005;16:76–9.

Head KA. Natural therapies for ocular disorders, part two: cataracts and glaucoma. *Altern Med Rev.* 2001 Apr;6(2):141–66.

Kodym A, Grzeskowiak E, Partyka D, Marcinkowski A, Kaczynska-Dyba E. Biopharmaceutical assessment of eye drops containing aloe (*Aloe arborescens* Mill.) and neomycin sulphate. *Acta Pol Pharm* 2002;59:181–186.

Kubo M, Matsuda H, Tokuoka K, Kobayashi Y, Ma S, Tanaka T. Studies of anti-cataract drugs from natural sources. I. Effects of a methanolic extract and the alkaloidal components from Corydalis tuber on in vitro aldose reductase activity. *Biol Pharm Bull* 1994a;17:458–459.

Liu SL. Therapeutic effects of borneol-walnut oil in the treatment of purulent otitis media. *Zhong Xi Yi Jie He Za Zhi.* 1990 Feb;10(2):93–5, 69.

Packer M, Brandt JD. Ophthalmology's botanical heritage. *Surv Ophthalmol.* 1992 Mar–Apr;36(5):357–65.

Pai ST, Platt MW. Antifungal effects of Allium sativum (garlic) extract against the Aspergillus species involved in otomycosis. *Lett Appl Microbiol.* 1995 Jan;20(1):14–8.

Ritch R. Complementary therapy for the treatment of glaucoma: a perspective. *Ophthalmol Clin North Am.* 2005 Dec;18(4):597–609.

Sarrell EM, Mandelberg A, Cohen HA. Efficacy of naturopathic extracts in the management of ear pain associated with acute otitis media. *Arch Pediatr Adolesc Med.* 2001 Jul;155(7):796–9.

Silver RJ. Ayurvedic veterinary medicine. In: Schoen AM, Wynn SG, eds. Complementary and Alternative Veterinary Medicine. St Louis, MO: Mosby, Inc. 1997:463–464.

Stoss M, Michels C, Peter E, Beutke R, Gorter RW. Prospective cohort trial of Euphrasia single-dose eye drops in conjunctivitis. *J Altern Complement Med* 2000;6:499–508.

Suryanarayana P, Saraswat M, Mrudula T, Krishna TP, Krishnaswamy K, Reddy GB. Curcumin and turmeric delay streptozotocin-induced diabetic cataract in rats. *Invest Ophthalmol Vis Sci.* 2005 Jun;46(6):2092–9.

Thiagarajan G, Chandani S, Sundari CS, Rao SH, Kulkarni AV, Balasubramanian D. Antioxidant properties of green and black tea, and their potential ability to retard the progression of eye lens cataract. *Exp Eye Res.* 2001 Sep;73(3):393–401.

Tomida I, Pertwee RG, Azuara-Blanco A. Cannabinoids and glaucoma. *Br J Ophthalmol.* 2004 May;88(5):708–13.

Treasure J. Urtica semen reduces serum creatinine levels. *J Am Herbalists Guild* 2003;4:22–25.

World Health Organization. Monographs on Selected Medicinal Plants, vol 1. Geneva, Switzerland: WHO; 1999.

Wynn S, Fougere B. Veterinary Herbal Medicine. Oxford: Elsevier, 2006.

Yamakoshi J, Saito M, Kataoka S, Tokutake S. Procyanidin-rich extract from grape seeds prevents cataract formation in hereditary cataractous (ICR/f) rats. *J Agric Food Chem* 2002;50:4983–4938.

Chapter Twenty-Five

Diseases of the Musculoskeletal System

HERBS FOR DISEASES OF THE MUSCULOSKELETAL SYSTEM

Disorders of the musculoskeletal system—including arthritis, hip and elbow dysplasia, ligament conditions such as anterior cruciate/luxating patellas, and spinal arthritis/spondylosis—generally present as altered gait or lameness caused by pain. These conditions benefit from physical therapies including acupuncture, chiropractics, physiotherapy, and massage, as well as weight reduction where appropriate. Chondroprotective agents should always be considered and conventional anti-inflammatory agents should be considered for acute injuries. Alternatives to nonsteroidal anti-inflammatories are often sought because of concerns over side effects of medications including continued degeneration of joints and gastrointestinal, hepatic, or renal effects.

Musculoskeletal conditions affect the whole body. Pain in one area leads to biomechanical changes elsewhere due to shifts in weight bearing and movement. The whole body must be evaluated, not just the affected limb or back. Frequently, muscle spasm, trigger points, myofascial pain, and joint pain are detected elsewhere in the body. Similarly, herbalists take a systemic approach to treating musculoskeletal disorders. The goal is to treat the condition, as well as the pain, possible depression, muscular spasms, and joint disease, as well as overall health of the patient.

One of the possible underlying conditions thought to contribute to inflammatory changes anywhere in the body is leaky gut. Animals that have been administered nonsteroidal drugs for long periods frequently have disordered digestive function, so questions about appetite; gastrointestinal symptoms; and feces quality, quantity, and frequency should be asked. Hence, herbalists frequently recommend a change in diet, treat the digestive tract, and use alteratives as part of the protocol. Herbs that may be beneficial in treating chronic musculoskeletal conditions include Burdock (*Arctium lappa*), Blue flag (*Iris versicolor*), Dandelion (Taraxacum officinale), Oregon grape

(*Mahonia aquifolium*), Yellow dock (*Rumex crispus*), and Sarsaparilla (*Smilax spp*).

The main herbs of interest are those that are anti-inflammatory or provide analgesic, antispasmodic action and those that improve circulatory function. Some of these herbs have already been discussed, so the emphasis here is on herbs with specific benefits in musculoskeletal disease.

ANTI-INFLAMMATORY HERBS

Withania (*Withania somnifera*)

Withania is a useful component of any musculoskeletal formula as both an adaptogen and an herb. It was traditionally recognized in Ayurvedic medicine for musculoskeletal disorders. Although the mechanism of action is not fully understood, it appears that Withania may involve cyclo-oxygenase inhibition (Mishra 2000, Somasundaram 1983) and a direct musculotropic action that accounts for the antispasmodic effects of Withania (Malhotra 1965a).

Devil's claw (*Harpagophytum procumbens*)

Devil's claw is a threatened plant species used in traditional African medicine for arthritis. In humans it has been investigated for the treatment of nonspecific lower back pain, arthritis, and rheumatism, and has been shown to be effective for pain relief when the extract provides more than 50 mg of harpagoside daily (Gagnier 2006, Chrubasik 2004, Wegener 2003). However, the effects of Devil's claw are not just due to the constituent harpagoside. In one in vitro study it was shown to suppress prostaglandin (PG)E$_2$ synthesis and nitric oxide production by inhibiting lipopolysaccharide-stimulated enhancement of cox2 and inducible nitric oxide synthase mRNA expression (Jang 2003). It has been included in a formula with Black currant (*Ribes nigrum*), Horsetail (*Equisetum arvense*), and White willow (*Salix alba*) and compared to phenylbutazone in a study conducted on 20 horses with bone spavin. The formula showed significant benefit for horses with bone spavin and scores for improvement were better for the formula over phenylbutazone (Montavon, 1994).

Withania dose: Dried herb, 50 to 125 mg/kg divided daily if extracted and dried; triple or quadruple dose for unprocessed herb; tincture, 1:2 to 1:3 : 1 to 2.5 mL per 10 kg (20 pounds) divided daily (Wynn 2006).

Boswellia (*Boswellia serrata*)

Boswellia may act as an anti-inflammatory and as an inhibitor of lipoxygenase activity (Ammon 1993). However, one study of 37 patients with rheumatoid arthritis showed no difference between treatment with Boswellia extract and the placebo in terms of reduced use of nonsteroidal anti-inflammatory drugs and in subjective, clinical, or laboratory measures (Sander 1998). In a prospective, open, multicenter clinical trial (not placebo-controlled), 24 dogs with osteoarthritis of the joints or spine were treated with a standardized Boswellia resin extract (50% triterpenic acids) at a dose of 400 mg/10 kg once daily in food for 6 weeks. Overall, 71% of the dogs were assessed with good or very good results at 2 and 6 weeks of treatment. The study claimed that 40% to 70% of the dogs were symptom-free after 6 weeks. While 11 of 29 dogs experienced adverse effects during the study, Boswellia was thought to be causative in only 1 dog (Reichling 2004).

Boswellia dose: Dried herb, 25 to 125 mg/kg divided daily if extracted and dried; triple or quadruple dose for unprocessed herb; tincture, 1:2 to 1:3 : 1.5 to 2.5 mL per 10 kg (20 pounds) divided daily (Wynn 2006).

Ginger (*Zingiber officinalis*)

Ginger is a common ingredient in natural anti-arthritic products for humans. It has anti-inflammatory effects as both a mild cyclo-oxygenase and lipoxygenase inhibitor and thromboxane synthase inhibitor (Sharma 1994). The potency was comparable to that of acetylsalicylic acid (Kawakishi 1994). A study of 113 patients with chronic lower back and rheumatic pain responded positively with full or partial relief of pain, reduced joint swelling, and improved joint function when injected with 5% to 10% Ginger extract into the painful areas (Ghazanfar 1994). Powdered Ginger administered to patients with rheumatism and musculoskeletal disorders has been shown to provide varying degrees of relief from pain and swelling (Srivastava 1992).

Ginger dose: Dried herb, 15 to 50 mg/kg divided daily if extracted and dried; triple or quadruple dose for unprocessed herb; tincture, 1:2 to 1:3 : 0.25 to 0.5 mL per 10 kg (20 pounds) divided daily (Wynn 2006).

Turmeric (*Curcuma longa*)

Turmeric may be beneficial in canine arthritis, although in a randomized, double-blind, placebo-controlled, parallel-group clinical trial using an extract of related species of Turmeric (*Curcuma domestica* and *Curcuma xanthorrhiza*), owners saw no difference from a placebo as a treatment for osteoarthritis of the canine elbow or hip. The investigators' assessment, however, showed a statistically significant treatment effect (Innes 2003). In a short-term double-blind, crossover study of 18 human patients with rheumatoid arthritis, treatment with Curcumin (1,200 mg/day) or phenylbutazone (30 mg/day) both produced significant improvement in morning stiffness, walking time, and joint swelling (Deodhar 1980). Turmeric can be added to food daily to palatability tolerance.

Turmeric dose: Dried herb, 50 to 150 mg/kg divided daily; OR curcumin, canine—50 to 250 mg TID, feline— 50 to 100 mg SID (Silver 1997); OR tincture, 1:2 to 1:3 : 1 to 3 mL per 10 kg (20 pounds) divided daily (Wynn 2006).

Other herbs with activity that supports their use as anti-inflammatory agents include Celery (*Apium graveolens*), a traditional remedy for gout; Meadowsweet (*Filipendula ulmaria*); Birch (*Betula* sp.); Willow bark (*Salix alba* and other salix sp.), which contains nonselective cox1 and cox2 inhibitor constituents; and Nettle (*Urtica dioca*) extracts, which were shown to suppress matrix metalloproteinase activity, thus reducing degradation of the extracellular matrix in joint cartilage (Schulze-Tanzil 2002). Other herbs used for musculoskeletal conditions include Angelica (*Angelica archangelica*), Boneset (*Eupatorium perfoliatum*), Celery (*Apium graveolens*), Blue cohosh (*Caulophyllum thalictroides*), Black cohosh (*Actea racemosa*), Guaiacum (*Guaiacum officinale*), Wintergreen (*Gaultheria procumbens*), Bogbean (*Menyanthes trifoliata*), Quaking aspen (*Populus tremuloides*), Yarrow (*Achillea millefolium*), and Arnica (*Arnica Montana*) topically.

SPASM-RELIEVING AND ANALGESIC (ANTIRHUEMATIC) HERBS

Skeletal muscle spasm may be relieved by spasmolytic herbs. Most of these herbs have demonstrated effects on smooth muscle, but rarely have they been investigated for their effects on skeletal muscle. Valerian (*Valeriana officinalis*) contains valerenic acid, which is spasmolytic and relaxes muscles (Wagner 1979, Bissett 1994) and may be useful for back pain associated with muscular spasm. Black cohosh (*Cimicifuga racemosa*) is a relaxing nervine, and is considered to be antirheumatic with the active cimicifugoside, which has been shown to inhibit N-acetylcholine receptor-mediated responses in vitro (Woo 2004). Wild yam (*Dioscorea villosa*) is also considered to be a traditional antirheumatic, anti-inflammatory, and spasmolytic. Cramp bark (*Viburnum opulus*) and other viburnum species have demonstrated antispasmodic activity in smooth muscle spasm (Cometa 1998, Calle 1999) and are useful for spasmodic muscular cramps.

More direct analgesia can be gained from using Corydalis (*Corydalis ambigua*), which is used in Traditional Chinese Medicine to invigorate the blood and alleviate pain, including back, abdominal, and arthritic pain (Bensky 1993). Tetrahydropalmatine (THP) is the most studied constituent, with demonstrated analgesic and sedative effects (Zhu 1998). In people with nerve pain, 75 mg THP daily was effective in 78% of patients tested (Lin 1990). Antidepressants are often used in human pain control. St. John's wort (*Hypericum perforatum*) has demonstrated analgesic and anti-inflammatory activity in laboratory animals (Viana 2003) and may be particularly helpful in neuralgia and post amputation conditions. Californian poppy (*Eschscholtzia californica*) has demonstrated peripheral analgesic effects (Rolland 1991, 2001). Passion flower (*Passiflora incarnate*) methanol leaf extract in mice (200 mg/kg) exhibited sedative analgesic and anti-inflammatory activities against induced pain and induced edema (Kamaldeep 2003).

Other traditional antirheumatic herbs include Blue cohosh (*Caulophyllum thalictroides*), Bladder wrack (*Fucus vesiculosus*) for rheumatoid arthritis, Lavender (*Lavendula officinalis*) topically, Parsley (*Petroselinum crispum*) for myalgia (orally and topically), and Poke root (*Phytolacca decandra*).

CIRCULATORY STIMULANTS

Another herbal strategy for treating arthritis is to enhance peripheral circulation. Two of the most commonly used circulatory stimulants for arthritis in animals are Ginger (*Zingiber officinalis*) and Prickly ash (*Zanthoxylum americanum*).

PRESCRIPTION FOR DEGENERATIVE JOINT DISEASES/ARTHRITIS

Strategy

Consider anti-inflammatory herbs to help reduce the dose of conventional anti-inflammatories or as an alternative to traditional drugs. Treat associated leaky gut with long-term NSAIDs or steroids. Reduce pain using spasmodic, antirheumatic, and analgesic herbs, improve circulation to joint and muscle tissues, and treat neuralgia if present. Consider adaptogens for chronic stress associated with pain.

Musculoskeletal

Use alcohol or glycetract tinctures for best results; alternatively, use teas.

Devil's claw: Anti-inflammatory, analgesic, bitter; 1 part.

Valerian: Antispasmodic, carminative, sedative; 1 part.

St. John's wort: Antidepressant, nervine tonic, anti-inflammatory, vulnery; 1 part.

Withania: Tonic, adaptogen, nervine, sedative, anti-inflammatory; 1 part.

Turmeric: Anti-inflammatory, antioxidant, antiplatelet, hepatoprotective, anticancer, cholagogue; one-half part.

Prickly ash: Antirheumatic, circulatory stimulant, carminative; one-half part.

For tinctures, give 1 ml per 10 pounds twice daily in food for 3 weeks. For teas, give 1 dessert spoon full twice daily in food for 3 weeks.

REFERENCES

Ammon HP, Safayhi H, Mack T, Sabieraj J. Mechanism of anti-inflammatory actions of curcumine and boswellic acids. *J Ethnopharmacol* 1993;38:113–119.

Bensky D, Gamble A, Kaptchuk T. *Chinese Herbal Medicine Materia Medica*. Vista, CA: Eastland Press; 1993:270.

Bermejo Benito, P. et al. In vivo and in vitro anti-inflammatory activity of saikosaponins. *Life Sciences*. 1998. 63:13, 1147–1156.

Bisset NG. *Herbal Drugs and Phytopharmaceuticals*. Wichtl M, ed. [German edition]. Stuttgart: Medpharm; 1994.

Calle J, Toscano M, Pinzon R, Baquero J, Bautista E. Antinociceptive and uterine relaxant activities of *Viburnum toronis* alive (Caprifoliaceae). *J Ethnopharmacol* 1999;66:71–73.

Chrubasik S, Conradt C, Roufogalis BD. Effectiveness of Harpagophytum extracts and clinical efficacy. *Phytother Res* 2004;18:187–189.

Cometa MF, Mazzanti L, Tomassini L. Sedative and spasmolytic effects of Viburnum tinus L. and its major pure compounds. *Phytotherapy Research* 1998; 12(S1): S89–S91.

Deodhar SD, Sethi R, Srimal RC. Preliminary study on antirheumatic activity of curcumin (diferuloyl methane). *Indian J Med Res* 1980;71:632–634.

Gagnier JJ, van Tulder M, Berman B, Bombardier C. Herbal medicine for low back pain. Cochrane Database Syst Rev. 2006 Apr 19;(2):CD004504.

Ghazanfar SA. Handbook of Arabian medicinal plants. Boca Raton, FL: CRC Press, 1994.

Innes JF, Fuller CJ, Grover ER, Kelly AL, Burn JF. Randomised, double-blind, placebo-controlled parallel group study of P54FP for the treatment of dogs with osteoarthritis. *Vet Rec* 2003;152:457–460.

Jang MH, Lim S, Han SM, et al. *Harpagophytum procumbens* suppresses lipopolysaccharide-stimulated expressions of cyclooxygenase-2 and inducible nitric oxide synthase in fibroblast cell line L929. *J Pharmacol Sci* 2003;93:367–371.

Kamaldeep D, Suresh K, Anupam S. Evaluation of central nervous system effects of *Passiflora incarnata* in experimental animals. *Pharmaceut Biol* 2003;41:2,87–91.

Kawakishi S, Morimitsu Y, Osawa T. Chemistry of ginger components and inhibitory factors of the arachidonic acid cascade. *American Chemical Society Symposium series,* 1994;547: 244–250.

Lin DZ, Fang YS. *Modern Study and Application of Materia Medica.* Hong Kong: China Ocean Press; 1990:323–325.

Malhotra CL, Mehta VL, Das PK, Dhalla NS. Studies on Withania-ashwagandha, Kaul. V. The effect of total alkaloids (ashwagandholine) on the central nervous system. *Indian J Physiol Pharmacol* 1965;9:127–136.

Mishra LC, Singh BB, Dagenais S. Scientific basis for the therapeutic use of *Withania somnifera* (ashwagandha): a review. *Altern Med Rev* 2000;5:334–346.

Montavon S. Efficacy of a phytotherapeutic preparation based on *Harpagophytum procumbens* in case of bone spavin of adult horses [in French]. *Prat Vet Equine* 1994;26:49–53.

Reichling J, Schmokel H, Fitzi J, Bucher S, Saller R. Dietary support with Boswellia resin in canine inflammatory joint and spinal disease. *Schweiz Arch Tierheilkd* 2004;146:71–79.

Rolland A, Fleurentin J, Lanhers MC, et al. Behavioural effects of the American traditional plant *Eschscholzia californica:* sedative and anxiolytic properties. *Planta Med.* 1991;5:212–216.

Rolland A, Fleurentin J, Lanhers MC, Misslin R, Mortier F. Neurophysiological effects of an extract of *Eschscholzia californica* Cham (Papaveraceae). *Phytother Res* 2001;15:377–381.

Sander O, Herborn G, Rau R. Is H15 (resin extract of Boswellia serrata, "incense") a useful supplement to established drug therapy of chronic polyarthritis? Results of a double-blind pilot study.] [In German] *Z Rheumatol* 1998;57:11–16.

Schulze-Tanzil G, de SP, Behnke B, Klingelhoefer S, Scheid A, Shakibaei M. Effects of the antirheumatic remedy hox alpha—a new stinging nettle leaf extract—on matrix metalloprotein-ases in human chondrocytes in vitro. *Histol Histopathol* 2002;17:477–485.

Sharma JN, Srivastava KC, Gan EK. Suppressive effects of eugenol and ginger oil on arthritic rats. *Pharmacology,* 1994;49:314–318.

Silver RJ Ayurvedic veterinary medicine. In: Schoen AM, Wynn SG, eds. Complementary and Alternative Veterinary Medicine. St Louis, MO: Mosby, Inc. 1997:463–464.

Somasundaram S, Sadique J, Subramoniam A. In vitro absorption of [14C]leucine during inflammation and the effect of anti-inflammatory drugs in the jejunum of rats. *Biochem Med* 1983;29:259–264.

Srivastava KC, Mustafa T. Ginger (*Zingiber officinale*) in rheumatism and musculoskeletal disorders. *Med Hypoth* 1992;39:342–348.

Viana AF, Heckler AP, Fenner R, Rates SM. Antinociceptive activity of *Hypericum caprifoliatum* and *Hypericum polyanthemum* (Guttiferae). *Braz J Med Biol Res* 2003;36:631–634. Epub April 22, 2003.

Wagner H, Jurcic K. On the spasmolytic activity of valeriana extracts. *Planta Med* 1979;37:84–86.

Wegener T, Lupke NP. Treatment of patients with arthrosis of hip or knee with an aqueous extract of devil's claw (*Harpagophytum procumbens* DC). *Phytother Res* 2003;17:1165–1172.

Woo KC, Park YS, Jun DJ, et al. Phytoestrogen cimicifugoside-mediated inhibition of catecholamine secretion by blocking nicotinic acetylcholine receptor in bovine adrenal chromaffin cells. *J Pharmacol Exp Ther* 2004;309:641–649. Epub February 2, 2004.

Wynn S, Fougere B. Veterinary Herbal Medicine. St. Louis: Elsevier, 2006.

Zhu YP. *Chinese Materia Media: Chemistry, Pharmacology, and Applications.* Australia: Harwood Academic Publishers; 1998a:445–448.

Zhu JS, Halpern GM, Jones K. The scientific rediscovery of an ancient Chinese herbal medicine: *Cordyceps sinensis.* Part II. *J Altern Complement Med* 1998b;4:429–457.

Chapter Twenty-Six

Diseases of the Respiratory System

HERBS FOR DISEASES OF THE RESPIRATORY SYSTEM

Herbs provide a number of actions that benefit both upper and lower respiratory diseases, including bronchitis (acute, allergic, and chronic), feline bronchial asthma, and sinusitis/rhinitis. Interestingly, some of the respiratory herbs are in the most commonly used, mass produced cough medicines available through pharmacies. These include cherry bark, Irish moss, and Licorice.

Several groups of herbal actions are useful in the treatment of chronic respiratory disorders, and many traditional respiratory herbs fall into more than 1 group. In terms of respiratory therapy, the major actions are as follows.

Antitussives

Antitussives reduce coughing either through demulcent action, by removing the irritation (expectorant) action, or by depressing the cough reflex. This group therefore includes expectorants, demulcents, and anticatarrhals. The best known antitussive herbs are Irish moss (*Chondrus crispus*), Wild cherry (*Prunus serotina*), and Licorice (*Glycyrrhiza glabra*). Licorice root contains a potent antitussive compound, liquilitin apioside, the antitussive effects of which may depend on both peripheral and central mechanisms. A 50% methanol extract of licorice (100 mg/kg PO) reduced by more than 60% the number of capsaicin-induced coughs (Kamei 2003).

Marshmallow (*Althaea officinalis*) and Burdock (*Articum lappa*) may also be useful. The antitussive capacity of marshmallow extract and its isolated polysaccharide were compared with the nonnarcotic drugs prenoxdiazine and dropropizine in cats. Unanesthetized cats were stimulated to cough through nylon fiber irritation of laryngopharyngeal and tracheobronchial mucus. Tracheal pressure was measured to determine the number of cough efforts. At 50 mg/kg PO, the polysaccharide inhibited the cough; and the cough was inhibited with 1,000 mg/kg PO of

althaea syrup. The whole plant extract was less effective than the polysaccharide (Nosal'ova 1992). Burdock was also tested for antitussive activity in cats. An inulin isolate (fructan) from *A. lappa* roots was found to be equally active as some nonnarcotic, synthetic preparations used in clinical practice to treat cough (Kardosova 2003).

Expectorants

Tenacious mucus can act as an airway irritant and invoke a cough reflex. Clearing mucus is a fundamental herbal principle for any respiratory disease characterized by excessive mucus production. Herbalists use expectorants to facilitate removal of secretions, either by reducing the tenacity of the mucus (catarrh), which can irritate airways, or by increasing expulsion. Expectorants are not indicated with a pharyngitis causing a cough; they are used when there is tracheal or lung involvement. They are best used for subacute or chronic inflammatory conditions. Depending on the constituents, expectorants can work by acting directly on goblet cells—these include the essential-oil-containing herbs such as Fennel (*Foeniculum vulgaris*) and Aniseed (*Pimpinella anisum*)—which might be useful if secretions are scant; by stimulating the vagus nerve and making secretions more watery—these include Lobelia (*Lobelia inflate*)—and by herbs that stimulate mucociliary transport, such as thyme (*Thymus vulgaris*).

There have been very few clinical studies on the benefits of expectorants; however, some studies show that saponin-containing herbs administered orally enhance production of respiratory tract fluid. In one study Senega root (*Polygala senega*) increased fluid output by 173% in cats in 3 to 4 hours (Boyd 1946). In another study the same herb caused a 10-fold increase in fluid output in dogs after 5 to 30 minutes when compared with a saline control (Misawa 1980). It should be noted that the doses used were extremely high.

Syrup of Thyme was compared to bromhexine in a double-blind, randomized study of 60 patients with productive cough, and there were no significant differences between the self-reported symptom relief (Leung 1996). Other commonly used expectorants include Licorice (*Glycyrrhiza glabra*), Grindelia (*Grindelia camporum*), White horehound (*Marrubium vulgare*), Elecampane (*Inula helenium*), and Malabar nut tree (*Adhatoda vasica*). Adhatoda is a source of vasicine from which the drug Bisolvin was developed. Expectorants are commonly prescribed with spasmolytic, anticatarrhal, and immune-stimulating herbs.

Demulcents

This group of herbs contains mucilage constituents, which have anti-inflammatory and soothing effects on the lower respiratory mucosa. They are ideal for acute coughs with very acute catarrh with inflammation and irritation. They include Marshmallow (*Althaea officinalis*), Irish moss (*Chondrus crispus*), and Slippery elm (Ulmus flava). Plantain (*Plantago major*), Mullein (*Verbascum thapsus*), Fenugreek (*Trigonella foenum-graecum*), and Coltsfoot (*Tussilago farara*) are other traditional demulcents.

Anticatarrhals

Anticatarrhals reduce excessive discharge from mucous membranes. They are particularly useful for nasal and sinus congestion and mucosal edema, and they can reduce airway hypersensitivity. Anticatarrhal herbs for the upper respiratory tract include Eyebright (*Euphrasia rostkoviana*), Elder flower (*Sambucus nigra*), Ribwort (*Plantago lanceolata*), Peppermint (*Mentha piperita*), Fenugreek (*Trigonella foenum-graecum*), Golden rod (*Solidago spp*), and Golden seal (*Hydrastis canadensis*). The latter two are particularly indicated for copious yellow to green discharge of a chronic nature. Sage (*Salvia officinalis*) has a drying effect that can be useful for copious watery discharges. Anticatarrhal herbs for the lower respiratory tract include Mullein (*Verbascum thaspus*) and Ribwort (*Plantago lanceolata*).

Antispasmodics

Respiratory spasmolytics help relax the bronchioles. These include Elecampane (*Inula helenium*), Lobelia (*Lobelia inflata*), Grindelia (*Grindelia camporum*), Thyme (*Thymus vulgaris*), Licorice (*Glycyrrhiza glabra*), Euphorbia (*Euphorbia hirta*), Celadine (*Chelodium majus*), and Ephedra. Lobeline, a constituent of Lobelia, induced hyperpnea due to both an increase in tidal volume and respiratory rate in ponies (Art 1991). Lobeline is also considered a Beta-adrenergic bronchodilator (Tyler 1994). Thymol, Carvacrol, and the essential oil from Thyme (Van den Broucke 1982, Reiter 1985), in sufficient doses, have tracheal relaxant activity.

Respiratory antiseptics

Most respiratory antiseptics have mild antimicrobial activity. This activity is usually related to volatile oil constituents. Steam inhalation of teas could be considered for small animals. These herbs include Thyme (*Thymus vulgaris*), Elecampane (*Inula helenium*), Garlic (*Allium sativum*), Hyssop (*Hyssopus officinalis*), Lavender (*Lavendula offincialis*), and Rosemary (*Rosmarinus officinalis*).

Anti-allergic herbs

The main herbs for respiratory tract allergies are Albizzia (*Albizzia lebbek*), Baical skullcap (*Scutellaria baicalensis*), Boswellia (*Boswellia serrata*), Ginkgo (*Ginkgo biloba*), Malabar nut tree (*Adhatoda vasica*), and Nettles (*Urtica* spp) for allergic rhinitis. Albizzia provided excellent reponses in an uncontrolled trial of patients with asthma of recent onset (less than 2 years), but the response was less predictable for chronic asthma (Tripathi 1979). Baicalin and Baicalein have demonstrated anti-allergic and anti-asthmatic activity in several animal models (Chang 1987).

Along with this classification of herbs, also consider the use of immune-regulating herbs such as Echinacea and Astragalus or antiviral herbs (see infectious diseases).

PRESCRIPTION FOR BRONCHITIS (ACUTE, ALLERGIC, AND CHRONIC)

Strategy

Warming tonics such as Astragalus or Panax ginseng are contraindicated in acute infection. In acute conditions consider antiseptic, antitussive, demulcent, expectorant, and immune-stimulating herbs. Consider perpetuating factors in chronic bronchitis such as pollution and airborne irritants. There is usually overactivity of secretory glands and goblet cells, so expectorant herbs are emphasized. Treat any chronic infection, and consider Ginger in cold patients to help diffuse the formula (circulatory stimulant). Antispasmodics, antimicrobials, expectorants, demulcents, and pulmonary tonics are indicated in chronic conditions. Bronchodialting herbs such as Lobelia may be helpful; also consider anti-inflammatory herbs such as Licorice. In chronic conditions, also consider cardiotonics such as Hawthorn and nervines such as Motherwort. Also consider immune stimulants such as Echinacea and Astragalus.

Herbal acute bronchitis support formula

Echinacea: Immunostimulant, anti-inflammatory, vulnery, antimicrobial; 1 part.

Marshmallow: Demulcent, vulnery, diuretic, antitussive; 1 part.

Elecampane: Expectorant, antitussive, antibacterial, diaphoretic; 1 part.

Licorice: Antispasmodic, antitussive, anti-inflammatory, adaptogen, expectorant; 1 part.

Thyme: Carminative, antitussive, antispasmodic, expectorant, antibacterial, astringent; 1 part.

For tinctures, give 1 ml per 10 pounds twice daily in food. For teas, give one-fourth cup per 10 pounds twice daily in food.

Herbal allergic bronchitis support formula

Polygala or Euphorbia: Expectorant, anti-asthmatic; 1 part.

Elecampane: Expectorant, antitussive, antibacterial, diaphoretic; 1 part.

Lobelia inflata: Respiratory stimulant, antispasmodic, anti-asthmatic, expectorant; 1 part.

Marshmallow: Demulcent, vulnery, diuretic, antitussive; 1 part.

Thyme: Carminative, antitussive, antispasmodic, expectorant, antibacterial, astringent; 1 part.

For tinctures, give 1 ml per 10 pounds twice daily in food. For teas, give one-fourth cup per 10 pounds twice daily in food.

Herbal chronic bronchitis support formula

Elecampane: Expectorant, antitussive, antibacterial, diaphoretic; 1 part.

Adhatoda: Expectorant, anti-asthmatic, bronchodilator; 1 part.

Astragalus: Immune-enhancing, tonic, cardiotonic; 1 part.

Mullein: Expectorant, demulcent, vulnery, mild sedative, mild diuretic; 1 part.

Thyme: Carminative, antitussive, antispasmodic, expectorant, antibacterial, astringent; 1 part.

Ribwort: Expectorant, vulnery, anti-inflammatory, astringent; 1 part.

For tinctures, give 1 ml per 10 pounds twice daily in food. For teas, give one-fourth cup per 10 pounds twice daily in food.

OR

Elecampane: Expectorant, antitussive, antibacterial, diaphoretic; 1 part.

Licorice: Antispasmodic, antitussive, anti-inflammatory, adaptogen, expectorant; 1 part.

Thyme: Carminative, antitussive, antispasmodic, expectorant, antibacterial, astringent; 1 part.

Lobelia inflata: Respiratory stimulant, antispasmodic, anti-asthmatic, expectorant; 1 part.

Grindelia: Anticatarrhal, antispasmodic, expectorant; 1 part.

Ginger: Antispasmodic, warming, circulatory stimulant, anti-inflammatory, diaphoretic, carminative; add 1/20 of total volume of rest of formula.

For tinctures, give 1 ml per 10 pounds twice daily in food. For teas, give one-fourth cup per 10 pounds twice daily in food.

PRESCRIPTION FOR FELINE BRONCHIAL ASTHMA

Strategy

Treatment depends on the severity and concurrent conventional treatment. For example, if the patient is on steroids, consider hepatoprotection and immune support. Inhalant drugs (bronchodilators and steroids) may be necessary for some patients. Consider inhalation therapy of inhaled steam from herbal teas. Avoid stressing cats if administering herbs is difficult. Consider herbs that stabilize mast cells and the herbs for allergic bronchitis.

The following simple formula for feline asthma support is easy to give and well tolerated (use glycetract).

Marshmallow: Demulcent, vulnery, diuretic, antitussive; 1 part.

Give one-half to 1 ml per 10 pounds 2 to 3 times daily in food or diluted and by mouth.

PRESCRIPTION FOR SINUSITIS/RHINITIS

Strategy

Determine whether inhaled allergens are involved (boarding the patient in a different environment for a few days might improve the condition) and reduce exposure to inhaled allergens (such as dust mites). Consider environmental irritants such as cigarette smoke, dust, and pollution, and consider elimination diets. Inhalation therapy may be useful. Consider immune-stimulating herbs such as Echinacea and Astragalus and anti-allergy herbs such as Albizzia and Baical skullcap. Nervines and adaptogens may be important if stress is a factor. Use anticatarrhal herbs such as Euprasia and Golden seal. Pain-relieving herbs might be helpful. Consider antimicrobial herbs. In chronic conditions consider alteratives and depuratives such as Poke root and Cleavers. In chronic rhinitis consider a T cell modulator such as Astragalus. For acute conditions, give more frequently and at higher doses.

Herbal allergic rhinitis support formula

Echinacea: Immunostimulant, anti-inflammatory, vulnery, antimicrobial; 1 part.

Baical skullcap: Anti-inflammatory, anti-allergy, antibacterial, bitter, mild sedative; 1 part.

Albizzia: Anti-allergic, antimicrobial; 1 part.

Eyebright: Anticatarrhal, astringent, anti-inflammatory; 2 parts.

For tinctures, give 1 ml per 10 pounds twice daily in food. For teas, give one-fourth cup per 10 pounds twice daily in food.

Herbal acute rhinitis/sinusitis support formula

Eyebright: Anticatarrhal, astringent, anti-inflammatory; 2 parts.

Golden seal: Mucous membrane trophorestorative, antimicrobial; 1 part.

Echinacea: Immunostimulant, anti-inflammatory, vulnery, antimicrobial; 1 part.

Golden rod: Anticatarrhal, anti-inflammatory, antiseptic, carminative; 1 part.

For tinctures, give 1 ml per 10 pounds twice daily in food. For teas, give one-fourth cup per 10 pounds twice daily in food.

Herbal chronic rhinitis/sinusitis support formula

Astragalus: Immune enhancing, tonic, cardiotonic; 1 part.

Albizzia: Anti-allergic, antimicrobial; 1 part.

Golden seal: Mucous membrane trophorestorative, antimicrobial; 1 part.

Eyebright: Anticatarrhal, astringent, anti-inflammatory; 2 parts.

Poke root: Anticatarrhal, immune-enhancing, lymphatic, alterative: 1/20th (5%) of formula. **Note:** Poke root is potentially toxic; use in small percentage of formula.

For tinctures, give 1 ml per 10 pounds twice daily in food.

REFERENCES

Art T, Desmecht D, Amory H, Lekeux P. Lobeline-induced hyperpnea in equids. Comparison with rebreathing bag and exercise. *Zentralbl Veterinarmed A.* 1991 Mar;38(2):148–52.

Boyd EM, Palmer ME. Effect of Quillaja, Senga, Grindelia, Saguinaria, Chionanthus and Dioscorea upon the output of respiratory tract fluid. *Acta Pharmacologia Toxicologia* 1946;2:235–239

Chang HM, But PPH. *Pharmacology and Applications of Chinese Materia Medica,* vol 2. Singapore: World Scientific Publishing; 1987.

Kamei J, Nakamura R, Ichiki H, Kubo M. Antitussive principles of *Glycyrrhizae radix*, a main component of the Kampo preparations Bakumondo-to (Mai-men-dong-tang). *Eur J Pharmacol* 2003;469:159–163.

Kardosova A, Ebringerova A, Alfoldi J, Nosal'ova G, Franova S, Hribalova V. A biologically active fructan from the roots of *Arctium lappa* L., var. Herkules. *Int J Biol Macromol* 2003;33:135–140.

Leung AY, Forster S. Encyclopedia of Common Natural Ingredients Used in Food, Drugs and Cosmetics, 2nd ed. NY: John Whiley 1996: p. 492–495

Misawa M, Yanaura S. Continuous determination of tracehobronchial secretory activity in dogs. *Japanese Journal of Pharmacology* 1980, 30:221–229.

Nosal'ova G, et al. Antitussive efficacy of the complex extract and the polysaccharide of marshmallow (*Althaea officinalis* L. var. Robusta*). Pharmazie* 1992;47:224–226.

Reiter M, Brandt W. Relaxant effects on tracheal and ileal smooth muscles of the guinea pig. *Arzneimittelforschung.* 1985;35(1A):408–14

Tripathi RM, Sen PC, Das PK. Further studies on the mechanism of the anti-anaphylactic action of Albizzia lebbeck, an Indian indigenous drug. *J Ethnopharmacol* 1979a;1:397–400.

Tyler VE. Herbs of Choice: The Therapeutic Use of Phytomedicinals. Binghamton, NY: Pharmaceutical Products Press; 1994:76–77.

Van den Broucke CO, Lemli JA. Antispasmodic activity of Origanum compactum. Part 2: Antagonistic effect of thymol and carvacrol. *Planta Med.* 1982 Jul;45(3):188–90.

Chapter Twenty-Seven

Diseases of the Urogenital System

HERBS FOR DISEASES OF THE UROGENITAL SYSTEM

Herbs can treat a number of diseases of the urogenital system, including acute and chronic nephritis, cystitis, FLUTD, urinary incontinence, prostate and ovarian conditions, and urolithiasis (calcium oxalate, struvite, and urate). Herbal actions of interest include the renal protective herbs that aid chronic renal disease, diuretics, urinary antiseptics, bladder tonics, antilithic herbs, and demulcents. Herbs that benefit prostate health are also discussed.

Renal-tonic and protective herbs

Several herbs may be beneficial for nephropathies. Astragalus (*Astragalus membranaceus*) has been shown to increase plasma and muscle protein and reduce urinary output of protein by improving dysfunctional protein metabolism in glomerulopathy. It can also prevent glomerular sclerosis (Zhou 1999). In rats with experimental nephritis, large doses of oral astragalus improved renal function, thus supporting the traditional use of large doses for the treatment of chronic nephritis in people (Chang 1987). In China, another species of Astragalus (*Astragalus mongholicus*) and Dong guai (*Angelica sinensis*) have been used to treat nephrotic syndrome. Both herbs together or enalapril were administered to rats with chronic induced nephrosis and compared with control rats. The treatment groups had significantly reduced deterioration of renal function and reduced histologic damage. The two herbs together retarded the progression of renal fibrosis and deterioration of renal function and were comparable to enalapril (Wang 2004).

Cordyceps (*Cordyceps sinensis*) is renal protective against gentamicin-induced nephrotoxicity in animals (Tian 1991). In a comparative, controlled clinical study, 28 of 51 patients with chronic renal failure received Cordyceps (3 to 5 g/day) and showed a significant improvement in renal function compared to the control group (Guan 1992). Nettle seed (*Urtica dioca*) may also be useful because it may lower creatinine, as reported in a case series of 2 human patients by North American herbalist David Winston. A hydroethanolic (1:5) tincture of Nettle seed, 5 ml TID, reduced serum creatinine in both patients (Treasure 2003).

Bladder tonics

Crataeva (*Crataeva nurvala*) has been shown to improve bladder tone in dogs (Deshpande 1982). In human studies, 50 ml decoction given twice daily for 3 months reduced incontinence, pain, and urine retention in prostatic hypertrophy with hypotonic bladder (Deshpande 1982).

Diuretic/aquaretic activity

Traditionally, conditions affecting the urogenital tract were treated with urinary diuretics, herbs given as teas and consumed in large volumes. The diuresis that was observed was thought to flush the tract and therefore aid in recovery. Diuretic action was also seen as alterative, aiding in the elimination of wastes and therefore improving overall health. Such herbs included Red clover (*Trifolium pratense*), Dandelion leaf (*Taraxacum officinale*), Cleavers (*Gallium aparine*), Burdock (*Arctium lappa*), and Celery (*Apium graveolens*).

On the other hand, some herbs have aquaretic activity, which is more closely aligned with our conventional view of diuretics. These herbs produce diuresis by acting directly on the glomerulus to increase urine production without impacting electrolytes (Werk 1994).

The diuretic and aquaretic herbs Nettle (*Urtica dioca*) and Cornsilk (*Zea Mays*) both have a high potassium content. Juniper (*Juniperus communis*) contains an essential oil that is reported to increase the glomerular filtration rate (Tyler 1993, Stanic 1998). Parsley (*Petroselinum crispum*) can inhibit the Na+-K+ pump, leading to an osmotic diuresis (Kreydiyyeh 2002). Couchgrass (*Agropyron repens*), which contains the constituent mannitol, also leads to osmotic diuresis. Lavender (*Lavendula officinalis*) contains the aqueous extract that can produce diuresis (Elhajili 2001). Dandelion (*Taraxacum officinalis*) leaf at a dose of 50 mL (equivalent to 2 g dried herb/kg body weight) in one study produced a comparable effect to furosemide (80 mg/kg) (Hook 1993); however, an ethanolic extract of the root did not produce a diuretic effect (Tita 1993). Pharmacological evaluation of Bearberry (*Arctostaphylos uva-ursi*) showed that it increases urine flow (Beaux 1999). Others include Celery (*Apium graveolens*) and Buchu (*Agathosma betulina*).

Urinary antiseptics

Urinary antiseptic herbs are perhaps most valuable for chronic infections, in those with resistant strains of bacteria, and for preventing infection in vulnerable patients. Some produce antiseptic metabolites which are excreted in urine. Others may improve the mucopolysaccharide layer produced by transitional cells coating the bladder wall (demulcents fall into this category as well). Yet others prevent adhesion of bacteria to the bladder wall.

Carbenoxolone derived from Licorice (*Glycyrrhiza glabra*) was shown to protect against laboratory-induced lower urinary tract infections in the rabbit model by influencing the mucopolysaccharide layer (Mooreville 1983). Cranberry (*Vaccinium macrocarpa*) inhibits bacterial adherence due to anti-adhesion agents in Cranberry juice (Reid 1987). This is most likely due to proanthocyanidins, which are shown to inhibit the adherence of P-fimbriated *E. coli* to uroepithelial cell surfaces (Howell 1998) and provide anti-adherence activity toward gram-negative rods including *Klebsiella*, *Enterobacter*, *Pseudomonas*, and *Proteus* (Schmidt 1988). Bearberry (*Arctostaphylos uva-ursi*) has the constituent arbutin, which is hydrolyzed to hydroquinone during excretion in urine. This metabolite is both antiseptic and astringent in action (Matsuda 1992). Arbutin works best in alkaline urine, and urinary acidifiers inhibit conversion of arbutin to active hydroquinone (De Smet 1993), so it can also modify bacterial adhesion. Others include Golden rod (*Solidago virgaurea*); Buchu (*Barosma betulina*), which has very low activity against Escherichia coli; *Saccharomyces cerevisiae* and *Staphylococcus aureus* (Lis-Balchin 2001), Couchgrass (*Agropyron repens*), Crataeva (*Crataeva nurvala*), and Saw palmetto (*Serenoa serrulata*).

Antilithics

Traditional antilithic herbs include Cornsilk (*Zea Mays*), Couchgrass (*Agropyron repens*), Stone root (*Collinsonia canadensis*), Gravel root (*Eupatorium purpureum*), and Hydrangea (*Hydrangea arborescens*). Uric stones have

benefited from the antiseptic action (tentatively to saponins) and possibly some solvent action by herbal infusions of Vervain (*Verbena officinalis*), Lithospermum (*Lithospermum officinale*), Dandelion (*Taraxacum officinale*), Horsetail (*Equisetum arvense*), Bearberry (*Arctostaphylos uva-ursi*), Burdock (*Arctium lappa*), and *Silene saxifrage*. In oxalate urolithiasis, Fenugreek seeds (*Trigonella foenum-graecum*) significantly decreased the quantity of calcium oxalate deposited in the kidneys in induced urolithiasis in rats (Ahsan 1989).

Crataeva (*Crataeva nurvala*) on calcium oxalate lithiasis has been studied in rats. A crude extract at 100 mg/kg PO in rats significantly reduced stone formation (81%) (Prabhakar 1997). It showed a regulatory action on endogenous oxalate synthesis and the decoction lowered stone-forming constituents in the kidneys of calculogenic rats (Varalakshmi 1990). Also in calcium oxalate kidney stones, Cranberry (*Vaccinium macrocarpa*) juice decreased oxalate and phosphate excretion, increased citrate excretion, and decreased the relative supersaturation of calcium oxalate. It was concluded that Cranberry juice has antilithogenic properties and may help manage calcium oxalate urolithiasis (McHarg 2003). On the other hand, cranberry juice contains oxalate and 5 healthy volunteers had significant increases in urinary oxalate while receiving cranberry tablets. However, inhibitors of stone formation, magnesium, and potassium, rose as well (Terris 2001).

Others

Traditional demulcents used to reduce pain and dysuria associated with mucosal inflammation include Marshmallow (*Althaea officinalis*), Cornsilk (*Zea mays*), Couchgrass (*Agropyron repens*), and Licorice (*Glycyrriza glabra*).

Spasmolytic herbs may be considered for urinary tract disorders. These include Saw palmetto (*Serenoa serrulata*), Cramp bark (*Viburnum opulus*), and Pumpkin seed (*Curcurbita pepo*). A formula consisting of uva–ursi, Hops, and Peppermint, administered for 6 weeks, improved symptoms in 70% of patients (915) suffering from compulsive strangury, enuresis, and painful micturition (Lenau 1984).

Astringents may be useful in hemorrhagic conditions. Two herbs traditionally used for this include Plantain (*Plantago major*) and Horsetail (*Equisetum arvense*).

PRESCRIPTION FOR NEPHRITIS

Strategy

Treat conventionally until the patient is stable in acute conditions. Treat the underlying etiology if known (infectious, immune complexes, etc.). Consider ACE inhibitors and conventional renal support, appropriate diet therapy, and thromboxane and PAF inhibitors.

Use alcohol or glycetract tinctures for best results; alternatively, use teas.

Astragalus: Immune enhancing, cardiotonic, diuretic, hypotensive; 1 part.

Dong guai: Blood tonic, circulatory stimulant, vasodilator; 1 part.

Siberian ginseng: Immune modulating, adaptogen; 1 part.

Hawthorn: Hypotensive, vasodilator, antioxidant, cardiotonic; 1 part.

Ginkgo: Inhibits platelet activating factor, antioxidant, circulatory stimulant; 1 part.

For tinctures, give 1 ml per 10 pounds twice daily in food. For teas, give one-fourth cup per 10 pounds twice daily in food.

Consider using Cordyceps as well: Dried herb, 25 to 100 mg/kg divided daily if extracted and dried; triple or quadruple dose for unprocessed herb; tincture, 1:2 to 1:3: 0.5 to 2 mL per 10 kg (20 pounds) divided daily and diluted or combined with other herbs (Wynn 2006).

Chinese herbal formulas including Rehmannia 6 and Rehmannia 8 are also useful.

PRESCRIPTION FOR CYSTITIS

Strategy

Treat conventionally until the patient is stable in acute conditions. Treat the underlying etiology if known (infectious, immune complexes, etc.). Consider ACE inhibitors and conventional renal support, appropriate diet therapy, and thromboxane and PAF inhibitors.

Use alcohol or glycetract tinctures for best results; alternatively, use teas.

Crataeva: Bladder tonic, anti-inflammatory, antilithic; 1 part.

Licorice: Anti-inflammatory, adaptogen, antispasmodic, taste improver, demulcent; 1 part.

Cornsilk: Diuretic, demulcent, antilithic; 1 part.

Golden rod: Anti-inflammatory, antiseptic, diuretic, carminative; 1 part.

Echinacea: Immune stimulant, anti-inflammatory, vulnery, antimicrobial; 1 part.

For tinctures, give 1 ml per 10 pounds twice daily in food. For teas, give one-fourth cup per 10 pounds twice daily in food.

Add Bearberry (*Archostaphylos uva-ursi*)(urinary antiseptic, astringent). Treat for 3 weeks, then take 1 week off, and repeat. Dose: Infusion, 5 to 30 gm per cup of water, administered at a rate of one-fourth to one-half

cup per 10 kg (20 pounds) divided daily; tincture, 1:2 to 1:3 : 1 to 2 mL per 10 kg (20 pounds) divided daily or combined with other herbs.

PRESCRIPTION FOR FLUTD/IC SUPPORT

Strategy

Consider treatment adjunctive to or instead of conventional treatment, depending on the severity and recurrence rate. Give moist diets only to increase water turnover. Consider a source of glycosaminoglycans and consider feline pheromones to reduce stress and ensure litter box hygiene. Anti-inflammatory herbs may be beneficial in treating cats with chronic interstitial cystitis; pain-relieving herbs may also help. Consider anxiolytic herbs or amitriptyline. Demulcents may be beneficial. Use alcohol or glycetract tinctures for best results; alternatively, use teas.

Marshmallow: Demulcent, vulnery, diuretic; 1 part.

Saw palmetto: Diuretic, spasmolytic, anabolic; 1 part.

Bilberry: Antioxidant, astringent, anti-inflammatory; 1 part.

Crataeva: Bladder tonic, anti-inflammatory, antilithic; 1 part.

St. John's wort or Kava kava: Nervine tonic, anti-inflammatory, vulnery; 1 part.

For tinctures, give 1 ml per 10 pounds twice daily in food. For teas, give one-fourth cup per 10 pounds twice daily in food.

PRESCRIPTION FOR URINARY INCONTINENCE SUPPORT

Strategy

Treat the underlying etiology if known (chiropractic, acupuncture may help). Improve bladder and sphincter tone. Prevent infection and urolithiasis. Consider Cranberry capsules to help deodorize urine and help prevent infection. Use alcohol or glycetract tinctures for best results; alternatively, use teas.

Crataeva: Bladder tonic, anti-inflammatory, antilithic; 2 parts.

Chaste tree: Regulates female hormonal activity, dopaminergic; 1 part.

OR

Saw palmetto: Diuretic, spasmolytic, anabolic; 1 part.

Marshmallow: Demulcent, vulnery, diuretic; 1 part.

Bilberry: Antioxidant, astringent, anti-inflammatory; 1 part.

For tinctures, give 1 ml per 10 pounds twice daily in food. For teas, give one-fourth cup per 10 pounds twice daily in food.

PRESCRIPTION FOR PROSTATE SUPPORT

Strategy

Treat the underlying etiology if known (chiropractic, acupuncture may help). Improve bladder and sphincter tone and prevent infection and urolithiasis. Consider Cranberry capsules to help deodorize urine and help prevent infection. Use alcohol or glycetract tinctures for best results; alternatively, use teas.

Crataeva: Bladder tonic, anti-inflammatory, antilithic; 2 parts.

Saw palmetto: Diuretic, spasmolytic, anabolic; 1 part.

Nettle root: Antihyperprostatic; 1 part.

Hydrangea: Diuretic, antihyperprostatic, antilithic; 1 part.

For tinctures, give 1 ml per 10 pounds twice daily in food. For teas, give one-fourth cup per 10 pounds twice daily in food.

PRESCRIPTION FOR PROSTATITIS SUPPORT

Echinacea: Anti-inflammatory, vulnery, immune stimulant, antimicrobial; 1 part.

Cornsilk: Diuretic, demulcent, antilithic; 1 part.

Bearberry: Urinary antiseptic, astringent; 1 part.

Corydalis: Analgesic, sedative, cardioprotective; 1 part.

Meadowsweet: Mild urinary antiseptic, anti-inflammatory, mildly diuretic, anti-ulcerogenic, astringent; 1 part.

For tinctures, give 1 ml per 10 pounds twice daily in food. For teas, give one-fourth cup per 10 pounds twice daily in food.

PRESCRIPTION FOR UROLITHIASIS SUPPORT

Strategy

Identify composition of uroliths and implement appropriate conventional treatment if needed (surgical removal may be required). Increase water intake, using broths and moist food. Implement an appropriate diet if needed. Struvite can be managed medically; initiate herbs to prevent cystitis. Consider the underlying metabolic disorder or infection. The goal of herbal therapy is to minimize recurrence by minimizing infection or urolith formation. Use alcohol or glycetract tinctures for best results; alternatively, use teas.

Calcium oxalate

Crataeva: Bladder tonic, anti-inflammatory, antilithic; 1 part.

Fenugreek: Demulcent, laxative, contains saponins; 1 part.

Cornsilk: Diuretic, demulcent, antilithic; 1 part.

Marshmallow: Demulcent, vulnery, diuretic; 1 part.

Echinacea: Immune stimulant, vulnery, anti-inflammatory, antimicrobial; 1 part.

For tinctures, give 1 ml per 10 pounds twice daily in food. For teas, give one-fourth cup per 10 pounds twice daily in food.

Urate

Crataeva: Bladder tonic, anti-inflammatory, antilithic; 1 part.

Bearberry: Urinary antiseptic, astringent; 1 part.

Burdock: Alterative, diuretic, mild laxative, mild antiseptic; 1 part.

Dandelion: Diuretic, laxative, chologogue; 1 part.

Echinacea: Immune stimulant, vulnery, anti-inflammatory, antimicrobial; 1 part.

For tinctures, give 1 ml per 10 pounds twice daily in food. For teas, give one-fourth cup per 10 pounds twice daily in food.

REFERENCES

Ahsan SK, Tariq M, Ageel AM, al-Yahya MA, Shah AH. Effect of Trigonella foenum-graecum and Ammi majus on calcium oxalate urolithiasis in rats. *J Ethnopharmacol* 1989 Oct; 26(3):249–54.

Beaux D, Fleurentin J, Mortier F. Effect of extracts of *Orthosiphon stamineus* Benth., *Hieracium pilosella* L., *Sambucus nigra* L. and *Arctostaphylos uva-ursi* (L.) Spreng. in rats. *Phytother Res* 1999;13:222–225.

Chang HM, But PPH. Pharmacology and Applications of Chinese Materia Medica, vol 2. Singapore: World Scientific Publishing; 1987.

Deshpande P, Sahu M, Kumar P. *Crataeva nurvala* Hook and Forst (Varun): the Ayurvedic drug of choice in urinary disorders. *Indian J Med Res* 1982;76(suppl):46–53.

De Smet PAGM, Keller K, Hänsel R, et al. *Adverse Effects of Herbal Drugs*. Berlin: Springer Verlag; 1993.

Guan YJ, Hu Z, Hou- Chung-Kuo Chung Hsi i Chieh Ho Tsa Chih M, [Effect of Cordyceps sinensis on T-lymphocyte subsets in chronic renal failure.] *Chinese J Integrated Med* 1992;12:323,338–339.

Hook I, et al. Evaluation of dandelion for diuretic activity and variation in potassium content. *Int J Pharmacog* 1993;31: 29–34.

Howell AB, Vorsa N, Der Marderosian A, Foo LY. Inhibition of the adherence of P fimbriated *Escherichia coli* to uroepithelial-cell surfaces by proanthocyanidin extracts from cranberries. *N Engl J Med* 1998;339:1085–1086.

Kreydiyyeh SI, Usta J. Diuretic effect and mechanism of action of parsley. *J Ethnopharmacol* 2002;79:353–357.

Lenau H, Muller A, Maier-Lewz H. Efficacy and tolerance of a mixture of plant extracts and alpha tocopherol acetate in patients with irritable bladder and or urinary incontinence. *Therapiewoche* 1984;34:6054–6059.

Lis-Balchin M, Hart S, Simpson E. Buchu *(Agathosma betulina* and *A. crenulata,* Rutaceae) essential oils: their pharmacological action on guinea-pig ileum and antimicrobial activity on microorganisms. *J Pharm Pharmacol* 2001;53:579–582.

Matsuda H, Nakamura S, Tanaka T, Kubo M. Pharmacological studies on leaf of *Arctostaphylos uva-ursi* (L.) Spreng. V. Effect of water extract from *Arctostaphylos uva-ursi* (L.) Spreng. (bearberry leaf) on the antiallergic and anti-inflammatory activities of dexamethasone ointment. *Yakugaku Zasshi* 1992;112:673–677.

McHarg T, Rodgers A, Charlton K. Influence of cranberry juice on the urinary risk factors for calcium oxalate kidney stone formation. *BJU Int* 2003;92:765–768.

Mooreville M, Fritz RW, Mulholland SG. Enhancement of the bladder defense mechanism by an exogenous agent. *J Urol* 1983;130:607–609.

Prabhakar Y, Kumar S. *Crataeva nurvala:* an Ayurvedic remedy for urological disorders. *Br J Phytother* 1997;4:103–109.

Reid G, Sobel JD. Bacterial adherence in the pathogenesis of urinary tract infection: a review. *Rev Infect Dis* 1987;9:470–487

Schmidt D, Sobota A. An examination of the anti-adherence activity of cranberry juice on urinary and nonurinary bacterial isolates. *Microbios* 1988;55:173–181.

Stanic G, Samarzija I, Blazevic N. Time dependent diuretic response in rats treated with juniper berry preparations. *Phytotherapy Research* 1998;12 494–497.

Terris MK, Issa MM, Tacker JR. Dietary supplementation with cranberry concentrate tablets may increase the risk of nephrolithiasis. *Urology* 2001;57:26–29.

Tian J, Yang JY, Li LS. Observation of effects of *Cordyceps sinensis* in isolated perfused kidney of gentamicin nephrotoxic rats. *J Am Soc Nephrol* 1991;2:671.

Tita B, et al. BMC complementary and alternative medicine: pharmacological effect of ethanol extract. *Pharmacol Res* 1993;27:23–24.

Treasure J. Urtica semen reduces serum creatinine levels. *J Am Herbalists Guild* 2003;4:22–25.

Tyler VE. The Honest Herbal. 3rd ed. Philadelphia: Strickley; 1993.

Varalakshmi P, Shamila Y, Latha E. Effect of *Crataeva nurvala* in experimental urolithiasis. *J Ethnopharmacol* 1990;28:313–321.

Wang H, Li J, Yu L, Zhao Y, Ding W. Antifibrotic effect of the Chinese herbs, *Astragalus mongholicus* and *Angelica sinensis,* in a rat model of chronic puromycin aminonucleoside nephrosis. *Life Sci* 2004;74:1645–1658.

Werk W., Wasser ausleiten: elektrolytneutral, *Erfahrungsheilkunde,* vol. 11, 1994 pp. 712–714

Wynn S, Fougere B. Veterinary Herbal Medicine. Oxford, UK: Elsevier, 2006.

Zhou Q. *Journal of Chinese Materia Medica.* 1999;30(5):386–388.

Chapter Twenty-Eight

Metabolic and Endocrine Diseases

HERBS FOR METABOLIC AND ENDOCRINE DISEASES

Herbal medicine can play an important role in veterinary endocrine medicine. The metabolic and endocrine diseases that can be treated with herbs include Cushing's disease, diabetes mellitus, and hypothyroid and hyperthyroid diseases. While herbs do not replace the hormones that are frequently used to treat endocrine diseases, they can treat the metabolic derangements that can occur as a result of these disorders. The adaptogens are an important group of herbs that have a direct impact on the endocrine system, and they should be considered for any patient in which stress is a contributing or perpetuating factor in the pathogenesis.

HERBS THAT INFLUENCE ADRENAL ACTIVITY

Some of the key herbs that influence adrenal activity are the adaptogens, which act directly on the adrenal gland or on the pituitary hypothalamic adrenal axis. *Panax ginseng* is a classic adaptogen and the activity of the ginsenosides has been attributed to an indirect action on the pituitary, leading to an augmentation of adrenal steroidgenesis (Ng 1987). Animal studies have shown that Ginseng increases resistance to irradiation, temperature stress, hyperbaric stress, physical exercise, and viral and tumor load (Nocerino 2000). Licorice (*Glycyrrhiza glabra*) is considered to have steroid–type action, and 2 of its constituents, glycyrrhizin and glycyrrhetinic acid (GA), are reported to bind to glucocorticoid and mineralocorticoid receptors with moderate affinity, and weakly to corticosteroid–binding globulin (Tamaya 1986; Armanini 1983, 1985).

One recent case study on the treatment of a hyperkalemic dog with Addison's disease reported that Licorice use normalized potassium after administration (Jarrett 2005). Cordyceps (*Cordyceps sinensis*) induced a dose-dependent increase in corticosterone production in vitro

in rat adrenal cells, and the effect was different from that of adrenocorticotropic hormone (Wang 1998). In stressed mice, Withania (*Withania somnifera*) extract has been shown to increase levels of corticoids (Singh 2000). *Ginkgo biloba* is not considered to be a classic adaptogen; however, constituents of Ginkgo inhibit stress-induced cortisone hypersecretion and at the hypothalamic level appear to reduce corticotrophic-releasing hormone expression and secretion (Marcilhac 1998). It has been suggested that Ginkgo could help control excess glucocorticoid production (Amri 2003). Eluethero or Siberian ginseng (*Eleutherococcus senticosis*) showed a protein anabolic effect (Kaemmerer 1980) and attenuated the rise on blood corticosterone in stressed rats (Kimura 2004).

PRESCRIPTION FOR HYPERADRENOCORTICISM

Strategy

Reduce endogenous production of cortisol and improve adrenal function and systemic health. Treat symptoms and improve immunity. If using concurrent mitotane, ketoconazole, or L-deprenyl, minimize side effects.

Use alcohol or glycetract tinctures for best results; alternatively, use teas.

Milk thistle: Hepatotonic, antioxidant, hepatoprotective; 1 part.

Ginkgo: Antioxidant, circulatory stimulant, cognition enhancer, may reduce corticosteroid production; 1 part.

Panax ginseng: Adaptogen, anti-inflammatory, anti-allergic, immune enhancing, hepatorestorative; 1 part.

Withania: Tonic, antitumor, adaptogen, nervine, sedative, anti-inflammatory; 1 part.

Astragalus: Immune modulating, tonic, cardiotonic, diuretic, hypotensive, antitumor; 1 part.

For tinctures, give 1 ml per 10 pounds twice daily in food. For teas, give one-fourth cup per 10 pounds twice daily in food.

PRESCRIPTION FOR HYPOADRENOCORTICISM

Strategy

Improve adrenal and systemic health and signs of Addison's disease. Supply corticosteroid activity and correct electrolyte abnormalities.

Siberian ginseng: Adaptogenic, immunomodulatory; 1 part.

Astragalus: Immune modulating, tonic, cardiotonic, diuretic, hypotensive, antitumor; 1 part.

Licorice: Anti-inflammatory, adaptogen, mineralocorticoid- and corticoid-like activity; 1 part.

Withania: Tonic, adaptogen, nervine, anti-inflammatory, antitumor; 2 parts.

For tinctures, give 1 ml per 10 pounds twice daily in food. For teas, give one-fourth cup per 10 pounds twice daily in food.

HERBS FOR DIABETES

Many herbs affect blood glucose, and a few herbs have been studied for their effects on diabetes per se. One of the most useful herbs is Gymnema (*Gymnema sylvestre*), which has been shown in (induced) diabetic animal studies to double the number of insulin-secreting beta cells in the pancreas and normalize blood sugar (Prakash 1986, Shanmugasundaram 1990). Ginseng (*Panax ginseng*) has been shown to increase insulin receptors in bone marrow (Yushu 1988) and ginsenosides promote an insulin release that uses a different mechanism than that of glucose (Goudong 1987), both of which contribute to Ginseng's antidiabetic action.

Cordyceps (*Cordyceps sinensis*) attenuated diabetes-induced weight loss, polydipsia, and hyperglycemia in an animal study (Lo 2004). Ginger (*Zingiber officinalis*) juice (4 ml/kg PO daily) given for 6 weeks to rats with induced diabetes increased insulin levels and decreased fasting glucose levels. It also reduced serum cholesterol, serum triglyceride, and blood pressure in diabetic rats (Akhani 2004).

Herbs that reduced blood sugar in induced-diabetic rabbit studies include Fenugreek (*Trigonella foenumgraceum*), Damania (*Turnera diffusea*), and Prostrate spurge (*Euphorbia prostrata*) (Alarcon-Aguilara 1998); Madagascar periwinkle leaf juice (*Catharanthus roseus*), and seed powder of Fenugreek (*Trigonella foenumgraecum*) (Satyanarayana 2003). Fenugreek (*Trigonella foenum-graecum*) and its constituents reduce both blood glucose and cholesterol; it is thought that this is mainly due to its dietary fiber and high saponin content (Madar 2002). Seed fractions were given to normal and diabetic dogs (treated with insulin) for 8 days. The defatted fraction reduced hyperglycemia and glycosuria in the diabetic dogs (Ribes 1986).

Bilberry (*Vaccinium myrtillus*) (bilberry leaf tea) also reduced hyperglycemia in normal and diabetic dogs when given concurrent intravenous glucose (Allen 1927). Other herbs that reduce blood sugar include Agrimony (*Agrimonia eupatoria*), Alfalfa (*Medicago sativa*), Bugleweed (*Lycopus virginicus*), Burdock (*Arctium lappa*), Celery (*Apium graveolens*), Corn silk (*Zea mays*), Dandelion (*Taraxacum officinalis*), Garlic (*Allium sativa*), Goats rue (*Galega officinalis*), Java tea (*Ortosiphon stamineus*), Marshmallow (*Althaea officinalis*), Nettle (*Urtica dioica*), Sage (*Salvia officinalis*), and Siberian ginseng (*Eleutherococcus senticosus*) (Brinker 1997), as well as Aloe and Rehmannia.

Other herbs have little effect on insulin or blood glucose, yet they may help treat diabetes. Bearberry (*Arctostaphylos uva ursi*), Golden seal (Hydrastis *canadensis*), Mistletoe (*Viscum album*), and Tarragon (*Artemisia dracunculus*) reduced hyperphagia and polydipsia associated with induced diabetes in mice but did not affect insulin or glucose (Swanston-Flatt 1989).

PRESCRIPTION FOR DIABETES MELLITUS

Strategy

Adapt diet appropriately. Insulin doses or oral hypoglycemic drugs may need to be reduced; monitoring is important. Improve systemic health and pancreatic health and prevent complications.

Gymnema: Hypoglycemic, pancreatic trophorestorative, astringent, mildly diuretic; 2 parts.

Panax ginseng: Adaptogenic, tonic, hypoglycemic, immunostimulant, hepatoprotective, cardioprotective; 1 part.

Rehmannia: Hypoglycemic, renal protective, adaptogen; 1 part.

Bilberry: Vasoprotective, antioxidant, anti-inflammatory, astringent; 1 part.

Use alcohol tinctures for best results; alternatively, use teas. Glycetracts may be used but careful monitoring is required. If the glycetract is only a small part of the formula, then the effect is negligible.

For tinctures, give 1 ml per 10 pounds twice daily in food. For teas, give one-fourth cup per 10 pounds twice daily in food.

HERBS FOR HYPOTHYROID FUNCTION

Because hypothyroid disease can be immune-mediated, degenerative, or caused by neoplastic processes, the underlying disease process should be treated. One of the first herbs many people think of for an underactive thyroid is kelp. However, neither kelp nor bladder wrack (*Fucus vesiculosus*) has research to support this use. It may be used as a source of iodine in iodine-deficient states, which are rare in dogs. Increased iodine intake is associated with initiation of autoimmune thyroiditis in genetically predisposed people (Lorini 2003, Ruwhof 2001). Because immune-mediated thyroiditis is a common form of hypothyroidism in dogs, kelp supplementation may be detrimental in some dogs.

Some herbs have been shown to stimulate thyroid production, including Withania, Bacopa, and Licorice. Withania (*Withania somnifera*) has been shown to increase thyroxine (T4) in rats (Panda 1999). Brahmi (*Bacopa monniera*) (200 mg/kg) leaf extracts also have a thyroid-stimulating effect; in mice they increased T4 concentration by 41%. They also may be beneficial in hypothyroidism (Kar 2002). Rats given Licorice (*Glycyrrhiza glabra*) for 15 days had dose-dependent increases of thyroxine, triiodothyronine, and thyrotrophic hormone (Al-Qarawi 2000).

PRESCRIPTION FOR HYPOTHYROIDISM

Strategy

Use thyroxine replacement, but monitor because the doses that are needed may be lower than expected. Consider herbs that stimulate the thyroid, but also consider herbs that modulate the immune system if thyroiditis plays a role. Treat the symptoms; use tonics, bitters, and circulatory stimulants; and consider whether alteratives and nervines may be beneficial.

Withania: Tonic, adaptogen, nervine, anti-inflammatory, antitumor; 2 parts.

Milk thistle: Hepatotonic, antioxidant, hepatoprotective; 1 part.

Bupleurum: Anti-inflammatory, hepatoprotective, renal protective, tonic; 1 part.

Bacopa: Nervine, mild sedative, spasmolytic, mental tonic; 1 part.

For tinctures, give 1 ml per 10 pounds twice daily in food. For teas, give one-fourth cup per 10 pounds twice daily in food.

HERBS FOR HYPERTHYROID FUNCTION

Aloe vera inhibited both T(3) and T(4) in mice and may be useful in the regulation of hyperthyroidism (Kar 2002). Bugleweed (*Lycopus virginicus*) is perhaps the most extensively studied herb for its effects on thyroid function. It reduced both thyroid-stimulating hormone and thyroxine (T4) (Wagner 1970) and inhibited both the extra-

thyroidal enzymic T4-5′-deiodination to T3 and the T4-5′-deiodination (Auf'mkolk 1984). *Lycopus europaeus* caused a long-lasting T3 reduction in rats and a reduction in T4 and thyroid-stimulating hormone (TSH) 24 hours after administration (Winterhoff 1994). However, administration of *Lycopus europaeus* did not affect thyroid hormone levels in rats in a more recent study but did reduce heart rate (Vonhoff 2006).

PRESCRIPTION FOR HYPERTHYROIDISM

Strategy

Conventional radioactive iodine, surgery or chemical ablation may be preferred. Oral agents may be effective and herbs may be used to minimize side effects. Herbs may assist in management in early cases. Consider using nervines, adaptogens, and cardioprotective herbs.

Bugleweed: Cardioactive, diuretic, reduces heart rate, sedative, thyroxine antagonist; 1 part.

Motherwort: Sedative, cardiotonic; 1 part.

Hawthorn: Cardiotonic, hypotensive, antioxidant; 1 part.

Passion flower: Sedative, nervine, antispasmodic; 1 part.

Rehmannia: Adaptogen, renal protective; 1 part.

Use glycetracts if available. Give 1 ml per 10 pounds twice daily in food or diluted and given by mouth.

For teas, give one-fourth cup per 10 pounds twice daily in food.

REFERENCES

Akhani SP, Vishwakarma SL, Goyal RK. Anti-diabetic activity of Zingiber officinale in streptozotocin-induced type I diabetic rats. *J Pharm Pharmacol.* 2004 Jan;56(1):101–5.

Alarcon-Aguilara FJ, Roman-Ramos R, Perez-Gutierrez S, et al. Study of the anti-hyperglycemic effect of plants used as anti-diabetics. *J Ethnopharmacol.* 1998 Jun;61(2):101–10.

Allen FM. Blueberry leaf extract: physiologic and clinical properties in relation to carbohydrate metabolism. *JAMA* 1927;89:1577–1581.

Al-Qarawi AA, Abdel-Rahman HA, Ali BH, El Mougy SA. Liquorice (Glycyrrhiza glabra) and the adrenal-kidney-pituitary axis in rats. *Food Chem Toxicol.* 2002 Oct;40(10):1525–7.

Amri H, Drieu K, Papadopoulos V. Transcriptional suppression of the adrenal cortical peripheral-type benzodiazepine receptor gene and inhibition of steroid synthesis by ginkgolide B. *Biochem Pharmacol* 2003;65:717–729.

Armanini D, Karbowiak I, Funder JW. Affinity of liquorice derivatives for mineralocorticoid and glucocorticoid receptors. *Clin Endocrinol* 1983;19:609–612.

Armanini D, Strasser T, Weber PC. Binding of agonists and antagonists to mineralocorticoid receptors in human peripheral mononuclear leucocytes. *J Hypertens* 1985; 3(3): S157–159.

Auf'mkolk M, Kohrle J, Gumbinger H, et al. Antihormonal effects of plant extracts: iodothyronine deiodinase of rat liver is inhibited by extracts and secondary metabolites of plants. *Horm Metab Res* 1984;16:188–192.

Brinker FJ. Herb Contraindications and Drug Interactions. Oregon: Eclectic Institute; 1997:104–106.

Guodong L, Zhongqi L. Effects of ginseng saponins on insulin release from isolated pancreatic islets of rats. *Chin J Integr Trad Western Med* 1987;7:326.

Jarrett RH, Norman EJ, Squires RA. Liquorice and canine Addison's disease. *N Z Vet J* 2005;53:214.

Kaemmerer K, Fink J. Untersuchungen von Eleutherococcus-Extrakt auf trophanabole Wirkungen bei Ratten. *Der praktische Tierarzt* 1980;61:748–753.

Kar A, Panda S, Bharti S. Relative efficacy of three medicinal plant extracts in the alteration of thyroid hormone concentrations in male mice. *J Ethnopharmacol* 2002;81:281–285.

Kimura Y, Sumiyoshi M. Effects of various *Eleutherococcus senticosus* cortex on swimming time, natural killer activity and corticosterone level in forced swimming stressed mice. *J Ethnopharmacol* 2004;95:447–453.

Lo HC, Tu ST, Lin KC, Lin SC. The anti-hyperglycemic activity of the fruiting body of *Cordyceps* in diabetic rats induced by nicotinamide and streptozotocin. *Life Sci* 2004;74:2897–2908.

Lorini R, Gastaldi R, Traggiai C, Perucchin PP. Hashimoto's Thyroiditis. *Pediatr Endocrinol Rev.* 2003 Dec;1 Suppl 2:205–11; discussion 211.

Madar Z, Stark AH. New legume sources as therapeutic agents. *Br J Nutr* 2002;88(suppl 3):S287–S292.

Marcilhac A, Dakine N, Bourhim N, et al. Effect of chronic administration of *Ginkgo biloba* extract or Ginkgolide on the hypothalamic-pituitary-adrenal axis in the rat. *Life Sci* 1998;62:2329–2340.

Ng TB, Li WW, Yeung HW, Li TB, *et al.* Effects of ginsenosides, lectins and *Momordica charantia* insulin–like peptide on corticosterone production by isolated rat adrenal cells. *J Ethnopharmacol* 1987; 21: 21–29

Nocerino E, Amato M, Izzo AA. The aphrodisiac and adaptogenic properties of ginseng. *Fitoterapia* 2000;71(suppl 1): S1–S5.

Panda S, Kar A. *Withania somnifera* and *Bauhinia purpurea* in the regulation of circulating thyroid hormone concentrations in female mice. *J Ethnopharmacol* 1999;67:233–239.

Prakash AO, Mather S, Mather R. Effect of feeding *Gymnema sylvestre* leaves on blood glucose in berylliumnitrate treated rats. *J Ethnopharmacol* 1986;18:143–146.

Ribes G, Sauvaire Y, Da Costa C, Baccou JC, Loubatieres-Mariani MM. Anitidiabetic effects of subfractions from fenugreek seeds in diabetic dogs. *Proc Soc Exp Biol Med* 1986;182:159–166.

Ruwhof C, Drexhage HA. Iodine and thyroid autoimmune disease in animal models. *Thyroid.* 2001 May;11(5):427–36.

Satyanarayana S, et al. Evaluation of herbal preparations for hypoglycemic activity in normal and diabetic rabbits. *Pharmaceut Biol.* 2003;41:6,466–472.

Shanmugasundaram ER, et al. Possible regeneration of the islets of Langerhans in streptozotocin-diabetic rats given *Gymnema sylvestre* leaf extracts. *J Ethnopharmacol* 1990;30:265–279.

Singh A, Saxena E, Bhutani KK. Adrenocorticosterone alterations in male, albino mice treated with *Trichopus zeylanicus*, *Withania somnifera* and *Panax ginseng* preparations. *Phytother Res.* 2000;14:122–125

Swanston-Flatt SK, Day C, Bailey CJ, Flatt PR. Evaluation of traditional plant treatments for diabetes: studies in streptozotocin diabetic mice. *Acta Diabetol Lat* 1989;26:51–55

Tamaya MD, et al. Possible mechanism of steroid action of the plant herb extracts glycyrrhizin, glycyrrhetinic acid, and paeoniflorin: Inhibition by plant herb extracts of steroid protein binding in the rabbit. *Am J Obstet Gynecol* 1986;155:1134–1139.

Vonhoff C, Baumgartner A, Hegger M, et al. Extract of Lycopus europaeus L. reduces cardiac signs of hyperthyroidism in rats. *Life Sci.* 2006 Feb 2;78(10):1063–70

Wagner H, Horhammer L, Frank U. Lithospermic acid, the antihormonally active principle of *Lycopus europaeus* L. and *Symphytum officinale* L. *Arzneimittelforschung* 1970;20:705–712.

Wang SM, Lee LJ, Lin WW, Chang CM. Effects of a water-soluble extract of *Cordyceps sinensis* on steroidogenesis and capsular morphology of lipid droplets in cultured rat adrenocortical cells. *J Cell Biochem* 1998;69:483–489.

Winterhoff H, Gumbinger HG, Vahlensieck U, et al. Endocrine effects of *Lycopus europaeus* L. following oral application. *Arzneimittelforschung* 1994;44:41–45.

Yushu H, Yuzhen C. The effect of *Panax ginseng* extract (GS) on insulin and corticosteroid receptors. *J Trad Chin Med* 1988;8:293–295.

Chapter Twenty-Nine

Neurological Disorders

HERBS FOR NEUROLOGICAL DISORDERS

Traditional herbalists employ nervine herbs to treat disorders of the nervous system, including cognitive dysfunction, degenerative myelopathy, epilepsy, and paresis/paralysis (IV disc disease). Any plant that affects the nervous system is called a nervine. Perhaps one of the most useful classes of traditional nervines are the nerve tonics. These include the adaptogens (for example, *Panax ginseng*, *Withania somnifera*, and *Elutherococcus senticosus*), which can reduce the impact of stress on the body; nervine trophorestoratives, which can directly improve the functioning of nerve tissue (such as *Ginkgo biloba*, *Bacopa monniera*, *Centella asiatica*, *Hypericum perforatum*, and *Scutellaria lateriflora*); and most of the herbs that reduce anxiety and stress discussed in the herbs for behavioral conditions section.

Cognitive enhancers

Several herbs have been investigated for their potential as cognition enhancers. Ginkgo (*Ginkgo biloba*) is perhaps one of the most commonly prescribed in human herbal medicine. Note that 2 case reports in humans suggest a possible role of Ginkgo in precipitating seizures in previously controlled epileptic patients (Granger 2001). Ginkgo improves peripheral and central circulation and protects the brain from oxidative damage. A Cochrane meta analysis showed that despite some methodological issues with earlier studies, overall Ginkgo is beneficial for treating dementia and cognitive decline in people; it benefits cognition, activities of daily living, mood, and emotional function with no difference from placebo in terms of adverse effects (Birks 2002).

Lemon balm (*Melissa officinalis*) was investigated for the treatment of Alzheimer's disease. Sixty drops of an extract/day was administered to patients with mild to moderate Alzheimer's disease for 4 months. Compared to the placebo, the Melissa extract significantly improved

cognitive function (Akhondzadeh 2003). *Withania somnifera*, an important adaptogen, has shown memory-improving and cognition-enhancing effects in animals and humans (Schliebs 1997). Gotu kola (*Centella asiatica*) has also been used as a cognitive enhancer. In rat models of human Alzheimer's disease and epilepsy, it decreased the markers of oxidative stress and improved cognitive measures (Veerendra 2002, Veerendra 2003, Gupta 2003).

Bacopa (*Bacopa monniera*) was traditionally used in Ayurvedic medicine as a brain tonic to improve learning, concentration, and memory development, and was used to treat seizure and anxiety (Chopra 1958). It also has adaptogenic activity in stressed rats (Rai 2003). It may play a role in the treatment of epilepsy; in rats, it reduced cognitive impairment associated with phenytoin treatment (Vohora 2000).

Nervine trophorestoratives

Herbs that are considered to have an affinity for neurological tissue and are used for neuralgias and nerve trauma include Ginkgo (*Ginkgo biloba*), Bacopa (*Bacopa monniera*), Gotu kola (*Centella asiatica*), St. John's wort (*Hypericum perforatum*), Dan shen (*Salvia miltiorrhiza*), and Skullcap (*Scutellaria lateriflora*). One interesting herb, Dan shen (*Salvia miltiorrhiza*), has been used in China for cerebrovascular disease, including stroke in people. One constituent, tanshinone I, has demonstrated in vivo anti-inflammatory activity (Kim 2002). The tanshinones penetrated the blood–brain barrier readily and reduced brain infarct volume by one-third 24 hours following treatment. The reduction in brain infarct volume was associated with improvements in observed neurologic deficit (Lam 2003). Rabbits with induced spinal cord injury and impacted vertebrae were injected with Dan Shen and showed histologically less serious damage compared with controls. The study concluded that Dan shen has a protective effect on spinal cord injury in the early stages (Ni 2002). Anti-inflammatory, antistress, immunomodulatory, and antioxidant activity explains how trophorestoratives probably exert their effects on neurological disorders.

Anticonvulsants

Many herbs have traditionally been used to treat epilepsy and seizure disorders, and more have been investigated to ascertain their activity. For example, Gastrodia (*Gastrodia elata*) and Uncaria (*Uncaria rhyncophylla*) are both commonly incorporated into Chinese formulas for epilepsy. Both reduced seizure activity in induced epilepsy rats (Hsieh 2001, 1999). Corydalis (*Corydalis ambigua*) contains an active THP (tetrahydropalmatine), which is an effective anti-epileptogenic and anticonvulsant agent (Lin 2002). It may act by inhibiting amygdaloid dopamine release during an epileptic attack (Chang 2001).

Epilepsy was induced in rats, which were then given 1 of 3 herbs in their water supply for 30 days. Compared to controls, which were not seizure free, rats that received either Skullcap (*Scutellaria lateriflora*), Gelsemium (*Gelsemium sempervirens*), or Jimson weed (*Datura stramonium*) did not display any seizures during treatment. Once the herbal treatment was removed the rats displayed equivalent seizure activity to the nontreated rats, suggesting that herbal compounds may be helpful (Peredery 2004). Chinese skullcap (*Scutellaria baicalensis*) may also have anticonvulsant effects. Most recently, Devil's claw (*Harpagophytum procumbens*), which has traditionally been used for childhood convulsions, has been shown to have anticonvulsant activity in mice. AH procumbens secondary root aqueous extract (HPE, 100–800 mg/kg IP) delayed the onset of and antagonized induced seizures, possibly by enhancing GABA-ergic neurotransmission and/or facilitating GABA-ergic action in the brain (Mahomed 2006).

It is important to note that nervine relaxants (such as Kava, Valerian, Chamomile, and Passion flower) may potentiate the effects of anti-epileptic drugs, and nervine stimulants (such as ephedra or ma huang and caffeine in tea, for example) have the potential to exacerbate seizures in epileptics. Ginkgo and Ginseng may also exacerbate seizures (although the evidence for this is uncertain). St. John's wort also has the potential to affect the seizure threshold (Spinella 2001).

Analgesics

A number of herbs have demonstrated analgesic activity from mild to moderate activity. Also consider the herbs with anti-inflammatory activity in the musculoskeletal section such as Willow (*Salix alba*), Boswellia (*Boswellia serrata*), Devil's claw (*Harpagophytum procumbens*), Prickly ash (*Zanthoxylum spp*), Ginger, and others. The needs of the patient must be considered, and conventional pain relief, where needed, may be more effective and predictable. However, for long-term pain minimization herbs may help reduce the dosage or need for conventional analgesia. Corydalis reduced pain from inflammation in a rat model (Wei 1999) and has demonstrated dose-related analgesic effects in a clinical trial in people (Yuan 2004). California Poppy (*Eschscholtzia californica*) has a long history of use for pain relief in people. St. John's wort has shown analgesic effects in laboratory animal studies (Kumar 2001, Trovato 2001, Viana 2003, Rieli 2002).

PRESCRIPTION FOR COGNITIVE DYSFUNCTION

Strategy

Address any underlying primary medical diseases and discuss behavioral management with the owner. Recommend a balanced diet with fresh vegetables. Consider drug therapy as well as herbs to improve circulation and herbs with antioxidant activity. Also consider herbs to improve cognitive function and adaptogenic herbs for stress reduction.

Use alcohol or glycetract tinctures for best results; alternatively, use teas.

Withania: Tonic, adaptogen, nervine, sedative, anti-inflammatory; 1 part.

Hawthorn: Cardiotonic, antioxidant, vasodilator, hypotensive; 1 part.

Ginkgo: Antioxidant, circulatory stimulant, cognitive enhancer; 1 part.

Lemon balm: Anxiolytic, sedative, carminative, antispasmodic; 1 part.

Bacopa: Nervine tonic, mild sedative, mental tonic, spasmolytic; 1 part.

For tinctures, give 1 ml per 10 pounds twice daily in food. For teas, give one-fourth cup per 10 pounds twice daily in food.

DEGENERATIVE MYELOPATHY

Degenerative myelopathy is a slowly progressive disease of the spinal cord. Acupuncture and chiropractic are the treatments of choice, and ongoing physical therapy and maintaining mobility are critical to patient wellbeing.

Strategy

A balanced diet rich in antioxidants and supplementation with essential fatty acids may be beneficial. The underlying pathogenesis is still unknown; however, immunosuppressive treatment does not seem to be beneficial. Despite this, herbs that are beneficial in autoimmune disease such as Dan shen, Albizzia, Baical skullcap, and Bupleurum may be useful. Herbs rich in antioxidants may help delay the degenerative process. Reduce stress and possible inflammation and improve circulation with appropriate herbs.

Use alcohol or glycetracts for best results; alternatively, use teas.

Withania: Tonic, adaptogen, nervine, sedative, anti-inflammatory; 1 part.

Hawthorn: Cardiotonic, antioxidant, vasodilator, hypotensive; 1 part.

Ginkgo: Antioxidant, circulatory stimulant, cognitive enhancer; 1 part.

Dan shen: Neuroprotective; 1 part.

Bilberry: Vasoprotective, antioxidant, anti-edema, astringent, anti-inflammatory; 1 part.

For tinctures, give 1 ml per 10 pounds twice daily in food. For teas, give one-fourth cup per 10 pounds twice daily in food.

EPILEPSY

Seizure disorders are common in dogs, and despite several possible etiologies, most are idiopathic epilepsy. Many animals can be managed with conventional treatment, but a quarter to a third of cases can be challenging when they either don't respond or are refractory. Herbs can augment conventional treatment and reduce medication use. Conventional treatment should always be tried; however, in cases where only 1 seizure has been observed or the intra-seizure period is extended, herbs might be used as an alternative.

Strategy

Rule out food hypersensitivity by using an elimination diet. If using conventional drugs, consider adding hepatoprotective herbs. Also consider antioxidant herbs.

Skullcap: Anxiolytic; 1 part.

Baical skullcap: Anxiolytic; 1 part.

Milk thistle: Antioxidant, hepatoprotective, hepatotonic; 1 part.

Bilberry: Anti-inflammatory, antioxidant, astringent; 1 part.

Bacopa: Nervine tonic, mild sedative, mental tonic, spasmolytic; 1 part.

For tinctures, give 1 ml per 10 pounds twice daily in food. For teas, give one-fourth cup per 10 pounds twice daily in food.

PRESCRIPTION FOR INTERVERTEBRAL DISK DISEASE (CERVICAL AND THORACOLUMBAR)

Where conservative treatment is the treatment of choice, rest and physical therapy are essential. Chiropractics and acupuncture can be very helpful when applied appropriately. Nonsteroidal drugs and analgesics may be necessary. Corticosteroid treatment, while common, is controversial. Pain relief may result in increased exercise and further damage. Surgical intervention may result in clinical improvement; however, some dogs deteriorate, possibly because of the inflammatory cascade that may occur following decompression. The main goals are to relieve pain and inflammation.

Strategy

Support the animal with adaptogens to reduce the impact of stress. Use herbal antioxidants to reduce free radical damage. Use circulatory herbs to improve blood flow and oxygenation of inflamed tissues. Use herbal anti-inflammatory and analgesic herbs. Bladder support herbs may be important to reduce the risk of cystitis and improve bladder tone.

Dan shen: Neuroprotective; 2 parts.

Corydalis: Reduces visceral and back pain; 1 part.

Kava kava or Cramp bark: Anxiolytic, sedative, anti-spasmodic; 1 part.

Ashwaganda: Nervine, sedative, anti-inflammatory; 1 part.

Prickly ash: Antirheumatic, carminative; 1 part.

For tinctures, give 1 ml per 10 pounds twice daily in food. For teas, give one-fourth cup per 10 pounds twice daily in food.

REFERENCES

Akhondzadeh S, Noroozian M, Mohammadi M, Ohadinia S, Jamshidi AH, Khani M. *Melissa officinalis* extract in the treatment of patients with mild to moderate Alzheimer's disease: a double blind, randomised, placebo controlled trial. *J Neurol Neurosurg Psychiatry* 2003;74:863–866.

Birks J, Grimley EV, Van Dongen M. *Ginkgo biloba* for cognitive impairment and dementia. Cochrane Database Syst Rev 2002;4:CD003120.

Chang CK, Lin MT. DL-Tetrahydropalmatine may act through inhibition of amygdaloid release of dopamine to inhibit an epileptic attack in rats. *Neurosci Lett* 2001;307:163–166.

Chopra RN. Indigenous Drugs of India. 2nd ed. Calcutta: U.N. Dhur and Sons; 1958:341.

Granger AS. Ginkgo biloba precipitating epileptic seizures. *Age Ageing.* 2001 Nov;30(6):523–5.

Gupta YK, Veerendra Kumar MH, Srivastava AK. Effect of Centella asiatica on pentylenetetrazole-induced kindling, cognition and oxidative stress in rats. *Pharmacol Biochem Behav.* 2003 Feb;74(3):579–85.

Hsieh CL, Tang NY, Chiang SY, Hsieh CT, Lin JG. Anticonvulsive and free radical scavenging actions of two herbs, *Uncaria rhynchophylla* (MIQ) Jack and *Gastrodia elata* Bl., in kainic acid-treated rats. *Life Sci* 1999;65:2071–2082.

Hsieh CL, Chiang SY, Cheng KS, et al. Anticonvulsive and free radical scavenging activities of *Gastrodia elata* Bl. in kainic acid-treated rats. *Am J Chin Med* 2001;29:331–341.

Kim SY, Moon TC, Chang HW, Son KH, Kang SS, Kim HP. Effects of tanshinone I isolated from Salvia miltiorrhiza bunge on arachidonic acid metabolism and in vivo inflammatory responses. *Phytother Res.* 2002 Nov;16(7):616–20.

Kumar V, Singh PN, Bhattacharya SK. Anti-inflammatory and analgesic activity of Indian *Hypericum perforatum* L. *Indian J Exp Biol* 2001;39:339–343.

Lam BY, Lo AC, Sun X, Luo HW, Chung SK, Sucher NJ. Neuroprotective effects of tanshinones in transient focal cerebral ischemia in mice. *Phytomedicine* 2003;10:286–291

Lin MT, Wang JJ, Young MS. The protective effect of dl-tetrahydropalmatine against the development of amygdala kindling seizures in rats. *Neurosci Lett* 2002;320:113–116.

Mahomed IM, Ojewole JA. Anticonvulsant activity of Harpagophytum procumbens DC [Pedaliaceae] secondary root aqueous extract in mice. *Brain Res Bull.* 2006 Mar 15;69(1):57–62. Epub 2005 Nov 15.

Ni JD, Ding RK, Lu GH. Protective effect of dansheng injection on experimental rabbits' spinal cord injury. Hunan Yi Ke Da Xue Xue Bao 2002;27:507–508.

Peredery O, Persinger MA. Herbal treatment following post-seizure induction in rat by lithium pilocarpine: *Scutellaria lateriflora* (Skullcap), *Gelsemium sempervirens* (Gelsemium) and *Datura stramonium* (Jimson Weed) may prevent development of spontaneous seizures. *Phytother Res* 2004;18:700–705.

Rai D, Bhatia G, Palit G, Pal R, Singh S, Singh HK. Adaptogenic effect of *Bacopa monniera* (Brahmi). *Pharmacol Biochem Behav* 2003;75:823–830.

Rieli Mendes F, Mattei R, de Araujo Carlini EL. Activity of *Hypericum brasiliense* and *Hypericum cordatum* on the central nervous system in rodents. *Fitoterapia* 2002;73:462–471.

Schliebs R, Liebmann A, Bhattacharya SK, Kumar A, Ghosal S, Bigl VLC, Singh BB, Dagenais S. Systemic administration of defined extracts from *Withania somnifera* (Indian Ginseng) and Shilajit differentially affects cholinergic but not glutamatergic and GABAergic markers in rat brain. *Neurochem Int* 1997;30:181–190.

Spinella M. Herbal Medicines and Epilepsy: The Potential for Benefit and Adverse Effects. *Epilepsy Behav.* 2001 Dec;2(6):524–532.

Trovato A, Raneri E, Kouladis M, Tzakou O, Taviano MF, Galati EM. Anti-inflammatory and analgesic activity of *Hypericum empetrifolium* Willd. (Guttiferae). *Farmaco* 2001;56:455–457.

Veerendra Kumar MH, Gupta YK. Effect of different extracts of Centella asiatica on cognition and markers of oxidative stress in rats. *J Ethnopharmacol.* 2002 Feb;79(2):253–60.

Veerendra Kumar MH, Gupa YK. Effect of *Centella asiatica* on cognition and oxidative stress in an intracerebroventricular streptozotocin model of Alzheimer's disease in rats. *Clinical and Experimental Pharmacology and Physiology* Volume 30 Issue 5-6 Page 336.

Viana AF, Heckler AP, Fenner R, Rates SM. Antinociceptive activity of *Hypericum caprifoliatum* and *Hypericum polyanthemum* (Guttiferae). *Braz J Med Biol Res* 2003;36:631–634. Epub April 22, 2003.

Vohora D, Pal SN, Pillai KK. Protection from phenytoin-induced cognitive deficit by *Bacopa monniera*, a reputed Indian nonropic plant. *J Ethnopharmacol* 2000;71:383–390.

Wei F, Zou S, Young A, Dubner R, Ren K. Effects of four herbal extracts on adjuvant-induced inflammation and hyperalgesia in rats. *J Altern Complement Med* 1999;5:429–436.

Yuan CS, Mehendale SR, Wang CZ, et al. Effects of *Corydalis yanhusuo* and *Angelicae dahuricae* on cold pressor-induced pain in humans: a controlled trial. *J Clin Pharmacol* 2004;44:1323–1327.

Chapter Thirty

Infectious Diseases

HERBS FOR INFECTIOUS DISEASES

Herbs can deactivate viruses, bacteria, or fungi directly (this may involve altering membranes or enzyme systems) and are considered to be antimicrobial or to have antiseptic action. Others act indirectly via stimulation of phagocytosis, natural killer cells, lymphocytes, or other immune cells. For example, Andrographis (*Andrographis paniculata*) was originally thought to have direct antibacterial activity but was later found to exert its effect though immune stimulation. On the whole, treatment for infectious diseases is symptomatic. Apart from feline interferon-omega, there are currently no antiviral medications registered for veterinary use. Human antiviral drugs are available but are largely uneconomical or untested and complete elimination of virus is also not usually achieved. Herbal medicine management offers great potential to provide strategic immune modulatory action for infectious diseases. Herbs can also provide antiviral, antibacterial, antifungal, and antiprotozoal activity as well as symptom support for various infections.

Some general principles apply with any infectious disease. Provide conventional therapy as required and according to the severity of the symptoms. Support the immune system with immune-enhancing herbs. Provide systemic support. Focus particularly on the digestive system, which aids immune regulation via gut activated lymphoid tissue (GALT). Consider bitter herbs and alteratives that support elimination. Use adaptogens, particularly because stress can be a contributing or compounding problem associated with infectious diseases. Support the particular organs or systems affected by the infection. For example, Milk thistle is an obvious choice as a hepatoprotective herb in liver infections. Consider Golden seal (*Hydrastis canadensis*) for the gastrointestinal system and Uva ursi (*Arctostaphylos uva-ursi*) for the bladder. Use organ-specific antimicrobial, antiseptic, antifungal, antiprotozoal, or antiviral herbs.

HERBS WITH IMMUNE-MODULATING ACTIVITY

A key strategy when dealing with any infection is to support inherent immunity by incorporating immune-modulating herbs into any formula. These include medicinal mushrooms, Astragalus (*Astragalus membranaceus*), Cat's claw (*Uncaria tomentosa*), Echinacea *spp*, Pau D'arco (*Tabebuia avellanedae*), and Siberian ginseng (*Elutherococcus senticosus*), among others. Because most acute infections are accompanied by fever, warming tonic herbs such as Astragalus (*Astragalus membranaceus*), Asian ginseng (*Panax ginseng*), and Siberian ginseng (*Eleutherococcus senticosus*) are contraindicated. They are suitable for chronic infections. For recurrent or persistent infections, immune-enhancing herbs are fundamental to any prescription.

Medicinal fungi include Reishi (*Ganoderma lucidum*), Maitake (*Grifola frondosa*), Cordyceps (*Cordyceps sinensis*), Shitake (*Lentinula edode*), Turkey tail (*Trametes versicolor*), and others. Most of the medicinal fungi contain polysaccharide complexes and sterols that appear to enhance cell-mediated immune functions (Ooi 2000, Wasser 1999, Zhu 1998). Astragalus (*Astragalus membranaceus*) has antiviral, antineoplastic, and anti-inflammatory effects and has been shown to improve the immunity of mice with solid tumors (Kurashige 1999). It increases T-cell–mediated immune functions, increases macrophage numbers, and enhances phagocytosis (Zhao 1990, Yoshida 1997), and raises the levels of antibodies, activity of natural killer cells, and possibly interferon. It is ideal for prevention of infection during epidemics or for chronic immune incompetence.

Echinacea (*Echinacea spp*) has nonspecific immune-modulating activity, mainly by improving phagocytosis and therefore immune surveillance. It takes about 3 days for Echinacea to reach peak activity in people. Constituents have been shown to stimulate natural killer cell,

699

neutrophil, and B-lymphocyte activity and macrophage cytokine production in vitro; to inhibit hyaluronidase activity; and to have anti-inflammatory, antibacterial, antiviral, and mild local anesthetic activity (Wynn 2006). Cat's claw (*Uncaria tomentose*) or Una de Gato contains alkaloid constituents that have anti-inflammatory and immune stimulant activity and antimicrobial and antiviral properties (Williams 2001).

Panax ginseng polysaccharides and saponins have shown immunostimulating activity (Kitts 2000). In one study, rats with *Pseudomonas aeruginosa* had chronic lung infections. Rats treated with *Panax ginseng* showed higher bacterial clearance and lower serum immunoglobulin levels than those treated with the placebo, suggesting that cell-mediated immunity was enhanced (Song 1998).

Other herbs used to support immunity include Siberian ginseng (*Eleutherococcus senticosis*), Andrographis (*Andrographis paniculata*), Poke root (*Phytolacca decandra*), Picrorrhiza (*Picrorrhiza kurroa*), and Thuja (*Thuja occidentalis*). Picrorrhiza is ideal for acute febrile states and works well with Echinacea. It also works well with Milk thistle (*Silybum marianum*) for infectious liver disease. Thuja (*Thuja occidentalis*) is a particularly interesting herb. It demonstrates activity against several viruses, including enveloped and nonenveloped viruses with DNA and RNA nucleic acids from the following families: Papovaviridae (responsible for warts), poxviridae and picornaviridae, and herpes virus. With activity on this range of virus structures, it is likely the antiviral action of Thuja can be extended to other viral diseases. St. John's wort (*Hypericum perforatum*) is another antiviral herb against enveloped viruses such as herpes viruses, poxviruses, paramyxoviruses (*Morbillivirus*), retroviruses, and coronaviruses. Many other herbs and constituents have been reported to have strong antiviral activity and some of them have already been used to treat animals and people who suffer from viral infection (Jassim 2003).

When prescribing a formula for an individual patient with an infectious disease, it is most important to treat the patient, not the diagnosis. Provide immune support, adaptogens, and herbs to support the systems affected by the disease. In addition, biomedical actions of herbs can be exploited, and particular herbs can be incorporated for particular infectious agents.

CORONAVIRUS INFECTIONS

Coronavirus infections are most often associated with acute, self-limiting, enteric, and respiratory infections, but they can become chronic in infected animals. The low virulence enteric coronaviruses in cats and disease-causing feline infectious peritonitis are closely related and may represent differences in virulence. Coronaviruses do not usually cause disease in adult dogs but can cause mild gastrointestinal disease in puppies unless there is concurrent infection with parvovirus occurs.

Strategy

Use immune-supporting herbs such as Echinacea (*Echinacea spp.*) or Astragalus (*Astragalus membranaceus*). Use adaptogenic herbs such as Withania (*Withania somnifera*), which also assists gastrointestinal function. For mild gastrointestinal disease consider the gastrointestinal herbs that can be used to alleviate symptoms; alternatively, consider the respiratory herbs if that system is affected. St. John's wort (*Hypericum perforatum*) has activity against coronaviruses.

CANINE DISTEMPER

Canine distemper virus (CDV) is a morbillivirus, which induces multifocal demyelination in the central nervous system in dogs. Part of the pathogenesis includes noninflammatory demyelination and viral-induced immunosuppression.

Strategy

Use immune-supporting herbs such as Echinacea (*Echinacea spp.*) and Picrorrhiza (*Picrorrhiza kurroa*). Use adaptogenic herbs such as Withania (*Withania somnifera*), which is also a relaxing nervine. For neurological disease consider the neurological herbs that can alleviate symptoms and neurorestorative herbs such as Dan shen (*Salvia miltiorrhiza*). St. John's wort (*Hypericum perforatum*) also has activity against morbillivirus. Also consider Thuja (*Thuja occidentalis*) for immune stimulation and antiviral effects.

Distemper in dogs is considered to be a model for multiple sclerosis. Medical cannabis is often used by patients with multiple sclerosis (MS) for muscle spasm and pain, and in an experimental model of MS low doses of cannabinoids alleviated tremor (Williamson 2000).

FELINE UPPER RESPIRATORY TRACT INFECTIONS

Feline upper respiratory disease (FURD) complex may be caused by viral or bacterial organisms, or concurrent infections of calicivirus, herpes virus, chlamydia, bordetella, and mycoplasma. Treatment is mainly supportive (a high level of nutrition, adequate hydration, and good nursing care). Herpes virus 1 (rhinotracheitis) and calicivirus are the most common viral causes of upper respiratory tract infection in cats, and can be recurrent and chronic with or without secondary bacterial infection. There are no consistently effective treatments in conventional medicine. Lysine at 250 mg PO BID may be beneficial but is unproven, and interferon may help some cats with suspected herpes virus 1 infection, but neither are likely to cure the disease. Anti-inflammatory medications such as piroxicam can assist with chronic lymphocytic-plasmacytic rhinitis but side effects are possible. Herbal medicine rarely cures chronic disease but can reduce severity and increase disease-free periods, in the author's experience.

Strategy

In cats, use medicinal mushrooms, particularly Reishi (*Ganoderma lucidum*), Maitake (*Grifola frondosa*), Cordyceps (*Cordyceps sinensis*), and Shitake (*Lentinula edode*) combinations, to support immunity and help treat respiratory infection. Echinacea (*Echinacea* spp.) is ideal for respiratory tract infections. For nonsymptom periods consider Astragalus (*Astragalus membranaceus*) as a preventative. For herpes, consider herbal steam nebulizers to deliver St. John's wort (*Hypericum perforatum*), or for calcivirus use Astragalus or both as teas to deliver direct activity to the nares and mucosal membranes. Consider the respiratory demulcents to reduce inflammation in the mucous membranes; Marshmallow (*Althaea officinalis*) is ideal in cats. If using conventional anti-inflammatory medications consider herbs that reduce the potential for side effects such as renal protective herbs (Astragalus is ideal).

Carrier status is common and stress induces disease; therefore, adaptogens play an important role in prevention.

FELV, FIV, FIP

These feline diseases present with different signs and severity and cats should be treated individually based on their needs. Immune-modulating herbs are a strategic part of therapy. With appropriate care, FeLV- or FIV-infected cats can live well with retroviruses. Reducing stress and providing a high level of nutrition are essential.

Use the medicinal mushrooms, in particular Reishi (*Ganoderma lucidum*), Maitake (*Grifola frondosa*), Cordyceps (*Cordyceps sinensis*) and Shitake (*Lentinula edode*) combinations, to support immunity.

Feline leukemia

Echinacea purpurea was given to mice with induced leukemia (powdered leaves, 7.5 mg/mouse/week). Survival was significantly prolonged and enlargement of thymic lymphoma was significantly suppressed compared with controls. The suppressive effects on the leukemia may depend on enhancement of nonspecific immune or cellular

immune systems (or both) by Echinacea (Hayashi 2001).

Compared to the control mice, of which none survived past 3 months after induction of leukemia, all of the *E. purpurea*–treated mice were alive 3 months after tumor onset. The survival advantage provided by *E. purpurea* to these leukemic mice vs. untreated mice was highly significant (Currier 2001).

In an uncontrolled study of leukemic cats, acemannan from *Aloe vera* gel was given for 6 weeks intraperitoneally to clinically symptomatic cats. It significantly improved both quality of life and survival rate. It was noted that 12 weeks after initiation of treatment, 71% of the treated cats were alive and in good health (Sheets 1991). This trial included historical controls because participating clients refused to allow placebo treatment in their sick cats. Treated cats showed nonsignificant rises in hematocrit and hemoglobin concentrations, and leukocyte and lymphocyte counts tended to normalize over the course of the trial.

FIV

In South Africa, the effects of betasterol (BSS), a major phytosterol in plants, along with Betasitosterolin (BSSG) on FIV in cats and HIV in humans were studied. Domestic cats infected with the retrovirus FIV (which induces the same pathogenic mechanisms of CD4 cell loss, immunosupression, and opportunistic infections) were examined. A group of 33 infected cats was divided into a treatment group (n = 16) or a placebo group (n = 17) (Bouic 1997). The results of the study revealed that the treated cats maintained stable CD4 immune cell numbers, had a reduction of CD4 lymphocyte apoptosis, had decreased IL-6 levels, had possibly decreasing viral replication rates and viral load over a period of 168 weeks, compared to the placebo group, which showed disease progression with the typical CD4 cell loss over the same period of time. At the end of the study, the treated cats exhibited 20% mortality compared to 75% in the nontreated group. This combination of sterols is patented in a product called Moducare, and the plant sterols are considered to be very safe to use.

Acemannan, an extract of *Aloe vera*, was investigated by Yates (1992) in 49 FIV-infected symptomatic cats; 23 had severe lymphopenia. Cats were given acemannan by oral, subcutaneous, or intravenous routes, once weekly for 12 weeks. Over the treatment time there was a significant increase in lymphocytes and a decrease in neutrophils and infections. The route of administration was not significant. Cats that had lymphopenia had a 235% increase in lymphocytes compared to nonlymphopenic cats (42%). In this uncontrolled trial, the rates of survival for all 3 groups was 75% up to 19 months after the trial began, which is to be expected because FIV-infected cats are expected to live 8 years or more without treatment (Wynn 2006).

In a study reported by Jones (1995), Cat's claw (*Uncaria tomentosea*) as a proprietary root extract called Krallendorn was given by injection (0.3 mg IM on days 1, 3, 5) to FIV-infected cats. Eighty-five percent of symptomatic cats were reported to improve and 44% of cats "with leukemia" were aviremic by 20 weeks.

Herbs and constituents that have demonstrated activity against human immunodeficiency virus include various sulphated polysaccharide groups extracted from seaweed, Baicalein from Skullcap (*Scutellaria baicalensis*), anti-HIV flavonoids such as quercetin, and myricetin and andrographolide extracted from *Andrographis paniculata* (Jassim 2003).

St. John's wort (*Hypericum perforatum*) has activity against HIV retrovirus.

FIP

FIP is associated with vascular and perivascular inflammation, possibly immune-mediated. The inflammation leads to leakage of fluid and accumulation of thoracic and abdominal exudate.

Strategy

In addition to appropriate symptomatic care, the overall goal is to modulate rather than stimulate the immune system. To improve blood vessel integrity, consider rutin-containing herbs and herbs such as Bilberry (*Vaccinium myrtillus*). Herbs that have activity against coronavirus are also suggested.

CANINE INFECTIOUS HEPATITIS

Acute canine infectious hepatitis has been associated with canine hepatitis virus (canine adenovirus type-1), *Helicobacter canis* infection, leptospirosis, Rocky Mountain spotted fever, and other agents. Infections can lead to chronic liver disease.

Strategy

Use immune-stimulating herbs. *Andrographis paniculata* is immune stimulating and has been used to treat leptospirosis (Chang 1987). In people with infective hepatitis a majority of 20 patients showed marked improvement after the equivalent of 40 grams of andrographis were given each day for an average of 24 days. Overall, 80% were cured and 20% improved (Chaturvedi 1983). *Picrorrhiza kurroa* may be valuable in viral hepatitis. In clinical trials using Picrorrhiza to treat infectious hepatitis, rapid decreases in bilirubin and quick clinical recoveries were observed (Chaturvedi 1966). Echinacea is another good choice. Use adaptogens. If the patient is not excessive, consider *Panax ginseng*, which aids liver regeneration and hepatic function. Herbs that support liver function, including Milk thistle (*Silymarin marianum*), and in combination with Picrorrhiza are particularly well suited to the treatment of infectious or immune-mediated liver damage.

FELINE HERPES: STOMATITIS, KERATITIS, CORNEAL ULCERS

The ocular syndromes caused by herpes in cats include ophthalmia neonatorum in the newborn, bilateral keratoconjunctivitis in young cats, and ulcerative keratoconjunctivitis in young and adult cats. Topical medications with specific antiviral activity such as Trifluridine may be beneficial. L-Lysine (500 mg twice daily) may also help.

Strategy

Consider the options under Feline Upper Respiratory Tract Infections. Consider the options under herbs for eye and ear disorders. Use immune-supporting, adaptogenic, antiviral, and symptom-alleviating herbs. Topical herbal teas may be helpful. Teas should be made daily with boiled water to which 2 teaspoons of herb and 1 teaspoon of salt have been added. The tea should be filtered through a coffee filter to remove impurities that could irritate the eye. Lemon balm (*Melissa officinalis*) is the tea of choice for cats. It has topical efficacy against human herpes virus (Gaby 2006). Consider adjunctive care and pain-relieving herbs if blepharospasm is evident.

PARAINFLUENZA/INFECTIOUS TRACHEOBRONCHITIS

Infectious tracheobronchitis (ITB) is often a mixed infection (viral, bacterial, mycoplasma). Canine parainfluenza virus, canine adenovirus-2, and *Bordetella bronchiseptica* are considered to be primary pathogens. Other bacteria and *Mycoplasma spp.* may be primary or secondary. Paroxysmal coughing can be hacking, dry, or productive, but is usually self-limiting. Complicated cases may benefit from antibiotic therapy to treat or prevent secondary infections.

Strategy

Uncomplicated ITB can be treated symptomatically using respiratory herbs, mainly antitussives. Use preventative measures for dogs that are in contact with one another;

for example, oral doses or nose drops of Astragalus (*Astragalus membranaceus*) decoction protected mice from parainfluenza virus type 1 infection (Chang 1987). Use immune-supporting herbs such as Echinacea (*Echinacea spp.*), Astragalus (*Astragalus membranaceus*), or Holy basil (*Ocimum sanctum*). Chronic upper respiratory infection in dogs may benefit from Echinacea. In an open, multicenter trial, 41 dogs not previously treated that had various conditions including kennel cough, bronchitis, pharyngitis, and tonsillitis were given powdered *Echinacea purpurea* root extract (1:3). Although there was no proof of diagnosis or control in this trial, 92% of the dogs had a good or very good improvement at 4 weeks and 95% showed the same results at 8 weeks (Reichling 2003). Use adaptogenic herbs such as Siberian ginseng (*Eluthero-coccus senticosus*), which is particularly indicated for infections due to stress that may occur in boarding situations. Note that it should not be used in acute infections. Use respiratory herbs such as demulcents, antitussives, and respiratory antimicrobials.

CANINE PARVOVIRUS AND FELINE PANLEUKOPENIA

These infectious diseases lead to hemorrhagic diarrhea and mucosal sloughing with breakdown of the gastrointestinal mucosal barrier. This in turn can lead to bacterial translocation and endotoxemia, as well as sepsis, which is made worse by a concurrent neutropenia. Antibiotics are indicated in these patients, along with fluid therapy, pain relief, and supportive nursing. Vomiting may preclude treatment with herbal medicine but gastrointestinal herbs should be used when recovering, or administered via enema using teas in the hospital. During the acute phase, if possible administer Slippery elm (*Ulmus rubra*) powder, which acts as a mucilage and demulcent and nutritive herb.

Herbs such as Agrimony (*Agrimonia eupatoria*) and Tormentil (*Potentilla erecta*) contain tannins, which can denature surface proteins and lead to reduced pain and bleeding. However, they must to be given orally, which may be counterproductive in the acute phase. Berberine-containing herbs such as Golden seal (*Hydrastis canadensis*) can reduce endotoxemia.

In the recovery phase, probiotics are important to help gastrointestinal repair. Also consider glucosamine, glutamine, and fructooligosaccharides. Once vomiting has stopped consider formulas presented under gastrointestinal herbs. Three to 4 weeks of gastrointestinal repair should be expected. Herbs such as Meadowsweet, Marshmallow, Dandelion, and Withania (*Withania somnifera*) may be helpful.

In one report by Jones (1995), 2 veterinarians treated 15 dogs with parvovirus using Cat's claw (*Uncaria tomen-*

tosa) as a distilled preparation (1 mL/kg twice daily). They reported that 10 of the 15 dogs recovered.

TICK-BORNE DISEASES: LYME, EHRLICHIOSIS, ROCKY MOUNTAIN SPOTTED FEVER

Tick-borne diseases should be treated conventionally with appropriate antibiotics and supportive therapy. Depending on the diagnosis and signs, more than 1 disease-causing agent may be present at the same time. The spirochete *Borrelia burgdorferi* is responsible for the clinical syndromes of Lyme disease, which include arthritis, nephritis, carditis, and neurological changes. Canine ehrlichiosis is an acute to chronic disease characterized by infection of monocytes and lymphocytes, with anemia, lucopenia, and thrombocytopenia as common sequelae. Secondary immune-mediated hemolytic anemia may also be triggered by infection. In the chronic stage, pancytopenia and lymphocytois may occur. Rocky Mountain spotted fever is caused by *Rickettsia rickettsii*, which invade vascular endothelium and cause necrotizing vasculitis and petechiae, ecchymoses, and edema. Respiratory and neurological signs and lymphadenopathy may be seen. Conventional therapy may also include whole blood transfusions, fluid therapy, and sometimes corticosteroids. Herbs can be used to support the patient during the acute stages but are more strongly indicated for convalescence and for chronic disease. Herbal treatment is based on the individual patients and their symptoms.

Strategy

Fundamentally immune-enhancing herbs are the most important part of treating these infections, acute or chronic. Prescribe herbs to support the organs and tissues affected by the infection; herbs that treat anemia may be useful. Provide herbs that alleviate symptoms such as nervines and musculoskeletal or respiratory herbs as needed. Consider restoring bowel flora following antibiotic therapy, particularly if extended treatment is needed.

Traditionally, spirochete infections (syphilis) in people were treated with Sarsparilla (*Smilax ornata*), Stillingia (*Stillingia sylvatica*), and Guaiacum resin (*Guaiacum officinalis*), and may have applications in the treatment of persistent Lyme disease.

REFERENCES

Bouic PJD. Immunomodulation in HIV/AIDS: the Tygerberg/Stellenbosch University experience. *AIDS Bull* 1997;6:18–20.

Chang HM, But PPH, eds. Pharmacology and Applications of Chinese Materia Medica, vol 2. Singapore: World Scientific Publishing; 1987.

Chaturvedi GN, Singh RH. Jaundice of infectious hepatitis and its treatment with an indigenous drug, *Picrorhiza kurrooa* [sic]. *J Res Ind Med* 1966;1:1–13.

Chaturvedi GN, Tomar GS, Tiwari SK, et al. Clinical studies on Kalmegh (Andrographis paniculate) in infectious hepatitis. *J Int Inst Ayurveda* 1983;26:423–38

Currier NL, Miller SC. *Echinacea purpurea* and melatonin augment natural-killer cells in leukemic mice and prolong life span. *J Altern Complement Med* 2001;7:241–251.

Gaby AR. Natural remedies for Herpes simplex. *Altern med rev* 2006, Jun ; 11(2) 93–101.

Hayashi I, Ohotsuki M, Suzuki I, Watanabe T. Effects of oral administration of *Echinacea purpurea* (American herb) on incidence of spontaneous leukemia caused by recombinant leukemia viruses in AKR/J mice. *Nihon Rinsho Meneki Gakkai Kaishi* 2001;24:10–20.

Jassim SAA, Naji MA. Novel antiviral agents: a medicinal plant perspective. *Journal of Applied Microbiology* 2003. 95 (3), 412–427.

Jones K. Cat's Claw: Healing Vine of Peru. Seattle: Sylvan Press; 1995:90–97.

Kitts D, Hu C. Efficacy and safety of ginseng. *Public Health Nutr* 2000;3:473–485.

Kurashige S, Akuzawa Y, Endo F. Effects of astragali radix extract on carcinogenesis, cytokine production, and cytotoxicity in mice treated with a carcinogen, N-butyl-N′-butanolnitrosoamine. *Cancer Invest* 1999;17:30–35.

Ooi VE, Liu F. Immunomodulation and anti-cancer activity of polysaccharide-protein complexes. *Curr Med Chem* 2000;7: 715–729.

Reichling J, Fitzi J, Furst-Jucker J, Bucher S, Saller R. Echinacea powder: treatment for canine chronic and seasonal upper respiratory tract infections. *Schweiz Arch Tierheilk* 2003;145: 223–231.

Sheets MA, Unger BA, Giggleman GF Jr, Tizard IR. Studies of the effect of acemannan on retrovirus infections: clinical stabilization of feline leukemia virus-infected cats. *Mol Biother* 1991;3:41–45.

Song Z, Kharazmi A, Wu H, et al. Effects of ginseng treatment on neutrophil chemiluminescence and immunoglobulin G subclasses in a rat model of chronic *Pseudomonas aeruginosa* pneumonia. *Clin Diagn Lab Immunol* 1998;5:882–887.

Wasser SP, Weis AL. Therapeutic effects of substances occurring in higher Basidiomycetes mushrooms: a modern perspective. *Crit Rev Immunol* 1999;19:65–96.

Williams JE. Review of antiviral and immunomodulating properties of plants of the Peruvian rainforest with a particular emphasis on Una de Gato and Sangre de Grado. *Altern Med Rev.* 2001 Dec;6(6):567–79.

Williamson EM, Evans FJ. Cannabinoids in clinical practice. *Drugs* 2000 Dec:60 (6): 1303–14

Wynn S, Fougere B. Veterinary Herbal Medicine. Oxford: Elsevier, 2006.

Yates KM, Rosenberg LJ, Harris CK, et al. Pilot study of the effect of acemannan in cats infected with feline immunodeficiency virus. *Vet Immunol Immunopathol* 1992;35:177–189.

Yoshida Y, Wang MQ, Liu JN, Shan BE, Yamashita U. Immunomodulating activity of Chinese medicinal herbs and *Oldenlandia diffusa* in particular. *Int J Immunopharmacol* 1997;19: 359–370.

Zhao KS, Mancini C, Doria G. Enhancement of the immune response in mice by *Astragalus membranaceus* extracts. *Immunopharmacology* 1990;20:225–233.

Zhu YP. Chinese Materia Media: Chemistry, Pharmacology, and Applications. Australia: Harwood Academic Publishers; 1998a:445–448.

Zhu JS, Halpern GM, Jones K. The scientific rediscovery of an ancient Chinese herbal medicine: *Cordyceps sinensis*. Part II. *J Altern Complement Med* 1998b;4:429–457.

Chapter Thirty-One

Western Herbal Cancer Treatment

WESTERN HERBAL CANCER PROTOCOLS

The herbal protocols discussed in this chapter can be used in the treatment of the following cancers:

Adenocarcinoma
Chondrosarcoma
Fibrosarcoma
Hemangiosarcoma
Histiocytoma
Leiomyosarcoma
Lymphoma/lymphosarcoma
Mammary cancer
Mast cell formula
Melanoma
Meningioma
Osteosarcoma
Pheochromocytoma
Spindle cell sarcoma
Transitional cell carcinoma
Thyroid carcinoma

Herbal medicine offers veterinary patients a variety of benefits in the integrative treatment of cancer. It can reduce toxicity of treatment; support the patient through surgery, chemotherapy, or radiation; or provide a palliative option when conventional treatment is declined. Many chemotherapeutic drugs currently in use in human (and some in veterinary) medicine were first identified in plants, including taxol, vinblastine and vincristine, and etoposide and teniposide (Boik 1996).

The use of herbal medicine for the treatment of cancer depends on a growing understanding of the biological mechanisms by which cancer cells proliferate, maintain life, and die. These include differentiation, angiogenesis, apoptosis, invasion, metastasis, mitosis, and evasion of the immune system. As these mechanisms have become elucidated, their weak points have been identified and have become the targets of research (Boik 1996).

An extremely comprehensive review of anticancer plants and natural compounds is provided in John Boik's book, *Natural Compounds in Cancer Therapy* (2001). This book reviews published literature and explains the mechanisms of actions for many plants and their constituents and their activity based on in vitro and in vivo research. The medicine is likely to inhibit procancer events by selecting compounds that have direct-acting, indirect-acting, and immune-stimulating activities (Boik 2001).

A number of strategies are available for the treatment and management of cancer when clients elect to use herbal medicine. When treating potentially life-threatening disease it behooves us as practitioners to either refer these cases to qualified veterinary herbalists or undertake additional study to gain an in-depth knowledge of herbal medicine for cancer treatment. Ideally, herbs are prescribed according to the patient's vitality, energetics, symptoms, concurrent treatment, prognosis, and diagnosis. The diagnosis is possibly the least important factor from an herbal medicine perspective, although it is useful from a prognostic point of view. Supporting the patient and improving vitality and immunity as well as incorporating herbs with anticancer activity are the fundamental principle.

Strategy

The primary goal of treatment is to improve systemic health. The nearer the patient's vitality is restored to normal, the better the expected outcome. Despite the poorest prognoses based on diagnosis, wellness and vitality are still achievable in some patients. In the author's experience, clients often remark on their pet being "more well" than they have been in years, despite the presence of cancer. Patients can go into remission; but more frequently, they can live with the chronic disease of cancer in a well state. It is important to normalize weight, provide a low-carbohydrate diet, reduce stress, ensure normal elimination processes, and provide exercise opportunities.

If the patient has an acute condition such as diarrhea, give that priority and treat it accordingly. Be strategic about herb selection; the more knowledge one has, the fewer herbs are needed to improve health.

ANTICANCER ACTION

Though research most often focuses on the activity of a given herb, a fraction of the herb, or a single chemical constituent, most herbs are actually used as part of a larger formula. When herbs are combined in moderate, nontoxic doses, targeting specific mechanisms, they have an additive or synergistic effect. The following list is just a sample of herbs with documented activity (Boik 2001).

Induce apoptosis: Greater celandine (*Chelidonium majus*), Baical skullcap (*Scutellaria baicalensis*), *Bupleurum spp.*

Induce differentiation: Burdock (*Articum lappa*), berberine-containing herbs, St. John's wort (*Hypericum perforatum*).

Cytotoxic: Mistletoe (*Viscum album*).

Inhibit angiogenesis: Horsetail (*Aesculus hippocastanum*), Garlic (*Allium sativum*).

Inhibit local invasion: *Crataegus spp.*, Nilberry (*Vaccinium myrtillus*).

Inhibit metastasis: Tea (*Camellia sinensis*), Dong guai (*Angelica sinensis*), Feverfew (*Tanacetum parthenium*).

Enhance vitality by using adaptogens: Herbs with adaptogens such as *Astragalus membranceous*, *Withania somnifera*, Siberian ginseng (*Eleutherococcus senticosis*), and *Panax ginseng* can strengthen body resistance and enhance vitality, particularly in debilitated animals. These herbs also have anticancer properties.

Enhance immune function: Most conventional veterinary chemotherapeutic agents (as well as radiation therapy) are immune-suppressing and cytotoxic in nature and are associated with short- and long-term side effects (McEntee 2006, McKnight 2003). Immune-modulating and immune-stimulating herbs may prevent or minimize the undesired adverse effects of these agents by strengthening resistance to the treatment's side effects or to the cancer, and they may have anti-neoplastic activity.

The two most important classes of herbs in the anticancer group are the immunomodulating medicinal fungi and immune herbs and the adaptogens.

It is important to focus on improving gut function, which impacts innate immunity, with appropriate diet and support (probiotics, Marshmallow, Licorice, Glutamine, fiber, antioxidants, or antioxidant herbs). Among the recommended medicinal fungi or other immune-

supporting herbs are Cat's claw, phytosterols, Astragalus, Echinacea, *Cordyceps sinensis*, and Withania.

Daily dietary administration of *E. purpurea* root extract to normal mice for as little as 1 week also resulted in significant elevations in natural killer cells. Such boosting of this fundamental immune cell population suggests a prophylactic role for this herb in normal animals (Currier 2001).

ALTERATIVES

Detoxification is an herbal medicine principle in cancer treatment because cancer is thought to be the end result of accumulated toxins in the body. While some may argue with this theory, the use of alteratives may be useful nonetheless, particularly in the early stages of cancer when vitality is still good. Essiac is a commonly used formula that consists of 4 herbs, 3 of which are considered to be mild alteratives. This formula is beneficial in palliative care of end-stage cancer patients. Other alteratives to consider include: Dandelion root *(Taraxacum radix)*; Yellow dock *(Rumex crispus)*; Poke root *(Phytolacca decandra)*, which is toxic and should only be used by experienced herbalists; Burdock (Articum lappa), Red clover (*Trifolium pretense*), and Sheep sorrel.

ANTIOXIDANTS

Antioxidants are important to treatment and palliation. Often the patient is subjected to free radical damage through treatment, and herbs with antioxidant activity can reduce the side effects of both chemotherapy and radiation, as well as the oxidative stress of general anesthesia. The literature includes several promising herbs whose antioxidant activity has been demonstrated in relation to anticancer properties, cancer prevention, and treatment.

These antioxidants include green tea (*Camellia sinensis*), which is an effective chemopreventive agent against the initiation, promotion, and progression of multistage carcinogenesis (Katiyar 1997); Milk thistle (*Silybum marianum*); and both Silymarin and Silibinin (silybin) with demonstrated anticancer effects (Gazak, et al. 2007). The cancer chemoprevention and anticarcinogenic effects of silymarin have been shown to be caused by silibinin, its major constituent (Bhatia 1999). Its antitumor effect occurs primarily at stage I tumor promotion; silymarin acts by inhibiting cyclo-oxygenase (cox-2) and interleukin (IL-1α) (Zhao 1999). Such effects may involve inhibition of promoter-induced edema, hyperplasia, the proliferation index, and the oxidant state (Lahiri-Chatterjee 1999). Turmeric (*Curcuma longa*) scavenges free radicals (Tilak 2004) and Curcumin halts carcinogenesis by inhibiting cytochrome P450 enzyme activity and increasing levels of glutathione-S-transferase (Chauhan 2002).

Dan shen (*Salvia miltiorrhiza*) is another potent antioxidant herb that demonstrates free-radical scavenging activity (Xia 2003). One of its tanshinone constituents possesses cytotoxic activity against many kinds of human carcinoma cell lines; it induces differentiation and apoptosis, and inhibits invasion and metastasis of cancer cells. Its mechanisms are believed to be inhibition of DNA synthesis and proliferation of cancer cells; regulation of the expression of genes related to proliferation, differentiation, and apoptosis; inhibition of the telomerase activity of cancer cells; and change in the expression of cellular surface antigen (Yuan 2003). Schisandra (*Schisandra chinensis*) lignans act as free radical scavengers (Lu 1992), and geranylgeranoic acid, a constituent of Schisandra, has been shown to induce apoptosis in a human hepatoma–derived cell line (Shidoji 2004).

Ginkgo biloba leaf extract has significant antioxidant activity because of its flavonoid and terpenoid components, and the anticancer properties of Ginkgo are related to its antioxidant, antiangiogenic, and gene-regulatory actions. For example, bladder cancer cells exposed to Ginkgo produce an adaptive transcriptional response that augments antioxidant status and inhibits DNA damage (DeFeudis 2003). Rosemary (*Rosmarinus officinalis*) has antioxidant activity (ESCP 1999); in rats, dietary supplementation with 1% Rosemary extract for 21 weeks reduced the development of induced mammary carcinoma in the treated group, compared with the control group (40% vs. 75%, respectively) (Singletary 1991).

SPECIFIC ORGAN SUPPORT

When a particular organ or system is impacted by cancer, consider herbs that support the functioning of that organ or the organs that detoxify metabolic wastes in the body. For example, consider Milk thistle and *Panax ginseng* for liver cancer; *Gynema slyvestre* and Feverfew for pancreatic cancer; St. John's wort (*Hypericum perforatum*) (Martarelli 2004) and Pau d'arco (*Tabebuia avellandedae*) for prostate cancer; and Black cumin (*Nigella sativa*) (Khan 2005), *Astragalus membranaceus*, and *Ligustrum lucidum* (Lau 1994) for kidney cancer. Refer to the individual herbs for different systems for herb choices.

SPECIFIC SYMPTOM SUPPORT

Alleviating symptoms is important to improving the patient's well being. Consider conventional treatment when analgesia is needed. Palliation can also be helped with analgesic herbs such as Devil's claw (*Harpagophytum procumbens*), Corydalis (*Corydalis ambigua*), Valerian (*Valeriana officinalis*), and Cramp bark (*Viburnum opulus*). Depression might be helped with St. John's wort (*Hypericum performatum*), Lavender (*Lavendula officinalis*), or *Panax ginseng*. Nausea may be alleviated with Ginger (*Zingiber officinalis*) (Sharma, et al. 1997) or Chamomile (*Chamomilla recutita*).

EVIDENCE FOR EFFICACY OF HERBS AS ADJUNCTIVE THERAPY

Withania somnifera has direct anticancer properties. It possesses cell cycle disruption and anti-angiogenic activity, which has been confirmed in vitro and in vivo and which may be a critical mediator for its anti-cancer action (Mathur 2006). It also protects against side effects of chemotherapy. Significant increases in hemoglobin, red blood cell, white blood cell, and platelet count as well as body weight were observed in cyclophosphamide-, azathioprine-, and prednisolone-treated mice that were given Withania (Ziauddin 1996). The antitumor and radiosensitizing effects of Withania have also been studied. The growth of induced carcinoma in mice was inhibited and survival increased with Withania treatment, especially when it was combined with radiation (Sharada 1996, Devi 1995). Complete regression of sarcoma in mice was observed with treatment by Withania root extract in another trial (Devi 1992). Likewise, it demonstrated antitumor properties in mice and protected against induced carcinogenic effects. It reversed the adverse effects of a carcinogen (urethane) on total leukocyte count, lymphocyte count, body weight, and mortality (Singh 1986).

Controlled, open-label clinical studies have shown that Cordyceps (*Cordyceps sinensis*) appeared to restore immune cell function in patients with advanced cancer who were given conventional cancer therapies (Zhou 1995, Zhu 1998a). Of 59 patients with advanced lung cancer, 95% were able to complete chemotherapy and radiotherapy with the use of Cordyceps compared with 64% of the control group. More than 85% of Cordyceps-treated patients showed more normal blood cell counts vs. 59% of the control group (Zhu 1998a). A study in patients with various types of tumors found that a cultured mycelium extract of cordyceps (6 g/d for more than 2 months) improved subjective symptoms in most patients. White blood cell counts were maintained and tumor size was significantly reduced in approximately half of the patients (Zhu 1998b).

The efficacy of Astragalus (*Astragalus membranaceus*) was investigated for its effects in enhancing quality of life and reducing the toxicity of chemotherapy in human patients with malignant tumors. One hundred twenty patients were randomly assigned to a control or treatment group; both groups received chemotherapy, and the treatment group received intravenously administered Astragalus. Astragalus was noted to inhibit the development of tumors, reduce the side effects of chemotherapy, improve immune function, and improve the quality of life of patients (Duan and Wang 2002).

POSSIBLE CONTRAINDICATIONS FOR ADJUNCTIVE USE OF HERBS IN CANCER TREATMENT

Despite evidence that shows the benefit of using adjunctive herbs with chemotherapy, concern has been raised about the concurrent use of antioxidants (plant-derived or nutritionally derived) with chemotherapy or radiotherapy. Chemotherapy and radiotherapy damage the DNA of both normal cells and cancer cells by causing free radical damage. Therefore, the theoretical concern is that antioxidants block free radical generation and reduce the efficacy of the treatment (Conklin 2004). Labriola and Livingston (1999), discussed at length the possible theoretical negative interactions between cancer chemotherapy drugs and concurrent use of antioxidants. However, the experimental evidence for such a hypothesis is lacking, and actually, in the majority of cases, shows the opposite. Block and Evans (2001) reviewed all of the English articles related to antioxidants and interactions with anticancer drugs or radiation that were listed in Index Medicus between the years 1990 and 2000. Their review concluded that "there is a rational basis for the continued use of antioxidant agents as a therapeutic adjunct in cancer therapy" (Block 2001).

HERBS AND CANCER AND METASTASES PREVENTION

Herbs may have a profound role in protecting some animals from developing cancer. Mice that received daily Echinacea (Echinacea purpurea) in their diets throughout their lives, from an early age until late middle age, had significant longevity/survival differences compared to controls, as well as differences in various populations of immune/hematopietic cells. Treated mice had significantly higher numbers of key immune cells, those that are the first line of defense against developing neoplasms as well as natural killer (NK) cells. It appeared in this study that regular dietary intake of Echinacea may be beneficial or prophylactic because it maintained elevated levels of NK cells, which are involved in immunosurveillance against spontaneously developing tumors (Brousseau 2005).

Consumption of green or black tea (Camellia sinensis) has been suggested to prevent cancer. Animal studies have shown that tea and its constituents inhibit carcinogenesis of the skin, lung, oral cavity, esophagus, stomach, liver, prostate, and other organs (Lambert 2003). For example, mice were given decaffeinated green or decaffeinated black tea in their drinking water before, during, and after treatment with a carcinogen. Mice that received 0.63% or 1.25% green tea or 1.25% black tea exhibited a reduction in liver tumors of 54%, 50%, and 63%, respectively, and a decrease in the mean number of lung tumors of 40%, 46%, and 34%, respectively (Cao 1996). Reduced tumor numbers and tumor size were also observed in other experiments employing tea (Yang 2005). Black tea preparations were noted to inhibit the progression of lung adenoma to adenocarcinoma. In many of these experiments, tea consumption resulted in reduced body fat and body weight; these factors may also contribute to the inhibition of tumor genesis (Yang 2005).

Flaxseed (Linum usitatissimum) is the richest source of lignans and α-linolenic acid and has been investigated regarding its effects on the growth and metastasis of established human breast cancer in a mouse model. Compared with controls, those mice supplemented with 10% Flaxseed showed a significant reduction in tumor growth rate and a 45% reduction in total incidence of metastasis. Lung metastasis incidence was 55.6% in the control group and 22.2% in the Flaxseed group and lymph node metastasis was 88.9% in controls and 33.3% in the Flaxseed group. The metastatic lung tumor number was reduced by 82% in the Flaxseed group. It was concluded that Flaxseed inhibits human breast cancer growth and metastasis in a mouse model, and that this effect is due in part to the down regulation of insulin-like growth factor I and epidermal growth factor receptor expression (Chen 2002).

HERBS AND THEIR EFFECTS ON SPECIFIC TYPES OF CANCER

A search for herbs with effects on particular cancers common in veterinary medicine revealed some interesting possibilities and applications. Many were based on in vitro cell line studies, but several were based on laboratory animals and cats and dogs. It is important to note, however, that herbal treatment of cancer is ideally prescribed for the individual patient and not the diagnosis per se.

Fibrosarcoma

Fibrosarcomas have been inhibited by Wormwood (Artemisia annua). The constituent artemisinin selectively kills cancer cells by inducing apoptosis in vitro and inhibits the growth of implanted fibrosarcoma tumors in rats (Singh 2004). Injection of acemannan from *Aloe vera* gel increased immune protection against implanted malignant tumor cells (Merriam 1995) and induced apoptosis in cancer cells (Ramamoorthy 1998). Acemannan is conditionally licensed by the U.S. Department of Agriculture (USDA) for the treatment of fibrosarcoma in cats and dogs (King 1995). In one uncontrolled study in 8 cats and dogs with confirmed fibrosarcoma, the researchers suggested that acemannan may be an effective adjunct to surgery and radiation therapy (King 1995). In another uncontrolled study, acemannan was administered by intraperitoneal and intralesional routes to 43 animals with various tumors. Five of 7 animals with fibrosarcoma had clinical improvement, as assessed by tumor shrinkage, tumor necrosis, or prolonged survival. It was suggested that acemannan activates macrophages and the release of tumor necrosis factor, interleukin (IL-1), and interferon (Harris 1991).

Lymphoma/Lymphosarcoma

Injections (subcutaneous) of Mistletoe (*Viscum album*) extract protected against metastasis of introduced lymphosarcoma and sarcoma cells in mice when given 3 times per week for 14 consecutive days. Doses greater than 20 µg reduced tumor weight and tumor volume (Braun 2002). Non-Hodgkin's lymphoma was induced in mice. Compared to controls, no evidence of a viable tumor was apparent in 4 of 15 mice fed a Mistletoe-supplemented diet (10 mg lectin daily) for 11 days. Results show that lectin exerts powerful antitumor effects when provided by the oral route (Pryme, et al. 2004).

Oral administration of crude extract of Gotu kola (*Centella asiatica L.*) retarded the development of solid and lymphoma ascites tumors and increased the life span of tumor-bearing mice (Babu 1995). Cordyceps (*Cordyceps sinensis*) extract was given orally to mice implanted with lymphoma cells; it reduced tumor size and prolonged mouse survival time. Mice treated with cyclophosphamide (100 mg/kg) 3 and 5 days after tumor transplantation had their immune suppression restored through treatment (Yamaguchi 1990). Ashwaganda (*Withania somnifera*), an ethanolic root extract, provided a significant increase in life span and a decrease in cancer cell numbers and tumor weight in lymphoma tumor–induced mice. Hematologic parameters were also corrected by Withania in tumor-induced mice (Christina 2004).

Mammary cancer

Following infusion of mammary tumor cells into the mammary glands, mice were fed a diet containing a

Calendula (*Calendula officinalis*) extract (high in the carotenoid lutein) for 3 weeks. Tumor latency increased and tumor growth was inhibited in a dose-dependent manner by dietary lutein. In addition, dietary lutein was reported to enhance lymphocyte proliferation (Chew 1996). In an in vitro study, organosulphur compounds from Garlic (*Allium sativum*) markedly inhibited growth of canine mammary cells in culture (Sundaram 1993).

Melanoma

Grapeseed extract, given orally, reduced the number of pulmonary metastatic melanoma nodules induced in mice by 26.07% compared with a control group treated with ethanol (Martinez 2005). Flaxseed was fed to mice as a supplement (0%, 2.5%, 5%, or 10% Flaxseed) for 2 weeks before and after an intravenous injection of melanoma cells. The median number of tumors in mice fed the 2.5%, 5%, and 10% Flaxseed-supplemented diets was 32%, 54%, and 63% lower, respectively, than that in controls (0%). The addition of Flaxseed to the diet also caused a dose-dependent decrease in tumor cross-sectional area and tumor volume. It was concluded that Flaxseed reduces metastasis and inhibits the growth of metastatic secondary tumors in animals (Yan 1998).

A pilot study of Poke weed (*Phytolacca americana*) mitogen immunotherapy in animals was conducted. One case reported a 3-year remission and an apparent cure of gum melanoma that was metastatic to regional and hilar lymph nodes and to the lungs in an aged dog following Poke weed mitogen therapy. A small total dose of 300 µg induced the remission. However, the authors state that it is possible that melanoma may be a uniquely responsive tumor (Wimer and Mann 2000).

Meningioma

Since brain tumors are rarely definitively identified in veterinary medicine, herbs that may benefit generic "brain tumors" are discussed. Two observational reports of patients undergoing treatment for brain tumor suggest that Boswellia (*Boswellia serrata*) extract may help reduce cerebral edema (Streffer 2001, Janssen 2000). Boswellia extract may slow growth and increase apoptosis of tumor cells in brain cells (Hostanska 2002). Several studies have shown that cannabinoids from *Cannabis sativa* and their derivatives slow the growth of gliomas. Cannabis induced apoptosis of glioma cells in culture and inhibited angiogenesis in vivo. Velasco, et al. (2004) remarkably claim that cannabinoids kill glioma cells selectively and can protect nontransformed glial cells from death. In another study, patients with malignant glioma were prospectively enrolled in a clinical trial and the treatment group received a galactoside-specific lectin from Mistletoe (*Viscum album*). Analyses of all patients revealed prolongation of relapse-free intervals and overall survival time for the treatment group as compared with the control group (Lenartz 2000).

Osteosarcoma

Extracts of Red clover (*Trifolium pretense L.*) were tested for their ability to stimulate the activity of osteoblastic osteosarcoma cells. Based on the in vitro study results, data suggest a role for Red clover isoflavonoids (chloroform extract) in the stimulation of osteoblastic cell activity and cellular differentiation (Wende 2004). Diosgenin (found in Trillium, Fenugreek, and Wild yam) was also investigated in vitro to determine its effects on proliferation rate, cell cycle distribution, and apoptosis in the human osteosarcoma cell line. Diosgenin treatment resulted in inhibition of cell growth, with a cycle arrest in G1 phase, apoptosis induction, and induced cyclooxygenase activity (Moalic 2001).

An antiviral protein was conjugated to Poke weed (*Phytolacca americana*) extract to produce an immunotoxin that was highly active against osteosarcoma. In vitro studies suggest that it may be useful in the treatment of patients with osteosarcoma and some soft tissue sarcomas (Anderson 1995). In vivo, the same immunotoxin elicits potent antitumor activity in a hamster cheek pouch model of human osteosarcoma. At nontoxic dose levels, it significantly delays the emergence and progression of leg tumors and markedly improves tumor-free survival in immunodeficient mice challenged with human osteosarcoma cells. Thus, it may be useful in the treatment of patients with osteosarcoma (Ek 1998).

Transitional cell carcinoma

Flavokawains identified in Kava (*Piper methysticum*) cause strong antiproliferative and apoptotic effects in human bladder cancer cells. The anticarcinogenic effects of flavokawain A were evident in the inhibiting of 57% of the bladder tumor cells in a nude mice model in vivo (Zi 2005). Garlic (*Allium sativum*) was investigated in induced transitional cell carcinoma in mice. Orally administered Garlic was tested at doses of 5 mg, 50 mg, and 500 mg per 100 mL of drinking water. Mice that received 50 mg oral Garlic demonstrated significant reductions in tumor volume when compared with the controls, and mice that received 500 mg oral Garlic exhibited signifi-

cant reductions in both tumor volume and mortality (Riggs 1997).

HERBS WITH NONSPECIFIC ACTIVITY FOR OTHER CANCERS

An aqueous extract of Mistletoe (*Viscum album*) was investigated in vivo for its effects on renal cell carcinoma, colon carcinoma, and testicular carcinoma. Significant tumor growth inhibition was observed with all 3 carcinomas at 30 and 300 ng mL/kg/d (Burger 2001).

Aloe vera may enhance the therapeutic results of melatonin in patients with advanced solid tumors (when conventional cancer treatment is not possible). Fifty patients with lung cancer, gastrointestinal tract tumors, breast cancer, or brain glioblastoma received melatonin alone (20 mg/d orally in the dark period) or melatonin plus *Aloe vera* tincture (1 mL twice/d). The percentage of non-progressing patients was significantly higher in the group treated with melatonin plus Aloe than in the melatonin group (14 of 24 vs. 7 of 26). The 1-year survival percentage was significantly higher in patients treated with melatonin plus Aloe (9 of 24 vs. 4 of 26). The combination may help in the stabilization of disease and survival in patients with advanced solid tumor, for whom no other standard effective therapy is available (Lissoni 1998).

Korean ginseng (*Panax ginseng*) consumption may play an important role in the prevention and treatment of cancers of the lip, oral cavity and pharynx, larynx, lung, esophagus, stomach, liver, pancreas, ovary, and colorectum. It did not seem to matter what the form of Ginseng was because cancer was reduced in users of fresh Ginseng extract, White ginseng extract, White ginseng powder, and Red ginseng. *Panax ginseng* has non–organ specific cancer preventive effects against various cancers primarily because of its ginsenosides (Yun 2003).

In hamsters with induced squamous cell carcinoma (SCC), 0.6% green tea (*Camellia sinensis*) powder added to drinking fluid or 10 μmol Curcumin from Turmeric or a combination or nothing (control) was applied topically to lesions 3 times weekly for 18 weeks. The combination decreased the incidence, number, and size of SCC and precursor tumors. This activity may be related to suppression of cell proliferation, induction of apoptosis, and inhibition of angiogenesis (Li 2002). Another study showed that Turmeric or Curcumin in the diet or applied as paint may have a chemopreventive effect on oral precancerous lesions (Krishnaswamy 1998).

Please the see Table 31.1 for a list of the herbs, as well as their ingredients, suppliers, and conditions treated.

Table 31.1. Western herbs by condition.

Condition	Supplier	Product	Herbal ingredients
Anemia	Genesis Resources D'Arcy Naturals World Herbs	Blood and Energy Formula Green Powder	Angelica sinensis, alfalfa powder, yellow dock, chlorella, lycium berry, ligusticum, red raspberry, red clover 100% organic, 20:1 concentrated juice powders: kamut, barley, oat, spirulina, spinach, carrot, powdered broccoli, parsley dandelion greens, sea kelp, sea dulse, oxyphyte
Emotional issues	Rx Vitamins	Nutricalm	Valerian, ashwaganda
	NaturVet	Quiet Moments	Chamomile, passion flower, ginger
	Herbalist and Alchemist	Serenity Compound	Eleuthero root, skullcap, chamomile flower, oat milky seed, linden flower
	D'Arcy Naturals World Herbs	Pet Calm	Zizyphus seed, poria sclerotium (hoelen), cnidium seed, licorice root, anemarrhena rhizome, valerian rhizome, chamomile flower, fo-ti root, biota seed, polygala root
		Separate Herbs	Chamomile, gingko, kava kava, passion flower, valerian in separate.
Cardiovascular issues	Rx Vitamins	CV Formula	Hawthorn berry
	D'Arcy Naturals World Herbs	Cardio Support	Asian ginseng root, polygala root, astragalus root, atractlodes root, poris, zizyphus seed, logan fruit, saussurea root, licorice root, Chinese angelica root, coleus rhizome, hawthorn berry, garlic bulb, ginkgo leaf, stevia
	Standard Process	Canine or Feline Cardiac Support	Hawthorn berry
	Herbalist and Alchemist	Healthy Heart Compound	Hawthorn fruit, leaf, flower; night blooming cereus stem; ginkgo leaf; prickly ash bark; tienchi ginseng root
Dermatological issues	Standard Process	Canine or Feline Dermal Support	Silymarin, alfalfa juice, carrot, black currant juice
	D'Arcy Naturals World Herbs	Hoxsey Formula	Oregon grape root, burdock root, red clover flower, alfalfa leaf, prickly ash bark, stillingia root, cascara sagrada bark, poke root, licorice root.
	Vetri-Science	Oli-Vet Olive Leaf Extract	Olive leaf extract
	D'Arcy Naturals World Herbs	Healthy Coat	Fo-ti root, horsetail herb, nettle leaf, dong quai root, kelp thalus, stevia leaf
	Designing Health Inc.	Missing Link Professional Strength Veterinary Formula	Flaxseed, barley grass, alfalfa, parsley, milk thistle, grapeseed, spirulina, kelp, burdock root, dandelion root, yucca schidigera
	NSA	Juice Plus+ for dogs	Beet root, flaxseed, garlic, alfalfa, barley juice, safflower petals, wheat grass
Topical for skin	D'Arcy Naturals World Herbs	Hot Spot	Gotu kola herb, eucalyptus leaf, barberry root, aloe, golden seal root
	Aveeno		Colloidal oatmeal
	Herbal Answers	Herbal Aloe Force® Skin Gel	Aloe, sheep sorrel, burdock root, slippery elm bark, rhubarb root, cat's claw, pau d'arco, hawthorn berry, chamomile, green tea
Gastritis/GI issues	Rx Vitamins	Nutrigest	Aloe extract, cat's claw, ginger root extract, fructooligosaccharide, Oregon grape root, garlic, psyllium seed, DGL (deglycerrhized licorice)
	Animal Essentials	Animals' Apawthecary Phytomucil	Marshmallow root (*Althaea officinalis*), Slippery elm inner bark (*Ulmus fulva*), Plantain (*Plantago major*), land licorice (*Glycyrrhiza glabra*)
	Standard Process	Canine or Feline Enteric Support™	Defatted wheat germ, alfalfa juice, mushroom, nutritional yeast, pea vine juice, carrot, rice bran, licorice, wheat germ oil, beet leaf juice, beet root, chlorophyll extract

Table 31.1. *Continued*

Condition	Supplier	Product	Herbal ingredients
Gastritis/GI issues *(continued)*	D'Arcy Naturals World Herbs	Pet Digest Tonic	Alfalfa leaf, Asian ginseng root, astragalus root, stevia leaf
	D'Arcy Naturals World Herbs	Dia-Relief	Plantain leaf, marshmallow root, fennel seed, bilberry leaf, golden seal root, barberry root, stevia
Hepatitis	D'Arcy Naturals World Herbs	Hoxsey Formula	Oregon grape root, burdock root, red clover flower, alfalfa leaf, prickly ash bark, stillingia root, cascara sagrada bark, poke root, licorice root.
	Natural Path Herb Company	Hoxsey Formula	Oregon grape root, burdock root, red clover flower, alfalfa leaf, prickly ash bark, stillingia root, cascara sagrada bark, poke root, licorice root
	Rx Vitamins	Hepato Support	Milk thistle
	Thorne Research	Hepagen C or Hepagen D	Milk thistle, tumeric
	Standard Process	Canine or Feline Hepatic Support	Emblica officinalis, buckwheat leaf, milk thistle, beet leaf, alfalfa, Rhizopus oryzae, beet root
	D'Arcy Naturals World Herbs	Liver Protect	Milk thistle seed, nettle leaf, bupleurum root, pinellia rhizome, baical skullcap root, Asian ginseng root, licorice root, ginger rhizome, zizyphus fruit, schisandra fruit, stevia leaf
	Animal Essentials	Animals' Apawthecary Senior Blend	Alfalfa, dandelion, milk thistle seed, oat tops, garlic, marshmallow, ethically wildcrafted Ginkgo biloba, hawthorn berries
	Animal Essentials	Animals' Apawthecary Dandelion/Milk Thistle	Dandelion, milk thistle seed
Eye issues	D'Arcy Naturals World Herbs	Eyebright Vision	Rehmannia root, dioscorea rhizome, alisma rhizome, cornus fruit, moutan root, bupleurum root, poria sclerotium (hoelen), dong quai root, lycii fruit, chrysanthemum flower, eyebright herb, bilberry leaf and fruit, nettles herb, schisandra fruit, ginkgo leaf
	Rx Vitamins	The Ocular Formula	Bilberry, grapeseed extract
	Animal Essentials	Animals' Apawthecary Eye and Nose Drops	Golden seal, eyebright herb, ethically wildcrafted Usnea barbata lichen
Otitis	NaturVet	Ear Wash with Tea Tree Oil	Witch hazel, tea tree oil, echinacea extract
	D'Arcy Naturals World Herbs	Ear Clear	Gentian root, bupleurum root, alisma rhizome, plantago leaf, clematis, rehmannia root, dong quai root, gardenia fruit, baical scutellaria root, licorice root, fo-ti root, eyebright herb, echinacea purpurea root, stevia leaf
	Animal Essentials	Animals' Apawthecary Herbal Ear Rinse	Cider vinegar, aloe vera, witch hazel extract, golden seal root, calendula and olive leaf
		Green tea in a 3 times concentration	Green tea
		Echinacea purpurea or angustifolia orally or as a rinse	
Musculoskeletal issues	Rx Vitamins	NutriFlex for Dogs and Cats	Sea cucumber, boswellian, yucca, bromelain, ginger, turmeric
	Standard Process	Canine Musculoskeletal Support™	Boswellia serrata, Perna canaliculus, Eleutherococcus senticosus, wheat germ, pea vine juice, oat flour, black currant juice, carrot
	Genesis Resources	Pain Plus	Yucca, boswellia, meadowsweet, cornus, licorice, ginger
	Genesis Resources	Joint Support Plus	Sea cucumber, angelica sinensis, rehmannia, alfalfa powder

Table 31.1. *Continued*

Condition	Supplier	Product	Herbal ingredients
Respiratory issues	D'Arcy Naturals World Herbs	First Defense	Honeysuckle flower, forsythia fruit, balloon flower root, burdock root, field mint, lophatherum stem and leaf, schizonepeta stem, licorice root, perilla seed, chrysanthemum flower, echinacea purpurea root, barberry bark, elderberry fruit and leaf, goldenseal root, stevia
	Source Naturals	Wellness Formula	Garlic clove powder, propolis powder, boneset leaf, polygonum odoratum rhizome, echinacea root and extract, isatis root and leaf, horehound stems, bioflavonoids, astragalus root, angelica root, mullein leaf, golden seal root, eleutherococcus senticosus root, hawthorn berry, Oregon grape root, pau d'arco bark extract, cayenne fruit
	D'Arcy Naturals World Herbs	Lung Sooth	Prepared rehmannia root, cornus fruit, dioscorea root, moutan bark, poria sclerotium, alisma rhizome, zizyphus seed, ophiopogonum tuber, wild cherry bark, eucalyptus leaf, schisandra fruit, stevia leaf
	D'Arcy Naturals World Herbs	Immune Prep	Asian ginseng root, atractylodes rhizome, poria sclerotium (hoelen), licorice root, ginger root, zizyphus fruit, astragalus root, Siberian ginseng root, baical skullcap root, schisandra fruit, dong quai root
	Vetriscience	Antiox	Grapeseed extract
Feline asthma	Vetriscience	Antiox	Grapeseed extract
Renal failure	Herbalist and Alchemist	Kidney Support Compound	Stinging nettle seed and leaf, rehmannia, pellitory of the wall, cordyceps
	Vetriscience	Renal Essentials	Astragalus root, rehmannia, nettle, cordyceps
Cystitis	NaturaVet	Cranberry Relief®	Cranberry extract, marshmallow root, echinacea, Oregon grape root
	Genesis Resources	Urinary Tract Support	Uva ursi, cranberry juice extract, marshmallow root powder, juniper berry, poria, kochia; polyporous extract feline formula has poria, corn silk, dandelion
	Vetriscience	UT Strength for Cats/Dogs	Uva ursi, chanca piedra, cranberry juice extract, marshmallow, corn silk, dandelion, olive leaf
Urinary incontinence	Genesis Resources	Incontinence	Wild yam root, bee pollen, rehmannia, angelica sinensis, psoralea, glandalai, licorice
	Vetriscience	Bladder Strength for Cats/Dogs	Wild yam, pumpkin seed, rehmannia, soy protein, corn silk, saw palmetto, olive leaf
Diabetes mellitus	Rx Vitamins	DB-7	Gymnema sylvestre
	Standard Process	Diaplex	Alfalfa, buckwheat, flaxseed oil extract
Hypothyroid	Standard Process	Canine Thyroid Support	Eleutherococcus senticosus, kelp, Tillandsia usneoides, mushroom, buckwheat leaf juice and seed, flaxseed oil
	D'Arcy Naturals World Herbs	Hypo-Thyro	Siberian ginseng root, kelp thalus, cayenne, Irish moss, gentian root
	D'Arcy Naturals World Herbs	Hyper-Thyrin	Prepared rehmannia root, cornus fruit, dioscorea root, poria sclerotium (hoelen), moutan bark, alisma rhizome, anemarrhena rhizome, phellodendron bark, kelp thalus, vervain rhizome, bugleweed leaf
Cognitive dysfunction	Animal Essentials	Animals' Apawthecary Senior Blend	Alfalfa, dandelion, milk thistle seed, oat tops, garlic, marshmallow; ethically wildcrafted Ginkgo biloba, hawthorn berries
	D'Arcy Naturals World Herbs	Alert	Ginseng root, ginkgo leaf, fo-ti root, astragalus root, codonopsis root, gotu kola herb, stevia leaf

Table 31.1. *Continued*

Condition	Supplier	Product	Herbal ingredients
Cancer	D'Arcy Naturals World Herbs	Hoxsey Formula	Oregon grape root, burdock root, red clover flower, alfalfa leaf, prickly ash bark, stillingia root, cascara sagrada bark, poke root, licorice root.
	Natural Path Herb Company	Hoxsey Formula	Oregon grape root, burdock root, red clover flower, alfalfa leaf, prickly ash bark, stillingia root, cascara sagrada bark, poke root, licorice root
	Genesis Resources	Canine CAS Options	Reishi, maitake, and shitake mushrooms; green tea
	D'Arcy Naturals World Herbs	Power Mushrooms	Organic maitake mushroom, organic reishi mushroom, organic shitake mushroom
	D'Arcy Naturals World Herbs	Green Powder	100% organic, 20:1 concentrated juice powders: kamut, barley, oat, spirulina, spinach, carrot, broccoli, parsley, dandelion greens, sea kelp, sea dulse, oxyphyte
	D'Arcy Naturals World Herbs	Petsiac	Burdock root, sheep sorrel herb, red clover aerial parts, reishi mushroom, slippery elm bark, turkey rhubarb root, stevia leaf
	Rx Vitamins	Immuno Support	Arabinogalactan, shitake, lutein

The chapters on Western herbal medicine address the treatment of various diseases with specific herbs that have been clinically proven to benefit those conditions. The above chart was compiled by Margo Roman, DVM. It lists specific products that contain Western herbs that are used as a component of her treatment protocols in her veterinary clinic for the listed conditions. It is intended as a product guide for the practitioner and is based solely upon Dr. Roman's experience with these products and their efficacy. This chart also was included at the request of the veterinarians who reviewed the initial manuscript of this book. There are many other reputable companies that are not included in this chart, some of which are listed in Section 8, the resources portion of this book.

REFERENCES

Anderson PM, Meyers DE, Hasz DE, Covalcuic K, Saltzman D, Khanna C, Uckun FM. In vitro and in vivo cytotoxicity of an anti-osteosarcoma immunotoxin containing pokeweed antiviral protein. *Cancer Research.* 1995;15;55(6):1321–7.

Babu TD, Kuttan G, Padikkala J. Cytotoxic and anti-tumour properties of certain taxa of Umbelliferae with special reference to *Centella asiatica* (L.) Urban. *J Ethnopharmacol* 1995;48:53–57.

Bhatia N, Zhao J, Wolf DM, Agarwal R. Inhibition of human carcinoma cell growth and DNA synthesis by silibinin, an active constituent of milk thistle: comparison with silymarin. *Cancer Lett* 1999;147:77–84.

Block JR, Evans S. A review of recent results addressing the potential interactions of antioxidants with cancer drug therapy. *JAMA* 2001;4:11–19.

Boik J. Cancer and Natural Medicine: A Textbook of Basic Science and Clinical Research. Princeton, MN: Oregon Medical Press; 1996.

Boik J. Natural Compounds in Cancer Therapy. Princeton, MN: Oregon Medical Press; 2001.

Braun JM, Ko HL, Schierholz JM, Beuth J. Standardized mistletoe extract augments immune response and down-regulates local and metastatic tumor growth in murine models. *Anticancer Res* 2002;22:4187–4190.

Brousseau M, Miller SC. Enhancement of natural killer cells and increased survival of aging mice fed daily Echinacea root extract from youth. *Biogerontology* 2005;6:157–163.

Burger AM, Mengs U, Schuler JB, Fiebig HH. Anticancer activity of an aqueous mistletoe extract (AME) in syngeneic murine tumour models. *Anticancer Research.* 2001;May–Jun;21(3B):1965–8.

Cao J, Xu Y, Chen J, Klaunig JE. Chemopreventive effects of green and black tea on pulmonary and hepatic carcinogenesis. *Fundam Appl Toxicol* 1996;29:244–250.

Chauhan DP. Chemotherapeutic Potential of Curcumin for Colorectal Cancer. Current Pharmaceutical Design. Hilversum, Netherlands: Bentham Science Publishers BV; 2002:1695–1706.

Chen J, Stavro PM, Thompson LU. Dietary flaxseed inhibits human breast cancer growth and metastasis and downregulates expression of insulin-like growth factor and epidermal growth factor receptor. *Nutr Cancer.* 2002;43(2):187–92.

Chew BP, Wong MW, Wong TS. Effects of lutein from marigold extract on immunity and growth of mammary tumors in mice. *Anticancer Res* 1996;16:3689–3694.

Christina AJ, Joseph DG, Packialakshmi M, et al. Anticarcinogenic activity of *Withania somnifera* Dunal against Dalton's ascitic lymphoma. *J Ethnopharmacol* 2004;93:359–361.

Conklin KA. Dietary antioxidants during cancer chemotherapy: impact on chemotherapeutic effectiveness and development of side effects. *Nutr Cancer* 2000;37:1–18.

Currier NL, Miller SC. *Echinacea purpurea* and melatonin augment natural-killer cells in leukemic mice and prolong life span. *J Altern Complement Med* 2001;7:241–251.

DeFeudis FV, Papadopoulos V, Drieu K. *Ginkgo biloba* extracts and cancer: a research area in its infancy. *Fundam Clin Pharmacol* 2003;17:405–417.

Devi PU, Sharada AC, Solomon FE, Kamath MS. In vivo growth inhibitory effect of *Withania somnifera* (Ashwagandha) on a transplantable mouse tumor, sarcoma 180. *Indian J Exp Biol* 1992;30:169–172.

Devi PU, Sharada AC, Solomon FE. In vivo growth inhibitory and radiosensitizing effects of withaferin A on mouse *Ehrlich ascites* carcinoma. *Cancer Lett* 1995;95:189–193.

Duan P, Wang ZM. Clinical study on effect of Astragalus in efficacy enhancing and toxicity reducing of chemotherapy in patients of malignant tumor. Zhongguo Zhong Xi Yi Jie He Za Zhi 2002;22:515–517.

Ek O, Waurzyniak B, Myers DE, Uckun FM. Antitumour activity of TP3 (anti-p80)-pokeweed antiviral protein immunotoxin in hamster cheek pouch and severe combined immunodeficient mouse xenograft models of human osteosarcoma. *Clinical Cancer Research*. 1998, Jul;4(7):1641–7

European Scientific Cooperative on Phytotherapy. Monographs on the Medicinal Uses of Plant Drugs, Fascicules 1 and 2 (1996), Fascicules 3, 4, and 5 (1997), Fascicule 6. 1999. Exeter. European Scientific Cooperative on Phytotherapy.

Gazak R, Walterova D, Kren V. Silybin and silymarin—new and emerging applications in medicine. *Curr Med Chem*. 2007; 14(3):315–38.

Harris C, Pierce K, King G, Yates KM, Hall J, Tizard I. Efficacy of acemannan in treatment of canine and feline spontaneous neoplasms. *Mol Biother* 1991;3:207–213.

Hostanska K, Daum G, Saller R. Cytostatic and apoptosis-inducing activity of boswellic acids toward malignant cell lines in vitro. *Anticancer Res*. 2002 Sep–Oct;22(5):2853–62.

Janssen G, Bode U, Breu H, Dohrn B, Engelbrecht V, Gobel U. Boswellic acids in the palliative therapy of children with progressive or relapsed brain tumors. *Klin Padiatr* 2000;212: 189–195.

Katiyar SK, Mukhtar H. Tea antioxidants in cancer chemoprevention. *J Cell Biochem Suppl* 1997;27:59–67.

Khan N, Sultana S. Inhibition of two stage renal carcinogenesis, oxidative damage and hyperproliferative response by *Nigella sativa*. *Eur J Cancer Prev* 2005;14:159–168.

King GK, Yates KM, Greenlee PG, et al. The effect of acemannan immunostimulant in combination with surgery and radiation therapy on spontaneous canine and feline fibrosarcomas. *J Am Anim Hosp Assoc* 1995;31:439–447.

Krishnaswamy K, Goud VK, Sesikeran B, Mukundan MA, Krishna TP. Retardation of experimental tumourigenesis and reduction in DNA adducts by turmeric and curcumin. *Nutrition and Cancer*. 1998. 30(2):163–6.

Labriola D, Livingston R. Possible interactions between dietary antioxidants and chemotherapy. *Oncology* (Williston Park). 1999 Jul;13(7):1003–8; discussion 1008, 1011–2.

Lahiri-Chatterjee M, Katiyar SK, Mohan RR, Agarwal R. A flavonoid antioxidant, silymarin, affords exceptionally high

protection against tumour promotion in the SENCAR mouse skin tumorigenic model. *Cancer Res* 1999;59:622–632.

Lambert JD, Yang CS. Mechanisms of cancer prevention by tea constituents. *J Nutr*. 2003 Oct;133(10):3262S–3267S.

Lau BH, Ruckle HC, Botolazzo T, Lui PD. Chinese medicinal herbs inhibit growth of murine renal cell carcinoma. *Cancer Biother* 1994;9:153–161.

Lenartz D, Dott U, Menzel J, Schierholz JM, Beuth J. Survival of glioma patients after complementary treatment with galactoside-specific lectin from mistletoe. *Anticancer Res* 2000;20: 2073–2076.

Li WG, Zhang XY, Wu YJ, Tian X. Anti-inflammatory effect and mechanism of proanthocyanidins from grape seeds. *Acta Pharmacol Sin*. 2001 Dec;22(12):1117–20.

Lissoni P, Giani L, Zerbini S, Trabattoni P, Rovelli F. Biotherapy with the pineal immunomodulating hormone melatonin versus melatonin plus aloe vera in untreatable advanced solid neoplasms. *Natural Immunology*. 1998, 16(1):27–33.

Lu H, Liu GT. Anti-oxidant activity of dibenzocyclooctene lignans isolated from Schisandraceae. *Planta Med* 1992;58: 311–313.

Martarelli D, Martarelli B, Pediconi D, Nabissi MI, Perfumi M, Pompei P. Hypericum perforatum methanolic extract inhibits growth of human prostatic carcinoma cell line orthotopically implanted in nude mice. *Cancer Lett*. 2004 Jul 8;210(1):27–33.

Martinez Conesa C, Vicente Ortega V, Yanez Gascon MJ, Garcia Reverte JM, Canteras Jordana M, Alcaraz Banos M. Experimental model for treating pulmonary metastatic melanoma using grape-seed extract, red wine and ethanol. *Clin Transl Oncol* 2005;7:115–121.

Mathur R, Gupta SK, Singh N, Mathur S, Kochupillai V, Velpandian T. Evaluation of the effect of *Withania somnifera* root extracts on cell cycle and angiogenesis. *Journal Ethnopharmacol*. 2006;May 24;105(3):336–41.

McEntee MC. Veterinary radiation therapy: review and current state of the art. *Journal American Animal Hospital Association*. 2006;Mar–Apr;42(2):94–109.

McKnight JA. Principles of chemotherapy. *Clinical Techniques Small Animal Practice*. 2003;May;18(2):67–72.

Merriam EA, Campbell BD, Flood LP, Welsh CJR, McDaniel HR, Busbee DL. Enhancement of immune function in rodents using a complex plant carbohydrate which stimulates macrophage secretion of immunoreactive cytokines. In: Advances in Anti-Aging Medicine, vol 1. Klatz RM, ed. Larchmont, NY: Mary Ann Liebert, Inc., 1995 pp 181–203.

Moalic S, Liagre B, Corbiere C, Bianchi A, Dauca M, Bordji K, Beneytout JL. A plant steroid, diosgenin, induces apoptosis, cell cycle arrest and COX activity in osteosarcoma cells. *FEBS Letters*. 2001;Oct 12;506(3):225–30.

Pryme IF, Bardocz S, Pusztai A, Ewen SW, Pfuller U. A mistletoe lectin (ML-1)-containing diet reduces the viability of a murine non-Hodgkin lymphoma tumor. *Cancer Detect Prev* 2004;28: 52–56.

Ramamoorthy L, Tizard IR. Induction of apoptosis in a macrophage cell line RAW 264.7 by acemannan, a β-(1,4)-acetylated mannan. *Molecular Pharma* 1998;53:415–421.

Riggs DR, DeHaven JI, Lamm DL. Allium sativum (garlic) treatment for murine transitional cell carcinoma. *Cancer.* 1997;May 15;79(10):1987–94.

Sharada AC, Solomon FE, Devi PU, Udupa N, Srinivasan KK. Antitumor and radiosensitizing effects of withaferin A on mouse Ehrlich ascites carcinoma in vivo. *Acta Oncol* 1996;35:95–100.

Shidoji Y, Ogawa H. Natural occurrence of cancer-preventive geranylgeranoic acid in medicinal herbs. *J Lipid Res* 2004;45(6):1092–1093. Epub April 1, 2004.

Singh N, Singh SP, Nath R, et al. Prevention of induced lung adenomas by Withania somnifera (L) Dunal in albino mice. *Int J Crude Drug Res* 1986 24:90–100.

Singh NP, Lai HC. Artemisinin induces apoptosis in human cancer cells. *Anticancer Res* 2004;24:2277–2280.

Singletary K. Inhibition of DMBA-induced mammary tumorigenesis by rosemary extract. *FASEB J* 1991;5:5A927.

Streffer JR, Bitzer M, Schabet M, Dichgans J, Weller M. Response of radiochemotherapy-associated cerebral edema to a phytotherapeutic agent, H15. *Neurology* 2001;56:1219–1221.

Sundaram SG, Milner JA. Impact of organosulfur compounds in garlic on canine mammary tumor cells in culture. *Cancer Lett* 1993;74:85–90.

Tilak JC, Banerjee M, Mohan H, Devasagayam TP. Antioxidant availability of turmeric in relation to its medicinal and culinary uses. *Phytother Res* 2004;18:798–804.

Velasco G, Galve-Roperh I, Sanchez C, Blazquez C, Guzman M. Hypothesis: cannabinoid therapy for the treatment of gliomas? *Neuropharmacology* 2004;47:315–323.

Wende K, Krenn L, Unterrieder I, Lindequist U. Red clover extracts stimulate differentiation of human osteoblastic osteosarcoma HOS58 cells. *Planta Medicine.* 2004;Oct;70(10):1003–5.

Wimer BM, Mann PL. Apparent pokeweed mitogen cure of metastatic gum melanoma in an older dog. *Cancer Biother Radiopharm* 2000;15:201–205.

Xia Z, Gu J, Ansley DM, Xia F, Yu J. Antioxidant therapy with *Salvia miltiorrhiza* decreases plasma endothelin-1 and thromboxane B2 after cardiopulmonary bypass in patients with congenital heart disease. *J Thorac Cardiovasc Surg* 2003;126:1404–1410.

Yamaguchi N, Yoshida J, Ren LJ, et al. Augmentation of various immune reactivities of tumor-bearing hosts with an extract of Cordyceps sinensis. *Biotherapy* 1990;2:199–205.

Yan L, Yee JA, Li D, McGuire MH, Thompson LU. Dietary flaxseed supplementation and experimental metastasis of melanoma cells in mice. *Cancer Lett* 1998;124:181–186.

Yang CS, Liao J, Yang GY, Lu G. Inhibition of lung tumorigenesis by tea. *Exp Lung Res* 2005;31:135–144.

Yuan SL, Wang XJ, Wei YQ. Anticancer effect of tanshinone and its mechanisms. *Ai Zheng* 2003;22:1363–1366.

Yun JH, Pang EK, Kim CS, et al. Inhibitory effects of green tea polyphenol (-)-epigallocatechin gallate on the expression of matrix metalloproteinase-9 and on the formation of osteoclasts. *J Periodontal Res* 2004;39:300–307.

Zhao J, Sharma Y, Agarwal R. Significant inhibition by the flavonoid antioxidant silymarin against 12-O-tetra-decanoylphorbol 13-acetate caused modulation of anti oxidant and inflammatory enzymes and cyclooxygenase 2 and interleukin-1 alpha expression in SENCAR mouse epidermis: implications in the prevention of stage I tumour promotion. *Mol Carcinogen* 1999;26:321–333.

Zhou DH, Lin LZ. Effect of Jinshuibao capsule on the immunological function of 36 patients with advanced cancer. *Chung-kuo Chung His I Chieh Ho Tsa Chih* 1995;15:476–478.

Zhu YP. *Chinese Materia Media: Chemistry, Pharmacology, and Applications.* Australia: Harwood Academic Publishers; 1998a:445–448.

Zhu JS, Halpern GM, Jones K. The scientific rediscovery of an ancient Chinese herbal medicine: *Cordyceps sinensis.* Part II. *J Altern Complement Med* 1998b;4:429–457.

Zi X, Simoneau AR. Flavokawain, a novel chalcone from kava extract, induces apoptosis in bladder cancer cells by involvement of Bax protein-dependent and mitochondria-dependent apoptotic pathway and suppresses tumour growth in mice. *Cancer Research.* 2005;Apr 15;65(8):3479–86.

Ziauddin M, Phansalkar N, Patki P, et al. Studies on the immunemodulatory effects of ashwagandha. *J Ethnopharmacol* 1996;50:69–76.

SECTION 5

Integrative Cancer Therapy Protocols: Therapeutic Nutrition, Chinese Herbal Medicine, and Homotoxicology

Chapter Thirty-Two

Integrative Cancer Therapy Protocols

DEFINITION AND CAUSE

The veterinary literature reports that the underlying cause and mechanism of cancer development in animals is unknown. What is known about cancer is that cells undergo a genetic change whereby they begin to divide and multiply in an uncontrolled manner, resulting in the cancerous growth. It is believed that one underlying cause for the uncontrolled cellular division is exposure to outside influences such as pesticides, herbicides, chemical toxins and pollutants, prolonged exposure to radiation, certain drugs or hormones, viruses (such as feline leukemia virus), prolonged nutritional deficiencies, and adverse reaction to vaccinations (see Chapter 35, Vaccinations). The literature also reports that the cumulative effects of these external factors over the life of the animal play a role and, therefore, age is considered one of the main factors in the development of cancer.

Also known about the development of cancer is that these aberrant cells have escaped the immune system's detection and can grow out of control and invade surrounding tissues. However, the specific reasons why the immune surveillance mechanism has failed to identify and destroy these cancer cells are unknown.

Breed susceptibility and genetic predisposition to cancer are well known by veterinarians. Breeds more at risk for developing cancer are Golden Retrievers, Rottweilers, Labrador Retrievers, Boxers, and German Shepherd dogs.

Surgically altering pets can affect their risk for cancer, but in many cases the relationship is not clear. For example, early surgical alteration is associated with lower risks for mammary neoplasia in both dogs and cats, but is associated with higher risks of hemangiosarcoma in female dogs (Ware and Hopper 1999). Neutering decreased the risk of leukemia in female cats by half, but was not associated with decreased risk in dogs (Schneider 1983). Neutering nearly doubled the risk of osteosarcoma in one study (Ru 1998).

The AVMA web site lists the 10 most common signs of cancer. This list is designed to give clients the ability of early detection thereby allowing for prompt therapy and an increased chance for remission or prolonged survival times (www.avma.org). These signs are:

Abnormal swellings that persist or continue to grow
Sores that do not heal
Weight loss
Loss of appetite
Bleeding or discharge from any body opening
Offensive odor
Difficulty eating or swallowing
Hesitation to exercise or loss of stamina
Persistent lameness or stiffness
Difficulty breathing, urinating, or defecating

Early diagnosis of cancer is extremely important for the effective treatment and longer remission time. Educating clients about the common signs and symptoms as listed by the AVMA is important for early diagnosis and greater effectiveness of the therapy.

CONVENTIONAL THERAPY RATIONALE

The accepted, conventional approach to cancer is entrenched in the use of chemotherapy, radiation therapy, surgery, and immunotherapies. This is based upon the underlying belief that cancers are made up of aggressively growing cells that the body can no longer control nor regulate in terms of normal cellular division. Conventional medical theory acknowledges that these cancer cells have been able to separate themselves from the body's immune regulatory system, allowing them to both grow and multiply out of control as well as invade and damage adjacent cells, tissues, and organs. However, the current literature clearly states that there is no evidence for this loss of control, nor is it known why or how this loss of control occurs.

As a result of this underlying belief system, the developed approach to treat cancer is to (1) surgically remove the cancer, (2) chemically destroy the cancer, (3) destroy the cancer cells with ionizing radiation, or (4) medically and nonspecifically stimulate the general immune system against the aberrant cancer cells. More recent research has expanded the approach into novel areas such as anti-angiogenesis (preventing blood supply to rapidly growing tumors) and genetic reprogramming of the cancer cells. These approaches hold much promise.

While exciting research is leading to alternative approaches to cancer treatment, the best strategy that is currently available to veterinarians is a multifaceted approach of surgery (removal or debulking), chemotherapy, and radiation therapy, depending upon the cancer type and the clinical condition of the animal.

At the North American Veterinary Conference in January 2006, the Iams Company published and distributed a booklet entitled *Nutrition and Cancer Regulation*. In that booklet Karen Cornell, DVM, (2006) stated:

> "Traditional therapeutic strategies for cancer of animals and people have been focused in three areas: surgery, radiation therapy and chemotherapy. When complete surgical resection is not possible, chemotherapy and radiation therapy are utilized to inhibit proliferating cancer cells of the primary tumor. Unfortunately these modalities are non-specific and inhibit normal proliferating cells as well. This general antiproliferative approach results in the normal tissue toxicity observed in cancer patients and limits the delivery of sufficient therapeutic doses to eradicate the tumor. Recently however, clinicians and researchers have shifted the focus away from the traditional plan of attack and have started to investigate novel anticancer strategies. . . . An example of these anticancer strategies is the use of chemoprevention compounds such as resveratol from grapes and sulforaphane from broccoli."

ANTICIPATED PROGNOSIS

Each of the following cancer protocols consists of a brief discussion of the anticipated prognosis when the patient is treated by conventional therapies such as surgery, chemotherapy, and/or radiation therapy. Knowing the anticipated prognosis gives veterinarians a point of reference for integrative therapies when discussing an animal's cancer with the client. While there currently are few published, evidenced-based studies on alternative therapies, this section gives clinicians not only treatment protocols, but also confirmation that their colleagues are using these therapies in the prevention and treatment of various cancer types. Further research is needed to validate these protocols and determine their worth in regard to increased survival times, improved clinical condition, and general efficacy so that clinicians can better answer client's questions.

INTEGRATIVE VETERINARY THERAPIES

Throughout the introductory section of this book we repeatedly referred to free radicals and antioxidants and their effects on aging and degeneration. This free radical/antioxidant theory was introduced by Harman in 1955. It states that free radicals, which are formed daily by the metabolic process or exposure to exogenous foreign substances, cause an expanding inflammatory process which, if left unchecked, will damage cells, tissues, and organs. This damage will lead to premature aging and degenerative diseases, particularly in the target organs. This theory is being proven by clinical trials in people and animals, confirming the direct effect on the aging process and the formation of chronic degenerative diseases and neoplasia (Harman 1992). In addition, this theory also integrates with modern research, which is demonstrating that these free radicals can alter DNA and cause mutations, which ultimately leads to neoplasia and other chronic degenerative diseases (Opara 1997, Harman 1992, Masoro 1993).

Degenerative diseases and neoplasia play a dominant role in modern veterinary practice, as confirmed by the 1998 survey by the Morris Animal Foundation, which found that cancer is a major concern for people and the leading cause of death in animals. For this reason it is important that veterinarians fully understand this theory of aging and neoplasia development so they can educate their clients in the methodology of cancer prevention and the maintenance of wellness.

As mentioned above in the introductory section, we as veterinary students have been taught how to treat disease when it is diagnosed. As practitioners, when dealing with chronic degenerative diseases, we mostly focus our attention upon the signs and symptoms of the disease and the alleviation of pain and suffering of our animals without doing any harm. The inherent problem with this approach is that many of the drugs we commonly use have adverse side effects that are counterproductive for the long-term wellness of our patients.

An important benefit of integrative veterinary medicine as it relates to cancer is offering patients nutritional, herbal, and homeopathic remedies that work with and help to reduce the reliance upon the chronic administration of medications. Besides reducing the need for medication, these natural remedies also help minimize free-radical-induced inflammation and the associated cellular damage.

What effects do these nutrients, herbs, and homeopathics have on the prevention of degenerative disease and the prevention of neoplasia? The important, often overlooked point is the oxidative damage and cellular inflammation caused by unencumbered free radicals that can alter cellular integrity and metabolism and weaken or destroy cells. This inflammatory process can cascade through tissues and organs, setting the stage for chronic degeneration, weakened organ function, and the development of cancer. The therapies outlined in this chapter can help to alleviate, by biological methods, this cellular and organ damage.

While many of the cancers that are addressed in this chapter are associated with "proven cause unknown," there is a mechanism, be it known or unknown, that starts the neoplastic process and many veterinarians and researchers believe that the basic underlying initiating process is related to an oxidative process involved with excessive free radicals.

Cancer and nutraceutical medicine and nutrition

General considerations/rationale

The list below includes the more common nutraceuticals and antioxidants that are recommended as part of cancer therapy protocols. For a complete list of all nutraceuticals please refer to the therapeutic nutraceuticals in Chapter 2. Specific therapeutic nutrients are recommended in each of the following cancer therapy protocols. However, because the treatment protocols also include Chinese herbs and biological remedies, therapeutic nutrition in these cancer protocols is (1) dosed at lower levels, (2) recommended in a support rather than therapeutic role, and (3) focused upon immune function support, and reduction of inflammation, while not interfering with the specific activity of the Chinese herbal formulations.

Appropriate nutrients

Vitamin A/beta carotene: Vitamin A is a retinoid and a potent antioxidant that is required for proper cell division and growth. It has also been shown to increase immune function and help to minimize chemotherapy side effects (Ehrenpreis 2005, McCullough 1999, Michels 2001, Russell 2000, Semba 1998, Thurnham 1999). Beta-carotene is a pigmented phytonutrient and a member of the carotenoid family. Carotenoids are potent antioxidants that have been associated with the reduction of the adverse side effects of chemotherapy and the cancer itself. While there is some indication that high levels of antioxidants can decrease the effectiveness of chemotherapy, the protocols presented in this book take the dosage consideration of antioxidants into consideration (Anon 1994, Baron 2003, Bohlke 1999, Greenberg 1994, Heinonen 1998, Keefe 2001, Lee 2002, Michaud 2002, Omenn 1996, Toma 2003, Zhang 1999).

Vitamin E (alpha-tocopherol): Vitamin E is one of the body's main antioxidants, and as a fat-soluble vitamin it is a protector of lipids and fats. Vitamin E has also been found to block the protein activity of kinase C, which is involved in the cell behaviors of the entire organism. In addition, vitamin E reduces inflammation and improves circulation by helping vessels to dilate and reduce the agglutination of blood platelets. In cancer, vitamin E has

been shown to induce apoptosis (Yu 2003, You 2002). It is also suggested that vitamin E inhibits tumor growth (Bohlke 1999; Helzlsouer 2000; Malafa 2000, 2002; Neuzil 2001; Weber 2002).

Vitamin C: Vitamin C is the most studied of all vitamins and their effects on cancer (Bendich 1995, Golde 2003, Hunter 1993, Jacobs 2002, Lee 2002, Moertel 1985). Early studies conducted by Linus Pauling stated that vitamin C, in high doses and given intravenously, helped to extend remission time and improved the day-to-day quality of life (Cameron, Pauling 1976). While many medical researchers have challenged Pauling's work stating it failed to prove conclusively that vitamin C has any effect whatsoever (Creagan, et al. 1979, Moertel et al. 1985), the American Cancer Society has recently claimed that vitamin C may enhance cancer cell growth by protecting cancer cells from free radical cells' killing effects produced by chemotherapy and radiation therapies (Golde 2003).

Recent research has shown that vitamin C inhibits the growth of a least 7 types of cancer and appears to be cytotoxic (Feiz 2002, Leung 1993). In a more recent study, Gonzales (2005) indicates that this anticancer effect is due to the antioxidant effects of vitamin C.

Intravenous vitamin C is also being studied for its cytotoxic effects (Riordan 1995). In one study, Riordan et al. (1995) used high dose IV vitamin C in a person with pancreatic cancer. CT scans 6 months post surgery did not show any tumor progression. However, the cancer did recur when the IV dose of vitamin C was reduced. These studies are encouraging; however, they do indicate that more good quality research is necessary.

Glandular therapy: Raw extracts of adrenal, lymph, spleen, bone marrow, and thymus tissue have been shown to be anti-inflammatory and tissue sparing on these gland systems (Craveri 1971, Hartleb 1997, Kang 1985, Kouttab 1989, Schulof 1985, Singh 1998, Volk 1991).

Maitake mushrooms: Maitake mushrooms have been used in Eastern herbal medicine for centuries. Studies have shown that properly extracted mushrooms, which are rich in beta-glucans, help support and enhance immune function, help the body to handle stressful conditions, and metabolically and physiologically help the organ systems maintain balance and homeostasis.

Numerous studies carried out in Japan and the United States confirm the health benefits and immune-enhancing abilities of maitake mushrooms. In addition, some recent studies indicate that maitake extracts may also be helpful as an adjunct to chemotherapy by not only enhancing the drugs' effectiveness but also in the ameliorization of the drugs' potential side effects (Adachi 1987, Nariba 1993, Wagner 1985).

Maitake mushroom are rich in beta-glucans, which help support and enhance immune function and can stimulate the production of natural killer (NK) cells (Kodama 2003, Nanba 1987).

Arginine: Studies on dogs with cancer determined that they had lower plasma levels of arginine and other amino acids, which did not change after the tumor was surgically removed, suggesting that protein metabolism changes in these dogs. It is also believed that the same is true for cats. Research indicates that the addition of arginine and essential fatty acids to the daily diet of dogs with cancer can improve the prognosis and remission times (Anderson 1997, Ogilvie 2000).

Glutamine: Glutamine is often depleted when cancer cachexia is occurring. Is has been suggested that supplementation with glutamine decreases tumor growth and improves immune function (Klimberg 1996). In addition to being the preferred nutrient of the intestinal cells, research has shown that glutamine is also tissue sparing and cellular regenerative. It is an intermediary for the antioxidant glutathione in its role of protecting against the adverse effects of radiation therapy (Klimberg 1996). When chemotherapy is being administered, glutamine helps reduce drug-induced inflammation in the bowel (Rombeau 1990, Fox 1988). In patients receiving chemotherapy, the addition of dietary glutamine has been shown to enhance the effectiveness of certain chemotherapeutics as well as increase patient survival times (Klimberg 1991, 1992).

Selenium: Selenium is an important antioxidant, functioning in this capacity along with the enzyme glutathione peroxidase. It is involved in the proper functioning of the pancreas and it helps the cells to absorb glucose. It is beneficial in animals with cancer. Selenium is an essential trace mineral (Burk 1999). There are many evidence-based studies demonstrating that the addition of selenium to the diet helps reduce the incidence of cancer in animals (Rayman 2000).

Fatty acids: Eicosapentaenoic acid (EPA) is an omega-3 fatty acid that helps to maintain the proper levels of eicosinoids, which in turn help mediate the body's immune response to cancer cells. EPAs are found in fish, flax, hemp, borage, and primrose oils. Research has shown that EPA can slow tumor growth and prevent metastasis. The addition of EPA to the diet can improve the response of cells to therapy such as chemotherapeutics (Sagaguchi 1990, Reich 1989) (see the diet restriction section for the recommended sources of fatty acids and EPA).

Phytonutrients or phytochemicals: New and growing research is proving that these nutrients, while not classified as essential nutrients nor required like foods and vitamins, can act as antioxidants and prevent oxidative damage and exert a positive and often dramatic effect on wellness, health, prevention, and treatment of disease and longevity (Broadhurst 2001, Duke 1992, Gaziano 1995, Shils 1994).

Categories of phytonutrients are now being discussed and are becoming more accepted according to their health benefits; these categories include: amines, bioflavonoids, carotenoids, lignans, organosulfurs, phenols, phytosterols, sterols, sterolins, and terpines, which are being clinically proven to exert a positive effect on health and well-being, reduce inflammation, and prevent degenerative diseases and can play a critical role in cancer treatment (Ames 1993, Block 1992, Carlton 2000, Duthie 1996).

Carotenoids: Besides helping to reduce inflammation as antioxidants do, research shows that carotenoids enhance immunity and regulate cellular communications and division (Agarwal 2000, Burri 2000, Gaziano 1995, Ito 1999, Nishino, 2000, Slattery, 2000, Zeegers 2001).

Flavonoiods: Several studies have indicated that flavonoids can help regulate the immune response and help control overreactivity of immune-mediated cells such as T- and B-lymphocytes, mast cells, and neutrophils (Middleton 1986, 1992, 1993; Myhrstad 2002; Panthong 1994; Roger 1988).

Lignans: Lignans are found in flax seed, fruits, and vegetables. Breast cancer research shows that these plant-derived compounds compete with the body's hormonal estrogen and help prevent hormonally influenced mammary cancers (Brooks 2005, Kleinsmith 2004, Wang 2002, Serraino 1992, Sung 1998, Thompson 1996, 1998).

Sterols and phytosterols: The most commonly known and well studied is betasitosterol. Pegel (1997) and Bouic (1996, 1999) feel that sterols are essential for a properly functioning immune system. In cancer patients, he feels that sterols can directly reduce the adverse immune-suppressing effects of both chemotherapy and radiation therapy.

Awad (1999a) proved that in the laboratory, sterols reduced the number of breast cancer cells as compared to the controls. In another study, Awad (1999b) proved that the sterols also enhanced intracellular communications, inhibiting cell growth and thus preventing the formation of cancer.

Coenzyme Q10: Coenzyme Q10, also known as CoQ10 or ubiquinone, helps reduce inflammation, strengthen cardiac function and output, and improve circulation (Folkers 1985, Gaby 1998, Shigeta 1966, Traber 2001). In cancer patients, CoQ10 has been proven to enhance immune function, is a potent antioxidant, and improves available metabolic energy required by the body to heal and prevent disease (Folkers 1982, Lockwood 1995).

N,N-Dimethylglycine (DMG): DMG, which is naturally produced by the body, enhances and modulates immune function and helps with cancer treatment protocols (Balch 1997, Mani 1999). DMG improves cellular oxygenation, which is important in the treatment of anaerobic cancer cells. DMG has been found to increase both tumor necrosis factor (TNF) and interferon production (Graber 1986; Mani 1999; Kendall 2000, 2003; Reap 1990; Wang 1988). In addition, DMG helps prevent metastasis to other organs (Reap 1988, Kendall 1991), repair DNA, regulate gene expression, and control cell division.

Kendall (2003) reports on research that suggests DMG can be cellular protective in animals that are receiving radiation therapy. Also, DMG is indicated as part of an overall therapy program for the prevention and potential treatment of cancer in animals (Balch 1997, Mani 1999). Recent work has shown that DMG is a potent antioxidant and anti-inflammatory agent (Yanez 2007).

Quercetin: Quercetin is in the flavonoid family (see phytonutrients in Chapter 2). Quercetin is also a phytoestrogen, which is a plant-derived compound that has estrogenic effects on the body. Miodini (1999) and Shoskes (1999) have demonstrated quercetin's positive effects in inhibiting breast cancer and reducing inflammation in men with prostatitis. Knekt (1997, 2002) has reported that quercetin has been proven to be beneficial in the inhibition of lung and other cancers.

Note: Because cancer can affect multiple organ systems and is often a systemic disease, a metabolic and physiological blood evaluation is recommended to assess general glandular and immune health. This information can help clinicians to formulate therapeutic nutritional protocols that address not only the cancer but associated organ disease and weaknesses that may be present (Cima 2000, Goldstein 2000) (see Chapter 2, Nutritional Blood Testing, for additional information).

Cancer and Chinese herbal medicine/acupuncture

General considerations/rationale
According to Traditional Chinese Medicine, a patient with cancer is considered to be in an overall deficient state. There is Qi and Blood stagnation. There may also be an accumulation of Phlegm, and there are excess pathological factors and toxin buildup.

The deficient state indicates that the body is simply not strong enough to overcome the disease process. The excess pathological factor is the tumor itself, or the viruses, toxin, radiation or other etiology of the cancer. The Qi and Blood stagnation can explain the mass lesions and the pain and inflammation associated with them. Phlegm accumulation is also a description of the mass lesions. Toxin buildup may be translated into paraneoplastic syndromes, tumor lysis syndromes, and any biochemical imbalance caused by the tumor.

Chinese herbal therapy
There are numerous benefits of herbal therapy for cancer. First, they can be combined with chemotherapy or surgery to decrease chemotherapy side effects or enhance the action of the chemotherapeutic agent. Often, the chemotherapy dose can be increased for greater efficacy without increasing the side effects. For example, when using Western agents alone, the chemotherapy dose must be decreased or treatment delayed due to neutropenia. If herbal therapy can be used to maintain the white blood cell count, the full course of Western chemotherapy can be administered.

An alternative approach to combining Western and Eastern protocols is to decrease the amount of chemotherapy given because the herbal therapy has an effect of its own. This allows for fewer side effects from chemotherapy simply due to decreased dose of the agent.

Herbal supplements can be used alone to ameliorate signs of neoplasia, prevent or slow progression, and in some instances induce remission. In some cases, notably osteosarcoma (AHVMA 2006) and hemangiosarcoma (unpublished data), life expectancy when herbs are given alone can be similar to that achieved by chemotherapeutic agents. In the author's experience, pathological fractures secondary to osteosarcoma can heal using herbal therapy, support bandages, and analgesics (AHVMA 2006). Human patients with lymphosarcoma treated with chemotherapy or radiation in conjunction with herbal therapy have fewer side effects from the chemotherapy or radiation. They also have longer remission times (Liu 2000).

There are 2 main criteria for selecting herbal preparations. Some supplements are organ- or location-based, while others are based on the type of cancer. Those based on organ or location are designed for any tumor type, be it sarcoma, carcinoma, etc., in a given location. Cancer-type herbs treat a specific cancer regardless of location. For example, mast cell tumors are treated with a cancer-type formula. The same formula is used regardless of the tumor's location on the body. For lymphosarcoma, however, the formula for nodal disease is different from that of nasal lymphoma. This is an example of a location-based formula. This explains why several formulas may be listed for one type of cancer. Years of study and practice allow a practitioner to formulate his or her own supplements. It is not possible to learn this from one book, or even one course.

Dosing
Capsules come in standard sizes from multiple manufacturers in the United States. The size "0" capsule holds approximately 0.5 g of powder. There is slight variation because some powders are finer than others. A coarse granule may not pack into the capsule as well as a fine powder will.

In this book, all doses are based upon a 1:5 extract powder. In other countries 1:10 and 1:15 extracts are available for some herbs. These are 2 and 3 times more concentrated, respectively. If the FDA does allow these powders into the country, the volume of the more concentrated herb required will decrease appropriately.

In general, the dose of herbal supplements for patients with neoplasia is 1 capsule per 8 to 10 pounds 3 times daily. Toy breeds and cats tend to use higher doses, i.e. 1 capsule per 8 pounds 3 times daily and the giant breeds use 1 capsule per 10 pounds 3 times daily. In less aggressive cancers, such as low-grade mast cell tumors or soft tissue cancers with complete excision and a tendency to recur locally rather than metastasize, twice daily dosing may be acceptable. Patients are treated as long as the cancer is present. If a patient has complete remission, in many cases herbal supplements may be discontinued after 2 years of treatment. Some clients elect to remain on the supplement for the rest of the animal's life for added protection. While rare, it is possible to see a recurrence once the herb is discontinued, even after 2 years.

Dietary restrictions are very important for optimal efficacy for almost all cancer patients. The protein portion of the diet can consist of beef, pork, venison, rabbit, buffalo, and cheese. Seafood, poultry (chicken, turkey, eggs, duck), and lamb should be avoided. These food items tend to interfere with the actions of the herbal supplements on the cancer cells. There is no restriction on vegetables.

Carbohydrates should make up less than 20% of the daily intake on a dry matter basis (Ming 1999). It is important not to oversupplement with antioxidants and vitamins when using traditional Chinese herbal medicine. Antioxidants (see above) may protect cancer cells from apoptosis induced by chemotherapy, herbal therapy, and radiation (Robinson 2006).

Appropriate Chinese herbs

Many herbs have been shown to have anti-neoplastic effects. Studies have shown tumor shrinkage, increased survival times, and enhanced well-being in terms of appetite and activity levels in cancer patients. Some herbs have been shown to increase immune function while simultaneously decreasing the side effects of chemotherapy. Other herbs have been shown to decrease leukocyte counts. Rather than using books, which only discuss TCM theory and herbs, the authors have tried to cite evidence of efficacy based upon modern scientific reports. The herbs mentioned below have shown anti-neoplastic effects in the laboratory or in animal or human studies.

Agrimony (Xian he cao): May have anti-neoplastic effects in mice (Shen Yang Yi Xue Yuan Xue Bao 1980).

Antler powder (Lu jiao shuang): Used as an adjunctive therapy to increase the immune functions in patients with cancer. It increases the phagocytic abilities of macrophages (Du 1981).

Apricot seed (Xing ren): Contains amygdalin, which increases the activity of NK cells (Zhao 1993).

Asparagus (Tian men dong): Has been used in a variety of tumors. It has demonstrated efficacy against sarcoma in mice (Yao Li Shi Yan Fang Fa Xue 1982) and breast cancer and lymphoma in humans (Jiang Su Yi Yao 1976, Xin Yi Xue 1975).

Astragalus (Huang qi): Improves the immunity of mice with tumors (Ying 1999). Furthermore, Huang Qi has an anti-neoplastic effect on GNM cells, which are a cell line derived from human oral squamous cell carcinoma (Liu 1999). Additionally, it inhibits S180 solid tumors (Shi 1999). Given the effect of astragalus on these tumors, it is possible it may have inhibitory effects on other solid tumors, such as fibrosarcomas.

Atractylodes (Bai zhu): Has demonstrated anti-neoplastic effects against esophageal cancer in in vitro studies (Zhong Liu Yu Zhi Tong Xun 1976). Atractylodes may have activity against other tumors as well.

Barbat skullcap (Ban zhi lian): Increases the phagocytic functions of macrophages and may inhibit tumor growth (Ren Min Wei Sheng Chu Ban She 1988).

Brucea seed (Ya dan zi): 388 patients with various cancers were treated with brucea seed (Yan dan zi). It prolonged life spans in 71% of the participants (Zhong Guo Yi Yao Bao 1985).

Bupleurum (Chai hu): Contains saikosaponin d (SSd), which has been shown to induce apoptosis in HL-60 (human leukemia) cells (Sun 1999). It may have similar effects on other neoplastic cells.

Burreed tuber (San leng): Has demonstrated some ability to inhibit neoplastic cells. In one study 31 patients with various terminal cancers were treated with a supplement containing burreed tuber (San leng) along with other herbs. Five improved significantly, 19 showed some improvement, and 7 did not respond (Zhe Jiang Zhong Yi Xue Yuan Xue Bao 1983). In a separate study, 30 patients with hepatic carcinoma were given burreed tuber as part of an herbal supplement. Three had significant improvement, 10 had some improvement, and 17 did not improve at all (Zhong Liu Yu Fang Yan Jiu 1973).

Centipede (Wu gong): Has demonstrated anti-neoplastic effects in vitro (Chang Yong Zhong Yao Cheng Fen Yu Yao Li Shou Ce 1994).

Cinnamon bark (Rou gui): Contains cinnamaldehyde, which can completely inhibit SV40-virus-induced tumors in mice (Higashikaze 1981). It may have anti-neoplastic activity against other tumors.

Codonopsis (Dang shen): Decreases lymphocyte counts (Zhong Yao Xue 1998), which may make this useful in cancers involving elevated leukocyte counts, such as lymphosarcoma.

Coix (Yi yi ren): Has been shown to inhibit the growth of hepatocarcinoma and S180 sarcomas in mice. It can also enhance the activity of NK cells in mice (Lu 1999).

Coptis (Huang lian): Inhibits human nasopharyngeal carcinoma cells (Tang 1995). Other studies have shown that coptis (Huang lian) has in vitro efficacy against hepatoma, gastric, colon, and breast cancer cells (Clin Exp Pharmacol Physiol. 2004).

Crataegus (Shan zha): Seems to protect the body from neoplastic transformations induced by chemicals. In one experiment, erinitrit and methyl phentolamine solution, which cause proliferative pathological changes in the lining of the esophagus, were given to rats and mice. The pathological changes did not occur when the animals were also given crataegus (Liu 1991). Crataegus seems to be able to prevent the proliferation of neoplastic cells without causing significant damage to normal cells (Liu 1994).

Cremastra (Shan ci gu): Has shown some antineoplastic efficacy in experiments involving mice (Chang Yong Zhong Yao Xian Dai Yan Jiu Yu Lin Chuan 1995).

Curcuma root (Yu jin): Contains curcumin A, which has antioxidant effects and can induce apoptosis and suppress cellular proliferation. It may prevent angiogenesis, thereby decreasing a tumor's blood supply (Singh 2006).

Dioscorea bulbifera bulb (Huang yao zi): Was used to treat 25 patients with thyroid tumors with an 80% efficacy rate (Fu Jian Yi Xue Yuan Xue Bao 1964).

Dittany bark (Bai xian pi): Contains obacunone, which potentiates chemotherapeutic agents such as vincristine, vinblastine, and paclitaxel (Planta Med 2000).

Earthworm (Di long): Has demonstrated the ability to inhibit the growth of various transplanted tumors in mice. It may do this either by improving the immune system or by scavenging free radicals (Wang 1991).

Ganoderma (Ling zhi): Has been shown to have antioxidant effects and can scavenge free radicals. It also increases the function of T cells, macrophages, and natural killer cells. It may induce apoptisis and may also have anti-angiogenic capabilities (Gao 2004).

Hornet's nest (Feng fang): Has been shown to inhibit the growth of S180 sarcomas and enhance the phagocytic activity of macrophages (Li Li 1999).

Kelp (Kun bu): Prevents the formulation of blood vessels and prevents the growth of RIF-1 tumors in rats (Xu 1999). It may inhibit the growth of other tumors by restricting angiogenesis.

Mastic (Ru xiang): Contains boswellic acids, which cause apoptosis in leukemia and meningioma cell lines in vitro (Shao 1998, Park 2002). These acids may also inhibit other cancer cells.

Milettia (Ji xue teng): Can help destroy tumor cells. When peripheral blood mononuclear cells are cultured with interleukin 2, they develop the ability to destroy tumor cells. This is termed lymphokine-activated killer or LAK activity. Milettia can increase LAK and NK cell activity in mice (Hu 1997, Xu 1996). It also helps to reduce the side effects of chemotherapy and radiation, both of which tend to cause decreases in red and white blood counts. Milettia can help prevent this unwanted side effect of Western therapy (Bo 1997, Chen 1999, Liu 1998).

Oldenlandia (Bai hua she cao): Has been shown to inhibit cellular proliferation of 8 types of cancer cell lines in vitro, and decreased the size of lung metastases in mice by approximately 70% (Gupta 2004).

Oyster shell (Mu li): Was administered to mice with hepatocarcinoma. The activity of NK cells was increased and the tumor size decreased as compared to a control group. The mice that received the oyster shell also lived longer (Wang 1997).

Pinellia (Ban xia): Pinellia, when processed with ginger, prevents the growth of tumor cell strain K_{562} (Wu 1996).

Polyporus (Zhu ling): Inhibits the growth of liver tumors in mice (Yao Xue Tong Bao 1985). In addition, it inhibited the tumor growth and enhanced the immune system in 200 people with lung cancer and 40 patients with leukemia (Zhong Xi Yi Jie He Za Zhi 1984).

Poria (Fu ling): Has anti-neoplastic properties. Experimentally, it was shown to significantly inhibit S180 cancers, which are normally very aggressive tumors in mice (Chen 1986). In addition, it can increase the phagocytic ability of macrophages in mice with cancer (Lu 1990). Poria decreases the side effects of chemotherapy and strengthens the immune system in patients with cancer. These patients then have better appetites and increased physical activity (Zhong Xi Yi Jia He Za Zhi 1985).

Pueraria (Ge gen): Can inhibit human leukemia 60 tumor cells (Modern TCM Pharmacology 1997).

Red peony (Chi shao): Inhibits local growth of Lewis pulmonary tumors and melanoma B16, and prevents hematogenous metastasis of those tumors in mice. In addition, it has synergistic activity with cyclophosphamide (Hu 1990).

Salvia (Dan shen): Has been shown to inhibit K562 and BCaP-37 tumor cells in vitro (Li Xu Fen 1999).

Scorpion (Quan xie): Inhibits sarcoma in mice (Jiang Su Yi Yao 1990).

Scutellaria (Huang qin): Contains baicalein, which has demonstrated the ability to cause apoptosis of human myeloma cells in vitro (Zi 2005).

Siler (Fang feng): Can prevent the growth of S180 tumors in mice and increase the phagocytic abilities of macrophages (Li Li 1999).

Subprostrata sophora root (Shan dou gen): Has antineoplastic effects, which are mediated by matrine, oxymatirine, and sophcarpine. It is especially effective in treating abdominal cancers (Zhong Guo Yi Xue Ke Xue Xue Bao 1988).

Wolfberry (Gou qi zi): Has been shown to inhibit the growth of cancer cells and enhance the immune system in mice (Zhong Guo Yao Li Xue Za Zhi 1985).

Wormwood (Yin chen): Can kill gastric carcinoma cells BGC-823 and can enhance the production of serum tumor necrosis factors (Zhang 1998, Du 1990).

Zedoaria (E zhu): Inhibits a range of cancers. Of 19 patients with various solid tumors who were treated with zedoaria, 1 patient recovered completely, 4 improved significantly, 3 improved somewhat, and 11 did not respond (Shan Dong Zhong Yi Xue Yuan Xue Bao 1980).

Acupuncture

Acupuncture can be used in cancer patients to relieve pain and inflammation. However, it is not routinely used for cancer treatment due to lack of response. In general, acupuncture points are chosen based upon the location of tumor, the etiology of the cancer (Cold, Heat, Phlegm, Stagnation, etc.), and the organ involved (Liver, Kidney, Heart, etc.). By convention, any patient with opened or infected tumors or septicemia should not receive acupuncture because this may promote the spread of the infection. Practitioners who are familiar with TCM pattern differentiation may find acupuncture to be beneficial. In general, practitioners who have not had this training are better off not administering acupuncture therapy.

Cancer and homotoxicology (as part of a combined integrative protocol with nutrition and Chinese herbal medicine)

Please refer to Chapter 34 for advanced homotoxicology and autosanguis treatment of cancer.

General considerations/rationale

Neoplastic, preneoplastic, and chronic diseases are commonly seen in veterinary practice. Due to the complex nature of these conditions, cure is often not possible, and a multimodality approach is often most successful in handling these conditions. The number of veterinarians practicing homotoxicology has increased substantially in the last 5 years, as clinicians become attracted to homotoxicology out of general interest and then usually continue after seeing a series of surprisingly good results. Research into mechanisms of action of low dose pharmacology is beginning to increase, and the results are interesting indeed. Because homotoxicology can be practiced at many different levels of sophistication, this section is intended to introduce veterinarians to the basic practices and techniques used in homotoxicology and its inclusion as a multimodality approach with therapeutic nutrients and Chinese herbal medicine. See Chapter 34 for advanced

homotoxicology and autosanguis protocols for the treatment of cancer.

As we have seen earlier in this text (Chapters 1 and 4), homotoxicology contains many useful agents for improving patient well being. Due to the low risks of serious side effects encountered with antihomotoxic therapy, clients readily accept and continue biological therapies that support organ function, drain toxins from the body, and improve patient condition and comfort. Antihomotoxic agents integrate nicely with many other forms of therapy commonly used to treat patients suffering from cancer or other chronic diseases. They are also environmentally friendly because patients using biological therapy excrete very few toxic metabolites into the environment.

A homotoxicologist's view of cancer

The scope of this introductory text is insufficient to address, other than very superficially, the topic of oncogenesis and biological oncologic therapies. Due to spatial constraints, we have divided this book's cancer section into a basic or introductory approach to cancer using antihomotoxic agents, in combination with therapeutic nutrition and Chinese herbal medicine (which follows here in this chapter). More data and protocols can be applied to patients in the Dedifferentiation Phase by use of autosanguis, and a deeper understanding of homotoxicology agents greatly facilitates that process. These areas are discussed in Chapter 34. The reader is also referred to the earlier discussion of the greater defense mechanisms in the homotoxicology (chapter 4), because this is the foundational material involved.

In homotoxicology, cancer is viewed simply as the body's expression of accumulated homotoxins and the damage that has been done to normally functioning systems. This represents the outcome of Dedifferentiation Phase disease. Very little data is formally published on the use of homotoxicology for cancer treatment in human or veterinary patients. However, a large body of anecdotal data and theories are available for investigation by those interested in the topic. Current efforts are beginning to correlate this data and present it in more useful form. Of particular interest is fundamental clinical research by Jarir Nakouzi, MD, who claims to have developed a new clinical approach to human patients suffering from Dedifferentiation Phase disease. Clinical impressions and approaches to human patients with chronic disease and cancer were presented in a seminar sponsored by Heel USA (Nakouzi, Smit, Shelton 2004). Interested parties should consider obtaining a copy of these lectures, which are available on CD from Heel.

Alterations in these defense mechanisms allow neoplastic cells to manifest. Heine (2006) of Germany has written extensively on this subject and is currently working on a new text. These theories seem to predict specific activities and give clinicians tools to address patients with disease in this phase, and the authors have found them intensely useful. Additional research is warranted. Several others are actively finding support for these applied theories, as well. Goldstein (1999, 2000) has assisted oncology and chronically diseased patients for years and routinely includes antihomotoxic medicines in the treatment plans of many of his patients. Joseph Demers (2005a, 2005b) has reported his approach to neoplasia and continues clinical work. Robert Goldstein (2006), the editing author of this text, is undertaking research projects in the United States involving homotoxicology and other integrative modalities in conjunction with a boarded oncologist on the subject of both canine lymphosarcoma and osteosarcoma. The results of these studies should prove intensely interesting.

The protocols that follow can be readily used in conjunction with other therapies, both conventional and complementary. Integration is the watchword of this new age in veterinary medicine. These therapies can be adjusted and customized into a nearly infinite set of possibilities as the clinician becomes more familiar and astute with biological therapy. The authors suggest that the reader simply begin by trying them on a few difficult cases, especially those that seem "hopeless." They are not intended to cure cancer in any case, but seeing pets respond with brighter eyes and higher energy makes both owner and veterinarian happier and makes these worth pursuing. As the clinician becomes more facile, and as cases presented become more difficult, the data in the latter chapters will be helpful. In the meanwhile, enjoy your journey into the new and exciting realm of biological therapy.

Appropriate homotoxicology remedies
Most protocols use a mixture of Galium-Heel, Lymphomyosot, Hepar compositum, Solidago compositum, Tonsilla compositum and/or Thyroidea compositum, Coenzyme compositum, and Ubichinon compositum. This combination covers many aspects of selecting phase remedies and establishing drainage and organ support in chronic disease cases. Commonly referred to as the modified deep detoxification formula, this combination generally assists cases in the Dedifferentiation Phase by supporting cellular repair of organelles and draining toxins from the cells into the matrix (Galium-Heel and Lymphomyosot). Once there, agents in the formula (Lymphomyosot and Thyroidea compositum) activate the clearing of the matrix and lymphatic system, support endocrine function, and strengthen the excretion and detoxification organs (liver, kidney, and bowel) (Hepar compositum and Solidago compositum).

Constant attention to cellular energy production is key to success in treating any chronic disease, and cancer is no exception. Catalysts, especially Coenzyme composi-

tum, Ubichinon compositum, and Glyoxal compositum, are critical to success, and they and make patients feel better very quickly. Start this formula out slowly, using it twice weekly for 2 weeks. If the patient feels better and is doing well, it can be continued at this level or given orally every other day. If excessive signs of homotoxin off-loading occur (diarrhea, vomiting, nasal discharge, aural discharge, ocular discharge, or coughing), then simply cut back on this formula or stop entirely for several days. Most patients recover quickly and feel better from the removal of their harmful homotoxins. This is usually not a problem if clients are properly prepared.

Alta Smit, MD, has recently recommended that Berberis homaccord be used daily in cancer patients. The system is bombarded daily by homotoxins, and Berberis homaccord helps support the adrenal glands, liver, gallbladder, renal tubules, and colon. Berberis homaccord contains Viscum album to support the Dedifferentiation Phase condition. This agent can be added to all of the cancer protocols in this book with good effect. This formula can also assist with rheumatic complaints and spasms that can accompany many chronic disease states.

Symptom remedies are used to manage signs that arise during therapy. The simplest approach is to note the main symptoms and look them up in the Biotherapeutic Index or in the medical protocol of this text. Then select agents that assist that problem and recheck the patient after a period of time. The clinician should always practice good medicine and ensure that patients have been adequately and properly diagnosed so that the patient's actual medical condition is known. In many cases it will be found that patients not responding to treatment have other undiscovered issues such as abscessed teeth, infected kidneys, allergies, food intolerances, or hidden viral conditions. Complementary medicine in no way replaces good diagnostic and proper conventional medicine. In fact, by properly integrating conventional practice and complementary modalities, the clinician will discover a whole host of new tools with which patient care can be improved.

Cancer treatment protocols
The protocols that follow can be readily used in conjunction with other therapies, both conventional and complementary. Integration is the watchword of this new age in veterinary medicine. These therapies can be adjusted and customized into a nearly infinite set of possibilities as the clinician becomes more familiar and astute with nutritional, herbal, and biological therapies. The authors suggest that the reader simply begin by trying them on a few difficult cases, especially those that seem "hopeless." They do not claim to cure cancer, but seeing pets respond with clear and brighter eyes, higher energy levels, and dramatically improved quality of life pleases animal

guardians and veterinarians and confirms the benefits of pursuing this integrative approach.

The following section lists treatment protocols for specific types of cancer. Each cancer treatment protocol will contain the following:

- General Western medical information, treatment options, and prognoses.
- General therapeutic nutritional information and the author's suggested treatment.
- General Chinese herbal information and the author's suggested treatment.
- General homotoxicology information and the author's suggested treatment (in abbreviated form).

Immediately following the above cancer treatment protocols are 2 additional chapters covering autosanguis therapy and advanced homotoxicology oncology protocols for practitioners who choose a more in-depth homotoxicology approach.

Diet and cancer

These dietary recommendations and restrictions apply to ALL of the following cancer protocols, which recommend using combinations of therapeutic nutrition, Chinese herbal medicine, and homotoxicology remedies.

It is important to address the matter of diet when using traditional Chinese herbal supplements for the treatment of neoplasia. Through years of study, it has been shown that the supplements are much more effective when the diet includes beef, pork, venison, rabbit, and/or cheese as the protein source. Lamb, poultry (chicken, turkey, eggs), and seafood (including fish oil) interfere with the action of the herbs. There are no restrictions on vegetables (Ming 1999).

Furthermore, *excessive* supplementation with vitamins, minerals, antioxidants, and herbs that have a strong tonifying or immune-stimulating effect can decrease the antineoplastic action of traditional Chinese herbal formulations. It is for this reason, in the following protocols, that nutrient doses have been reduced to levels that do not interfere with the effectiveness of the herbs but still supply important beneficial antioxidants. These antioxidants have the important function of supporting gland function and helping to reduce free radical load and inflammation. In cancer patients, free-radical-induced inflammation is increased due to the following factors:

- Chemotherapeutics or ionizing radiation
- Immune-suppressing drugs such as corticosteroids
- Toxic load from cellular debris (healthy and cancerous cells break down) and metabolites
- Inefficient metabolism due to weakened or diseased organ systems

Note: Fixed formula nutritional recommendations are listed in all of the following cancer treatment protocols.

Cancer is a systemic, immune-deficient disease, and therefore can affect all organ systems, even though the specific cancer is localized. It is for this reason that the authors recommend that when possible, as part of the medical work-up, a physiological blood analysis be performed to identify associated organ weaknesses. This is more important when dealing with systemic cancers such as lymphosarcoma or those that affect vital organs such as the liver, kidney, or heart. This analysis helps the clinician to match the nutritional support program specifically to the organ system, while still meeting the restrictions required for the use of the Chinese herbal remedies (see Nutritional Blood Testing in Chapter 2 for more details).

The typical sample diet shown below gives animal companions the ability to prepare food at home or use commercially prepared foods that meet the above criteria. The guidelines for the ratio of protein, fat, and carbohydrates generally follow those representative of the research carried out by the Hills Company for the formulation of their N/D® diet for cancer patients. Studies on feeding dogs with cancer have shown that adding essential amino and fatty acids improved not only the prognosis but also the remission times (Davenport 2000) (see fatty acids in Chapter 2 for more details). In addition to the elevated fatty acid content, it also has been shown that a low-carbohydrate diet is also beneficial for treatment cancer (Ming 1999).

For presentation purposes, a few brands with wide distribution are listed in each category. For a complete list of suppliers that formulate foods that meet the restrictive guidelines of these cancer protocols, please refer to Section 8.

Dietary restrictions

Do not use fish oil. Instead, use flax, hemp, evening primrose, and borage oils or AFA Algae (*Aphanizomenon Flos Aquae*). Do not use chicken, turkey, lamb, fish or eggs. Instead, use beef, venison, pork, or tofu.

Commercial choices

Sample raw food sources: Nature's Variety, Bravo, Primal, Northwest Naturals, Steve's Real Food, Farmore, Raw Advantage, Natural Balance, Earth Animal, and Wild Kitty Cat Food.

Sample canned choices: Natural Balance Canned Beef, Evangers Beef 100% Beef, Blue Buffalo Canned Beef, Wysong Canned Beef, and Evo 95% Beef or Venison.

Sample dry or premixes: Natural Balance Vegetarian, Dr. Harvey's Premix, Soujourner Farms Premix, Wysong Vegan, and Pet Guard Organic Vegetarian.

Guidelines for home cooking

Meat protein: 50% to 75%; complex carbohydrates: 10% to 20%; and fat (rich in omega-3 and 6; no chicken or fish oil): 20%.

Sample home-prepared diet

1 pound organic or free-range beef, tofu, venison, rabbit, or buffalo
One-half to 1 cup Dr. Harvey's or organic brown rice or oatmeal
2 tablespoons organic yogurt
1 tablespoon organic flaxseed oil (evening primrose, hemp, or borage oil OK)
One-half cup organic carrots or chopped greens
1 to 3 teaspoons chopped organic parsley
1 clove organic garlic

REFERENCES

Therapeutic nutrition

Adachi K, Nanba H, Kuroda H. Potentiation of Host-Mediated Antitumor Activity in Mice by Beta-glucan Obtained from Grifola frondosa (Maitake), *Chem. Pharm. Bull.* 1987;35; 262–270.

AHVMA. Proceedings of conference, 2006. Louisville, KY.

Agarwal S, Rao AV. Carotenoids and chronic diseases. *Drug Metab Drug Interact* 2000:17(1–4):189–210.

Ames BN, Shigenaga MK, Hagen T M. Oxidants, antioxidants and the degenerative diseases of aging. *Proc. Natl. Acad. Sci. U.S.A.* 1993; 90:7915–7922.

Anderson CR, Ogilvie GK, Fettman MJ, et al. Effects of fish oil and arginine on acute effects of radiation injury in dogs with nasal tumors: A double-blind, randomized study. In: Proceedings. Veterinary Cancer Society/American College of Radiology, Chicago, IL, December 1997, 33–34.

Anon. The effect of vitamin E and beta carotene on the incidence of lung cancer and other cancers in male smokers. The Alpha-Tocopherol, Beta Carotene Cancer Prevention Study Group. *N Engl J Med* 1994;330(15):1029–1035.

Awad A. Plant-based fat inhibits growth of breast-cancer cell line, UB researchers show. University of Buffalo press release, April 29, 1999a.

Awad A. Plant-based fat inhibits cancer-cell growth by enhancing cell's signaling system, UB researchers show. University of Buffalo press release, April 29,1999b.

Balch JF, Balch PA. Prescription for Nutritional Healing, New York: Avery Publishing Group, 1997.

Baron JA, Cole BF, Mott L, et al. Neoplastic and antineoplastic effects of beta-carotene on colorectal adenoma recurrence: results of a randomized trial. *J Natl Cancer Inst* 2003;95(10): 717–722.

Bendich A, Langseth L. The health effects of vitamin C supplementation: a review. *J Am Coll Nutr* 1995; 14:124–136.

Block G, Patterson B, Subar A. Fruit, vegetables and cancer prevention: a review of the epidemiological evidence. *Nutr. Cancer* 1992;18:1–29.

Bohlke K, Spiegelman D, Trichopoulou A, Katsouyanni K, Trichopoulos D. Vitamins A, C, and E and the risk of breast cancer: results from a case-control study in Greece. *Br.J.Cancer* 1999;79(1):23–29.

Bouic PJD, Etsebeth S, Liebenberg RW, et al. Beta-sitosterol and beta-sitosterol glycoside stimulate human peripheral blood lymphocyte proliferation: implications for their use as an immunomodulatory vitamin combination. *Int J Immunopharmacol* 1996:18:693–700.

Bouic PJD. Plant sterols and sterolins: a review of their immune-modulating properties. *Altern Med Rev* 1999;4:170–177.

Boynes C. A case of canine mast cell neoplasia. *Biological Therapy Journal of Natural Medicine* 1991. June;9(3):pp 155–6.

Broadhurst CL. *Nutrition Science News*, July 2001, Vol. 6, No. 7, p 262.

Brooks JD, Thompson LU. Mammalian lignans and genistein decrease the activities of aromatase and 17 beta-hydroxysteroid dehydrogenase in MCF-7 cells. *J Steroid Biochem Mol Biol.* 2005;94(5):461–467.

Burk RF, Levander OA. Selenium. In: Shils M, Olson JA, Shike M, Ross AC, eds. Nutrition in Health and Disease. 9th ed. Baltimore: Williams and Wilkins; 1999:265–276.

Burri BJ. Carotenoids and gene expression. *Nutrition* 2000 Jul-2000 Aug 31;16(7–8):577–8.

Cameron E, Pauling L. Supplemental ascorbate in the supportive treatment of cancer: Prolongation of survival times in terminal human cancer. *Proc Natl Acad Sci U S A.* 1976;73(10): 3685–3689.

Charlton CJ, Smith BHE, O'Reilly JD, Rock E, Mazur A, Treunov E, Harper EJ. Dietary carotenoid absorption in the domestic cat. *FASEB J.* 2000; 14:363.15.

Cima J. Biochemical Blood Chemistry Evaluation, Palm Beach Gardens, FL., March 2000.

Clin Exp Pharmacol Physiol. 2004 Jan–Feb;31(1–2):65–9.

Cornell KK. Cancer Biology: Targets for intervention, Nutrition and cancer regulation, The Iams Company, Dayton Ohio, 2006.

Craveri F, De Pascale V. Activity of orally administered adrenocortical extract. I. Effect on the survival test. *Boll Chim Farm* 1971;110:457–62.

Creagan ET, Moertel CG, O'Fallon JR, et al. Failure of high-dose vitamin C (ascorbic acid) therapy to benefit patients with advanced cancer. *N Engl J Med.* 1979;301(13):687–690.

Davenport D. Hill's Science and Technology Center. 2000, Topeka, KS, USA.

Davenport D. Hill's Science and Technology Center. Topeka, KS, USA. Ogilvie G. Comparative Oncology Unit College of Veterinary Medicine and Biomedical Sciences Colorado State University, Ft. Collins, CO, USA. 2000. The Management of Canine Cancer, Hills Pet Food, Topeka, KS.

Duke J. Handbook of biologically active phytochemicals and their activities. Boca Raton, FL: CRC Press; 1992. p 99, 131.

Duthie SJ, Ma A-G, Ross MA, Collins AR. Antioxidant supplementation decreases oxidative DNA damage in human lymphocytes. *Cancer Res* 1996; 56:1291–1295.

Ehrenpreis ED, Jani A, Levitsky J, Ahn J, Hong J. A prospective, randomized, double-blind, placebo-controlled trial of retinol palmitate (vitamin A) for symptomatic chronic radiation proctopathy. *Dis.Colon Rectum* 2005;48(1):1–8.

Feiz HR, Mobarhan S. Does vitamin C intake slow the progression of gastric cancer in Helicobacter pylori-infected populations? *Nutr Rev.* 2002;60(1):34–36.

Folkers K, et al. Biochemical Rationale and Mitochondrial Tissue Data on the Effective Therapy of Cardiomyopathy with Coenzyme Q10. *Proc. Nat'l. Acad. Sci.* 1985;82: 901.

Folkers K, Shizukuishi S, Takemura K, et al. Increase in levels of IgG in serum of patients treated with coenzyme Q10. *Res Commun Pathol Pharmacol* 1982;38:335–8.

Fox AD, et al. Effect of glutamine supplemented enteral diet on methotrexate induced enterocolitis, *JPEN* 1988;12:325–331.

Gaby AR. Coenzyme Q10. In: Pizzorno JE, Murray MT. *A Textbook of Natural Medicine*. Seattle: Bastyr University Press, 1998, V:CoQ10-1–8.

Gao YH, Zhou SF. Chemopreventive and Tumoricidal Properties of Ling Zhi Mushroom *Ganoderma lucidum* (W.Curt.: Fr.)Lloyd (Aphyllophoromycetideae). Part II. Mechanism Considerations (Review). *International Journal of Medicinal Mushrooms* 2004;vol 6 issue 3.

Gaziano JM, et al. A prospective study of consumption of carotenoids in fruits and vegetables and decreased cardiovascular mortality in the elderly. *Ann Epidemiol* 1995 Jul;5(4): 255–60.

Golde DW. Vitamin C in cancer. *Integr Cancer Ther* 2003;2(2):158–159.

Goldstein R, et al. The BNA Handbook: A Working Manual for Veterinarians, Westport, CT: Animal Nutrition Technologies, 2000.

González MJ, Miranda-Massari JR, Mora EM, Guzmán A, Riordan NH, Riordan HD, Casciari JJ, Jackson JA, Romá-Franco A. Orthomolecular oncology review: Ascorbic acid and cancer 25 years later. *Integ Cancer Ther* 2005.4(1):pp 32–44.

Graber G, Kendall R. N,N-Dimethylglycine and Use in Immune Response, US Patent 4,631,189, Dec 1986.

Greenberg ER, Baron JA, Tosteson TD, et al. A clinical trial of antioxidant vitamins to prevent colorectal adenoma. Polyp Prevention Study Group. *N Engl J Med* 1994;331(3): 141–147.

Harman D. Aging: A theory based on free radical and radiation chemistry. *Univ. Calif. Rad. Lab. Report No. 3078*, 1955.July 14.

Harman D. Free radical theory of aging. In: Emerit I, Chance B eds. Free Radicals and Aging. Birkhauser Verlag, Basel, 1992.

Hartleb M, Leuschner J. Toxicological profile of a low molecular weight spleen peptide formulation used in supportive cancer therapy. *Arzneimittelforschung* 1997;47:1047–51.

Heinonen OP, Albanes D, Virtamo J, et al. Prostate cancer and supplementation with alpha-tocopherol and beta-carotene: incidence and mortality in a controlled trial. *J Natl Cancer Inst* 1998;90(6):440–446.

Helzlsouer KJ, Huang HY, Alberg AJ, et al. Association between alpha-tocopherol, gamma-tocopherol, selenium, and subsequent prostate cancer. *J Natl Cancer Inst.* 2000;92(24): 2018–2023.

Hunter DJ, Manson JE, Colditz GA et al. A prospective study of the intake of vitamins C, E, and A and the risk of breast cancer. *N Engl J Med* 1993; 329:234–240.

Ito Y, et al. A study of serum carotenoids levels in breast cancer in Indian women in Chenni, India. *J Epidemiol* 1999 Nov: 9(5): 306–14.

Jacobs EJ, Connell CJ, McCullough ML, et al. Vitamin C, vitamin E, and multivitamin supplement use and stomach cancer mortality in the Cancer Prevention Study II cohort. *Cancer Epidemiol Biomarkers Prev* 2002; 11:35–41.

Kang SD, Lee BH, Yang JH, Lee CY. The effects of calf-thymus extract on recovery of bone marrow function in anticancer chemotherapy. *New Med J* 1985;28:11–5.

Keefe KA, Schell MJ, Brewer C, et al. A randomized, double blind, Phase III trial using oral beta-carotene supplementation for women with high-grade cervical intraepithelial neoplasia. *Cancer Epidemiol Biomarkers Prev* 2001;10(10):1029–1035.

Kendall R, Lawson J. Treatment of Melanoma Using N,N-Dimethylglycine, US Patent 4,994,492, Feb 1991.

Kendall RV. Building Wellness with DMG, Topanga, CA: Freedom Press, 2003.

Kendall R, Lawson JW. Recent Findings on N,N-Dimethylglycine (DMG): A Nutrient for the New Millennium. *Townsend Letter for Doctors and Patients*, 2000. May.

Kleinsmith LJ, Kerrigan D, Kelly J. Science Behind the News: Understanding Estrogen Receptors, Tamoxifen and Raloxifene. National Cancer Institute. January, 2003. http://press2.nci.nih.gov/sciencebehind/estrogen/estrogen01.htm. Accessed April 5, 2004.

Klimberg VS, et al. Does glutamine facilitate chemotherapy while reducing toxicity? *Surg Forum* 1991;42:16 *Jiangsu* 18.

Klimberg VS, et al. Effect of supplemental dietary glutamine on methotrexate concentration in tumors, *Arch Surg* 1992;127: 1317 *Jiangsu* 1322.

Klimberg VS, et al. Glutamine, cancer, and its therapy. *Am J Surg*, 1996;172:418–424.

Klimberg VS. How glutamine protects the gut during irradiation, *ICCN*, 1996;3:21.

Knekt P, Jarvinen R, Seppanen R, et al. Dietary flavonoids and the risk of lung cancer and other malignant neoplasms. *Am J Epidemiol* 1997;146:223 *Jiangsu* 30.

Knekt P, Kumpulainen J, Jarvinen R, et al. Flavonoid intake and risk of chronic diseases. *Am J Clin Nutr.* 2002;76(3): 560–568.

Kodama N, Komuta K, Nanba H. Effect of Maitake (Grifola fondosa) D-Fraction on the Activation of NK Cells in Cancer Patients, *J of Medicinal Foods*, 6(4) 2003, 371–377.

Kouttab NM, Prada M, Cazzola P. Thymomodulin: biological properties and clinical applications. *Med Oncol Tumor Pharmacother* 1989;6:5–9 [review].

Lee IM, Cook NR, Manson JE, et al. Randomized beta-carotene supplementation and incidence of cancer and cardiovascular disease in women: is the association modified by baseline plasma level? *Br J Cancer* 2002;86(5):698–701.

Lee KW, Lee HJ, Kang KS, et al. Preventive effects of vitamin C on carcinogenesis. *Lancet* 2002; 359:172.

Leung PY, Miyashita K, Young M, Tsao CS. Cytotoxic effect of ascorbate and its derivative on cultured malignant and nonmalignant cell lines. *Anticancer Research*. 1993;13:47–80.

Lockwood K, Moesgaard S, Yamamoto T, Folkers K. Progress on therapy of breast cancer with vitamin Q10 and the regression of metastases. *Biochem Biophys Res Commun* 1995;212: 172–7.

Malafa MP, Fokum FD, Mowlavi A, Abusief M, King M. Vitamin E inhibits melanoma growth in mice. *Surgery*. 2002;131(1):85–91.

Malafa MP, Neitzel LT. Vitamin E succinate promotes breast cancer tumor dormancy. *J Surg Res.* 2000;93(1):163–170.

Mani S, Lawson JW. Partial fractionation of Perna and the effect of Perna and Dimethylglycine on immune cell function and melanoma cells. South Carolina Statewide Research Conference, Charleston, SC 1999.Jan 3–5.

Mani S, Whitesides J, Lawson J. Role of Dimethylglycine in Melanoma Inhibition—Abstract from Nutrition and Cancer Prevention: American Institute for Cancer Research, 1999. Sept.

Masoro EJ. Theories of aging. In: Yu, BY, ed. Free Radicals in Aging, Boca Raton, FL: CRC Press, Inc. LJ 1993.

McCullough FS, Northrop-Clewes CA, Thurnham DI. The effect of vitamin A on epithelial integrity. *Proc. Nutr. Soc.* 1999;58(2):289–293.

Michaud DS, Pietinen P, Taylor PR, et al. Intakes of fruits and vegetables, carotenoids and vitamins A, E, C in relation to the risk of bladder cancer in the ATBC cohort study. *Br J Cancer* 2002;87(9):960–965.

Michels KB, Holmberg L, Bergkvist L, Ljung H, Bruce, A, Wolk A. Dietary antioxidant vitamins, retinol, and breast cancer incidence in a cohort of Swedish women. *Int.J.Cancer* 2-15-2001;91(4):563–567.

Middleton E Jr, Kandaswami C. The impact of plant flavonoids on mammalian biology: implications for immunity, inflammation and cancer; Chapter 15. In: Harbourne JB, ed. The flavonoids: advances in research since 1986. London: Chapman and Hall, 1993;619–652.

Middleton E Jr. Effect of flavonoids on basophil histamine release and other secretory systems. *Prog Clin Biol Res.* 1986;213:493–506.

Middleton E, Kandaswami C. Effects of flavonoids on immune and inflammatory cell functions. *Biochem Pharmacol* 1992;43(6):1167–1179.

Miodini P, Fioravanti L, di Fronzo G, Capelletti V. The two phyto-oestrogens genistein and quercetin exert different effects on oestrogen receptor function. Br J Cancer 1999;80: 1150–5.

Moertel CG, Fleming TR, Creagen ET, et al. High-dose vitamin C versus placebo in the treatment of patients with advanced cancer who have had no prior chemotherapy: a randomized double-blind comparison. *N Engl J Med* 1985; 312:137–141.

Myhrstad MC, Carlsen H, Nordstrom O, et al. Flavonoids increase the intracellular glutathione level by transactivation of the gamma-glutamylcysteine synthetase catalytical subunit promoter. *Free Radic Biol Med* 2002; Mar 1;32(5):386–93.

Nanba H, Hamaguchi AM, Kuroda H. The chemical structure of an antitumor polysaccharide in fruit bodies of *Grifola frondosa* (maitake). *Chem Pharm Bull* 1987;35:1162–8.

Nariba H. Antitumor Activity of Orally Administered "D-Fraction" from Maitake mushroom (Grifola frondosa), *J. of Nat. Med.* 1993.1(4):10–15.

Neuzil J, Weber T, Schroder A, et al. Induction of cancer cell apoptosis by alpha-tocopheryl succinate: molecular pathways and structural requirements. *FASEB J.* 2001;15(2):403–415.

Nishino H, et al. Cancer prevention by carotenoids. *Biofactors* 2000;13:89.

Ogilvie G. The Management of Canine Cancer. Topeka, KS: Hill's Pet Food, 2000.

Ogilvie GK, Vail DM. Advances in nutritional therapy for the cancer patient. *Veterinary Clinics of North America: Small Animal Practice* 1990; 20: 969–985.

Ogilvie GK, MJ Fettman, CH Mallinckrodt, JA Walton, RA Hansen, DJ Davenport, KL Gross, KL Richardson, QR Rogers, MS Hand. Effect of fish oil, arginine, and doxorubicin chemotherapy on remission and survival time in dogs with lymphoma. *Cancer* 2000;88:1916–1928.

Omenn GS, Goodman GE, Thornquist MD, Balmes J, Cullen MR, Glass A, Keogh JP, Meyskens FL, Valanis B, Williams JH, Barnhart S, Hammar S. Effects of a combination of beta carotene and vitamin A on lung cancer and cardiovascular disease. *N.Engl.J.Med.* 5-2-1996;334(18):1150–1155.

Opara EC. Antioxidants—The latest weapon in the war on smoking. *VRP Nutritional News* 1997; Vol 11 (July).

Panthong A, Kanjanapothi D, Tuntiwachwuttikul P, et al. Anti-inflammatory activity of flavonoids. *Phytomedicine* 1994;1:141–144.

Park YS, Lee JH, Bondar J, et al. Cytotoxic action of acetyl-11-keto-beta-boswellic acid (AKBA) on meningioma cells. *Planta Med.* 2002;68:397–401.

Pegel KH. The importance of sitosterol and sitosterolin in human and animal nutrition. *South African Journal of Science* 1997;June 93:263–268.

Planta Med, 2000 Feb; 66(1): 74–6.

Rayman MP, Clark LC. Selenium in cancer prevention. In: Roussel AM, ed. Trace elements in man and animals. 10th ed. New York: Plenum Press; 2000:575–580.

Reap E, Lawson J. The Effects of Dimethylglycine on B-16 Melanoma in Mice. Annual Meeting of the American Soc. of Microbiology, Oct. 1988.

Reap E, Lawson J. Stimulation of the Immune Response by Dimethylglycine, a non-toxic metabolite. *Journal of Laboratory and Clinical Medicine.* 1990;115:481.

Reich R, et al. Eicosapentanoic Acid Reduces the Invasive and Metastatic Activities of Malignant Tumor Cells. *Biochemical and Biophysical Res. Comm.* 1989.160:2, 59.

Riordan NH, Riordan HD, Meng X, LI Y, Jackson JA. Intravenous Ascorbate as a Tumor Cytotoxic Chemotherapeutic Agent. *Medical Hypotheses* 1995, March, Volume 44, Number 3, pp. 207–213.

Robinson N. Antioxidants' Effects on Cancer Therapy Unclear, *Veterinary Practice News* 2006; Oct p 20.

Roger CR. The nutritional incidence of flavonoids: some physiologic and metabolic considerations. *Experientia* 1988;44(9):725–804.

Rombeau J. A review of the effects of glutamine-enriched diets on experimentally induced enterocolitis. *J Parental and Enteric Nutrition* 1990;14 (4):100s–105s.

Ru G, Terracini B, Glickman LT. Host related risk factors for canine osteosarcoma. *Vet J.* 1998. Jul;156(1):31–9.

Russell RM. The vitamin A spectrum: from deficiency to toxicity. *Am.J.Clin.Nutr.* 2000;71(4):878–884.

Sakaguchi M, et al. Reduced Tumor Growth of Human Colonic Cancer Cell Lines COLO-320 and HT29- in Vivo by Dietary n-3 Lipids. *British J. of Cancer.* 1990;62:5, 742–747.

Schneider R. Comparison of age- and sex-specific incidence rate patterns of the leukemia complex in the cat and the dog. *J Natl Cancer Inst.* 1983. May;70(5):pp 971–7.

Schulof RS. Thymic peptide hormones: basic properties and clinical applications in cancer. *Crit Rev in Oncol Hematol* 1985;3:309–76.

Semba RD. The role of vitamin A and related retinoids in immune function. *Nutr.Rev.* 1998;56(1 Pt 2):S38–S48.

Serraino M, Thompson LU. The effect of flaxseed supplementation on the initiation and promotional stages of mammary tumorigenesis. *Nutr Cancer.* 1992;17:153–159.

Shigeta Y, Izumi K, Abe H. Effect of coenzyme Q7 treatment on blood sugar and ketone bodies of diabetics. *J Vitaminol* 1966;12:293–8.

Shils ME, et al. Modern nutrition in health and disease: 8th ed. Philadelphia: Lea and Febiger, 1994. p 290.

Shoskes DA, Zeitlin SI, Shahed A, Rajfer J. Quercetin in men with category III chronic prostatitis: a preliminary prospective, double-blind, placebo-controlled trial. *Urology* 1999;54: 960–3.

Singh VK, Biswas S, Mathur KB, et al. Thymopentin and splenopentin as immunomodulators. Current status. *Immunol Res* 1998;17:345–68 [review].

Singh S, Khar A. Biological effects of curcumin and its role in cancer chemoprevention and therapy. *Anticancer Agents in Medicinal Chemistry,* 2006;6(3):259–270.

Slattery ML, et al. Carotenoids and colon cancer. *Am. J. Clin. Nutr.* 2000 Feb: 71(2), 575–82.

Sung MK, Lautens M, Thompson LU. Mammalian lignans inhibit the growth of estrogen-independent human colon tumor cells. *Anticancer Res.* 1998;18:1405–1408.

Thompson LU. Experimental studies on lignans and cancer. *Baillieres Clin Endocrinol Metab.* 1998;12:691–705.

Thompson LU, Rickard SE, Orcheson LJ, et al. Flaxseed and its lignan and oil components reduce mammary tumor growth at a late stage of carcinogenesis. *Carcinogenesis.* 1996;17: 1373–1376.

Thurnham DI, Northrop-Clewes CA. Optimal nutrition: vitamin A and the carotenoids. *Proc.Nutr.Soc.* 1999;58(2):449–457.

Toma S, Bonelli L, Sartoris A, et al. beta-carotene supplementation in patients radically treated for stage I-II head and neck cancer: results of a randomized trial. *Oncol Rep* 2003;10(6):1895–1901.

Traber MG. Does vitamin E decrease heart attack risk? Summary and implications with respect to dietary recommendations. *J Nutr.* 2001;131(2):395S–397S.

Volk HD, Eckert R, Diamantstein T, Schmitz H. Immunorestitution by a bovine spleen hydrosylate and ultrafiltrate. *Arzneimittelforschung* 1991;41:1281–5.

Wagner H, Proksch A. Immunostimulatory Drugs of Fungi and Higher Plants, Ecorpomic and Medical Plant Research, New York: Academic Press, 1985.

Wang C, Lawson J. The Effects on the Enhancement of Monoclonal Antibody Production. Annual Meeting of the American Soc. of Microbiology, Oct. 1988.

Wang LQ. Mammalian phytoestrogens: enterodiol and enterolactone. *J Chromatogr B Analyt Technol Biomed Life Sci.* 2002;777(1–2):289–309.

Ware WA, Hopper DL. 1999. Cardiac tumors in dogs: 1982–1995. *J Vet Intern Med.* Mar-Apr;13(2):pp 95–103.

Weber T, Lu M, Andera L, et al. Vitamin E succinate is a potent novel antineoplastic agent with high selectivity and cooperatively with tumor necrosis factor-related apoptosis-inducing ligand (Apo2 ligand) in vivo. *Clin Cancer Res.* 2002;8(3):863–869.

Yanez J, et al. Pharmacological evaluation of Glycoflex III and its ingredients on canine chondrocytes, Washington State University, North American Veterinary Conference, Orlando FL, 2007.

You H, Yu W, Munoz-Medellin D, Brown PH, Sanders BG, Kline K. Role of extracellular signal-regulated kinase pathway in RRR-alpha-tocopheryl succinate-induced differentiation of human MDA-MB-435 breast cancer cells. *Mol Carcinog.* 2002;33(4):228–236.

Yu W, Sanders BG, Kline K. RRR-alpha-tocopheryl succinate-induced apoptosis of human breast cancer cells involves Bax translocation to mitochondria. *Cancer Res.* 2003;63(10): 2483–2491.

Zeegers MP. Are retinol, vitamin C, vitamin E, folate and carotenoids intake associated with bladder cancer risk? Results from the Netherlands Cohort Study. *Br. J Cancer* 2001 Sep 28:85(7): 977–83.

Zhang S, Hunter DJ, Forman MR, et al. Dietary carotenoids and vitamins A, C, and E and risk of breast cancer. *J Natl Cancer Inst* 1999;91(6):547–556.

Chinese herbal medicine

Bo X, et al. *Journal of Science and Technology of TCM.* 1997;4(3):153–154, 175.

Chang Yong Zhong Yao Cheng Fen Yu Yao Li Shou Ce (A Handbook of the Composition and Pharmacology of Common Chinese Drugs), 1994; 1725:1728.

Chang Yong Zhong Yao Xian Dai Yan Jiu Yu Lin Chuan (Recent study and Clinical Application of Common Traditional Chinese Medicine), 1995; 165:166.

Chen Chun Xia. *Journal of Chinese Materia Medica.* 1986;16(4):40.

Chen YH, et al. *China Journal of Pharmacy.* 1999;34(5):305–307.

Du DJ, et al. The effects of 30 Chinese patent herbal formulas on the generation of tumor necrosis factors. *Journal of Pharmacology and Clinical Application of TCM.* 1990;6(5):27–29.

Du YT. Lu Jiao Jiao injection's effect on the phagocytosis of macrophagocytes in patients of mammary cancer. *Journal of Traditional Chinese Medicine.* 1981;(3):36.

Fu Jian Yi Xue Yuan Xue Bao (*Journal of Fujian University of Medicine*), 1964; 2: 21.

Gupta S, Zhang D, Yi J, Shao J. Anticancer Activities of Oldenlandia diffusa. *Journal of Herbal Pharmacotherapy,* 2004 volume 4 (1):21–33.

Higashikaze M, et al. CA. 1981;94:16805k.

Hu SK, et al. *China Journal of Medicine.* 1990;5(3):22–23.

Hu LP, et al. *Journal of Zhejiang College of TCM.* 1997;21(6):29–30.

Jiang Su Yi Yao (*Jiang Su Journal of Medicine and Herbology*), 1990;16 (9):513.

Jiang Su Yi Yao (*Jiangsu Journal of Medicine and Herbology*), 1976; 4:33.

Li L, et al. *Journal of Beijing Medical University*. 1999;22(3): 38–40.

Li XF, et al. In vitro anti-tumor effects of Dan Shen and Dan Shen compound injection. *Zhejiang Journal of Integrated Medicine*. 1999;9(5):291–292.

Liu ZP, et al. Shan Zha extracts. *Journal of Henan Medical University*. 1991;26(4):349–352.

Liu ZP, et al. Suppressive effects of Shan Zha extracts on human fetus lung 2BS cell and related cancerous cells. *Henan Journal of Oncology*. 1994;7(3):173–174.

Liu P, et al. *Journal of Pharmacology and Clinical Application of TCM*. 1998;14(3)25–26.

Liu Hui. *Journal of Stomatology*. 1999;19(2):60–61.

Liu WS, Xu K. TCM in Oncology. People's Health Press Oct. 2000 p442.

Lu SC, et al. *Journal of No. 1 Military Academy*. 1990;10(3): 267.

Lu Y, et al. Yi Yi Ren oil's anti-tumor effects. *Journal of Pharmacology and Clinical Application of TCM*. 1999;15(6):21–23.

Ming LY, Xing ZX, Huang R. Chinese Famous Doctors Secret Formulas for Chronic Terminal Illness. Guang Xi Science and Technology Press House, July 1999, p 768.

Modern TCM Pharmacology. Tianjin: Science and Technology Press; 1997.

Ren Min Wei Sheng Chu Ban She (*Journal of People's Public Health*), 1988; 302.

Shan Dong Zhong Yi Xue Yuan Xue Bao (*Journal of Shandong University School of Chinese Medicine*), 1980;1:30.

Shao Y, Ho C-T, Chin C-K, et al. Inhibitory activity of boswellic acids from *Boswellia serrata* against human leukemia HL-60 cells in culture. *Planta Medica*. 1998;64:328–331.

Shen Yang Yi Xue Yuan Xue Bao (*Journal of Shenyang University of Medicine*), 1980; (12): 11.

Shi Ren Bing. *Journal of Beijing University of TCM*. 1999;22(2):63–64.

Sun JH, et al. *China Journal of Hematology*. 1999;20(1):354–356.

Tang FQ, et al. Research on killing effects of Huang Lian and its formulas on human nasopharyngeal carcinoma cells. *Journal of Hunan College of TCM*. 1995;15(4):41–44.

Wang KW. Forecast of research on anti-cancer effects of Di Long capsules (912). *China Journal of Clinical Research on Tumor*. 1991;18(3):131–132.

Wang K, et al. *China Journal of Ocean Medicinal Products*. 1997;16(1):18–22.

Wu H, et al. *Journal of Chinese Patented Medicine*. 1996;18(5): 20–22.

Xin Yi Xue (*New Medicine*), 1975;4:193.

Xu QL, et al. *Shanghai Journal of Immunology*. 1996;16(3):141.

Xu ZP, et al. *Journal of Chinese Materia Medica*. 1999;30(7): 551–553.

Yao Li Shi Yan Fang Fa Xue (Research Methodology of Herbal Medicine), 1982; 363.

Yao Xue Tong Bao (*Report of Herbology*), 1985; (2): 74.

Ying ZZ, et al. *Journal of Shizhen Medicine*. 1999;10(10): 732–733.

Zhang JH. Yin Chen extract's effect on tumor cells. *Journal of Traditional Chinese Medicine Material*. 1998;21(7):366–367.

Zhao SL, et al. Amygdalin's effects on the activity of mice's splenic NK cells. *Journal of Shanxi College of Medicine*. 1993;24(1):14–16.

Zhe Jiang Zhong Yi Xue Yuan Xue Bao (*Journal of Zhejiang University of Chinese Medicine*), 1983;3:31.

Zhong Guo Yi Xue Ke Xue Xue Bao (*Journal of Chinese Medical Science University*), 1988; 10(1): 39.

Zhong Guo Yi Yao Bao (*Chinese Journal of Medicine and Medicinals*), 1985.

Zhong Guo Yao Li Xue Za Zhi (*Journal of Herbology and Toxicology*), 1985; 2(2): 127.

Zhong Liu Yu Fang Yan Jiu (*Tumor Prevention and Research*), 1973;1:31.

Zhong Liu Yu Zhi Tong Xun (*Journal of Prevention and Treatment of Cancer*), 1976; 2:40.

Zhong Xi Yi Jie He Za Zhi (*Journal of Integrated Chinese and Western Medicine*), 1984;5:285.

Zhong Xi Yi Jia He Za Zhi (*Journal of Integrated Chinese and Western Medicine*), 1985; 2:115.

Zhong Yao Xue (*Chinese Herbology*) 1998; 739:741.

Zi Ma, Ken-ichiro Otsuyama, Shangqin Liu, Saeid Abroun, Hideaki Ishikawa, Naohiro Tsuyama, Masanori Obata, Fu-Jun Li, Xu Zheng, Yasuko Maki, Koji Miyamoto, and Michio M. Kawano. Baicalein, a component of *Scutellaria* radix from Huang-Lian-Jie-Du-Tang (HLJDT), leads to suppression of proliferation and induction of apoptosis in human myeloma cells. *Blood*. 2005; 105:3312–3318.

Homotoxicology

Demers J. A holistic approach to treatment of cancer. *J Am Hol Vet Med Assoc*. 2005a.Jan–Mar;(23)4:p 31.

Demers J. A holistic approach to cancer. In: proceedings of AHVMA Annual Conference, on CD, Ogden, Utah 2005b.

Goldstein M. The Nature of Animal Healing. New York: Ballantine Books, 1999. pp. 250.

Goldstein M. Understanding the Cancer Patient. In: proceedings of Wisdom of the Past/Wisdom of the Future, American Holistic Veterinary Association Annual Conference, Sept 9–12, Williamsburg, PA, 2000. pp 138–141.

Goldstein R. Canine osteosarcoma study in progress. 2006. Personal unpublished communication.

Heine H. *Lehrbuch der Biologische Medizin: Groundregulation und Extrazellulare Matrix* (Textbook of Biological Medicine: Ground Regulation and Extracellular Matrix) 3rd ed. Hippokrates: Stuttgard GMBH: 2006. pp 116–147.

Ming LY, Xing ZX Huang R. Chinese Famous Doctors Secret Formulas for Chronic Terminal Illness. Guang Xi Science and Technology Press House, July 1999, p 768.

Nakouzi J, Smit A, Shelton B. Cancer and Chronic Disease. Recorded lecture series on CD. October, 2004. Heel USA.

Ogilvie GK, Fettman MJ, Mallinckrodt CH, Walton JA, Hansen RA, Davenport DJ, Gross KL, Richardson KL, Rogers QR, Hand MS. Effect of fish oil, arginine, and doxorubicin chemotherapy on remission and survival time in dogs with lymphoma. *Cancer* 2000;88:1916–1928.

Chapter Thirty-Three

IVM Cancer Treatment Protocols Presented by Cancer Type

ANAL GLAND TUMOR

General comments

Anal gland adenocarcinomas arise from the apocrine glands of the anal sacs and can be locally invasive and can spread to the lymph glands, particularly the sublumbar lymph nodes. These tumors are also often associated with hypercalcemia and can affect renal function (Meuten 1981). The recommended therapy is surgical excision along with chemotherapy. Adjunctive radiation therapy is recommended when there is metastasis to the regional lymph nodes. The average survival time is 6 to 15 months, depending upon whether or not there is metastasis (Thomas 1998, Richardson 2003, Williams 1997).

Nutrition

Apocrine tumors of the anal gland are both locally invasive and can spread to the regional lymph glands. Nutritional therapy focuses on reducing inflammation in the rectum, improving stool formation with added fiber, and supporting lymph drainage and circulation.

Homotoxicology

Anal gland tumors represent the Dedifferentiation Phase. Adenocarcinoma is a common malignancy and is often associated with paraneoplastic syndromes involving elevated calcium levels. These tumors often spread to the regional lymph node and can remain silent for long periods of time.

They are generally best treated when detected early and by broad surgical excision with attention to the patient's homotoxin load. Radiation may be needed. If it is used, see the oncology section in Chapter 34. When complete excision is not possible, where metastasis has occurred, or in the event that caregivers do not desire surgery or more invasive therapies, then homotoxicology can be used to improve quality of life. See the additional data in Chapter 34.

Authors' suggested protocols

Nutritional/gland therapy
Intestines and lymph support formulas: One-half tablet for 25 pounds of body weight BID.

Probiotic MPF: One-half capsule per 25 pounds of body weight with food.

Glutamine: Supports intestinal heath. The authors recommend Glutimmune® at one-fourth scoop per 25 pounds of body weight SID.

Chinese herbal medicine
Uro-G Plus: Can be used if the tumor is nonresectable, but is more effective if the tumor has been removed or debulked. The dose is 1 capsule per 10 pounds TID regardless of whether or not the mass has been debulked.

The authors recommend Uro-G Plus along with appropriate analgesics such as opioids or NSAIDs. Uro-G Plus contains apricot seed (Xing ren), asparagus (Tian men dong), astragalus (Huang qi), atractylodes (Bai zhu), barbat skullcap (Ban zhi lian), centipede (Wu gong), cremastra (Shan ci gu), hornet's nest (Feng fang), kelp (Kun bu), mastic (Ru xiang), milettia (Ji xue teng), oldenlandia (Bai hua she cao), oyster shell (Mu li), poria (Fu ling), salvia (Dan shen), scorpion (Quan xie), and subprostrata sophora root (Shan dou gen).

In addition to the herbs mentioned above, Uro-G Plus also contains angelica root (Dang gui), arisaema/bile (Dan nan xing), Chinese sage (Shi jian chuan), codonopsis (Dang shen), corydalis (Yan hu suo), eupolyphaga (Tu bie cong), glehnia root (Sha shen), houttuynia (Yu xing cao), licorice (Gan cao), lily bulb (Bai he), myrrh (Mo yao), ophiopogon (Mai men dong), panicled swallowwort root (Xu chang qing), prunella (Xia ku cao), pseudodanum (Qian hu), pseudotellaria (Tai zi shen), rehmannia cooked (Shu di huang) and raw (Sheng di huang), sargassum (Hai zao), scrophularia (Xuan shen), selaginellae doederleini (Shi shang bai), stemona (Bai bu), tortoise shell (Bie jia), and trichosanthes (Gua lou). These additional herbs increase the efficacy of the formula.

Homotoxicology during chemotherapy (Dose: 10 drops for 50-pound dog; 5 drops for cat or small dog)

Galium-Heel, Lymphomyosot, Ginseng compositum, BHI-Hemorrhoid: PO BID. In addition, hemorrhoid suppositories may help to alleviate local pain and irritation.

Tonsilla compositum, Pulsatilla compositum, Coenzyme compositum, Ubichinon compositum: 10 drops PO every 3 days.

Glyoxal compositum: 1 vial orally every 2 weeks.

Homotoxicology if no chemotherapy (Dose: 10 drops for 50-pound dog; 5 drops for cat or small dog)

Galium-Heel, Lymphomyosot, Ginseng compositum, BHI-Hemorrhoid: PO BID.

Galium-Heel, Lymphomyosot, Thyroidea compositum, Hepar compositum, Solidago compositum, Tonsilla compositum, Coenzyme compositum, Ubichinon compositum, Mucosa compositum: 10 drops PO BID every 3 days.

Glyoxal compositum: 1 vial orally every 2 weeks.

Product sources

Nutritional/gland therapy

Intestines and lymph support formulas: Animal Nutrition Technologies. **Alternatives:** Enteric Support—Standard Process Veterinary Formulas; NutriGest—Rx Vitamins for Pets.

Probiotic MPF: Progressive Labs. **Alternative:** NutriGest—Rx Vitamins for Pets.

Glutimmune: Well Wisdom, LLC. **Alternative:** L-Glutamine Powder—Thorne Veterinary Products.

Chinese herbal medicine/acupuncture

Uro-G Plus—Natural solutions, Inc.

Homotoxicology

BHI/Heel Inc.

REFERENCES

De Simone C, Vesely R, Bianchi SB, et al. The role of probiotics in modulation of the immune system in man and in animals. *Int J Immunother* 1993;9:23–8.

Meuten DJ, Cooper BJ, Capen CC, et al. Hypercalcemia associated with adenocarcinoma derived from the apocrine glands of the anal sac. *Vet Pathol* 1981;18:454–471.

Richardson RC. Adenocarcinoma, Anal Sac/Perianal/Rectal. In: Tilley L, Smith F. The 5-Minute Veterinary Consult: Canine and Feline, Blackwell Publishing, 2003.

Thomas RC, Fox LE. Tumors of the skin and subcutis. In: Morrison WB, ed. Cancer in dogs and cats: medical and surgical management. Baltimore: Williams and Wilkins, 1998: 489–510.

Williams LE. Response to chemotherapy in dogs with adenocarcinomas of the perineum: retrospective study 1985–1995. Paper presented at the annual meeting of the Veterinary Cancer Society, Chicago, IL, 1997.

FIBROSARCOMA (NATURALLY OCCURRING AND VACCINE-INDUCED)

General comments

Fibrosarcoma occurs in both dogs and cats; the common sites are the gums, lips, nasal sinuses, and skin. These tumors are usually slow growing and locally invasive, and tend not to metastasize. In cats, vaccine-induced sarcomas are now the more common form. They are usually much more aggressive and often metastasize. These tumors are found at the site of the vaccine and are more common after repeated vaccinations. The vaccine-induced tumors are believed to be an inflammatory process at the vaccination site (Kass 1996, Thompson 2003). Therapy is usually wide excision surgery along with radiation therapy (Evans 1989, Hahn 2003). Chemotherapy is palliative for fibrosarcomas (Hahn 2003). Survival times are approximately 1 year or longer; however, nasal and vaccine-induced tumors often carry a more guarded prognosis of 3 to 9 months (Evans 1989, Hahn 2003).

Nutrition

Fibrosarcoma is a dense, fairly avascular tumor. A combination of biological therapies and surgery results in the best prognosis. The nutritional therapy focuses on the immune system. With vaccine-induced tumors it is important to remove and neutralize the effects of prior vaccinations (see Section 6, Vaccinations, for more detailed information).

Note: Fibrosarcomas are often resistant and recurrent, and require a balanced immune effort for control. A metabolic and physiological blood evaluation is recommended to assess general glandular and immune health. This can help clinicians to formulate therapeutic nutritional protocols that address not only the cancer but associated organ disease and weaknesses that may be present (Cima 2000, Goldstein 2000) (see Chapter 2, Nutritional Blood Testing, for additional information).

Homotoxicology

Fibrosarcomas represent Dedifferentiation Phase disease. They are generally best treated by early detection and broad surgical excision (amputation may be advised). Radiation and chemotherapy are often recommended. If radiation is used, see the oncology section of Chapter 34. In cases where complete excision is not possible or where metastasis has occurred, or in the event that caregivers do not desire surgery or more invasive therapies, then homotoxicology can be used to improve quality of life. Injections in the region of the tumor should be avoided. In cases of vaccine-related fibrosarcoma, carefully evaluate the need for injections before proceeding.

Authors' suggested protocols

Nutritional/gland therapy

Immune and lymph support formulas: One-half tablet for 25 pounds of body weight BID.

Betathyme: 1 capsule for each 25 pounds of body weight BID (maximum, 2 capsules BID).

Maitake DMG: 1 ml per 25 pounds of body weight BID.

Chinese herbal medicine/acupuncture

Formula H85 Sarcoma: 1 capsule per 10 pounds of body weight TID. H85 Sarcoma contains astragalus (Huang qi), atractylodes (Bai zhu), barbat skullcap (Ban zhi lian), bupleurum (Chai hu), burreed tuber (San leng), centipede (Wu gong), Kelp (Kun bu), oldenlandia (Bai hua she cao), oyster shell (Mu li), pinellia (Ban xia), poria (Fu ling), red peony (Chi shao), scorpion (Quan xie), and zedoaria (E zhu). It also contains buttercup roots (Mao zao cao), citrus (Chen pi), codonopsis (Dang shen), fritillary bulb (Zhe bei mu), prunella (Xia ku cao), sargassum (Hai zao), uncaria (Gou teng), and white peony (Bai shao) to increase efficacy. It is more effective after surgical debulking.

Homotoxicology during chemotherapy (Dose: 10 drops for 50-pound dog; 5 drops for cat or small dog)

Galium-Heel, Lymphomyosot, Ginseng compositum, Zeel: PO BID.

Tonsilla compositum, Pulsatilla compositum, Coenzyme compositum, Ubichinon compositum: 10 drops PO every 3 days.

Glyoxal compositum: 1 vial orally every 2 weeks.

Homotoxicology if no chemotherapy (Dose: 10 drops for 50-pound dog; 5 drops for cat or small dog)

Galium-Heel, Lymphomyosot, Ginseng compositum, Zeel PO BID.

Galium-Heel, Lymphomyosot, Thyroidea compositum, Hepar compositum, Solidago compositum, Tonsilla compositum, Coenzyme compositum, Ubichinon compositum, Mucosa compositum, Discus compositum: 10 drops PO BID every 3 days.

Glyoxal compositum: 1 vial orally every 2 weeks.

Product sources

Nutritional/gland therapy

Immune and lymph support formulas: Animal Nutrition Technologies. **Alternatives:** Immune System Support—Standard Process Veterinary Formulas; Immuno Support—Rx Vitamins for Pets; Immugen—Thorne Veterinary Products.

Betasitosterol: Betathyme; Best for Your Pet. **Alternative:** Moducare—Thorne Veterinary Products.

Maitake DMG: Vetri Science.

Chinese herbal medicine/acupuncture

Formula H85 Sarcoma: Natural Solutions Inc.

Homotoxicology

BHI/Heel Inc.

REFERENCES

Cima J. Biochemical Blood Chemistry Evaluation, Palm Beach Gardens, FL. March 2000.

Evans SM, Goldschmidt M, McKee LJ, Harvey CE. Prognostic factors and survival after radiotherapy for intranasal neoplasms in dogs: 70 cases (1974–1985). *J Am Vet Med Assoc* 1989;194:1460–1463.

Goldstein R, et al. The BNA Handbook: A Working Manual for Veterinarians, Westport, CT: Animal Nutrition Technologies, 2000.

Hahn KA. Fibrosarcoma, Nasal and Paranasal Sinus. In: Tilley L, Smith F. The 5-Minute Veterinary Consult: Canine and Feline, Blackwell Publishing, 2003.

Hahn KA. Fibrosarcoma, Nasal and Paranasal Sinus. In: Tilley L, Smith F. The 5-Minute Veterinary Consult: Canine and Feline, Blackwell Publishing, 2003.

Kass PH, Barnes WG, Spangler WL, et al. Epidemiologic evidence for a causal relation between vaccination and fibrosarcoma tumorigenesis in cats. *J Am Vet Med Assoc* 1993;203:396–405.

Kass PH. Epidemiologic issues in the study of vaccine-associated sarcomas in cats. *Feline Pract* 1996;24:33.

Kodama N, Komuta K, Nanba H. Effect of Maitake (Grifola fondosa) D-Fraction on the Activation of NK Cells in Cancer Patients, *J of Medicinal Foods*, 6(4) 2003, 371–377.

Nanba H, Hamaguchi AM, Kuroda H. The chemical structure of an antitumor polysaccharide in fruit bodies of Grifola frondosa (maitake). *Chem Pharm Bull* 1987;35:1162–8.

Thompson JP. Vaccine-Associated Sarcoma. In: Tilley L, Smith F. The 5-Minute Veterinary Consult: Canine and Feline, Blackwell Publishing, 2003.

GASTRIC ADENOCARCINOMA

General comments

Gastric adenocarcinoma is a tumor of glandular origin that arises from the epithelial lining of the stomach.

Treatment is usually surgical excision; chemotherapy is ineffective. The prognosis is poor, with most survival times less than 1 year (Morrison 1998, Richardson 2003).

Nutrition

Gastric adenocarcinomas are aggressive, and biological therapies should be done in combination with surgical excision if at all possible. Therapeutic nutrition focuses upon reducing pain and inflammation as well as providing general support and enhancing immune function.

Note: Gastric adenocarcinoma is an aggressive tumor that often affects digestion and assimilation and promotes wasting. It is recommended that a metabolic blood analysis be performed to confirm or rule out organ involvement and to add additional appropriate gland and organ support when indicated (Cima 2000, Goldstein 2000) (see Chapter 2, Nutritional Blood Testing, for additional information).

Homotoxicology

This is a Dedifferentiation Phase disorder. Homotoxicology does not cure this condition, but patients may benefit from support of their biological processes through drainage, detoxification, and cellular support. Also see the protocol for adenocarcinoma.

Authors' suggested protocols

Nutritional/gland therapy

Immune and esophageal/stomach support formulas: One-half tablet for each 25 pounds of body weight BID.

Glutimmune: One-fourth scoop per 25 pounds of body weight SID.

Betathyme: 1 capsule for each 25 pounds of body weight BID (maximum, 2 capsules BID).

Gluta-DMG: 3 level scoops per 25 pounds of body weight, divided BID.

Chinese herbal medicine/acupuncture

Gastric tumor formula: 1 capsule per 10 pounds TID. Gastric tumor formula contains astragalus (Huang qi), atractylodes (Bai zhu), barbat skullcap (Ban zhi lian), burreed tuber (San leng), centipede (Wu gong), crataegus (Shan zha), curcuma root (Yu jin), kelp (Kun bu), oldenlandia (Bai hua she cao), oyster shell (Mu li), pinellia (Ban xia), salvia (Dan shen), scorpion (Quan xie) and zedoaria (E zhu). It also contains aconite root/chuan (Chuan wu), ark shell (Wa leng zi), bletilla tuber (Bai ji), chicken gizzard lining (Ji nei jin), citrus (Chen pi), codonopsis (Dang shen), corydalis tuber (Yan hu suo), cuttlebone (Hai piao xiao), fleece flower root (He shou wu), haematite (Dai zhe shi), inula (Xuan fu hua), laminaria (Hai dai), leaven (Shen qu), malt (Mai ya), melia (Chuan lian zi), prunella (Xia ku cao), pteropus (Wu ling zhi), rehm-

annia (Shu di huang), sargassum (Hai zao), and saussurea (Mu xiang). These herbs increase the potency of the supplement.

Homotoxicology during chemotherapy (Dose: 10 drops for 50-pound dog; 5 drops for cat or small dog)

Galium-Heel, Lymphomyosot, Ginseng compositum, Gastricumeel: PO BID.

Tonsilla compositum, Pulsatilla compositum, Coenzyme compositum, Ubichinon compositum: 10 drops PO every 3 days.

Glyoxal compositum: 1 vial orally every 2 weeks.

Homotoxicology if no chemotherapy (Dose: 10 drops for 50-pound dog; 5 drops for cat or small dog)

Galium-Heel, Lymphomyosot, Ginseng compositum, Gastricumeel: PO BID.

Galium-Heel, Lymphomyosot, Thyroidea compositum, Hepar compositum, Solidago compositum, Tonsilla compositum, Coenzyme compositum, Ubichinon compositum, Mucosa compositum: 10 drops PO BID every 3 days.

Product sources

Nutrition/gland therapy

Immune and esophageal/stomach support formulas: Animal Nutrition Technologies. **Alternatives:** Immune System Support—Standard Process Veterinary Formulas; Immuno Support—Rx Vitamins for Pets; Immugen—Thorne Veterinary Products.

Glutamine: Well Wisdom, LLC. **Alternative:** L-Gutamine Powder—Thorne Veterinary Products.

Betathyme: Best for Your Pet. **Alternative:** Moducare—Thorne Veterinary Products.

Chinese herbal medicine/acupuncture

Gastric Tumor Formula: Natural Solutions Inc.

Homotoxicology

BHI/Heel Inc.

REFERENCES

Cima J. Biochemical Blood Chemistry Evaluation, Palm Beach Gardens, FL. March 2000.

Goldstein R, et al. The BNA Handbook: A Working Manual for Veterinarians, Westport, CT: Animal Nutrition Technologies, 2000.

Morrison WB. Nonlymphomatous cancers of the esophagus, stomach, and intestines. In: Morrison WB, ed. Cancer in dogs and cats: medical and surgical management. Baltimore: Williams and Wilkins, 1998:551–558.

Richardson RC. Adenocarcinoma, Stomach, Small and Large Intestine, Rectal. In: Tilley L, Smith F. The 5-Minute Veterinary Consult: Canine and Feline, Blackwell Publishing, 2003.

HEART BASE TUMOR (CHEMODECTOMA)

General comments

One of the common causes of pericardial effusion is heart base tumors and hemangiosarcoma (See hemangiosarcoma). Surgery can be beneficial, especially is there is associated pericardial effusion. Chemotherapy is not recommended (Hamilton 2003, Morrison 1998).

Nutrition

Heart base tumors respond best to surgery in combination with nutritional therapies. Surgery is directed at the tumor and the pericardial effusion. Nutritional therapy focuses upon the improvement of circulation and cardiac output as well as general support of immune function.

Note: Because heart base tumors can affect multiple organ systems, a medical and physiological blood evaluation is recommended to assess general glandular health. This helps clinicians to formulate therapeutic nutritional protocols that address the pituitary and thyroid glands as well as organ disease that may be present (Cima 2000, Goldstein 2000) (see Chapter 2, Nutritional Blood Testing, for additional information).

Homotoxicology

These tumors respond poorly to surgery and chemotherapy. There is no literature documenting the use of homotoxicology for these tumors.

Authors' suggested protocols

Nutritional/gland therapy

Cardiac and immune support formulas: Contain taurine and L-carnitine. One-half tablet for each 25 pounds of body weight BID.

Vitamin E: 50 IU for each 15 pounds of body weight SID.

Coenzyme Q10: 25 mgs for each 25 pounds of body weight SID.

Quercetin tablets: 50 mgs for each 10 pounds of body weight SID.

Beyond essential fats: One-half teaspoon for every 35 pounds of body weight with food or

Oil of evening primrose: 1 capsule for every 25 pounds of body weight SID or

Hemp oil: 1 teaspoon for every 25 pounds of body weight with food BID.

Chinese herbal medicine/acupuncture

H60 Anticancer/generic and H38 Pleural effusion/cardiac tumor: 1 capsule of each formula per 10 pounds BID. This condition is unique in that there are no dietary restrictions.

H60 Anticancer/generic contains antler powder (Lu jiao shuang), astragalus (Huang qi), barbat skullcap (Ban zhi lian), centipede (Wu gong), coix (Yi yi ren), hornet's nest (Lu feng fang), poria (Fu ling), Reishi mushroom (Ling zhi), salvia (Dan shen), and scorpion (Quan xie). H60 Anticancer/generic also contains arisaema (Dan nan xing), cornus (Shan zhu yu), dandelion (Pu gong ying), dioscoria (Shan yao), ginseng (Ren shen), honeysuckle (Jin yin hua), licorice (Gan cao), mugwort (Liu ji nu), rehmannia (Shu di huang), and tortoise shell (Bie jia).

H38 Pleural effusion/cardiac tumor contains astragalus (Huang qi) and scutellaria (Huang qin). It also contains angelica root (Dang gui), codonopsis (Dang shen), dianthus (Qu mai), fritillaria (Bei mu), lily bulb (Bai he), ophiopogon (Mai men dong), pharbitis (Qian niu zi), platycodon root (Jie geng), talc (Hua shi), trichosanthes root (Tian hua feng), and white peony (Bai shao). These additional components improve the function of the formula.

Homotoxicology

For chemodectoma, add *Berberis homaccord* and appropriate cardiac and blood pressure agents based upon clinical status. See hemangiosarcoma and use those treatment recommendations as a starting place.

Product sources

Nutrition

Cardiac and immune support formulas: Animal Nutrition Technologies. **Alternatives:** Cardio Strength; Vetri Science; Canine Cardiac and Immune System Support—Standard Process; Formula CV and Immuno Support—Rx Vitamins for Pets, Immugen—Thorne Veterinary Products.

Coenzyme Q10: Vetri Science; Rx Vitamins for Pets; Integrative Therapeutics.

Quercetin: Source Naturals; Quercitone—Thorne Veterinary Products.

Beyond essential fats: Natura Health Products.

Oil of evening primrose: Jarrow Formulas.

Hemp oil: Nature's Perfect Oil.

Chinese herbal medicine/acupuncture

Formula H60 Anticancer/generic and H38 Pleural effusion/cardiac tumor: Natural Solutions Inc.

Homotoxicology

BHI/Heel Inc.

REFERENCES

Cima J. Biochemical Blood Chemistry Evaluation, Palm Beach Gardens, FL. March 2000.

Folkers K, et al. Biochemical Rationale and Mitochondrial Tissue Data on the Effective Therapy of Cardiomyopathy with Coenzyme Q10. Proc. Nat'l. Acad. Sci., 198582: 901.

Goldstein R, et al. The BNA Handbook: A Working Manual for Veterinarians, Westport, CT: Animal Nutrition Technologies, 2000.

Hamilton TA. Chemodectoma. In: Tilley L, Smith F. The 5-Minute Veterinary Consult: Canine and Feline, Blackwell Publishing, 2003.

Lockwood K, Moesgaard S, Yamamoto T, Folkers K. Progress on therapy of breast cancer with vitamin Q10 and the regression of metastases. *Biochem Biophys Res Commun* 1995;212:172–7.

Morrison WB. Nonpulmonary intrathoracic cancer. In: Morrison WB, ed. Cancer in dogs and cats: medical and surgical management. Baltimore: Williams and Wilkins, 1998:537–550.

HEMANGIOSARCOMA

General comments

Hemangiosarcoma is a malignancy of the cellular lining of blood vessels; the most common sites are the spleen, liver, heart, and skin. It is more common in dogs than cats (Morrison 1988, Scavelli 1985). Surgery alone or in combination with chemotherapy is the recommended therapy (Hamilton 2003, Johnson 1989, Ward 1994). The prognosis for heart, spleen, and liver is poor, with estimated survival times of 1 to 9 months. For skin tumors treated with surgery, the prognosis is much better and is often 1 to 2 years (Elmslie 2003).

Nutrition

Because hemangiosarcoma is a vascular, endothelial tumor, nutritional therapy focuses on reducing inflammation in the blood vessel system, providing nourishment, and enhancing immune function. Nutritional remedies that are anti-angiogenic are also included.

Note: Hemangiosarcoma is an aggressive tumor that originates in blood vessels and can initiate or metastasize to any organ. Therefore, it is recommended that a metabolic blood analysis be performed to confirm or rule out organ involvement and to add appropriate gland and organ support when indicated (Cima 2000, Goldstein 2000) (see Chapter 2, Nutritional Blood Testing, for additional information).

Homotoxicology

Hemangiosarcoma represents Dedifferentiation Phase disease. Metastasis at the time of diagnosis is common. Surgery, radiation, and chemotherapy may be needed. If radiation is used, see the oncology section of Chapter 34. Homotoxicology can be used to improve the quality of life in cases in which complete excision is not possible, metastasis has occurred, or the caregivers do not desire surgery or more invasive therapies.

Authors' suggested protocols

Nutritional/gland therapy

Splenic and liver:—Liver and immune support formulas: One-half tablet for every 25 pounds of body weight BID.

Skin—Skin and immune support formulas: One-half tablet for each 25 pounds of body weight BID.

Heart—Cardiac and immune support formulas: One-half tablet for each 25 pounds of body weight BID.

Vascustatin (anti-angiogenic): 1 capsule (250 mgs) per 20 pounds of body weight divided BID.

Imm Kine (immune enhancement): 50 mgs for each 25 pounds of body weight SID.

Quercetin tablets: 50 mgs for each 10 pounds of body weight SID.

Chinese herbal medicine/acupuncture

For splenic hemangiosarcoma, the authors recommend H83 Abdominal tumor. It can be started before surgery and continued afterward. If the patient is not capable of surviving the surgery it may be used as a sole therapeutic option. The dose is 1 capsule per 10 pounds TID.

Formula H83 Abdominal tumor contains agrimony (Xian he cao), astragalus (Huang qi), atractylodes (Bai zhu), barbat skullcap (Ban zhi lian), burreed tuber (San leng), centipede (Wu gong), cinnamon bark (Rou gui), kelp (Kun bu), mastic (Ru xiang), oldenlandia (Bai hua she cao), oyster shell (Mu li), poria (Fu ling), red peony (Chi shao), scorpion (Quan xie), and zedoaria (E zhu). In addition, it contains achyranthes (Niu xi), amber (Hu po), angelica root (Dang gui), Chinese sage (Shi jian chuan), cnidium (Chuang xiong), codonopsis (Dang shen), corydalis tuber (Yan hu suo), licorice (Gan cao), myrrh (Mo yao), notoginseng (San qi), peach kernel (Tao ren), pteropus (Wu ling zi), rehmannia (Sheng di huang), and rhubarb (Da huang) to increase efficacy.

For cutaneous hemangiosarcoma, the authors recommend Lymph "K." The dose is 1 capsule per 10 pounds TID. Lymph "K" contains astragalus (Huang qi), atractylodes (Bai zhu), barbat skullcap (Ban zhi lian), burreed tuber (San leng), centipede (Wu gong), coix (Yi yi ren), hornet's nest (Feng fang), kelp (Kun bu), mastic (Ru xiang), oldenlandia (Bai hua she cao), poria (Fu ling), salvia (Dan shen), scorpion (Quan xie), wolfberry (Gou qi zi), and zedoaria (E zhu). In addition to the herbs mentioned above, Lymph "K" contains arisaema pulvis

(Dan nan xing), codonopsis (Dang shen), cornus (Shan zhu yu), dioscorea (Shan yao), eupolyphaga (Tu bie cong), forsythia (Lian qiao), fritillaria (Bei mu), house lizard (Bi hu, Tian long, or Shou gong), myrrh (Mo yao), prunella (Xia ku cao), rehmannia (Shu di huang), sargassum (Hai zao), Selaginellae doederleini (Shi shang bai), silkworm (Jiang can), Typhonium gigantium rhizome (Bai fu zi), and white peony (Bai shao). These additional herbs increase the efficacy of the formula.

For cardiac hemangiosarcoma, the authors recommend H60 Anticancer/generic and H38 Pleural effusion/cardiac tumor (see Heart-Based Tumors). The dose is 1 capsule of each for every 10 pounds twice daily.

H60 Anticancer/generic contains antler powder (Lu jiao shuang), astragalus (Huang qi), barbat skullcap (Ban zhi lian), centipede (Wu gong), coix (Yi yi ren), hornet's nest (Lu feng fang), poria (Fu ling), Reishi mushroom (Ling zhi), salvia (Dan shen), and scorpion (Quan xie).

Homotoxicology during chemotherapy (Dose: 10 drops for 50-pound dog; 5 drops for cat or small dog)

Galium-Heel, Lymphomyosot, Ginseng compositum, Phosphor homaccord (if bleeding or liver involvement): PO BID.

BHI-Bleeding: Every 15 minutes in acute hemorrhage and then BID to QID PRN.

Tonsilla compositum, Placenta compositum, Pulsatilla compositum, Coenzyme compositum, Ubichinon compositum: 10 drops PO every 3 days.

Glyoxal compositum: 1 vial orally every 2 weeks.

Homotoxicology if no chemotherapy (Dose: 10 drops for 50-pound dog; 5 drops for cat or small dog)

Galium-Heel, Lymphomyosot, Ginseng compositum, Phosphor homaccord (if bleeding or liver involvement): PO BID.

BHI-Bleeding: PRN.

Galium-Heel, Lymphomyosot, Thyroidea compositum, Hepar compositum, Solidago compositum, Tonsilla compositum, Coenzyme compositum, Ubichinon compositum, Mucosa compositum: 10 drops PO BID every 3 days.

Glyoxal compositum: 1 vial orally every 2 weeks.

Placenta compositum: Give at intervals (every 2 to 4 weeks).

Product sources

Nutrition

Cardiac, liver, skin, and immune support formulas: Animal Nutrition Technologies. **Alternatives:** Immune System, Cardiac, Hepatic, and Dermal Support—

Standard Process Veterinary Formulas; CV Formula, Immuno, Hepato Support—Rx Vitamins for Pets; Bio-Cardio, Immugen, Hepagen—Thorne Veterinary Products; Cardio-Strength, Derma Strength—Vetri Science Laboratories.

Vascustatin and Imm Kine: Allergy Research.

Quercetin: Source Naturals; Quercitone—Thorne Veterinary Products.

Chinese herbal medicine

Formula H60 Anticancer/generic, H38 Pleural effusion/cardiac tumor and H83 Abdominal tumor, and Lymph "K": Natural Solutions, Inc.

Homotoxicology

BHI/Heel, Inc.

REFERENCES

Cima J. Biochemical Blood Chemistry Evaluation, Palm Beach Gardens, FL., March 2000.

Goldstein R, et al. The BNA Handbook: A Working Manual for Veterinarians, Westport, CT: Animal Nutrition Technologies, 2000.

Elmslie R. Hemangiosarcoma, Skin. In: Tilley L, Smith F. The 5-Minute Veterinary Consult: Canine and Feline, Blackwell Publishing, 2003.

Hamilton TA. Hemangiosarcoma, Spleen and Liver. In: Tilley L, Smith F. The 5-Minute Veterinary Consult: Canine and Feline, Blackwell Publishing, 2003.

Johnson KA, Powers BE, Withrow SJ, et al. Splenomegaly in dogs: predictors of neoplasia and survival after splenectomy. *J Vet Intern Med* 1989;3:160–166.

Morrison WB. Blood vascular, lymphatic, and splenic cancer. In: Morrison WB, ed. Cancer in dogs and cats: medical and surgical management. Baltimore: Williams and Wilkins, 1998:705–715.

Morrison WB. Hemangiosarcoma, Heart. In: Tilley L, Smith F. The 5-Minute Veterinary Consult: Canine and Feline, Blackwell Publishing, 2003.

Scavelli TD, Patnaik AK, Melhaff CJ, et al. Hemangiosarcoma in the cat: retrospective evaluation of 31 surgical cases. *J Am Vet Med Assoc* 1985;187:817–819.

Ward H, Fox LE, Calderwood-Mays MB, et al. Cutaneous Hemangiosarcoma in 25 dogs: a retrospective study. *J Vet Intern Med* 1994:8:345–348.

HEPATIC ADENOCARCINOMA

General comments

While the cause is not known, it is believed that hepatocellular adenocarcinomas are related to chronic inflammation or toxicity. Viral disease may predispose to neoplastic changes, too. Surgery is recommended if the cancer is not diffuse and throughout all lobes. Chemotherapy is generally ineffective. Antioxidant vitamins such as E and C along, with omega-3 fatty acids, are recommended. Prognosis is generally considered to be guarded and survival is about 1 year (Morrison 2003).

Nutrition

Surgery in combination with nutritional therapies is recommended for the best prognosis for hepatocellular tumors that are confined to a lobe. The therapeutic nutrition focuses on reducing inflammation, protecting and nourishing liver cells, and enhancing immune and detoxification functions.

Note: Because the liver is so vital to many of the bodily functions, it is recommended that a metabolic blood analysis be performed to confirm or rule out other organ involvement and to add appropriate gland and organ support when indicated (Cima 2000, Goldstein 2000) (see Chapter 2, Nutritional Blood Testing, for additional information).

Homotoxicology

Hepatic adenocarcinomas represent the Dedifferentiation Phase. Chemotherapy is often not terribly helpful in these cases because the neoplastic cells contain detoxification systems, which render the chemotherapy drugs less effective. Such cases are generally best treated by early detection and broad surgical excision with attention to the patient's homotoxin load. These cases can do surprisingly well. In cases where complete excision is not possible, where metastasis has occurred, or if caregivers do not desire surgery or more invasive therapies, then homotoxicology can be used to improve the quality of life. See the additional data under the adenocarcinoma protocol in the advanced homotoxicology chapter in this section.

Authors' suggested protocols

Nutrition

Liver and immune support formulas: One-half tablet for each 25 pounds of body weight BID.

Lecithin/phosphatidylcholine: One-fourth teaspoon for each 25 pounds of body weight BID.

Vitamin E: 50 IU for every 25 pounds of body weight SID.

Alpha-lipoic acid: 20 mg per 10 pounds of body weight SID.

SAMe: 20 mg/kg SID.

Chinese herbal medicine/acupuncture

H8 Hepatic tumor and H83 Abdominal tumor: 1 capsule of each formula per 10 to 20 pounds of body weight TID.

H8 Hepatic tumor contains astragalus (Huang qi), atractylodes (Bai zhu), barbat skullcap (Ban zhi lian), bupleurum (Chai hu), burreed tuber (San leng), centipede

(Wu gong), cremastra (Shan ci gu), curcuma root (Yu jin), ganoderma (Ling zhi), kelp (Kun bu), oldenlandia (Bai hua she cao), oyster shell (Mu li), poria (Fu ling), red peony (Chi shao), salvia (Dan shen), scorpion (Quan xie), wormwood (Yin chen), and zedoaria (E zhu). In addition to the herbs mentioned above, H8 Hepatic tumor contains alisma (Ze xie), blue citrus (Qing pi), corydalis (Yan hu suo), ginseng (Ren shen), leaven (Shen qu), licorice (Gan cao), malt (Mai ya), melia (Chuan lian zi), notoginseng (San qi), prunella (Xia ku cao), tortoise plastron (Gui ban), tortoise shell (Bie jia), and white peony (Bai shao). These herbs increase the efficacy of the formula.

H83 Abdominal tumor contains agrimony (Xian he cao), astragalus (Huang qi), atractylodes (bai zhu), barbat skullcap (Ban zhi lian), burreed tuber (San leng), centipede (Wu gong), cinnamon bark (Rou gui), kelp (Kun bu), mastic (Ru xiang), oldenlandia (Bai hua she cao), oyster shell (Mu li), poria (Fu ling), red peony (Chi shao), scorpion (Quan xie), and zedoaria (E zhu). In addition, it contains achyranthes (Niu xi), amber (Hu po), angelica root (Dang gui), Chinese sage (Shi jian chuan), cnidium (Chuang xiong), codonopsis (Dang shen), corydalis tuber (Yan hu suo), licorice (Gan cao), myrrh (Mo yao), notoginseng (San qi), peach kernel (Tao ren), pteropus (Wu ling zi), rehmannia (Sheng di huang), and rhubarb (Da huang) to increase efficacy.

Homotoxicology during chemotherapy (Dose: 10 drops for 50-pound dog; 5 drops for cat or small dog)

Chelidonium homaccord, Phosphor homaccord, Lymphomyosot, Ginseng compositum: PO BID.

Galium-Heel, Tonsilla compositum, Pulsatilla compositum, Coenzyme compositum, Ubichinon compositum: 10 drops PO every 3 days.

Glyoxal compositum: 1 vial orally every 2 weeks.

Homotoxicology if no chemotherapy (Dose: 10 drops for 50-pound dog; 5 drops for cat or small dog)

Chelidonium homaccord, Phosphor homaccord, Lymphomyosot, Ginseng compositum: PO BID.

Galium-Heel, Lymphomyosot, Thyroidea compositum, Hepar compositum, Solidago compositum, Tonsilla compositum, Coenzyme compositum, Ubichinon compositum, Mucosa compositum: 10 drops PO BID every 3 days.

Glyoxal compositum: 1 vial orally every 2 weeks.

Product sources

Nutrition

Liver and immune support formulas: Animal Nutrition Technologies. **Alternatives:** Hepatic and Immune System

Support—Standard Process Veterinary Formulas; Hepato and Immuno Support—Rx Vitamins for Pets; Hepagen, Immugen—Thorne Veterinary Products.

Alpha-lipoic acid: Progressive Labs.

SAMe: Nutramax Laboratories, Inc.

Lecithin/phosphatidylcholine: Designs for Health.

Chinese herbal medicine

H8 Hepatic tumor and H83 Abdominal: Natural Solutions, Inc.

Homotoxicology

BHI/Heel Corporation.

REFERENCES

Cima J. Biochemical Blood Chemistry Evaluation, Palm Beach Gardens, FL. March 2000.

Goldstein R, et al. The BNA Handbook: A Working Manual for Veterinarians, Westport, CT: Animal Nutrition Technologies, 2000.

Morrison WB. Hepatocellular Carcinoma (HCCA). In: Tilley L, Smith F. The 5-Minute Veterinary Consult: Canine and Feline, Blackwell Publishing, 2003.

LEIOMYOSARCOMA

General comments

Leiomyosarcoma is classified as a malignancy of the smooth muscle of the stomach or intestinal tract. This cancer may be locally invasive but it is a slow-growing malignancy. The treatment of choice is surgical excision.

Nutrition

Surgical excision along with nutritional therapy gives the best results for leiomyosarcomas. Nutritional therapy focuses on reducing inflammation, providing cellular protection, and enhancing immune function.

Note: Because cancer can affect multiple organ systems and is often a systemic disease, a metabolic and physiological blood evaluation is recommended to assess general glandular and immune health. This can help clinicians to formulate therapeutic nutritional protocols that address not only the cancer but associated organ disease and weaknesses that may be present (Cima 2000, Goldstein 2000) (see Chapter 2, Nutritional Blood Testing, for additional information).

Homotoxicology

Leiomyosarcomas represent the Dedifferentiation Phase. They are generally best treated by early detection and broad surgical excision.

Authors' suggested protocols

Nutritional/gland therapy

Immune, esophageal/stomach, or intestinal support formulas: One-half tablet for each 25 pounds of body weight BID.

Glutimmune: One-fourth scoop per 25 pounds of body weight SID.

Betasitosterol: 1 capsule for each 25 pounds of body weight BID (maximum, 2 capsules BID).

Gluta-DMG: 3 level scoops per 25 pounds of body weight, divided BID.

Chinese herbal medicine/acupuncture

Lymph "K": 1 capsule per 10 pounds of body weight TID. If the patient cannot tolerate surgery, Lymph "K" can be used as the sole therapy. The prognosis is better with surgical debulking.

Lymph "K" contains astragalus (Huang qi), atractylodes (Bai zhu), barbat skullcap (Ban zhi lian), burreed tuber (San leng), centipede (Wu gong), coix (Yi yi ren), hornet's nest (Feng fang), kelp (Kun bu), mastic (Ru xiang), oldenlandia (Bai hua she cao), poria (Fu ling), salvia (Dan shen), scorpion (Quan xie), wolfberry (Gou qi zi), and zedoaria (E zhu). In addition to the herbs mentioned above, Lymph "K" contains arisaema pulvis (Dan nan xing), codonopsis (Dang shen), cornus (Shan zhu yu), dioscorea (Shan yao), eupolyphaga (Tu bie cong), forsythia (Lian qiao), fritillaria (Bei mu), house lizard (Bi hu, Tian long, or Shou gong), myrrh (Mo yao), prunella (Xia ku cao), rehmannia (Shu di huang), sargassum (Hai zao), Selaginellae doederleini (Shi shang bai), silkworm (Jiang can), Typhonium gigantium rhizome (Bai fu zi), and white peony (Bai shao). These additional herbs increase the efficacy of the formula.

Homotoxicology during chemotherapy (Dose: 10 drops for 50-pound dog; 5 drops for cat or small dog)

Galium-Heel, Lymphomyosot, Ginseng compositum: PO BID to TID. Add Gastricumeel, Duodenoheel, or Nux vomica homaccord if gastrointestinal upset is present.

Tonsilla compositum, Pulsatilla compositum, Coenzyme compositum, Ubichinon compositum: 10 drops PO every 3 days.

Glyoxal compositum: 1 vial orally every 2 weeks.

Homotoxicology if no chemotherapy (Dose: 10 drops for 50-pound dog; 5 drops for cat or small dog)

Galium-Heel, Lymphomyosot, Ginseng compositum: PO BID to TID. Add Gastricumeel, Duodenoheel, or Nux vomica homaccord if gastrointestinal upset is present.

Galium-Heel, Lymphomyosot, Thyroidea compositum, Hepar compositum, Solidago compositum, Tonsilla compositum, Coenzyme compositum, Ubichinon compositum, Mucosa compositum: 10 drops PO BID every 3 days.

Product sources

Nutrition

Immune, esophageal/stomach, and intestinal support formulas: Animal Nutrition Technologies. **Alternatives:** Nutrigest—Rx Vitamins for pets; GI Complex—Professional Complementary Health.

Betathyme: Best for Your Pet; Moducare—Thorne Veterinary Products.

Gluta-DMG: Vetri Science.

Glutamine: Well Wisdom, LLC. **Alternative:** L-Gutamine Powder—Thorne Veterinary Products.

Chinese herbal medicine/acupuncture

Lymph X: Natural Solutions Inc.

Homotoxicology

BHI/Heel Inc.

REFERENCES

Cima J. Biochemical Blood Chemistry Evaluation, Palm Beach Gardens, FL. March 2000.

Goldstein R, et al. The BNA Handbook: A Working Manual for Veterinarians, Westport, CT: Animal Nutrition Technologies, 2000.

Morrison WB. Nonlymphomatous cancers of the esophagus, stomach, and intestines. In: Morrison WB, ed. Cancer in dogs and cats: medical and surgical management. Baltimore: Williams and Wilkins, 1998:551–558.

Richardson RC. Leiomyosarcoma, Stomach, Small and Large Intestine. In: Tilley L, Smith F. The 5-Minute Veterinary Consult: Canine and Feline, Blackwell Publishing, 2003.

LYMPHOMA/LYMPHOSARCOMA

General comments

Lymphosarcoma is one of the most common cancers of dogs and cats. Commonly affected breeds are Golden Retrievers, German Shepherds, Boxers, Scottish Terriers, and West Highland Whites. Suspected causes include genetic predisposition, viral, radiation, herbicides, and compromised immune function. Scientific references list lymphosarcoma as cause unknown.

The rationale for medical therapy is to achieve remission via a combination of cytotoxic chemotherapeutics and anti-inflammatory drugs such as cortisone. The goal is to kill off the cancer cells, thereby allowing normal, healthy cells to grow and repopulate the lymph system and tissues. Dietary recommendations include a low-carbohydrate diet with adequate and appropriate amounts of protein, essential n-3 fatty acid, and specific amino acids such as arginine (Anderson, Ogilvie 1997; Davenport, Ogilivie 1998). Hills has since introduced their Prescription Diet N/D, which follows the guidelines for protein, fat, carbohydrates, and amino acids described in this study (Hills Pet).

Remission is defined as the elimination of all detectable cancer. Most dogs that receive chemotherapy achieve a remission; the average remission time is reported to be 9 months and the average survival time is 1 year (Morrison 2002, 2004; Mutsaera 2002; Ogilvie 2000).

Integrative veterinary therapies

The lymph system, by definition, is a system of cells, tissue, and organs that protects the body from foreign invasion, and therefore is continually functioning in this capacity for the body. As the front line of protection, this system is often overworked and continually exposed to infectious organisms and toxins that can lead to continual inflammation, degeneration, and ultimately loss of control of cellular division.

While chemotherapeutics and cortisone are the recommended treatment, they are intended to destroy the cancer cells; they do not support the assimilation of nutrients, cellular metabolism, or the elimination of chemical and metabolic wastes and detoxification, nor are they intended to. These are the areas in which integrative veterinary therapies help improve the response to medication, protect the cells from chemicals and toxins, improve the day-to-day quality of life, and enhance remission probability and time.

Nutrition

Nutrition, antioxidants, and phytonutrients often are afterthoughts when it comes to the treatment of lymphoma. Lymphoma is a systemic cancer whereby the immune system is overwhelmed and loses its ability to control cell division. The supply of vital nutrients, replenishment of the antioxidants reserves, and proper diet are critical for long-term survival and improved quality of life. Lymphoma responds to chemotherapy and prednisone; therefore, offsetting and minimizing the side effects of chemotherapy and immune suppression helps with long-term remission and improved quality of life.

Note: Because lymphoma is systemic and can affect multiple organ systems, a metabolic and physiological blood evaluation is recommended to assess general glandular and immune health. This information helps clinicians to formulate therapeutic nutritional protocols that address not only the cancer but associated organ disease and weaknesses that may be present (Cima 2000, Goldstein 2000) (see Chapter 2, Nutritional Blood Testing, for additional information). Currently a clinical trial is being conducted to evaluate the benefits (day-to-day quality of life and longevity) of adding nutritional, biological, and herbal support to chemotherapy protocols for lymphoma (Goldstein, Post 2006).

Homotoxicology

Lymphosarcoma is a Dedifferentiation Phase disorder. Because this condition is right of the biological division, therapy is generally palliative. In lymphosarcoma, homotoxins have accumulated and damaged the cellular regulation processes sufficiently that neoplastic alterations manifest (Reckeweg 2000). Therapy is directed at removing cancer cells, reconditioning cellular organelles (especially energy production systems), draining toxic materials away from the diseased area, improving the microenvironment of the matrix, and improving detoxification and repair capabilities. Detoxification should not take place while a patient is receiving chemotherapy because this can reduce chemotherapy agent blood levels, and thus reduce killing of the targeted cancer cells (Smit 2004). Caution should be exercised when considering administration of agents, which could cause progressive vicariation. Overvaccination of these patients is not advised because it can cause the immune system to be overwhelmed, resulting in a sudden worsening of the patient's condition.

Authors' suggested protocols

Nutritional/gland therapy

Diet: See the dietary restrictions associated with the Chinese herbal medicine protocols in Chapter 32.

Lymph and blood/bone marrow support formulas: One-half tablet for each 25 pounds of body weight BID.

Maitake-DMG: 1 ml per 25 pounds of body weight, BID. For animals 15 pounds or less, one-half ml BID.

Betathyme: 1 capsule for each 35 pounds of body weight BID (maximum, 2 capsules BID).

Selenium: 20 micrograms for each 20 pounds of body weight SID (maximum, 100 mcg).

Quercetin tablets: 50 mgs for each 10 pounds of body weight SID.

Chinese herbal medicine

The authors use Lymphoma "AA" for nodal lymphoma. The dose is 1 capsule per 10 pounds of body weight TID. Lymphoma "AA" contains astragalus (Huang qi), atractylodes (Bai zhu), codonopsis (Dan shen), oyster shell (Mu li), poria (Fu ling), and wolfberry (Gou qi zi). It also contains alisma (Ze xie), angelica root (Dang gui), chry-

santhemum (Ju hua), cnidium (Chuan xiong), codonopsis (Dang shen), cornus (Shan zhu yu), dioscorea (Shan yao), lycium bark (Di gu pi), moutan (Mu dan pi), prunella (Xia ku cao), rehmannia/cooked (Shu di huang), rehmannia/ raw (Sheng di huang), tortoise plastron (Bie jia), and white peony (Bai shao) to increase the efficacy of the formula.

For cutaneous, gastrointestinal, or ocular lymphosarcoma, the authors use Lymph "K." The dose is 1 capsule per 10 pounds of body weight TID. Lymph "K" contains astragalus (Huang qi), atractylodes (Bai zhu), barbat skullcap (Ban zhi lian), burreed tuber (San leng), centipede (Wu gong), coix (Yi yi ren), hornet's nest (Feng fang), kelp (Kun bu), mastic (Ru xiang), oldenlandia (Bai hua she cao), poria (Fu ling), salvia (Dan shen), scorpion (Quan xie), wolfberry (Gou qi zi), and zedoaria (E zhu). It also contains arisaema pulvis (Dan nan xing), codonopsis (Dang shen), cornus (Shan zhu yu), dioscorea (Shan yao), eupolyphaga (Tu bie cong), forsythia (Lian qiao), fritillaria (Bei mu), house lizard (Bi hu, Tian long, or Shou gong), myrrh (Mo yao), prunella (Xia ku cao), rehmannia (Shu di huang), sargassum (Hai zao), Selaginellae doederleini (Shi shang bai), silkworm (Jiang can), Typhonium gigantium rhizome (Bai fu zi), and white peony (Bai shao) to increase the efficacy of the formula.

For nasal lymphosarcoma, the authors use H112 Nasal tumor. The dose is 1 capsule per 10 pounds of body weight TID. H112 Nasal tumor contains atractylodes (Bai zhu), barbat skullcap (Ban zhi lian), Dioscorea bulbifera bulb (Huang yao zi), oldenlandia (Bai hua she cao), oyster shell (Mu li), pinellia (Ban xia), and poria (Fu ling). In addition to the herbs listed above, H112 Nasal tumor includes buttercup herb (Mao zao cao), citrus (Chen pi), codonopsis (Dang shen), fritillary bulb (Bei mu), globe thistle (Lou lu), peach kernel (Tao ren), and prunella (Xia ku cao). These herbs increase the efficacy of the formula.

Homotoxicology during chemotherapy (Dose: 10 drops for 50-pound dog; 5 drops for cat or small dog)

Galium-Heel, Lymphomyosot: PO BID.

Tonsilla compositum, Pulsatilla compositum, Coenzyme compositum, Ubichinon compositum: 10 drops PO every 3 days.

Glyoxal compositum: 1 vial orally every 2 weeks.

Homotoxicology after chemotherapy (Dose: 10 drops for 50-pound dog; 5 drops for cat or small dog)

Galium-Heel, Lymphomyosot, Thyroidea compositum, Hepar compositum, Solidago compositum, Tonsilla compositum, Coenzyme compositum, Ubichinon compositum: 10 drops PO BID every 3 days.

Products

Nutrition

Lymph and blood/bone marrow support formulas: Animal Nutrition Technologies. **Alternative:** Immunstim Complex—Professional Complementary Health.

MAITAKE-DMG Liquid: Vetri Science.

Betathyme: Best for Your Pet. **Alternative:** Moducare—Thorne Veterinary Products.

Quercetin tablets: Source Naturals; Quercitone—Thorne Veterinary Products.

Chinese herbal medicine

Formulas Lymphoma AA, Lymph K, and H112 Nasal tumor: Natural Solutions Inc.

Homotoxicology

BHI/Heel Inc.

REFERENCES

Anderson CR, Ogilvie GK, Fettman MJ, et al. Effects of fish oil and arginine on acute effects of radiation injury in dogs with nasal tumors: A double-blind, randomized study. In: Proceedings. Veterinary Cancer Society/American College of Radiology, Chicago, IL, December 1997, 33–34.

Cima J. Biochemical Blood Chemistry Evaluation, Palm Beach Gardens, FL. March 2000.

Davenport D. The Management of Canine Cancer, Hills Pet Food, Topeka, KS.

Goldstein R, et al. The BNA Handbook: A Working Manual for Veterinarians, Westport, CT. Animal Nutrition Technologies, 2000.

Goldstein R, Post G. A clinical trial to evaluate chemotherapy in combination with an antioxidant rich nutritional program for the treatment of Lymphosarcoma and Osteosarcoma in dog, 2006.

Morrison WB. Cancer in Dogs and Cats: Medical and Surgical Management, Teton New Media; 2nd ed, September 1, 2002.

Morrison WB. Lymphoma in Dogs and Cats, Teton New Media, June 2004.

Mutsaers AJ, Glickman NW, DeNicola DB, Widmer WR, Bonney PL, Hahn KA, Knapp DW. Evaluation of treatment with doxorubicin and piroxicam or doxorubicin alone for multicentric lymphoma in dogs, *J Am Vet Med Assoc* 2002 Jun 15;220(12):1813–7.

Ogilvie GK, Fettman MJ, Mallinckrodt CH, Walton JA, Hansen RA, Davenport DJ, Gross KL, Richardson KL, Rogers QR, Hand MS. Effect of fish oil, arginine, and doxorubicin chemotherapy on remission and survival time in dogs with lymphoma. *Cancer* 2000;88:1916–1928.

MAMMARY ADENOCARCINOMA

General comments

Mammary adenocarcinoma is a common tumor of both dogs and cats; its cause is unknown. Hormonal influence may be causally involved because the incidence is lower in spayed females (Downing 2003; Hahn 1992; MacEwen 1996; Morrison 1998, 2003). The treatment of choice is wide surgical excision. Metastasis to the lungs should be ruled out in advance. Chemotherapy is more commonly recommended in cats than dogs (Jeglum 1985). The prognosis is often good with surgery; however, recurrences are common, especially in cats (Allen 1989).

Nutrition

Mammary adenocarcinoma (ductal and glandular) should be approached with a combination of surgical excision and nutritional support. Therapeutic nutrition focuses on reducing inflammation, helping to balance gland and hormonal function, and enhancing the immune system.

Mammary cancer frequently metastasizes to the lungs, making such animals poor surgical candidates. If this is the case and surgery is not an option, nutritional and biological therapies are still indicated.

Note: It is recommended that a metabolic blood analysis be performed to confirm or rule out organ involvement and to add appropriate gland and organ support when indicated (Cima 2000, Goldstein 2000) (see Chapter 2, Nutritional Blood Testing, for additional information).

Homotoxicology

Mammary adenocarcinomas represent the Dedifferentiation Phase. They are generally best treated by early detection and broad surgical excision. Early ovarectomy has been linked to reduced incidence of this tumor in dogs and cats. Ovariohysterectomy is commonly recommended by clinicians to reduce the number of cases encountered. Radiation may be needed; if so, see the oncology section of Chapter 34. In cases where complete excision is not possible, where metastasis has occurred, or when caregivers do not desire surgery or more invasive therapies, then homotoxicology can be used to improve quality of life.

Authors' suggested protocols

Nutritional/gland therapy

Lymphatic and female support formulas: One-half tablet for each 25 pounds of body weight BID.

Bronchus/lung support formula: One-half tablet for each 25 pounds of body weight SID.

Coenzyme Q10: 25 mgs for each 25 pounds of body weight SID.

Quercetin tablets: 50 mgs for each 10 pounds of body weight SID.

Chinese herbal medicine/acupuncture

H86 Mammosol: 1 capsule per 10 pounds of body weight TID. This formula may be used alone if the tumor is nonresectable, but it is more effective if the tumor has been debulked. Mammosol contains astragalus (Huang qi), barbat skullcap (Ban zhi lian), burreed tuber (San leng), centipede (Wu gong), coix (Yi yi ren), crataegus (Shan zha), cremastra (Shan ci gu), kelp (Kun bu), mastic (Ru xiang), milettia (Ji xue teng), oldenlandia (Bai hua she cao), oyster shell (Mu li), scorpion (Quan xie), wolfberry (Gou qi zi), and zedoaria (E zhu). In addition to the herbs mentioned above, H86 Mammosol contains angelica root (Dang gui), buffalo horn shavings (Shui niu jiao), citron fruit (Xiang yuan), epimedium (Yin yang huo), fleece flower root (He shou wu), leaven (Shen qu), malt (Mai ya), myrrh (Mo yao), notoginseng (San qi), prunella (Xia ku cao), pseudotellaria root (Tai zi shen), sargassum (Hai zao), and viola (Zi hua di ding). These herbs help improve the actions of the formula.

Homotoxicology during chemotherapy (Dose: 10 drops for 50-pound dog; 5 drops for cat or small dog)

Galium-Heel, Lymphomyosot, Ginseng compositum, Hormeel: PO BID.

Tonsilla compositum, Pulsatilla compositum, Coenzyme compositum, Ubichinon compositum: 10 drops PO every 3 days.

Glyoxal compositum: 1 vial orally every 2 weeks.

Homotoxicology if no chemotherapy (Dose: 10 drops for 50-pound dog; 5 drops for cat or small dog)

See additional data in the oncology section of Chapter 34.

Galium-Heel, Lymphomyosot, Ginseng compositum, Hormeel: PO BID.

Galium-Heel, Lymphomyosot, Thyroidea compositum, Hepar compositum, Solidago compositum, Tonsilla compositum, Coenzyme compositum, Ubichinon compositum, Mucosa compositum: 10 drops PO BID every 3 days.

Glyoxal compositum: 1 vial orally every 2 weeks.

Product sources

Nutrition
Lymphatic, female, and bronchus/lung support formulas (contain acceptable levels of antioxidant vitamins): Animal Nutrition Technologies.

Coenzyme Q10: Vetri Science; Rx Vitamins for Pets; Integrative Therapeutics.

Quercetin tablets: Source Naturals; Quercitone—Thorne Veterinary Products.

Chinese herbal medicine/acupuncture
Formula H86 Mammosol: Natural Solutions Inc.

Homotoxicology
BHI/Heel Inc.

REFERENCES

Allen SW, Mahaffey EA. Canine mammary neoplasia: prognostic indicators and response to surgical therapy. J Am Anim Hosp Assoc 1989;25:540–546.

Cima J. Biochemical Blood Chemistry Evaluation, Palm Beach Gardens, FL. March 2000.

Downing S. Mammary Gland Tumors—Cats. In: Tilley L, Smith F. The 5-Minute Veterinary Consult: Canine and Feline, Blackwell Publishing, 2003.

Goldstein R, et al. The BNA Handbook: A Working Manual for Veterinarians, Westport, CT: Animal Nutrition Technologies, 2000.

Hahn KA, Richardson RC, Knapp DW. Canine malignant mammary neoplasia: biological behavior, diagnosis, and treatment alternatives. J Am Anim Hosp Assoc 1992;28:251–256.

Jeglum KA, DeGuzman E, Young KM. Chemotherapy of advanced mammary adenocarcinoma in 14 cats. J Am Vet Med Assoc 1985;187:157–160.

MacEwen EG, Withrow SJ. Tumors of the mammary gland. In: Withrow SJ, MacEwen EG, eds. Small animal clinical oncology. 2nd ed. Philadelphia: Saunders, 1996;365–372.

Morrison WB. Canine and feline mammary tumors. In: Morrison WB, ed. Cancer in dogs and cats: medical and surgical management. Baltimore: Williams and Wilkins, 1998:591–598.

Morrison WB, Hahn KA. Mammary Gland Tumors–Dogs. In: Tilley L, Smith F. The 5-Minute Veterinary Consult: Canine and Feline, Blackwell Publishing, 2003.

MAST CELL TUMOR

General comments

Mast cell tumor is a malignancy that can occur in multiple locations in the body; the common sites are the skin, spleen, and gastrointestinal tract (Elmslie 2003, Molander-McCray 1998). The treatment of choice is wide surgical excision, chemotherapy, radiation therapy, and prednisone (McCaw 1984). The prognosis is always guarded with grade III tumors. Grade I and II tumors often respond well to the above therapies (Elmslie 2003, Fox 1998, Patnaik 1984).

Nutrition

Grade I and II mast cell tumors respond well to integrative therapies and surgical excision. Grade III tumors require a much more intensive integrative program. Because mast cell tumors are made up of one of the body's normal cellular components, nutritional therapies focus on the immune system and reducing inflammation.

Note: Mast cell tumors, and particularly grade III tumors, can be locally aggressive and can spread both locally around the primary site as well as to other organs and tissues. Therefore, it is recommended that a metabolic blood analysis be performed to confirm or rule out organ involvement and to add appropriate gland and organ support when indicated (Cima 2000, Goldstein 2000) (see Chapter 2, Nutritional Blood Testing, for additional information).

Homotoxicology

Mast cell tumors represent the Dedifferentiation Phase. They are generally best treated by early detection and broad surgical excision. Radiation may be needed; if so, see the section on biotherapeutics and remedies in radiotherapy in the oncology section of Chapter 34. Homotoxicology can be used to improve quality of life when complete excision is not possible, where metastasis has occurred, or if caregivers do not desire surgery or more invasive therapies.

A single case is reported to have gone into remission on simple, single injections of Ubichinon compositum (Boynes 1991). Palmquist had a case of canine multiple cutaneous mastocytoma that resolved on combination therapy, and another that responded favorably to combination therapy and repeated cryosurgery. Interestingly, these cases involve brachycephalic breeds (English Bulldog and Pug).

Authors' suggested protocols

Nutritional/gland therapy

Immune and blood/bone marrow support formulas: One-half tablet for each 25 pounds of body weight BID.

Maitake-DMG: 1 ml per 25 pounds of body weight, BID. For animals 15 pounds or less, give one-half ml SID.

Betasitosterol: Betathyme—1 capsule for each 25 pounds of body weight BID.

Quercetin tablets: 50 mgs for each 10 pounds of body weight SID.

Chinese herbal medicine/acupuncture

Lymph "K": 1 capsule per 10 pounds of body weight BID for grade II mast cell tumors and TID for grade III tumors. It can be used after surgical debulking or as a sole therapy; however, it is more effective after surgical excision of the tumor.

Lymph "K" contains astragalus (Huang qi), atractylodes (Bai zhu), barbat skullcap (Ban zhi lian), burreed tuber (San leng), centipede (Wu gong), coix (Yi yi ren), hornet's nest (Feng fang), kelp (Kun bu), mastic (Ru xiang), oldenlandia (Bai hua she cao), poria (Fu ling), salvia (Dan shen), scorpion (Quan xie), wolfberry (Gou qi zi), and zedoaria (E zhu). In addition to the herbs mentioned above, Lymph "K" contains arisaema pulvis

(Dan nan xing), codonopsis (Dang shen), cornus (Shan zhu yu), dioscorea (Shan yao), eupolyphaga (Tu bie cong), forsythia (Lian qiao), fritillaria (Bei mu), house lizard (Bi hu, Tian long, or Shou gong), myrrh (Mo yao), prunella (Xia ku cao), rehmannia (Shu di huang), sargassum (Hai zao), Selaginellae doederleini (Shi shang bai), silkworm (Jiang can), Typhonium gigantium rhizome (Bai fu zi), and white peony (Bai shao). These additional herbs increase the efficacy of the formula.

Homotoxicology (Dose: 10 drops for 50-pound dog; 5 drops for cat or small dog)

Also see Chapter 34 for more advanced treatment ideas.

Psorinoheel, Apis compositum, BHI-Allergy, Cutis compositum: Orally BID.

Traumeel: Indicated at intervals.

Galium-Heel, Lymphomyosot, Hepar compositum, Solidago compositum, Tonsilla compositum, Coenzyme compositum, Ubichinon compositum: Orally 3 to 7 times weekly.

Product sources

Nutrition

Immune and blood/bone marrow support formulas: Animal Nutrtion Technologies. **Alternatives:** Immune System Support—Standard Process Veterinary Formulas; Immuno Support—Rx Vitamins for Pets; Immugen—Thorne Veterinary Products.

Maitake-DMG: Vetri Science.

Betathyme: Best for Your Pet. **Alternative:** Moducare—Thorne Veterinary Products.

Quercetin tablets: Source Naturals; Quercitone—Thorne Veterinary Products.

Chinese herbal medicine/acupuncture

Lymph K: Natural Solutions Inc.

Homotoxicology

BHI/Heel Inc.

REFERENCES

Cima J. Biochemical Blood Chemistry Evaluation, Palm Beach Gardens, FL. March 2000.

Elmslie RE. Mast Cell Tumors. In: Tilley L, Smith F. The 5-Minute Veterinary Consult: Canine and Feline, Blackwell Publishing, 2003.

Fox, LE. Mast Cell Tumors. In: Morrison WB, ed. Cancer in dogs and cats: medical and surgical management. Baltimore: Williams and Wilkins, 1998:479–488.

Goldstein R, et al. The BNA Handbook: A Working Manual for Veterinarians, Westport CT: Animal Nutrition Technologies, 2000.

McCaw DL, Miller MA, Ogilvie GK, et al. Response of canine mast cell tumors to treatment with oral prednisone. *J Vet Intern Med* 1994;8:406–408.

Molander-McCray H, Henry CJ, Potter K, et al. Cutaneous mast cell tumors in cats: 32 cases (1991–1994). *J Am Anim Hosp Assoc* 1998;34:281–284.

Patnaik AK, Ehler WN, MacEwen EG. Canine cutaneous mast cell tumors: morphologic grading and survival time in 83 dogs. *Vet Pathol* 1984;21:469–474.

MELANOMA

General comments

Malignant melanomas commonly occur in the mouth, skin, and digits and have no reported cause. Oral melanomas are common to both dogs and cats, are locally invasive to the bone and surrounding lymph nodes, and can cause considerable pain (Hahn 2003). Melanomas of the skin and digit are also locally invasive and can spread to local and regional lymph nodes (Graham 2003, Miller 1993). Surgery is recommended, with wide margins on the skin or amputation of the affected digit. In oral tumors, removal of one side of the mandible or maxilla is advised. In addition, radiation and chemotherapy are often recommended, especially if the surgical excision is incomplete (Bateman 1994). The prognosis for skin and digit melanoma is good with surgery and can be 1 to 2 years. The prognosis is usually poor with cats, especially with the oral form (Bostick 1979, Thomas 1998).

Nutrition

Melanoma is an aggressive and invasive tumor that can cause considerable pain and inflammation, especially in the mouth. Nutritional therapy focuses on reducing inflammation and pain, providing general nourishment, and enhancing immune function.

Note: Because they are aggressive and can spread via the lymph system, melanomas can cause tissue and organ damage. It is recommended that a metabolic blood analysis be performed to confirm or rule out additional organ involvement and damage and add specific and appropriate gland and organ support when indicated (Cima 2000, Goldstein 2000) (see Chapter 2, Nutritional Blood Testing, for additional information).

Homotoxicology

Malignant melanomas represent the Dedifferentiation Phase. These tumors spread rapidly when located in the oral or other mucocutaneous areas. Cutaneous melanomas may be less aggressive. Early and aggressive surgery is advised. See the additional data for this disease in the oncology section of Chapter 34.

Authors' suggested protocols

Nutritional/gland therapy
Immune support formula: One-half tablet for each 25 pounds of body weight BID.

Maitake-DMG: 1 ml per 25 pounds of body weight BID. For animals 15 pounds or less, one-half ml BID.

Betathyme: 1 capsule for each 25 pounds of body weight BID.

Evening primrose, hemp, and flax oils: 1 teaspoon per 25 pounds of body weight SID.

Chinese herbal medicine/acupuncture
Lymph "K": 1 capsule per 10 pounds of body weight TID. This is more effective after surgical debulking of the tumor.

Lymph "K" contains astragalus (Huang qi), atractylodes (Bai zhu), barbat skullcap (Ban zhi lian), burreed tuber (San leng), centipede (Wu gong), coix (Yi yi ren), hornet's nest (Feng fang), kelp (Kun bu), mastic (Ru xiang), oldenlandia (Bai hua she cao), poria (Fu ling), salvia (Dan shen), scorpion (Quan xie), wolfberry (Gou qi zi), and zedoaria (E zhu). In addition to the herbs mentioned above, Lymph "K" contains Arisaema pulvis (Dan nan xing), codonopsis (Dang shen), cornus (Shan zhu yu), dioscorea (Shan yao), eupolyphaga (Tu bie cong), forsythia (Lian qiao), fritillaria (Bei mu), house lizard (Bi hu, Tian long, or Shou gong), myrrh (Mo yao), prunella (Xia ku cao), rehmannia (Shu di huang), sargassum (Hai zao), Selaginellae doederleini (Shi shang bai), silkworm (Jiang can), Typhonium gigantium rhizome (Bai fu zi), and white peony (Bai shao). These additional herbs increase the efficacy of the formula.

Homotoxicology (Dose: 10 drops for 50-pound dog; 5 drops for cat or small dog)
Also see Chapter 34 for more advanced treatment ideas.

Cutis compositum: Alternated every week with Glyoxal compositum.

Galium-Heel, Lymphomyosot, Thyroidea compositum, Hepar compositum, Solidago compositum, Tonsilla compositum, Coenzyme compositum, Ubichinon compositum: 10 drops PO BID every 3 days.

Product sources

Nutrition
Immune support formula: Animal Nutrition Technologies. **Alternatives:** Immune System Support—Standard Process Veterinary Formulas; Immuno Support—Rx Vitamins for Pets; Immugen—Thorne Veterinary Products.

Maitake-DMG: Vetri Science.

Betathyme: Best for Your Pet. **Alternative:** Moducare; Thorne Veterinary Products.

Evening primrose oil: Jarrow Formulas.

Chinese herbal medicine/acupuncture

Lymph "K": Natural Solutions Inc.

Homotoxicology

BHI/Heel Inc.

REFERENCES

Bateman KE, Catton PA, Pennock PW, Kruth SA. 0–7–21 radiation therapy for the treatment of canine oral melanoma. *J Vet Intern Med* 1994;8:267–272.

Bostock DE. Prognosis after surgical excision of canine melanomas. *Vet Pathol* 1979;16:32–40.

Cima J. Biochemical Blood Chemistry Evaluation, Palm Beach Gardens, FL. March 2000.

Goldstein R, et al. The BNA Handbook: A Working Manual for Veterinarians, Westport, CT: Animal Nutrition Technologies, 2000.

Graham, JC. Melanocytic Tumors, Skin and Digit. In: Tilley L, Smith F. The 5-Minute Veterinary Consult: Canine and Feline, Blackwell Publishing, 2003.

Hahn KA. Melanocytic Tumors, Oral. In: Tilley L, Smith F. The 5-Minute Veterinary Consult: Canine and Feline, Blackwell Publishing, 2003.

Hahn KA, DeNicola DB, Richardson RC, Hahn EA. Canine oral malignant melanoma: prognostic utility of an alternative staging system. *J Small Anim Pract* 1994;35:251–256.

Miller WH, Scott DW, Anderson WI. Feline cutaneous melanocytic neoplasms: a retrospective analysis of 43 cases (1979–1991). *Vet Dermatol* 1993;4:19–26.

Thomas RC, Fox LE. Tumors of the skin and subcutis. In: Morrison WB, ed. Cancer in dogs and cats: medical and surgical management. Baltimore: Williams and Wilkins, 1998:489–510.

MENINGIOMA

General comments

The cause of meningioma is unknown. It generally causes slow-growing tumors in both dogs and cats. They are space-occupying masses that cause local inflammation and compression of surrounding healthy brain tissue (Braund 1986, Joseph 2003). Therefore, the clinical picture is often related to the compression; it includes seizures, circling, neurological deficits, and personality changes (Morrison 1998). Depending on the location, surgical removal is recommended along with radiation therapy. Medical management of the inflammation with corticosteroids and the seizures with anticonvulsants is beneficial. Chemotherapy is generally not recommended. The prognosis with surgery can be 1 to 2 years (Joseph 2003, Morrison 1998).

Nutrition

Meningomas generally cause clinical signs of personality changes or neurological deficits; and therefore, surgery, if it can be done, often offers an improved prognosis. Nutritional therapy focuses upon reducing inflammation and swelling, improving mental function, and providing basic support for the immune system. Nutritional therapies also can offset the side effects of corticosteroids if they are used to control symptoms. Nutritional support also may be added to help reduce and control seizures.

Note: Menigiomas can affect multiple organ systems. It is recommended that blood be analyzed both medically and physiologically to determine associated organ involvement and disease. This allows for a more specific gland and nutritional support protocol (Cima 2000, Goldstein 2000) (see Chapter 2, Nutritional Blood Testing, for more information).

Homotoxicology

Meningioma is a Dedifferentiation Phase disorder. No specific references to successful management of this tumor exist in the veterinary literature. Because this condition is right of the biological division, therapy is generally palliative. In this disorder, homotoxins accumulate and damage the cellular regulation processes sufficiently that neoplastic alterations manifest (Reckeweg 2000). Therapy is directed at removing cancer cells, reconditioning cellular organelles (especially energy production systems), draining toxic materials away from the diseased area, improving the microenvironment of the matrix, and improving detoxification and repair capabilities. Detoxification should not be done while a patient is receiving chemotherapy because this can reduce chemotherapy agent blood levels, and thus reduce killing of the targeted cancer cells (Smit 2004). Caution should be exercised when considering administration of agents that could cause progressive vicariation. Overvaccination of these patients is not advised because it can cause the immune system to be overwhelmed, resulting in a sudden worsening of the patient's condition.

Authors' suggested protocols

Nutritional/gland therapy

Brain/nerve and immune support formulas: 1/2 tablet for each 25 pounds of body weight BID.

Coenzyme Q10: 25 mgs for each 15 pounds of body weight SID.

Phosphatidyl serine: 20 mgs for each 15 pounds of body weight SID.

Phosphatidyl choline: One-fourth teaspoon for each 25 pounds of body weight BID.

Betathyme: 1 capsule for each 25 pounds of body weight BID.

Chinese herbal medicine/acupuncture

H5 Brain tumor: 1 capsule per 10 pounds of body weight TID. Occasionally, a patient may also need a low dose of steroid to control the signs. H5 Brain tumor contains astragalus (Huang qi), barbat skullcap (Ban zhi lian), burreed tuber (San leng), centipede (Wu gong), earthworm (Di long), kelp (Kun bu), oldenlandia (Bai hua she cao), oyster shell (Mu li), pinellia (Ban xia), polyporus (Zhu ling), poria (Fu ling), scorpion (Quan xie), and zedoaria (E zhu). It also contains angelica root (Dang gui), arisaema (Dan nan xing), Chinese sage (Shi jian chuan), chrysanthemum (Ju hua), eupolyphaga (Tu bie chong), gastrodia (Tian ma), grass-leave sweet-flag root (Shi chang pu), peach kernel (Tao ren), polygala root (Yuan zhi), prunella (Xia ku cao), safflower (Hong hua), sargassum (Hai zao), silkworm (Jiang can), and uncaria (Gou teng). These additional herbs increase the efficacy of the formula.

Homotoxicology

In cases of brain swelling and brain tumors, begin with Apis homaccord, Galium-Heel, Lymphomyosot, Thalamus compositum, Cerebrum compositum, Viscum compositum, Ginseng compositum, and Molybdan compositum.

Homotoxicology during chemotherapy (Dose: 10 drops for 50-pound dog; 5 drops for cat or small dog)

See the additional data for this disease in Chapter 34.

Galium-Heel, Lymphomyosot: PO BID.

Tonsilla compositum, Pulsatilla compositum, Coenzyme compositum, Ubichinon compositum: PO every 3 days.

Glyoxal compositum: 1 vial orally every 2 weeks.

Homotoxicology after chemotherapy (Dose: 10 drops for 50-pound dog; 5 drops for cat or small dog)

Galium-Heel, Lymphomyosot, Thyroidea compositum, Hepar compositum, Solidago compositum, Tonsilla compositum, Coenzyme compositum, Testis compositum, Ubichinon compositum: PO BID every 3 days. Remove the Testis compositum from the formula if strong detoxification reactions occur.

Product sources

Nutrition

Brain/nerve and immune support formulas: Animal Nutrition Technologies. Alternatives: Immune System Support—Standard Process Veterinary Formulas; Immuno Support—Rx Vitamins for Pets; Immugen—Thorne Veterinary Products.

Coenzyme Q10: Vetri Science; Rx Vitamins for Pets; Integrative Therapeutics.

Phosphatidyl choline: Designs for Health.

Phosphatidyl serine: Progressive Labs.

Betathyme: Best for Your Pet. Alternative: Thorne Veterinary Products.

Chinese herbal medicine/acupuncture

Formula H5 Brain tumor: Natural Solutions Inc.

Homotoxicology

BHI/Heel Inc.

REFERENCES

Braund KG, Ribas JL. Central nervous system meningiomas. *Compend Contin Educ Pract Vet* 1986;8:241–248.

Cima J. Biochemical Blood Chemistry Evaluation, Palm Beach Gardens, FL. March 2000.

Goldstein R, et al. The BNA Handbook: A Working Manual for Veterinarians, Westport, CT: Animal Nutrition Technologies, 2000.

Joseph, RJ. Meningioma. In: Tilley L, Smith F. The 5-Minute Veterinary Consult: Canine and Feline, Blackwell Publishing, 2003.

Morrison W. Cancer Affecting the Nervous System. In: Morrison WB, ed. Cancer in dogs and cats: medical and surgical management. Baltimore: Williams and Wilkins, 1998:479–488.

NASAL TUMORS

General comments

The most common tumors of the nasal and paranasal sinuses are fibrosarcoma, squamous cell carcinoma, chondrosarcoma, and adenocarcinoma. Nasal tumors are common in dogs and cats (Cox 1991). In most instances these are slowly progressive and sometimes locally invasive, and they usually begin unilaterally and spread to both cavities. The cause for nasal tumors is unknown; however, there is a belief that exposure to environmental pollutants may incite tumor growth (Hahn 2003, Patnaik 1989). Surgical removal of the tumor alone often results in recurrences. The addition of radiation or chemotherapy can improve the prognosis (Adams 1987, Frazier 1995, Hahn 2003, Theon 1994). The prognosis is guarded, and if left untreated usually results in survival times of 3 to 5 months. With surgery, radiation, and/or chemotherapy, the prognosis improves to 1 to 2 years (Evans 1989, Hahn 2003).

Nutrition

These tumors are confined to the sinus and are often painful and/or infected. The authors recommend surgical debulking of the tumor in combination with nutritional and biological therapies, resulting in a better prognosis. In addition, the use of controlled cryosurgery after the tumor has been debulked and before surgical closure appears to further improve the prognosis (DeAngelis, Goldstein 2006, Goldstein 1974).

Note: A metabolic blood analysis is recommended because nasal tumors have an inherent ability to cause discomfort, loss of appetite, and general health decline. This nutritional evaluation can confirm or rule out organ involvement and serve as the basis for adding specific and appropriate gland and organ support when indicated (Cima 2000, Goldstein 2000) (see Chapter 2, Nutritional Blood Testing, for additional information).

Homotoxicology
Nasal tumors represent the Dedifferentiation Phase. Adenocarcinomas are most common, but other forms exist. Most conventional and alternative therapy is considered palliative. Palmquist has treated several of these cases with integrative programs of homotoxicology and nutritional therapy and has seen longer survival times than expected. High-dose intravenous vitamin C can cause apparent sudden tumor shrinkage and resulting epistaxis. Tumor growth seemed to slow following regular use of this treatment. While such cases are generally best treated following early detection, the nature of this disease means that many cases are very advanced before they are properly diagnosed. Surgical removal is not successful in most circumstances. Radiation may be very useful; if it is used, see the oncology section in Chapter 34. Homotoxicology can be used to improve the quality of life when complete excision is not possible, metastasis has occurred, or if the caregivers do not desire surgery or more invasive therapies. See the additional data in the adenocarcinoma protocol in the advanced homotoxicology chapter.

Authors' suggested protocols

Nutritional/gland therapy
Immune and bronchus/lung support formulas: 1 tablet for each 25 pounds of body weight BID.

Probiotic MPF: One-half capsule per 25 pounds of body weight with food.

Maitake DMG: 1 ml per 25 pounds of body weight BID.

Bee propolis: 1 capsule for each 25 pounds of body weight, divided.

Chinese herbal medicine/acupuncture
H112 Nasal tumor: 1 capsule per 10 pounds of body weight TID. H112 Nasal tumor contains atractylodes (Bai zhu), barbat skullcap (Ban zhi lian), Dioscorea bulbifera bulb (Huang yao zi), oldenlandia (Bai hua she cao), oyster shell (Mu li), pinellia (Ban xia), and poria (Fu ling). It also includes buttercup herb (Mao zao cao), citrus (Chen pi), codonopsis (Dang shen), fritillary bulb (Bei mu), globe

thistle (Lou lu), peach kernel (Tao ren), and prunella (Xia ku cao) to increase the efficacy of the formula. This formula is more effective after surgical debulking of the tumor.

Homotoxicology during chemotherapy (Dose: 10 drops for 50-pound dog; 5 drops for cat or small dog)
Galium-Heel, Lymphomyosot, Ginseng compositum, BHI-Sinus, BHI-Infection, Echinacea compositum forte: PO BID.

BHI-Bleeding: PRN.

Tonsilla compositum, Pulsatilla compositum, Coenzyme compositum, Ubichinon compositum: 10 drops PO every 3 days.

Glyoxal compositum: 1 vial orally every 2 weeks.

Homotoxicology if no chemotherapy (Dose: 10 drops for 50-pound dog; 5 drops for cat or small dog)
Galium-Heel, Lymphomyosot, Ginseng compositum, BHI-Sinus, BHI-Infection, Echinacea compositum forte: PO BID.

BHI-Bleeding: PRN.

Galium-Heel, Lymphomyosot, Thyroidea compositum, Hepar compositum, Solidago compositum, Tonsilla compositum, Coenzyme compositum, Ubichinon compositum, Mucosa compositum: 10 drops PO BID every 3 days.

Glyoxal compositum: 1 vial orally every 2 weeks.

Product sources

Nutrition
Immune and bronchus/lung support formulas: Animal Nutrition Technologies. **Alternatives:** Immune System Support—Standard Process Veterinary Formulas; Immuno Support—Rx Vitamins for Pets; Immugen—Thorne Veterinary Products.

Probiotic MPF: Progressive Labs.
Maitake DMG: Vetri Science.
Bee Propolis: Best for Your Pet.

Chinese herbal medicine/acupuncture
Formula H112 Nasal tumor: Natural Solutions Inc.

Homotoxicology
BHI/Heel Inc.

REFERENCES

Adams WM, Withrow SJ, Walshaw R, et al. Radiotherapy of malignant nasal tumors in 67 dogs. *J Am Vet Med Assoc* 1987;191:311–315.

Cima J. Biochemical Blood Chemistry Evaluation, Palm Beach Gardens, FL. March 2000.

Cox NR, Brawner WR, Powers RD, Wright JC. Tumors of the nose and paranasal sinuses in cats: 32 cases with comparison to a national database (1977 through 1987). *J Am Anim Hosp Assoc* 1991;27:339–347.

Deangelis M, Goldstein M. Personal communication 2005.

Evans SM, Goldschmidt M, McKee LJ, Harvey CE. Prognostic factors and survival after radiotherapy for intranasal neoplasms in dogs: 70 cases (1974–1985). *J Am Vet Med Assoc* 1989;194:1460–1463.

Frazier DL, Hahn KA. Cancer chemotherapeutics. In: Hahn KA, Richardson RC, eds. Cancer chemotherapy—a veterinary handbook. Baltimore: Williams and Wilkins, 1995:77–150.

Goldstein R, et al. The BNA Handbook: A Working Manual for Veterinarians, Westport, CT: Animal Nutrition Technologies, 2000.

Goldstein R. Handbook of Veterinary Cryosurgery, Santa Clara, CA: Spembly Inc. 1974.

Hahn KA, Knapp DW, Richardson RC, Matlock CL. Clinical response of nasal adenocarcinoma to cisplatin chemotherapy in 11 dogs. *J Am Vet Med Assoc* 1992;200:355–357.

Hahn KA. Squamous Cell Carcinoma, Nasal and Paranasal Sinuses. In: Tilley L, Smith F. The 5-Minute Veterinary Consult: Canine and Feline, Blackwell Publishing, 2003.

Hahn KA. Fibrosarcoma, Nasal and Paranasal Sinus. In: Tilley L, Smith F. The 5-Minute Veterinary Consult: Canine and Feline, Blackwell Publishing, 2003.

Hahn KA. Adenocarcinoma, Nasal. In: Tilley L, Smith F. The 5-Minute Veterinary Consult: Canine and Feline, Blackwell Publishing, 2003.

Hahn KA. Chondrosarcoma, Nasal and Paranasal Sinus. In: Tilley L, Smith F. The 5-Minute Veterinary Consult: Canine and Feline, Blackwell Publishing, 2003.

Patnaik AK. Canine sinonasal neoplasms: soft tissue tumors. *J Am Anim Hosp Assoc* 1989;25:491–497.

Theon AP, Peaston AE, Madewell BR, Dungworth DL. Irradiation of nonlymphoproliferative neoplasms of the nasal cavity and paranasal sinuses in 16 cats. *J Am Vet Med Assoc* 1994;204:78–83.

NERVE SHEATH TUMOR (SCHWANNOMA/NEUROFIBROSARCOMAS)

General comments

Nerve sheath tumors arise from Schwann cells. They grow slowly and can cause inflammation, neuropathy, neurological deficits, and muscle wasting, particularly of the limbs. These tumors can occur in dogs but less commonly in cats; the cause is not known. Therapy is most often surgical excision. In some cases amputation or laminectomy is required based upon the location of the tumor. Chemotherapy is generally not effective. Anti-inflammatories and corticosteriods can help to reduce inflammation. Prognosis is about 8 months to 1 year because recurrences are common and pain and neurological deficits can be serious (Morrison 1998, Rhodes 2003).

Nutrition

Pain and discomfort are often the primary concern with nerve sheath tumors. Combined with motor nerve deficits, often the clinical picture outweighs the fact that this is a malignancy. Surgery to relieve pain and inflammation is recommended when possible. Nutritional and biological therapies focus on reducing pain and inflammation, minimizing the potential side effects of pain medication and corticosteroids, and enhancing immune function.

Note: Nerve sheath tumors can be painful and involve multiple organs of the immune system. It is recommended that blood be analyzed both medically and physiologically to determine associated organ involvement and disease. This allows for a more specific gland and nutritional support protocol to be developed (Cima 2000, Goldstein 2000) (see Chapter 2, Nutritional Blood Testing, for additional information).

Homotoxicology

Nerve sheath tumors are frustrating entities. Homotoxicology does not cure them. Therapy is aimed at the patient's Dedifferentiation Phase condition. Early aggressive surgery and radiation therapy are useful in managing this condition. No reports of cure of from biological therapy can be located in the literature.

Authors' suggested protocols

Nutritional/gland therapy

Brain/nerve and immune support formulas: One-half tablet for each 25 pounds of body weight BID.

Phosphatidyl serine: 20 mgs for each 10 pounds of body weight SID.

Phosphatidyl choline: One-fourth teaspoon for each 25 pounds of body weight BID.

Betathyme: 1 capsule for each 25 pounds of body weight BID.

Essential fatty acids (hemp or flax oil): 1 teaspoon for every 25 pounds of body weight with food.

Chinese herbal medicine/acupuncture

H85 Sarcoma: 1 capsule per 10 pounds of body weight TID. H85 Sarcoma contains astragalus (Huang qi), atractylodes (Bai zhu), barbat skullcap (Ban zhi lian), bupleurum (Chai hu), burreed tuber (San leng), centipede (Wu gong), kelp (Kun bu), oldenlandia (Bai hua she cao), oyster shell (Mu li), pinellia (Ban xia), poria (Fu ling), red peony (Chi shao), scorpion (Quan xie), and zedoaria (E zhu). In addition to the herbs mentioned above, it contains buttercup roots (Mao zao cao), citrus (Chen pi), codonopsis (Dang shen), fritillary bulb (Zhe bei mu), prunella (Xia ku cao), sargassum (Hai zao), uncaria (Gou teng), and white peony (Bai shao) to increase efficacy. It is more effective after surgical debulking. It may be used as the sole therapy or as an adjunctive treatment after surgical removal of the mass.

Homotoxicology during chemotherapy (Dose: 10 drops for 50-pound dog; 5 drops for cat or small dog)

Galium-Heel, Lymphomyosot, Ginseng compositum, Zeel: PO BID.

Tonsilla compositum, Pulsatilla compositum, Coenzyme compositum, Ubichinon compositum: 10 drops PO every 3 days.

Glyoxal compositum: 1 vial orally every 2 weeks.

Homotoxicology if no chemotherapy (Dose: 10 drops for 50-pound dog; 5 drops for cat or small dog)

Galium-Heel, Lymphomyosot, Ginseng compositum, Zeel: PO BID.

Neuralgo-rheum, Neuroheel, and/or Spigelia, Discus compositum, Mezereum homaccord: BID to TID as indicated.

Galium-Heel, Lymphomyosot, Thyroidea compositum, Hepar compositum, Solidago compositum, Tonsilla compositum, Coenzyme compositum, Ubichinon compositum, Mucosa compositum, Discus compositum: 10 drops PO BID every 3 days.

Glyoxal compositum: 1 vial orally every 2 weeks.

Product sources

Nutrition
Brain/nerve and immune support formulas: Animal Nutrition Technologies. Alternatives: Immune System Support—Standard Process Veterinary Formulas; Immuno Support—Rx Vitamins for Pets; Immugen—Thorne Veterinary Products.

Phosphatidyl serine: Progressive Labs.
Phosphatidyl choline: Designs for Health.
Betathyme: Best for Your Pet. Alternative: Moducare—Thorne Veterinary Products.
Flax oil: Barlean's Organic Oils, Spectrum.
Hemp oil: Natures Perfect Oil.

Chinese herbal medicine/acupuncture
Formula H85 Sarcoma: Natural Solutions Inc.

Homotoxicology
BHI/Heel Inc.

REFERENCES

Cima J. Biochemical Blood Chemistry Evaluation, Palm Beach Gardens, FL. March 2000.

Goldstein R, et al. The BNA Handbook: A Working Manual for Veterinarians, Westport, CT: Animal Nutrition Technologies, 2000.

Rhodes KH. Schwannoma. In: Tilley L, Smith F. The 5-Minute Veterinary Consult: Canine and Feline, Blackwell Publishing, 2003.

Morrison WB. Tumors Affecting the Nervous System. In: Morrison WB, ed. Cancer in dogs and cats: medical and surgical management. Baltimore: Williams and Wilkins, 1998:655–665.

ORAL TUMORS

General comments

Oral tumors are common in both dogs and cats. The more common oral tumors are osteosarcoma, melanoma, squamous cell carcinoma, and fibrosarcoma (see these specific tumor types for more detailed protocol information). In this section we present a general protocol for oral tumors. Please review other sections for more specific protocols based upon biopsy results and the tumor type.

Nutrition
Oral tumors, depending upon the type, are usually invasive and painful, and they become infected and often negatively affect the appetite. Surgical debulking or removal or cryosurgical ablation is always indicated along with nutritional and biological therapies (Goldstein 1974).

Note: Because oral tumors are often painful, can affect appetite, can spread to local lymph nodes, and affect multiple organ systems, a metabolic and physiological blood evaluation is recommended to assess general glandular and immune health. This can help clinicians to formulate therapeutic nutritional protocols that address not only the cancer but also associated organ disease and weaknesses that may be present (Cima 2000, Goldstein 2000) (see Chapter 2, Nutritional Blood Testing, for additional information).

Homotoxicology
See the remarks for specific malignant tumor types such as melanoma, squamous cell carcinoma, osteosarcoma, and fibrosarcoma. These Dedifferentiation Phase disorders represent end-stage homotoxicoses and can progress very rapidly. In the case of fibrosarcoma, Palmquist and Goldstein have used early cryosurgery in conjunction with biological therapy to control tumors of moderate aggressive character. In one unpublished instance, an aged feline

has survived more than 4 years with repeated cryosurgery. More benign oral tumors such as epulis can be addressed surgically and with radiation. Good dental hygiene is an important part of prevention and therapy in these cases, because unattended poor oral health leads to massive invasion of the body by homotoxins, which can lead to weakening of the host's greater defenses.

Authors' suggested protocols

Nutritional/gland therapy

Immune support formula: One-half tablet for each 25 pounds of body weight BID.

Maitake-DMG: 1 ml per 25 pounds of body weight twice daily. For animals 15 pounds or less, one-half ml BID.

Betasitosterol: 1 capsule for each 25 pounds of body weight BID.

Evening primrose oil: 1 capsule (500 mgs) per 25 pounds of body weight SID.

Corydalis PIS (botanical cox2 inhibitor): 1 tablet for each 25 pounds of body weight SID.

Chinese herbal medicine/acupuncture

Tumor "K": 1 capsule per 10 pounds of body weight TID. Tumor "K" contains barbat skullcap (Ban zhi lian), burreed tuber (San leng), coptis (Huang lian), dittany bark (Bai xian pi), oldenlandia (Bai hua she cao), oyster shell (Mu li), poria (Fu ling), red peony (Chi shao), siler (Fang feng), and zedoaria (E zhu). In addition, Tumor K contains angelica (Bai zhi), angelica root (Dang gui), belamcanda (She gan), citrus (Chen pi), cicada (Chan tui), Dioscorea bulbifera root (Huang yao zi), forsythia (Lian qiao), fritillaria (Bei mu), kochia (Di fu zi), licorice (Gan cao), magnolia (Hou po), prunella (Xia ku cao), and white mustard seed (Bai jie zi) to improve the formula's efficacy.

Homtoxicology

See the protocols for specific tumor types (osteosarcoma, fibrosarcoma, melanoma, squamous cell carcinoma).

Product sources

Nutrition

Immune support formula: Animal Nutrition Technologies. **Alternatives:** Immune System Support—Standard Process Veterinary Formulas; Immuno Support—Rx Vitamins for Pets; Immugen—Thorne Veterinary Products.

Maitake-DMG: Vetri Science.

Betathyme: Best for Your Pet. **Alternative:** Moducare; Thorne Veterinary Products.

Evening primrose oil: Jarrow Formulas.

Corydalis PIS: Natura Health Products.

Chinese herbal medicine/acupuncture
Tumor "K": Natural Solutions Inc.

Homotoxicology
BHI/Heel Inc.

REFERENCES

Goldstein R. Handbook of Veterinary Cryosurgery, Santa Clara, CA: Spembly, 1974.

Cima J. Biochemical Blood Chemistry Evaluation, Palm Beach Gardens, FL. March 2000.

Goldstein R, et al. The BNA Handbook: A Working Manual for Veterinarians, Westport, CT: Animal Nutrition Technologies, 2000.

OSTEOSARCOMA

General comments

Osteosarcoma is a common bone tumor seen most frequently in dogs and less commonly in cats (Botettp 1987). The underlying cause is unknown; however, chronic inflammation is suspected. Osteosarcoma can affect any limb, and the primary recommended therapy is surgical amputation followed by chemotherapy (Chun 2003, Morrison 1998, Waters 1989). When the client chooses against amputation or when tumors are inoperable, radiation therapy can be helpful in controlling the pain (Chun 2003). Metastasis to the chest is common. The prognosis without any therapy is guarded at about 4 months. With surgery and amputation the prognosis is about 9 months to 1 year. In cats the prognosis is up to 2 years because the tumor is less aggressive (Chun 2003, Waters 1989).

Nutrition

Therapeutic nutrition focuses on reducing pain and inflammation, providing general nourishment, and enhancing immune function.

Note: Osteosarcoma is an aggressive, often painful tumor that spreads to regional lymph nodes and metastasizes to the lungs. A metabolic and physiological blood evaluation is recommended to assess general glandular and immune health. This can help clinicians to formulate therapeutic nutritional protocols that address not only the cancer but also associated organ disease and weaknesses that may be present (Cima 2000, Goldstein 2000) (see Chapter 2, Nutritional Blood Testing, for additional information). Currently a clinical trial is being conducted to evaluate the benefits (day-to-day quality of life and longevity) of adding nutritional, biological, and herbal support to chemotherapy protocols for osteosarcoma (Goldstein, Post 2006).

Homotoxicology

Osteosarcoma is a commonly encountered Dedifferentiation Phase disorder. Because this condition is to the right of the biological division, therapy is generally palliative. Metastasis has usually occurred by the time the tumor is diagnosed. Amputation does not prolong survival time, but it does increase patient comfort and is commonly discussed for extremity tumors. In osteosarcoma, homotoxins have accumulated and damaged the cellular regulation processes sufficiently that neoplastic alterations manifest (Reckeweg 2000). Therapy is directed at removing cancer cells, reconditioning cellular organelles (especially energy production systems), draining toxic materials away from the diseased area, improving the microenvironment of the matrix, and improving detoxification and repair capabilities. Pain management is important in these patients because they frequently have severe pain. Detoxification should not be done while a patient is receiving chemotherapy because this can reduce chemotherapy agent blood levels, and thus reduce killing of the targeted cancer cells (Smit 2004). Caution should be exercised when considering administration of agents that could cause progressive vicariation. Overvaccination of these patients is not advised because it can cause the immune system to be overwhelmed, resulting in a sudden worsening of their condition.

Authors' suggested protocols

Nutritional/gland therapy

Immune and cartilage/ligament/muscle/skeletal support formulas: One-half tablet for 25 pounds of body weight BID.

Bronchus/lung/sinus support formula: One-half tablet for 25 pounds of body weight SID.

Betathyme: 1 capsule for each 25 pounds of body weight BID (maximum, 2 capsules BID.)

Maitake DMG: 1 ml per 25 pounds of body weight BID.

Evening primrose oil: 1 capsule (500 mgs) per 25 pounds of body weight SID.

Corydalis PIS (botanical cox2 inhibitor): 1 tablet for each 25 pounds of body weight SID.

Quercetin tablets: 50 mgs for each 10 pounds of body weight SID.

Chinese herbal medicine/acupuncture

Uro-G Plus: 1 capsule per 10 pounds of body weight TID, along with appropriate analgesics such as opioids or NSAIDs. In some cases the patient lives longer without amputation of the limb. Pathological fracture may heal with proper support bandages, exercise restriction, and analgesics.

Uro-G-Plus contains apricot seed (Xing ren), asparagus (Tian men dong), astragalus (Huang qi), atractylodes (Bai zhu), barbat skullcap (Ban zhi lian), centipede (Wu gong), cremastra (Shan ci gu), hornet's nest (Feng fang), kelp (Kun bu), mastic (Ru xiang), milettia (Ji xue teng), oldenlandia (Bai hua she cao), oyster shell (Mu li), poria (Fu ling), salvia (Dan shen), scorpion (Quan xie), and subprostrata sophora root (Shan dou gen). In addition to the herbs mentioned above, Uro-G Plus also contains angelica root (Dang gui), arisaema/bile (Dan nan xing), Chinese sage (Shi jian chuan), codonopsis (Dang shen), corydalis (Yan hu suo), eupolyphaga (Tu bie cong), glehnia root (Sha shen), houttuynia (Yu xing cao), licorice (Gan cao), lily bulb (Bai he), myrrh (Mo yao), ophiopogon (Mai men dong), paniculed swallowwort root (Xu chang qing), prunella (Xia ku cao), pseudodanum (Qian hu), pseudotellaria (Tai zi shen), rehmannia/cooked (Shu di huang) and raw (Sheng di huang), sargassum (Hai zao), scrophularia (Xuan shen), Selaginellae doederleini (Shi shang bai), stemoma (Bai bu), tortoise shell (Bie jia), and trichosanthes (Gua lou). These additional herbs increase the efficacy of the formula.

Homotoxicology

Autosanguis therapy is advised, due to the aggressive and difficult nature of this disease. See the autosanguis section of Chapter 34.

Homotoxicology during chemotherapy (Dose: 10 drops for 50-pound dog; 5 drops for cat or small dog)

Galium-Heel, Lymphomyosot, and Osteoheel: PO BID.

Tonsilla compositum, Pulsatilla compositum, Coenzyme compositum, Ubichinon compositum: 10 drops PO every 3 days.

Glyoxal compositum: 1 vial orally every 2 weeks.

Homotoxicology after chemotherapy (Dose: 10 drops for 50-pound dog; 5 drops for cat or small dog)

Glyoxal compositum: 1 vial orally every 2 weeks.

Osteoheel: TID PO.

Galium-Heel, Lymphomyosot, Thyroidea compositum, Hepar compositum, Solidago compositum, Tonsilla compositum, Coenzyme compositum, Ubichinon compositum: 10 drops PO BID every 3 days.

For pain: There are many alternative handlings for pain in biological therapy. Discus compositum, Zeel, Osteoheel, and Traumeel are commonly used. Catalysts such as Coenzyme compositum, Glyoxal compositum, and Ubichinon compositum can bring relief in some instances. Apis compositum, Aconitum homaccord, Euphorbium compositum, Neuralgo-Rheum-Injeel, and Ferrum homaccord are also useful. Mixing herbal formulas with mainstay homotoxicology remedies can give surprising results in some patients, and dismally ineffective results in others. The authors feel that narcotics are superior to nonsteroidal anti-inflammatory agents if drugs are needed for pain management.

Product sources

Nutritional/gland therapy

Immune, cartilage, and bronchus/lung support formulas: Animal Nutrition Technologies. **Alternatives:** Immune System and Musculoskeltal Support—Standard Process Veterinary Formulas; Immuno Support, Nutriflex Vet—Rx Vitamins for Pets; Immugen—Thorne Veterinary Products; Cosequin—Nutramax Labs; Glycoflex—Vetri Science; Arthragen—Thorne Veterinary Products.

Betathyme: Best for Your Pet. **Alternative:** Moducare—Thorne Veterinary Products.

Maitake DMG: Vetri Science.

Evening primrose oil: Jarrow Formulas.

Corydalis PIS: Natura Health Products.

Quercetin: Source Naturals; Quercitone—Thorne Veterinary Products.

Chinese herbal medicine/acupuncture

Uro-G Plus: Natural Solutions Inc.

Homotoxicology

BHI/Heel Inc.

REFERENCES

Botettp WV, Patnaik AK, Schrader SC, et al. Osteosarcoma in cats: 22 cases (1974–1984). *J Am Vet Med Assoc* 1987;190:91–93.

Cima J. Biochemical Blood Chemistry Evaluation, Palm Beach Gardens, FL. March 2000.

Chun R. Osteosarcoma. In: Tilley L, Smith F. The 5-Minute Veterinary Consult: Canine and Feline, Blackwell Publishing, 2003.

Goldstein R, et al. The BNA Handbook: A Working Manual for Veterinarians, Westport, CT: Animal Nutrition Technologies, 2000.

Goldstein R, Post G. A clinical trial to evaluate chemotherapy in combination with an antioxidant rich nutritional program in the treatment of Lymphosarcoma and Osteosarcoma in dog, 2006.

Morrison WB. Cancer drug pharmacology and clinical experience. In: Morrison WB, ed. Cancer in dogs and cats: medical and surgical management. Baltimore: Williams and Wilkins, 1998:359–385.

Waters DJ, Cooley DM. Skeletal neoplasms. In: Morrison WB, ed. Cancer in dogs and cats: medical and surgical management. Baltimore: Williams and Wilkins, 1998:639–654.

PANCREATIC ADENOCARCINOMA

General comments

Pancreatic adenocarcinomas arise in the duct or acinar cells and are often aggressive and can metastasize. The cause of these tumors is unknown. Treatment is limited and a subtotal pancreatectomy is the best option. The prognosis is guarded and it is fatal because no therapies are available (Harari 1993; Morrison 1998, 2003).

Nutrition

Pancreatic adrenocarcinmoas are locally aggressive and can spread. These tumors can cause considerable pain and inflammation. Nutritional therapy focuses on the reducing inflammation and pain, providing general nourishment, and enhancing immune function. Surgery may be beneficial if diagnosed early.

Note: Because they are aggressive and can spread, pancreatic adenocarcinomas can cause tissue and organ damage. It is recommended that a metabolic blood analysis be performed to confirm or rule out additional organ involvement and damage and add specific and appropriate gland and organ support when indicated (Cima 2000, Goldstein 2000) (see Chapter 2, Nutritional Blood Testing, for additional information).

Homotoxicology

Pancreatic tumors represent the Dedifferentiation Phase. This aggressive form of neoplasia carries a very poor long-term prognosis with current therapy. Homotoxicology can be used to improve quality of life when complete excision is not possible, metastasis has occurred, or if caregivers do not desire surgery or more invasive therapies. See the oncology section of Chapter 34.

These patients seem easily unbalanced, and a very gentle approach with all orally administered agents is recommended, because they seem very prone to sudden progressive vicariation reactions.

Authors' suggested protocols

Nutritional/gland therapy

Immune and pancreas support formulas: One-half tablet for 25 pounds of body weight BID.

Betathyme: 1 capsule for each 25 pounds of body weight BID.

Maitake DMG: 1 ml per 25 pounds of body weight BID.

Corydalis PIS (botanical cox2 inhibitor): 1 tablet for each 25 pounds of body weight SID.

Chinese herbal medicine/acupuncture

H83 Abdominal tumor: 1 capsule per 10 pounds of body weight TID. H83 Abdominal tumor contains agrimony

(Xian he cao), astragalus (Huang qi), atractylodes (bai zhu), barbat skullcap (Ban zhi lian), burreed tuber (San leng), centipede (Wu gong), cinnamon bark (Rou gui), kelp (Kun bu), mastic (Ru xiang), oldenlandia (Bai hua she cao), oyster shell (Mu li), poria (Fu ling), red peony (Chi shao), scorpion (Quan xie), and zedoaria (E zhu). In addition, it contains achyranthes (Niu xi), amber (Hu po), angelica root (Dang gui), Chinese sage (Shi jian chuan), cnidium (Chuang xiong), codonopsis (Dang shen), corydalis tuber (Yan hu suo), licorice (Gan cao), myrrh (Mo yao), notoginseng (San qi), peach kernel (Tao ren), pteropus (Wu ling zi), rehmannia (Sheng di huang), and rhubarb (Da huang) to increase efficacy.

Homotoxicology (Dose: 10 drops for 50-pound dog; 5 drops for cat or small dog)

See Chapter 34 for more advanced treatment ideas.

Ginseng compositum, BHI-Enzyme, Momordica compositum, BHI-Pain-Spasm: PO BID.

Galium-Heel, Lymphomyosot, Thyroidea compositum, Hepar compositum, Solidago compositum, Tonsilla compositum, Coenzyme compositum, Ubichinon compositum, Mucosa compositum: 10 drops PO BID every 3 to 7 days PRN.

If stable, consider Glyoxal compositum and do not repeat until case further stabilizes.

Product sources

Nutritional/gland therapy

Immune and pancreas support formulas: Animal Nutrition Technologies. **Alternatives:** Immune System Support—Standard Process Veterinary Formulas; Immuno Support—Rx Vitamins for Pets; Immugen—Thorne Veterinary Products.

Betathyme: Best for Your Pet. **Alternative:** Moducare—Thorne Veterinary Products.

Maitake DMG: Vetri Science.

Corydalis PIS (botanical cox2 inhibitor): Natura Health Products.

Chinese herbal medicine/acupuncture

Formula H83 Abdominal tumor: Natural Solutions Inc.

Homotoxicology

BHI/Heel Inc.

REFERENCES

Cima J. Biochemical Blood Chemistry Evaluation, Palm Beach Gardens, FL. March 2000.

Goldstein R, et al. The BNA Handbook: A Working Manual for Veterinarians, Westport, CT: Animal Nutrition Technologies, 2000.

Harari J, Lincoln J. Surgery of the exocrine pancreas. In: Slatter D, ed. Textbook of small animal surgery. Philadelphia: Saunders, 1993:678–691.

Morrison WB. Primary cancers and cancer-like lesions of the liver, biliary epithelium, and exocrine pancreas. In: Morrison WB, ed., Cancer in dogs and cats: medical and surgical management. Baltimore: Williams and Wilkins 1998:559–568.

Morrison WB. Adenocarcinoma, Pancreas. In: Tilley L, Smith F. The 5-Minute Veterinary Consult: Canine and Feline, Blackwell Publishing, 2003.

PHEOCHROMOCYTOMA

General comments

Pheochromocytomas arise from the chromaffin cells of the adrenal gland and are malignant in about 50% of the cases. Common side effects are local invasion of adjacent structures such as the vena cava or those secondary to increased production of epinephrine and norepinephrine. Metastasis to other parts of the body can occur. The treatment of choice is surgical removal, and medical therapy is used for side effects such as hypertension and arrhythmias (Gilson 1994). Survival times postoperatively are more than 2 years; however, the prognosis becomes more guarded when there are complicating side effects (Gilson 1994, Maher 1997, Tyler 2003).

Nutrition

If diagnostic testing reveals invasion of the vena cava or there are complicating side effects such as hypertension, then surgery in combination with nutritional and biological therapies can offer an improved prognosis. Nutritional therapy focuses upon reducing inflammation and hyperactivity as well as enhancing the immune system.

Note: With pheochromocytomas that cause secondary effects such as local invasion and hypertension and arrhythmias, a metabolic blood analysis is recommended to identify and help support other organ function such as the heart (Cima 2000, Goldstein 2000) (see Chapter 2, Nutritional Blood Testing, for additional information).

Homotoxicology

Pheochromocytoma is a Dedifferentiation Phase disorder. No cases in the veterinary literature are known to have been successfully handled, so therapy must be supportive and viewed as experimental. Adrenal constituents of the basic support program of Thyroidea compositum and Tonsilla compositum indicate their use in these cases as part of the usual therapy for most Dedifferentiation Phase cases.

Authors' suggested protocols

Nutritional/gland therapy

Adrenal support formula: One-half tablet for each 25 pounds of body weight BID.

Heart and immune support formulas: One-half tablet for every 25 pounds of body weight SID.

Phosphatidyl serine: 25 mgs for each 25 pounds of body weight BID.

Coenzyme Q10: 25 mgs for each 15 pounds of body weight SID.

Vetri DMG: Liquid—one-half ml per 25 pounds of body weight (maximum, 2 mls); tablets—125 mg–1 tablet for every 40 pounds of body weight (maximum, 3 tablets).

Chinese herbal medicine/acupuncture

H83 Abdominal tumor: 1 capsule per 10 pounds of body weight TID. It is more effective after surgical debulking, but can be used as the sole therapy when surgery is not possible.

H83 Abdominal tumor contains agrimony (Xian he cao), astragalus (Huang qi), atractylodes (bai zhu), barbat skullcap (Ban zhi lian), burreed tuber (San leng), centipede (Wu gong), cinnamon bark (Rou gui), kelp (Kun bu), mastic (Ru xiang), oldenlandia (Bai hua she cao), oyster shell (Mu li), poria (Fu ling), red peony (Chi shao), scorpion (Quan xie), and zedoaria (E zhu). In addition, it contains achyranthes (Niu xi), amber (Hu po), angelica root (Dang gui), Chinese sage (Shi jian chuan), cnidium (Chuang xiong), codonopsis (Dang shen), corydalis tuber (Yan hu suo), licorice (Gan cao), myrrh (Mo yao), notoginseng (San qi), peach kernel (Tao ren), pteropus (Wu ling zi), rehmannia (Sheng di huang), and rhubarb (Da huang) to increase efficacy.

Homotoxicology during chemotherapy (Dose: 10 drops for 50-pound dog; 5 drops for cat or small dog)

Galium-Heel, Lymphomyosot, Ginseng compositum, Ypsiloheel: PO BID.

Tonsilla compositum, Pulsatilla compositum, Coenzyme compositum, Ubichinon compositum: 10 drops PO every 3 days.

Glyoxal compositum: 1 vial orally every 2 weeks.

Homotoxicology after chemotherapy (Dose: 10 drops for 50-pound dog; 5 drops for cat or small dog)

Ypsiloheel: BID as needed.

Galium-Heel, Lymphomyosot, Thyroidea compositum, Hepar compositum, Solidago compositum, Tonsilla compositum, Coenzyme compositum, Ubichinon compositum: 10 drops PO BID every 3 days.

Product sources

Nutritional/gland therapy

Adrenal, heart, and immune support formulas: Animal Nutrition Technologies. **Alternatives:** Adrenal, Cardiac,

Immune System Support—Standard Process Veterinary Formulas; Immuno Support, CV Formula—Rx Vitamins for Pets; Bio Cardio, Immugen—Thorne Veterinary Products; Cardio-Strength—Vetri Science.

DMG: Vetri Science.

Phosphatidyl serine: Progressive Labs.

Coenzyme Q10: Vetri Science; Rx Vitamins for Pets; Integrative Therapeutics.

Chinese herbal medicine/acupuncture

H83 Abdominal tumor: Natural Solutions Inc.

Homotoxicology

BHI/Heel Inc.

REFERENCES

Cima J. Biochemical Blood Chemistry Evaluation, Palm Beach Gardens, FL. March 2000.

Gilson SD, Withrow SJ, Orton EC. Surgical treatment of pheochromocytoma: technique, complications, and results in six dogs. *Vet Surg* 1994;23:195–200.

Gilson SD, Withrow SJ, Wheeler SL, Twedt DC. Pheochromocytoma in 50 dogs. *JVIM* 1994;8:228–232.

Goldstein R, et al. The BNA Handbook: A Working Manual for Veterinarians, Westport, CT: Animal Nutrition Technologies, 2000.

Maher ER, McNeil EA. Pheochromocytoma in dogs and cats. *Vet Clin North Am Small Anim Pract* 1997;27:359–380.

Tyler JW. Pheochromocytoma. In: Tilley L, Smith F. The 5-Minute Veterinary Consult: Canine and Feline, Blackwell Publishing, 2003.

RENAL ADENOCARCINOMA

General comments

Renal adenocarcinomas are common in dogs. They usually affect both kidneys, are highly aggressive, and tend to metastasize. The cause is unknown. When unilateral, the treatment of choice is surgical removal of the affected kidney because chemotherapy use has not been reported to be effective. The prognosis is poor, with survival estimated at 6 to 9 months (Chun 2003, Morrison 1998).

Nutrition

Renal tumors, which are highly aggressive, should be approached with a combination of surgical excision and nutritional and biological support. The therapeutic nutritional focus is on reducing inflammation and enhancing the immune system.

Note: Renal adenocarcinoma often metastasizes to the lungs and other organs, making the animal less of a candidate for surgery. If this is the case and surgery is not an option, nutritional and biological therapies are still indicated. It is recommended that a metabolic blood analysis be performed to confirm or rule out other organ involvement and to add appropriate gland and organ support when indicated (Cima 2000, Goldstein 2000) (see Chapter 2, Nutritional Blood Testing, for additional information).

Homotoxicology

Renal tumors represent end-stage homotoxicoses in the Dedifferentiation Phase. Therapy is not anticipated to reverse diseases in this phase; however, these patients can be positively influenced by gentle support of metabolism, detoxification, drainage, and organ support. Such tumors are not commonly seen in clinical practice and no papers could be located involving their treatment by homotoxicology.

Authors' suggested protocols

Kidney and immune support formulas: 1 tablet for 25 pounds of body weight BID.

Bronchus/lung formula: 1 tablet for each 25 pounds SID.

Essential fatty acids (hemp or flax oil): 1 teaspoon for every 25 pounds of body weight with food.

Maitake DMG: 1 ml per 25 pounds of body weight BID.

Chinese herbal medicine/acupuncture

Formula Kidney tumor: 1 capsule per 10 pounds of body weight TID. This formula can be used with or without surgical removal of the affected kidney.

Formula Kidney tumor contains apricot seed (Xing ren), barbat skullcap (Ban zhi lian), burreed tuber (San leng), centipede (Wu gong), kelp (Kun bu), oldenlandia (Bai hua she cao), oyster shell (Mu li), red peony (Chi shao), salvia (Dan shen), scorpion (Quan xie), and zedoaria (E zhu). In addition, Kidney tumor also contains angelica root (Dang gui), areca peel (Da fu pi), blue citrus (Qing pi), bulrush (Pu huang), carthamus (Hong hua), cirsium (Da xiao jie), melia (Chuan lian zi), peach kernel (Tao ren), pteropus (Wu ling zhi), rehmannia (Sheng di huang), sargassum (Hai zao), saussurea (Mu xiang), and tortoise shell (Bie jia). These additional herbs increase the efficacy of the formula.

Homotoxicology during chemotherapy (Dose: 10 drops for 50-pound dog; 5 drops for cat or small dog)

Galium-Heel, Lymphomyosot, Ginseng compositum, Berberis homaccord: PO BID.

Tonsilla compositum, Pulsatilla compositum, Coenzyme compositum, Ubichinon compositum: 10 drops PO every 3 days.

Glyoxal compositum: 1 vial orally every 2 weeks.

Homotoxicology if no chemotherapy (Dose: 10 drops for 50-pound dog; 5 drops for cat or small dog)

Galium-Heel, Lymphomyosot, Ginseng compositum, Berberis homaccord: PO BID.

Galium-Heel, Lymphomyosot, Thyroidea compositum, Hepar compositum, Solidago compositum, Tonsilla compositum, Coenzyme compositum, Ubichinon compositum, Mucosa compositum: 10 drops PO BID every 3 days.

Glyoxal compositum: 1 vial orally every 2 weeks.

If normotensive or hypertensive: Consider Rauwolfia compositum twice weekly for its glandular content and ability to control blood pressure, and the Ren suis, which is a kidney supportive suis organ preparation.

Product sources

Nutritional/gland therapy

Kidney, immune, and bronchus/lung support formulas: Animal Nutrition Technologies. **Alternatives:** Immune System and Renal Support—Standard Process Veterinary Formulas; Immuno Support—Rx Vitamins for Pets; Immugen—Thorne Veterinary Products; Renal essentials—Vetri Science.

Maitake DMG: Vetri Science.

Flax oil: Barlean's Organic Oils, Spectrum.

Hemp oil: Nature's Perfect Oil.

Chinese herbal medicine/acupuncture

Formula Kidney tumor: Natural Solutions Inc.

Homotoxicology

BHI/Heel Inc.

REFERENCES

Chun R. Adenocarcinoma, Renal. In: Tilley L, Smith F. The 5-Minute Veterinary Consult: Canine and Feline, Blackwell Publishing, 2003.

Cima J. Biochemical Blood Chemistry Evaluation, Palm Beach Gardens, FL. March 2000.

Goldstein R, et al. The BNA Handbook: A Working Manual for Veterinarians, Westport, CT: Animal Nutrition Technologies, 2000.

Morrison WB. Cancers of the urinary tract. In: Morrison WB, ed. Cancer in dogs and cats: medical and surgical management. Baltimore: Williams and Wilkins 1998:569–579.

SQUAMOUS CELL CARCINOMA (CUTANEOUS)

General comments

Squamous cell carcinoma (SCC) is a common malignancy in cats and dogs. Oral SCC is described under oral tumors, above. In this section we present general protocols for SCC of the skin, digits, and genital area.

Cutaneous SCC is commonly found on the skin, digit, and ear. It is usually locally invasive but it does not usually metastasize. The reported cause is unknown; however, an inciting cause is believed to be exposure to sunlight. The treatment for an affected digit is amputation (O'Brien 1992). Surgery is also recommended for SCC of the skin and ear pinnae. Vitamin E is recommended for the ear pinnae to slow progression of precancerous lesions. Chemotherapy is recommended when there is metastasis (Graham 2003, Elmslie 2003). The prognosis is generally good unless there is metastasis. Survival times are 1 to 2 years (Graham 2003, Elmslie 2003).

Nutrition

Squamous cell carcinoma should be approached with a combination of surgical excision and nutritional support. Therapeutic nutrition focuses on reducing inflammation and enhancing the immune system.

Note: Squamous cell carcinomas can be locally invasive, spread to regional lymph glands, and affect multiple organ systems. A metabolic and physiological blood evaluation is recommended to assess general glandular and immune health. This can help clinicians to formulate therapeutic nutritional protocols that address not only the cancer but associated organ disease and weaknesses that may be present (Cima 2000, Goldstein 2000) (see Chapter 2, Nutritional Blood Testing, for additional information).

Homotoxicology

Squamous cell carcinoma represents the Dedifferentiation Phase because malignant transformation occurs following damage to the patient's greater defenses. Ultraviolet exposure from solar radiation is a common predisposing cause, and these tumors are frequently seen in white or light pigmented areas with solar exposure—ear tips, face, and the ventrum of dogs that sleep on their backs in sunlight. An oral form is particularly common and aggressive in cats. The tumor can involve other sites such as nail beds and nasal tissue as well.

As with most tumors, they are generally best treated by early detection and broad surgical excision, with attention to the patient's homotoxin load. Radiation is helpful; if it is used, see the oncology section in Chapter 34. Palmquist has published case reports involving the use of photoacupuncture in these cases and has seen some limited but startlingly good results in a few cases. These cases were all extremely aged cats and had remissions that lasted longer than expected (Palmquist 2000). One was suspicious for squamous cell carcinoma and the other was confirmed by incomplete surgical biopsy. This may represent a new modality for use in these cases. Homotoxicol-

ogy can be used to improve quality of life when complete excision is not possible, metastasis has occurred, or if caregivers do not desire surgery or more invasive therapies. A large amount of data exists in classical homeopathic literature about these tumors. See the additional data in Chapter 34.

Authors' suggested protocols

Nutritional/gland therapy
Skin and immune support formulas: 1 tablet for every 25 pounds of body weight BID.

Vitamin E: 50 IU for each 20 pounds of body weight SID.

Chinese herbal medicine/acupuncture
For squamous cell carcinoma of the skin and digital area, the authors use Lymph "K." The dose is 1 capsule per 10 pounds of body weight TID. Lymph "K" contains astragalus (Huang qi), atractylodes (Bai zhu), barbat skullcap (Ban zhi lian), burreed tuber (San leng), centipede (Wu gong), coix (Yi yi ren), hornet's nest (Feng fang), kelp (Kun bu), mastic (Ru xiang), oldenlandia (Bai hua she cao), poria (Fu ling), salvia (Dan shen), scorpion (Quan xie), wolfberry (Gou qi zi) and zedoaria (E zhu). In addition to the herbs mentioned above, Lymph "K" contains arisaema pulvis (Dan nan xing), codonopsis (Dang shen), cornus (Shan zhu yu), dioscorea (Shan yao), eupolyphaga (Tu bie cong), forsythia (Lian qiao), fritillaria (Bei mu), house lizard (Bi hu, Tian long, or Shou gong), myrrh (Mo yao), prunella (Xia ku cao), rehmannia (Shu di huang), sargassum (Hai zao), Selaginellae doederleini (Shi shang bai), silkworm (Jiang can), Typhonium gigantium rhizome (Bai fu zi), and white peony (Bai shao). These additional herbs increase efficacy of the formula.

The authors recommend Tumor "K" for oral squamous cell carcinoma. See Oral Tumors, above.

For genital areas the authors use H 83 Abdominal tumor. The dose is 1 capsule per 10 pounds of body weight TID. H83 Abdominal tumor contains agrimony (Xian he cao), astragalus (Huang qi), atractylodes (bai zhu), barbat skullcap (Ban zhi lian), burreed tuber (San leng), centipede (Wu gong), cinnamon bark (Rou gui), kelp (Kun bu), mastic (Ru xiang), oldenlandia (Bai hua she cao), oyster shell (Mu li), poria (Fu ling), red peony (Chi shao), scorpion (Quan xie), and zedoaria (E zhu). In addition it contains achyranthes (Niu xi), amber (Hu po), angelica root (Dang gui), Chinese sage (Shi jian chuan), cnidium (Chuan xiong), codonopsis (Dang shen), corydalis tuber (Yan hu suo), licorice (Gan cao), myrrh (Mo yao), notoginseng (San qi), peach kernel (Tao ren), pteropus (Wu ling zi), rehmannia (Sheng di huang), and rhubarb (Da huang) to increase efficacy.

Homotoxicology during chemotherapy (Dose: 10 drops for 50-pound dog; 5 drops for cat or small dog)

Galium-Heel, Lymphomyosot, Ginseng compositum, Causticum compositum: PO BID.

Tonsilla compositum, Pulsatilla compositum, Coenzyme compositum, Cutis compositum and Ubichinon compositum: 10 drops PO every 3 days.

Glyoxal compositum: 1 vial orally every 2 weeks.

Homotoxicology if no chemotherapy (Dose: 10 drops for 50-pound dog; 5 drops for cat or small dog)

Galium-Heel, Lymphomyosot, Ginseng compositum, Causticum compositum: PO BID.

BHI-Body Pure: BID for detoxification of environmental factors.

Galium-Heel, Lymphomyosot, Thyroidea compositum, Hepar compositum, Solidago compositum, Cutis compositum, Tonsilla compositum, Coenzyme compositum, Ubichinon compositum, Mucosa compositum: 10 drops PO BID every 3 days.

Glyoxal compositum: 1vial orally every 2 weeks.

Product sources

Nutritional/gland therapy

Skin and immune support formulas: Animal Nutrition Technologies. **Alternatives:** Immune System and Canine Dermal Support—Standard Process Veterinary Formulas; Immuno Support—Rx Vitamins for Pets; Immugen—Thorne Veterinary Products; Derma Strength—Vetri Science.

Chinese herbal medicine/acupuncture

Lymph "K," Tumor "K," and H83 Abdominal tumor: Natural Solutions Inc.

Homotoxicology

BHI/Heel Inc.

REFERENCES

Cima J. Biochemical Blood Chemistry Evaluation, Palm Beach Gardens, FL. March 2000.

Dorn CR, Taylor D. Sunlight exposure and the risk of developing cutaneous and oral squamous cell carcinoma in white cats. *J Natl Cancer Inst* 1971;46:1073–1078.

Elmslie RE. Squamous Cell Carcinoma—Digit. In: Tilley L, Smith F. The 5-Minute Veterinary Consult: Canine and Feline, Blackwell Publishing, 2003.

Elmslie RE. Squamous Cell Carcinoma—Ear. In: Tilley L, Smith F. The 5-Minute Veterinary Consult: Canine and Feline, Blackwell Publishing, 2003.

Goldstein R, et al. The BNA Handbook: A Working Manual for Veterinarians, Westport, CT: Animal Nutrition Technologies, 2000.

Graham JC. Squamous Cell Carcinoma—Skin. In: Tilley L, Smith F. The 5-Minute Veterinary Consult: Canine and Feline, Blackwell Publishing, 2003.

O'Brien MG, Berg J, Engler SJ. Treatment by digital amputation of subungual squamous cell carcinoma in dogs: 21 cases (1987–1988). *J Am Vet Med Assoc* 1992;201:759–761.

Thomas RC, Fox LE. Tumors of the skin and subcutis. In: Morrison WB, ed. Cancer in dogs and cats: medical and surgical management. Baltimore: Williams and Wilkins, 1998:489–510.

THYMOMA

General comments

Thymoma is a tumor of thymic epithelial origins that is generally locally invasive and can occur in dogs and cats. If possible, surgical excision is the preferred treatment. Radiation therapy may be beneficial, especially if the mass is nonresectable. Corticosteroids may also help shrink the mass. Surgically removed masses offer the best prognosis; nonresectable masses offer a guarded prognosis (Arwater 1994, Morrison 1998, Hamilton 2003).

Nutrition

There are few reported results for thymoma with medical management alone; therefore, chemotherapy or radiation therapy and surgery remains the best option. Nutritional therapy has been used in combination with medicinal Chinese herbal therapy to support and enhance immune function, reduce inflammation and swelling, and improve the process of elimination of toxins via the lymph system. In addition, nutraceuticals protect the cells from medication of radiation therapy and help to improve the day-to-day quality of life and extend remission time.

Note: In thymomas that are not surgical candidates and that are locally invasive to surrounding organs, it is recommended that a metabolic blood analysis be performed to confirm or rule out organ involvement and to add appropriate gland and organ support when indicated (Cima 2000, Goldstein 2000) (see Chapter 2, Nutritional Blood Testing, for additional information).

Homotoxicology

Biologically, this is a frustrating tumor to deal with. Therapy is usually unrewarding in the author's experience. Damage to the foundation of the immune system is too severe to reverse; therefore, therapy is directed at general support of defenses and organs. As with most Dedifferentiation Phase diseases, no established protocols exist and the practitioner should note the patient's response to select appropriate remedies. The foundational therapy is based upon the approach to lymphosarcoma.

Authors' suggested protocols

Nutritional/gland therapy

Immune and lymph support formulas: One-half tablet for each 25 pounds of body weight BID.

Maitake-DMG: 1 ml per 25 pounds of body weight BID. For animals 15 pounds or less, one-half ml BID.

Betasitosterol: Betathyme—1 capsule for each 25 pounds of body weight BID.

Selenium: 20 micrograms for each 20 pounds of body weight SID.

Quercetin tablets: 50 mgs for each 10 pounds of body weight SID.

Chinese herbal medicine/acupuncture

Formula Thymoma: 1 capsule per 10 pounds of body weight TID. Thymoma contains astragalus (Huang qi), atractylodes (Bai zhu), barbat skullcap (Ban zhi lian), bupleurum (Chai hu), burreed tuber (San leng), centipede (Wu gong), cremastra (Shan ci gu), earthworm (Di long), kelp (Kun bu), oldenlandia (Bai hua she cao), oyster shell (Mu li), pinellia (Ban xia), pueraria (Ge gen), red peony (Chi shao), salvia (Dan shen), scorpion (Quan xie), and zedoaria (E zhu). In addition, it contains carthamus (Hong hua), cuttlebone (Hai piao xiao), codonopsis (Dang shen), dioscorea (Shan yao), platycodon root (Jie geng), sargassum (Hai zao), and white peony (Bai shao) to improve the efficacy of the formula.

Homtoxicology during chemotherapy (Dose: 10 drops for 50-pound dog; 5 drops for cat or small dog)

Galium-Heel, Lymphomyosot: PO BID.

Tonsilla compositum, Pulsatilla compositum, Coenzyme compositum, Ubichinon compositum: 10 drops PO every 3 days.

Glyoxal compositum: 1 vial orally every 2 weeks.

Homotoxicology after chemotherapy (Dose: 10 drops for 50-pound dog; 5 drops for cat or small dog)

Galium-Heel, Lymphomyosot, Thyroidea compositum, Hepar compositum, Solidago compositum, Tonsilla compositum, Coenzyme compositum, Ubichinon compositum: 10 drops PO BID every 3 days.

Glyoxal compositum: Every 2 weeks.

Product sources

Nutritional/gland therapy

Immune and lymph support formulas: Animal Nutrition Technologies. **Alternatives:** Immune System Support—Standard Process Veterinary Formulas; Immuno Support—Rx Vitamins for Pets; Immugen—Thorne Veterinary Products.

Maitake-DMG: Vetri Science.

Betathyme: Best for Your Pet. **Alternative:** Moducare—Thorne Veterinary Products.

Quercetin tablets: Source Naturals; Quercitone—Thorne Veterinary Products.

Chinese herbal medicine/acupuncture

Formula Thymoma: Natural Solutions Inc.

Homotoxicology

BHI/Heel Inc.

REFERENCES

Arwater SW, Powers BE, Park RD, et al. Thymoma in dogs: 23 cases (1980–1991). *J Am Vet Med Assoc* 1994;205:1007–1013.

Cima J. Biochemical Blood Chemistry Evaluation, Palm Beach Gardens, FL. March 2000.

Goldstein R, et al. The BNA Handbook: A Working Manual for Veterinarians, Westport, CT: Animal Nutrition Technologies, 2000.

Morrison WB. Nonpulmonary intrathoracic cancer. In: Morrison WB, ed. Cancer in dogs and cats: medical and surgical management. Baltimore: Williams and Wilkins, 1998:537–550.

Hamilton TA. Thymoma. In: Tilley L, Smith F. The 5-Minute Veterinary Consult: Canine and Feline, Blackwell Publishing, 2003.

TRANSITIONAL CELL CARCINOMA

General comments

Transitional cell carcinoma is a malignant tumor of the epithelial of the urogenital system, most commonly in the bladder and ureters. One of the possible underlying causes is believed to be adverse reactions to flea control products and cyclophosphamide in dogs. This form of cancer rarely occurs in cats. Surgical excision, when possible, is the treatment of choice. The associated medical therapy is piroxicam and sometimes chemotherapy. The prognosis is guarded. With surgery and piroxicam, the average survival time is 6 to 12 months.

Nutrition

Transitional cell tumors that can be removed surgically respond to integrative therapies. For those that are inoperable (trigone and ureter infiltration), aggressive nutritional and biological therapies are indicated. Because of the potential underlying cause of exposure to pesticides, chemicals, and drugs that increase free radical production and secondary inflammation which propagate the disease, nutritional and biological therapies should address under-lying inflammation as well as immune system enhancement. In addition, botanically based cox2 inhibiting supplements are added at a level that supports additional inflammation reduction (usually in combination with piroxicam) without adding additional chemicals.

Note: Because of the potential for associated kidney involvement, a metabolic blood analysis is recommended to confirm or rule out not only kidney, but also other organ involvement. This helps clinicians to more specifically add appropriate nutritional, gland, and organ support when indicated (Cima 2000, Goldstein 2000) (see Chapter 2, Nutritional Blood Testing, for additional information).

Homotoxicology

Transitional cell carcinoma is an aggressive and difficult to treat Dedifferentiation Phase disorder. Because this condition is right of the biological division, therapy is generally palliative. Tumors may be excised if found early, but surgery frequently fails. In this type of cancer, homotoxins have accumulated and damaged the cellular regulation processes sufficiently that neoplastic alterations manifest (Reckeweg 2000). Therapy is directed at removing cancer cells, reconditioning cellular organelles (especially energy production systems), draining toxic materials away from the diseased area, improving the microenvironment of the matrix, and improving detoxification and repair capabilities. Detoxification should not be done while a patient is receiving chemotherapy because this can reduce chemotherapy agent blood levels, and thus reduce killing of the targeted cancer cells (Smit 2004). Caution should be exercised when considering administration of agents that could cause progressive vicariation. Over-vaccination of these patients is not advised because it can overwhelm the immune system, resulting in a sudden worsening of their condition.

Authors' suggested protocols

Nutritional/gland therapy

Urinary support formula: 1 tablet for each 25 pounds of body weight BID.

Kidney and immune support formulas: One-half tablet for each 25 pounds of body weight SID.

Zyflamend: One-half dropper for each 25 pounds of body weight BID.

Note: Botanical cox2 inhibitors have been shown to induce apoptosis, as well as having anti-oxidative and anti-inflammatory effects (Bemis 2005).

Chinese herbal medicine/acupuncture

H58 Uro-G Plus: 1 capsule per 10 pounds of body weight TID, with or without surgery. The authors recommend

Uro-G Plus along with appropriate analgesics such as opioids or NSAIDs.

Uro-G Plus contains apricot seed (Xing ren), asparagus (Tian men dong), astragalus (Huang qi), atractylodes (Bai zhu), barbat skullcap (Ban zhi lian), centipede (Wu gong), cremastra (Shan ci gu), hornet's nest (Feng fang), kelp (Kun bu), mastic (Ru xiang), milettia (Ji xue teng), oldenlandia (Bai hua she cao), oyster shell (Mu li), poria (Fu ling), salvia (Dan shen), scorpion (Quan xie), and subprostrata sophora root (Shan dou gen). In addition to the herbs mentioned above, it contains angelica root (Dang gui), arisaema bile (Dan nan xing), Chinese sage (Shi jian chuan), codonopsis (Dang shen), corydalis (Yan hu suo), eupolyphaga (Tu bie cong), glehnia root (Sha shen), houttuynia (Yu xing cao), licorice (Gan cao), lily bulb (Bai he), myrrh (Mo yao), ophiopogon (Mai men dong), panicled swallowwort root (Xu chang qing), prunella (Xia ku cao), pseudodanum (Qian hu), pseudotellaria (Tai zi shen), rehmannia/cooked (Shu di huang) and raw (Sheng di huang), sargassum (Hai zao), scrophularia (Xuan shen), Selaginellae doederleini (Shi shang bai), stemoma (Bai bu), tortoise shell (Bie jia), and trichosanthes (Gua lou). These additional herbs increase the efficacy of the formula.

Homotoxicology during chemotherapy (Dose: 10 drops for 50-pound dog; 5 drops for cat or small dog)

Galium-Heel, Lymphomyosot, Engystol N, Ginseng compositum, Reneel: PO BID.

Tonsilla compositum, Pulsatilla compositum, Coenzyme compositum, Ubichinon compositum: 10 drops PO every 3 days.

Glyoxal compositum: 1 vial orally every 2 weeks.

Homotoxicology after chemotherapy (Dose: 10 drops for 50-pound dog; 5 drops for cat or small dog)

Galium-Heel, Lymphomyosot, Thyroidea compositum, Hepar compositum, Solidago compositum, Tonsilla compositum, Coenzyme compositum, Ubichinon compositum, Mucosa compositum: 10 drops PO BID every 3 days.

Reneel: PRN for symptomatic relief.

BHI-Body Pure: BID for detoxification of environmental factors.

Glyoxal compositum: 1 vial orally every 2 weeks.

Product sources

Nutritional/gland therapy

Urinary, kidney, and immune support formulas: Animal Nutrition Technologies. Alternatives: Immune System, Renal Support—Standard Process Veterinary Formulas; Immuno Support—Rx Vitamins for Pets; Immugen—

Thorne Veterinary Products; Renal Essentials, UT and Bladder Strength—Vetri Science.

Zyflamend: New Chapter. **Alternative**: Botanical Treasures—Natura Health Products.

Chinese herbal medicine/acupuncture
Uro-G Plus: Natural Solutions Inc.

Homotoxicology
BHI/Heel Inc.

REFERENCES

Bemis DL, Capodice JL, Anastasiadis AG, Katz AE, Buttyan R. Zyflamend®, a Unique Herbal Preparation With Nonselective COX Inhibitory Activity, Induces Apoptosis of Prostate Cancer Cells That Lack COX-2 Expression, *Nutr Cancer*. 2005;52(2):202–12.

Chun R, Knapp DW, Widmer WR, et al. Cisplatin treatment of transitional cell carcinoma of the urinary bladder in dogs: 18 cases (1983–1993). *J Am Vet Med Assoc* 1996;209:1588–1591.

Chun R. Transitional cell carcinoma, Renal, Bladder, Urethra. In: Tilley L, Smith F. The 5-Minute Veterinary Consult: Canine and Feline, Blackwell Publishing, 2003.

Cima J. Biochemical Blood Chemistry Evaluation, Palm Beach Gardens, FL. March 2000.

Goldstein R, et al. The BNA Handbook: A Working Manual for Veterinarians, Westport, CT: Animal Nutrition Technologies, 2000.

Morrison WB. Cancers of the urinary tract. In: Morrison WB, ed. Cancer in dogs and cats: medical and surgical management. Baltimore: Williams and Wilkins, 1998:569–579.

THYROID CARCINOMA

General comments

Thyroid carcinoma is a malignant growth of the thyroid gland that is locally aggressive and invasive and can metastasize to the lymph nodes and the lungs (Fineman 2003, Waters 1998). The treatment of choice is surgical excision, either alone or in combination with chemotherapy (Fineman 1998, 2003; Jeglum 1983; Klein 1995). Radiotherapy with activated iodine may shrink the tumor, and thyroid hormone replacement therapy may be indicated. The prognosis depends upon the local and metastatic picture. The prognosis is poor when the cancer has spread to the regional lymph nodes and lungs (Fineman 2003, Waters 1998).

Nutrition

Thyroid carcinoma is most often locally aggressive and therefore should be approached with a combination of surgical excision and nutritional support. The therapeutic nutritional focus is on reducing inflammation, helping to balance gland and hormonal function, and enhancing the immune system.

Note: Thyroid carcinoma can metastasize, making the animal a poor candidate for surgery. If this is the case and surgery is not an option, nutritional and biological therapies are still indicated. It is recommended that a metabolic blood analysis be performed to confirm or rule out organ involvement and to add appropriate gland and organ support when indicated (Cima 2000, Goldstein 2000) (see Chapter 2, Nutritional Blood Testing, for additional information).

Homotoxicology

Thyroid carcinoma is a Dedifferentiation Phase disorder of the thyroid tissue. Because this condition is to the right of the biological division, therapy is generally palliative. Homotoxins have accumulated and damaged the cellular regulation processes sufficiently that neoplastic alterations manifest (Reckeweg 2000). Surgical or radioisotope therapy is commonly recommended. Therapy is directed at removing cancer cells, reconditioning cellular organelles (especially energy production systems), draining toxic materials away from the diseased area, improving the microenvironment of the matrix, and improving detoxification and repair capabilities. Caution should be exercised when considering administration of agents that could cause progressive vicariation. Overvaccination of these patients is not advised because it can cause the immune system to be overwhelmed, resulting in a sudden worsening of their condition.

Authors' suggested protocols

Nutritional/gland therapy

Thyroid and immune support formulas: One-half tablet for each 25 pounds of body weight BID.

Pituitary/hypothalamus/pineal support formula: One-half tablet for each 25 pounds of body weight SID.

Coenzyme Q10: 25 mgs for each 15 pounds of body weight SID.

Maitake DMG: 1 ml per 25 pounds of body weight BID.

Hemp oil: 1 tsp for each 20 pounds of body weight with food.

Quercetin tablets: 50 mgs for each 10 pounds of body weight SID.

Chinese herbal medicine/acupuncture

H83 Abdominal tumor: 1 capsule per 10 pounds of body weight TID, with or without surgery, regardless of whether it is metastatic or localized.

H83 Abdominal tumor contains agrimony (Xian he cao), astragalus (Huang qi), atractylodes (bai zhu), barbat skullcap (Ban zhi lian), burreed tuber (San leng), centipede (Wu gong), cinnamon bark (Rou gui), kelp (Kun bu), mastic (Ru xiang), oldenlandia (Bai hua she cao), oyster shell (Mu li), poria (Fu ling), red peony (Chi shao), scorpion (Quan xie), and zedoaria (E zhu). In addition, it contains achyranthes (Niu xi), amber (Hu po), angelica root (Dang gui), Chinese sage (Shi jian chuan), cnidium (Chuang xiong), codonopsis (Dang shen), corydalis tuber (Yan hu suo), licorice (Gan cao), myrrh (Mo yao), notoginseng (San qi), peach kernel (Tao ren), pteropus (Wu ling zi), rehmannia (Sheng di huang), and rhubarb (Da huang) to increase the formula's efficacy.

Homotoxicology during chemotherapy (Dose: 10 drops for 50-pound dog; 5 drops for cat or small dog)

Galium-Heel, Lymphomyosot, Ginseng compositum: PO BID.

Tonsilla compositum, Pulsatilla compositum, Coenzyme compositum, Ubichinon compositum, Strumeel: 10 drops PO every 3 days.

Thyroidea compositum: Weekly.

Glyoxal compositum: 1 vial orally every 2 weeks.

Homotoxicology after chemotherapy (Dose: 10 drops for 50-pound dog; 5 drops for cat or small dog)

Galium-Heel, Lymphomyosot, Thyroidea compositum, Hepar compositum, Solidago compositum, Tonsilla compositum, Coenzyme compositum, Ubichinon compositum: PO BID every 3 days.

Strumeel: PRN for symptomatic control.

Glyoxal compositum: 1 vial orally every 2 weeks.

Product sources

Nutritional/gland therapy

Immune, thyroid and pituitary/hypothalamus/pineal support formulas: Animal Nutrition Technologies.

Alternatives: Immune System, Thyroid Support—Standard Process Veterinary Formulas; Immuno Support—Rx Vitamins for Pets; Immugen—Thorne Veterinary Products.

Coenzyme Q10: Vetri Science; Rx Vitamins for Pets; Integrative Therapeutics.

Maitake DMG: Vetri Science.

Quercetin: Source Naturals; Quercitone—Thorne Veterinary Products.

Hemp oil: Nature's Perfect Oil.

Chinese herbal medicine/acupuncture

Formula H83 Abdominal tumor: Natural Solutions Inc.

Homotoxicology

BHI/Heel Inc.

REFERENCES

Cima J. Biochemical Blood Chemistry Evaluation, Palm Beach Gardens, FL. March 2000.

Fineman, LS. Adenocarcinoma, Thyroid—Dogs. In: Tilley L, Smith F. The 5-Minute Veterinary Consult: Canine and Feline, Blackwell Publishing, 2003.

Fineman LS, Hamilton TA, de Gortari A, et al. Cisplatin chemotherapy for treatment of thyroid carcinoma in dogs: 13 cases. *J Am Anim Hosp Assoc* 1998;34;109–112.

Goldstein R, et al. The BNA Handbook: A Working Manual for Veterinarians, Westport, CT: Animal Nutrition Technologies, 2000.

Jeglum KA, Whereat A. Chemotherapy of canine thyroid carcinoma. *Compend Contin Educ Pract Vet* 1983;5:96–98.

Klein MK, Powers BE, Withrow SJ, et al. Treatment of thyroid carcinoma in dogs by surgical resection alone: 20 cases (1981–1989). *J Am Vet Med Assoc* 1995;206:1007–1009.

Waters CB, Scott-Moncrieff JCR. Cancer of endocrine origin. In: Morrison WB, ed. Cancer in dogs and cats: medical and surgical management. Baltimore: Williams and Wilkins, 1998:599–637.

Chapter Thirty-Four

Advanced Homotoxicology: Autosanguis Therapy, Oncology, and Cancer Protocols

AUTOSANGUIS THERAPY

Therapy using the patient's own blood, which has received special treatment for the purpose of activating specific and nonspecific immunity, is the basis of autosanguis therapy. The term literally means "auto" (self) and "sanguis" (blood). It represents a powerful tool for healthcare professionals in addressing both acute and chronic diseases.

Medical practitioners have been interested in blood therapy for centuries, and modern medicine continues to recognize the importance of blood elements in normal healing. A related procedure, autohemotherapy, has long been used in human medicine, and has a very good safety record. It involves the use of one's own blood, which is often treated by radiation with ultraviolet light or ozone infusion and then reinfused. It is commonly practiced in human clinics in central Europe (Klemparskaya, et al. 1986).

It has only been in the last few decades that data has emerged to explain the precise mechanisms at work in the simple but powerful tool of autosanguis therapy. Blood therapies have historically been associated with superstitious practices and the occult, and have not been favored by conventional medicine in the United States. However, as physicians and veterinarians begin to understand the actual mechanisms of action of blood therapy, they are becoming more interested in its use in clinical practice (Broadfoot 2005).

Immunology for the homotoxicologist

Although veterinarians graduate from veterinary school with a basic understanding of immune mechanisms and inflammation, the understanding of immunology is advancing so rapidly that many healthcare professionals cannot be expected to stay current in this fascinating arena of scientific enquiry. One need not be an immunologist to do autosanguis therapy, but it is helpful to have a basic understanding of immune events when discussing this with medical professionals or clients.

Immune cellular elements such as macrophages, neutrophils, and monocytes phagocytize foreign material and present it to the lymphatic system for processing. Plasma proteins also coat foreign invaders with plasma proteins, which promote adhesion of the opsonized bacteria and the macrophage (McHeyzer-Williams, Malherbe, McHeyzer-Williams 2006). Inflammatory reactions are regulated by a wide variety of cytokines, such as interleukins (IL-1, IL-2, IL-6, etc.) and tumor necrosis factor (TNF-alpha). These cytokines act as biochemical mediators and provide information and cellular instruction for regulating immune cell function.

Macrophages present larger proteins to the lymphatic system, and, as demonstrated in the homotoxicology chapter, they participate in the immunological bystander reaction (see Figure 34.1).

A specialized type of macrophage called the dendritic cell (DC) has recently provided much exciting information about how the immune system regulates and controls its functions (Kumar, Jack 2006). DCs appear in low frequency in tissues that contact the environment (skin, nasal, pulmonary, and gastrointestinal mucosae). They also circulate in the blood in the immature state. There are two types of dendritic cells:

MDC: Myeloid dendritic cells, which are most similar to monocytes.

PDC: Plasmacytoid dendritic cells, which look like plasma cells but have characteristics similar to myeloid dendritic cells. These are interferon-producing cells (IPC) and they can produce high amounts of interferon-alpha.

MDC probably form from monocytes and, depending on the right biological signal, can transform into either dendritic cells or macrophages. They have a lifespan of only a few days. Activated dendritic cells, with some variation with type and origin, also have a lifespan that is usually only a few days in length. However, immature dendritic cells seem to be able to exist in an inactivated state for much longer.

Once activated, these cells migrate to lymphoid tissues (spleen, lymph node, Peyer's patches, skin, mucosal

767

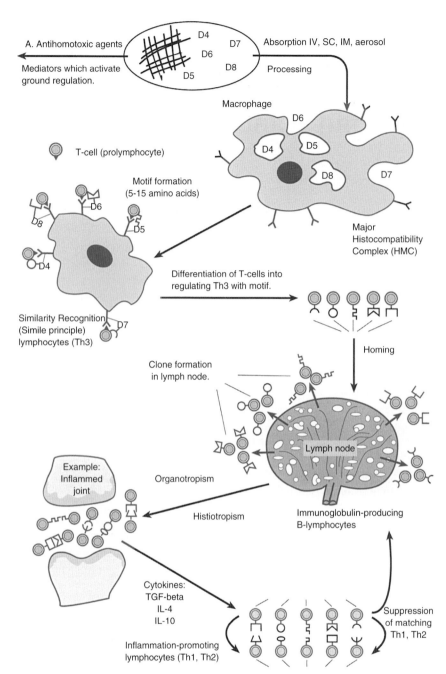

Figure 34.1. The immunological bystander reaction and its relationship to low-dose antihomotoxic formulas (A). Macrophages are stimulated by low-potency homeopathic dilutions in the D1 to D14 dilution range. These agents can be presented by administration via several routes including subcutaneous (SC), intravenous (IV), intramuscular (IM), and across respiratory mucosal membranes (aerosol). Upon uptake of these antihomotoxic agents, the macrophages form antigen motifs, which are prerequisites for the response by lymphocytes (Th3). These Th3 lymphocytes find chemotactically phlogogenic lymphocytes (T4, Th1, Th2) with similar antigen motifs and suppress these by releasing cytokines. (Image used courtesy of Prof Heine, all rights reserved 1997).

tissues, and bone marrow), where they interact with T-cells and B-cells to initiate and shape immune responses. In doing so they regulate both the cell-mediated and humeral immune responses. DCs have large cellular processes—dendrites—that extend from the central cell body. These dendrites provide the cell with a high surface-to-volume ratio, which allows for a single cell to contact many other cells at one time.

Lymphocytes literally migrate in and through a complex interdigitating network and receive instruction that leads them to differentiate appropriately to maintain immune integrity. In the gut, the bulk of this instruction appears to be to convey tolerance to foreign antigens that have gained access to the gut as products of digestion (Xiao, Huang, Link 2006). This process is only marginally understood (the surface antigens that characterize DCs were only identified in 2000), but the discovery of these cells explains many immune functions. It also supports the work by Heine (1997, 1998) that explains the primary mode of operation seen in patients experiencing rapid recovery following autogenous blood therapy, a procedure that has been actively used in alternative medicine since 1951 (Broadfoot 2005).

Dendritic cells also have a role in cancer (Woo, et al. 2006; Kim, Emi, Tanabe 2006; Shurin, et al. 2006). Cytotoxic T-lymphocyte (CTL) soldiers come in contact with neoplastic cells that have the same surface antigens as the original cancer cell and bind to it. They then release a chemical that destroys the cell membrane of the tumor cell, which deflates and dies, releasing further antigen for immune processing.

The principal function of dendritic cells is to act as the generals of the immune response, instructing the adaptive arms to respond to invading pathogens and directing the most effective type of response. Altered intestinal mucosal permeability, also known as leaky gut syndrome, is a factor of immune function. There are three layers of defense in the GI tract:

- The outermost layer, furthest from the bloodstream, contains about 400 species of bacteria. Some are beneficial; others are dangerous. They compete for dominance, and chemicals produced by the bacteria can make the environment antagonistic for the competing species or enable another species to proliferate.
- The next layer is made up of epithelial cells with Toll receptors on their surface. These receptors pick up chemical signals from the battle zone to help the immune system stay prepared to respond to potential transgressors.
- Behind the epithelial layer, directly protecting the bloodstream, is a compact layer of immune cells (lymphocytes, microphages, monocytes, and dendritic cells), some of which bear Toll receptors themselves.

The primary mechanism for immune activation is signaling through the Toll receptors. The proximity of the compact immune cell layer to the bloodstream implies a potentially global response. Oral antibiotics profoundly influence the enteric population dynamics, and therefore have a comparably profound influence on the signaling system (Kabelitz, Wesch, Oberg 2006). Some of the effects of antibiotics on the immune system are well understood. Many more remain insufficiently investigated. One effect that is fairly well understood is a form of malnutrition resulting from an overstimulated signaling system. Overstimulation of signaling can cause a hypersensitivity of the intestinal tract's immune response.

This hypersensitivity can result in an allergic-type response to certain foods and the nutrients they contain. Generally speaking, the more hyperactive this immune cell layer, the fewer nutrients will be properly absorbed. Suppression of this immune response is critical to avoid malnutrition.

Dendritic cell dysfunction, then, can play a major role in allergy and autoimmune diseases such as systemic lupus erythematosus and others. Allergy is a pathologically overblown reaction to an outside allergen, and autoimmune diseases are erroneous immune reactions to self-antigen (Broadfoot 2005, Howard 2006).

Progressive autosanguis therapy according to Reckeweg

Dr. Hans-Heinrich Reckeweg coined the term "progressive autosanguis therapy" and theorized that using a patient's blood assisted the autocontrol mechanisms of the patient's greater defense mechanisms. Reckeweg felt that because the blood is actually an intercellular matrix (mesenchymal connective tissue), it would contain elements of immune recognition as well as homotoxins involved in the patient's specific disease process. He theorized that healing could be initiated in accordance with basic homeopathic theory and the Arndt-Schultz principle of dilution, through serially diluting and homeopathically potentizing a patient's blood while mixing it with certain antihomotoxic agents. This process of removing some blood from the patient, mixing it with antihomotoxic drugs, potentizing it homeopathically, and then readministering it in a series of injections is the basis of Reckeweg's progressive autosanguis therapy. Researchers later began to theorize how this phenomenon works, and today macrophages and lymphocytes explain and support the theory (Heel 2000).

Homotoxicologists use many procedures when performing autosanguis (Broadfoot, Demers, Palmquist 2004). Each clinician has slight differences in technique, and no controlled studies have evaluated differences in results. From a practical, clinical basis, at this time, all commonly performed procedures seem to give good results. It is probably more important to perform this procedure in chronically weakened patients than to argue over precise procedural theories. Diluting homotoxins, presenting diluted homotoxins to immune elements in conjunction with appropriate antihomotoxic drugs, and allowing for initiation of normal immune functions are the key actions in all of the commonly used techniques. The following procedural technique is commonly used by Broadfoot, including demonstrations. It is relatively simple.

Progressive Autosanguis Therapy According to Reckeweg

✔ Exploitation of the immunomodulatory capabilities.
✔ Addition of appropriate antihomotoxic preparations at each stage.
✔ Used mainly in patients with weakened immune responses.

Progressive autosanguis procedure and protocols

Remedies are selected according to the illness/disease process that is clinically presented, and arranged in accordance with the principles set forth in the *Biotherapeutic Index* and elsewhere. Strict sterility is maintained and new materials are used in each patient. Because of the possibility of bloodborne diseases and zoonoses, operators must strictly follow personal and patient protection advisories. When these advisories are followed, the procedure is exceptionally safe and simple to perform (Webster, et al. 2000).

Antihomotoxic agents are generally administered in this order:

1. Symptom therapy
2. Drainage remedy
3. Organ (suis) remedy
4. Nosodes
5. Enzyme (catalyst) therapy

To prepare for the procedure, arrange the antihomotoxic agents in order, and set up a corresponding number of sterile vials to mix and store the therapies (e.g., the sterile water vials left over from vaccine diluents, which the authors save for this purpose). Number these according to the number of dilutions that will be used. Obtain blood from the patient using a 3-cc syringe, and then depress the plunger to empty the syringe of all but the traces of blood that are left coating the syringe and needle. The first dilution antihomotoxic agent is drawn into this blood-coated syringe, succussed (strike the mixture against the palm of your hand to activate it homeopathically) 10 to 20 times, and then injected into the sterile vial labeled #1.

Using the same syringe, draw up the second remedy, succuss it thoroughly, and inject it into sterile vial #2.

Note: The authors frequently put more than 1 remedy in the vial, to make a total volume of 2.2 ml per vial (i.e., some remedies are 1.1 ml, others are 2.2 ml). This process is repeated with all of the dilutions, using the same syringe for all of the remedies.

When all of the dilutions are mixed, then injection therapy can be given to the patient. Generally 0.5 to 1 ml of each vial is administered by subcutaneous injection. Depending on the size and tolerance of the animal (and owners!), the authors may use the acupuncture points at the lateral crease of the elbows (LI11) for the first 2 dilutions. When injecting acupuncture points, do not give more than 0.1 ml per point, or the volume may overwhelm the acupuncture point and cause discomfort for several days after therapy.

If the injections are met with patient resistance, simply use the subcutaneous tissue over the dorsal and lateral neck, where larger injections will be well tolerated. For those not trained in acupuncture, Joseph Demers, a well known American veterinary homotoxicologist and clinical instructor, recommends the use of acupuncture belts, which simply means injecting the material in the area near the target organ. Starting with vial #1, draw up the dose and inject it. Repeat this, in order, for the remaining vials. This is all done in one sitting and takes only a few minutes.

The vials that have remaining blood dilutions can be used in 2 ways. In some cases, the authors have drawn up all of the remaining vials and put them into a Heel formula or combination of formulas, which are referred to as a "cocktail"—e.g., a combination of the *Detox Kit Lymphomyosot, Nux vomica homaccord*, and *Berberis homaccord* in chronic disease states, or a combination of *Lymphomyosot* and *Galium-Heel* in cancer cases. This cocktail is simply mixed together in a glass dropper bottle of approximately 1 to 2 ounces. When treating animals it is recommended that one choose dropper bottles with plastic droppers to prevent accidental injury from broken glass if the patient bites the dropper. There are also some very nice "drip lip" bottles on the market, similar to the Heel tincture bottles, and of course, the authors recycle the Heel glass bottles as well.

Dosing varies according to the patient's medical diagnosis, constitutional strength, and biological response. This procedure can be readily modified as needed. The possibilities are endless, and are left to the discretion of the practitioner. Demers prefers to separate the symptom remedies and drainage/detoxification agents into separate oral cocktails. This allows the clinician to adjust the therapy without having to dispense another bottle of antihomotoxic medicines. This is especially useful when patients begin detoxification that is too aggressive and suffer from diarrhea, vomiting, or depression. If separate bottles have been dispensed, then the clinician can simply stop the detoxification remedy for several days and then restart it at a lower dose and frequency.

After the remedies have been added to the tinctures in the oral cocktail, the entire mixture is succussed 10 to 20 times and sent home with the client as an oral support formula. Formulas containing autogenous blood should be refrigerated and discarded if an off-color develops. Because Heel oral formulas are stabilized in 60% alcohol, most of these mixtures are stable for 30 days when refrigerated properly.

The second option, which is used clinically more frequently by Broadfoot, is to have the owners administer the remedies at home, starting with vial #1, giving a decreased dose on a daily basis, until the remedy is finished. Approximately 0.4 ml is administered per day. Specifically, administer 0.4 ml of remedy #1 daily until it is gone, then administer vial #2 at a dose of 0.4 ml a day until gone, etc. This generally takes a few weeks to finish. The remedies may be given by injection or orally, depending on the expertise of the caregiver. The therapy may be repeated several times, but it is advised that the practitioner give a break between therapies to allow the patient's system a chance to respond. Broadfoot often interposes Glyoxal compositum administration between rounds of therapy, and this appears to improve the patient's energetics in a majority of cases. Clients in these cases often report obvious improvement in vitality.

When treating horses, obtain the drop of blood in a syringe, draw up the first vial as in the above protocol, succuss it, and inject it subcutaneously. Then, using the same syringe, draw up the second remedy, succuss it, and inject. Repeat this down the lineup of remaining antihomotoxic formulas being used. If a send home therapy is desired, then prepare a tincture, or so-called "oral cocktail," for maintenance therapy. The procedure is to simply draw some of the oral tincture into the autosanguis syringe when finished with the injections, empty the contents of the syringe back into the tincture bottle, succuss it, and send it home to be given at the rate of 1 to 2 ml, 2 to 6 times per day, as needed. Broadfoot frequently puts a daily dose into the horse's water bucket.

Palmquist follows a simpler procedure for performing progressive autosanguis therapy. He simply selects the agents desired for injection, arranges them in order of administration, and then draws a blood sample from the patient. The appropriate amount of blood is left in the syringe (see below for discussion of large blood and small blood autosanguis therapy). The entire vial of antihomotoxic agent is drawn into the syringe, succussed, and then HALF the amount is injected into the patient and the other half goes into a bottle for an oral cocktail. This is repeated for each remedy stage in the autosanguis procedure. The oral cocktail is mixed and the resulting combination is succussed and dispensed for oral administration. Palmquist generally places the autosanguis solutions in the detoxification cocktail and dispenses this every 3 days to the patient. In acutely ill, very sick animals, it can be placed in the symptom cocktail and given 2 to 5 times daily.

General therapeutics used in autosanguis therapy

Drainage:

Galium-Heel: Provides cellular drainage and supports greater defenses.

Hepar compositum: Provides liver drainage and supports hepatic tissues.

Lymphomyosot: Provides lymph drainage and immune and endocrine support.

Nux vomica homaccord: Provides hepatic and gastrointestinal drainage.

Solidago compositum: Provides urinary tract drainage and supports urinary tissues.

Strengthening organ function:

Suis organ preparations: Tissue extracts of specific organs.

Compositae preparations: Combinations of animal, mineral, and plant agents.

Catalysts: Agents that support metabolism. *Coenzyme compositum* supports cytoplasmic energy production; *Ubichinon compositum* supports mitochondrial functions; and *Glyoxal compositum* depolymerizes trapped homotoxins.

Immunostimulation/immunomodulation:

Nosodes: Disease-causing agents in dilution (i.e., influenza virus, Staph aureus).

Heteronosodes

Autonosodes: Autologous blood, urine, autovaccines; immunostimulant homeopathic remedies.

Echinacea compositum: Used for bacterial infections.

Euphorbium compositum: Used for viral infections.

Engystol: Stimulates immune responses in viral and allergic cases. It is often combined with *Gripp-Heel* for phagocytic synergism.

The following examples illustrate how homotoxicologists can address commonly encountered pathologies using progressive autosanguis therapy.

Disorders of the immune system: possible remedies

Supportive agents: *Engystol, Gripp-Heel.*

Treatment of immune dysfunction: *Galium-Heel; Tonsilla compositum.*

Treatment of metabolism—catalyst: *Coenzyme compositum.*

Treatment of the constitution: *Tonico-Injeel Neuro-Injeel* ampules.

Stage 1: Symptom remedies

Cutis compositum: Treats chronic skin problems.

Echinacea compositum: Treats chronic bacterial disease.

Engystol: Treats viral diseases, cancer, and allergies.

Euphorbium compositum: Treats recurrent respiratory disease.

Gripp-Heel: Used for fevers.

Traumeel: Used for inflammation.

Viscum compositum: Treats neoplastic conditions.

Stage 2: Drainage remedies

Galium-Heel: Drains cellular debris.

Hepar compositum and *Hepeel*: Drain the liver.

Lymphomyosot: Drains the matrix.

Phosphor homaccord: Drains the liver, lungs, and parenchymous organs, and is used in bleeding issues.

Psorinoheel: Drains the cutaneous structures and central nervous system.

Solidago compositum, Reneel, and *Berberis homaccord*: Drain the kidneys and urinary tract.

Stage 3: Organ (suis) remedies

Cerebrum compositum: Used for the cerebral cortex, embryo, liver, and placenta.

Cor compositum: Treats the heart and liver.

Discus compositum: Treats the intervertebral disc, cartilage, bone marrow, embryo, and adrenal cortex.

Hepar compositum: Used for the liver, duodenum, thymus, colon, gallbladder, and pancreas.

Mucosa compositum: Used for the mucosa (respiratory, gastrointestinal, gall bladder, urinary, and conjunctival) and pancreas.

Ovarium compositum: Treats the ovary, placenta, uterus, fallopian tube, and pituitary gland.

Placenta compositum: Used for vascular elements, the placenta, vein, artery, embryo, umbilicus, and pituitary gland.

Solidago compositum: Treats kidneys, ureter, and bladder.

Testis compositum: Used for testicle, embryo, and adrenal.

Thalamus compositum: Treats thalamus, pineal gland, and adrenal gland.

Thyroidea compositum: Used for thyroid, adrenal, thymus, spleen, bone marrow, liver, and umbilicus.

Tonsilla compositum: Treats tonsil, lymph node, bone marrow, umbilicus, spleen, hypothalamus, liver, and adrenal gland.

Zeel: Used for cartilage, umbilicus, and placenta.

Stage 4: Nosode therapy

Atropinum compositum: Contains Medorrhinum-nosode. Not currently available in the injectable form, but a marvelous remedy nonetheless, which can be used in tablet oral form in combined remedy formulas. The tablet form cannot be injected for autosanguis therapy, however.

Cerebrum compositum: Contains Medorrhinum-nosode.

Cutis compositum: Contains Pyrogenium-nosode.

Echinacea compositum: Contains Influenza-nosode, Streptococcus-nosode, Staphylococcus-nosode.

Galium-Heel: Contains Pyrogenium-nosode.

Mucosa compositum: Contains E. coli bacterium-nosode.

Psorinoheel: Contains Vaccininum-nosode.

Solidago compositum: Contains E. coli-nosode, Coxsackie virus-A9-nosode, Pyrogenium-nosode.

Tartephedreel: Contains Medorrhinum-nosode.

Tonsilla compositum: Contains Pyrogenium-nosode, Psorinum-nosode.

Stage 5: Catalysts

Coenzyme compositum: Works with superficial cytosol metabolism receptors.

Ubichinon compositum: Has mitochondrial elements and helps with energy production.

Glyoxal compositum: Depolymerizes homotoxins, unblocking enzymes and receptors. Helpful in viral conditions and many chronic diseases, but is used less frequently than other catalysts.

Catalysts are also in the following compositae products from Heel: *Cor compositum, Cutis compositum, Discus compositum, Hepar compositum, Placenta compositum, Tonsilla compositum,* and *Zeel.*

Protocols for specific disease types

Chronic musculoskeletal pain

Stage 1: Traumeel.

Stage 2: Spascupreel plus Lymphomyosot.

Stage 3: Discus compositum or Zeel.

Stage 4: Psorinoheel or Tonsilla Compositum.

Stage 5: Coenzyme compositum plus Ubichinon compositum (Galium-Heel can be used intermittently between cycles).

Chronic skin diseases

Stage 1: Echinacea compositum or Tonsilla compositum.

Stage 2: Lymphomyosot plus Engystol N.

Stage 3: Hepar compositum with or without Solidago compositum.

Stage 4: Cutis compositum or Psorinoheel.

Stage 5: Coenzyme compositum plus Ubichinon compositum (Galium compositum can be used intermittently between cycles).

Chronic vaccinosis—neuro form

Stage 1: Traumeel.

Stage 2: Spigelon plus Gelsemium homaccord.

Stage 3: Cerebrum compositum plus Lymphomyosot.

Stage 4: Thalamus compositum plus Galium-Heel.

Stage 5: Coenzyme compositum plus Ubichinon compositum (Galium compositum can be used intermittently between cycles).

Small blood autosanguis versus large blood autosanguis therapy

Large blood autosanguis may be helpful in acute cases. This is a simple procedure involving drawing a larger blood sample from the patient. Draw up the first antihomotoxic drug into a new syringe of adequate capacity. Inject half the quantity intravenously, where allowed by law, and then draw 1 to 5 ml of blood back into the syringe, mixing it with the remaining antihomotoxic drug. Succuss the mixture 10 to 20 times against the palm of the hand, and then inject this mixture subcutaneously or intramuscularly if possible in several sites.

Large blood autosanguis may engage a larger number of matrix elements, and it seems to bring about better results in many cases. This procedure can be very helpful in managing allergy patients that are undergoing acute flare-ups of their symptoms. The usual procedure for Reckeweg's progressive autosanguis therapy is a small blood technique, meaning that a small amount of blood is serially diluted and given to the patient in multiple sites, which may include acupuncture points. By administering the remedies intravenously, subcutaneously, and intra-muscularly, a maximum surface area of the matrix is stimulated. The remaining amounts from the last dose go into the oral cocktail remedy to be sent home with the client, and this mixture is used to stimulate the mucosa-associated lymphoid tissue (MALT)/gut-associated lym-phoid tissue (GALT) system of the gastrointestinal tract's immune system. Recall that macrophages respond better to agents presented in dilution, a fact that according to Immune Bystander Theory may explain why autosanguis serves to activate macrophages that are complacent in the blood of patients with much higher levels of homotoxins (Heine 1998). Agitation occurring in the process of suc-cussion may serve to further this process but this data is not known at this time and is only speculation on the part of the authors.

A compelling observation is that patients receiving autosanguis report similar experiences. First, they often experience a sudden brightening immediately upon injec-tion. This is an instantaneous response similar to Di Chi seen in acupuncture therapy. They next experience cell-mediated phenomena as the local lymph node is recruited and responds over the next 18 to 24 hours. Such responses are compatible with known data about the function of inflammation and other immune processes. Discharges and off-loading of homotoxins often occur within 24 to 48 hours of autosanguis therapy. Such discharge may involve soft stools, mucus discharge, sinus congestion, epiphora, or rhinitis, and occasionally, vomiting. All of these commonly fade rapidly if properly handled and they usually cause little discomfort. Human patients usually report feeling more alive and vital, even in the face of such discharges. If patients experience such effects, especially when they are observed to appear brighter, the symptoms/signs usually fade within 72 hours, and should not be much cause for alarm if all parties have been properly educated prior to undergoing therapy.

Autosanguis therapy provides clinicians with a wonder-ful, simple tool to assist patients in recovering from illness and feeling better more quickly. As further research is done, this form of therapy will no doubt be seen as quite advanced immunotherapy.

Autosanguis therapy is very rewarding in chronic disease patients, and treating cancer without autosanguis is not nearly as beneficial, based upon patient response rates. The reader is referred to the introductory and advanced homotoxicology chapters for further discussion of autosanguis and its application in treating neoplasia.

REFERENCES

Broadfoot P. Autosanguis Therapy: New Insights into an Ancient Therapeutic Tool, proceedings from 1st Veterinary Congress, Memphis, TN. 2005. May 11–13. Heel USA.

Broadfoot PJ, Demers J, Palmquist R. Autosanguis Therapy, in proceedings of the AHVMA/Heel Homotoxicology Seminar, Denver, CO, 2004.May 15–16, pp 1–17 and group discus-sion/demonstration following.

Heel. Biotherapeutic Index: Ordinatio Antihomotoxica et Materia Medica, 5th ed. Baden-Baden, Germany: Biologische Heilmittel Heel GMBH, 2000. pp. 42–8.

Heine H. Neurogene entzundung als basis chronischer schmer-zen. *Beziehungen zur Antihomotoxischen Therapie*. Vortrag 31. Med. Woche Baden-Baden, 1997. Nov 1 (*Bio. Medzin*, in Druck).

Heine H, Schmolz M. Immunologische bystander reaction durch pflanzliche extrakte in anti-homotoxischen preparationen. *Biol Med*. 1998. 27(1):pp 12–4.

Howard Oz. Autoantigen signalling through chemokine recep-tors. *Curr Opin Rheumatol*. 2006. Nov;18(6):pp 642–6.

Kabelitz D, Wesch D, Oberg HH. Regulation of regulatory T cells: role of dendritic cells and toll-like receptors. *Crit Rev Immunol*. 2006. 26(4):pp 291–306.

Kim R, Emi M, Tanabe K. Functional roles of immature den-dritic cells in impaired immunity of solid tumour and their targeted strategies for provoking tumour immunity. *Clin Exp Immunol*. 2006. Nov;146(2):pp 189–96.

Klemparskaya NN, Shalnova GA, Ulanova AM, Kuzmina TD, Chuhrov AD. Immunomodulating effect of autohaemotherapy (a literature review). *J Hyg Epidemiol Microbiol Immunol*. 1986. 130(3):pp 331–6.

Kumar S, Jack R. Origin of monocytes and their differentiation to macrophages and dendritic cells. *J Endotoxin Res*. 2006. 12(5):pp 278–84.

McHeyzer-Williams L, Malherbe L, McHeyzer-Williams M. Helper T cell-regulated B cell immunity. *Curr Top Microbiol Immunol*. 2006. 311:pp 59–83.

Shurin MR, Shurin GV, Lokshin A, Yurkovetsky ZR, Gutkin DW, Chatta G, Zhong H, Han B, Ferris RL. Intratumoral cytokines/chemokines/growth factors and tumor infiltrating dendritic cells: friends or enemies? *Cancer Metastasis Rev*. 2006. Sep 23; [Epub ahead of print].

Webster GJ, Hallett R, Whalley SA, Meltzer M, Balogun K, Brown D, Farrington CP, Sharma S, Hamilton G, Farrow SC, Ramsay ME, Teo CG, Dusheiko GM. Molecular epidemiol-ogy of a large outbreak of hepatitis B linked to autohaemo-therapy. *Lancet*. 2000. Jul 29;356(9227):pp 379–84.

Woo CY, Osada T, Clay T, Lyerly H, Morse M. Recent clinical progress in virus-based therapies for cancer. *Expert Opin Biol Ther*. 2006. Nov;6(11):pp 1123–34.

Xiao BG, Huang YM, Link H. Tolerogenic dendritic cells: the ins and outs of outcome. *J Immunother*. 2006. Sep–Oct;29(5): pp 465–71.

ONCOLOGY

Approaching the patient

When approaching a patient with neoplasia, the clinician must clarify the purpose and goals of therapy for that specific patient's disease process. While clients presenting their pets to integrative veterinarians frequently seek a cure, it is inappropriate at this time to promise that in more advanced cases. Instead, the discussion should center on quality of life and support of the systemic organs and immune systems that are under stress from the primary disease and in response to the iatrogenic pressures of cancer treatment.

An integrative approach is often much appreciated by clients as they navigate the confusions of neoplastic disorders. Such patients require a wide variety of modalities to properly assist them in their pursuit of improved health and well being. Simply excising or destroying the primary tumor mass (i.e., laser and cryosurgery) may not lead to cure, but early and aggressive surgery is an important part of therapy in nearly all cases of neoplasia. Counseling, allopathic medications and chemotherapeutics, radiation, and the gamut of natural therapies such as those discussed herein are also used as needed in conjunction with surgery.

Integrative veterinarians must work with the client and possibly other specialists such as internists, surgeons, and oncologists. Every effort is made to coordinate the therapy so that maximum survival and quality of life are obtained within the client's budget. Frank discussions need to occur about the expectancy of results of various types of therapies available.

A proper diagnosis is essential in selecting therapy for Dedifferentiation Phase patients. Tumor type, location, and grade are all critical factors needed to properly program these cases. Consultation and use of specialists can greatly improve outcomes.

According to Reckeweg, the clinician is concerned with: "(1) the location and extent of the tumor; (2) the growth velocity of the tumor; and (3) the metastatic ability of the tumor" (Reckeweg 2000).

All Dedifferentiation Phase patients suffer from damage to cellular and genetic components. Homotoxins may be bound to elements such as receptors and enzymes, and can actually block or activate oncogenes and their expression. Damage to enzymes and receptors can prevent proper cellular aging and apoptosis, as well as hinder repair of DNA. When the matrix is damaged in content and constituency, it cannot properly allow for diffusion of waste products, oxygen, and nutrients. Cellular damage results when homotoxins accumulate, and vicious cycles ensue favoring the development of neoplastic cell populations. A diseased matrix blocks proper cellular immunity and further favors tumor development. The presence of tumor elements anywhere in the body affects a wide sphere of health, and a tumor's location cannot be viewed to be the sum total of a patient's disease.

Successful management depends utterly on the treatment of the Dedifferentiation Phase as a systemic disease process. Reckeweg and others have emphasized that neoplasia develops as the immune system fails and free radicals do further cellular damage. As tissue acidosis increases, leading to a host of negative cellular events, proteolytic enzyme activity is increased, and tissue regulation fails. All elements must be addressed in a balanced fashion to improve the conditions of patients with this category of pathology; however, this is not always possible (Reckeweg 2000).

Dedifferentiation Phase remedies

As in all forms of biological therapy, the clinician must treat the patient for the correct phase of homotoxicosis for maximum benefit. Phase remedies allow for appropriate repair and drainage to occur so that the patient can move to the left on the Six-Phase Table of Homotoxicology (see Chapter 4, Homotoxicology—The Modern Approach to Homeopathy for further data on the Six-Phase Table). An examination of the ingredients in antihomotoxic agents used as phase remedies in Dedifferentiation Phase cases reveals that many of the factors discussed in prior paragraphs may be addressed with gentle stimulatory therapy of low-dose antihomotoxic drugs. The Dedifferentiation Phase remedies are summarized below:

Galium-Heel: An incredible compositum remedy and useful drainage and cellular support formula for all cellular phase cases. It is also useful in viral issues. Its 18 balanced constituents are indicated for glomerular and renal tubular disorders, mucosal catarrh, gastritis, vomiting, diarrhea, chronic otitis, allergy, polyp formation, eczema, itching, sneezing, exhaustion, nosebleeds, hemorrhage, otitis media, swelling and redness, cystitis, joint pain, and urticaria. It is commonly used in geriatric cases and is part of the Deep Detoxification formula (Heel 2005). Among *Galium-Heel*'s constituents are Galium aparine (common to *Cutis compositum, Ginseng compositum, Thyroidea compositum, Tonsilla compositum, Ubichinon compositum, BHI-Gastro-Cleanse*, et al.), which has been used both internally and externally against cancer and glandular swellings and ulcers. It is said to be able to suspend or modify the further development of a carcinoma.

Its use in cancerous ulcers and nodular tumors of the tongue has been clinically verified, and it has a powerful effect in favor of regressive vicariation. When suppression into cellular phases and in Degeneration and incipient neoplasm phases has occurred, it can reverse them in a biologically correct way. Galium-Heel has proven itself to be extremely important in geriatrics, and in precancerous states, where it regulates numerous basic autonomic functions.

It also contains Calcium fluoratum (*Abropernol, Cutis compositum, and Thyroidea compositum*, et al.) for swelling and fistulae of bones and glandular swellings that are stony-hard and suggest carcinoma. The main action is on connective structures, such as elastic tissue and the periosteum. It promotes the resorption of indurated exudates and also is used in mammary tumors. Nitricum acidum (*Abropernol, Galium-Heel, Hormeel, Lamioflur, Reneel*, et al.) is potentized nitric acid, which is one of the most important polychrests in classical homeopathy. It has a wide therapeutic range, especially in chronic Impregnation Phases that are brought about by deficiencies or retoxications. It is used for hypertrophy of the prostate, benign and malignant proliferation of tissue (hyperblastosis), and illness associated with excessive loss of weight, such as is seen in cases of tumor cachexia.

Sedum acre (also in *Thyroidea compositum*) is used in pre-cancerous states. Sempervivum tectorum (also in *Ginseng compositum, Thyroidea compositum*) is mainly indicated for preneoplastic and Dedifferentiation (formally known as Neoplasm phases) conditions, and it has a particular affinity for nodular hardening in the skin, tongue, and breast, as well as warts. Thuja (also in *Cerebrum compositum, Cutis compositum, Echinacea compositum, Psorinoheel, Thuja compositum*, and others) is a remedy for the most varied range of retoxic Impregnation Phases, and is indicated in vaccination reactions. The Thuja patient gives an impression of being ill, particularly in the emaciation of cancer, with a yellowish or often pale, cachectic complexion. It is also used in skin diseases within the context of Deposition or Inflammation phases, developing out of Impregnation phases, especially warts, condylomata, papilloma, and other excrescences. The constituent Caltha palustris is said to have been useful in uterine cancer. Echinacea angustifolia (*Aesculus compositum, Arnica homaccord, Belladonna homaccord, Echinacea compositum, Tonsilla compositum, Traumeel*, et al.) was used as for complications of vaccination or when a malignant degeneration began in the course of acute or subacute illnesses (Reckeweg 2002). Phytotherapy represents a beneficial form of adjuvant therapy for cancer patients. Echinacea will be covered in more detail, later in this section. In sarcomas, *Galium-Heel*, orally and parenterally, has sometimes proved effective in slowing the advance of the disease.

Glyoxal compositum: This remedy's main ingredients are Glyoxal and Methylglyoxal, which stimulate the general defenses through uncoupling of homotoxins that have become bound to receptors and enzymes (Heel 2005). Patients with neoplasia who receive this agent may become very sleepy and rest thoroughly for 24 to 48 hours after administration. Discharge of mucus or other signs of regressive vicariation may then follow this deep restfulness. Owners need to be advised of this effect in advance, so that it is understood as desirable healing. The agent should not be repeated until recovery has waned. The process of enzyme damage creates the Impregnation Phase, and in serious cases or in repeated retoxications it may even result in progressive vicariation to the Degeneration or Neoplasm phases. The body seeks to compensate for damage by means of a regressive vicariation, in which the retoxins (particularly histamine) are conducted away through reaction phases, which, in severe iatrogenic damage—particularly in Degeneration or even Neoplasm phases—may possibly take on the nature of evasive phases, e.g., suppurative fistulae, chronic skin conditions, etc. These evasive phases allow intermediate homotoxins to be eliminated, thus relieving the toxic state that corresponds to the cellular phase.

Glyoxal has a catalytic effect on damaged respiratory enzymes and unblocks toxin-loaded processes, making it useful in cellular phases, especially in Neoplasm phases. Glyoxal and Methylglyoxal, according to W. Frederik Koch, have deep-reaching actions on a wide variety of degenerative diseases. They contain carbonyl groups, which free blocked energy-producing systems of the cells, and they dissolve cancerous tissue that is in the process of formation by depolymerization of homotoxins and carcinotoxins. This can be influenced by quinones and by free carbonyl groups, provided that they are suitably diluted in homeopathic potency. In their nonpotentized form, they are carcinogenic homotoxins (Reckeweg 2002). The Impregnation Phase is to a certain extent broken up by their free carbonyl groups and quinones, which remove hydrogen (Reckeweg 1967).

Methylglyoxal is produced in small quantities during metabolic processes, and it has a carbonyl group and an aldehyde group. It is suited for transfer of hydrogen and catabolism of toxic amino groups from azomethin compounds, and it is indicated in cellular phases, and particularly in Degeneration and Neoplasm phases (Reckeweg 2002). Methylglyoxal has been studied as a potential treatment for cancer since 1958. Doctors in India recently concluded a 10-year study, including clinical trials, which proved that Methylglyoxal kills cancer tumors in human beings. Methylglyoxal inhibits both mitochondrial respiration and glycolysis in malignant cells, which critically reduces their ATP levels and starves them to death. Methylglyoxal was effective against a wide variety of cancers.

The subjects who returned to excellent health included patients in very advanced stages of colon cancer; acute myeloid leukemia; non-Hodkin's lymphoma; and cancers of the ovary, breast, liver, lung, bone, gall bladder, pancreas, and oral cavity. The researchers noted that concern in some quarters about the safety of Methylglyoxal were not borne out from the clinical trials, which showed that when it was administered in combination with protective agents such as ascorbic acid and vitamins, the drug had no major toxic effects (Ray 2001).

Methylglyoxal is a normal metabolite (Ray and Ray 1981, 1987, 1998; Cooper 1984; Murata et al. 1986). It has the potential to act specifically against malignant cells (Szent-Gyorgyi 1979). Recent research has indicated that Methylglyoxal is tumoricidal (Biswas, et al. 1997). It inhibits both glyceraldelyde-3-phosphate dehydrogenase and mitochondrial complex I of specifically malignant cells. Due to the catalytic activities of these 2 enzymes, nearly 85% of the cellular ATP is generated. The inhibitory effect of Methylglyoxal on these enzymes of malignant cells depletes their ATP pool, rendering these cells nonviable. In contrast, Methylglyoxal has no inhibitory effect on these enzymes of normal cells (Biswas, et al. 1997; Ray, Biswas, Ray 1997). These findings also suggest the possibility of alternation of these 2 enzymes in malignant cells.

Methylglyoxal in combination with ascorbic acid is quite effective in arresting tumor growth, and in some cases could completely eliminate the malignant tissues. Previous in vitro research from Ray's laboratory using human tissue had shown that the anticancer effect of methylglyoxal was significantly augmented in the presence of ascorbic acid (Ray et al. 1991). There is a strong similarity between the mitochondria of malignant and cardiac cells, which poses a serious challenge for the development of an effective anti-cancer drug. This is because the drug in question that will effectively kill cancerous cells by its selective ability to attack mitochondria of malignant cells will also have a deleterious effect on cardiac mitochondria and hence on cardiac functions. However, experimental results suggest that in intact cardiac cells the mitochondria's outer coating acts as a protective device that counteracts the inhibitory effect of methylglyoxal.

It was observed that GSH [N-(N-L-gamma-glutamyl-L-cysteinyl)glycine], commonly called Glutathione, also has a protective function. The results presented in Ray's paper show clearly that this post-mitochondrial supernatant of cardiac cells could almost completely protect the cardiac mitochondria from the potential deleterious effect of methylglyoxal (Ray, et al. 1991). Moreover, it appears that creatine present in high amounts in cardiac cells is mainly responsible for this protective effect. Glutathione is a tripeptide formed from the amino acids cysteine, glycine, and glutamic acid. Reduced levels are always found in cancer patients, as well as those affected by other oxidative stress-induced diseases such as AIDS. GSH also has some protective effect. There may be other unidentified compounds that have some protective ability.

Lymphomyosot: Provides lymph drainage and supports endocrine function (thyroid) and the immune system. May assist with pain by reducing edematous swelling (particularly in combination with antihomotoxic complexes containing Apis, such as *Apis homaccord* and *Traumeel S*). Scrophularia nodosa, one of the main components, has specific indications for breast tumors and is a supporting remedy in neoplasm phases, for general weakness and debilitation, hardening of the glands, and rectal inflammation (Reckeweg 2002).

Procainum compositum: This remedy is not available in the United States at this time. It assists with membrane potentials associated with loss of autoregulatory controls, particularly the pituitary, adrenal cortex, and sympathetic nervous system. It is used in precancerous and neoplastic states. It contains Viscum album, which is useful in headache, dizziness, and hypertonia. Ginseng and China are included for weakness and disability. Artemesia abrotanum addresses emaciation, Berberis vulgaris supports joints and urogenital organs and assists in detoxification, and Procainum hydrochloricum assists peripheral circulation and neuralgia/pain issues (Reckeweg 2000).

Tonsilla compositum: A major phase remedy that is used in all cancer patients and deeply supports immune constituents, endocrine, and central neural controls. It assists with passage of mucus and clearance of homotoxins through mucosal elements (Conium maculatum, Dulcamara, Aesculus hippocastanum, Antimonium tartaricum, Coccus cacti, and Gentiana lutea). Sarcolactum acidum assists in elements of pharyngeal irritation. Calcarea phosphorica and Ferrum phosphoricum both assist with issues involving the chest. Cellular, matrix, and lymphatic drainage is provided through Galium aparine and Glandula lymphatica suis. Ascorbic acid in dilution supports enzyme function as a cofactor. Sulfur activates blocked enzymes, Pulsatilla assists in regulation rigidity cases, and Baryta carbonica assists in glandular swelling. Tonsilla suis, Hepar suis, Funiculus umbilicus suis, Hypothalamus suis, Medulla ossis suis, Splen suis, Adrenal cortex suis, and Embryo suis all support organs that are critical to immune response (Heel 2005).

Glandula lymphaticas suis is included for lymphadenopathy, exudative diathesis, malignant lymphoma, and agranulocytosis, and as a supporting remedy in lymphosarcoma and reticuloses (in company with Galium and Psorinum). Conium (also in *Cerebrum compositum, Cocculus compositum, Ginseng compositum, Rauwolfia compositum, Testis compositum, Thyroidea compositum, Ubichinon compositum, BHI-Prostate*, et al.) addresses glandular swelling and induration that is stony-hard to the touch, which occurs especially after contusions and bruises, sometimes starting as a lump in the breast. Thus, Conium is also given in cancerous conditions of the breasts and the womb, as well as in hypertrophy of the prostate and stomach pains with vomiting, thirst, and craving for sour things, such as is often found in cancer of the stomach. It is considered to be a constitutional treatment in neoplasm phases, and is used for tissue neoformation in various organs.

Funiculus umbilicalis suis (also in *Cutis compositum, Discus compositum, Placenta compositum, Thyroidea compositum,* and *Zeel*) is a connective tissue remedy indicated in almost all chronic diseases, particularly those with damage to connective tissue, such as collagen diseases, scleroderma, and fibromas. It can be used for conditions that result from radiation damage, e.g., sarcomas and carcinomas. It is also useful in auto-immune and general iatrogenic damage. This remedy should always be given in combination with suitable biotherapeutic remedies and other sarcodes (such as pituitary and adrenal gland, particularly with suitable catalysts and combination remedies).

L(+)-lacticum acidum (*Ginseng compositum, Placenta compositum, Thyroidea compositum, Ubichinon compositum, BHI-Rendimax,* et al.) is included for disturbed cell respiration, pre-cancerous conditions, and neoplasm phases. Splen suis (*Cutis compositum* and *Thyroidea compositum*) is used for leukemia, anemia, and agranulocytosis, and in carcinoma for general revitalization. Sulphur (also in *Causticum compositum, Cerebrum compositum, Coenzyme compositum, Cutis compositum, Discus compositum, Echinacea compositum, Engystol N, Ginseng compositum, Hepar compositum, Molybdan compositum, Mucosa compositum, Psorinoheel, Pulsatilla compositum, Sulfur-Heel, Thyroidea compositum, Ubichinon compositum, Zeel, BHI-Enzyme, BHI-Gastro-Cleanse, BHI-Intestine, BHI-Skin,* and many others) achieves its effects by reactivating enzyme-based detoxification. Sulphur is the major remedy in practically all cellular phases. Numerous enzymes become active through sulphide groups, such as Coenzyme A, the cytochromes, and others, and synthetic drugs and heavy metals easily block SH-groups, resulting in subclinical, iatrogenic damage. Thus, Sulphur, which is contained in many compositae-class remedies in a suitable attenuation appropriate to the biological milieu, may reverse damage in many cases. It should always be given intercurrently in high potencies if well-indicated remedies do not act, even in Degeneration or Neoplasm phases (i.e., the further to the right of the Biological Divide, the higher the potency).

Thyroxine has particular importance for the functioning of the interstitial mesenchyme, which is generally accelerated and activated by Thyroxine, Thyroidinum, or other thyroid hormones. Doses of the hormone are given not in substitutive dosage, but in excitative dosage (higher homeopathic potencies, which are lower dosages in milligrams), and are used to activate the mesenchyme to help purge the terrain of homotoxins (Reckeweg 2002). This remedy also contains Galium aparine and Echinacea (see *Galium homaccord,* above).

Viscum compositum: Functions best when given by injection due to digestion of active ingredients by the gastrointestinal system. Viscum album (mistletoe) is a semi-parasitic botanical, native to Europe and Asia, that is found on almost all deciduous trees. It contains several lectins, which are cytotoxic (mouse ascites tumor; human tumor cells). Several parenteral preparations of mistletoe exist such as Iscador, Plenosol, Helixor, and others. Mistletoe extract in a mother tincture and is available in 10 X, 28 X, and 198 X dilutions. Viscum album is an herb that has been used safely by herbalists, holistic doctors, and veterinarians for more than 80 years. It lowers blood pressure and heart rate (through altered nitrogen oxide levels) and may slow the growth of certain neoplastic elements (Tenorio Lopez, et al. 2006).

This agent has been determined to have immunomodulatory and antiangiogenesis effects, and active research is currently under way to determine its method of action (Huber, et al. 2005, Yance and Sagar 2006). The exact tumor-inhibiting action of the extract of Viscum is controversial. The mechanism of action on tumor cells by mistletoe may be due to enhanced cytokine release (Interleukin-1, Interleukin-6, and Tumor Necrosis Factor-alpha), which affect fibroblastic activity in the matrix, amongst other actions. Its effect may be due to the lectins contained in plant extracts (Hostanska 1993) or carbohydrates (Schink 1997). Mistletoe lectin has been reported to induce apoptosis in different cancer cell lines in vitro and has shown antitumor activity against a variety of tumors in animal models by inhibiting telomerase activity and inducing apoptosis that resulted from dephosphorylation of Akt in the survival signaling pathways. Viscum album triggers molecular changes that inhibit cell growth and induce apoptotic cell death of cancer cells (Choi, et al. 2004).

A recent PubMed search under this agent resulted in more than 400 hits, indicating the quantity of work currently under way (Hajto, et al. 2006). Viscum has been found to reduce ascites accumulation in advanced cancer patients in humans (Bar-Sela, et al. 2006, Harmsma, et al. 2006). Viscum album is also a key ingredient in *Aesculus compositum, Ginseng compositum, Thalamus compositum,* and *Thyroidea compositum.* The main indications are Impregnation Phases, precancerous states, and neoplastic phases (Reckeweg 2002). The ingredient cyclic AMP (cAMP), which is also in *Thalamus compositum,* stimulates cellular enzyme and regulatory systems (Heel

2005). cAMP has become known as a significant intracellular regulating factor that is produced in the cell membrane as the result of stimuli, which are generated in the surrounding connective tissue and engender cell differentiation. It is antagonistic toward cGMP (cyclic guanosine monophosphate), through which undifferentiated cell growth is promoted, i.e., cancerous growths, which are distinguished by disturbances in respiration and mutation and unlimited growth of undifferentiated cells. cAMP is used principally for stimulative reactivation in enzyme blocks in cellular phases and in iatrogenic damage. It may be tried experimentally in virus diseases and as a supportive treatment in cancer; it can be given in higher potencies in cancer, e.g., 12 X to 20 X dilution (Reckeweg 2002).

Extracts of mistletoe combined with homeopathic treatment also seem to help small cell lung carcinoma (Bradley 1999). Palmquist has used Viscum compositum to lower chronically elevated serum calcium levels associated with paraneoplastic syndrome in an aged dog suffering from advanced, metastatic anal gland carcinoma. Giving *Viscum compositum forte* subcutaneously 4 days weekly resulted in a marked decline of serum calcium levels, and an interruption in therapy resulted in a return of hypercalcemic states, which regressed upon resumption of the injection series. This application deserves much deeper investigation, and will be published once survival data is available (Palmquist 2005).

Activation of cell metabolism (catalyst therapy)

Cancer is a disorder of deranged metabolic function. Catalysts improve cellular metabolism by activating enzymes. Several remedies are specifically designed for metabolic support:

Coenzyme compositum: Contains *cis-Aconiticum acidum* (also in *BHI-Enzyme*). As with all catalysts of the citric acid cycle, aconitic acid shows an affinity for internal respiration. It is very effective when combined with Succinicum acidum and Natrum oxalaceticum, and can be used for pain in the bones, in the spine between T3 and T4, in C7, and in the sacrum. It is also indicated in disturbances of the citric acid cycle, Impregnation Phases, precancerous states, and in Dedifferentiation Phases (especially in the early stages) to improve cell respiration. It also contains Baryta oxalsuccinica (*BHI-Enzyme*). This compound has an affinity for mesenchymal structures and it improves the function of the citric acid cycle and redox systems. It has a regenerative effect on cell respiration and is useful in debilitated patients. It works well in combination with the sarcodes (pituitary, testis, oophorinum, and brain) and with Hydrastis, Lachesis, Kali carbonicum, Calcium carbonicum, Agaricus, petroleum, and Thuja. It is recommended for lung cancer with congestion extending to the head and nasal polyps, prostate and bladder cancer, kidney diseases, and uremia.

The constituent Beta vulgaris rubra reactivates cell respiration and can regenerate blocked respiratory enzymes, and is therefore indicated in all cellular phases. This remedy also includes Cerium oxalicum, which is common to *Molybdan compositum* and *BHI-Enzyme*. It should also be tried as an anti-emetic in cancer patients that can no longer keep down any food. Cerium salts promote the use of oxygen in the tissues, and thus may be used as an intercurrent remedy in the treatment of neoplasms and precancerous states, and in Degeneration Phases.

Citricum acidum (common to *BHI-Enzyme, BHI-Exhaustion, BHI-UriCleanse*) is also included. Citric acid has a close affinity for respiratory disturbances when there are tumors, and is also indicated for cancer pain (Boericke 1927). Citric acid is also helpful in certain complaints arising from vitamin C deficiency. As noted in the section on *Glyoxal compositum*, vitamin C has a protective effect on normal cells. Cysteinum, an SH-group-containing factor of redox potentials (e.g., glutathione), is used in retoxic and iatrogenic damage of all kinds, and used intercurrently in all cellular phases, especially in liver damage, leukemia, pre-cancerous states, and neoplastic phases. Fumaricum acidum (*Causticum compositum, Hepar compositum, Thyroidea compositum, BHI-Enzyme*, et al.) is very similar in indications to the aforementioned citric acid cycle catalysts. Malic acid and fumaric acid should always be injected together to avoid disturbances in the chain of the citric acid cycle. Alpha-Ketoglutaricum acidum (also in *Causticum compositum, Hepar compositum, Thyroidea compositum, BHI-Enzyme*, et al.) has the same indications as other catalysts in this remedy, along with the feeling of utter exhaustion, general glandular hypofunction, after excision of tumors, stomach atony, prostate patients, and post-amputation pain (causalgia). DL-Malicum acidum (*Hepar compositum, Thyroidea compositum, BHI-Enzyme*, et al.) is used as above, and has a diuretic action.

This is one of the main remedies for general detoxification as well as for oxygenation of glandular and muscular tissues. It also plays a dominant role in neoplastic processes. It is indicated in fevers of unknown origin, serious infectious diseases, chronic respiratory disease, intestinal cancers, and cancer of the bladder, and as a supporting remedy in bronchial cancer. Natrum oxalaceticum (*Causticum compositum, Ginseng compositum, Hepar compositum, Mucosa compositum, Thyroidea compositum, Ubichinion compositum, Zeel, BHI-Enzyme*, et al.) is another component. Like all catalysts of the citric acid cycle, oxaloacetic acid—a product of the dehydration of malic acid—has an affinity for the internal respiration of the tissues and is useful in Dedifferentiation Phase homotoxicoses (especially initially) to improve cell respiration.

When used as a supporting remedy with Fumaricum acidum, Natrum oxalaceticum can accelerate patient response considerably; the 6 X should be given in acute cases, and the 12 X should be given in chronic cases. Consider its use in acute and chronic inflammations of the naso-pharynx, lungs and bronchi, duodenal ulcer and other inflammatory illnesses of the stomach and intestinal tract, prostatitis, and neoplasms.

Natrum pyruvicum (*Placenta compositum, Solidago compositum, BHI-Enzyme*) has certain similarities to the indications for Sulphur because pyruvic acid is situated at a focal point in the citric acid cycle and Sulphur-like symptoms occur when there is an accumulation of pyruvates, e.g., in iatrogenic damage. Natrum pyruvicum can be advantageously combined with *Engystol, Sulphur-Heel*, and possibly *Hepar compositum*; with all sarcodes and numerous nosodes, particularly in cellular phases of all kinds; and in pre-cancerous states and neoplasm phases. The homotoxins that require Natrum pyruvicum do not depend so much on disorders of the direct energy extraction and use, as they do in respiratory disorders, but rather they concern an integral part of the energy extraction, which precedes the introduction of the decomposing carbohydrates into the citric acid cycle. Alpha-lipoic acid can be useful in combination with sodium pyruvate. Pyruvic acid stands at the dividing line between respiration and fermentation, and a study of Warburg's oxygen deprivation theories of cancer gives a glimpse into the critical aspect of these processes.

Succinicum acidum (*BHI-Enzyme, BHI-Prostate*) is another active factor in the citric acid cycle and in redox systems. It is used from the Impregnation Phase throughout the Neoplasm Phases, particularly early in the pathological process. Succinic acid is related to blood formation and should therefore be used in cases of anemia and leukemia, duodenal ulcers which do not heal, enteritis and colitis with a sensation of weakness in the whole abdomen, and carcinoma of the colon (Reckeweg 2002). Recent work at the University of Glasgow has highlighted the critical importance of succinic acid. This work discovered how mitochondria can sustain and even create a cancerous state. Mitochondria are complex structures that exist in cells to generate energy for growth and activity. It was recently discovered that the excessive build-up of a simple metabolic molecule in mitochondria can trigger a sequence of events that leads to tumor growth. The study looked at one of the known tumor suppressor genes, SDH, which codes for succinate dehydrogenase. When the SDH gene is damaged, succinic acid accumulates in cells. This then causes the levels of a protein called HIF-1 to rise, which is activated in response to low oxygenation because it encourages the growth of blood vessels to help cells get more oxygen. If the SDH gene mutates, the succinic acid blocks the degradation of HIF-1, and blood vessel pro-duction goes unchecked, thereby feeding the tumor. Mutations in SDH can predispose to cancer of the kidney, adrenal gland, and thyroid gland, as well as stomach and bowel cancer. This study is the first to find a molecular mechanism that links mitochondrial mutations to tumor formation (Thompson, Gottlieb 2005).

Sulphur (common to *Causticum compositum, Cerebrum compositum, Echinacea compositum, Engystol N, Ginseng compositum, Hepar compositum, Molybdan compositum, Mucosa compositum, Psorinoheel, Pulsatilla compositum, Thyroidea compositum, Tonsilla compositum, Ubichinon compositum, Zeel, BHI-Gastro-Cleanse*, and many, many others) is also a component. For more data on this component, see *Tonsilla compositum*, above.

Glyoxal compositum: See above.

Pulsatilla compositum: A fairly simple remedy for activation of the host defensive system—particularly the function of detoxicating connective tissues containing Pulsatilla for catarrhs of the mucosa—and general support in regulation rigidity type II, wherein the body seems to be incapable of mounting an adequate or appropriate response. Sulfur is included for chronic diseases (see *Tonsilla compositum*, above) and cortisone acetate is included for damage to the adrenal cortex, pituitary gland, and connective tissue. This combination stimulates the defensive system, especially connective tissue function. It is synergistic with nosodes for the treatment of cancer, as well as for the therapy of cellular phases in general. It can help to reactivate damaged defensive systems, e.g., bone marrow, interior lobe of the pituitary gland, and adrenal, and help with liver damage. It can also be considered in retoxic/iatrogenic damage from antibiotics, phenylbutazone, etc.

Pulsatilla compositum can be used to try to achieve regressive vicariation or to convert Degenerative Phases into Inflammation Phases. Because inflammation is a biologically advantageous defensive process against toxins, any defensive reactions that are increased by *Pulsatilla compositum* should not be suppressed with antibiotics or chemotherapeutics unless they are critical to the patient's survival. Most feverish conditions that arise in the course of the biological treatment of neoplasia must not be treated with any anti-inflammatory or antipyretic measures. These measures would interfere with the vegetative organization's attempts to bring about the degradation and decomposition of defective cell groups or cellularly fixed Degeneration phases through immune reactions and subsequent connective tissue reactions with inflammation and fever.

Fresh cell therapy with the most damaged organs of the defensive system (thymus, liver, spleen, bone marrow, thalamus, and pineal gland) should also be tried. Antibiotics should be reserved for life-threatening circumstances.

Pulsatilla compositum, for all its simplicity, has a great scope of action and diverse applications from the aspect of activating the defensive function, especially that of the connective tissue (Reckeweg 2000).

Thyroidea compositum: Contains Glandula thymi suis (also in *Hepar compositum*) for disorders of growth and development as well as for neoplasm phases. Glandula thyroidea suis is indicated in thyroid tumors, neoplastic phases, adiposity, and liver and kidney diseases. Fucus vesiculosus is indicated for enlarged lymph glands and benign tumors. In addition, there are many other components that are common to previously mentioned combinations, including Colchicum, Conium, L(+)-lacticum acidum (see *Ubichinon compositum*), Corpus pineale suis (see Thalamus compositum), Calcium fluoratum, Galium aparine, Sempervivum tectorum, Sedum acre (see *Galium-Heel*), Graphites, Funiculus umbilicalis suis, Splen suis, Sulphur (see *Tonsilla compositum*), DL-Malicum acidum, Natrum oxalaceticum, alpha-Ketoglutaricum acidum, and Fumaricum acidum (see *Coenzyme compositum*).

Tonsilla compositum: See above.

Ubichinon compositum: This combination resembles *Coenzyme compositum*, and shares many remedies. It is considered to be a deeper acting remedy and it has strong indications in Dedifferentiation Phases. Anthrachinon is one of its many useful components. According to W. F. Koch, it regenerates blocked cell respiration by burning away accumulated toxins (amines and others), and is therefore indicated in cellular phases, e.g., Impregnation, Degeneration, and neoplastic disease (Reckeweg 2000). It acts on the regulation of the respiratory chain function. It is particularly indicated in cancer of the prostate and in cancer of the uterus when there is watery, brown discharge with great tiredness and possibly ascites.

The component para-Benzochinonum has a comprehensively regenerative action on cell respiration in many cases (citric acid cycle) because it diminishes the effect of free radicals and mutative damage. It is indicated in all cellular phases, especially leukemia, asthma, organic diseases of the nerves, precancerous states, neoplasias, hepatitis, et al. It is similar to Hydroquinone in its structure and action; however, it is substantially more specific and deeper-acting. para-Benzochinonum has been used for cancer patients with almost hopeless cachexia and totally wrecked metabolism. The most important indications for para-Benzoquinone are cancers of the lower sections of the intestines, papilloma of the bladder, condylomata on the penis—which are often hard and strongly pigmented—and faulty hormone function (pituitary or adrenals). It is essential to cleanse the body of its whole homotoxic state by using nosodes, and especially remedies that stimulate elimination. Otherwise, the homotoxic material which is set in motion by the para-Benzoquinone may give rise to

considerable extension of reaction phases, e.g., to abscess-formation which, under the circumstances, must be seen as a biologically favorable channel of elimination. It is expedient to give it in combination with whichever of the other remedies is also indicated, especially with the corresponding nosodes and sarcodes of the tissues or organs in question. For expediency in parenteral treatment it should always be given singly, with the other remedies being given alongside it.

Colchicum (common to *Aesculus compositum, Arnica-Heel, Ginseng compositum, Thyroidea compositum*, et al.) acts on individual areas of the mucosa (stomach and small intestine), serous membranes (pleura, peritoneum and pericardium), fibrous tissues (ligaments and tendons, especially of the smaller joints), and muscle fibers (especially the intercostal muscles and the diaphragm), where inflammatory processes predominate. Colchicum has also proved effective in neoplasm phases, especially when there is lack of appetite. This has been supported by the results of pharmacological trials which have shown that colchicine, the active principle of the meadow saffron, is a typical mitosis poison. It has a blocking effect that prevents cancer cells from further division.

Conium (also in *Cerebrum compositum, Ginseng compositum, Testis compositum, Thyroidea compositum, Tonsilla compositum, BHI-Prostate*, et al.) is a component; see *Tonsilla compositum*, above. Galium aparine (see *Galium-Heel*, above) is another constituent. Hydrastis canadensis (also in *Ginseng compositum, Lamioflur, Mucosa compositum, Ovarium compositum, Ubichinon compositum*, et al.) is used principally in serious disorders of the autonomic nervous system. It is also used in cancer and septic states, gastrointestinal ulceration, liver conditions with jaundice, cystitis, illnesses of the uterus with vaginal discharge, breast lumps, and when there is great weakness. The clinical picture includes cachexia with suspected neoplasm, especially where there is complete failure of the stomach, resulting in emaciation. It is useful in acrid, raw, excoriating discharges when a general deterioration of energy is present, e.g., in cancer and cancerous degeneration and tumors in various organs and parts of the body, including the mammary tissue.

Hydrochinon is included for disturbances in oxygen utilization from Impregnation Phases with a characteristic disturbance in the respiratory chain. It is used alongside alpha-ketoglutaric acid and Benzoquinone to compensate for side effects of allopathic drugs on the respiratory center. It may be useful in progressive dyspnea and cardiac weakness of lung cancer. Hydroquinone obviously has a similar action on the vascular system to that of rutin, and can be used in cases of hemorrhage. In the course of relapses of cancer in the breast or abdomen, and if hemorrhages of short duration which improve the general state of health are observed, then Hydroquinone must be given at short intervals—approximately every 2 days—to cleanse the toxicity of the body. L(+)-lacticum acidum and sarcolactic acid (see *Tonsilla compositum*) are also components of this remedy. The component Myrtillus exerts a catalytic action on cell respiration; thus it is indicated in neoplasm phases and viral diseases, which are, by definition, cellular phase diseases.

Naphthoquinone has carbonyl group functions, and thus, according to Koch, can metabolize toxic amino groups from azomethine compounds. It should be used in all cellular phases, viral diseases, and toxic infections (reaction phases), and particularly in neoplasms. Serious forms of carcinoma in the areas of the intestines and genitalia are the main indications, especially when radiotherapy follows surgical removal of the carcinoma. It is particularly useful in carcinoma of the uterus and the prostate, and it helps with the pain associated with these cancers. It is also recommended for rapidly growing brain tumors that occur with no premonitory signs. Other indications are diseases of the air passages and from severe sinusitis associated with intestinal sluggishness, laryngeal cancer with very hard nodes, lung cancer, and cancer of the oral cavity. Naphthoquinone is indicated in stomach cancer with complete emaciation, degenerative kidney diseases, chronic nephritis with albumen excretion and increasing residual nitrogen, and cancer of the bladder with agonizing pain and suppurating inflammations of the renal pelvis. In severe cases of cancer, lymphatic congestion may also be present. The deficient adrenalin function is suited to the cachectic patient, whose whole vital activity is exclusively directed to the rapidly multiplying cancer cells; thus, Naphthoquinone should be tried. Because it has particular affinities for the tonsils and the appendix, i.e., for the secondary defenses of the lymphatic mechanism, Naphthoquinone should also be used after tonsillectomy or appendectomy, and in adenoma of the pancreas.

Podophyllum (*Leptandra, Momordica compositum, Podophyllum compositum, BHI-Pancreas*, et al.) may be used in a wide range of potencies in the treatment of pancreatic problems. In recent years it has been found to be important in cancer treatment, particularly in the colitis that occurs after radiotherapy. Podophyllum's characteristic conditions can affect the entire gastrointestinal tract, from the mouth (dental caries) to the anus. Podophyllum is a remedy of limited therapeutic range, but of great importance in gastrointestinal and biliary illnesses, particularly in pancreatic conditions and cancer. Because it is very likely that the pancreas plays a part—the exact nature of which is not yet known—in the genesis of neoplasms, Podophyllum may well have relationships to cancer therapy (Reckeweg 2002). For more data on the pancreatic role in cancer, study John Beard's work, and the *Trophoblastic Theory of Cancer*.

General support remedies and viral implications of cancer

Viral infection can predispose patients to secondary local and systemic bacterial and fungal diseases. Progressive vicariation is linked to a direct effect of viruses on the tissues, as well as alterations in cells involved in immune surveillance. A number of viruses have been shown to suppress various functions of polymorphonuclear leukocytes, which are critical for controlling bacterial and viral infections and can predispose toward some cancers, particularly when we interfere with normal body defense mechanisms by suppressing defense symptoms. The alteration in functions of polymorphonuclear leukocytes includes abnormalities of adherence, chemotaxis, phagocytosis, oxidation, secretion, and bactericidal activities (Abramson 1988).

Molecular analysis of viruses associated with cancer has revealed that they function in part by encoding proteins with which they can associate and subvert the function of the host-cell-encoded tumor suppressor proteins, which regulate pathways of growth arrest and apoptosis (Morris 1995). Infections such as gastritis, hepatitis, and colitis are recognized risk factors for human cancer. The progression of conditions from viral infection to bacterial infection to neoplastic processes follows the chart of homotoxicology. A large number of complementary methods have been proposed, such as mistletoe preparations, organotherapeutics (cell cytoplasmic, and thymus therapy), and enzyme therapy (Malafronte 1996). Chronic viral infections have been documented in mice that become carriers for life-harboring viruses in many tissues such as the thymus, kidney, testes, and brain. However, the thymus retains the ability to restore immunocompetence to the host and protect against re-infestation (Jamieson 1991).

The following remedies can help improve the patient's condition by supporting organs, improving immune status, and providing drainage therapy:

BHI-Chelidonium complex: Also known as *Gall Bladder*, this remedy contains Chelidonium majus, Belladonna, and Lycopodium. According to Reckeweg (2002), Lycopodium and Belladonna complement Chelidonium for improving the liver function and reducing spastic and inflammatory symptoms. Cholesterinum (also in Hepar compositum and BHI-Body-pure) have indications for experimental use in liver cancer and hepatomegaly (Reckeweg 2002).

Causticum compositum: An excellent combination for exhaustion and debility. It is particularly indicated in cases that are undergoing radiotherapy, because it is specifically protective in radiation burns. It contains many useful components, including Embryo suis as a regenerative therapy, Arsenicum album (see the above protocols section), Fumaricum acidum, alpha-Ketoglutaricum acidum, Natrum oxalaceticum (see *Coenzyme compositum*), and Sulphur (see *Tonsilla compositum*).

Chelidonium homaccord: Contains the remedy Chelidonium majus (also in *Hepar compositum*, *Hepeel*, and others). This remedy helps to promote the discharge of toxins, much like the similar remedies. Celandine has a healing action in liver and biliary conditions, and is indicated when the stools are clay-colored or golden yellow, or when the urine is lemon-yellow or dark brown, because of the presence of biliary coloring. Crude extracts, as well as purified compounds of Chelidonium majus, have been reported to exhibit antiviral, anti-inflammatory, antitumor, and antimicrobial properties both in vitro and in vivo. Chelidonium is a homeopathic drug that is routinely used against various liver disorders, including cancer in humans. The homeopathic dilutions exhibited antitumor and antigenotoxic activities and also favorably modulated activities of several marker enzymes. Thus, nanopharcological doses of Chelidonium may be effectively used in cancer of the liver (Biswas 2002).

Echinacea compositum forte: Stimulates the general defense mechanisms, and is a complementary treatment for system immune surveillance. Phytotherapy represents a beneficial form of adjuvant therapy for cancer patients; evidence proves that Echinacea is effective in this context. Polysaccharide extracts from Echinacea purpurea activate macrophages against tumor cells and microbes (Luettig 1989), with the primary action directed toward the nonspecific cellular immune system (Bauer 1996).

Engystol: This remedy, particularly when combined with *Gripp-Heel*, must be used along with conventional methods of treatment such as chemotherapy or immunotherapy, because there are no controlled studies on the exclusive use of these complex homeopathic preparations. Because of the association of lymphoma with viral diseases such as Epstein-Barr in humans and feline leukemia in cats, a complex homeopathic formula with demonstrated anti-infectious activity, such as *Engystol*, can be selected. *Engystol* is a combination preparation containing Vincetoxicum hyrundinaria (swallowwort) and Sulphur, which has other effects that stimulate a mesenchymal purge. It has been the subject of extensive studies, including a few on the efficacy and mode of action in immunoprophylaxis in cancer patients with neoplastic disease. The primary focus of these particular studies was the use of the remedies to reduce complications of infection peri-operatively in cancer patients, and they demonstrated an increase in both cellular defense numbers and phagocytic activity. This is critically important in immunosuppressed individuals, bacterial and viral defense, and oncotic recognition (Siewerska 1999).

Ginseng compositum: Indicated in exhaustion cases and used for general revitalization. Extracts of Panax ginseng enhance cellular immune function of peripheral blood mononuclear cells from healthy individuals as well as from patients with depressed cellular immunity (Broumand 1997). Kreosotum (also in *Lamioflur*, *Mucosa compositum*, *Ovarium compositum*, *Populus compositum SR*, *BHI-Skin*, and others) is a component. Creosote is a carcinogen, and has effects that are similar to those of pure phenol (carbolic acid), with an excoriating effect on the skin and mucosa, followed by deeper destruction of the tissue. Thus, it should engender significant curative action by reversal effect. Excoriating, fetid, and burning discharges are characteristic indications, as are hemorrhages and ulcers.

This remedy is useful in mammary tumors, catarrhs of the lungs, cachexia, and weakness. It is said to complement Arsenicum album, Phosphorus, and Sulphur in malignant illnesses. Can be used in hypertrophy of the prostate gland and carcinoma of the uterus. This remedy also contains Colchicum, Conium, Hydrastis, L(+)-lacticum Acidum (see *Ubichinon compositum*), Galium aparine and Sempervivum tectorum (see *Galium Heel*), Natrum oxalaceticum (see *Coenzyme compositum*), and Sulphur (see *Tonsilla compositum*). ATP is contained for critical mitochondrial support of the energy-consuming systems, along with Nadidum (NAD), a biocatalyst that stimulates end oxidation in the respiratory chain. *Ginseng compositum* is useful when serious endogenous toxin levels are present in degenerative diseases, particularly cancer, which cannot be overcome without medical aid. Ginseng acts by strengthening the anterior lobe of the hypophysis cortex of the suprarenal gland system, and Acidum L(+)-lacticum, particularly in neoplasia, counteracts the pronounced acidosis of the affected tissue by the reversal effect. Sulphur, Psorinum, and Pulsatilla all possess a constitutional action to mobilize and eliminate toxins, while Hydrastis, Conium, Colchicum, Kreosotum, Viscum album, Galium aparine, and Sempervivum tectorum reduce the tendency toward neoplasia.

The enzyme systems, always deranged in the cellular phases, are stimulated by the intermediary catalysts Natrium oxalaceticum, Coenzyme A, adenosine triphosphate, and NAD, particularly when combined with compositae formulas such as the catalysts *Coenzyme compositum* and *Ubichinon compositum* the *suis*-containing remedies such as *Hepar compositum* and *Mucosa compositum*, or specific organ compounds. *Engystol* and *Pulsatilla compositum* are also good adjuncts, along with *Galium-Heel* and *Thalamus compositum* for faulty neural control. *Ginseng compositum* is an auxiliary therapeutic agent in neoplasia, leukemia, lymphogranulomatosis, precancerous states, adrenal exhaustion, and cases of toxic overload. In addition, *Molybdan compositum* should always be administered concurrently, as a trace element donor-regulator (Reckeweg 2000).

Gripp-Heel: This is a useful antiviral formula used traditionally for cold and flu-like symptoms (Rabe, Weiser, Klein 2004). *Gripp-Heel* is mentioned in medical literature as early as 1954. The total effect theoretically corresponds to an acceleration of mesenchymal immune reaction(Till 1986). *Gripp-Heel* combines nicely with *Engystol N*; they appear to work synergistically to enhance immune function. In vitro tests have demonstrated that *Engystol* stimulates the phagocytic activity of human granulocytes up to 33%. This effect was further enhanced to 41% by combining *Engystol* and *Gripp-Heel* (Wagner, et al. 1993).

Patients suffering from Dedifferentiation homotoxicoses often harbor virus particles in their tissues, and as they undergo regressive vicariation, these viruses may emerge and manifest clinical symptoms. Such viruses may be oncogenic or simply just be present in affected tissues. *Gripp-Heel* is useful in management of these symptoms (particularly upper respiratory, sinus, and pulmonary signs with or without fever and myalgia).

Another phenomenon frequently noted in responsive cancer patients is the accumulation of so-called toxic fluids. These congest the matrix as the homotoxins move out of cells and into the intercellular space, where they are diluted and processed. Because these patients often have thickened lymph and reduced lymphatic function, not to mention reduced nutrition and physical activity, such accumulations often cause clinical distress, febrile response, discomfort, pain, and even dyspnea or coughing. Using adequate drainage (*Lymphomyosot, Apis compositum* or *homaccord*, and *Galium-Heel*) greatly assists these individuals through their discomfort.

There is some evidence that *Gripp-Heel* may function to reduce pain (most likely not by suppression but by reducing homotoxins associated with the genesis of discomfort). People frequently report reduction in myalgia from influenza in response to *Gripp-Heel*, and the authors have experienced this directly. Placebo effect could be a factor because no larger studies have been conducted; however, one study carried out on 170 German soldiers compared acetylsalicylic acid to a combination preparation, *Gripp-Heel*, and found that the homeopathic preparation was comparable to acetylsalicylic acid with respect to the beneficial changes in the clinical findings and in the length of time the patients were unable to work (Maiwald 1993).

The ingredients of *Gripp-Heel* address a wide number of symptoms commonly associated with influenza in humans. The Aconitum fraction acts specifically against cold symptoms (see *Aconitum homaccord*), while Eupatorium perfoliatum (see *FluPlus*) assists with symptoms of cough, pain in the extremities and chest, as well as headaches. Lachesis (see *Echinacea compositum*) is useful for hot flushes, sore throat, and sepsis; Bryonia is useful for pleuritis, dry cough and thirst; and Phosphorus (see

Echinacea compositum) is helpful when there is a risk of pneumonia or bronchopneumonia. Phosphorus also is supportive of hepatic function, a fact that makes this useful for patients suffering from toxicity related to neoplastic disorders as well as cytotoxic therapy.

Gripp-Heel is most effective if given early in the disease process. Endogenous immunity can no longer be adequately activated once the illness has advanced. In uncomplicated cases the viral infection lasts only a few days, unless secondary infections arise, which may result in persistence, particularly with immunosuppressed patients. These viremia periods can be longer in patients with neoplastic disease, due to their immunosuppressed status, and longer periods of *Gripp-Heel* therapy are often indicated.

Palmquist recently treated a difficult feline lymphosarcoma case which developed long-term upper respiratory signs, and *Gripp-Heel* was needed to control the symptoms. This cat had suffered from extensive upper respiratory viral problems earlier in its life, supporting Hering's Law of Cure (disease signs appear in reverse order of occurrence when natural healing is progressing in a desirable fashion). It is advantageous to handle fevers and other signs that occur in these patients through biological therapy as opposed to suppressive pharmaceuticals. Healing will be found to be deeper and more long lasting. Antiphlogistic and antipyretic medicines repress the symptoms but delay healing, because they interfere with normal biological functions.

Hepar compositum: Contains Glandula thymi suis (see *Thyroidea compositum* and other *suis* organs, such as Hepar, Duodenum, Colon, and Vesica fellea). Also contains Pancreas suis, which is useful in cachectic states. Additional support comes from Lycopodium, Chelidonium, Carduus marianus, and catalysts in the form of Natrium oxalaceticum, Acidum a-ketoglutaricum, Acidum DL-malicum, (see *Coenzyme compositum* and *Ubichinon compositum* in the catalysts section below). These remedies also stimulate the functions of the liver cells and the gall bladder. The action of *Hepar compositum* can be increased by the intermediate administration of *Ubichinon compositum* ampules, *Coenzyme compositum* ampules, and possibly *Thyroidea compositum* (antineoplastic action). In addition, consider the comcomitant use of *Podophyllum compositum* as well as *Viscum compositum* (*mite, medium*, and *forte* concentrations) (Reckeweg 2000).

Molybdan compositum: Serves as a mineral and catalyst donor. It has a broad range of potentized remedies, some of which have specific notations in neoplastic phases. Dietary deficiency of trace metals is becoming a health problem, due to consumption of highly refined and heavily processed foods and soil deficiencies. The higher trace element requirements of chronic disease further contribute to states of marginal trace metal deficits, which can lead to altered immunologic function. Furthermore, trace metal deficits have been implicated in initiation and progression of a large variety of neoplasias. Studies on the effect of trace metal deficiency and cancer are inconsistent in methodology and quantification of host alterations in response to neoplastic challenge (Beach, et al. 1982).

Molybdan compositum helps to moderate these deficits, contributing a number of known and as yet unknown co-factors to metabolic function. The component Natrum molybdaenicum-molybdenum is an important trace element and co-factor in enzyme functions. It is found in xanthine oxidase as an active factor, and used for long-term treatment of neoplasms, in which there is almost always a deficit in *molybdenum* level. Nitrate reductase, a flavoprotein enzyme, also contains molybdenum in a complex compound and many bacterial and fungal forms, e.g., Escherichia coli, Clostridium, Neurospora, and Aspergillus. It has been suggested that this is valuable in dysbiosis, especially when combined with Sulphur.

Zincum gluconicum (zinc gluconate) is a constituent of cells and tissue fluids; it is important for the normal course of numerous metabolic processes. Zinc has many trace element functions, and after iron, is the trace element present in the largest quantities in the body. Zinc deficiency has many influences upon the process of neoplasias, e.g., in the blood supply of neoplasms there is practically always a zinc deficiency, resulting in faulty enzyme function. The deaminases of the lymphocytes only work in the presence of zinc; therefore, zinc is critical to immune function. Thus, zinc compounds can influence important enzyme functions, e.g., in anemia, liver damage, kidney diseases, degeneration phases, and particularly neoplastic phases. Zincum metallicum showed a 55% increase in the of life span of female tumor-bearing Swiss albino mice at the 200 X potency (Thobias 1987).

Magnesium asparaginicum, next to potassium, is the most important intracellular cation and it is critical to the activation of a wide variety of enzyme systems, ossification processes, muscle metabolism, membrane permeability, and erythropoiesis. The component Cerium oxalicum (see *Coenzyme compositum*) is useful in stages of cancer in which undigested food is vomited. The cerium salts promote oxygen utilization in the tissues, and are therefore valuable in neoplastic states. The component Manganum gluconicum has particular influence on the respiration of the epidermal cells. Sulphur (covered extensively elsewhere in this chapter) acts as a reagent in all chronic diseases. Phosphorus is a remedy for affections of the parenchyma, particularly of the liver.

Molybdan compositum can regulate the mineral balance and augment body stores when there are deficiencies (including in degenerative diseases and neoplasia). The effect is intensified by the synergism of the individual constituents according to Burgi's principle, i.e., through the combination effect of the contained minerals when coupled to organic acids (aspartic acid, gluconic acid, fumaric acid, etc.). This favors the transfer into the cells or into the region of the enzymes. The use of catalysts, such as *Coenzyme compositum* and *Ubichinon compositum*, and the compositae, which are directed toward similar dysfunctions, intensify the effects of this remedy (Reckeweg 2000).

Thyroidea compositum: See the remedies listed in the Activation of Cell Metabolism section, above.

Approaching the patient's specific case

Dedifferentiation Phase patients are usually treated in stages according to specific goals. Many of these pets are in advanced states of weakness and their excretion and elimination systems are overloaded by homotoxins. If detoxification therapy is begun suddenly in such patients, they may become easily overloaded by the release of homotoxins into the peripheral circulation. Therefore, the first stage of therapy often concerns support of cellular function, particularly the main organs of excretion (bowel, liver, and kidney). Dedifferentiation Phase cases generally suffer from mitochondrial damage, and neoplastic cells function on anaerobic metabolism. Anaerobic metabolism yields far fewer ATP molecules and generates larger quantities of metabolic toxins, which then must be handled by the surrounding cells of the body. Assisting aerobic metabolism through catalyst therapy provides for improved cellular energetics.

The initial holistic and conventional treatment is usually surgery or tumor ablation by direct surgical removal (cold knife, laser surgery, cryosurgery, or irritant herbal substances). Because of the possibility of tumor cells surviving elsewhere in the body, or the induction and development of further tumor by aberrant stem cells affected by neoplastic processes, Dedifferentiation Phase patients may require chemotherapy and/or radiation therapy in addition to surgical ablation of primary tumor. Surgery that is done properly, with wide margins and gentle tissue handling, is critical to success because most tumors are best treated by complete resection at the primary surgical approach.

The next step involves complementary therapy, which supports the immune system, drains the matrix, improves circulation and energetics, and assists with cellular repairs. This step can be quite extensive in scope and varies from case to case depending upon the specific aspects of the particular case. While most cases are treated as part of a larger, more integrative approach to neoplasia, a few have gone into remission in the author's practice (multiple mast cell tumor) with only biological therapy. This aspect of medicine needs investigation to determine the circumstances that lead to such improvements, and which are simply spontaneous remissions.

In human medicine, the final stage deals with psychological/spiritual factors. While this is often not addressed in veterinary medicine, it must be remembered that homotoxins can include psychical and emotional elements. The immune system in its entirety cannot be removed from the psychoneuroendocrine influences that surround it. An entire area of specialized study is arising around psychoneuroendocrine-immune (PNEI) physiological and regulation medicine. Psychological aspects of veterinary cases involve both the afflicted pet as well as the mental states of all people in the pet's environment. The collective state of mind of the owner and the environment where the pet is housed can be very influential in the outcome of the case. In many instances this is as simple as emotional states and attitudes determining whether an animal caregiver will continue to seek treatment or simply let the pet go through euthanasia or hospice. Effective clinicians address this on a regular basis, whether they be conventional or CAVM practitioners.

Biological therapy deals with excretion and detoxification, drainage, diet, and improved immune system function. Establishing improved autoregulation of the patient is highly desirable, and the clinician and owner will observe that the patient cycles through Inflammation Phases when improving. In fact, a significant goal of the biological therapist is to re-establish normal physiological oscillations, as discussed in the greater defense section of homotoxicology chapter. The low pH period necessary for collagen removal and matrix liquefaction, and corresponding cleansing, must give way to the higher pH period and its gelification of the matrix, which marks repair and healing. This regular diurnal cycle of action, which has been significantly inactivated or inhibited in chronic disease states, must be respected and re-initiated if healing is to occur.

Pharmaceutical drugs such as corticosteroids fix the patient in the gel state and block regular matrix cleansing. Other drugs block the enzymes needed for the inflammatory pH cycle and thus prevent homotoxin removal, creating regulation rigidity and poorly responding cases. In both circumstances, before a patient can begin to respond to biological therapy, it is necessary to unblock enzymes, re-establish energy production, and allow for the normal oscillations of pH to be regained. Initial efforts by the body to do this may be extreme, and it takes some time and management for these conditions to stabilize.

Generally speaking, the normal control systems of the body do this in a fashion that does not present serious danger to the patient. Mild diarrhea, productive coughing, nausea, vomiting, and mucus discharges are commonly encountered and they signal desirable regressive vicariation. However, sometimes acute medical care is required to stabilize patients suffering from chronic diseases. During life-threatening emergencies, any and all conventional and alternative agents should be used.

Because of the deeper state of degeneration that is present in many chronic disease cases, it is impossible to stop using allopathic drugs and still preserve patient comfort and even life. Therefore, the biological therapy program is usually begun without changing the existing drug therapy. As improvement occurs these drugs may be minimized or removed under the guidance of an experienced veterinarian. It may be necessary for the biological therapist to coordinate the treatment with an internist/ oncologist. This coordination is encouraged so that a cooperative and supportive professional environment be promoted and maintained at all times. Suddenly removing a necessary drug, or one that has led to substantial suppression of the natural defenses, can seriously destabilize a patient and cause undesirable progressive vicariation.

While detoxification and much of the excretion of homotoxins occur as a result of physiologic inflammation reactions, they may lead to damage and pathology if they are carried to excess. Chronic inflammation is strongly associated with certain types of cancer (Dalgleish, O'Byrne 2006; Moss, Blaser 2005). One of the best methods for down-regulating chronic, excessive inflammation is to re-establish naturally occurring bioregulation. A properly functioning PNEI system is vital to healing any chronic disease. Heel phase remedies, such as *Tonsilla compositum*, address this area. In addition, an Italian company called GUNA, known for their physiological regulating medicine (PRM), produces complex homeopathic medicines that contain inflammatory mediators such as homeopathically diluted cytokines, hormones, and homeopathic neurotransmitters, which may help to manage patients in any phase, including Dedifferentiation (GUNA 2006a). The authors have just begun to use these agents and can make no major claims or offer any advice at this time. However, GUNA is conducting several excellent university studies and appears to be quite serious in its approach to biological therapy (GUNA 2006b).

To reach the goal of down-regulating chronic inflammation, a number of biological agents can and should be integrated as is appropriate for each case. Biological therapies often supplement each other, but the clinician must be aware of interactions between herbs and drugs. Such interactions are not usually an issue in selecting antihomotoxic agents, but certain homeopathic agents are thought to be inimical to one another, and so it is theoretically possible to decrease the efficacy of a protocol if such agents are given simultaneously or in succession. This topic is controversial, and there is little science to guide the practitioner (Boericke 1927). Surely, future work will bring clarity to this subject, but from practical experience it does not seem to be a major concern for those using balanced combination homeopathic remedies, and it may be a larger issue in the classical practice of homeopathy.

Approach to cases not on chemotherapy

Providing gentle detoxification and elimination is the first step in cases in which chemotherapy is not used. Support begins with the organs of elimination (liver, kidney, and gastrointestinal). Adequate clean air and water are important, and a clean and toxin-free diet that is easily digested and absorbed is essential. Patients with neoplasia require special attention to the nutritional aspects of their care. It is important to avoid unnecessary chemical additives and preservatives, because these substances can readily cause further damage to an already compromised system. For example, in human medicine the consumption of cured luncheon meats has recently been shown to raise the risk of chronic obstructive pulmonary disease (COPD) by 71%, perhaps from nitric-oxide-mediated damage to the lungs (Daniells 2006). Peters, et al. (1994) studied the relationship between the intake of certain foods and the risk of leukemia in children and found that children who eat more than 12 hot dogs per month have 9 times the normal risk of developing childhood leukemia. Children born to mothers who consumed hot dogs once or more per week during pregnancy have almost double the risk of developing brain tumors. Children who ate hot dogs once or more per week also have a higher risk of brain cancer (Sarasua 1994).

Preservatives can disrupt metabolism, but it has not been adequately determined whether or not this is a significant risk to pets with cancer. Ethoxyquin, a common preservative in pet foods, has been shown to damage human lymphocytes and inhibit the electron transport chain in mitochondria, particularly those in cells of the renal cortex (Reyes 1995, Blaszczyk 2006). Ogilvie (1998) and others have demonstrated clear benefits to survival in certain types of cancer associated with feeding proper levels of dietary protein and fatty acids. For many years holistic veterinarians have routinely encouraged clients to feed patients in the Dedifferentiation Phase higher protein diets, and there appears to be scientific support of this practice. The Hills Company produces a unique prescription diet, N/D, which has been shown to increase the survival times of canine patients with mammary gland neoplasia and lymphosarcoma. Other toxins such as aflatoxins, heavy metals, pesticides, and even drug residues may lie hidden in food and cause progressive vicariation in patients already overwhelmed by homotoxins.

Numerous antihomotoxic drugs are applicable in treating patients in the Dedifferentiation Phase. Galium-Heel is indicated as a cellular agent in all cases of neoplasia. This remedy is quite complex and contains many agents that help with cellular repair and matrix drainage. *Sempervivum tectorium* (also in Ginseng compositum and

Thyroidea compositum) is a classical remedy with a long use in neoplasia cases (Boericke 1927).

The antihomotoxic drug *Lymphomyosot* drains and supports the immune and lymphatic system, allowing for the movement of homotoxins. Exercise and massage can move vast quantities of toxins, but it must be done gently, or signs of illness such as depression can occur as these toxins gain access to the peripheral blood. *Nux vomica homaccord* drains the liver and gastrointestinal system, while *Berberis homaccord* (or *Hepeel* and *Reneel* tablets) drains the liver, gallbladder, and kidney. *Berberis homaccord* also supports weakened adrenal glands and assists with the stress of chronic disease. Use of the aforementioned agents for 30 days or more begins the process of tissue cleansing.

Another approach, according to Leimbach, involves giving *Galium-Heel* (6 times daily for 8 weeks) and then *Lymphomyosot* (QID), *Psorinoheel* (once daily), and *Phosphor homaccord* (TID) (Reckeweg 2000). Mitochondrial dysfunction is associated with defects in neuronal oxidative phosphorylation within the central nervous system. A trigger of impressive potency is phosphorylation, because only one phosphate molecule is needed for every 300 molecules of kinase in a cell, resulting in massive reaction (Pollack 2001). Phosphorylation is constitutionally indicated for phosphorus deficiency and for too rapid growth (*Calcoheel*, *Cruroheel* and *Osteoheel* are auxiliary remedies), precancerous dermatitis, and neoplasm phases.

Hepar compositum supports and drains the liver and gallbladder, while *Solidago compositum* supports and drains the kidney and can be readily given by injection or orally.

BHI-Body Pure has many components in the sphere of environmental toxicities, which often serve as a trigger for neoplastic cell changes. *Coenzyme compositum* and *Ubichinon compositum*, as well as *Glyoxal compositum*, support metabolic energy production and they activate enzyme systems and receptors. Para-Benzochinon-Injeel D30 and cAMP D30 are also useful in this area and are often alternated. Standard therapy involves detoxification for approximately 1 month, at which time the patient's progress is evaluated and other treatment can ensue to improve immune function, repair organ systems, and target tumor cells for removal (Reckeweg 2000). Carefully controlled studies must be conducted to determine which protocols are best in each case, but to date none have been performed.

Thalamus compositum is an interesting therapeutic adjunct in neoplasias. To some degree it maintains central regulatory control because it controls arousal and excitatory states. A brief search of the Internet reveals many scientific articles concerning the use of thalamic function to moderate the pain caused by cancer. It also contains cAMP, a significant intracellular regulating factor produced in the cell membrane that is antagonistic toward cGMP (cyclic guanosine monophosphate), through which undifferentiated cell growth is promoted (i.e., cancerous tumors).

Corpus pineale suis (also contained in *Thyroidea compositum*) slows down neoplasm phases, and it has some specific indications for papilloma of the bladder (Reckeweg 2002). The pineal gland and the major hormone it produces, melatonin, seem to play a role in immune modulation, and it has been described as an "oncostatic gland." Melatonin in physiologic concentrations suppresses the growth of some breast cancer cell lines, and conversely pinealectomy increases the growth and proliferation of certain cancers. In some studies, melatonin has shown oncostimulatory activity, but the oncostatic or oncostimulation appears to be diurnal in nature. Melatonin antagonizes the immunosuppressive effects of corticosteroids, increases the cytotoxic activity of natural killer (NK) cells, and stimulates T-lymphocytic responses by acting on opioid receptors. Melatonin is reportedly cytotoxic as well as oncostatic for in vitro cultures of breast, ovary, and bladder cancer cells. The circadian rhythm of melatonin secretion is altered in some human cancer patients. In those with prostate cancer, the amplitude of the melatonin circadian rhythm is significantly lower than is found in healthy men. Patients with primary breast cancer have a decreased melatonin level, inversely correlated with tumor size and increased pineal gland calcification with age may partially account for the increase in breast cancer with age. Electromagnetic fields can affect pineal gland function if they act below the threshold of perception as "synchronizers" or "stimuli." The greatest amount of energy absorption occurs in the hypothalamus and thalamus regions, near the pineal gland. The selective absorption of energy in this region could functionally disturb the pineal-hypothalamus network (Ronco 1996). *Thalamus compositum* also contains Viscum album (see above).

Besides the Heel remedies, there are other possible biological therapies, e.g., large-dose, long-term therapy with enzyme preparations. High doses of vitamin C (ascorbic acid) have been shown to be very useful in many types of cancer. For more information, see the pioneering work by Dr. Hugh Riordan (Gonzalez, et al. 2005) on vitamins A and E (vitamin E must not be administered in cases of hormonally active tumors, such as ovarian cancer, certain kinds of carcinomas of the breast, testicular carcinomas, etc.). Restoration of an intact and functioning intestinal tract, with attention to repopulation of the microbial flora, should be attempted. Selenium ampules or Selenium homaccord is indicated for daily oral use as a long-term therapy, along with routine detoxification as detailed elsewhere in this text. Enzyme therapies are also interesting, and can be very valuable as an adjunctive treatment. Enzymes are given between meals so that they can be absorbed and used outside the gastrointestinal tract. The rationale for this approach can be more appreciated by a detailed study of the work of John Beard, William Donald Kelley, and more recently Nicholas Gonzales, who have studied the use of enzymes in a variety of cancers (Gonzalez 2005).

Case programming for patients on chemotherapy

When chemotherapy is used, the clinician must avoid detoxification therapy because it may remove levels of the chemotherapeutic needed to kill aberrant neoplastic cells. In these cases, *Galium-Heel* can be used for cellular support, and *Hepar compositum*, *Solidago compositum*, and catalysts (*Glyoxal compositum*, *Ubichinon compositum*, and *Coenzyme compositum*) can be used intermittently (Hu, Kit 2005). These agents can be given 2 to 7 times weekly, orally or by injection. Each case must be tailored to the particular patient and the specific therapy. Treatments that supplement chemotherapy include mistletoe formulas such as *Viscum compositum*; digestive enzymes (proteolytic enzymes); *Molybdan compositum* (trace minerals); and nutraceutical agents such as selenium, vitamin C, vitamin E, and beta-carotene.

In cases of radiation therapy, the catalysts (*Coenzyme compositum*, *Ubichinon compositum*, and *Glyoxal compositum*) and especially *Causticum compositum* (1 to 3 times weekly) are supportive and helpful. As discussed earlier in this text, *Traumeel S* has been shown to reduce radiation-induced stomatitis in children and should be considered in radiation-induced mucositis in animals as well (Oberbaum 2001).

Broadfoot's general Dedifferentiation Phase protocol

All cancer patients may receive this autosanguis as a first step of therapy. There are many protocols for treating neoplastic conditions. For the sake of brevity, this text only presents one such technique. As research progresses it may be that other successful protocols surface, and the reader is instructed to actively search for such information as it becomes available. Broadfoot recommends the following general protocol in approaching Dedifferentiation Phase patients:

Initial therapy
Week 1

- Day 1: *Lymphomyosot* plus *Engystol*, one-half to 1 ampule each, mixed together and given IV.
- Days 2 through 5: One-fourth to one-half vial daily PO.

Week 2

- Day 1: *Galium-Heel* plus *Lymphomyosot* plus *Engystol*, one-half to 1 ampule each, mixed together and given IV.
- Days 2 through 5: *Lymphomyosot* plus *Engystol*, one-fourth to 1 vial daily PO.

Autosanguis
Weeks 3 through 5

- Day 1: Perform a full-run autosanguis, in this order, at one-half cc per injection, saving the remaining vials for oral support:
  1. *Viscum compositum* medium
  2. *Galium-Heel* plus *Engystol N*
  3. *Psorinoheel* plus *Lymphomyosot*
  4. *Tonsilla compositum*
  5. *Coenzyme compositum*
  6. *Ubichinon compositum*
- Day 2: *Viscum compositum medium*, one-fourth to 1 vial by subcutaneous injection where legally allowed. Where not legal, give PO.
- Day 3: *Galium-Heel* plus *Engystol N*, one-fourth to 1 vial each by subcutaneous injection or PO.
- Day 4: *Lymphomyosot* and *Psorinoheel*, one-fourth to 1 vial each by subcutaneous injection or PO.
- Day 5: *Tonsilla compositum*, one-fourth to 1 vial each by subcutaneous injection or PO.
- Day 7: *Coenzyme compositum*, one-fourth to 1 vial each by subcutaneous injection or PO.
- Day 8: *Ubichinon compositum*, one-fourth to 1 vial each by subcutaneous injection or PO.
- Days 9 through 11: Rest; no remedies given.
- Day 12: *Glyoxal compositum*, one-half vial each by subcutaneous injection or PO.
- Days 13 through 15: Rest; no remedies given.
- Day 16: Repeat the protocols for Days 3 through 15 until the remaining vials from Week 3/Day 1 are gone.

Continued therapy

This therapy continues as long as necessary through the use of tinctures and/or tablets. There are a number of possible therapeutic strategies, including liver repair/regeneration with Hepar compositum and Hepeel; continued catalyst support of mitochondrial function with Coenzyme compositum, Ubichinon compositum, and Glyoxal compositum; Detox Kit (Nux vomica homaccord, Lymphomyosot, and Berberis homaccord); and Galium-Heel for ongoing cellular support. Ginseng compositum can be tremendously valuable for exhaustion phases. Also consider Solidago compositum to reduce stress on the renal system and help patients that move into regressive vicariation.

Active biotherapeutics specific to organ conditions

Therapy can be individualized to address specific organ conditions. Previously published texts from Heel have suggested the following general therapeutics, in a simplified form:

Apis compositum: Hypernephroma.

Bronchalis-Heel: Carcinoma of the lung (also *Droperteel*, *Phosphor homaccord*, *Husteel*, and *Tartephedreel*).

Chelidonium homaccord: Liver and gallbladder conditions (see general support remedies).

Duodenoheel and **Spascupreel**: Duodenum and pancreas conditions.

Graphites homaccord: Pylorus.

Gynacoheel, Lamioflur, Hormeel: Uterine cancer, cancer of the adnexa, etc.

Hormeel: Carcinoma of the glands and genitals.

Lamioflur: Carcinoma of the nose, mouth, and genitals.

Mezereum homaccord: Carcinoma of the mucous membranes in general.

Mucosa compositum: Cancer of mucosal tissues.

Nux vomica homaccord, Veratrum homaccord: Cancer of the intestine.

Veratrum homaccord: Contains aloe vera, which, when used in low potency, increased the life span of induced cancer (Dalton's lymphoma ascites) in mice by 21% (Thobias 1990).

Phosphor homaccord: Laryngeal neoplasia.

Reneel, Spascupreel: Urinary passage conditions.

Schwef-Heel: Epithelioma.

Ubichinon compositum: Neoplasias of the lower intestinal tract (via para-Benzochinon).

Continual attack by intermediary homotoxins (oncogenic agents, tumor antigens, lactic acid, chemotherapeutic agents, etc.) occurs in neoplasias and cancer therapies, engendering a chronic state of stress exhaustion of the adrenal cortex. *Berberis homaccord* and possibly *Strumeel* and *Thyroidea compositum* may be used to stimulate the functions of the thyroid gland. They should be given once daily.

Preparations indicated according to symptoms

Just as specific organs can be addressed, individual symptoms can be addressed as well. Patients suffering from neoplasia may have a wide variety of concurrent signs, and use of symptom formulas can provide tremendous relief. The readers should also refer to individual protocols for medical conditions in this text.

Arsuraneel: Has a generally calming action on the toxin level; likewise, *Cruroheel* calms the connective tissue structures. These preparations should be interpolated daily in frequent doses.

Colocynthis homaccord: Used in neuralgiform disorders, ischialgia.

Drosera homaccord, Husteel, Droperteel, Bronchalis-Heel, Tartephedreel: Used for coughs.

Gelsemium homaccord, Spigelon: Used for headaches and neuralgiform disorders.

Ginseng compositum, Molybdan compositum: Used for weakness and exhaustion at the start of the treatment. Give 1 to 2 tablets 3 times daily for 2 to 3 weeks, then once daily, and subsequently 1 tablet 2 to 3 times weekly (every second or third day).

Mercurius-Heel, Traumeel tablets: Used for ulcerating carcinomas. *Traumeel* ointment also can be used.

Nux vomica homaccord, Veratrum homaccord: Used in tenesmus (cancer of the rectum).

Rendimax: Used for latent acidosis that is characteristic of neoplasias (cancer thrives in an acidic environment).

Spascupreel, Atropinum compositum: Used for shooting pains and spasms.

Biotherapeutics and remedies in radiotherapy

The following protocol has been designed for patients undergoing radiotherapy. This protocol must be completed 4 days before the start of radiotherapy treatment when it is used as a protective adjunctive therapy:

- Day 1: Ubichinon compositum with Traumeel, Engystol, and Hepeel.
- Day 2: Galium-Heel, Traumeel, Engystol, and Hepeel.

The reader should be aware of several issues related to the use of antihomotoxic drugs during radiotherapy. *Reneel* tablets are alternated with *Causticum compositum* on the day of the radiation to prevent disorders of the bladder (cystitis) after radiation. They should be given every 15 to 30 minutes. Opiates may be given to ease the pain. *Ubichinon compositum* is indicated, possibly daily, and particularly after each application of radiotherapy. It can assist with the side effects (depressed breathing) and should possibly be given at the dose of 1 vial daily. *Ubichinon compositum* helps with the pain that result from the cancerous condition. It has been used with some success in painful cancers such as osteosarcomas. *Traumeel* ointment has proved effective in the treatment of skin damage from radiotherapy (Heel).

REFERENCES

Abramson JS, Mills EL. Depression of neutrophil functions induced by viruses and its role in secondary microbial infections. *Rev Infect Dis.* 1988. Mar–Apr; 10(2): pp 326–341.

Bar-Sela G, Goldberg H, Beck D, Amit A, Kuten A. Reducing malignant ascites accumulation by repeated intraperitoneal administrations of a Viscum album extract. *Anticancer Res.* 2006. Jan–Feb; 26(1B): pp 709–13.

Bauer R. Echinacea drugs—effects and active ingredients. *Z Arztl Fortbild.* (Jena) 1996. Apr; 90(2): pp 111–115.

Beach RS, Gershwin ME, Hurley LS. Zinc, copper, and manganese in immune function and experimental oncogenesis *Nutr Cancer.* 1982. 3(3): pp 172–91.

Biswas SJ, Khuda-Bukhsh AR. Effect of a homeopathic drug, Chelidonium, in amelioration of p-DAB induced hepatocarcinogenesis in mice BMC. *Complement Altern Med.* 2002. Apr 10; 2(1): p 4.

Biswas S, Ray M, Misra S, Dutta DP, Ray S. Selective inhibition of mitochondrial respiration and glycolysis in human leukemia leukocytes by methylglyoxal. 1997. *Biochem J* 323, 343–348.

Blaszczyk A. DNA damage induced by ethoxyquin in human peripheral lymphocytes. *Toxicol Lett.* 2006.May 5; 163(1): pp 77–83.

Boericke W. Materia Medica with Repertory, 9th ed. Santa Rosa, CA: Boericke and Tafel, Glossary, 1927. p 845.

Bradley GW, Clover A. Apparent response of small cell lung cancer to an extract of mistletoe and homoeopathic treatment. *Thorax.* 1989; 44(12): pp 1047–1048.

Broumand DM, Sahl N, Tilles L. In vitro studies of Echinacea and Ginseng on natural killer and antibody-dependent cell cytotoxicity in healthy subjects and chronic fatigue syndrome or acquired immuno-deficency syndrome patients. *Immunopharmacology.* 1997. Jan; 35(3): pp 229–235.

Choi SH, Lyu SY, Park WB. Mistletoe lectin induces apoptosis and telomerase inhibition in human A253 cancer cells through dephosphorylation of Akt. *Arch Pharm Res.* 2004.Jan; 27(1): pp 68–76.

Cooper RA. Methylglyoxal metabolism in microorganisms. *Annu Rev Microbiol.* 1984:38, pp 49–68.

Dalgleish A, O'Byrne K. Inflammation and cancer: the role of the immune response and angiogenesis. *Cancer Treat Res.* 2006. 130: pp 1–38.

Daniells S. Nitrites in Cured Meat Linked to Lung Disease. MeatProcess.com: Breaking News on Prepared Food and Meat Processing, 2006. December 9. http://www.meatprocess.com/news/ng.asp? n = 70484.

González MJ, Miranda-Massari JR, Mora EM, Guzmán A, Riordan NH, Riordan HD, Casciari JJ, Jackson JA, Romá-Franco A. Orthomolecular oncology review: Ascorbic acid and cancer 25 years later. *Integ Cancer Ther* 2005. 4(1): pp 32–44.

GUNA. GUNA-Method-Physiological Regulating Medicine: How to treat diseases and cure patients with clinically proven natural medicines. Hand-out from GUNA Method Opinion Leaders Conference, Santa Fe, NM. 2006(a) pp 6–8.

GUNA. Welcome to GUNA. 2006(b). http://www.gunainc.com.

Hajto T, Berki T, Palinkas L, Boldizsar F, Nemeth P. Effects of mistletoe extract on murine thymocytes in vivo and on gluco-corticoid-induced cell count reduction. *Forsch Komplementarmed.* 2006. Feb; 13(1): pp 22–7.

Harmsma M, Ummelen M, Dignef W, Tusenius KJ, Ramaekers FC. Effects of mistletoe (Viscum album L.) extracts Iscador on cell cycle and survival of tumor cells. *Arzneimittelforschung*. 2006. Jun; 56(6A): pp 474–82.

Heel. Routine Therapy: The Practitioner's Handbook of Homotoxicology. Albuquerque, NM: Heel Inc 2005. pp 137–8, 179, 185.

Heel Medical Department. Homotoxicology: Theoretical Concepts and Therapeutic Applications: International Correspondence Course on CD.

Hostanska K, Hajto T, Herrmann R. Immunomodulatory potency of mistletoe lectins in cancer patients: results of a dose finding study. Meeting abstract: Molecular Biology of Hematopoiesis, 8th Symposium; 1993. July 9–13. Basel, Switzerland: p 27.

Hu C, Kitts DD. Dandelion (Taraxacum officinale) flower extract suppresses both reactive oxygen species and nitric oxide and prevents lipid oxidation in vitro. *Phytomedicine*. 2005. Aug; 12(8): pp 588–97.

Huber R, Rostock M, Goedl R, Ludtke R, Urech K, Buck S, Klein R. Mistletoe treatment induces GM-CSF- and IL-5 production by PBMC and increases blood granulocyte- and eosinophil counts: a placebo controlled randomized study in healthy subjects. *Eur J Med Res*. 2005.Oct 18; 10(10): pp 411–8.

Jamieson BD, Somasundaram T, Ahmed R. Abrogation of tolerance to a chronic viral infection. *J Immunol*. 1991. Nov 15; 147(10):pp 3521–3529.

Luettig B, Steinmuller C, Gifford GE, Wagner H, Lohmann-Matthes ML. Macrophage activation by polysaccharide arabinogalactan isolates from plant cell cultures of Echinacea Purpurea. *J Natl Cancer Inst*. 1989. May 3; 81(9): pp 669–675.

Maiwald L. The therapy of the common cold. *Bio Ther*. 1993. Jan; 11(1): pp 2–8.

Malafronte B, Dunais B, Mondain V, Durant J, Carles M, Dellamonica P. Use of unconventional medicine among HIV positive patients: survey of 3 care-providing centres. *Int Conf AIDS*. 1996. Jul 7–12; 11(2): p 432(abstract no. Th. D.5183).

Morris JD, Eddleston AL, Crook T. Viral infection and cancer. *Lancet*. 1995.Sep16; 346(8977): pp 754–8.

Moss S, Blaser M. Mechanisms of disease: Inflammation and the origins of cancer. *Nat Clin Pract Oncol*. 2005. Feb; 2(2): pp 90–7.

Murata K, Saikusa T, Fukuda Y, Watanabe K, Inoue Y, Shimosaka M, Kimura A. Metabolism of 2-oxoaldehydes in yeasts. Possible role of glycolytic bypath as a detoxification system in L-threonine catabolism by Saccharomyces cerevisiae. *Eur J Biochem*. 1986:157, pp 297–301.

Oberbaum M, Yaniv I, Ben-Gal Y, Stein J, Ben-Zvi N, Freedman L, Branski D. A randomized, controlled clinical trial of the homeopathic medication TRAUMEEL S® in the treatment of chemotherapy-induced stomatitis in children undergoing stem cell transplantation. *Cancer*. 2001. 92(3): pp 684–690.

Ogilvie G. Nutrition and Cancer: Frontiers for Cure! In: Proceedings American Holistic Veterinary Association Annual Conference, New Orleans, LA, 1998. pp 69–73.

Palmquist R. Unpublished clinical history of use of Viscum compositum in management of paraneoplastic induced hypercalcemia in an aged mixed breed dog with advanced metastatic anal gland carcinoma. 2005.

Peters J, et al. Processed meats and risk of childhood leukemia (California, USA) *Cancer Causes and Control 5*: 1994. 195–202.

Pollack GH. Cells, Gels, and the Engines of Life. Ebner and Sons Publishers, 2001. p 127.

Rabe A, Weiser M, Klein P. Effectiveness and tolerability of a homeopathic remedy compared with conventional therapy for mild viral infections. *International Journal of Clinical Practice*, 2004. 58(9): pp 827–832.

Ray M, Ghos S, Kar M, Datta S, Ray S. Implication of the bioelectronic principle in cancer therapy: treatment of cancer patients by methylglyoxal-based formulation. *Indian J. Phys.* 2001.75B: pp 73–77.

Ray M, Ray S. Methylglyoxal: From a putative intermediate of glucose breakdown to its role in understanding that excessive ATP formation in cells may lead to malignancy. *Current Sci.* 1998: pp 75, 103–113.

Ray S, Biswas S, Ray M. Similar nature of inhibition of mitochondrial respiration of heart tissue and malignant cells by methylglyoxal. A vital clue to understand the biochemical basis of malignancy. *Mol Cell Biochem*. 1997.171: pp 95–103.

Ray M, Halder J, Dutta SK, Ray S. Inhibition of respiration of tumor cells by methylglyoxal and protection of inhibition by lactaldehyde. *Int J Cancer*. 1991:47, 603–609.

Ray M, Ray S. Aminoacetone oxidase from goat liver. Formation of methylglyoxal from aminoacetone. *J Biol Chem*. 1987: pp 262, 5974–5977.

Ray S, Ray M. Isolation of methylglyoxal synthase from goat liver. *J Biol Chem*. 1981: pp 256, 6230–6233.

Reckeweg HH. Neue Gesichtspunkte der antihomotoxischen Therapie bei zellulären Phasen [New view on anti-homotoxic therapy in cellular phases]. *Homotoxin-Journal*. 1967.6: pp 285–395.

Reckeweg H. Biotherapeutic Index: Ordinatio Antihomotoxica et Materia Medica, 5th ed. Baden-Baden, Germany: Biologische Heilmittel Heel GMBH, 2000. pp 49–52, 340–2, 347–9, 366–7, 389, 424.

Reckeweg H. Homoeopathia Antihomotoxica Materia Medica, 4th ed. Baden-Baden, Germany: Aurelia-Verlag GMBH, 2002. pp 118–20, 136–7, 153, 158, 169–70, 176–8, 182, 197, 201–2, 213–4, 226–7, 235, 241–2, 249–51, 254, 257, 271–2, 307–9, 310–12, 324, 325, 327–8, 335–6, 344–5, 346–8, 373–5, 377–9, 383, 422, 433, 437–40, 442, 446–9, 450–2, 458, 460, 495–6, 497, 508, 509, 525, 528, 530, 542, 552–4, 555–60, 574–5, 576, 591, 598, 609–10.

Reyes JL, Hernandez ME, Melendez E, Gomez-Lojero C. Inhibitory effect of the antioxidant ethoxyquin on electron transport in the mitochondrial respiratory chain. *Biochem Pharmacol*. 1995.Jan 31;49(3): pp 283–9.

Ronco AL, Halberg F. The pineal gland and cancer. *Anticancer Res*. 1996.16(4A):pp 2033–40.

Sarasua S, Savitz D. Cured and broiled meat consumption in relation to childhood cancer: Denver, Colorado (United States), *Cancer Causes and Control* 1994.5:141–8.

Schink M. Mistletoe therapy for human cancer: the role of the natural killer cells. *Anticancer Drugs.* 1997. Apr;8(S1): pp S47–51.

Siewierska K, Denys A. Efficacy of preoperative immunoprophylaxis in patients with neoplastic diseases. *Int. Rev. Allergol. Clin. Immunol.* 1999. 5(1):pp 39–45.

Szent-Gyrgyi A. The living state and cancer. *Ciba Found Symp* 1979. 67:pp 3–18.

Tenorio Lopez F, del Valle Mondragon L, Zarco Olvera G, Torres Narvaez J, Pastelin Hernandez G. Viscum album aqueous extract induces inducible and endothelial nitric oxide synthases expression in isolated and perfused guinea pig heart. Evidence of the coronary vasodilation mechanism. *Arch Cardiol Mex.* 2006. Apr–Jun;76(2): pp 130–9. In Spanish.

Thobias MP. Antineoplastic effects of 4 homoeopathic medicines. *Brit Homeo J.* 1987. April;86: pp 90–91.

Thobias MP. An experimental homeopathic application of Aloe Vera Linn on mice bearing induced cancer. *Homeopath Herit.* 1990. Feb: pp 67–69.

Till MW. The effective principle of gripp-heel. *Biol Ther.* 1986. 4(3/4):pp 47, 52.

Thompson CB, Gottlieb E. Succinate links TCA cycle dysfunction to oncogenesis by inhibiting HIF-a prolyl hydroxylase. *Cancer Cell.* 2005. 7: pp 77–85.

Wagner H, Jurcic K, Doenicke A, Behrens N. Influence of homeopathic drug preparations on the phagocytosis capability of granulocytes. *Biol Ther* 1993; XI(2): pp 43–9.

Yance D Jr, Sagar S. Targeting angiogenesis with integrative cancer therapies. *Integr Cancer Ther.* 2006. Mar;5(1): pp 9–29.

PROTOCOLS FOR SPECIFIC TUMORS

These treatment protocols supplement proper surgical, radiation, and necessary medical therapies. They should not be represented as curative of cancer, but rather as supportive of patient defenses. Owners should be fully informed of the experimental nature of alternative approaches in handling Dedifferentiation Phase patients.

A general 3-point format for therapy is followed for each cancer type. All cancer patients require the first step, which includes Broadfoot's general Dedifferentiation Phase protocol (see above). Because oncologic patients are all individual, the general protocol for cancer must be adjusted to the particular cancer tissue type, as well as the patient's particular biological type. Steps 2 and 3 of the program involve the specific antihomotoxic agents. Use Table 5.1 to locate tissue-specific remedies.

Adenocarcinoma

Step 1: Follow Broadfoot's general Dedifferentiation Phase protocol, above.

Step 2: Select at least 1 agent representing the tissue of origin from Table 34.1. As an example, in the case of jejunal adenocarcinoma, one could select *Mucosa com-*

Table 34.1. Summary of glandular- and epithelial-containing tissues and antihomotoxic medications containing suis organ glandular elements. Identify a carcinoma's tissue of origin and select at least 1 organ preparation.

Organ/tissue	Suis organ preparation
Adrenal cortex	*Tonsilla compositum*
Adrenal gland	*Cutis compositum, Discus compositum Testis compositum, Thalamus compositum*
Bladder	*Solidago compositum*
Brain	*Cerebrum compositum, Thalamus compositum*
Colon	*Hepar compositum*
Duodenum	*Hepar compositum*
Embryo	*Causticum compositum, Cerebrum compositum, Discus compositum, Placenta compositum Testis compositum, Tonsilla compositum, Zeel*
Epidermis	*Cutis compositum*
Fallopian tube	*Ovarium compositum*
Gallbladder	*Hepar compositum*
GI mucosa	*Mucosa compositum*
Kidney	*Solidago compositum, Rauwolfia compositum*
Liver	*Hepar compositum*
Nasal mucosa	*Mucosa compositum*
Ocular mucosa	*Mucosa compositum*
Ovary	*Ovarium compositum*
Pancreas	*Hepar compositum, Mucosa compositum Syzygium compositum*
Pituitary gland	*Ovarium compositum, Placenta compositum*
Teste	*Testis compositum*
Thyroid gland	*Thyroidea compositum*
Umbilicus	*Cutis compositum, Discus compositum Placenta compositum, Thyroidea compositum Tonsilla compositum, Zeel*
Ureter, urethra	*Solidago compositum*
Urinary mucosa	*Mucosa compositum*

positum and/or *Hepar compositum* or *Duodenoheel* as part of the treatment plan. Note that because this is a Degeneration Phase disorder, *Mucosa compositum* is an excellent selection because it is a phase remedy, as well.

Step 3: Consider special single remedies based upon the location of the neoplasm and the patient's individual symptoms. The clinician should attempt to identify any single remedies which seem appropriate and make an effort to include a combination remedy that contains these:

Acidum aceticum: Contained in *Arsuraneel*; classically indicated for consideration in epithelial cancers. This remedy is very valuable in cases of chronic disease, and has particular use in cancer of the stomach.

Arsenicum iodatum: Contained in *Tartephedreel*, et al.; treats skin cancer and mammary tumors.

Asterias rubens: In *Lamioflur*; used in mammary tumors (particularly those with tendency toward ulceration) and uterine diseases.

Baryta oxalsuccinica: In *Coenzyme compositum* and *BHI-Enzyme*. Treats lung cancer with congestion, cancer of the prostate, cancer of the bladder.

Calcium fluoratum: In *Galium-Heel, Thyroidea compositum*, et al. Has indications for swelling or fistula and glandular swellings. Is suggestive of carcinoma, and has action on connective structures (including elastic tissue) and the periosteum. These aforementioned qualities make it worth considering in cases of osteosarcoma, chondrosarcoma, and other connective tissue neoplasias.

Caltha palustris: In *Galium-Heel*; used for uterine cancer.

Cartilago suis: In *Discus compositum, Zeel*; used for muscle, bone and joint diseases, and cartilaginous degenerations.

Chelidonium: In *BHI-Chelidonium complex, Hepar compositum, Hepeel, BHI-Gallbladder*. Used for liver cancer.

Cholesterinum: In *Hepar compositum, BHI-Body pure, BHI-Chelidonium complex*. Used in gallbladder and liver cancer.

Colchicum: In *Aesculus compositum, Diarrheel, Ginseng compositum, Thyroidea compositum, Ubichinon compositum, Vomitusheel*. Used for stomach cancer.

Condurango (Marsdenia condurango): In *Arsuraneel, Mucosa compositum*, and *BHI-Headache II*. Useful in stomach issues and cancer of the stomach as well as other forms of cancer, such as epitheliomas, mucocutaneous fissures, ulcerative cancers.

Conium: In *Cerebrum compositum, Ginseng compositum, Testis compositum, Thyroidea compositum, Tonsilla compositum, Ubichinon compositum, BHI-Prostate, BHI-Saw palmetto*. Used for mammary and uterine neoplasias.

DL-Malicum acidum (malic acid): In *Coenzyme compositum, Cor compositum, Hepar compositum, Thyroidea compositum, BHI-Enzyme*. Should always be considered in intestinal cancers, cancer of the bladder, bronchial cancer.

Euphorbium: In *Euphorbium compositum, Echinacea compositum, BHI-Sinus*. In high concentrations has been shown to be an irritant of skin and mucosa, with possible carcinogenic effects (Zayed 2001). Homeopathic dilutions appear to be safe for long-term use. Protein kinase C enzymes represent the receptor for various xenobiotics, and some phorbol esters are tumor promoters in the mouse, whereas others are anticarcinogenic by stimulating the differentiation of leukemic cells (Nakao 1982). There is epidemiologic evidence to suggest that exposure to diterpene esters may be a risk factor for the development of esophageal cancers in humans (Szallasi 1999). Several species of Euphorbium have been shown to be of value in multidrug resistance in mouse lymphoma (Hohmann 2002). *Euphorbium compositum* is a remedy that can be used as a pain management agent in many forms of neoplasia. This agent commonly assists with intense pain in limbs, paralytic pain in joints, and irritant problems and pain and ulceration of the skin. *Galium-Heel, Lymphomyosot, Apis homaccord, Traumeel S*, and *Zeel* are also helpful for pain management and are commonly used in elderly pets with Dedifferentiation Phase disease. Because pain is a sign of homotoxin presence and/or damage, properly handling the homotoxins in a patient may give surprisingly good results in pain management. In advanced cases use narcotic agents as needed and avoid nonsteroidal anti-inflammatory drugs if possible because they interfere with intestinal function and damage organs of elimination such as kidney and liver.

Fuligo ligni: Not contained in any Heel or BHI formulas, but historically recommended by classical homeopaths when signs match. Used for rectal adenocarcinoma.

Funiculus umbicalis suis: In *Cutis compositum, Discus compositum, Placenta compositum, Thyroidea compositum, Tonsilla compositum*, and *Zeel*. Generally used in carcinomas and sarcomas. May be of particular value in osteosarcomas with attendant bone pain.

Germanium robertianum: In *Lymphomyosot* and *Tonsilla compositum*, which are part of the therapy for all cancer patients. Indicated for gastric tumors.

Glandula thyroidea suis: In *Thyroidea compositum*. Treats thyroid tumors and liver and kidney diseases.

Graphites: In *BHI-Skin, Cutis compositum, Placenta compositum, Discus compositum, Thyroidea compositum, Tonsilla compositum*, and *Zeel*; used for precancerous conditions in the pyloric region.

Hekla lava: In *Osteoheel, BHI-Bone*. Treats osteosarcoma, osteitis, and exostosis.

Hydrastis canadensis: In *Ginseng compositum, Lamioflur, Mucosa compositum, Ovarium compositum*, and *Ubichinon compositum*. Used for tumors in the breasts and other organs, especially mucosal pathology.

Kali cyanatum: Not contained in any Heel or BHI remedies, but may be obtained from other suppliers of homeopathic medicines. Classically indicated for cancer of the rectum and tumors of the tongue if signs align with the agent's proving.

Kreosotum: In *Bronchalis, Ginseng compositum, Lamioflur, Mucosa compositum, Ovarium compositum, Populus compositum, BHI-Prostate, BHI-Saw palmetto, BHI-Skin*; used for mucosal masses, uterine carcinoma, and prostatic hypertrophy.

Naphthoquinone: In *Ubichinon compositum*. For serious forms of carcinoma in the areas of the intestines and genitalia, particularly in carcinoma of the uterus and the prostate. Also used for rapidly growing brain tumors, laryngeal cancer with very hard nodes, lung cancer, cancer of the oral cavity, stomach cancer with complete emaciation, cancer of the bladder with agonizing pain, and adenoma of the pancreas and adrenals.

Natrum oxalaceticum: In *Causticum compositum, Coenzyme compositum, Cutis compositum, Discus compositum, Ginseng compositum, Hepar compositum, Mucosa compositum, Thyroidea compositum, Ubichinion, BHI-Enzyme*; treats prostatic neoplasms.

Podophyllum: In *Diarrheel, Leptandra compositum, Momordica compositum, Podophyllum compositum, Ubichinon compositum, BHI-Diarrhea, BHI-Pancreas*; used for pancreatic cancer.

Ranunculus bulbosus: In *Discus compositum, Ranunculus homaccord*; treats epithelioma and skin cancer.

Rectum suis: In *Mucosa recti* and *Mucosa compositum*; treats carcinoma of the rectum.

Ruta graveolens: In *Aesculus compositum* and *Cerebrum compositum*. Indicated for rectal adenocarcinoma.

Scrophularia Nodosa: In *Lymphomyosot, Populus compositum*. Used for mammary tumors.

Selenium: In *Cerebrum compositum, Cutis compositum, Selenium homaccord, Testes compositum,* and *Tonico-Injeel*. Protects colon tissue (Jacobs, et al. 2004) and is used in prostatic adenoma and many other neoplasms. The trace mineral selenium inhibits cancer development in a variety of experimental animal models. In a study on DNA damage in prostate tissue and on apoptosis in prostate epithelial cells, the extent of DNA damage in prostate cells and in peripheral blood lymphocytes was lower among the selenium-supplemented dogs than control dogs (Waters, et al. 2003).

Sempervivum tectorum: *Galium Heel, Ginseng compositum, Thyroidea compositum*; used for nodular hardening in the skin, tongue, and breast; warts.

Splen suis: In *Cutis compositum, Thyroidea compositum, Tonsilla compositum*. Treats leukemia, anemia, agranulocytosis. Should be used in carcinoma for general support and revitalization.

Ubiquinone: In *Ubichinon compositum*. Used for cancer of the genitalia, breast cancer with ulceration, and after cancer surgery if healing is delayed.

Ventriculus suis (stomach): In *Mucosa compositum*. Used for precancerous state of the stomach, with ulcers and gastric achylia.

Chondrosarcoma

Step 1. Follow Broadfoot's general Dedifferentiation Phase protocol, above.

Step 2. Select at least 1 agent representing cartilaginous tissue (*Discus compositum* or *Zeel*) and include this in the individualized health program.

Step 3. Consider special single remedies based upon location and symptoms:

Conium maculatum: In *Ginseng compositum*. A powerful detoxicating agent that may strengthen the anterior lobe of the pituitary. Conium maculatum in dilution is historically used for glandular swellings and cancerous conditions. It is also contained in several other agents commonly used in neoplasia including *Cerebrum compositum, Colchicum compositum, Rauwolfia compositum, Testis compositum, Thyroidea compositum, Tonsilla compositum, Vertigoheel,* and *Ubichinon compositum*. When used concurrently with catalysts, this gives a powerful boost to patients that are weakened and tired.

Pain: In *BHI-Inflammation, BHI-Bone, BHI-Injury, BHI-Spasm-Pain, Spascupreel, Atropinum compositum, Bryaconeel,* and *Cruroheel*. All are excellent for localized pain. *Belladonna homaccord* may assist with throbbing pain. *Euphorbium compositum* is a remedy that can be used as a pain management agent in many forms of neoplastic related pain management. Commonly assists with intense pain in limbs, paralytic pain in joints, irritant problems, and pain and ulceration of the skin. *Galium-Heel, Lymphomyosot, Apis homaccord, Traumeel S,* and *Zeel* are also helpful for pain management and are commonly used in elderly pets with Dedifferentiation Phase disease. Because pain is a sign of homotoxin presence and/or damage, properly handling the homotoxins in a patient may give surprisingly good results in pain management. Pain may suddenly appear in a Degeneration Phase case that is undergoing desirable regressive vicariation. This requires skillful biological therapy to move the disease process toward healing (inflammation and excretion) rather than forcing it back into progressive vicariation by suppressive pharmaceutical agents. Use narcotic agents as needed in advanced cases and avoid nonsteroidal anti-inflammatory drugs if possible because they interfere with intestinal function and damage organs of elimination such as kidney and liver.

Hemangiosarcoma

Step 1. Follow Broadfoot's general Dedifferentiation Phase protocol, above.

Step 2. Select at least 1 agent representing splenic tissue (*Tonsilla compositum, Cutis compositum*—for cutaneous hemangiosarcoma—*Thyroidea compositum*) and include this in the individualized health program. Note that these are part of the basic autosanguis and deep detoxification formulas that are so commonly used in advanced diseases such as neoplasia. Because of the vascular nature of these tumors it may prove helpful to include vein and artery tissues as well; these are contained in *Aesculus compositum* (artery only) and *Placenta compositum* (both artery and vein).

Step 3. Consider special single remedies based upon location and symptoms:

Aurumheel N: Treats hypotension and circulatory arrythmias.

Berberis homaccord: Provides adrenal cortex support in stressful conditions.

BHI-Bleeding: In *Crotalis horridus*. Helps control hemorrhages. Very useful due to its complement of agents; a favorite remedy used by the authors for acute hemorrhage as well as maintenance therapy of hemangiosarcoma patients.

Carbo compositum: Supports circulatory failure during shock.

China homaccord: Used for debility and weakness following blood loss. Useful in treating shock from blood loss.

Cinnamomum compositum: Used for active bleeding cases. Not currently available but a very useful remedy during acute hemorrhagic crises. In the absence of this formula consider *BHI-Bleeding*.

Crotalis-Injeel: Used for dark hemorrhages from viscous organs. Not readily available in the United States.

Ginseng compositum: A powerful detoxicating agent that may strengthen the anterior lobe of the pituitary. *Conium maculatum* in dilution is historically used for glandular swellings and cancerous conditions. It is also contained in several other agents commonly used in neoplasia including *Cerebrum compositum, Colchicum compositum, Rauwolfia compositum, Testis compositum, Thyroidea compositum, Tonsilla compositum, Vertigoheel*, and *Ubichinon compositum*. Used concurrently with catalysts, this gives a powerful boost to patients that are weakened and tired.

Hamamelis homaccord: Used for venous stasis and varicosities of extremities (cutaneous hemangiosarcomas may fit this picture).

Phosphor homaccord: Used for hemorrhages that are typically more petechial in nature.

Veratrum homaccord: Treats shock.

Leiomyosarcoma

Step 1. Follow Broadfoot's general Dedifferentiation Phase protocol, above.

Step 2. Use *Jejunum-suis-Injeel* (if available) for jejunal tumors, *Uterus suis-Injeel* for uterine diseases, or *Myoma-Uteri-Injeel* (if available) for uterine myoma. In the United States, *Mucosa compositum* is presently available and will suffice in most issues for this purpose.

Step 3. Consider special single remedies based upon location and symptoms:

Condurango: In *BHI-Headache II* and *BHI-Migraine Rx*, but in no Heel formulas. Used for stomach issues and cancer of the stomach, other forms of cancer, mucocutaneous fissures, and ulcerative cancers.

Duodenoheel: Treats vomiting, nausea, and disease of the duodenum.

Gastricumeel: Treats nausea stemming from gastric diseases.

Gynacoheel: Treats myomas, uterine inflammation, ovarian diseases, ovarian pain.

Klimakt-Heel: Treats uterine polyps, debility.

Metro-Adnex-Injeel: Treats uterine diseases.

Nux vomica homaccord: Supports entire gastrointestinal tract.

Mammary cancer (also see adenocarcinoma)

Step 1. Follow Broadfoot's general Dedifferentiation Phase protocol, above.

Step 2. Consider Mamma-suis-Injeel (if available) or Carcinosin (see below).

Step 3. Consider special single remedies, or combination formulas containing these agents, based upon location and symptoms:

Acidum aceticum: In *Arsuraneel*. Classically indicated for epithelial cancers; very valuable in chronic diseases.

Arsenicum album: In many Heel products commonly used for advanced homotoxicoses, such as *Arsuraneel, Atropinum compositum, Cantharsis compositum, Cor compositum, Cerebrum compositum, Diarrheel S, Echinacea compositum, Gastricumeel, Leptandra compositum, Mezereum homaccord, Solidago compositum, Strophanthus compositum, Sulfur-Heel*, and *Syzygium compositum*. Used for mammary tumors; discharges that are putrid and/or green in color; fear, fright, and worry; and when symptoms are worse at night with debility and weakness.

Asterias rubens: In *Lamioflur*; contains another commonly indicated remedy for mammary cancer. Used for ulceration with sharp pain (worst in the left), mammary swelling, indurated swelling. History may include epilepsy and skin may have ulcers with fetid discharge.

Calcarea fluorica: In *Galium-Heel, Cutis compositum, Thyroidea compositum, Abropernol*. Used for hard, stony glands; knots in the breast; induration that appears in transition to suppuration; and indolent ulcerations that weep thick, yellow pus.

Calcarea idodata: In *Strumeel* and *Barijodeel*. Used for its association with enlarged glands. Classically indicated for thyroid masses near puberty and enlarged tonsils with cryptic formation.

Carcinosin: Not contained in any Heel or BHI products but can be obtained from reputable homeopathic companies. Classically used for mammary cancer (Macleod 1983).

Chimaphilia umbellate: Not contained in any Heel remedies, but contained in *BHI-Prostate Rx* and *BHI-Saw palmetto complex*. Used for inflamed labia, painful mammary tumors that are not ulcerated but may secrete milk, and sharp pain in the tumor (Heel 2002).

Conium maculatum: In *Cerebrum compositum, Colchicum compositum, Ginseng compositum, Rauwolfia compositum, Thyroidea compositum, Tonsilla compositum, Ubichinon compositum* and *Vertigoheel*. Used for mammary cancer. Conium is a classical remedy that can be used singly at appropriate intervals.

Hydrastis: In *Ginseng compositum, Lamioflur, Mucosa compositum, Ovarium compositum*, and *Ubichinon compositum*. Cases are often typified with yellowish, ropey discharges from mucous membranes and aged, weak, easily tired, cachectic patients. Treats cancer states before ulceration and painfulness, vulvar pruritus, mammary tumors. Most cancer patients receive this agent because of the frequency of use of the particular combination remedies.

Phosphorus: In a wide variety of antihomotoxic formulas, including some that are commonly used in Degeneration Phase cases such as *Bryaconeel, Echinacea compositum, Galium-Heel, Hepeel, Molybdan compositum, Mucosa compositum, Phosphor homaccord*, and *Testis compositum*. It is a constitutional remedy of great importance. Patients may have thinner body types and be prone to hemorrhagic disorders in their health history. Treats suppurative mammary tumors.

Phytolacca: In *Echinacea compositum* and *Mercurius-Heel S*. Used for mammary swellings with abscess formation, and possibly mastitis history cases. Useful if given early in the course of tumor development (Macleod 1983).

Plumbum iodatum: In *Placenta compositum*. Used for breast tumors.

Thuja occidentalis: In many remedies, including *Cutis compositum, Echinacea compositum, Galium-Heel*, and *Psorinoheel*. Used for a wide variety of deep homotoxicoses. Used for warty masses and cutaneous protuberances and spongy tumors; warts on vulva and perineum; and polyps and fleshy growths. May help reverse some undesirable side effects stemming from vaccinosis.

Melanoma

Melanoma is a neoplasm with typical history of rapid and aggressive metastasis. Immunotherapy with a vaccination may prove very helpful in the future management of melanoma. Such success indicates that techniques that manage the patient's immune system may be advantageous in this disease. Autosanguis, through its action of macrophages,

dendritic cells, and lymphocytes, may prove particularly useful in this disease.

Palmquist and Broadfoot have 3 cases of canine oral melanosarcoma, one which metastasized rapidly following oral surgery (lumpectomy and biopsy). The owners of all cases declined advanced oncologic handling and elected only homotoxicology (as outlined above) and nutraceutical support. One dog has lived more than 2 years with overt metastasis to regional lymph nodes being resolved. This case series has been accepted for publication in the Journal of the American Holistic Veterinary Medical Association. Palmquist feels higher dose, preservative-free IV ascorbic acid plays an important part in the therapy of this disease. The basic protocol:

Step 1. Follow Broadfoot's general Dedifferentiation Phase protocol, above.

Step 2. Specific immunotherapy for melanoma has been administered to several thousand patients since 1972, using an irradiated whole-cell preparation (Slingluff 1992). Hersey (1993) performed immunotherapy with a vaccine made from vaccinia lysates of an allogenic melanoma cell following surgical removal of lymph node metastases. Modern variants of this medical approach have used buffy coat (a layer of the blood cells) to treat melanoma, creating an artificial hematoma to reactivate the immune system, as well as other strategies for treatment. A homotoxicological variation of these procedures is to use a large blood autosanguis in combination with appropriate remedies, and given as a series of injections.

Step 3. Consider special single remedies, or combination formulas containing these agents, based upon location and symptoms:

Arsenicum album: In many Heel products commonly used for advanced homotoxicoses, such as *Arsuraneel, Atropinum compositum, Cantharsis compositum, Cor compositum, Cerebrum compositum, Diarrheel S, Echinacea compositum, Gastricumeel, Leptandra compositum, Mezereum homaccord, Solidago compositum, Strophanthus compositum, Sulfur-Heel*, and *Syzygium compositum*. Helpful in cases manifesting signs including discharges that are putrid and/or green in color; fear, fright, and worry; and symptoms that are worse at night with debility and weakness. A related remedy, Arsenicum iodatum, is indicated for skin cancers and mammary tumors, and is found in several respiratory remedies including *Tartephedreel, Husteel*, and *BHI-Chest* (Reckeweg 2002). A recent study, broadcasted by the BBC, revealed that an Iranian research team suggested arsenic trioxide as a first-line treatment for acute promyeloctytic leukemia; the survival rate in their study was 88.5% of patients after 34 months. Multiple myeloma may also be a candidate for this therapy. Arsenic trioxide works by causing changes in cancer cells, which induce apoptosis (programmed cell death). It appears to correct the gene responsible for making a flawed protein that causes leukemia. It may be particularly valuable for treating the elderly, who often die earlier in the treatment process due to cumulative toxicity from standard forms of chemotherapy (BBC 2004). A homeopathic trial showed a 33% increase in the survival rate in induced cancer (Dalton's lymphoma ascites) in mice treated with Arsenicum album 30 X (Thobias 1991).

Asterias rubens: In *Lamioflur*. Used to treat cancer.

Carbo animalis: Contained in no Heel or BHI remedy formulas. Used in elderly patients with lowered vitality. Used for indurated glands, offensive secretions, vaginal dermatitis with painful indurations in the breast of females, uterine cancer, and flatulence.

Curare: In *Arsuraneel, Circulo-Injeel, Syzygium compositum, Testis compositum, BHI-Headache,* and *BHI-Migraine Rx*. Used in human melanoma cases (Reckeweg 2002).

Chimaphilla umbellate: In *BHI-Prostate Rx* and *BHI-Saw palmetto complex*. Used in cases with a history of catarrhal bladder issues, glandular enlargements, vaginitis, and diabetes mellitus.

Clematis erecta: In *Galium-Heel* and *Atropinum compositum*. Treats swollen meibomian glands, iritis, blepharospasm, submaxillary gland swelling, and mammary tumors.

Condurango: Found in no Heel formulas but is in *BHI-Headache II* and *BHI-Migraine Rx*. Used in stomach issues and cancer of the stomach as well as other forms of cancer, mucocutaneous fissures, and ulcerative cancers.

Fuligo: Is in no Heel or BHI formulas; comes from soot. Classically used for many forms of cancer.

Galium aparine: In *Galium-Heel*. A powerful agent for suspending or modifying cancerous processes. Useful for general cancers and nodules of the tongue.

Hydrastis: In *Ginseng compositum, Lamioflur, Mucosa compositum, Ovarium compositum,* and *Ubichinon compositum*. Cases are often typified with yellowish, ropey discharges from mucous membranes and aged, weak, easily tired, cachetic patients. Treats cancer before ulceration that is painful, vulvar pruritus, and mammary tumors. Most cancer patients receive this agent because of its frequency of use of the particular combination remedies.

Kreosotum: In *Mucosa compositum, Ginseng compositum, Lamioflur,* and *Ovarium compositum*. Due to the phenolic compounds, this is a potent carcinogen in larger amounts and is associated with a wide variety of neoplasms. It is used for many forms of neoplastic phase disease.

Lachesis: In a large number of formulas, most notably *Gripp-Heel, Mucosa compositum,* and *Ovarium compositum*. This remedy is useful for management of symptoms associated with several types of tumors. These include masses or precancerous conditions of the mammary gland (with purplish coloration), larynx, ovary, uterus, vagina, skin, and thyroid. Gangrenous paraneoplastic situations and draining tracts may be indications as well.

Tarentula cubensis: Not in any Heel or BHI formulas but available from homeopathic pharmacies. Should be considered in melanoma. Indications are malignant suppuration and purplish hue. Also used for genital pruritus.

Thuja occidentalis: In many remedies, including *Cutis compositum, Echinacea compositum, Galium-Heel,* and *Psorinoheel*. Used for a wide variety of deep homotoxicoses. Used for warty masses, cutaneous protuberances, spongy tumors, warts on vulva and perineum, polyps, and fleshy growths. May help reverse some undesirable side effects stemming from vaccinosis.

Viscum album: In *Aesculus compositum, Arteria-Heel, Ginseng compositum, Procainum compositum* (not available in the USA), *Rauwolfia compositum,* and *Viscum compositum (mite, medium, forte)*. It has been studied in Europe as a potential therapy for melanoma.

Meningioma

No reports of resolution of meningioma can be found in the literature. The goal of therapy in such cases is improving immune function and removing homotoxins, with the goals of slowing the growth of the existing mass and reducing the swelling of the tissue surrounding the tumor. A very small reduction in swelling can lead to markedly improved clinical status in patients suffering from intracranial masses. The basic protocol:

Step 1. Follow Broadfoot's general Dedifferentiation Phase protocol, above.

Step 2. Brain tissue is contained in *Cerebrum compositum* (Cerebrum suis), *Testes compositum* (Diencephalon suis), and *Thalamus compositum* (Thalamus opticus suis and Corpus pineale suis). No Heel products available in the USA contain meningeal tissue; however, there are specific injeel remedies available in Europe: Meningeoma-Injeel, Glioma-Injeel, and Neurofibroma-Injeel. As a basic protocol for brain tumors and cerebral compression, consider *Apis homaccord, Galium-Heel, Lymphomyosot, Thalamus compositum, Cerebrum compositum, Viscum compositum, Ginseng compositum,* and *Molybdan compositum*.

Step 3. Consider special single remedies, or combination formulas containing these agents, based upon location and symptoms:

Apomorphia: No homotoxicology remedies contain this agent, which is best known for its emetic qualities. It is listed as a remedy for brain tumors in humans by Boericke (1927).

Baryta carbonica: In *BHI-Ginko complex*. Commonly used in degenerative conditions involving elderly people. Treats cerebral issues, senile dementia, vertigo, bashful personality; tonsilar swelling may have been common in juvenile periods.

Calcarea carbonicum: In *Hepar compositum*, *Hormeel*, and *Graphites homaccord*. Used for pituitary and thyroid disorders.

Conium maculatum: In *Cerebrum compositum*, *Colchicum compositum*, *Ginseng compositum*, *Rauwolfia compositum*, *Thyroidea compositum*, *Tonsilla compositum*, *Ubichinon compositum*, and *Vertigoheel*. Treats geriatric pets with ascending paralysis or weakness with accompanying urinary problems. Conium is a classical remedy that can be used singly at appropriate intervals.

Glonoinum: In *Ypsiloheel* and several other cardiac remedies such as *Cactus compositum*, *Cardiacum-Heel*, and *Cor compositum*. Used for high blood pressure, headache, angiospastic neuralgia, and vertigo. Ypsiloheel is used to rekindle central autoregulation.

Graphites: In *Graphites homaccord* and *Paeonia homaccord*. Used in overweight patients and those with excessive cicatrixal formation; dry, flaky skin; brittle nails; perianal fissures; and constipation.

Hydrastis: In *Ginseng compositum*, *Lamioflur*, *Mucosa compositum*, *Ovarium compositum*, and *Ubichinon compositum*. Cases are often typified by yellowish, ropey discharges from mucous membranes and aged, weak, easily tired, cachetic patients. Used for cancer before ulceration and that is painful, vulvar pruritus, and mammary tumors. Because of the frequency of use of the particular combination remedies, most cancer patients receive this agent.

Kali iodatum: In *Osteoheel* and *BHI-Sinus*. Used for bone inflammation, periosteal disease, or bone pain.

Plumbum metallicum: In *Syzygium compositum*. Used for a wide variety of neurological disorders, including paresis.

Sepia: In several formulas, including *China homaccord*, *Discus compositum*, *Hormeel*, *Nervoheel*, and *Ovarium compositum*. A classical female remedy that is associated with sadness, anxiety, and vertigo.

Traumeel **S**: Reduces inflammation and activates blocked enzyme systems. Contains Apis for swelling and Belladonna for inflammation and seizures. *Traumeel* solution was studied in a randomized, controlled clinical trial for the treatment of chemotherapy-induced stomatitis in children undergoing stem cell transplantation. This study indicated that *Traumeel* may significantly reduce the severity and duration of stomatitis in children undergoing bone marrow transplantation (Oberbaum 2001).

Pheochromocytoma

Broadfoot's general Dedifferentiation Phase protocol, above, can be used for these cases, because its normal constituents include the adrenal components that support patients with this disease.

Spindle cell sarcoma

See Fibrosarcoma, above.

Transitional cell carcinoma

See Adenocarcinoma, above.

Step 1. Follow Broadfoot's general Dedifferentiation Phase protocol, above.

Step 2. Include *Solidago compositum* and *Mucosa compositum* in the individualized health program.

Step 3. Select remedies for symptom relief as for other bladder issues (see the cystitis section). Consider special single remedies based upon location and symptoms:

Taraxacum officinale: In *Hepar compositum* and *Injeel-Chol*. Relieves some signs in cases of bladder cancer.

Berberis homaccord: Relieves stress and supports urinary tissues. Useful for most cancer patients for purpose of adrenal support.

REFERENCES

BBC News: Arsenic could be suitable as first-line treatment in rare type of leukaemia. 2004/09/29 http://news.bbc.co.uk/go/pr/fr/-/1/hi/health/3699962.stm

Boericke W. Materia Medica with Repertory, 9th ed. Glossary. Santa Rosa, CA: Boericke and Tafel, 1927. p 845.

Heel. BHI Homeopathic Therapy: Professional Reference. Albuquerque, NM: Heel, Inc. 2002. p 112.

Hersey P. Evaluation of vaccinia viral lysates as therapeutic vaccines in the treatment of melanoma. *Ann NY Acad Sci*. 1993. Aug 12;690:pp 167–177.

Hohmann J, Molnar J, Redei D, Evanics F, Forgo P, Kalman A, Argay G, Szabo P. Discovery and biological evaluation of a new family of potent modulators of multidrug resistance: reversal of multidrug resistance of mouse lymphoma cells by new natural jatrophane diterpenoids isolated from euphorbia species. *J Med Chem*. 2002. Jun 6;45(12):pp 2425–31.

Jacobs ET, Jiang R, Alberts DS, Greenberg ER, Gunter EW, Karagas M, Lanza E, Ratnasinghe L, Reid ME, Schatzkin A, Smith-Warner SA, Wallace K, and Martnez ME. Selenium and colorectal adenoma: results of a pooled analysis. *J Natl Cancer Inst*. 2004. Nov 17;96(22): pp 1669–1675.

Macleod G. A Veterinary Materia Medica and Clinical Repertory with a Materia Medica of the Nosodes. Safron, Walden: CW Daniel Compositumany, LTD. 1983. pp 127, 172.

Nakao Y, Matsuda S, Kimoto H. Paradoxical anti-leukemic effects of plant-derived tumor promoters on a human thymic lymphoblast cell line. *Int J Cancer*. 1982. 30:pp 687—695.

Oberbaum M, Yaniv I, Ben-Gal Y, Stein J, Ben-Zvi N, Freedman L, Branski D. A randomized, controlled clinical trial of the homeopathic medication TRAUMEEL S® in the treatment of chemotherapy-induced stomatitis in children undergoing stem cell transplantation. *Cancer*. 2001.92(3):pp 684–690.

Reckeweg, H. Homoeopathia Antihomotoxica Materia Medica, 4th ed. Baden-Baden, Germany: Aurelia-Verlag GMBH, 2002. pp 118–20, 136–7, 153, 158, 169–70, 176–8, 182, 197, 201–2, 213–4, 226–7, 235, 241–2, 249–51, 254, 257, 271–2, 295 307–9, 310–12, 324, 325, 327–8, 335–6, 344–5, 346–8, 373–5, 377–9, 383, 422, 433, 437–40, 442, 446–9, 450–2, 458, 460, 495–6, 497, 508, 509, 525, 528, 530, 542, 552–4, 555–60, 574–5, 576, 591, 598, 609–10.

Slingluff CL Jr, Seigler HF. Immunotherapy for malignant melanoma with a tumor cell vaccine. *Ann Plast Surg.* 1992. Jan;28(1):pp 104–107.

Szallasi A. Active substances in euphorbium and their risk for causing acute and/or chronic toxicity. *Biomedical Therapy.* 1999. 27(3):pp 95–98.

Thobias MP. The Homeopathic Heritage 1991; March:119–\120.

Waters DJ, Shen S, Cooley DM, Bostwick DG, Qian J, Combs G, Glickman G, Oteham C, Schlittler D, Morris JS. Effects of dietary selenium supplementation on DNA damage and apoptosis in canine prostate. *J Nat Cancer Inst.* 2003. Feb 5;95(3): pp 237–241.

Zayed SM, Farghaly M, Soliman SM, Gotta H, Sorg B, Hecker E. Dietary cancer risk from conditional cancerogens (tumor promoters) in produce of livestock fed on species of spurge (Euphorbiaceae). V. Skin irritant and tumor-promoting diterpene ester toxins of the tigliane and ingenane type in the herbs Euphorbia nubica and Euphorbia helioscopia contaminating fodder of livestock. *J Cancer Res Clin Oncol.* 2001. Jan;127(1):pp 40–7.

SECTION 6

Vaccinations

Chapter Thirty-Five

Vaccinations

VACCINATION ISSUES

Any veterinarian who administers vaccinations knows the difficulties encountered when a puppy or kitten suddenly collapses due to an acute hypersensitivity reaction resulting from the administration of a routine vaccination given with the intention of increasing its health and well being. A feline practitioner presented with a persistent mass at the site of prior vaccination is acutely aware of the despair and regret that can come from finding and diagnosing a feline vaccine-related fibrosarcoma.

Immunization is an important tool used to protect these young animals from the ongoing presence of devastating viral diseases, such as canine parvovirus, canine distemper virus, feline panleukopenia, feline viral rhinotracheitis, feline leukemia virus, and rabies virus, as well as other diseases that may threaten human and animal health. Veterinarians across the nation are beginning to give careful consideration to their routine vaccination recommendations due to the possibility of adverse events (AE) associated with vaccination. Despite this reduction in the number of vaccinations recommended for veterinary patients, AEs still occur, and some diseases, like leptospirosis, create difficult issues for patient, client, and clinician when they make honest efforts to decide upon a best and safest course of prevention for a particular pet. Our ability to predict AEs is poor, and our understanding of more complex interactions between patient, environment, and vaccination content leaves much room for investigation and improvement.

Since the 1950s, veterinary medicine has done an excellent job of educating pet owners on the importance of vaccination. There is no doubt that millions of dogs and cats have been protected against life-threatening infections. Human health has also been improved thanks to the development and widespread use of rabies vaccination. Decades ago, the American Veterinary Medical Association (AVMA) recommended annual revaccination of all dogs, a practice still common today. This recommendation was based on the assumption that immunity would dwindle in some pets, so that frequent revaccina-

tion was required to ensure immunity in the population. Recommendation for annual revaccination of all canine and feline patients with multivalent or "combo" vaccines assumes that every pet is at significant risk for exposure to every infectious agent in the vaccine, and that each agent in the vaccine will stimulate the same degree of immunity that lasts the same amount of time (Greene 2001). Today, we know that these assumptions are neither rational nor scientifically justified.

Vaccination should not be a regimented, one-size-fits-all procedure. The objective of vaccination is simply to give the right vaccine at the right time to the right individual to protect that individual from an infectious disease. To accomplish this objective, each patient should be evaluated with regard to age, lifestyle, disease prevalence in the community, potential for exposure to infected animals and environments, and the severity of clinical disease, if any, after infection (Ford 2001). Vaccination is a medical procedure and deserves the same level of consideration and concern as any other serious healthcare decision.

There are 3 types of vaccines: killed vaccines, modified live vaccines, and recombinant vaccines (Greene 2001, Van Kampen 2001). Vaccines that contain killed viruses or bacteria are usually adjuvanated with agents such as aluminum hydroxide, which function as nonspecific immune boosters, thus improving patient response to the vaccination. Because the vaccine is killed, there is no replication or reversion to virulence, and these are considered safer in breeding bitches and the immunosuppressed. However, there is a higher incidence of adverse reactions to the killed organisms suspended in adjuvant (Tater 2005), and killed vaccines confer lower immunity and shorter duration of protection. Leptospirosis, bordetella, Lyme, giardia, and rabies vaccines can all be found in killed form.

Modified live vaccines (MLV) contain live viruses that have been attenuated to allow replication in the host without causing clinical disease, and they stimulate a more long-lasting, physiological type of humoral and cell-mediated immune response. Some of these can be given at the site where the pathogen normally invades, e.g., intranasal vaccinations for bordetella, parainfluenza, and feline viral rhinotracheitis, which induce a localized immune response. Distemper, parvovirus, hepatitis, parainfluenza, and bordetella are available as MLV vaccines.

Recombinant vaccines are genetically engineered by inserting selected genes from an infectious agent into a nonpathogenic carrier agent that serves as a production factory. The proteins then produced are critical in stimulating specific immunity to the infectious agent, and thus focus the immune response. Lyme vaccine now comes as a recombinant, and there are a number of newer vaccines in this genre, e.g., distemper vaccine (Crawford 2002).

The clinician must consider the proper timing for vaccination administration in order that optimum immunity results. High levels of maternal antibodies acquired from ingestion of colostrums protect puppies and kittens from disease for the first 6 to 8 weeks of life. Thereafter a window of susceptibility to infection is created because maternal antibodies are high enough to interfere with the vaccine-induced response, but not high enough to protect the pup from infection and disease. This is the most common cause of vaccine failure in puppies. Therefore, immunizations are repeated at timed intervals to ensure development of a protective immune response. The pediatric series includes the core vaccines for distemper, parvovirus, and infectious canine hepatitis starting with an initial immunization at 6 to 8 weeks of age, followed by boosters every 3 to 4 weeks until 12 to 14 weeks old. Improved vaccine technology as is present in Recombitek© canine distemper vaccination helps to overcome this issue. This advance makes such vaccines highly desirable for use in shelters and other high-risk environments.

Concurrent environmental or medical factors may affect patient response to vaccination. Many vaccines carry the statement in their packaging "for use in healthy animals only." This is sage advice, as vaccination during periods of illness may negatively affect patient response. It is not known if administration of vaccines during illness increases the risk of other adverse events, such as immune imbalance, but basic homotoxicology phase theory would predict that administration of homotoxins to biological systems under duress would be more likely to lead to progressive vicariation. Bearing in mind that MLV vaccines create an Impregnation Phase (already to the right of the biological divide), it would be sensible to be as certain as possible that the patient's health was good before administering any vaccine (see Chapter 4 for an in-depth discussion of homotoxicology).

The use of steroids concurrently with vaccination has long been discussed in our profession. Newer drugs such as cyclosporin should be evaluated as well. Nonsteroidal anti-inflammatory drugs (NSAIDs) are commonly used agents in veterinary medicine. They are common in geriatric patients and also commonly used by veterinarians as post-operative pain management. They are known to decrease healing and may cause other negative effects on the host's greater defenses. A recent study involving mice seems to indicate that concurrent drug therapy with cox2-inhibiting NSAIDs can negatively affect immune response. Mice were pretreated with a cox2 inhibitor and then vaccinated with a model vaccine against human papillomavirus (HPV). The mice in the control group responded well to this new product recently released for human protection against HPV, an agent responsible for early-onset cervical cancer in women. The cox2 inhibitor group responded poorly. This group showed 70% less anti-HPV 16 immunoglobulin, 50% fewer antibody-secreting cells, and one-tenth of the neutralizing antibodies to HPV 16 than the control group (Ryan 2006). This powerful data may explain in part why elderly human patients respond more poorly than younger ones to influenza vaccination, and this information gives veterinarians cause to consider routine use of NSAIDs on yet another level. Further study of this issue is warranted in our profession.

Recent challenge studies performed by independent research groups have demonstrated that modified live virus vaccines for distemper, parvo, canine infectious hepatitis, and parainfluenza induced immunity for 5 to 7 years. Considering that annual revaccination in these challenge studies did not provide any increased strength in the humoral immune response elicited or duration of immunity, nor did it improve resistance to disease (Ford 2001, Greene 2002), the practice of annual revaccination needs to be seriously reconsidered, especially given that the incidence of clinical disease from distemper, hepatitis, and parvovirus in dogs older than 1 year of age is virtually nil.

Dr. R.D. Schultz at the University of Wisconsin proposed an ideal canine vaccination program to consist of 1 booster vaccination given 1 year after completion of the pediatric series, with subsequent vaccinations given at 3-year intervals thereafter (Greene 2002). This recommendation is consistent with that of the American Animal Hospital Association. In a recent survey of holistic veterinarians attending the annual meeting of the American Holistic Veterinary Medical Association, the majority of survey respondents were currently following this protocol (Palmquist 2007).

For some diseases, such as canine distemper and canine parvovirus, it may be possible to assess the adequacy of protection through use of vaccination titers. Practitioners using this method report a high success in prevention of these diseases and have reported that they feel they are encountering a reduced incidence of other autoimmune diseases, such as immune hemolytic anemia and idiopathic thrombocytopenia. No formal studies have been published comparing rates of these diseases before and after adopting titering and reducing dependency upon yearly boosters. Such a study would shed light on this area and would be welcomed data. Such practitioners reported this observed trend seemed to follow their decision to reduce vaccination by use of vaccine titers. In human medicine, vaccine titers are routinely used in evaluating patients for their need of rabies revaccination. It may be possible to do something similar with veterinary patients, but at this time most states do not recognize rabies vaccine titers as a legal substitution for required rabies vaccination boosters.

Use of canine vaccine titers is still a controversial subject among veterinarians. Researchers have reported that canine distemper and canine parvovirus antibody titers may not always correspond to protection against disease (Ford 2001, Greene 2002). A high-antibody titer does not guarantee immune protection, and a low or negative-antibody titer does not indicate guaranteed susceptibility to infection. There is a breed predisposition for low titering among the Rottweiler, Doberman Pinscher, Labrador Retriever, Alaskan sled dog, Pomeranian, and American Staffordshire Terriers. These dogs may remain healthy, presumably via vaccine stimulation of other important immune system arms, such as cell-mediated immunity, mucosal immunity, and immune memory cells.

In a recent study, serum antibody titers to distemper and parvovirus were measured in 1,441 dogs of various ages and breeds located across the U.S. and Canada, with more than 95% showing adequate titers to distemper and parvo. In the study, 468 dogs with known vaccination histories had a vaccine 1 to 2 years before the testing (60%), 2 to 7 years before (30%), and less than 1 year (10%) (Twark 2000).

Palmquist has routinely titered for canine distemper and parvo viruses in his inner-city practice population of 15,000 pets. He surveyed U.S. veterinarians responsible for more than 136,000 dogs. In this study no clinical cases of canine parvovirus or distemper were reported in dogs properly vaccinated as puppies and then booster vaccinated only when they were determined to have inadequate antibody levels on vaccine titer testing (Palmquist 2003). This study indicates that titering patients can be used as a tool to reduce unnecessary vaccinations, and although not all diseases lend themselves to this practice, it is useful to consider when developing preventive medicine programs for the companion animal veterinarian. Palmquist feels that the incidence of autoimmune diseases such as AIHA and ITP have decreased dramatically in his practice since implementing such protocols. In 2006 only 2 cases of AIHA and only 1 case of ITP were reported to occur in his practice of 15,000 dogs and cats. More study is indicated.

In cats, vaccination titers may not be that useful. Lappin has shown that cats vaccinated for the feline herpes virus, type 1 (FHV-1), are protected by vaccination against clinical infections, even though their vaccine titer levels have declined over time. This makes titering less useful in determining need of revaccination in cats, but also establishes that we may be administering unnecessary vaccination for FHV-1. Lappin states, "Because most client-owned cats had detectable serum antibodies suggestive of resistance to infection, use of arbitrary booster vaccination intervals is likely to lead to unnecessary vaccination of some cats" (Lappin 2002). Veterinarians are just beginning to appreciate the relationship of herpes virus and its implication in difficult to diagnose and treat feline dermatoses. The possibility of impregnation by vaccine strain herpes virus in cats would be predicted to cause chronic, refractory inflammatory conditions by basic homotoxicology phase theory, and it is compatible with what we already know about the biological behavior of feline herpes virus.

Just as no vaccine confers 100% immunity, no vaccine is 100% free of adverse events, which consist of any undesirable consequence, including illness or a reaction, whether or not a cause-and-effect relationship can be established. The most commonly recognized AEs are nonspecific: fever, anorexia, and stiffness for 24 to 36 hours after vaccination. The most frequently reported AE associated with killed vaccines is immediate hypersensitivity or anaphylaxis, indicated by urticaria (hives), pruritus of the face and ears, and possibly vomiting and/or diarrhea in some dogs (Meyer 2001). These may occur immediately after vaccination or several hours later. Vaccines containing killed coronavirus combined with killed leptospirosis bacteria targeted for use in puppies should not be used due to increased frequency of hypersensitivity reactions. Canine leptospirosis is a bacterial infection that causes kidney and liver failure in dogs of all ages. There are several different serovars, which are antigenically distinct from each other, and strains may not be cross protective. The killed bacteria suspended in adjuvant are responsible for many hypersensitivity reactions, particularly in Dachshunds and other small breeds, and only induce a short-lived immunity of 6 to 8 months (Greene 2002).

Type-1 (immediate) hypersensitivity reactions involve antigen-specific IgE or IgG on the surface of a mast cell or basophil, resulting in degranulation and release of vasoactive substances. These can be seen within minutes in most cases or can be delayed up to 24 hours post exposure. In some cases these reactions are generalized and in others they are localized. In dogs, the primary manifestations are facial pruritus and edema, hives, and urticarial lesions. More severe cases can show hypotension, dyspnea, diarrhea, and collapse. Cats suffer more respiratory signs, including dyspnea, shock, salivation, and pulmonary edema. Miniature Dachshunds are overrepresented in the literature. Death can occur quickly in such situations, and emergency care is warranted.

The authors report a disproportionate number of young canines that react, represented by Dachshunds, Pugs, and Boston Terriers, with a smattering of other breeds. Interestingly, we also see a fair number of these breeds presented for atopic issues as well. Vaccination has been found to exacerbate the immune response of dogs with preexisting inhalant allergies. Vaccine antigens may potentially exceed the immunologic tolerance threshold of some animals with atopy. The more antigens administered in a vaccine, the greater the chance of inducing hypersensitivity. Often it is difficult to link this kind of tissue damage to vaccination, but this may be due to the fact that damage tends to be caused by the accumulation of many antigens from many vaccines over years of a dog's life, rather than from any one given vaccine. We most assuredly see a link between worsening of allergy symptoms within 2 to 4 weeks post vaccination in sensitized dogs.

A more minor reaction, yet one of concern to owners, is a very localized reaction, in the form of a subcutaneous mass at the injection site. These swellings may be occasionally painful and tend to be transient in nature. We have considered the possibility that the development of such lesions may suggest increased sensitivity in the affected patients, but no proof of this exists at this time. The granuloma may not appear for several weeks post vaccination, and it is thought that this is a local reaction to the adjuvants in vaccine. Such swellings that persist for more than 6 to 8 weeks should be examined by cytology or biopsy for neoplasia. Other reactions can be local swelling, pain, and alopecia at the injection site (Broadfoot 2006). Alopecia at the site of rabies vaccination is a well-known and frustrating complaint seen by veterinary dermatologists, and although not life threatening, such lesions can cause extremely disgruntled clients, especially when occurring on show dogs.

Other less-recognized AEs include abortions, stillbirths, and birth defects due to vaccination of pregnant dogs, and illness in neonates (Crawford 2002). There are approximately 12,000 reports of AEs annually for human vaccines, all of which must be forwarded to the FDA. In contrast, animal vaccine manufacturers are neither required to list possible adverse reactions on vaccine labels, nor keep records of adverse events reported directly to them, nor forward reports to the USDA or FDA. There are approximately 10,000 reports of adverse events associated with animal vaccines annually in the U.S., communicated directly to the manufacturers (Meyer 2001).

Because reporting of AEs is not required, this most likely represents a markedly low figure, as most veterinarians do not take time to file AE reports. One of the best-developed surveillance schemes in the world for monitoring veterinary vaccine AEs is in the United Kingdom, where vaccine manufacturers are legally required to record reports of adverse reactions and submit the reports to a regulatory agency (Gaskill 2002). Veterinarians in the United States interested in practicing evidence-based medicine would welcome such data.

There is a growing awareness of health problems that may be associated with vaccine administration, both in the short term, and in the prevalence of chronic "vaccinosis." This term was created in holistic medical circles to describe disease states that may arise from vaccination. There is increasing evidence suggesting that vaccination, particularly overvaccination, meaning the administration of unnecessary vaccinations, is associated with development or aggravation of immune-mediated disorders and chronic diseases in individuals that are genetically predisposed.

There appears to be a breed predisposition for developing adverse reactions and immune-mediated diseases, including the Old English Sheepdog, Akita, American Cocker Spaniel, Standard Poodle, Scottish Terrier, Shetland Sheepdog, Shih Tzu, Vizsla, Weimaraner, Irish Setter, Doberman Pinscher, and Dachshund (Dodds 2001). There are 2 published studies that linked vaccination and development of immune-mediated hemolytic anemia (David 1996, Hogenesch 1999). More recent reports have suggested vaccine-induced development of hypertrophic osteodystrophy in Weimaraner puppies that were genetically predisposed to the disease (Dodds 2001, Harrus 2002). To date, there are no controlled scientific studies that prove a cause and effect relationship between vaccination and development of immune-mediated diseases or chronic diseases (Gaskell 2002).

Homeopathic veterinarians have long charged that a relationship between rabies vaccination and onset of neurological disease exists. There are studies that have linked neurological disease with vaccines, particularly the rabies component. A canine study (Rehulova 1971) and a human report of four cases of neurological complications following vaccination with cerebral-type lyophilized vaccine from the Province of Poznan have been profiled in journals. The latter reported cases occurring in middle-aged men that exhibited the following syndromes: Landry's ascending paralysis, polyradiculoneuritis, polyneuritis, and encephalopolyradiculoneuritis (Kowal 1986).

In the Hayward Study on Vaccines, William R. LaRosa, M.D., (Trustee of the Hayward Foundation) states that a number of autoantibodies to several critical proteins and DNA were identified in the vaccinated group. Identifying these autoimmune antibodies and monitoring their titers may lead to better understanding of the thyroiditis conditions, as well as to a better understanding of the role of vaccines in soliciting adverse events that contribute to problematic conditions observed in the Great Dane, such as cardiomyopathy and various bone-related disorders. One control group was not vaccinated and the other group was vaccinated with a commercial multivalent vaccine at 8, 10, 12, 16, and 20 weeks of age and with a rabies vaccine at 16 weeks of age.

Some autoimmune diseases that may be considered in this spectrum are: diseases of the pancreas (diabetes), thyroid (Hashimoto's disease), collagen and fibronectin (scleroderma, lupus), cardiolipin (cardiomyopathy), and so on. The body literally attacks itself to cause the autoimmune disease. In this study, the vaccinated group developed significant levels of autoantibodies against fibronectin, laminin, DNA, albumin, cytochrome c, transferrin, cardiolipin, and collagen. The responses varied among individual animals, probably reflecting genetic differences. It is surmised that something in the vaccines is one of the etiologies (in the genetically susceptible dog) of such diseases as cardiomyopathy, lupus erythematosus, glomerulonephritis, and so on (Hogenesch 1997).

A recent research project studied 20 healthy research Beagles and 16 healthy pet dogs. The research Beagles were split into several groups. Five dogs were vaccinated with a multivalent vaccine and a rabies vaccine, five dogs received only the multivalent vaccine, five dogs received only the rabies vaccine, and five dogs were unvaccinated controls. The multivalent vaccine was administered at 8, 10, 12, 16, 20, 26, and 52 weeks of age and every 6 months thereafter. The rabies vaccine was administered at 16 and 52 weeks of age and then once per year. Assays for antibodies directed against bovine and canine thyroglobulin were performed prior to and 2 weeks after each yearly vaccination. In the pet dogs, blood was collected prior to and 2 weeks after 1 vaccination. A significant increase in antibovine thyroglobulin antibodies in all vaccinated dogs was found, compared with control dogs. There was a significant increase in anticanine thyroglobulin antibodies in the 2 groups of dogs that received the rabies vaccine but not in the group that received the multivalent vaccine alone. In the pet dogs, there was a significant increase in anticanine thyroglobulin antibodies after vaccination but no significant change in antibovine thyroglobulin antibodies (Scott-Moncrief 2002). Once again no one has proven that these rises in anticanine thyroglobulin result directly in clinical hypothyroidism, but this study coupled with other observations suggests that veterinarians use caution when designing preventive medicine programs for their patients.

Vaccines are sometimes grown in cell cultures containing same-species antigens. This is done to reduce unwanted reactions to foreign proteins, and it is the case for FVRCP vaccination, which is propagated in Crandall-Reese feline kidney (CRFK) cells. There has been concern over vaccination with autogenous species antigen and its ability to sensitize the immune system toward "self-antigens."

Lappin reported the presence of autoantibodies to feline renal tissue following routine vaccination, but has been careful to state that there is no positive research link between vaccination and the incidence of chronic renal disease (CRD) in cats. Because CRD is such a common disease in cats, this relationship deserves further investigation. Autoantibody production occurred in both subcutaneously administered killed and MLV FVRCP vaccinations, but did not result from intranasal vaccination. Veterinarians may wish to explore further which route they select for routine protection.

In 1983, a study showed that allergies (such as atopic dermatitis) develop in dogs when vaccinated with distemper, hepatitis, and leptospirosis vaccines just before, but not after, exposure to pollen extracts. Dogs predisposed to atopy produce excess amounts of IgE antibodies in response to antigens, resulting in chronically irritating skin inflammations. Other organs may exhibit signs of hypersensitivity, causing, for example, conjunctivitis or rhinitis, as exhibited in further studies by this group (Frick 1983).

In humans, hemophilus influenza B (HIB) vaccination appeared to be a risk factor and was shown to induce diabetes-related autoantibodies in 1-year-old children. Researchers concluded that HIB vaccination may have an unspecific stimulatory polyclonal effect, altering beta cell-related immune response (Wahlberg et al. 2003).

Vaccines may contain many other ingredients besides the attenuated pathogen. Substances such as heavy metals, antibiotics, antifungals, preservatives, and other chemicals may be present, along with biological protein and cellular extracts, and even the possibility of other unknown disease agents. Little is known about the long-term effects of these agents. For years we have operated on the idea that these small amounts of chemicals were simply too little to cause significant disease phenomena, but with the advent of discoveries into the field of nanopharmacology, we now know that small quantities of substance can cause stimulation of various bodily functions. The presence of heavy metals is one such concern, and although many manufacturers have removed one such substance (thimerosal), it is not known what other similar substances may be contained in the patented formulas of current products. Most pharmaceutical companies will not disclose the exact contents of their products.

A study conducted at the University of Maryland School of Medicine finds that exposure to low levels of mercury can speed up and worsen the symptoms of an induced lupus-like disease in mice, even when the exposure occurs before the development of the disease. In this study, healthy mice that were not genetically susceptible to mercury-induced autoimmune disease were given injections of low-dose inorganic mercury over the course of 2 weeks. The levels of mercury and the length of exposure chosen were much lower than the range commonly used in mouse studies of mercury toxicity. Five days later, the mice were given cells from the lupus-inclined mouse strain to induce lupus-like chronic graft-versus-host disease, a well-established mouse model of acquired autoimmunity. Mercury exposure accelerated the deaths of the lupus-induced mice and sped up the course of a kidney disease associated with lupus. Further, antibodies, or markers characteristic of lupus-like autoimmunity, were significantly elevated in the mice that had been pretreated with mercury.

Mercury exposure in animals can exacerbate preexisting autoimmune disease and even induce autoimmune disease in susceptible animals (Via 2003). Because thimerosal is still present in some veterinary vaccines, this may be an issue in vaccinosis, and furthermore, this fact should alert consumers and professionals about the possibility of chemical exposure and vaccines in relation to onset of chronic disease states.

HOMOTOXICOLOGY AND NOSODES

Due to concerns about vaccination overload of the immune system with development of autoimmune diseases and "vaccinosis," there has been a proliferation of anti-vaccination Web sites offering alternatives to conventional vaccinations. One of the alternatives is the use of "nosodes" to convey immunity. A nosode is defined in Dorland's Medical Dictionary as any disease product used as a remedy. In the *Homeopathic Pharmacopoeia of the United States* (HPUS), which is recognized by the FDA, a nosode is defined as "A homeopathic attenuation of pathological organs or tissues, causative agents such as ova, bacteria, fungae, parasites, virus particles, yeast, of diverse products or excretions." To get new nosodes officially recognized in the *Homeopathic Pharmacopoeia*, these nosodes have to have a track record and be written about in homeopathic literature. An official nosode has to be in the homeopathic literature before 1960 (Wilson 1990).

Microdoses of a medication can be used to stimulate the body's defense systems. Classical homeopathy may use single remedies, homotoxicology may use complex remedies, and others may use a great deal of isopathy, which consists of using small amounts of the same thing as the patient's pathologic process. Yet each branch of homeopathy is guided by this principle in conjunction with the Law of Similars. This concept is, of course, not unique to homeopathy; vaccination against smallpox is an isopathic example of this principle dating back to about 800 BC, when Chinese doctors prevented smallpox by sniffing pox lesion secretions. In 1,400 tuberculosis patients, they used some of their own diluted sputum. Then, in 1796, Jenner developed a smallpox vaccination by dilution of cowpox lesions, as a "similar." In 1820,

Wilhelm Lux, a veterinarian, cured very sick animals that had distemper symptoms using auto-nosodes, by taking various discharges from the animals and giving those discharges back to them as a treatment. (We do this procedure, in a modified fashion, when we employ autosanguis techniques, which are reviewed elsewhere in this text.) In 1825, Samuel Hahnemann proved a Psorinum (scabies) pustule, and it is the first mention in the homeopathic literature of using diseased product. Hering coined the term "nosode" in 1831, when he proved an important nosode, Lyssin, which is made from the saliva of a rabid dog. By 1900, bacteriology was rapidly evolving, and nosodes could be made from specific bacteria, viruses, protozoa, and fungi.

Nosodes are generally diffuse immune stimulators. Allopathic literature cites the experimental use of low-dose typhoid vaccine as an immune stimulant for AIDS patients in March of 1989. This study used five-hundredths of a milliliter, injected weekly into AIDS patients, and found that this nosode raised the lymphocyte count in patients that were not currently on AZT. There is also ongoing research using BCG (an attenuated TB bacterium) in the management of superficial bladder cancer, in which researchers instilled BCG vaccine inside the bladder once a week for 6 weeks. This therapy had a fairly high success rate, at 75% (Soloway 1988). Pyrogen is an interesting nosode, based on placenta, which has immune stimulant activity. It is useful for septic fevers, especially if the pulse is low and the fever is high, or vice versa.

Colibacillinum (E. coli) was introduced in 1933, and it was used in diarrheas and meningitis, as well as for bladder infections. In an epidemic outbreak of meningitis in 1974 in Brazil, a 10 CH nosode was made from meningitis types A and C and given as a preventive, due to a lack of adequate allopathic therapeutics. This reduced the incidence markedly. Though this wasn't double blinded, it was a compelling report, given that 18,000 children were treated, with only 7 active cases and 4 deaths.

On the basis of their composition, nosodes act on the basis of the microvaccines that they contain. Nosodes may function to eliminate the antigenic stimuli initiated by bacteria and viruses. As a result of the products of disease that they also contain, nosodes additionally act to bind the autoantigens created by decomposition of the body's cells. Nosodes may also enable reactivation of the partially inhibited mesenchyme by dissolution of the stable bond of the antigen to the micelles. They thereby affect the accelerated discharge of disease toxins that, because of their great molecular weight of more than twenty thousand, can be transported away only by lymphogenic channels and not through the blood. Optimal effects are developed here by nosodes in attenuation of D6 to D200, such as those found in Psorinoheel (Neuner 1988).

Nosodes have a long history of safety. Thus far, in the track record of 150 years of using nosodes, there have been no diseases caused by using them. The HPUS states that no nosodes can be dispensed in a concentration below 6 X. The first attenuation must be rendered sterile. The manufacturers must sterilize the first attenuation, usually with alcohol or ethanol, or they pass it through a millipore filter (Wilson 1990). There are few or no controlled studies in animals that support the use of nosodes, though nosodes do have a long track history of usage.

Nosodes are often offered as a substitute for conventional vaccinations, and further research may show varying success or lack thereof for this practice as it relates to each specific pathogen. There are many research opportunities involving nosodes, but at this time there is not sufficient evidence to recommend that nosodes be used in this manner. Some veterinarians recommend using conventional vaccinations and then using nosodes for annual boosters. Because most vaccinations last more than 1 year, this may not be needed, but it should not prove harmful to most patients.

Author's note

In an outbreak of disease, it is worthwhile to make a "herd" nosode, e.g., in a recent outbreak of warts in a goat herd, we obtained a scraping of a wart, crushed and suspended it in alcohol, and added a ml of the alcohol admixture to a 2-oz. cocktail of Galium plus Engystol and Thuja compositum tablets. This remedy was administered to the entire herd in their drinking water. The entire herd cleared within a very short time, and an individual animal that had just started with early lesions had rapid regression. This same system can be used in an outbreak of kennel cough or other viral disease, as it is disease- and species-specific. We use it routinely in herds of horses that have had a West Nile case, or in strangles outbreaks as well (Broadfoot).

Primary remedy selections with specific indications in vaccine-related issues

Echinacea compositum is a compound formula that contains several useful components, including:

Echinacea angustifolia (also in *Aesculus compositum, Arnica-Heel, Belladonna compositum, Galium-Heel, Mercurius-Heel, Tonsilla compositum, Traumeel, Echinacea PC, BHI-Infection,* and *BHI-Injury*). It is useful in fever, sepsis, and inflammations of every kind, as it acts on the lymphatic system. Echinacea has been used as well for the bad consequences of vaccination (Hamalcik 1989).

Aconitum napellus (also in *Aconitum homaccord, Cerebrum compositum, Gripp-Heel, Spascupreel, BHI-*

Chamomilla, BHI-FluPlus, BHI-Injury, Traumeel, and so on) is one of the important homoeopathic remedies for fever, great anxiety, rapid and tense pulse, strong and possibly irregular heartbeat, alternating fever and chills, and possible hyperthermia. Low potencies are normally given in pyrexia, in neuralgic symptoms with paraesthesia, as well as with post-vaccinial encephalitis or meningo-encephalitis.

Influenzinum, which is a nosode of influenza vaccine (also in *Ginseng compositum*), has been recommended for the general tendency to corpulence and adiposity that arises from thyroid hypofunction. This has some intriguing possibilities, given the emerging data on thyroiditis and hypothyroidism related to vaccinosis. It has excellent action in exhaustion phases. It is used as a prophylactic measure in patients with a tendency to catch viral diseases. It is also used in bronchial asthma, chronic polysinusitis and other sequelae of influenza, and iatrogenic damage.

Thuja occidentalis (also in *Atropinum compositum, Cerebrum compositum, Cutis compositum, Galium-Heel, Psorinoheel, Thuja compositum, Ypsiloheel, BHI-Allergy, BHI-Hair and Skin, -Inflammation,* and *Neuralgia, Sinus*) is indicated in cases of poisoning or in adverse reactions to vaccination, especially smallpox. Retoxically caused impregnations, whether caused by the introduction of deep-acting toxins, such as bacterial toxins and so forth, or by the medical inhibition of reaction phases and also the suppression of a fever, influenza, throat infection, and so on, become the object of attempts by the body to redirect them into regressive vicariation, eliminating the toxins via skin eruptions of various descriptions or other excretion phases. This remedy is selected when signs of the patient match the proving symptoms of Thuja.

Zincum metallicum (also in *Discus compositum, Testis compositum,* and *FluPlus*) is a great nerve remedy, exerting action both on the brain and on the autonomic centers, as well as the sympathetic and the parasympathetic nervous systems. When eruptions have been suppressed, or if symptoms of cerebral irritation occur after vaccination, or in cases of viral encephalitis, this component may provoke a regressive vicariation, inducing a release of the homotoxins from the nervous system. Among the chronic symptoms of Zinc are nerve pains, muscular twitching, and hyperesthesia (Reckeweg 2002).

Galium Heel contains Thuja occidentalis and Echinacea angustifolia.

Inflammation contains Echinacea purpurea (also in *Traumeel, BHI-Echinacea PC, Inflammation, Infection, Injury*), which has the same indications as Echinacea angustifolia. (See *Echinacea compositum*.)

Mercurius is indicated in cases that may have damage from low-level mercury exposure, and its brief use may assist with handling of symptoms. Also contains Echinacea angustifolia. (See *Echinacea compositum*.)

Psorinoheel named for its content of Psorinum-nosode contains many nosodes. Of particular note is Medorrhinum (Gonococcinum). The proving of Psorinoheel was first published by Hering in 1891. It is well indicated in skin diseases (especially when they alternate with asthma), and in infectious, chronic, protracted illnesses (Impregnation phases). It is indicated as a constitutional remedy in vaccinosis, in alternation with Thuja, Natrum sulphuricum, and Vaccininum, and in chronic rheumatism. Vaccininum is also known as Vaccinotoxinum (Julian).

Smallpox vaccine nosode (also in the discontinued formula *Lymphatic*) is used in cases of overreaction following smallpox vaccination, for example, and in post-vaccinial nephritis with albuminuria and haematuria, and thus should be considered in chronic renal failure of cats, which may occur secondary to vaccine autoimmunity. It may be used generally in severe toxic states and in septic illnesses (Reckeweg 2002).

Traumeel contains Echinacea angustifolia and purpurea (which has the same indications). It is useful in a wide range of inflammatory conditions, and in regulation rigidity cases, where there is chronicity of the Inflammation Phase.

Ubichinon compositum contains para-Benzochinonum, which has certain protective functions against viral infections and may also help with paresis occurring after poliomyelitis, encephalitis, or vaccinations, when there is a disturbance in neuromuscular coordination, or in conditions such as multiple sclerosis, which has been suggested to be a vaccine-induced condition in some patients. It is helpful in autoimmune illnesses, which may be iatrogenic in origin. It is also of use in cellular phases, viral diseases, and in toxic infections (reaction phases). Particularly helpful in neoplasm phases is Naphthoquinone, which is also indicated in epilepsy with a brief aura and in threatened vaccinial encephalitis. Ubiquinone may change the course of vaccinial damage following severe reaction to vaccination (Reckeweg 2002).

HOMOTOXICOLOGY TREATMENT OPTIONS AND IMMEDIATE HYPERSENSITIVITY REACTIONS

In an acute health crisis, standard emergency medications such as antihistamine and corticosteroids are appropriate. Antihomotoxic agents can be used along with these agents or in cases where animal stewards decline drug therapy (Reckeweg 2002).

Because the signs of immediate hypersensitivity syndrome are reminiscent of bee sting hypersensitivity, we treat symptomatically with a combination of *Apis homaccord* and *Lymphomyosot*. The dose varies from one-fourth vial to 1 vial each, depending on the size of the patient. Puppies under 10 pounds receive one-fourth vial,

dogs that are 10 to 30 pounds get one-half vial, and larger dogs get a full vial. In many cases, we give the remedies combined and administer half the dose in an intravenous injection, for rapid response. The remaining half, which contains a small amount of blood from the injection IV, is succussed and given subcutaneously.

Apis homaccord and *Lymphomyosot* drops can be mixed together as a take-home cocktail, and given at the rate of one-fourth to one-half cc per dose. Advise the owners to give as needed until the swelling subsides.

Palmquist has used *Schwef-Heel* successfully in several puppies presenting in acute collapse following vaccination. This is likely due to the effect of sulphur, as it "shocks" the system back into autoregulation. This remedy may be used in conjunction with or following *Apis homaccord* and *Lymphomyosot* when response is poor.

Engystol has had good effects on various skin diseases, such as neurodermitis, urticaria, eczema, and furunculosis, as well as on diseases of the respiratory organs, especially asthma and cardiac and circulatory diseases, and therefore should be considered in feline vaccine reactions (including cutaneous herpetic dermatitis), as there is a strong respiratory component to their manifestations of hypersensitivity. *Enygstol* is dosed at one-half cc in acute feline asthma cases or vaccine sensitivity reactions. We frequently give part of this intravenously. The remedy is succussed in the syringe, and then the remainder is given as a subcutaneous injection, in the manner of an autosanguis therapy. Acute cases, such as the "lumpy puppies," generally respond quite dramatically, and they seldom require ongoing therapy, although the atopic, pruritic skin patients may need long-term support. For atopic cases, refer to the section in this text on atopy.

If thyroiditis is suspected, give *Thuja-Injeel* (for the vaccinosis), *Thyroidea compositum* to support thyroid and matrix, *Traumeel* for inflammation, *Hepar compositum* to dispose of the toxins, *Galium-Heel* and *Lymphomyosot* for drainage, and possibly *Cutis compositum* for skin. See also protocols for hypothyroidism.

The following can be used as deep detoxification remedies: *Galium-Heel, Lymphomyosot, Hepar compositum, Solidago compositum, Thyroidea compositum* ideally as an autosanguis, followed by oral therapy at 5 to 8 drops every 3 days. This should take 90 to 120 days minimum in many cases.

Ubichinon compositum and *Coenzyme compositum*, 1 tablet on alternate days, or these can be mixed into the main formula above and given as directed.

In the case of mercury issues, e.g. Thimerosal, Thuja containing formulas may be used (*Atropinum compositum, Cerebrum compositum, Cutis compositum, Echinacea compositum, Galium-Heel, Psorinoheel, Spigelon,* and *Ypsiloheel*) according to patient symptoms, and remedies containing Mercurius may be selected to try to offset the mercury damage. Both of these are contained in *BHI-Inflammation* tabs, along with many other useful components contained in *Traumeel* and *Belladonna homaccord*, *Osteoheel*, and *BHI-Bone*. Note also that these remedies may be helpful in cases manifesting bone inflammation and bone pain.

Engystol is an important agent for immunoprophylaxis, particularly in conjunction with *Gripp-Heel*.

Psorinoheel, *Tonsilla*, and *Echinacea compositum* can be used as indicated for general support, but not as a substitute for vaccination.

REFERENCES

Broadfoot, P. 2006. Puppyatrics. *J Biomed Ther*. Winter:14–15.

Crawford, C. 2002. *The Current Status of Canine Vaccinations: Are We Vaccinating Dogs with Too Many Vaccines Too Often?* Dog Owners and Breeders Symposium. University of Florida College of Veterinary Medicine.

David, D., and U. Giger. 1996. Vaccine-associated immune-mediated hemolytic anemia in the dog. *JVIM*. 10:290–295.

Dodds, W.J. 2001. Vaccination protocols for dogs predisposed to vaccine reactions. *JAAHA*. 37:211–214.

Ford, R.B. 2001. Vaccines and vaccination: The strategic issues. In: North American Veterinary Clinics. Ford, R.B., ed. 31(3):439–453.

Frick, O.L., and D.L. Brooks. 1983. Immunoglobulin E antibodies to pollens augmented in dogs by virus vaccines. *Am J Vet Res*. 44:440–445.

Gaskell, R.M., G. Gettinby, and S.J. Graham, et al. 2002. Veterinary Products Committee working group report on feline and canine vaccination. *Vet Rec*. 150:126–134.

Greene, C.E., R.D. Schultz, and R.B. Ford. 2001. Canine Vaccination. In: North American Veterinary Clinics. Ford, R.B., ed. 31(3):473–492.

Hamalcik, P. 1989. Echinacea angustifolia. *Biological Therapy*. 7(2):40–42.

Harrus, S., Wainer, T., and Aizenberg, I., et al. 2002. Development of hypertrophic osteodystrophy and antibody response in a litter of vaccinated Weimaraner puppies. *J Small Animal Practice*. 43: 27–31.

Hogenesch, H., Azcona-Olivera, J., and Scott-Moncrieff, C., et al. 1999. Vaccine-induced autoimmunity in the dog. *Adv Vet Med*. 41:733–747.

Hogenesch, H., and Glickman, L.T. 1997. Effects of Vaccination on the Endocrine and Immune Systems of Dogs Phase II. Purdue University International Veterinary Vaccines and Diagnostics Conference, July 27-31, in Madison, WI.

Kowal, P. 1986. Neurological complications after vaccination against rabies as exemplified by 4 cases from Poznan province. *Neurol Neurochir Pol*. 20(2):132–136. Polish.

Lappin, M., Andrews, J., and Simpson, D., et al. 2002. Use of serologic tests to predict resistance to Feline Herpesvirus 1, Feline Calicivirus, and Feline Parvovirus infection in cats. *JAVMA*. 220(1):38–42.

Meyer, E.K. 2001. Vaccine-associated adverse events. In: North American Veterinary Clinics. Ford, R.B., ed. 31(3):493–514.

Moncrieff, S., Catharine, J., Azcona-Olivera, J., et al. 2002. Evaluation of antithyroglobulin antibodies after routine vaccination in pet and research dogs. *JAVMA*. 221(4):515–521.

Otto, N. 1988. Pathological processes of rheumatoid nature as caused by focal disorders, and the possibilities of their therapy by biological means. *Biol Ther*. 6(1):19.

Palmquist, R. 2003. A survey of canine vaccine practices in contemporary veterinary clinics in the U.S. *JAHVMA*. 22:27–29.

Palmquist, R. 2007. Attitudes and practices of attendees of the 2006 AHVMA annual meeting. *JAHVMA*. [Accepted for publication.]

Reckeweg, H. in Homeopathia Antihomotoxica Materia Medica, 4th ed. Baden-Baden, Germany:Aurelia-Verlag, 2002. 121, 177–178, 285, 358, 407, 437, 572–575, 589, 611.

Rehulova, E., and Sykora, I. 1971. Neural complications after preventive vaccination of beagles against rabies. *Vet Med (Praha)*. 16(9):571–574. [Czech]

Ryan, E.P., Malboeuf, C.M., Bernard, M., et al. 2006. Cyclo-oxygenase-2 inhibition attenuates antibody responses against human papillomavirus-like particles. *J Immunol*. 177(11): 7811–7819.

Soloway, M.S. 1988. Introduction and overview of intravesical therapy for superficial bladder cancer. *Supplement to Urology*. 31(3):5–16.

Tater, K.C., Jackson, H.A., Paps, J., et al. 2005. Effects of routine prophylactic vaccination or administration of aluminum adjuvant alone on allergen-specific serum IgE and IgG responses in allergic dogs. *Amer J Vet Res*. 66(9), 1572–1577.

Twark, L., and Dodds, W.J. 2000. Clinical use of serum parvovirus and distemper virus antibody titers for determining revaccination strategies in healthy dogs. *JAVMA*. 217:1021–1024.

Van Kampen, K.R. 2001. Recombinant vaccine technology in veterinary medicine. In: North American Veterinary Clinics. Ford, R.B., ed. 31(3):535–538.

Via, C.S., Silbergeld, E.K., and Nguyen, P., et al. 2003. University of Maryland School of Medicine. Study Suggests Low-Dose Mercury Accelerates Autoimmune Disease. In: *Environmental Health Perspectives*, published by the National Institute of Environmental Health Sciences, part of the National Institutes of Health.

Wahlberg, J., Fredriksson, J., and Vaarala, O., et al. 2003. Vaccinations may induce diabetes-related autoantibodies in one-year-old children. *Ann. N.Y. Acad. Sci*. 1005:404–408.

Wilson, J. 1990. Nosodes and their role in homeopathic therapy. *Biol Ther*. 8(1): 1–6. Reprinted July 27, 2002, pp. 22–31.

SECTION 7

Glossary

Acrid (pungent): An herb that promotes circulation of Qi or blood or causes sweating.

Acupoint: A specific area on the body that, when stimulated by pressure, current, or a needle, has a physiologic effect upon the body.

Acupressure: The application of pressure, usually digital, to the acupuncture point.

Acupuncture: The introduction of a needle into a specific area of the body to elicit a physiological response in a patient.

Adaptogens: Herbs that increase resilience and resistance to stress. They act via the hypothalamic-pituitary-adrenal axis on endocrine, nervous, or immune function. One definition of an adaptogen is a plant that (a) increases nonspecific responses to stress, (b) is mild in action, without strong adverse effects, and (c) can be taken for extended periods.

Adjutant (assistant, zuo) herbs: Herb(s) in a formula that either treat less bothersome symptoms of a disease, decrease toxicity of other herbs, or counteract some of the actions of the major herbs to prevent overcorrection of the problem. For example, in a formula with a very cold chief herb, the adjutant may be warm to prevent excessive cooling action of the chief.

Allopathic: Using an agent that works against a symptom or pathogen, such as an antibiotic, anti-inflammatory medication, and so on; also, the method of treating disease with medications that produce effects differing from those produced by the disease itself.

Alterative: An herb that restores proper functioning of the body by improving physiologic processes of digestion and elimination. Alteratives are commonly referred to as depuratives, blood cleaners, or purifiers, because of their effects on altering the excretion of metabolites. They are most useful in chronic disease states.

Amplitude: The intensity of the electrical stimulation of an acupoint.

Antagonism: The use of 2 herbs with opposing actions to prevent overcorrection. For example, when using a very cold herb in a formula, the herbologist may add a warm herb to prevent the formula from being too cold.

Anticatarrhal: Herbs with this action help to remove excess mucus from the body, such as the sinuses, but may reduce secretions, inflammation, and congestion on any mucous membrane.

Antioxidants (free radical scavengers): Prevent oxidation and neutralize reactive free radicals, preventing the initiation of the inflammatory process. This inflammatory response is often responsible for organ degeneration and cell death.

Antispasmodic: Relieves muscle spasms, especially smooth muscle spasms.

Aperient: An herb with mild laxative action.

Aquapuncture: The injection of a fluid, such as vitamin C, vitamin B, or medication, into acupuncture points to achieve an effect in the body.

Arndt-Schulz Principle: A pharmacologic principle stating that different doses of a substance result in different responses by the body. Very low doses stimulate, moderately strong doses accelerate, stronger doses act to suppress metabolic functions, and still higher doses suspend life functions and result in toxic reactions.

Assistant (adjutant, zuo) herbs: Herb(s) in a formula that either treat less bothersome symptoms of a disease, decrease toxicity of other herbs, or counteract some of the actions of the major herbs to prevent overcorrection of the problem. For example, in a formula with a very cold chief herb, the adjutant may be warm to prevent excessive cooling action of the chief.

Astringent: An herbal action referring to the plant actives that astringe tissues and reduce secretions and discharges.

Autosanguis: The use of a patient's own blood and the homotoxins contained therein to stimulate the greater defense toward healing.

Biological therapy: Use of agents that gently work with the body's greater defense to stimulate and bring about improved function and repair of the organism. These agents assist the body in eliminating homotoxins, draining homotoxins, repairing cellular and humoral elements, and re-establishing autocontrol of the body. Another form of biological therapy refers to use of biological agents (such as monoclonal antibodies) in cancer treatment.

Biological value of food: The level of activated or intact nutrients present in food that helps to create health and maintain wellness. This is called "life force" in human food circles and is found in the highest content in fresh, uncooked fruits and vegetables.

Bitter: An herb with a bitter taste. Herbs that are bitter constituents tend to increase tone and activity of gastric mucosa, improve appetite, and stimulate gastric juices. The term covers a number of different types of phytochemicals.

Bitter (TCM usage): An herb that dries and clears pathogens.

Bladder: Urinary bladder. It combines fluids with toxins from the body and eliminates them.

Bland: An herb capable of promoting urination.

Blood: Both the fluid within the blood vessels and the substance that nourishes the mind and carries the Qi throughout the body. When capitalized, it generally refers to the Traditional Chinese Medicine definition.

Calmative: An herb that relieves nervous tension.

Carminative: An herb that contains volatile oils that promote proper intestinal function through relieving bloating, aiding expulsion of gas, and reducing inflammation.

Carotenoids: A large category of phytonutrients that are synthesized by plants and impart the yellow, red, or orange pigment color to fruits and vegetables. The most common and well known are alpha, beta, and gamma carotene, as well as lutein, lycopene, and xanthophylls.

Chen (deputy): The herb(s) in a formula designed to enhance the function of the main, or king, herb.

Chief (king) herb: The herb in a formula that treats the main symptom of a disease.

Cholagogue: An herb that stimulates release and flow of bile already formed in the liver; generally a property of bitters, but produced by other plant constituents as well.

Choleretics: Stimulate bile production by hepatocytes, and most have effective cholagogue properties as well.

Classical homeopathy: The method of treatment developed by Samuel Hahnemann, as detailed in his text, *The Organon*. It consists of using a single agent in miniscule dilution to treat disease conditions by finding the agent, which predictably creates signs of toxicity most similar to a patient's current disease symptoms.

Clear: To rid the body of a pathogen.

Cold: A pathogenic force that interrupts the normal flow of Qi. It can cause pain by causing Qi stagnation, interrupt breathing leading to coughs, interfere with digestion causing diarrhea or vomiting, and so on. In general, if discharges are present, they are clear or white.

Compositae (singular: compositum): Combination anti-homotoxic agents that contain a combination of suis-organ and homeopathic dilutions of various agents to assist recovery from more chronic disease types.

Conception vessel: A meridian running along the ventral midline.

Counteraction: The use of a second herb to decrease or eliminate the toxicity of a primary herb.

Damp: A sticky, wet, heavy pathogen. It is manifested as mucus or leucorrhea.

Decoction: An herbal preparation made by boiling plant material and reducing the liquid to make it more concentrated. It is used with hard parts of plants like seeds, roots, and bark.

Dedifferentiation Phase: Damage to the genetic material leading to development of undifferentiated, nonspecialized cell lines that can take on malignant behavior.

Deficiency: An imbalance in the body caused by insufficiency. For example, a patient who is dehydrated may have a Yin deficiency.

Degeneration Phase: Homotoxin damage that is severe enough to cause sufficient disruption of cell function and tissue disruption and to result in organ degeneration.

Demulcent: An herb that is rich in mucilage, which helps to soothe and protect irritated or inflamed tissue.

Deposition Phase: A phase wherein the homotoxins accumulate in the matrix with little response by the body, and they have not done major structural damage.

Depurative: Herbs that help to remove impurities (metabolites) from the blood and organs (gastrointestinal tract, urine, skin, or lungs), thereby performing "blood purifying."

Deputy (chen): The herb(s) in a formula designed to enhance the function of the main, or king, herb.

Diaphoretic: Promotes perspiration, usually via vasodilation of blood vessels.

Dry: A pathogen that damages fluids. It can result in dry eyes, dry skin, or a dry cough.

Dry needling: The insertion of solid acupuncture needles into an acupoint.

Electroacupuncture: The act of attaching acupuncture needles to a machine, which generates a current at the desired frequency and amplitude to achieve the desired effect.

Emollient: Protects, smoothes, and softens external tissue.

Endogenous and exogenous free radicals: Endogenous free radicals result from normal day-to-day bodily and immune functions. Exogenous free radicals are from exposure to environmental chemicals and toxins.

Endogenous homotoxins: Agents that are generated through normal physiological processes by the body itself.

Enhancement: The addition of a secondary herb to help increase the effect of a primary herb in a formula.

Envoy (shi) herbs: The herb(s) in a formula that direct the herbal formula to work on a specific part of the body or harmonize the functions of the herbs in a formula.

Essence: The substance that forms the basis for birth, development, and reproduction. It is similar to genetic potential in Western parlance.

Evidence-based veterinary medicine (EBVM): "The incorporation of evidence-based medicine (EBM) principles into veterinary practice." EBM relies upon the principle that "the practice of medicine should be based on valid, clinically relevant research data" with a footnote that states "to be accurate, this definition should include the phrase, 'whenever possible,' as medical ethics precludes conducting research that includes inhumane circumstances" (EBVMA 2000).

Excess: The state of having too much of a substance in the body in relation to a steady state. For example, a patient with a fever can have excess heat in the body.

Excretion Phase: Phase of homotoxicosis wherein the body attempts to excrete homotoxins by a wide variety of means, including such routes as sweating, urination, defecation, vomiting, coughing, and sebum formation.

Exogenic or exogenous homotoxins: Homotoxins that are introduced into the body from exterior to the organism, such as pollutants or other chemical exposures.

Expectorant: Soothes bronchial spasm and promotes the removal of mucus from lungs and bronchi.

Fire: Extreme heat. It may cause a very high fever, severely painful red throat, petechiae, and so on.

Flavonoids: A large family of plant-derived chemicals discovered in the 1930s by Albert Szent-Gyorgyi, who originally classified them as vitamin P. The more commonly known flavonoids are flavones, isoflavones, anthocyanins, anthocyanidins, and flavonols. Commonly named flavonoids are rutin, heseridin, and quercetin. Flavonoids help to regulate the immune response and help to control the reactivity of immune-mediated cells, such as T and B lymphocytes, mast cells, and neutrophils. As antioxidants, they help to reduce inflammation.

Fluid extract: A plant extracted as one part plant to one part solvent 1:1 (i.e., 1 ml of liquid equals 1 g of herb).

Fluids: All the moisture substances in the body, including blood, tears, urine, joint fluid, digestive enzymes, and so on.

Free radicals: Molecules or atoms containing additional electrons that make the substance into a reactive and potentially damaging molecule. Formed on exposure to oxygen, free radicals can initiate a local cellular inflammation and death.

Frequency: The number of electrical impulses generated per second to an acupuncture point.

Fu: Tubular organs such as intestines or the bladder. Sometimes also referred to as Yang organs.

Gallbladder: Stores bile and assists the liver with control of sinews and joints. It also "cleans" the blood that the liver stores.

Generalities: General signs, such as "hot in the morning," that are used in homeopathy to help make up the patient's symptom picture.

Gland therapy: Also known as organ, glandular, or cellular therapy, gland therapy is the use of raw glands and organ concentrates to achieve therapeutic results. Glandular extracts have been proven to possess an affinity for similar tissues and contain many chemicals, hormones, enzymes, and co-factors that can exert significant physiological, metabolic, and therapeutic effects on cells and organ systems.

Glycetract: An herb extracted in glycerine and sometimes an herb extracted in alcohol but preserved in glycerine with the alcohol removed.

Governing vessel: A meridian that runs along the dorsal midline.

Greater defense mechanisms: The entire defense system of an organism.

Ground regulation system: The multisystemic components responsible for autocontrol and regulation of the matrix/ground substance and its contents.

Ground substance: Composed of polymerized sugars plus structural and meshing glycoproteins, this is commonly referred to as "the gel between cells," mesenchyme, or matrix. It is regulated by cellular, humoral, and nervous components of the organism.

Harmonize: The action of blending the function of multiple herbs to decrease toxicity and improve function. The action of integrating functions of the body to promote optimal health.

Heart: The organ that governs blood and circulation and also houses the mind.

Heat: A warm pathogen. It can be thought of as inflammation or infection.

Hemoacupuncture: The process of inserting needles into a blood vessel to promote bleeding.

Homaccords: Combination antihomotoxic agents that contain multiple homeopathic potencies of the same agent in one formula.

Homotoxicology: The study of agents toxic or destructive to biological systems, and the organism's biological response to those toxins in the manifestation of disease and pathologic processes. The field uses combination homeopathic and herbal agents to drain, detoxify, and stimulate healing through natural means. Originally coined by its founder, German physician Dr. Hans-Heinrich Reckeweg, the term homo-toxicology originates from "Homo sapiens" and "toxicology."

Homotoxicosis (plural: homotoxicoses): "A non-physiological condition which arises after reaction of a homotoxin on cells and tissues. A homotoxicosis occurs as a humeral or cellular appearance and can be followed by morphological changes on tissues. The homotoxicosis leads to defensive measures of the organism whose goal is to eliminate the homotoxins and to restore the physiological conditions when possible" (Reckeweg 2000).

Homotoxins: "All of those substances (chemical/biochemical) and non-material influences (physical, psychical) which can cause ill health in humans. Their appearance results in regulation disorders in the organism. Every illness is due therefore to the effects of Homotoxins. Homotoxins can be introduced from exterior (exogenic homotoxins) or originate in the body itself (endogenic homotoxins)" (Reckeweg 2000).

Homotoxones: Chemical compounds that are combined to reduce the toxicity of homotoxins.

Impregnation Phase: A phase consisting of homotoxin incorporation into matrix structures and subsequent damage to their functions. This results in cellular damage and dysfunction.

Incompatibility: Two (or more) herbs that cannot be mixed together without causing severe side effects.

Inflammation Phase: A phase of homotoxicoses marked by the use of inflammatory mediators and cells to remove homotoxins.

Infusion: An herbal preparation made by steeping (not boiling) the herb parts in water, usually for soft plant parts like leaves and flowers.

Injeels and Injectable Homeopathics: Injectable homeopathic agents from Heel (**INJ**ectable-**HEEL**). Many of these are not available in the United States.

Integrative Veterinary Medicine (IVM): Combines natural and alternative approaches with conventional veterinary practice methods for the benefit of the patient.

Jing: Essence.

Jing luo: A web of pathways that connect the acupuncture points on the body with the internal organs, one side of the body to the other and one organ to the other.

Jun (king): The main ingredient in a formula. It is used to control the major symptom.

Kidney: The kidneys store the body's essence and provide all the warmth needed for all physiological processes within the body. They also produce the marrow that fills the bones.

King (jun): Main ingredient in a formula. It is used to control the major symptom.

Large blood autosanguis: The use of larger quantities of blood, usually combined with homotoxicology formulas, ostensibly to create a hematoma, which deposits larger volumes of cytokines, markers, defense cells, such as white blood cells, particularly macrophage elements, such as dendritic cells, into the muscle tissue, to encourage a more pronounced body defense response.

Large intestine: The organ system involved in reabsorbing water from ingesta and sending it to the kidney.

Laser therapy: The application of low-intensity lasers to the acupuncture points.

Lignans: Naturally occurring chemicals found in flax seed, fruits, vegetables, and seeds. Lignans are considered phytoestrogens; they mimic animal estrogen and are being studied in breast cancer and heart disease.

Liver: The organ responsible for ensuring the smooth flow of Qi in the body. This function integrates the body into one unit, ensuring that all organs have the energy required to function. It stores blood and regulates circulation and menstruation. Finally, it controls the joints and sinews.

Lung: The organ responsible for respiration, control of the skin, and sweating.

Materia Medica: A textbook listing the various components of a medical modality and their appropriate uses. Literally, it translates from Latin as "the materials of medicine."

Matrix: The ground substance that serves as a meshwork for cellular basement membranes. It also comprises a bioactive space for communication and metabolism of mesenchymal structures.

Mentals: Mental symptoms that are used in homeopathy to help to make up the patient's symptom picture.

Meridian: A pathway through which energy flows.

Metabolic analysis of blood (nutritional blood testing [NBT]): Nutritional blood testing evaluates blood chemistries physiologically. This metabolic interpretation of blood focuses upon organ system function by tracing chemical values toward their underlying physiology, i.e., the biochemical processes that produced these blood chemicals. This type of analysis serves as the basis for determining organ functionality as well as determining the required vitamins, minerals, enzymes, co-factors, and nutrients.

Modern: Being done in recent times and not necessarily indicating a superior nature to prior methods.

Moxibustion: The burning of moxa (Artemesia vulgaris) directly over acupuncture points or on the top of an acupuncture needle to achieve a physiological effect.

Mucilage: An herb containing constituents that are gelatinous, such as mucins (complex carbohydrates) that are demulcent or emollient in effect.

Nanopharmacology: The study of the effects of low doses of material on the body.

Nervine: Herbs that have an affinity for the nervous system. They may be relaxing, sedative, or stimulating, or they may nourish and support the nervous system.

Neural segmental gate theory: A proposed mechanism to explain the efficacy of acupuncture. In this model, the theory states that acupuncture stimulates the afferent A-delta fibers. These send impulses to the substantia gelatinosa and synapse on inhibitory neurons. This prevents pain impulses traveling on more slowly conducting C fibers from reaching the higher nervous system and being perceived.

Nutritive: Having the action to supply nutrients that aid in normal physiology and thereby nourish the body. Constituents that supply minerals, vitamins, fats, oils, or amino acids.

Nutraceutical: A combination of terms describing nutrition or the use of nutrients and "ceutical" (from pharmaceutical), simply meaning nutrients that have a therapeutic effect on the body.

Pathogen: Cause of disease. There are six external pathogens that come from the environment. These include Heat, Dry, Cold, Wind, Summerheat, and Damp. There are also internal pathogens, such as emotional distress, stress, anger, and so on, which can cause disease.

Patterns: Instead of an etiologic diagnosis, TCM diagnoses are patterns. The pattern is then treated. Excess heat conditions are cooled. Deficient conditions are tonified, and so on.

Pericardium: Bag that encloses the heart, similar to Western terminology. However, in TCM terms, it may also be manipulated to treat emotional disorders.

Phase 1, or the Excretion Phase: A phase of homotoxicosis wherein the body attempts to excrete homotoxins by a wide variety of means, including such routes as sweating, urination, defecation, vomiting, coughing, and sebum formation.

Phase 2, or the Inflammation/Reaction Phase: A phase of homotoxicosis marked by the use of inflammatory mediators and cells to remove homotoxins.

Phase 3, or the Deposition Phase: A phase wherein the homotoxins accumulate in the matrix with little response by the body and have not done major structural damage.

Phase 4, or the Impregnation Phase: A phase consisting of homotoxin incorporation into matrix structures and subsequent damage to their functions. This results in cellular damage and dysfunction.

Phase 5, or the Degeneration Phase: Homotoxin damage that is severe enough to cause sufficient disruption of cell function and tissue disruption that results in organ degeneration.

Phase 6, or the Dedifferentiation Phase: Damage to the genetic material leading to development of undifferentiated, nonspecialized cell lines that can take on malignant behavior.

Phase Theory: The predictable response of the body to homotoxins as they are contacted and penetrate into the body, doing damage, and the use of this information to predict course, prognosis, and treatment planning.

Phlegm: A pathogen created in the body from dampness. It is an accumulation of damp leading to nodules or masses, such as lipomas.

Physicals: Symptoms of the physical body that are used in homeopathy to help to make up the patient's symptom picture.

Physiological range: Marker used to identify and localize organ and metabolic function. It is based upon a physiological/homeostasis model stating that changes occur in the blood and organ systems and can be identified before pathology occurs and symptoms of disease appear. Results that are outside of the physiological range are not indicative of disease but may present an indication that a particular organ system is weak or becoming imbalanced, thereby affecting the overall homeostasis.

Phytonutrients: Chemical compounds that are produced by and help in the performance of many of the metabolic functions of the plant. New and growing research is proving that these nutrients, although they are not classified as essential nor required like foods and vitamins, can act as antioxidants and prevent oxidative damage and exert a positive and often dramatic effect on wellness and health and longevity, as well as prevention and treatment of disease.

Phytotherapy: The modern use of science and tradition in employing plants as medicines.

Potentiation: The combination of herbs with similar taste and temperature to increase the effect on the body.

Progressive vicariation: Undesirable observed course of the patient's homotoxicosis, moving from upper left to lower right on the Six-Phase Table of Homotoxicology. It signifies worsening of the patient's condition and can be associated with sudden worsening and even death.

Pulse diagnosis: The palpation of the quality of a pulse to reach a diagnosis. It takes into consideration the rate, strength, location, and characteristics of the pulse to differentiate patterns of illness.

Pungent (acrid): An herb that promotes circulation of blood and Qi or causes sweating.

Purgative: Laxative or cathartic action.

Qi (chi): Energy, life force. It is the force that warms the body, defends the body, and provides the energy needed to activate all processes within the body.

Qi gong: A series of movements designed to promote physical and mental well being. Used in human therapy only.

Reaction Phase or Inflammation Phase: A phase of homotoxicosis marked by the use of inflammatory mediators and cells to remove homotoxins.

Reference range: A measurement defined as the values that 95% (or two standard deviations) of the population fall into.

Regressive vicariation: The desirable observed course of the patient's homotoxicosis moving from lower right to upper left of the Six-Phase Table of Homotoxicology. It is significant because it indicates biological improvement of the case.

Regular meridians: Main meridians. There are 14, one for each zang fu organ along with the conception vessel and the governing vessel.

Restorative: An herb that helps to strengthen tissue and restores normal function.

Retoxins (residual toxins): "Residual poisons," which "consist of deposits of homotoxins and endogenic substances that cannot be eliminated." Glucosylation of normal proteins by excess glucose in diabetic patients is an important example (Reckeweg 2000).

Salty: Herbs that soften hardness and therefore may be used in cases of mass lesions. They may be used to guide formulas into the kidney to treat kidney disorders, and they have purgative actions and may be used in conditions such as constipation.

San jiao: See Triple Heater.

Sedate: To diminish a symptom.

Sedative: An herb or constituent that reduces functional activity; it calms or tranquilizes.

Shen: The mind (as opposed to the brain, which is an organ).

Shi (envoy) herbs: The herb(s) in a formula that direct the herbal formula to work on a specific part of the body or harmonize the functions of the herbs in a formula.

Shu xue: Acupuncture point.

Sialagogue: An herb that promotes the secretion of saliva.

Single effect: The use of a single herb to treat a patient.

Six-Phase Table of Homotoxicology: A table demonstrating the six phases of homotoxicosis (consisting of Excretion, Reaction/Inflammation, Deposition, Impregnation, Degeneration, and Dedifferentiation/Neoplasia), and their relationship to tissue and organ types. This table can be used to identify response to therapy and worsening of disease patterns, as well as for the selection of appropriate antihomotoxic agents.

Small blood autosanguis: Therapy that uses very small amounts of blood, usually in combination with anithomotoxic medicines. They are often given in stepwise dilutions. Often employed in chronic, unresponsive disease states.

Small intestine: A digestive organ. It separates fluid from the ingesta and passes the rest down to the large intestine.

Sour: Herbs that prevent leakage of fluids; for example, they may decrease perspiration or treat polyuria.

Spasmolytic: See antispasmodic.

Spleen: The organ responsible for extracting the energy from food for the nourishment of the body. It also holds the substances in the body in place. For example, a weak spleen allows blood to leak from vessels or organs to prolapse.

Stagnation: An interruption in the normal flow of Qi, digestion, breath, blood flow, and so on. It often leads to a feeling of fullness or pain.

Sterols: Plant-based lipid compounds that are chemically similar to, and that compete with, cholesterol. The most commonly known and well studied is betasitosterol. It is felt that the phytosterols reduce inflammation, are immune modulators, and affect cell membranes in tumor growth.

Stomach: The organ involved in transporting food.

Stomachic: An herb that is a digestive aid or tonic or that improves appetite.

Suis: The Latin term for glandular or organ therapy originating from swine. Useful in stimulating repair of diseased organ(s) and contained in many compositae remedies.

Summerheat: The only pathogen restricted to a season. It is a combination of heat and damp and is manifested by signs that Western-trained physicians classify as heatstroke.

Sweet: An herb that is tonifying and moistening. These herbs can decrease toxicity of other herbs in a formula.

Symptom-based therapeutic formulas: Antihomotoxic agents used to address a particular symptom set.

Symptom picture: A list of the patient's symptoms used in homeopathy to match a proper remedy as precisely as possible. The symptom picture includes mentals, physicals, and generalities (see specific definitions).

Taste (of an herb): The effect of the herb upon the body, as opposed to the sensation it provokes on the tongue. See bland, salty, acrid/pungent, sweet, bitter, and sour.

Temperature (of an herb): The action of an herb on the body. A warm herb counteracts a cool pathogen, whereas a cool herb counteracts a warm pathogen or condition.

Therapeutic nutrition: Broadly defined as the use of various nutrients, such as vitamins, minerals, amino acids, essential fatty acids, co-factors, enzymes, antioxidants, and phytonutrients, to support the body's immune and healing systems, thereby altering the course and outcome of a disease process.

Tonic: An herb that works to restore and strengthen the functioning or structure of the body, organ, or system; it enhances or normalizes function.

Tonify: To strengthen.

Toxins: Pathogens that harm the body. In Western terms, toxins would be inflammatory mediators, bacteria endotoxins, metabolic byproducts, and so on.

Traditional Chinese Medicine (TCM): An integral system of diagnosis and treatment of ill health using acupuncture and moxibustion, diet and herbs, physiological manipulation, and, in human medicine, Qi gong.

Triple Heater: The three functional divisions of the body. The first is from the head to the diaphragm, the second from the diaphragm to the navel, and the third from the naval to the feet. Each section is assigned a function. The upper section is concerned with respiration, the middle section is involved with digestion, and the lower section controls excretion.

Trophorestorative: An herb that has an affinity for restoring function and morphology of a specific organ or tissue.

Urinary bladder: The organ that combines fluids with toxins from the body and eliminates them.

Vermicide: A constituent or herb that kills intestinal worms.

Vermifuge: A constituent or herb that is used to expel intestinal worms.

Vicariation: "The transition of the indicating signs of an illness within one phase to another organ system, or the change of the fundamental symptoms and signs into another phase, with or without a change of the organ system" (Reckeweg 2000).

Vital force: The principle that energy or a life force is inherent in the growth and function of the cells and tissues of the body.

Vulnerary: An herb that aids in the healing of wounds or ulcers, particularly of the skin, but it can also apply to stomach ulcers. Usually applied externally.

Wild peptides: Wild peptides are formed when molecules or substances are conjugated to body proteins, thus forming a new, potentially antigenic complex. These complexes can create autoimmunity, when the body recognizes them as a foreign antigen, followed by extension of this immune response to self-antigens.

Wind: Movement such as tremors or seizures. It is also a pathological force that can blow a second pathogen into the body to allow a disease to develop.

Yang: The active warm aspect of an entity that complements Yin.

Yin: The cooler restful aspect of an entity that complements the Yang aspect. It can also refer to fluids or moisture.

Zang: Solid organs such as the spleen or liver. Sometimes also referred to as Yin organs.

Zang fu organs: A pairing of one zang (Yin) and one fu (Yang) organ.

Zuo (adjutant, assistant) herbs: Herb(s) in a formula that either treat less bothersome symptoms of a disease, decrease toxicity of other herbs, or counteract some of the actions of the major herbs to prevent overcorrection of the problem. For example, in a formula with a very cold chief herb, the adjutant may be warm to prevent excessive cooling action of the chief.

REFERENCES

Evidence-Based Veterinary Medicine Association (EBVMA), http://www.ebvma.org. Accessed from Web site Dec. 2006.

Reckeweg, Hans-Heinrich. *Biotherapeutic Index: Ordinatio Antihomotoxica et Materia Medica.* Baden-Baden, Germany: Biologische Heilmittel Heel GMBH, 2000, p. 10.

Reckeweg, Hans-Heinrich. *Biotherapeutic Index: Ordinatio Antihomotoxica et Materia Medica.* Baden-Baden, Germany: Biologische Heilmittel Heel GMBH, 2000, p. 12.

SECTION 8

Resources, Product Suppliers, Suggested References, and Readings

ORGANIZATIONS

The Academy of Veterinary Homeopathy
P.O. Box 9280
Wilmington, DE 19809
(866) 652-1590 (Voice and Fax, United States and Canada)
www.theavh.org

American Holistic Veterinary Medical Association
Carvel Tiekert, DVM, Executive Director
2218 Old Emmorton Road
Bel Air, MD 21015
(410) 569-0795
Fax (410) 569-2346
www.ahvma.org
E-mail: office@ahvma.org

American Veterinary Chiropractic Association
442154 E 140 Road
Bluejacket, OK 74333
(918) 784-2231
Fax (918) 784-2675
www.animalchiropractic.org

Veterinary Botanical Medicine Association
Jasmine C. Lyon, Executive Director
1785 Poplar Drive
Kennesaw, GA 30144
www.vbma.org

The American Academy of Veterinary Acupuncture
100 Roscommon Drive, Suite 320
Middletown, CT 06457
(860) 632-9911 8:30 a.m. to 6 p.m. EST
www.AAVA.org

International Veterinary Acupuncture Society
P.O. Box 271395
Fort Collins, CO 80527
(970) 266-0666
www.ivas.org
E-mail: Offica@IVAS.org

COLLEGES OFFERING TRAINING IN VETERINARY TCM/ACUPUNCTURE

Chi Institute
9700 West Highway 318
Reddick, FL 32686
(352) 591-5385 and (800) 891-1986, ext. 101
www.tcvm.com
E-mail: Barbara@tcvm.com

International Veterinary Acupuncture Society
P.O. Box 271395
Fort Collins, CO 80527
(970) 266-0666
www.ivas.org
E-mail: Offica@IVAS.org

USEFUL TEXTS

Chinese herbal medicine

Bensky, Dan, and Randall Barolet, comp. Chinese Herbal Medicine Formulas and Strategies. Seattle: Eastland Press, 1990.

Bensky, Dan, Steven Clavey, and Erich Stoger, comp. Chinese Herbal Materia Medica, 3rd ed. Seattle: Eastland Press, 2004.

Chen, John K. and Tina T. Chen. Chinese Medical Herbology and Pharmacology. City of Industry, CA: Art of Medicine Press, 2001.

Huisheng, Xie. Traditional Chinese Veterinary Medicine. Beijing: Beijing Agricultural University Press, 1994.

Maciocia, Giovanni. The Foundations of Chinese Medicine. Edinburgh: Churchill Livingstone, 1989.

Schoen, Alan. Veterinary Acupuncture Ancient Art to Modern Medicine. Goleta, CA: American Veterinary Publications, Inc., 1994.

Schwartz, Cheryl. Four Paws, Five Directions. Berkeley, CA: Celestial Arts Publishing, 1996.

General books; complementary veterinary medicine

Schoen, A., and S. Wynn, eds. Complementary and Alternative Veterinary Medicine: Principles and Practice. St Louis: Mosby, 1998.

Wynn, Susan, and Steve Marsden. Manual of Natural Veterinary Medicine: Science and Tradition. St Louis: Mosby, 2003.

Homotoxicology

Hamilton, D. Homeopathic Care for Cats and Dogs. Berkeley, CA: North Atlantic Books, 1999.

Heine, Harmut. Homotoxicology and Ground Regulation System (GRS). Baden-Baden, Germany: Aurelia Verlag, 2000.

Herzberger, Gabriele. Fundamentals of Homotoxicology. Baden-Baden, Germany: Aurelia Verlag, 2001.

Reckeweg, Hans-Heinrich. Biotherapeutic Index, 5th revised ed. Baden-Baden, Germany: Biologische Heilmittel Heel GmbH 1, 2000.

Reckeweg, Hans-Heinrich. Materia Medica Homeopathia Anti-homotoxica, 4th ed. Baden-Baden, Germany: Aurelia-Verlag, 2002.

Van Brandt, Bruno. Inflammation Means Healing. Belgium: Inspiration, 2002.

Consumer-oriented; alternative medicine

Appleton, N. Rethinking Pasteur's Germ Theory. Berkeley, CA: Forg Ltd., 2002.

Appleton, N. Stopping Inflammation. Garden City, NY: Square One Publications, 2005.

Billinghurst, Ian. Give Your Dog a Bone. Lithgow N.S.W. Australia: Ian Billinghurst, 1993.

Cusick, W.D. Canine Nutrition. Wilsonville, OR: Doral Publishing, 1997.

Erasmus, U. Fats That Heal Fats That Kill. Vancouver, British Columbia, Canada: Alive Books, 1993. The complete lecture is available at www.udoerasmus.com.

Flam, D. The Holistic Dog Book. Housem, NY: Howell Book, 2003.

Goldstein, M. The Nature of Animal Healing. New York: Ballantine Book, published by the Random House Publishing Group, 1999.

Goldstein, R., and S. Goldstein. The Goldstein Wellness and Longevity Program. Neptune City, NJ: TFH Publication, 2005.

Kendall, R. Building Wellness with DMG. Topanga, CA: Freedom Press, 2003.

Martin, A.N. Foods Pets Die For. Troutdale, OR: New Sage Press, 1997.

Messonier, S. Natural Health Bible for Dogs and Cats. Roseville, CA: Prima Publications, 2001.

Mindell, E., and E. Renaghan. Earl Mindell's Nutrition and Health for Dogs. Roseville, CA: Prima Publications, 1998.

Murray, M.T. Encyclopedia of Nutritional Supplements. Roseville, CA: Prima Publications, 1996.

Murray, M., and N.D. Pizzorno. Encyclopedia of Natural Medicine, revised 2nd ed. Roseville, CA: Prima Publications, 1998.

Pitcairn, R., and S. Pitcairn. Dr. Pitcairn's Complete Guide to Natural Health for Dogs and Cats. Emmaus, PA: Rodale Press, 2005.

Pottenger, F.M. Pottenger's Cats—A Study in Nutrition. The Price Pottenger Nutrition Foundation, Inc., P.O. Box 2614, La Mesa, CA 92041.

Puotinen, C.J. The Encyclopedia of Natural Pet Care. New Canaan, CT: Keats Publ., 1998.

Werbach, M.R. Nutritional Influences on Illness. Tarzana, CA: Third Line Press, 1996.

Western medicine

Cunningham, J.G. Textbook of Veterinary Physiology. St. Louis, MO: WB Saunders and Co., 1992.

Guyton, A.C. Textbook of Medical Physiology. Philadelphia: WB Saunders and Co., 1961.

Hand, M.S., C.D. Thatcher, and R.L. Remillard, et al., eds. Small Animal Clinical Nutrition: Making Pet Foods at Home, 4th ed. Topeka, KS: Mark Morris Institute, 2000.

Linder, M.C. Nutritional Biochemistry and Metabolism. New York: Elsevier, 1991.

Morrison, W.B. Cancer in Dogs and Cats. Baltimore, MD: Lippincott, Williams and Wilkens, 1998.

Ogilvie, G. Nutritional Therapy for the Cancer Patient. Fort Collins, CO: College of Veterinary Medicine, Colorado State University, 2002.

Strombeck, Donald R. Home-prepared Dog and Cat Diets, The Healthful Alternative. Ames, IA: Iowa State University Press, 1999.

Western herbs

Mowrey, D.B. The Scientific Validation of Herbal Medicine. New Canaan, CT: Keats Publishing, 1986.

Rotblatt, M., and I. Ziment. Evidence Based Herbal Medicine. Philadelphia: Hanlet and Belfus, 2002.

Yance, D.R. Herbal Medicine Healing and Cancer. Chicago: Keats Publishing, 1999.

MEDICATIONS

Natural Hydrocortisone
Pet Health Pharmacy
12012 N. 111th Avenue
Youngtown, AZ 85363
(800) 742-0516
www.PetHealthPharmacy.com

CHINESE HERBAL REMEDIES

Blue Light, Inc.
631 W. Buffalo Street
Ithaca, NY 14850-3317
(607) 275-9700

Blue Poppy Enterprises
5441 Western Avenue, #2
Boulder, CO 80301
(303)447-8372
(800) 487-9296
Fax: (303) 245-8362

Four Seasons Herbs Co.
16-A Goddard
Irvine, CA 92618
(949) 450 1188

Jing Tang Herbals
9700 West Highway 318
Reddick, FL 32686
(352) 591-5385
(800) 891-1986, ext. 101
www.tcvm.com
E-mail: Barbara@tcvm.com

Mayway
1338 Mandela Parkway
Oakland, CA 94607
(800) 2MAYWAY
E-mail: info@mayway.com

Natural Solutions, Inc.
P.O. Box 493
176 Montauk Highway
Speonk, NY 11972
(631) 325 2047

Thorne Research, Inc.
25820 Highway 2 West
Dover, ID 83825
www.Thorne.com
Products: Chinese herbs

HOMEOPATHICS

BOIRON BORNEMAN, Inc.
Ludovic RASSAT
6 Campus Boulevard
Building A
Newtown Square, PA 19073
(610) 325-7464
Fax: (610) 325-7480
E-mail: info@boiron.com
Products: Classical homeopathic remedies

Hahnemann Pharmacy
(888) 427-6422
Custom remedies
Vaccine nosodes—Rabies nosode (Lyssinum), Canine
    Distemper virus, Canine Parvo virus, DHLPP
    combination, Feline vaccines
Heartworm nosode

Heel, Inc.
10421 Research Road SE
Albuquerque, NM 87123-3376
(800) 621-7644
www.HeelUSA.com
Products: Antihomotoxic medications

Helios
01144-189-251511 (English company)
Good selection of remedies

Natural Health Supply
6410 Avenida Christina
Santa Fe, NM 87505
Contact: Jim Klemmer
(888) 689-1608
a2zhomeopathy.com

Standard Homeopathic Co.
(800) 624-9659
Single remedies and combination remedies

Washington Homeopathic Products, Inc.
Contact: Joe Lillard
(800) 336-1695

FLOWER ESSENCES

Anaflora Flower Essences
Earth Animal Inc.
606 Post Road East
Westport CT 06880
800-622-0260
www.earthanimal.com

Bach Flower Essences and Rescue Remedy
Ellon Bach USA
Traditional Flower Remedies
400 Oak Hill Drive
Winona Lake, IN 46590
tel: 1-800-423-2256
fax: 1-574-269-4060
E-mail:info@traditionalflowers.com

NUTRACEUTICALS

Allergy Research Group®
2300 North Loop Road
Alameda, CA 94502
(800) 545-9960 or (510) 263-2000
Fax: (800) 688-7426 or (510) 263-2100
www.AllergyResearchGroup.com
Products: Imm Kine, Vascustatin

Animal Nutrition Technologies
1175 Post Road East
Westport, CT 06880
(888) 533-5162
(203) 341-8875
www.animalnutritiontechnologies.com
Products: Adrenal, behavioral/emotional, blood/bone
    marrow, bone, brain nerve, bronchus/lung/sinus,
    cardiac, cartilage, ear, female, esophageal/gastric, eye,

gingival/mouth, immune/autoimmune/cancer, intestinal/IBD, kidney, liver/gall bladder, male, pancreas/endocrine/exocrine, pituitary/hypothalamus/ pineal, skin, thyroid, urinary bladder support formula, nutritional blood testing (NBT)

Best for Your Pet
Doctors Mutual Service Corp.
P.O. Box 4136
Newport Beach, CA 92661
(800) 952 9568
http://bestforyourpet.com/
Products: Betathyme, megalipotrophic, liquid glandulars

Designs for Health
2 North Road
E. Windsor, CT 06088
(800) 847-8302
Products: Lecithin/phosphatidyl choline

4Life Research
9850 S. 300 W.
Sandy, UT 84070
(800) 667-8176
www.4Life.com
Products: Transfer factor-related supplements

NZYMES.COM
A Division of Biopet Inc.
P.O. Box 94347
Las Vegas, NV 89193-4347
(702) 228-0097
Fax: (702) 252-7988
Toll Free: (877) 816-6500

Biovet International
5152 Bolsa Avenue, Suite 101
Huntington Beach, CA 92649
(714) 899-3477
(800) 788-1084
Fax: (714) 899-0078
E-mail: info@PetWafer.com

Gerizyme Vitamins
Nutritech, Inc.
6283 Dean Martin Drive, Suite F
Las Vegas, NV 89118

GUNA, Inc.
1520 Tramway Blvd. NE, Suite 150
Albuquerque, NM 87112
(888) GUNA-TEL (486-2835)
http://www.gunausa.com
Products: Physiological regulation medicines

Jarrow Formulas
1824 S. Robertson Blvd.
Los Angeles, CA 90035

(800) 726-0886 and (310) 204-6936
Fax: (800) 890-8955 and (310) 204-2520
http://www.jarrow.com/
Products: Evening primrose oil

Liquid Health Inc.
Murrieta, CA 92562
(800) 995-6607
www.liquidhealth.com
Products: Canine liquid health

McGuff Company, Inc.
3524 West Lake Center Drive
Santa Ana, CA 92704
(800) 854-7220
Fax: (714) 540-5614
info@mcguff.com

Natura Health Products
249 A Street, Suite A
Ashland, OR 97520
(541) 488-0210
www.naturahealthproducts.com

New Life Foods, Inc.
2150 Northwest Parkway, Suite J
Marietta, GA 30067
(770) 988-0222
(888) 777-0468
Fax: (770) 956-9099
Products: Bovine colostrum

Pavia
3505 Ranier Lane N
Plymouth, MN 55447
www.PaviaSalesGroup.com
Products: Pavia shampoo, wipes, and wound cream

Kinetic Technologies, Inc.
P.O. Box 12388
Lexington, KY 40583
www.KineticTech.net
Products: Hyaluronic acid eye drops, Hy-Optik Eye Drops

Integrative Therapeutics
(800) 376-7889
www.phytopharmica.com
Products: N-acetylcysteine, coenzyme Q10

Life Extension Foundation
P.O. Box 229120
Hollywood, FL 33022
Health Advisors: (800) 226-2370
Customer Service: (800) 678-8989
Orders: (800) 544-4440
Fax: (954) 761-9199
www.lef.org
Products: Cat mix, dog mix

New Chapter
90 Technology Drive
Brattleboro, VT 05301
(800) 543-7279
Fax: (800) 470-0247
E-mail: info@new-chapter.com
Products: Zyflamend

Nutramax Laboratories, Inc.
2208 Lakeside Blvd.
Edgewood, MD 21040
(410) 776-4000
(800) 925-5187 (in United States and Canada)
Fax: (410) 776-4009
Products: Cosequin, Denosyl, Denamarin

PhytoPharmica, Inc.
Customer Service Department
825 Challenger Drive
Green Bay, WI 54311
Retailers: (800) 553-2370
Consumers: (800) 376-7889
Fax: (888) 311-5657
Products: Energizing iron

Professional Complementary Health Products
P.O. Box 80085
Portland, OR 97280
(800) 952-2219
www.professionalformulas.com

Progressive Laboratories, Inc.
1701 W. Walnut Hill Lane
Irving, TX 75038
(800) 527-9512
www.progressivelabs.com
Products: Utract (D-Mannose Powder), Pan 5
Plus, Probiotic MPF, lutein, folic acid, phosphatidyl
serine

Prozyme Digestive Enzyme
Prozyme Products, LTD
Sold by distributors
(800) 522-5537

Pure Encapsulations, Inc.
490 Boston Post Road
Sudbury, MA 01776
(800) 753-2277
Fax: (888) 783-2277

Resources Genesis
Genesis, Ltd.
P.O. Box 2568
Valley Center, CA 92082
(877) PETS-4-LIFE
(877) 738-7454

http://www.genesispets.com
Products: Blood and Energy, Pain Plus, Joint Support
Plus, urinary tract support, incontinence

Saskatoon Colostrum Company Ltd.
3319 Wells Avenue
Saskatoon, Sakatchewan
Canada S7K 5W6
(306) 242-3185
(866) 242-3185
E-mail: support@colostrum.sk.ca

Simplexity (formerly Cell Tech International)
P.O. Box 609
Klamath Falls, OR 97601
Order Line: (800) 800-1300
Order Fax: (800) 797-8228
Customer Service: (800) 687-1107
Customer Service Fax: (541) 884-1869
TDD (hearing impaired): (541) 885-4330
Corporate Office: (541) 882-5406
www.SimplexityHealth.com
Products: Blue green algae, Stemplex, probiotics,
enzymes, antioxidants, bone health support, skin care,
soil amendments

Source Naturals
19 Janis Way
Scotts Valley, CA 95066
(831) 438-1144
(800) 815-2333
Fax: (831) 438-7410
http://www.sourcenaturals.com/
Products: Quercetin, wellness formula

Standard Process Veterinary Formulas
1200 West Royal Lee Drive
Palmyra, WI 53156
(800) 848-5061
www.standardprocess.com
Products: Adrenal support, cardiac support, dermal
support, enteric support, hepatic support, immune
system support, musculoskeletal support, renal
support, thyroid support, Diaplex

Thorne Research, Inc.
25820 Highway 2 West
Dover, ID 83825
www.Thorne.com
Products: Nutraceuticals, vitamins, Chinese herbs,
Moducare, Mediclear, Lithogen, Gastrogen, Quercetone,
Hepagen

Tyler Encapsulations
825 Challenger Drive
Green Bay, WI 54311
(800) 931-1709

Integrativeinc.com
Product: Eskimo fish oil

Vetri Science
20 New England Drive
Essex Jct., VT 05453
(800) 882-9993
Fax: (802) 878-0549
E-mail: info@vetriscience.com
http://www.vetriscience.com
Products: Glycoflex, Acetylator, Coenzyme Q10, Gluta
   DMG, Maitake DMG, Oli Vet, Antiox, Renal
   essentials, UT strength, Bladder strength, Acetylator,
   Cardiostrength, Dermal strength, Jointegen, Omega
   3,6,9

Vetoquinol USA, Inc.
101 Lincoln Avenue
Buena, NJ 08310
www.vetoquinol.com
Product: Azodyl

Rx Vitamins, Inc.
150 Clearbrook Road, Suite 149
Elmsford, NY 10523
(800) 792-2222
(914) 834-1804
www.RxVitamins.com
Products: Liquid Immuno, Ultra EFA, Liquid Immuno,
   Nutrigest, Nutricalm, CV Formula, Hepato support,
   Ocular formula

Vitamin Research Products
4610 Arrowhead Drive
Carson City, NV 89706
(800) 877-2447
http://www.vrp.com

Wellwisdom, LLC
P.O. Box 191047
San Diego, CA 92159
(800) 735-1003
Fax: (800) 705-7441
http://www.wellwisdom.com/
Products: Glutimmune

Xymogen® Inc.
Exclusive Professional Formulas
725 S. Kirkman Road
Orlando, FL 32811
(800) 647-6100

Zymox
Pet King Brands, Inc.
710 Vandustrial Drive
Westmont, IL 60559
www.PetKingBrands.com

OILS (FATTY ACIDS)

Barlean's Organic Oils, L.L.C.
4936 Lake Terrell Road
Ferndale, WA 98248
(360) 384-0485
Customer Service: (800) 445-3529
Product: Flax seed oil

Natures Perfect Oil
Hemp Oil
103 Hillsboro Drive
Galena, MO 65656
(417) 538-9077
Fax: (417) 538-9078

Natura Health Products
249 A Street, Suite A
Ashland, OR 97520
(541) 488-0210
www.naturahealthproducts.com
Products: Beyond essential fats

WESTERN HERBS

Animal Apothecary
Animal Essentials
P.O. Box 131388
Carlsbad, CA 92013
Retail: (888) 463-7748
Wholesale: (888) 551-0416
Fax: (888) 273-9233
E-mail: info@animalessentials.com
Products: Phytomucil, senior blend, dandelion milk
   thistle, herbal ear rinse

Buck Mountain Botanicals, Inc.
HC 30
Miles City, MT 59301
(406) 232-1185
Fax: (406) 232-4491
www.buckmountainbotanicals.com/
E-mail: buckmountainherbs@hotmail.com

Herbalist and Alchemist
David Winston Herbalist
51 S. Wandling Avenue
Washington, NJ 07882
(800) 611-8235
Fax: (908) 689-9071
E-mail: herbalist@nac.net
Products: Serenity compound, healthy heart compound

Gia herbs
Pure Encapsulations, Inc.
490 Boston Post Road

Sudbury, MA 01776
Tel: (800) 753-2277
Fax: (888) 783-2277
http://www.purecaps.com

Mountain Health Products
(800) MHP-0074
(303) 823-9338
Fax: (303) 823-9359

Natura Health Products
Donald Yance, Master Herbalist
249 A Street, Suite A
Ashland, OR 97520
(541) 488-0210
www.naturahealthproducts.com
Products: Botanical treasures, Vital Adapt, Power
    Adapt, Botanibol, ImmunoCare

Naturvet
The Garmon Corporation
27461-B Diaz Road
Temecula, CA 92590
(888) 628-8783 or (951) 296-6308
Fax: (951) 296-6329
E-mail: naturvet@naturvet.com
Products: Ear wash, Quiet moments

World Herbs
Geoff D'Arcy Lic.Ac., D.O.M.
(800) RXDARCY (800-793-2729) M-F, 9 a.m. to
    5 p.m. EST
63 South Main Street
Natick, MA 01760
(508) 652-1975
Fax: (508) 653-3283
http://darcynat.com
Products: Hoxey formula, Healthy coat, Green Powder,
    Pet Calm, Cardio Support, Hot Spot, Pet Digest, Dia-
    relief, Lung soothe, Immune prep, Alert, Hypo-Thyro,
    Hyper-Thyrin

GLANDULARS

Animal Nutrition Technologies
606 Post Road East
Westport, CT 06880
(888) 533-5162
(203) 341-8875
www.animalnutritiontechnologies.com

Professional Complementary Health Products
P.O. Box 80085
Portland, OR 97280
(800) 952-2219
www.professionalformulas.com

Progressive Labs, Inc.
1701 W. Walnut Hill Lane
Irving, TX 75038
(800) 527-9512
www.ProgressiveLabs.com

Standard Process of Southern California
981 Park Center Drive
Vista, CA 92801
(800) 372-7218
www.customerserviceSPocal.com
Products: Glandulars and whole food supplements

OTICS

Maxiguard Zinc Otic
Addison Biological Lab, Inc.
507 North Cleveland Avenue
Fayette, MO 65248
www.AddisonLabs.com

DOG AND CAT FOODS THAT MEET THE DIETARY RESTRICTIONS FOR THE CANCER PROTOCOLS

The Blue Buffalo Co.
P.O. Box 770
Wilton, CT 06897
(800) 919-2833

Bravo
1084 Hartford Tpke.
Vernon, CT 06066
(866) 922-9222
Fax: 860.896.1256
http://www.bravorawdiet.com/

Dr. Harveys
180 Main Street
Keansburg, NJ 07734
(866) Doc H 123 (866-362-4123)
(732) 787-2445
http://www.drharveys.com/contact.asp

Evanger's Dog and Cat Food Company, Inc.
221 S. Wheeling Road
Wheeling, IL 60090
Toll Free: (800) 288-6796
Office: (847) 537-0102
Fax: (847) 537-0179
http://www.evangersdogfood.com/contact/

FarMore® Manufacturing Ltd.
5900 Trietsch
Sanger, TX 76266
http://www.farmoredogfood.

Northwest Naturals Inc.
4050 NE 158th Ave.
Portland, OR 97230
Customer Service: (866) 637-1872
www.nw-naturals.net

Natura Pet Products
P.O. Box 271
Santa Clara, CA 95052-0271
(800) 532-7261
(408) 261-0770
E-mail: custserv@naturapet.com

Natural Balance Pet Foods, Inc.
12924 Pierce Street
Pacoima, CA 91331
(800) 829-4493
http://www.naturalbalanceinc.com/

Oma's Pride
Miller Foods, Inc.
308 Arch Road
Avon, CT 06001
Tel: (800) 678-6627
Tel: (860) 673-3256
Fax: (860) 673-6454
www.omaspride.com

Primal Pet Foods, Inc.
1120 Illinois Street
San Francisco, CA 94107
(866) 566-4652
(415) 642-7400 (within the San Francisco Bay area)
http://www.primalpetfoods.com/about/contact.htm

Raw Advantage
P.O. Box 837
Stanwood, WA 98292
Customer Service: (360) 387-5185
Fax: (360) 387-8966
http://www.rawadvantagepetfood.com/

Sojourner Farms
1723 Adams Street NE
Minneapolis, MN 55413
(888) 867-6567
(612) 343-7262
Fax: (612) 343-7263
http://www.sojos.com/contactus.html

Stella and Chewy's
Tel: (718) 522-9673
Fax: (718) 522-9675
http://www.stellaandchewys.com/

Steve's Real Food For Pets
1848 Pearl Street
Eugene, OR 97401
Tel: (541) 683-9950
Fax: (541) 683-2035
(888) 526-1900
http://www.stevesrealfood.com/

Wild Kitty Cat Food
1272 Portland Road
Arundel, ME 04046
(888) 733-1033
Fax: (207) 985-3038
http://www.wildkittycatfood.com/

Wysong
7550 Eastman Avenue
Midland, MI 48642-7779
Customer Service: (989) 631-0009
Ordering: (800) 748-0188
Fax: (810) 496-4589
http://www.wysong.net/

Appendix

ACUPUNCTURE POINTS MENTIONED

BL 10: In the indentation at the caudolateral margin of the atlas lateral to the space between C1 and C2.

BL 11: Midway between the medial border of the scapula and the caudal border of the dorsal spine of T1. It is in the intercostal space between the 1st and 2nd ribs.

BL 13: Lateral to the longissimus thoracicis muscle at the level of the 3rd intercostal space.

BL 14: Lateral to the longissimus thoracicis muscle at the level of the 4th intercostal space.

BL 15: Lateral to the longissimus thoracicis muscle at the level of the 5th intercostal space.

BL 17: Lateral to the longissimus thoracicis muscle at the level of the 7th intercostal space.

BL 18: Lateral to the longissimus thoracicis muscle at the level of the 9th intercostal space.

BL 19: Lateral to the longissimus thoracicis muscle at the level of the 10th intercostal space.

BL 20: Lateral to the longissimus thoracicis muscle at the level of the 11th intercostal space.

BL 21: Lateral to the longissimus thoracicis et lumborum muscle caudal to the last rib and cranial to the transverse process of the 12th lumbar vertebra.

BL 22: Lateral to the longissimus lumborum muscle cranial to the transverse process of the 2nd lumbar vertebra.

BL 23: Lateral to the longissimus lumborum muscle cranial to the transverse process of the 3rd lumbar vertebra.

BL 25: Lateral to the longissimus lumborum muscle cranial to the transverse process of the 5th lumbar vertebra.

BL 26: Lateral to the longissimus lumborum muscle cranial to the transverse process of the 6th lumbar vertebra.

BL 28: Lateral to the longissimus lumborum muscle caudal to the transverse process of the 7th lumbar vertebra. It is craniolateral to Bai hui.

BL 37: On the caudal surface to the thigh midway between the tuber ishium and popliteal crease.

BL 40: On the caudal midline of the hind leg at the level of the popliteal crease.

BL 54: Dorsal to the greater trochanter.

BL 60: Cranial to the attachment of the Achilles tendon to the calcanian tuber in the indentation between the insertion of the Achilles tendon and the lateral malleolus.

CV 3: On the ventral midline four-fifths of the distance from the umbilicus to the pubis.

CV 4: On the ventral midline three-fifths of the distance from the umbilicus to the pubis.

CV 6: On the ventral midline three-tenths of the distance from the umbilicus to the pubis.

CV 12: On the ventral midline midway between the umbilicus and xiphoid process.

CV 13: On the ventral midline one-fourth of the distance from the xiphoid process to the umbilicus.

CV 17: On the ventral midline at the 4th intercostal space.

CV 22: On the ventral midline just cranial to the manubrium.

CV 23: On the ventral surface of the chin just caudal to the mandibular symphasis.

HT 7: On the caudolateral surface of the carpus between the tendons of the flexor carpi ulnaris and the superficial digital flexor.

GB 2: With the mouth open, it is the depression in front of the intertragic notch dorsal to the condyloid process of the mandible.

GB 20: On the dorsocranial aspect of the neck just caudal to the occipital condyles between the sternooccipitalus and cleidocervicalis.

GB 21: The midpoint between GV 14 and the acromion.

GB 29: Craniodorsal to the hip joint.

GB 30: Caudodorsal to the greater trochanter.

GB 34: In the indentation cranioventral to the head of the fibula.

GV 3: On the dorsal midline between the dorsal processes of L4 and L5.

GV 4: On the dorsal midline between the dorsal processes of L2 and L3.

GV 11: On the dorsal midline between the dorsal processes of T5 and T6.

GV 12: On the dorsal midline between the dorsal processes of T3 and T4.

GV 14: On the dorsal midline between the dorsal processes of C7 and T1.

GV 15: On the dorsal midline between C1 and C2.

GV 16: On the dorsal midline between C1 and the skull.

GV 20: On the dorsal midline on a line drawn between the tips of the ears.

GV 25: On the dorsal midline of the snout where the nose meets the hairline.

GV 26: On the midline between the nose and the lips, approximately one-third of the distance from the nose to the lips.

KI 1: On the plantar surface of the foot under the metatarsal pad between metatarsals 2 and 3.

KI 3: On the medial surface of the hock between the medial epicondyle of the tibia and the Achilles tendon.

KI 4: Caudoventral to KI 3.

LI 3: On the medial surface of the distal 2nd metacarpal bone.

LI 4: On the medial surface of the second metacarpal bone at the level of the junction with the 1st digit.

LI 10: On the lateral surface of the forearm one-sixth of the distance from the elbow between the extensor carpi radialis and the common digital extensor.

LI 11: On the lateral surface of the elbow at the lateral aspect of the crease when the elbow is fully flexed.

LI 18: On the ventrolateral surface of the neck between the sternocephalicus and brachicephalicus at the midpoint.

LIV 3: The position of this point is controversial in animals. Some claim that it is in the indentation on the dorsal surface of the hind foot where the 2nd and 3rd metatarsal bones meet. Others say it is on the medial surface of the 2nd metatarsal bone at the same level.

LU 1: In the first intercostal space in the depression medial to the greater tubercle of the humerus.

LU 7: On the medial surface of the paw caudal to the styloid process of the radius medial to the tendon of the extensor carpi radialis.

PC 5: One-fourth the distance from the carpal joint to the elbow, proximal to PC6 in the same groove.

PC 6: On the caudal surface of the forelimb at the distal junction of the radius and ulna.

PC 7: On the caudal surface of the forelimb in the center of the crease of the flexed carpal joint.

SI 9: Sometimes called "Qiang feng"; in the indentation at the meeting point of the lateral head of the triceps, the long head of the triceps, and the deltoideus.

SI 10: Just caudal to the shoulder joint ventral to the scapula.

SP 6: On the medial surface of the hindlimb one-fifth of the distance from the hock to the stifle tibia just caudal to the tibia.

SP 9: Caudodistal to the medial condyle of the tibia.

SP 10: On the medial surface of the hindlimb proximal and cranial to the distal femoral epicondyle.

ST 6: Rostral to the angle of the mandible, on the belly of the masseter muscle.

ST 7: Ventral to the caudal aspect of the temporomandibular joint with the mouth closed.

ST 25: In the muscle groove of the rectus abdominus lateral to the umbilicus.

ST 28: Three-fifths of the distance from the umbilicus to the pubis in the same sagittal plane as ST 25.

ST 35: In the lateral depression distal to the patella.

ST 36: Cranial to the proximal tibia one-fourth the distance from the stifle to the hock.

ST 40: Between the long digital extensor and the tibialis cranialis halfway between the stifle and the hock just lateral to the fibula.

ST 44: Just distal and lateral to the 2nd metatarso-phalangeal joint.

TH 5: On the cranial surface of the forelimb between the radius and ulna opposite PC 6.

TH 6: Three-fourths of the distance from the elbow to the wrist in line with PC 6.

TH 14: Just caudal to the shoulder joint and ventral to the acromion process.

Bai hui: On the dorsal midline at the lumbosacral junction.

Ding-chuan: At the lateral margin of the vertebrae at the level of the junction between C7 and T1.

Hua tuo jia ji: A series of points on the lateral edges of the vertebral bodies.

Index

Page references in *italics* denote figures; page references followed by t denote tables.

Ginkgo *(Ginkgo biloba)*
  for cancer, 707
  for cardiovascular system diseases, 654, 655
  description, 660
  for endocrine diseases, 691
  for eye diseases, 673–674, 675
  for neurological disorders, 695, 696, 697
  for respiratory system diseases, 682
  for skin diseases, 661
  for urogenital system diseases, 687
Ginseng. *See Panax ginseng;* Siberian ginseng *(Eleutherococcus senticosus)*
Ginseng (Ren shen)
  for granulomatous meningoencephalitis (GME)/peripheral
      neuropathies, 563
  for megaesophagus, 339
  for pericardial effusion, 233
Ginseng compositum
  for Addison's disease, 510
  for blood and lymph diseases
    chylothorax, 157
    Hemobartonella felis, 161
  for cancer
    hemangiosarcoma, 794
    overview, 782
    symptomatic therapy, 789
  for corneal ulcers, 401
  for diarrhea/enteritis, 297
  for digestive system diseases
    acute gastric dilitation/bloat, 325
    gastritis, 320
    inflammatory bowel disease, 331
    megacolon, 343
    vomiting, 316
  for infectious diseases
    feline upper respiratory diseases, 617
    tick-borne diseases, 635
  for myasthenia gravis, 149
  for neurological disorders
    cognitive dysfunction, 541
    degenerative myelopathy, 547
    granulomatous meningoencephalitis (GME)/peripheral
        neuropathies, 565
    vestibular syndromes, 585
Gland therapy. *See also specific indications; specific organs*
  for cancer, 721
  definition, 813
  effectiveness of, 21–22
  historic use, 18
  organ specificity, 19–20
  overview, 18
  processing of gland extracts, 20
  scientific basis of, 19
  tissue sparing effects, 20–21
    adrenal extracts, 20
    cartilage extracts, 21
    heart extracts, 21
    liver extracts, 20–21
    pancreas extracts, 20
    phospholipids, 21
Glandula thyroidea suis
  for adenocarcinoma, 792
Glaucoma
  definition and cause, 402–403

drug(s) of choice, 403
integrative veterinary therapies
  acupuncture, 404, 408
  Chinese herbal medicine, 404, 408
  homotoxicology, 404–407, 408
  nutrition, 403–404, 407–408
  overview, 403
  product sources, 408
  suggested protocols, 407–408
medical therapy rationale, 403
nutritional recommendations, 403
prognosis, 403
Western herbal medicine, 674–675
Glaucoma formula, 407, 408
Glechoma (Jin qian cao)
  for cystitis, 491
  for feline lower urinary tract disease syndrome (FLUTDS),
      496
  for urolithiasis, 504–505
Globe artichoke *(Cynara scolymus)*
  for digestive system diseases, 668, 669
  for skin diseases, 660
Globulin, blood test, 45
Glonoin (nitroglycerin)
  for cardiovascular system diseases
    cardiac arrhythmias, 212
    heart disease, 219–220
    hypertension, 230
  for glaucoma, 406
Glonoin homaccord
  for glaucoma, 406
  for hyperthyroidism, 533
Glonoinum
  for meningioma, 797
Glucagon, 41
Glucocorticoids, 37
Glucosamine
  for arthritis, 424
  in cartilage extracts, 21
  for feline lower urinary tract disease syndrome (FLUTDS),
      496, 498
  for immune-mediated arthritis, 132
  for osteochondrosis, 434
Glucose, blood test, 44
Glucosilization, 84, 86
Gluta-DMG
  for gastric adenocarcinoma, 738
  for leiomyosarcoma, 743
Glutamine
  for cancer, 722, 735
  description, 24
  for digestive system diseases
    acute gastric dilitation/bloat, 323, 325
    colitis, 307, 310
    diarrhea/enteritis, 294, 298
    inflammatory bowel disease, 329, 332
    irritable bowel syndrome, 301, 304
    malabsorption syndrome, 382, 385
    megacolon, 342, 344
    megaesophagus, 339, 340
  for infectious diseases
    canine coronavirus diarrhea, 592
    canine parvovirus, 601–602, 603
Glutathione, 355, 362, 776